MOSBY'S COMPREHENSIVE REVIEW OF NURSING

MOSBY'S COMPREHENSIVE REVIEW OF NURSING

ELEVENTH EDITION

Illustrated

MOSBYSYSTEMS

ST. LOUIS   TORONTO   1984

Editor: Alison Miller
Assistant editors: Susan R. Epstein, Terry Young
Manuscript editor: George B. Stericker, Jr.
Design: Diane Beasley
Production: Susan Trail

ELEVENTH EDITION

Library of Congress Cataloging in Publication Data

Main entry under title:

Mosby's Comprehensive review of nursing.

  Bibliography: p.
  Includes index.
    1. Nursing—Examinations, questions, etc.
2. Nursing—Outlines, syllabi, etc. I. C.V. Mosby
Company. II. Title: Comprehensive review of nursing.
[DNLM: 1. Nursing—Examination questions. 2. Nursing
—Outlines. WY 18 M8944]
RT55.M64 1984   610.73'076   83-13229
ISBN 0-8016-3551-9

C/VH/VH 9 8 7 6 5 4 3 2 1   03/B/308

Editorial Panel

Editor

DOLORES F. SAXTON, R.N., B.S. in Ed., M.A., Ed.D.

Professor, Department of Nursing, Nassau Community College, Garden City, New York

Associate editors

PATRICIA M. NUGENT, R.N., A.A.S., B.S., M.S.

Assistant Professor, Department of Nursing, Nassau Community College, Garden City, New York

PHYLLIS K. PELIKAN, R.N., A.A.S., B.S., M.A.

Professor, Department of Nursing, Nassau Community College, Garden City, New York

Contributing authors

JUDITH BEYER, R.N., B.S.N.E., M.S., Ph.D.

Assistant Professor of Nursing, University of Virginia, Charlottesville, Virginia; Robert Woods Fellow, 1983-1984

ALBERT E. DONOR, B.S., M.S., Ph.D.

Vice-President, Academic Affairs, Nassau Community College, Garden City, New York

JOANN FESTA, R.N., A.A.S., B.S., M.S.

Assistant Professor, Department of Nursing, Nassau Community College, Garden City, New York

MARYANN HELLMER, R.N., A.A.S., B.S., M.S.

Assistant Professor, Department of Nursing, Nassau Community College, Garden City, New York

MILDRED L. MONTAG, R.N., B.A., B.S., M.A., Ed.D., LL.D.

Professor Emeritus, Teachers College, Columbia University, New York, New York

THERESA A. MORAN, R.N., A.A.S., B.S., Ed.M.

Instructor, Department of Nursing, Nassau Community College, Garden City, New York

Preface

The material in *Mosby's Comprehensive Review of Nursing* has been revised and updated for this eleventh edition. The progression of subject matter in each area reflects the consistent approach that has been used throughout the book. Selected information incorporates the latest knowledge, newest trends, and current practices in the profession of nursing.

The medical-surgical, maternity, pediatric, and psychiatric chapters incorporate material from the basic sciences, nutrition, pharmacology, and rehabilitation. Chapter 6, Historical and Legal Aspects of Nursing in the United States and Canada, provides a concise overview of the background, law, and trends that today's nurse must know to practice nursing effectively. Chapter 1 gives directions on how to study and use the review to prepare for the licensing examination.

We have continued to present the material in the traditional clinical groupings, for we still believe that, even in preparing for the comprehensive examination, the average student will study all the distinct parts before attempting to put them together.

In this edition we have added, for every question in the book, the reasons why the incorrect answers are incorrect as well as why the correct answer is correct. We have also included two additional 120-question comprehensive examinations and have analyzed each of the questions in the six comprehensive examinations as to the step in the nursing process, the level of cognitive ability required, the responsibility for decision making, and the clinical area involved.

The comprehensive tests at the back of the book give the reader an opportunity to apply material from the specific clinical areas to any nursing situation. With both Canada and the United States using comprehensive examinations, these tests will help the student prepare for this experience. The movement from specific learning to general application is educationally sound, and the reader should follow this approach in studying.

All the questions used in this book have been submitted by outstanding educators and practitioners of nursing. Initially the editorial panel reviewed all questions, selecting the most pertinent for inclusion in a mass field-testing project. Students graduating from baccalaureate, associate degree, and diploma nursing programs in various locations in the United States and Canada provided a diverse testing group. The results were statistically analyzed. This analysis was used to select questions for inclusion in the book and to provide the reader with a general idea of each question's level of difficulty.

We would like to take this opportunity to express our sincere appreciation to our many colleagues for their contributions and support: to Winifred Hennessy, Arleen Glamkowski, and Chris Dorn for their careful typing of the manuscript; to Kelly and Heather Nugent for their clerical help; and last, but not least, to our families, who survived without our assistance for a prolonged period of time.

Dolores F. Saxton
Patricia M. Nugent
Phyllis K. Pelikan

Contents

1

Introduction for Students Preparing for the Licensing Examination

The licensing examinations in the United States and Canada have been integrated and comprehensive for a number of years. Nursing candidates in both countries are required to answer questions that necessitate a recognition and understanding of pertinent principles from the physiologic, biologic, and social sciences, as well as the specific nursing skills and abilities involved in a given client situation.

Both tests contain approximately 500 objective multiple-choice questions. To answer the questions appropriately, a candidate needs to understand and correlate certain aspects of anatomy and physiology, the behavioral sciences, basic nursing, the effects of medications administered, the client's attitude toward illness, and other pertinent factors (e.g., legal responsibilities). Most questions are based on nursing situations similar to those with which candidates have had experience since both the United States and Canada emphasize the nursing care of clients with representative common national health problems. Some questions, however, require candidates to apply basic principles and techniques to clinical situations with which they have had little if any actual experience.

To prepare adequately for an integrated comprehensive examination, it is necessary to understand the discrete parts that comprise the universe under consideration. This is one of the major principles of learning on which *Mosby's Comprehensive Review of Nursing* has been developed.

1

Using this principle, the text first presents a review of each of the major clinical areas. Each review is followed by related questions that test the student's knowledge of principles and theories underlying nursing care in a variety of situations (acute, critical, and long term), in a variety of settings (acute care hospitals, nursing homes, and the community), and with a variety of nursing goals (preventive, curative, palliative, and restorative).

The correct answer to each question as well as a rationale supporting this answer is provided. Explanations are also presented to document why a specific answer is inappropriate as a response to the question. By reviewing the rationales the student is able to verify information and reinforce knowledge.

The text concludes with a series of integrated comprehensive examinations of 120 questions reflecting those that make up the licensing examinations. In other words, the questions require the student to cross clinical disciplines and respond to individual needs, as well as specific needs, associated with given health problems. Rationales are also provided for each question.

Similar to those in the comprehensive licensing examinations, the questions in the comprehensive tests have been classified by four separate categories: (1) phases of the nursing process; (2) cognitive level; (3) locus of decision making; and (4) clinical area.

The following descriptions with examples are presented to assist the reader in understanding these classifications:

Phases of the nursing process
1. Assessment. The assessment phase requires the nurse to obtain objective and subjective data from primary and secondary sources, to identify and group significant data, and to communicate this information to other members of the health team. The information necessary for making nursing decisions is obtained through assessment. Question no. 1 is an *assessment* question.
2. Analysis. This phase requires the nurse to interpret data gathered during the assessment phase. A nursing diagnosis must be made, client and family needs identified, and both short-term and long-term goals set to meet the identified needs. Question no. 2 is an *analysis* question.
3. Planning. The planning phase requires the nurse to design a regimen with the client and family to achieve the goals set during the analysis phase. It also requires the setting of priorities for nursing intervention. Question no. 3 is a *planning* question.
4. Implementation. The implementation phase requires the nurse to provide care designed during the planning phase. The client may be given total care or may be assisted and encouraged to perform activities of daily living or follow the regimen prescribed by the physician. Implementation also includes activities such as counseling, teaching, and supervising. Question no. 4 is an *implementation* question.
5. Evaluation. This phase requires the nurse to determine the effectiveness of nursing care. The goals of care are reviewed, the client's response to intervention identified, and a consideration made as to whether the client has achieved the predetermined goals. Evaluation also includes appraisal of the client's compliance with the health plan. Question no. 5 is an *evaluation* question.

Cognitive levels
1. Knowledge. The knowledge level of the intellectual process requires the recollection of facts about principles, theories, terms, or procedures. Knowledge questions, which require the examinee to define, identify, or select, involve the ability to recall information (a basic cognitive skill). Question no. 2 is a *knowledge* question.
2. Comprehension. The comprehension level of the intellectual process requires the demonstration of some understanding or interpretation of the subject matter presented. It is much more than just the recall of information. The examinee is required to interpret, explain, distinguish, and/or predict. Question no. 1 is a *comprehension* question.
3. Application. The application level of the intellectual process requires the examinee not only to know and understand information but also to apply it in a new situation. When applying comprehended information, the examinee must show, solve, modify, change, manipulate, use, demonstrate, or teach in a specific client situation. Question no. 4 is an *application* question.
4. Analysis. The analysis level of the intellectual process requires the recognition of inherent structure and the relationship between component parts as well as an understanding of the underlying concepts or principles. If the examinee is required to analyze, evaluate, select, differentiate, or interpret data from a variety of sources prior to responding, the question is an analysis question. Question no. 5 is an *analysis* question.

Locus of decision making
1. Decision rests with the nurse. When the client is prevented from taking part in decision making by nature of the physical or psychologic status or the developmental level, the nurse must compensate

by assuming total responsibility for decisions relative to care. Under these conditions the client is usually (a) in a life-threatening situation, (b) an infant or young child, (c) unconscious or confused, or (d) out of touch with reality. In question no. 5 the decision rests with the *nurse*.

2. Decision rests with the client. When the client is able to assume responsibility for care and the nurse supports and encourages independence, provides health guidance, maintains an environment that fosters client decision making, and acts as a consultant, the decision for care rests with the client. In question no. 3 the decision rests with the *client*.

3. Decision shared between the client and nurse. When the client's abilities are limited and the nurse must assist, guide, teach, or support the client, the act of decision making is shared. In questions 1, 2, and 4 the decision rests with both *the client and the nurse*.

Clinical area

1. Medicine. The medical specialty is involved in the care of adult clients who have health problems that do not require surgical intervention or invasive techniques. Question no. 1 is a *medical* nursing question.

2. Surgery. This specialty is utilized in the care of adult and child clients with health problems that require surgical intervention or invasive techniques. Question no. 5 is a *surgical* nursing question.

3. Obstetrics. This area deals with the care of clients preparing for or experiencing childbirth. Question no. 2 is a *maternity* nursing question.

4. Pediatrics. This specialty is involved in caring for clients from birth to young adulthood. Question no. 4 is a *pediatric* nursing question.

5. Psychiatry. This specialty is called upon to care for clients experiencing emotional stress with or without overt psychiatric behavior. Question no. 3 is a *psychiatric* nursing question.

1 Mr. Evere, a 69-year-old retired musician, was admitted to the intensive care unit with a diagnosis of Adams-Stokes syndrome. Symptoms most likely include:
1. Syncope and low ventricular rate
2. Flushing and slurred speech
3. Cephalagia and blurred vision
4. Nausea and vertigo

2 Miss Daley has decided to go through with her pregnancy and keep her baby. Now the crisis intervention worker's primary responsibility is to:
1. Support her for making a wise decision
2. Make an appointment for her to see a physician for prenatal care

3. Explore other problems she may be experiencing
4. Provide information about other health resources where she may receive additional assistance

3 When monoamine oxidase (MAO) inhibitors are prescribed, the patient should be cautioned against:
1. The use of medications with an elixir base
2. Prolonged exposure to the sun
3. Ingesting wines and cheeses
4. Engaging in active physical exercise

4 Jamey, age 4, has been hospitalized for fever of undetermined origin (FUO). He screams and becomes uncontrollable as his mother leaves after visiting hours. The best approach is to:
1. Ignore this outburst
2. Sit quietly at his bedside
3. Hold and pat him even though he struggles
4. Give him a favorite toy to hold

5 Following surgery, while receiving a blood transfusion, Mr. Manning develops chills and headache. The nurse's best action is to:
1. Stop the transfusion immediately
2. Lightly cover the patient
3. Notify the physician STAT
4. Slow the blood flow to keep vein open

HOW TO USE THIS BOOK IN STUDYING

A. Start in one area. Study the material covered by the section. Refer to other textbooks to find additional details if you are unsure of a specific fact.

B. Take the test following the area. As you answer each of the questions, write a few words about why you think that answer was correct; in other words, simply justify why you selected the answer you did. If you guess at an answer in this book you should make a special mark to identify the answer as a "guess." This will permit you to recognize areas that need further review. It will also help you to see how correct your "guessing" can be. Remember on the licensing examination you should guess at answers rather than leave blank spaces.

C. Record the answer in the space and manner specified.

D. Compare your answers with the answers in the back of the book. If you answered the item correctly, check your reason for selecting the answer with the rationale presented. If you answered the item incorrectly, read the rationale to determine why the distractor you selected was incorrect. In addition, you should review the correct answer and rationale for each item answered incorrectly. If you still do not understand your mistake, look up and reread the theory pertaining to these questions. You should carefully review all questions and rationales for items you identified as guesses, since you did not have mastery of the material being questioned.

E. Following the correct answer you will find a letter—a, b, or c—in parentheses. These letters indicate the difficulty of the question and can serve as a guide in your studying. The letter a signifies that more than 75% of the graduating students in the testing group answered this question correctly; b signifies that between 50% and 75% answered it correctly; and c that 25% to 50% answered it correctly.

F. For the comprehensive examinations, in addition to the difficulty level of the question (a, b, c), you will find a grouping of letters that classify the question by phases of the nursing process (AS for assessment, AN for analysis, PL for planning, IM for implementation, and EV for evaluation); cognitive level (KN for knowledge, CP for comprehension, AP for application, AN for analysis); locus of decision making (NU for nurse, CL for client, SH for shared); and clinical area (ME for medicine, SU for surgery, OB for obstetrics, PE for pediatrics, PS for psychiatry). This series of letters will always appear in the same order for each question on the comprehensive examinations.

G. A few days later, review the area again and retake the test following it. If you miss the same questions again, you should recognize that you need further study of the material.

H. After you have completed all the area tests, begin taking the comprehensive tests, since they will assist you in applying knowledge and principles from the specific clinical area to any nursing situation. Take each of these examinations under conditions as closely approximating those of the licensure examination as possible.
   1. Arrange a quiet, uninterrupted, 2-hour time span for each of the Comprehensive Tests.
   2. Pace yourself during the testing period.
   3. Do not rush.
   4. Make educated guesses.
   5. Read carefully and answer the question asked.
   6. Try putting questions and answers in your own words to test your comprehension.

I. To help you analyze your mistakes on the comprehensive examinations and to provide a data base for making future study plans, two types of worksheets have been included. One is designed to aid you in identifying and recording errors in the way you process information. The other is to help you identify and record gaps in knowledge. (See pp. 637 and 638 for these worksheets.)

J. After completing your worksheets, do the following:

1. Use Worksheet I to identify the frequency with which you made particular errors. As you review material in class notes or this review book, pay special attention to correcting your most common problems.
2. Use Worksheet II to identify the topics you want to review. It might be helpful to set priorities; review the most difficult topics first so that you will have time to review them more than once.

GENERAL CLUES FOR ANSWERING MULTIPLE-CHOICE QUESTIONS

On a multiple-choice test the question and all possible answers are called a *test item*. The part of the item that asks the question or poses a problem is called the *stem*. All of the answers presented are called *options*. One of the options is the correct answer whereas the remainder are incorrect. The incorrect options are called *distractors* because their major purpose is to distract the test taker from the correct answer.

A. Read the question carefully before looking at the answers.
   1. Attempt to determine what the question is really asking; look for key words.
   2. Read each answer thoroughly and see if it completely covers the material asked by the question.
   3. Narrow the choices by immediately eliminating those answers which you know are incorrect.

B. Because few things in life are absolute without exceptions, avoid selecting answers that include words such as *always, never, all, every,* and *none,* since they are rarely correct.

C. Attempt to select the answer that is most complete and includes the other answers within it. An example might be as follows:
   A child's intelligence is influenced by
   1. Heredity and environment
   2. Environment and experience
   3. A variety of factors
   4. Education and economic factors
   The most correct answer is 3 because it includes all the other answers.

D. Make certain that the answer you select is reasonable and obtainable under ordinary circumstances and that the action can be carried out in the given situation.

E. *Watch for grammatical inconsistencies.* If one or more of the options is not grammatically consistent with the stem, the alert test taker can identify a probable distractor. When the stem is in the form of an incomplete sentence, each option should complete the sentence in a grammatically correct way.

F. Avoid selecting answers that state hospital rules or regulations as a reason or rationale for action.

G. Look for answers that focus on the patient or are directed toward feelings.

H. If the question asks for an immediate action or response, all the answers may be correct, so base your selection on identified priorities for action.

I. Do not select answers that contain exceptions to the general rule, controversial material, or degrading responses.

J. Reread the question if the answers do not seem to make sense, since you may have missed the word *not* or *except* in the statement.

K. Do not worry if you select the same numbered answer repeatedly, since there is usually no pattern to the answers.

L. Make certain you mark the correct space on the answer sheet for the question you are answering.

M. Mark the space completely with a dark line but do not extend your answer over the lines.

PREPARING FOR THE LICENSURE EXAMINATION

A few individuals can improve their scores significantly by a highly concentrated period of study immediately before taking an examination. The majority, however, profit more by spreading their review over a much longer period of time, and the best time to begin studying for state boards is the first class attended in the school.

After you have completed studying this book, you may wish to try Mosby's *AssessTest* before you take the licensing examination. *AssessTest* is a computer-scored, multiple-choice examination designed to test essential nursing knowledge and evaluate ability to apply that knowledge in various clinical situations. The extensive computer analysis of your performance, which is the most oustanding feature of this test, will help you de-sign effective and efficient plans for further study and review. Identification of your own *specific* strengths and weaknesses ought to eliminate much of the anxiety connected with deciding what material to study by giving you a sense of direction and a means of setting priorities.

TAKING THE LICENSURE EXAMINATION

The most crucial requisite for doing well on the licensure examination is to bring to it a sound understanding of the subject and a high level of reading comprehension. Determination to do well and a degree of confidence will further enhance the well-prepared individual's chances of earning high scores.

At least three other requirements must be met if an individual's performance is to accurately reflect professional competence. First, the candidate must follow explicitly all the directions given by the examiner and those printed at the beginning of each test, as well as any that refer to a specified group of questions. Second, the candidate must read each question carefully before deciding how to answer it. Third, the candidate must record the answers in the space and manner specified. Some candidates find it helpful to glance over a test before starting to answer the questions. This enables them to answer the questions in the order most efficient and comfortable for them. Others find it more efficient to go through the test answering all questions they are sure of first, then going back to the more difficult questions.

The score candidates earn on each test is the number of questions answered correctly; there is no deduction for incorrect answers. You are not penalized for guessing. Do not leave an answer blank. You have a 1 in 4 (25%) chance of guessing the correct answer. Do not mark more than one answer on your answer sheet, for questions with more than one answer will be scored as incorrect.

The licensing examination is given over a 2-day period and one overall score is reported.

2

Medical-Surgical Nursing

Medical-surgical nursing is concerned with those aspects of nursing care that are related to the physical and emotional needs of patients with specific types of health problems. The concepts, principles, and skills included here will assist the practitioner in all aspects of nursing care.

Medical-surgical content has been developed by using a systems approach with examples of major diseases. The areas covered include a general conceptual introduction, preoperative and postoperative care, and cardiovascular, respiratory, gastrointestinal, genitourinary, endocrine, neurologic, musculoskeletal, and integumentary systems. The format for each section follows a similar pattern, beginning with a review of anatomy and physiology, related pharmacology, and related procedures and moving into the major diseases. Etiology and pathophysiology, subjective and objective symptomatology, treatment, and nursing care are included for each disease presented.

Conceptual Introduction

THE HEALTH-ILLNESS CONTINUUM
Introduction

A. Health is a generally accepted right; well-being is the norm toward which most governments and all health personnel direct their efforts
B. One of the primary functions of the nursing and medical professions is to help individuals, families, and groups reach the highest level of wellness of which they are capable

Definition

A. The World Health Organization states, ''Health is a state of complete physical, mental, and social well-being and not just the absence of disease or infirmity''
B. This definition implies that there is
   1. Interaction between self and environment
   2. Preservation of structure and function
   3. Maintenance of adaptive potential
C. Significance of definition
   1. Accepted right of all rather than a privilege
   2. Reciprocal relationships between individual health and community health
   3. Increasing public expectation of government support for health services and the extent of care provided
   4. Need for nursing and medical practice to move toward maintenance and promotion of health and rehabilitation of the ill rather than merely to focus on provision of episodic care

Basic Concepts

A. Health—a continually changing phenomenon
1. Moves on a continuum between optimal wellness (where potential is maximized and used with purpose) and death
2. Change may be gradual or abrupt
3. Level attainable depends on adaptive energy and on genetic and environmental factors
   a. Fluctuates throughout life cycle
   b. Varies among individuals
4. Individual may or may not be aware of change
5. Person's position on the continuum determined by
   a. Ability to adapt
   b. Level of adaptation
   c. Culture's view of health
   d. Ability to carry out social, family, and job responsibilities
B. Stresses affect physical, emotional, and social health
1. May be internal or external
2. Can be beneficial or detrimental to life
   a. Tension essential to life
   b. Stress of life and living causes wear and tear
      (1) Produces a nonspecific response that Hans Selye identifies as the general adaptation syndrome (GAS)
      (2) Three stages—alarm, resistance, and exhaustion
3. Elicit some response from or change in the individual
4. Sources vary widely for different individuals and within the same individual at different times
5. Tolerance is individual
6. May be
   a. Physical—thermal, acoustical
   b. Chemical—gas, hormonal, nutrient
   c. Microbiologic—viral, bacterial
   d. Physiologic—neoplasmic, hypofunctional, hyperfunctional
   e. Developmental—genetic, aging
   f. Psychologic—values, self-image
C. Rehabilitation assists people in attaining their maximum level of wellness on the continuum
1. Particularly concerned with establishing function that is lost while at the same time expanding, maintaining, and supporting the limited remaining function
2. Immediate or potential needs exhibited in all health problems
3. The patient is the primary rehabilitator—professional health team members only assist the patient and family with the process of self-rehabilitation
4. Not an isolated process; rehabilitation involves the patient, family, health team, community, and society
5. Concerned with all levels of prevention—primary, secondary, and tertiary
6. Health problems that cause disabilities are socially significant because of the number of people affected, the economic cost and loss, the distress of personal suffering, and the conditions in society that increase their incidence
D. Ability to maintain and return to a level of health is influenced by the availability of health resources

Principles Related to Needs of the Adult

THE YOUNG ADULT (25 TO 45 YEARS)
Growth and Development

A. Physiologic development
1. Physical maturation occurs
2. Muscle strength and coordination peak
3. Biorhythms become established
4. Sexuality
   a. Established sex drive remains high for men
   b. Female sex drive reaches a peak during later phase of young adulthood
   c. Physiologically optimal period for childbearing
B. Psychosocial development
1. Mental abilities reflect formal operations (see growth and development of the adolescent in pediatric nursing)
2. Resolving the developmental crisis of intimacy versus isolation
3. Establishing new family relationships and parenting patterns
4. Establishing the self in, and advancing in, a chosen occupation

Health Promotion

A. Health problems
1. Accidents—leading cause of death in the United States
2. Periodontal disease
3. Cancer involving the reproductive organs
4. Hypertension
5. Suicide
6. Alcoholism
7. Spouse abuse

8. Fertility regulation
9. Divorce
B. Preventive interventions
  1. Encourage attendance at safety programs to promote accident prevention (e.g., defensive driving programs)
  2. Encourage dental checkups
  3. Teach self-examination techniques and encourage regular medical checkups
  4. Stress weight control through diet and physical activity
  5. Increase public awareness of problems and availability of crisis counseling, support groups, and other community resources (e.g., "hot lines," Alcoholics Anonymous, family planning clinics)

THE MIDDLE ADULT (45 TO 65 YEARS)
Growth and Development

A. Physiologic development
  1. Greater diversity in physiologic conditioning resulting from established life-style
  2. Early signs of aging (e.g., wrinkling, thinning hair, decreased muscle tone and nerve function)
  3. Decreased BMR with subsequent weight gain
  4. Decreased production of sexual hormones
    a. Menopause (see maternity nursing)
    b. Male climateric; may pass unnoticed, especially in those with high self-esteem; symptoms may include less forceful ejaculation, hot flashes, dizziness, headache, and depression
B. Psychosocial development
  1. Cognitive abilities enhanced because of motivation and past experiences
  2. Resolving developmental crisis of generativity versus stagnation
  3. Adjusting to changes in family caused by aging parents and teenage to adult children
  4. Maintaining satisfactory status of one's career
  5. Accepting physical changes associated with advancing age
  6. Developing social and civic activities that are personally satisfying

Health Promotion

A. Health problems
  1. Cardiovascular disease
  2. Cancer
  3. Presbyopia
  4. Accidents
  5. Respiratory disease
  6. Sexual dysfunction
  7. Death of spouse

B. Preventive interventions
  1. Encourage individuals to maintain a schedule of regular medical, dental, and visual examinations to control or prevent health problems
  2. Assess living conditions for possible hazards that could cause accidents
  3. Refer widows and widowers to appropriate self-help groups as necessary
  4. Encourage individuals to anticipate and plan for retirement

THE OLDER ADULT (65+ YEARS)
Growth and Development

A. Physiologic development
  1. Diminished sensation and reaction time (e.g., narrowed visual field, hearing loss)
  2. Increased sensitivity to cold because of decreased subcutaneous tissue and thyroxin utilization as well as impaired circulation
  3. Decreased enzyme secretion in and motility of the GI tract
  4. Decreased glomerular filtration rate
  5. Decreased cardiac output
  6. Arteriosclerotic changes with diminished elasticity of blood vessels
  7. Decreased lung capacity
  8. Demineralization and other degenerative skeletal changes, particularly in weight-bearing bones
  9. Muscle atrophy
B. Psychosocial development
  1. Cognitive abilities not necessarily affected by age; but may be impaired as a result of disease, leading to diminished awareness
  2. Resolving the developmental crisis of ego integrity versus despair
  3. Adjusting to the death of important others
  4. Adapting to decreased physical capacity and changes in body image
  5. Adjusting to the economic burden of a fixed income
  6. Recognizing the inevitability of death
  7. Reminiscing increasingly about the past

Health Promotion

A. Health problems
  1. Cardiovascular disease
  2. Cataracts, glaucoma, hearing loss
  3. Accidents (e.g., falls resulting in hip fractures)
  4. Resistance to changes in environment
  5. Respiratory disease
  6. Cerebral vascular insufficiency
  7. Impaired nutritional intake
  8. Death

B. Preventive interventions
1. Encourage individuals to maintain a schedule of regular medical supervision
2. Assess the individual's ability to cope with the environment
3. Promote maximum degree of independence
4. Initiate appropriate referrals for individuals requiring assistance with activities of daily living
   a. Home health aides
   b. Health-related facilities
   c. Skilled nursing facilities
   d. Acute care hospitals
5. Open channels of communication for reality orientation and emotional support
6. Refer to social service and other channels that can provide economic assistance when necessary
7. Ensure that prosthetic devices (e.g., dentures, contact lenses, eye prosthetics, braces, limbs) fit comfortably and do not cause irritation; teach proper care of such devices

HEALTH RESOURCES

A. Government agencies
1. Definition—associations functioning at the international, national, state, and local levels, providing a variety of services to meet the health, education, and welfare needs of the people; these programs are funded by the government, and services are rendered by professionals
2. Examples
   a. International—World Health Organization
   b. National
      (1) United States—Department of Health and Human Services, United States Public Health Service
      (2) Canada—Department of National Health and Welfare
   c. State or provincial
      (1) United States—state health departments
      (2) Canada—provincial departments of health
   d. Local—county or city department of health, fire department, police department
B. Voluntary agencies
1. Definition—organizations consisting of lay and professional persons dedicated to the prevention and solution of health problems by providing educational, research, and service programs; these agencies are dependent on voluntary donations for funds, are often concerned with specific health problems, and are national organizations that function through state and/or provincial and local chapters
2. Examples
   a. International—Rockefeller Foundation, international branches of professional organizations
   b. National—American Heart Association, American Cancer Society, National Multiple Sclerosis Society
   c. State and/or provincial—chapters of national organizations
   d. Local—branches of national voluntary organizations, community hospitals, volunteers (e.g., a league of women supporting a community hospital, a Girl Scout troop visiting a nursing home, a church group visiting an orphanage)
C. Crisis intervention groups
1. Services
   a. Provide assistance for people in crises—clients' previous methods of adaptation are inadequate to meet present needs
   b. The focus of some groups is specific (e.g., poison control, drug addiction centers, suicide prevention) or general (e.g., walk-in mental health clinics, hospital emergency rooms)
   c. Depending on the community's needs and facilities, these services can be offered by the government (e.g., state hospitals, state health departments) or voluntary organizations (e.g., community hospitals, community drug councils)
   d. Some crisis intervention groups provide service over the phone (e.g., poison control, suicide prevention centers), others help those who are physically present (e.g., hospital emergency rooms, walk-in mental health clinics)
2. Success factors
   a. The client or family seeking help
   b. Immediate opportunity for exploring feelings
   c. Assistance in investigating alternative approaches to solving the problem
   d. Information about other health resources where the client may receive additional assistance
D. Self-help groups
1. Services
   a. Organized by patients or their families to provide services that are not adequately supplied by previous organizations
   b. Meet the needs of patients and families with chronic problems requiring intervention over an extended period of time

c. Focus of some is specific (e.g., Gamblers Anonymous); others deal with a range of problems (e.g., Association for Children with Learning Disabilities)

d. Some are nonprofit (e.g., Alcoholics Anonymous); others are profit making (e.g., Weight Watchers International)

e. Provide services to people who frequently are not accepted by society (e.g., a drug addict, an alcoholic, a child abuser, one who is mentally ill, obese, or brain injured)

2. Success factors

a. All members accepted as equals

b. All members have experienced similar problems

c. Dealing with behavior and changes in behavior rather than with underlying causes of the behavior

d. Ready supply of human resources available
   (1) Personal resources
   (2) Assistance from peers
   (3) Finally, extension of self to others

e. Each member has identified the problem and wants help in meeting needs—self-motivation

f. Ritual and language specific to the group and specific to the problems

g. Leadership remains with the membership

h. Group interaction
   (1) Identification with peers—sense of belonging
   (2) Group expectations—discipline required of members
   (3) Small steps encouraged and, when attained, reinforced by the group

i. As a member achieves success within the group, he or she frequently starts to receive reinforcement from outside the group

E. Acute care facilities—these are general hospitals and provide care for the short-term ill patient undergoing treatment for a health problem

1. Intensive care—services and equipment to meet the needs of the acutely ill patient undergoing intensive treatment for a health problem (e.g., intensive care unit, coronary care unit, burn unit, psychiatric unit)

2. Intermediate care—services for the moderately ill patient who is overcoming a health crisis but still has special needs that cannot be adequately met in a general unit (e.g., intermediate care unit, progressive coronary care unit, isolation units)

3. Self-care—services for the patient and family who need little assistance with health care but have a greater need for teaching, motivation, and control over their own care

F. Extended care facilities—these provide services to persons who are either short-term or long-term convalescents; such patients need a wide range of services beyond acute care (nursing care, physical therapy, social and psychologic services); extended care facilities can be self-contained or can function as an extension of a hospital that offers its facilities when needed; the expense of extended care services is usually less than that for hospital care because of larger nursing units, less building support systems, increased paramedical personnel, and smaller range of services

G. Long-term facilities—these provide services over an extended period; most deal with chronic or long-term health problems

1. Skilled nursing facility—agency in which the residents require a relatively large degree of physical care and technical intervention

2. Health-related facility—agency in which the residents require minimal to moderate technical intervention and are supervised by nursing and ancillary staff

3. Adult facility—residence where an individual goes to live; meals and recreational programs may often be supplied; however, medical and nursing supervision are generally not provided on a full-time basis

4. Rehabilitation center—institution that provides multiple services and facilities which assist a patient and family to make an adjustment to living; the patient can obtain an optimal level of health by developing personal abilities to their fullest potential and utilizing the following resources
   a. Medical and nursing—total health assessment and planning, physical therapy, occupational therapy, and speech therapy
   b. Psychosocial—personal counseling, social service, and psychiatric service
   c. Vocational—work evaluation, vocational counseling, vocational training, trial employment in sheltered workshops, terminal employment in sheltered workshops, and placement

5. Continued care facility—agency that provides services for people with health needs who are living at home
   a. Outpatient or ambulatory care—diagnosis, treatment, and follow-up on an outpatient basis (e.g., emergency room, outpatient clinics, mobile health units)
   b. Home care—comprehensive services for people who do not need to be hospitalized

and yet require more care than an outpatient facility can provide (e.g., public health nurses, homemaker services, medical home care programs)

   c. Community resources—special services by organizations to meet specific client needs (e.g., Meals on Wheels, FISH)

   d. Day-care facilities—supervised activities and other services to individuals on a daily basis; the individual comes to the center for the day and returns home each evening

H. Health services personnel
1. Roles and functions
   a. Multiplicity of health professionals can result in overlapping and/or fragmentation of patient care (e.g., nurse, physician, therapist, nutritionist, social worker, physician's assistant, paramedic)
   b. Requirements for quality care
     (1) Clarification of role and function
     (2) Development of standards for licensure
     (3) Better utilization of personnel
     (4) Enforcement of present health practice acts
2. Team approach often used—provides optimal, unified care to the patient who is the focus of the team
   a. Professional health team includes registered professional nurse and physician as colleagues
   b. Other members—social worker, nutritionist, therapists, chaplains, etc.—are utilized as necessary
   c. The registered nurse leads the nursing team

THE NURSE'S ROLE
Introduction

A. General responsibilities
1. Recognize the right of persons to receive necessary help
2. Know and understand self as a person, including personal attitudes, values, and exhibited behavioral responses
3. Understand the pathophysiologic and psychosocial processes involving the patient's and family's health problem
4. Encourage and preserve the patient's individuality, self-identity, and inalienable right to be the center of the health team
5. Utilize the problem-solving approach to meet patient needs in achieving full potential
6. Function as collaborator with team members
B. Methods of delivery of nursing care
1. Functional—specific tasks (e.g., medicine ad-

ministration, treatments, vital signs) assigned to individual nurses
2. Team nursing—patient assigned to specific group of nurses responsible for that patient's total care
3. Primary nursing—specific nurse responsible for a specific patient's total care

Problem-Solving Approach

A. Introduction
1. Basis of personalized patient care is planned rather than intuitive intervention
2. Most efficient way to accomplish this in a time of exploding knowledge and rapid social change is by the problem-solving process
   a. Theoretical framework used by the nurse
   b. Assists in solving or alleviating both simple and complex nursing problems
3. Changing, expanding, more responsible role demands knowledgeably planned, purposeful, and accountable action by nurses
4. Better-prepared health professionals and more efficient use of health facilities can meet increasing demands for health care
5. Decision making that systematically selects and uses relevant information is a requisite for individualized patient care
6. Cognitive, affective, and activity components that are nursing can best be integrated by the problem-solving process
7. Process consists of assessing, planning, implementing, and evaluating a problem
B. Steps in the process
1. Assessment
   a. Collection of personal, social, medical, and general data
     (1) Sources—primary (patient, family, and chart) and secondary (colleagues, Kardex, literature)
     (2) Methods
       (a) Interviewing formally (nursing health history) or informally during various nurse-patient interactions
       (b) Observation
       (c) Review of records
   b. Classification of data—screening, organizing, and grouping significant and related information
   c. Definition of problem—making a nursing diagnosis that is the scientific identification of patient problems
     (1) Use of judgment
       (a) Inductive reasoning—specific data to generalizations

        (b) Deductive reasoning—generalizations to specific data

    (2) Identification of stresses in environments (external and internal)

    (3) Awareness of the patient's reactions to stress

2. Intervention
   a. Making a hypothesis or formulating a nursing care plan—a blueprint for action
      (1) Individualized prescription for care
      (2) Synonymous with nursing orders
   b. Implementation of plan or chosen solution
      (1) Actual administration of planned care
      (2) Adjusted as necessary to immediate needs
   c. Awareness that nursing functions are both independent and interdependent
3. Evaluation and revision include nursing prognosis as to effectiveness of and response to care

C. Advantages of the process
1. Makes allowance for individual responses to problems
2. Determines priority of care, permitting organization of individual needs in order of importance
3. Permits independent, creative, and flexible nursing intervention
4. Facilitates team cooperation by promoting
   a. Communication between team members
   b. Contribution of team members
   c. Coordination of care
   d. Continuity of approach
5. Provides for patient input

D. Extension to medical records
1. Problem-oriented medical record (POMR) consists of standardized data base, problem list, assessment and plan for each problem, and progress notes
   a. Updated by appropriate team members on a single progress note
   b. Each problem described according to specific format, which includes *s*ubjective data, *o*bjective findings, *a*ssessment, and a *p*lan for diagnosis, therapy, or teaching (SOAP)
2. Problem-oriented records have become the basis for peer review
3. Justifies nursing function
4. Focuses on the patient rather than the task
5. Improves patient care

Maintenance of Effective Communication

A. Introduction
1. The need to communicate is universal
2. People communicate to satisfy needs

3. Recognition of what is communicated is basic for the establishment of a therapeutic nurse-patient relationship
4. Clear and accurate communication among members of the health team, including the patient, is vital to support the patient's welfare

B. Nursing responsibilities in promotion of productive communication
1. Be aware that effective communication requires skill in both sending and receiving messages
   a. Verbal—words, tone of voice, etc.
   b. Written
   c. Nonverbal—facial expression, eye contact, posture, tension, etc.
2. Recognize the high stress–anxiety potential of most health settings created in part by
   a. Health problem itself
   b. Treatments and procedures
   c. Exclusive behavior of personnel
   d. Foreign environment
   e. Change in life-style, body image, and self-concept
3. Recognize the intrinsic worth of each person
   a. Listen, consider wishes when possible, explain when necessary
   b. Avoid stereotyping, snap judgments, unjustified comparisons
   c. Be nonjudgmental and nonpunitive in response and behavior
4. Be aware that each individual must be treated as a whole person
5. Recognize that all behavior has meaning and usually results from coping with stress or anxiety
   a. Be aware of importance of value systems
   b. Be aware of significance of cultural differences
   c. Be sensitive to personal meaning of experiences to patients
   d. Recognize that giving information may not alter the patient's behavior
   e. Recognize the defense mechanisms that the individual is using
   f. Recognize own anxiety and cope with it
   g. Search for patterns of adaptation on which to base action
   h. Recognize that adequate behavior patterns may become inadequate under stress
      (1) Health problems may produce a change in family or community constellations
      (2) Health problems may lead to change in self-perception and role identity

     i. Be aware that behavioral changes are possible only when the individual has a replacement behavior to maintain equilibrium

6. Help the patient to accept the health problem and its consequences

7. Identify the individual's needs and determine their priority for care

8. Maintain an accepting, open environment
   a. Be permissive rather than authoritarian
   b. Identify and face problems honestly
   c. Value the expression of feelings
   d. Be nonjudgmental

9. Where possible, encourage patient participation in decision making

10. Recognize the patient as a person
    a. Use names rather than labels such as room numbers or diagnoses
    b. Maintain the patient's dignity
    c. Be courteous toward the patient, family, and visitors
    d. Protect the patient's privacy by use of curtains, avoidance of probing
    e. Permit personal possessions where practical (e.g., own nightclothes, pictures, toys)
    f. Explain at the patient's level of understanding and tolerance
    g. Encourage expression of feelings
    h. Approach the patient as a person with difficulties, not as a ''difficult'' person

11. Support a social environment that focuses on patient needs
    a. Use problem-solving techniques in assessment, intervention, and recording
    b. Be flexible in carrying out routines and policies
    c. Be discreet in use of power
    d. Recognize that use of medical jargon can isolate the patient

C. Patient factors influencing communication
   1. Hierarchy of needs
      a. Need to survive—physiologic needs for air food, water, etc.
      b. Need for safety and comfort—physical and psychologic security
      c. Interpersonal needs—social needs for love, acceptance, status, and recognition
      d. Intrapersonal needs—self-esteem, self-actualization
   2. Developmental level
      a. Infant—must adapt to a totally new environment; the stress from this culture shock is compounded for the infant with a congenital defect
      b. Child—maturation involves physical, functional, and emotional growth; it is an ever changing process that produces stress; disabilities will provide additional factors that may quantitatively or qualitatively affect maturation
      c. Adolescent—is experiencing a physical, psychologic, and social growth spurt; the individual is asking: ''Who am I?'' on the way to developing a self-image; limitations provide additional stress during identity formation
      d. Adult—is expected to be independent and productive, to provide for self and family; if one cannot assume this role totally or partially, it can cause additional stress
      e. Aged—our society tends to venerate youth and deplore old age; all elderly persons are experiencing multiple stresses (loss of loved ones, changes in usual life-style, loss of physical vigor, and, for many, the thought of approaching death) at a time when their ability to adapt is compromised by the anatomic, physiologic, and psychologic alterations that occur during the aging process

3. Type of condition affecting the patient
   a. Acute illness—caused by a health problem that produces signs and symptoms abruptly, runs a short course, and from which there is usually a full recovery; an acute illness may leave an individual with a loss of a body part or function and may develop into a long-term illness
   b. Chronic illness—caused by a health problem that produces signs and symptoms over time, running a long course, and from which there is only partial recovery
      (1) Exacerbation—period when a chronic illness becomes more active and there is a recurrence of pronounced signs and symptoms of the disease
      (2) Remission—period when a chronic illness is controlled and signs and symptoms are reduced or not obvious
      (3) Degenerative—continuous deterioration or increased impairment of a person's physical state
   c. Terminal illness—no cure possible; death is inevitable in the near future
   d. Primary health problem—original condition, developing independently of another health problem
   e. Secondary health problem—direct result of another health problem

4. Personal resources
   a. Level of self-esteem—attitude that reflects the individual's perception of self-worth; it is a personal subjective judgment of oneself
   b. Experiential background—knowledge derived from one's own actions, observations, or perceptions; maturation, culture, and environment influence the individual's experiential foundation
   c. Intelligence
      (1) Genetic intellectual potential
      (2) Amount of formal and informal education
      (3) Level of intellectual development (e.g., child versus adult)
      (4) Ability to reason, conceptualize, and translate words into actions
   d. Level of motivation—internal desire or incentive to accomplish something
   e. Values—factors that are important to the individual
   f. Religion—deep personal belief in a higher force than humanity
5. Extent of actual or perceived change in body image
   a. Obvious reminder of disability to self and others
      (1) Loss of a body part
      (2) Need for a prosthesis (e.g., breast, leg, eye)
      (3) Need for hardware (e.g., pacemaker, braces, hearing aid, wheelchair)
      (4) Extent of disability or limitation
      (5) Need for medication
   b. Value placed on loss by self or society
      (1) "No longer whole," "a cripple"
      (2) Type of loss—perceptions of body part or function as being good, pleasing, repulsive, clean, dirty, etc.
         (a) Symbols of sexuality—breast, uterus, prostate, heart
         (b) May lack social acceptability—colostomy, mental illness, incontinence, cancer, tuberculosis
         (c) Impairment of senses and/or ability to communicate—laryngectomy, stroke, deafness, blindness
         (d) Altered body image resulting from anatomic changes—amputation of limb or breast, colostomy
6. Patient's and family's stage of adaptation
   a. Self-protection—disbelief, denial, avoidance, and/or intellectualization; with developing awareness of implications of illness the individual defends the self further—anger, depression, and/or joking
   b. With developing realization of implications of illness the individual reorganizes self-feelings and restructures relationships with family and society
   c. As the losses are resolved, the individual begins to accept the consequences of the illness and acknowledges feelings about the self and further changes that must be made
7. Patient's previous history
   a. Health history
      (1) Physiologic—what physical adaptations were manifested in the past
      (2) Psychologic—what psychologic methods of adaptation were exhibited in the past
   b. Sociocultural history
      (1) Religion—particular denomination, specific belief (e.g., agnostic, atheist, "energy force")
      (2) Ethnic group
      (3) Occupation
      (4) Economic status
      (5) Family members and their personal resources
      (6) Race
      (7) Educational background
      (8) Environment—urban versus rural, private home versus apartment
      (9) Social status

Establishment of a Teaching-Learning Environment

A. Definitions
   1. Teaching is communication especially structured and sequenced to produce learning
   2. Learning is the activity by which knowledge, attitudes, and skills are acquired, resulting in a change in behavior
   3. Goals of learning
      a. Understanding or acquiring knowledge—cognitive learning (e.g., What is diabetes and how does it affect me?)
      b. Feeling or developing attitudes—affective learning (e.g., What does this health problem mean to me?)
      c. Doing or developing psychomotor skills—conative learning (e.g., How do I give myself an injection?)
B. Principles of the teaching-learning process and related nursing approaches
   1. Learning occurs best when there is a felt need or readiness to learn

a. Identify the patient's emotional or motivational readiness—is the person ready to put forth the effort necessary to learn
b. Identify the patient's experiential readiness—does the person have the necessary background of experience, skills, attitudes, and ability to learn what is needed
c. Determine the patient's level of adaptation—it is usually difficult to teach during the beginning stages of adaptation because the patient is expressing denial, anger, and/or depression; once the initial defensive compensatory reactions have passed, the individual is more receptive to teaching
d. Assess the patient's level of human needs; the patient whose physical and safety needs are not met will not be concerned with interpersonal and intrapersonal needs
e. Specific signs of the patient's readiness to learn
    (1) The patient is adapting to the initial crisis
    (2) The patient has a developing awareness of the health problem and its implications
    (3) The patient is asking direct questions
    (4) The patient is presenting clues that indicate indirect seeking of information
    (5) The patient's physical condition or behavior invites the nurse to intervene through teaching
f. Once a need has been recognized, readiness has been determined, and the time and place are appropriate, develop a plan and teach
2. The method of presentation of material influences the patient's ability to learn
a. A tentative teaching plan should be developed and communicated to all members of the health team
b. Information presented should be organized, accurate, and concise (e.g., simple to the complex, general to the specific)
c. Appropriate teaching methods should be instituted
    (1) Concepts are best taught with lectures, audiovisual materials, and discussion
    (2) Attitudes are taught by exploring feelings, role models, discussions, and an atmosphere of acceptance
    (3) Skills are taught by illustrations, models, demonstration, return demonstration, and practice
d. Teaching tools should be used when indicated (e.g., models, filmstrips, illustrations)

e. The patient and family should be encouraged to ask questions, which should be answered directly
f. Opportunities should be provided for evaluation
3. Learning is made easier when material to be learned is related to what the learner already knows
a. Find out what the patient knows about the problem
b. Begin the teaching program at the patient's level of understanding
c. Avoid the use of technical terminology; use simple terms or ones with which the patient feels comfortable
4. Learning is purposeful; short- and long-term goals are important because they identify the behavior to be attained
a. With the patient, set short- and long-term goals
b. Goal should meet the following criteria:
    (1) Specific—state exactly what is to be accomplished
    (2) Measurable—set a minimum acceptable level of performance
    (3) Realistic—must be potentially achievable
5. Learning is an active process and takes place within the learner
a. Utilize a teaching approach that includes the learner (e.g., programed instruction books, discussion, questions and answers, return demonstration)
b. Provide opportunities for the patient to practice motor skills
c. Encourage self-directed activities
6. Every individual has capabilities and strengths (physical strengths, emotional maturity, a supportive family) that can be utilized to help the patient learn
a. Identify the patient's personal resources
b. Build on the identified strengths
c. Utilize these personal resources when and where appropriate
7. Energy and endurance levels will affect the patient's ability to learn and perform
a. During instructions, balance teaching with sufficient rest periods
b. Provide teaching at opportune times (e.g., earlier in the day rather than at night, after periods of rest)
c. Present instruction in a manner the patient can comprehend and at a pace that can be maintained

d. Be flexible and adjust the plan according to the patient's rest and activity needs

8. Learning does not always progress on a straight line forward and upward; the patient may experience plateaus and remissions with a resulting change in adaptation and needs
   a. Accept the patient's feelings regarding lack of progress
   b. Point out progress that has been made
   c. Be patient and do not cause additional stress for the learner
   d. Try alternative approaches for achieving goals
   e. Identify short-term objectives for meeting goals
   f. Alter long-term goals as necessary

9. Learning from previous experience can be transferred to new situations
   a. When teaching something new, relate the commonalities or similarities of previously learned experiences
   b. Base the plan of instructions on the foundation of the patient's knowledge
   c. Once the known is reinforced, then the unknown can be explored and the differences taught

C. Motivation
   1. Definition—motivation is the process of stimulating a person to assimilate certain concepts or behavior
   2. Principles of motivation and related nursing approaches
      a. People are complex products of self, family, and culture; the nurse must care for the patient as a unified being
         (1) Respect the patient as a person
         (2) Accept the patient's feelings without minimizing them
         (3) Assist the patient and family in accepting that the person's individuality and wholeness continue despite the changed physical or emotional state
         (4) Involve the patient in deciding what to do and how to do it
         (5) The patient must take precedence over the purpose of the lesson
      b. Learning is fostered when the plan of instruction is designed to operate within the individual's personal attitude and value system
         (1) Provide an atmosphere that allows for acceptance of differing value systems
         (2) Let the patient explore personal values, attitudes, and feelings concerning the health problem and its implications
         (3) Explore with the family the possibilities of carrying out instruction and how to individualize it so it is acceptable and practical for the patient and family
      c. Motivated learner assimilates what is learned more rapidly than does one who is not motivated
         (1) The patient needs an opportunity to explore and discover personal learning needs and feelings concerning them
         (2) Awareness of a need to know can cause mild anxiety, which in itself is motivating
         (3) Motivation that is too intense may reduce the effectiveness of learning
         (4) Determine the patient's readiness for learning
      d. Intrinsic motivation (stimulated from within the learner) is preferable to extrinsic motivation (stimulated from outside the learner)
         (1) Identify factors that are essential for the individual to have a feeling of meaningful achievement (e.g., being able to care for own health needs, respect and appreciation from others, acquiring new knowledge, receiving a reward)
         (2) Satisfaction with learning progress promotes additional learning; therefore design nursing care that will assist the patient in attaining a feeling of meaningful achievement
         (3) Encourage the patient to participate as a member of the health team and to be self-directed
      e. Information is learned more readily when it is relevant and meaningful to the learner
         (1) Help the patient interpret why the information is important and how the information gained will be useful
         (2) Relate the information by building the teaching plan on the patient's foundation of knowledge, experience, attitudes, and feelings
      f. Learning motivated by success or rewards is preferable to learning by failure or punishment
         (1) Help the patient set realistic goals within the motivation zone (goals set too high may be too challenging, whereas goals set too low may lead to no action)
         (2) Focus on the patient's strengths and abilities rather than on failures and disabilities

(3) Select learning tasks in which the patient is likely to succeed

(4) Assist the patient to master or feel successful at one stage of instruction before moving on to the next

(5) Errors must be accepted as part of the learning process

(6) Tolerance for failure is best taught through providing a backlog of success that compensates for experienced failure

g. Planned reinforcement is essential for learning; operant conditioning is based on the theory that satisfaction motivates learning and that those events which occur together are associated

(1) For each patient, identify and utilize factors that are stimulants or incentives for action (e.g., praise, smile, rewards, rest, specific privileges, being able to care for self)

(2) Provide visible reinforcements (e.g., progress charts, graphs)

(3) Repetition is a form of reinforcement; therefore repeated activities tend to become habitual

(a) Provide opportunities for the patient to practice old and new skills

(b) Review information previously taught before introducing new information

(4) Involve the patient in groups with people who have the same health problems but are at various stages of convalescence

(a) To be successful, it is helpful for the patient to associate with successful people

(b) Individuals can often learn more by teaching others

h. Evaluation of performance aids in learning

(1) Purpose

(a) To measure and interpret results with regard to what degree the set goals are being attained

(b) To reinforce correct behavior

(c) To help the learner realize how to change incorrect behavior

(d) To help the teacher determine the adequacy of the teaching

(2) Together the teacher and learner should observe and evaluate the learner's response in light of the desired behavior

(3) Explain the "whys" of a good or poor evaluation

(4) Value judgments, especially "poor" or "inadequate," must relate to the performance rather than to the individual

Leadership

A. Definition—process of influencing the actions of an individual or group toward specific goals in a particular situation

B. Styles of leadership

1. Three basic styles

a. Autocratic—leader does not seek input from the group but sets the goals, plans, makes the decisions, and evaluates the action taken

b. Democratic—leader seeks input from the group, and responsibilities for action taken are shared between the leader and the group

c. Laissez-faire—leader's input and control of the group are minimal, permitting each individual to set independent goals

2. Leadership styles influenced by the leader, the environment, and the cultural climate of the organization

3. The effective leader modifies his or her style to fit changing circumstances, problems, and people (e.g., autocratic style of leadership is appropriate in an emergency situation)

C. Principles of leadership

1. Interpersonal influence is dependent upon a knowledge of human behavior and a sensitivity to others in terms of feelings, values, and problems

a. Explore and understand attitudes, feelings, and personal values about self

b. Project self into the place of the individuals being led

c. Know how you appear to subordinates

2. Communication is an essential component of leadership

a. Effective communication dependent upon use of the appropriate medium

(1) Communication may be verbal, written, and/or nonverbal

(2) Communication may be formal or informal

(3) Communication should have two directions: up and down; to and from

b. Communication style can affect the person or persons with whom the leader communicates

(1) Meanings or ideas communicated should be received or intended without distraction

(a) People react to communication differently

(b) Written communication should be in language that is understood by the person or persons intended (e.g., ancillary personnel should have a written assignment which does not require them to make judgments)

(c) Verbal communication can be influenced by facial expressions, body movement, and tone of voice

c. Effectiveness of communication can be influenced by inappropriate timing; the information communicated may be correct, but the time may be wrong (ascertain readiness)

3. Leader's success is influenced by the perception of those being led as to the leader's ability to respond to group needs effectively

a. A role is composed of a number of expectations for the behavior of an individual in a specific position or status classification

(1) Any individual's role consists of a number of expectations and relationships

(2) Nurse leader, by virtue of behavior and status, can influence the perceptions of peers, patients, and colleagues

b. Power is a leader's source of influence

c. Power may be professional or positional

(1) *Positional power*—acquired through position the leader has in the hierarchy of the organization

(2) *Professional power*—acquired through the knowledge or expertise displayed by the leader and/or perceived by the followers

4. Leadership moves from one person to another as changes occur in the work situation

a. Nurse's expertise about a specific patient care problem along with the availability of other resources can place the nurse in the position of providing leadership for a group

b. Member of another discipline may assume the role of leadership in specific situations (e.g., the physician leads the cardiac arrest team; the nurse coordinates physical rehabilitation and nutrition for the patient)

5. Leadership process requires the utilization of actions associated with problem solving: decision making, relating, influencing, and facilitating

a. Decision making requires knowledge about and skill in solving the problem; participative decision making lends itself to the quality of the decision made, improves relationships, and influences the readiness of an individual or group to accept change (e.g., the patient

or the family should have the opportunity to participate in the development of the patient's plan of care; unit staff may decide which primary nurse or team leader should care for a newly admitted patient)

b. Effective delegation of responsibilities is inherent in effective leadership; delegation of work requires matching the task with the appropriate position (e.g., a nursing assistant should not be providing care that requires the expertise of a registered nurse; utilizing a registered nurse for housekeeping duties is wasteful)

6. Need for change should be understood by those effecting the change as well as those affected by the change

a. Movement from goal setting to goal achievement involves change

b. Process of changing includes communication, planning, participation, and evaluation by the individual or group affected

c. Change is more acceptable when

(1) It has not been dictated but follows a sequence of impersonal principles

(2) Individuals or groups affected have participated it its creation

(3) It has been planned

(4) It follows a number of successful rather than unsuccessful series of changes

(5) It is initiated after other changes have been absorbed, not during the confusion of a major change

(6) It does not threaten security

7. Effective use of leadership is conducive to accomplishing the goals of the group; an evaluation process is necessary if the results of efforts to attain the goals are to be interpreted accurately

a. Goals should be identified as short term and long term

b. Evaluation process should be ongoing

c. Climate in which the evaluation process occurs influences its success

Administration of Medications

A. Introduction

1. Scientific age has introduced an increasing number of pharmaceuticals appropriate for relief of stress symptoms, for support of defense systems, and as adjuncts to other supplemental and curative therapies

2. Increasingly, as part of nursing care, the nurse is assuming the responsibility of administering

these medications, either singly or in combinations

3. In the interest of patient welfare and safety, it is imperative that the independent and collaborative responsibilities inherent in this function be understood and practiced

B. Basic concepts

1. Legally, administration of medications is a dependent function requiring a physician's written order and knowledge of cause and effect
2. Legally, morally, and ethically, independent judgment is required before prescribed medications are administered
3. Certain chemical agents alter, inactivate, or potentiate other medications when mixed either prior to or after administration
4. Medications may be given for local or systemic effects
5. Pharmacologic actions of drugs tend to stimulate or depress physiologic activity
6. Medications may be given in a variety of ways, depending on factors such as the effect desired, rapidity of action desired, or the effect of the chemical on the tissues

C. Common terms

1. Chemotherapy—use of drugs to destroy invading organisms or abnormal tissue in the host
2. Drug—chemical agent that interacts with living systems and is employed to prevent, diagnose, or treat disease
3. Drug legislation—laws that provide the standards for drug manufacture and distribution and protect the public against fraudulent claims about drug action (e.g., Federal Controlled Substances Act, regulations of the Federal Bureau of Narcotics and Dangerous Drugs, regulations by specific states)
4. Drug standards—criteria for drug composition established by chemical or bioassay and published in official publications (e.g., *United States Pharmacopeia, National Formulary, Pharmacopoeia Internationalis*)
5. Pharmacodynamics—biochemical and physiologic effects of drugs and their mechanisms of action on living tissue
6. Pharmacology—analysis of properties of chemicals that have a biologic action
7. Pharmacotherapeutics—planned use and evaluation of the effect of drugs employed to prevent and treat disease
8. Toxicology—analysis of poisons and poisonings caused by drugs

D. Terms that describe drug effects

1. Adverse effect—action differing from the planned effect that is undesirable
2. Side effect—often predictable outcome that is unrelated to the primary action of the drug
3. Toxic effect—pathologic extension of the primary action of the drug
4. Cumulation—elevation of circulating levels of a drug consequent to slowing of metabolic pathways or excretory mechanisms
5. Drug dependence—driving need for continued use of a behavior- or mood-altering drug that leads to abuse
   a. Psychic dependence—craving requiring periodic or continued use of a drug for pleasure or relief of discomfort
   b. Physical dependence—appearance of characteristic symptoms when drug use is suspended or terminated (withdrawal or abstinence symptoms)
6. Hypersusceptibility—response to a drug action which is higher than that occurring when the same dosage is given to 90% of the population
7. Idiosyncrasy—unpredictable, highly individualized response; genetically conditioned enzymatic or receptor responsiveness that interferes with metabolic degradation of a drug
8. Paradoxical response—action of a drug producing a response that contrasts sharply with the usual therapeutic effect obtained with the same dosage of the drug
9. Receptor—cellular site where union between a drug and a cellular constituent produces a reversible action
10. Tolerance—lowering of effect obtained from an established dosage of a drug that necessitates raising the dosage to maintain the effect
11. Tachyphylaxis—rapidly developing tolerance to a drug
12. Drug allergy—response occurring when drugs are from protein sources or combine with body protein and induce an allergen-antibody reaction which releases vasoactive intermediates that cause fluid transudation into tissues
    a. Anaphylaxis—life-threatening episode of bronchial constriction and edema which obstruct the airway and cause generalized vasodilation that depletes circulating blood volume; occurs when a drug allergen is administered to an individual having antibodies produced by prior use of the drug
    b. Urticaria—generalized pruritic skin eruptions or giant hives; occurs when a drug is

administered to an individual having antibodies produced by prior use of the drug

  c. Angioedema—fluid accumulation in periorbital, oral, and respiratory tissues with lengthening of the expiratory phase and wheezing as bronchial constriction gradually progresses; occurs when a drug is administered to an individual having antibodies produced by prior use of the drug

  d. Serum sickness—gradually emerging intermittent episodes of dyspnea, hypotension, generalized edema, joint pain, rash, swollen lymph glands; occurs 7 or more days after initial administration of a drug causing gradual low-level (titer) production of antibodies that interact with circulating drug to produce symptoms as long as the drug remains in the body

  e. Arthus reaction—localized area of tissue necrosis caused by disruption of blood supply; occurs when spasticity, occlusion, and degeneration of blood vessels are precipitated by injection of a drug into a site having large quantities of bivalent antibodies

  f. Delayed-reaction allergies—rash and fever occurring during drug therapy

E. Drug actions
  1. Local—drug acts at the site of application
  2. Systemic—drug is distributed to selected internal receptor sites after being absorbed from tissues following administration; these routes include oral, sublingual, buccal, rectal, parenteral (intradermal, subcutaneous, intramuscular, intravenous, intraspinal, intracardiac)

F. Mechanisms
  1. Replacement—e.g., administration of insulin required for cellular utilization of glucose
  2. Interruption—e.g., antimetabolic drugs tricking the cell into utilizing an inactive component in building protein
  3. Potentiation—e.g., sulfonylurea group of oral hypoglycemic agents stimulating pancreatic beta cells to produce insulin

G. Factors influencing dosage-response relationships
  1. Age, weight, sex, size, physiologic status and genetic and environmental factors affect responses and dosage required for therapeutic effect
  2. The ratio between the median toxic dose and the median effective dose (TD50/ED50) of a drug provides the therapeutic index (T.I.), which is used as a guide to the safe dosage range; a low T.I., provides a narrow margin of safety, and the patient's status is monitored closely for evidence of drug-related adverse effects (e.g., antineoplastic drugs)

  3. Concentration of active drug at receptors and duration of drug action are affected by
    a. Characteristics of the drug and the rate of absorption, distribution, biotransformation, and excretion
    b. Drug affinity for particular tissues, immaturity of enzymes required for metabolism of the drug, or depressed function of tissues naturally metabolizing or excreting the drug
  4. Membrane barriers, placental or blood-brain barrier, may block or selectively pass the drug from the circulating fluids to protected areas
  5. Plasma protein binding of drugs maintains tissue levels by liberating the drug when stores are lowered and by slowing renal clearance until the drug is freed from binding sites

H. Drug interactions
  1. Drugs and foods may interact to affect the therapeutic plan adversely (e.g., ingestion of foods or vitamin preparations containing vitamin K may inhibit the hypothrombinemic effect of oral anticoagulants)
  2. Drug antagonism—opposing effects of 2 drugs at receptor sites in body tissues
    a. Chemical antagonism—combining or binding of 2 drugs causing inactivation of the chemicals
    b. Pharmacologic antagonism—competition of 2 drugs for a receptor that may allow the weaker drug to block access by the more potent drug
    c. Physiologic antagonism—opposing action on physiologic systems that allows cancellation of action by either drug
  3. Drug action summation—combined or concurrent action of drugs that increases therapeutic effects or incidence of adverse effects
    a. Synergism—interaction of drugs at common receptor sites that alters metabolism or excretion and enhances the effect of drugs
    b. Addition—action of 2 drugs at different receptors which produces an effect twice that possible when either drug is used alone
    c. Potentiation—intensified action occurring when 2 drugs are administered concurrently that is greater than when either drug is administered alone

I. General information
  1. Drug nomenclature
    a. Official name (generic, nonproprietary)—designated title under which a drug is listed in offical publications

b. Chemical name—descriptive name identifying chemical composition and placement of atoms

c. Trade name (brand, proprietary)—manufacturer's registered and legally owned name for a drug

2. Sources of drugs

a. Active constituents of plants—alkaloids, glycosides, gums, resins, tannins, waxes, volatile or fixed oils

b. Animal sources of biologic products—enzymes, sera, vaccines, antitoxins, toxoids, hormones

c. Mineral sources—iron, iodine, Epsom salt

3. Drug dosage forms

a. Prepared by manufacturers in units for convenience of administration

b. Forms used include capsules, extended-release capsules, tablets (enteric-coated, extended-release), troches, pills, suppositories, powders, ampules, vials, delayed-release (repository) suspensions, prefilled cartridges, liniments, lotions, creams, ointments, pastes

c. Chemical preparations—solutions (waters, true solutions, syrups), aqueous suspensions (mixtures, emulsions, magmas, gels), spirits, elixirs, tinctures, fluidextracts, extracts

J. Nursing responsibilities

1. Ascertain the presence and correctness of a physician's order

2. Know the common symbols and equivalents in the apothecary and metric systems

3. Know the common abbreviations denoting frequency and route of administration

4. Know the usual dosage of a drug, the usual route of administration, and the expected, unusual, untoward, or toxic effects of drug

5. Use independent judgment before administering a medication by assessing

a. The patient's need relative to factors such as p.r.n. medications and expected effects of the medication (e.g., diuresis or sleep)

b. Untoward or toxic manifestations of prior doses (e.g., pruritus following an antibiotic, bradycardia below 60, visual disturbances with digoxin)

c. Compatibility of medications administered at the same time

(1) The presence of clouding or a precipitate when mixing injectables (e.g., phenobarbital [Luminal Sodium] and meperidine [Demerol])

(2) Inhibition of medication (e.g., antacids or milk given with tetracycline interferes with absorption, resulting in decreased serum levels of the antibiotic)

(3) Potentiation of another medication (e.g., A.S.A. given when a patient is receiving anticoagulants intensifies the anticoagulant effect)

d. Effects on living tissues

(1) Iron can discolor tissue and must be given through a straw in liquid form or by the Z-track method intramuscularly

(2) Abscess formation can occur when the same area is used too frequently for intramuscular administration; thus rotation of site is necessary

(3) Pain, irritation, or inflammation can occur during intravenous administration and may necessitate adjustments such as greater dilution or slower flow rate

6. Help the patient accept ordered medications by independent actions such as

a. Crushing tablets that cannot be swallowed

b. Disguising unpalatable tastes with fruit juices

c. Reinforcing the need for medication

7. Ensure that the right medication is given to the right patient at the right time in the right dose and by the right route

a. Verify orders

b. Read labels

c. Calculate the dosage accurately when prescribed dose is not available

d. Pour or draw up correct amounts

e. Identify the patient correctly by checking the arm band

f. Prepare the patient psychologically by providing explanations as needed

g. Prepare the patient physically by

(1) Positioning appropriately for oral and parenteral medications

(2) Disinfecting the skin when it is to be punctured

h. Use clean or sterile technique as indicated by route of administration

i. Use the route specified as appropriate for the ordered medication and dosage

8. For assistance with calculation of solutions and dosages refer to a programed text (see Bibliography)

9. Use the appropriate technique for administration

a. Preparations such as tablets, capsules, pills, powders, or liquids may be swallowed; in addition

(1) Tablets (e.g., nitroglycerine) may be held sublingually
(2) Powders (e.g., cromolyn sodium) may be inhaled with a Medihaler
(3) Liquids may be nebulized and inhaled or may be swabbed, sprayed, or instilled
b. Parenteral preparations such as ampules or vials containing the dose in solution or powder to which sterile water or saline must be added may be given in several ways
(1) Subcutaneously or hypodermically in small volume (0.5 to 2 ml)
(a) Pinch the tissue on the outer surface of the upper arm or the anterior aspect of the thigh or the abdomen
(b) Insert a 25- to 26-gauge needle ⅝ to 1 inch in length at a 45-to-60-degree angle, aspirate slightly, and inject the medication if there was no blood return (aspiration not indicated when heparin is administered)
(c) Massage to increase absorption (contraindicated when giving heparin)
(2) Intramuscularly in slightly larger volume (up to 5 ml)
(a) Spread the tissue taut or pinch if necessary
(b) Use the upper outer quadrant of the buttock or ventral gluteal muscle, the lateral aspect of the thigh, or the deltoid area of the arm
(c) When using the gluteal muscle, promote relaxation of the muscle whenever possible by placing the patient in a prone position with toes pointing inward or on the side with the upper leg flexed
(d) Insert a 19- to 22-gauge needle 1 to 2 inches in length at a 90-degree angle quickly and smoothly
(e) Depth of insertion depends on factors such as weight of the patient and size of the muscle used
(f) Aspirate when the needle is in place and tissue is released (unless giving a substance such as iron-dextran [Imferon], for which it is contraindicated)
(1) If no blood returns, continue injection

(2) If blood is aspirated, withdraw and prepare a fresh dose
(g) Apply pressure or massage area after injection as required (unless contraindicated, e.g., Z-track technique)
(3) Intradermally with very small volume for local effect
(a) Use syringe with appropriate calibrations; e.g., tuberculin
(b) Inject at a 15-degree angle using a 26-gauge needle, ⅜ to ½ inch in length with the bevel up
(4) Piggyback administration using intravenous tubing in place
(a) Dilute medication according to directions—usually with 50 to 150 ml of fluid
(b) Remove air from tubing of piggyback
(c) Cleanse diaphragm on intravenous tubing already in place with alcohol
(d) Insert needle in rubber diaphragm on tubing leading from the infusion that is keeping the vein open
(e) Stop flow of or lower the primary solution below level of the piggyback
(f) Adjust rate of flow on piggyback medication to complete absorption in time designated—usually about 30 minutes
(g) Remove the piggyback and readjust flow rate
10. Clearly and accurately record and report the administration of medications and the patient's response

Preoperative and Postoperative Care

REVIEW OF MICROBIOLOGY
Bacteria

A. Definition—bacteria are unicellular microbes without chlorophyll
B. Some examples of medically important bacteria
1. Eubacteriales ("true bacteria")—typically unicellular microbes having a rigid cell wall; the morphologic types are
a. Rod-shaped bacilli—variations of the rod shape may be curved or clubbed (some of the gram-positive rods form endospores)
b. Spherical cocci

c. Eubacteriales are divided into 5 families based on shape, Gram stain, and endospore formation
   (1) Gram-positive cocci include
      (a) Diplococci—occurring predominantly in pairs (e.g., *Diplococcus pneumoniae*)
      (b) Streptococci—occurring predominantly in chains (e.g., *Streptococcus pyogenes*)
      (c) Staphylococci—occurring predominantly in grapelike bunches (e.g., *Staphylococcus aureus*)
   (2) Gram-negative cocci include *Neisseria gonorrhoeae* and *Neisseria meningitidis*
   (3) Gram-negative rods include enterobacteria such as *Escherichia*, *Salmonella*, and *Shigella* species
   (4) Gram-positive rods that do not produce endospores include *Corynebacterium diphtheriae*
   (5) Gram-positive rods producing endospores include *Bacillus anthracis, Clostridium botulinum,* and *Clostridium tetani*
2. Actinomycetales (actinomycetes)—moldlike microbes with elongated cells, frequently filamentous (e.g., *Mycobacterium tuberculosis* and *Mycobacterium leprae*)
3. Spirochaetales (spirochetes)—flexuous, spiral organisms (e.g., *Treponema pallidum*)
4. Mycoplasmatales (mycoplasmas)—delicate, nonmotile microbes displaying a variety of sizes and shapes
   a. Commonly referred to as pleuropneumonia-like organisms (PPLO)
   b. Mycoplasmas are the smallest organisms known that are capable of growth and reproduction outside living cells

C. Bacterial cell
1. Size—from 0.5 to 15 mm
2. Cell wall—gram-positive species are rich in muramic acid and low in lipids; the opposite is true of the gram-negative species
3. Capsule—a thickened protective material (generally a polysaccharide) that is secreted by the cell, thereby protecting it from being phagocytized and increasing its virulence (e.g., *Diplococcus pneumoniae*)
4. Spores—the inactive resistant structures into which bacterial protoplasm can transform under adverse conditions (under favorable conditions a spore germinates into an active and growing vegetative cell)
   a. The endospores are resistant to heat, desiccation, and other antimicrobial agents
   b. Spore formers *Clostridium tetani* and *Clostridium botulinum* are difficult to destroy; therefore their destruction is used to set the standards of sterilization for the hospital and food industries
5. Flagella—organelles of locomotion possessed by all motile bacteria; some species have 1 flagellum (monotrichous), whereas others have flagella over their entire surface (peritrichous)
6. Reproduction—bacteria reproduce by binary fission, an asexual process dividing the cell into new daughter cells; bacteria are also able to conjugate and exchange genetic material (recombination)

D. Growth needs
1. Nutrition
   a. Autotrophic organisms—may do well on simple diet of carbon dioxide, inorganic salts, and water
   b. Heterotrophic organisms—demand organic nutrients
      (1) Saprophytes—derive nourishment from dead or decaying organic matter
      (2) Parasites—derive nourishment from living tissue; obligate parasites cannot be cultured except in living tissue
2. Culturing
   a. Culture—growth of large numbers of microbes on suitable food media (e.g., broth, agar, milk)
   b. Culture media—food substances in or on which cultures are grown
   c. Colony—cluster of millions of microbes, presumably all descendants from a single bacterium, visible to naked eye
   d. Ways in which cultures are studied
      (1) Smears made and organisms studied microscopically either with or without staining
      (2) Cultural characteristics observed
         (a) Media most favorable to growth
         (b) Appearance of colonies—color, shape, and texture, whether large or small, smooth or rough, opaque or translucent
         (c) Molecular oxygen requirement—anaerobic, aerobic, or facultative

E. Biochemical reactions
1. Fermentation—anaerobic oxidation reactions by which some organisms use carbohydrates to generate energy-rich adenosine triphosphate

(ATP) molecules; various kinds of fermentation reactions are useful for identifying different groups of microorganisms
   a. Nonfermenters
   b. Fermenters that produce only acid
   c. Fermenters that produce acid and gas (e.g., *Escherichia coli,* a normal inhabitant of the intestinal tract)
   d. Lactose fermenters (e.g., *Escherichia coli* and other nonpathogens in the intestinal tract)
   e. Nonlactose fermenters (e.g., *Shigella* and *Salmonella* pathogens in the intestinal tract)
  2. Urea-splitting reaction—identifies organisms as
   a. Urease-positive organisms (contain enzyme urease, which catalyzes conversion of urea to ammonia) (e.g., *Proteus bacilli* [gram-negative, normal inhabitants of the intestinal tract])
   b. Urease-negative organisms—do not contain urease so cannot convert urea to ammonia (e.g., *Salmonella* and *Shigella,* pathogens in the intestinal tract)
F. Hydrogen ion concentration (pH)—majority of bacteria grow and are cultured best at a pH of about 7.5; most fungi (molds and yeasts) are cultured best at a pH of about 5
G. Oxygen utilization
  1. Obligate aerobes—organisms that cannot grow without free (molecular) oxygen
  2. Obligate anaerobes—organisms that cannot grow in the presence of free (molecular) oxygen
  3. Facultative—organisms that can grow with or without free oxygen
H. Temperature
  1. Psychrophiles—organisms growing best at low temperatures (10° to 20° C [50° to 68° F])
  2. Mesophiles—organisms growing best at "middle temperatures" (20° to 45° C [68° to 113° F]); this range includes human pathogens that have an optimum temperature of 37° C (98.6° F)
  3. Thermophiles—organisms growing best at high temperatures (45° to 65° C [113° to 149° F])
I. Staining—artificial coloration to facilitate visualization and identification of tissues and microorganisms.
  1. Gram stain—gram-positive organisms retain the crystal violet color when treated with ethyl alcohol; gram-negative organisms are decolorized with ethyl alcohol
  2. Acid-fast stain—after being stained with carbol-fuchsin, acid-fast organisms resist decolorization with dilute acid alcohol and do not take counterstain (usually methylene blue); non-acid-fast organisms decolorize and take counterstain
J. Pathogenicity—some 2000 species of bacteria, most of which are harmless; those causing disease (pathogens) are usually heterotrophic mesophiles

Viruses

A. Definition—obligate intracellular parasite of unknown relationship to other forms of life
B. Characteristics—virions (virus particles)—range in size from 1 to 350 nanometers (nm); 1 nm equals 1 billionth of a meter or $\frac{1}{1000}$ of a millimeter; some cuboidal and others rod shaped; unlike rickettsiae and chlamydiae, composed of either ribonucleic acid (RNA) or deoxyribonucleic acid (DNA), not both
C. Classification
  1. Animal viruses—some contain RNA and others DNA; divided into 14 categories on the basis of particle size, symmetry, and nucleic acid content
  2. Plant viruses—contain RNA
  3. Bacterial viruses—most contain DNA; those which destroy bacterial cells called bacteriophages
D. Culturing—being obligate parasites, viruses demand living tissues such as embryonated hen's eggs, tissue cultures, and animal inoculation
E. Pathogenicity—viruses cause cancer in animals and Burkitt's lymphoma, mumps, rubeola, rubella, smallpox, chickenpox, herpes simplex, encephalitis, yellow fever, and many other infections in humans

Fungi

A. Definition—higher protists; include morels, truffles, cup fungi, mildews, mushrooms, puffballs, smuts, rusts, molds, and yeasts (molds and yeasts are of medical concern)
B. Molds—fuzzy growths of intertacing filaments called hyphae
  1. Hyphae—filaments of a mold; in some species hyphae are divided by partial septa and appear to be multicellular, whereas in others they are nonseptate
  2. Mycelium—tuft of interwoven hyphae
  3. Spores—means by which molds reproduce; a single spore in the proper environment gives rise to a new mycelium; spores produced sexually and asexually
C. Yeasts—organisms that usually are single celled and usually reproduce by budding
  1. Yeast cell—round or ovoid and much larger and more complex than bacterial cell
  2. Reproduction—usually by the asexual process of budding, but many species also reproduce sexually by means of ascospores

3. True yeasts—reproduce sexually as well as asexually (by budding); many species, such as *Saccharomyces cerevisiae* (baker's yeast), convert glucose into alcohol and carbon dioxide (alcoholic fermentation); *Candida albicans,* another type of yeast, causes "thrush" in humans (this yeast is part of the normal flora but may become an opportunistic pathogen in persons with low resistance)

4. Pathogenicity—certain species of molds cause infection, particularly those belonging to the class Fungi Imperfecti (Deuteromycetes), which account for diseases such as athlete's foot, ringworm of the scalp and axillary regions, and systemic mycosis

Microbial Control

A. Definitions
1. Disinfection—removal of or destruction of pathogenic microbes
2. Sterilization—removal or destruction of all microbes

B. Physical methods
1. Heat sterilization
   a. Moist heat
      (1) Steam under pressure (autoclave)—usually operated at 121° C (250° F) (15 lb pressure per square inch); time needed for procedure depends on material(s) being sterilized
      (2) Boiling water—object(s) to be sterilized immersed in water and boiled for 15 minutes; because some spores resist boiling, this procedure is not suitable for surgical instruments
   b. Dry heat (hot-air oven)
      (1) Operating temperature—160° to 170° C (310° to 338° F) (usually for 2 hours)
      (2) Items sterilized—petrolatum gauze dressings and other items that might be damaged by steam or water
   c. Pasteurization—disinfection of milk and other substances by moderate heat; pathogenic organisms killed and microbial development considerably delayed (thus retarding spoilage)
      (1) Holding method—heating to 63° C (145° F) for 30 minutes, followed by rapid cooling
      (2) Flash method—heating to 71.7° C (161° F) for not less than 15 seconds, followed by rapid cooling
2. Radiation—all types of radiation injurious to microbes

   a. Gamma rays—used to sterilize food and drugs
   b. Ultraviolet light—used to inhibit the microbial population of air in operating rooms, nurseries, laboratories, school rooms, and food establishments (the disadvantage of ultraviolet light is that it has little penetration power)
3. Filtration—removal of microbes from liquids by means of porous materials (diatomaceous earth, asbestos, porcelain); used to sterilize drugs, culture media, and certain other heat-sensitive substances
4. Refrigeration—low temperature inhibits microbial multiplication; used for food preservation
5. Hypertonicity—by their osmotic effects hypertonic solutions inhibit microbial multiplication (e.g., brine and syrups)
6. Desiccation (drying)—removal of water; bacterial spores and certain vegetable cells are resistant to such treatment; commonly used in food preservation

C. Chemical agents (for body surfaces and inanimate objects)
1. Definitions—many terms used to describe action of chemical agents on microorganisms; in actual practice such terms often have little meaning because of variables
   a. Antiseptic—inhibits microbial growth
   b. Disinfectant—destroys pathogenic microbes
   c. Germicide—destroys pathogenic microbes
   d. Bactericide—destroys bacteria
   e. Fungicide—destroys fungi
   f. Viricide—destroys viruses
2. Conditions (variables) affecting action of chemical agents
   a. Type and number of microbes—microbes respond differently to different agents; spores are resistant to most agents
   b. Concentration—typically the greater the concentration of chemical, the greater the effect
   c. Time—a certain time needed for maximum effect
   d. Temperature—a rise usually hastens action
   e. Organic matter—presence inhibits action
3. Evaluation—various tests used to evaluate antiseptics and disinfectants; all have limitations
   a. Phenol coefficient—bactericidal activity of a chemical agent in relation to the bactericidal action of phenol
   b. Culture inhibition—filter paper disks impregnated or saturated with chemical agent placed on agar plates previously inoculated

with test organism; clear zone observed around disk (following incubation) if agent is inhibitory to organism (this is the same procedure used in determining the sensitivity of a culture to chemotherapeutic agents)

4. Commonly used chemical agents
    a. Ethyl alcohol (70%)
    b. Isopropyl alcohol (80%)
    c. Benzalkonium chloride (Zephiran) (1:1000)
    d. Hydrogen peroxide (3%)
    e. Silver nitrate (1%)
    f. Iodine and iodine-releasing compounds
    g. Chlorine and chlorine-releasing compounds
    h. Substituted phenols
    i. Cresols
    j. Ethylene oxide

D. Chemotherapy—the systemic use of chemical agents (antiinfectives) in the treatment of infection
    1. Anti-infectives
        a. Antibiotics
        b. Sulfonamides
        c. Anthelmintics
        d. Antiprotozoals
        e. Tuberculostatics
    2. Antibiotic sensitivity—determined by 2 general techniques
        a. Paper disks—multilobed disk impregnated with different antibiotics placed on surface of inoculated plate; zones of inhibition (following incubation) surround lobes containing antibiotics to which microbe is sensitive
        b. Tube dilution—antibiotic in question diluted out in growth broth and tubes then inoculated with the organisms in question; minimal inhibitory concentration (MIC) determined (following incubation) by noting minimal concentration preventing growth

Infection

A. Definition—invasion of the body by pathogenic microorganisms (pathogens) and the reaction of the tissues to their presence and to the toxins generated by them

B. Types
    1. Local, focal, or systemic
        a. Local infection—one in which etiologic agent is limited to one locality of the body, such as a boil; often a local infection may have systemic repercussions such as fever and malaise
        b. Focal infection—a local infection such as an abscess from which the organisms themselves spread to other parts of body (e.g., a tooth abscess that continues to seed organisms into the blood)
        c. Systemic infection—one in which the infectious agent is spread throughout the body (e.g., typhoid fever)
    2. Acute or chronic
        a. Acute infection—one that develops rapidly, usually resulting in a high fever and severe sickness
        b. Chronic infection—one that develops slowly, with mild but longer-lasting symptoms; sometimes an acute infection may become chronic and vice-versa
    3. Primary or secondary
        a. Primary infection—initial infection, unrelated to other health problems
        b. Secondary infection—occasioned when invaders (or opportunists) take advantage of the weakened defenses resulting from the primary infection (e.g., staphylococcal pneumonia as a sequela of measles)
    4. Bacteremia—presence of nonmultiplying bacteria in the blood
    5. Septicemia—bacterial cells actively multiplying in the blood
    6. Toxemia—presence of microbial toxins in the blood
    7. Viremia—presence of viruses in the blood

C. Proof of etiology (Koch's postulates)—4 requirements must be fulfilled to establish a given microbe as the etiologic agent of a given disease
    1. Particular microbe must be found in every case of the particular disease
    2. Particular microbe must be isolated and grown in pure culture
    3. Particular microbe must cause particular disease when inoculated into susceptible animal
    4. Particular microbe must be recovered from inoculated animal and its identity established

D. Source and transmission of pathogens
    1. Source—ultimate source (or reservoir) of almost all pathogens is humans or animals; human sources include
        a. Persons exhibiting symptoms of disease
        b. Carriers—persons who harbor a pathogen in the absence of a discernible clinical disease
            (1) Types of carriers
                (a) Healthy carriers—those who have never had the disease in question
                (b) Incubatory carriers—those in the incubation period of a disease
                (c) Chronic carriers—those who have recovered from a disease but continue to harbor pathogens

(2) Diseases commonly spread by carriers
   (a) Typhoid fever
   (b) Diphtheria
   (c) Meningitis
   (d) Pneumonia
   (e) Dysentery
2. Transmission
   a. Direct
      (1) Body contact
      (2) Droplets (droplet infection)
   b. Indirect
      (1) Food
      (2) Water
      (3) Air
      (4) Soil
      (5) Fomites
      (6) Vectors (insects)
         (a) Mechanical transfer—insects' feet
         (b) Biologic transfer—microbe undergoes part of its life cycle in the insect's body
3. Portals of entry and exit
   a. Portal of entry—where microbes enter the body
      (1) Nose
      (2) Mouth
      (3) Urogenital tract
      (4) Skin: wounds, abrasions, and insect bites
   b. Portal of exit—where microbes leave the body
      (1) Nose
      (2) Mouth
      (3) Feces
      (4) Urine
      (5) Vaginal discharges
      (6) Pus and exudates
      (7) Vomitus
      (8) Blood
E. Development
   1. Definitions
      a. Pathogenicity—ability of a microbe to cause disease
      b. Virulence—degree of pathogenicity
   2. Determinants of pathogenicity
      a. Chemical products
         (1) Exotoxins—heat-labile proteins readily released from bacterial cell; most deadly of all biologic poisons (e.g., botulism, tetanus, and diphtheria)
         (2) Endotoxins—heat-stable lipopolysaccharide-protein complexes released from gram-negative bacteria; less deadly than exotoxins (e.g., typhoid fever and dysentery)
         (3) Other toxic products
            (a) Hemolysins—these destroy the red cells (erythrocytes)
            (b) Leukocidins—these destroy the white cells (leukocytes)
            (c) Coagulase—clots blood plasma
            (d) Hyaluronidase—dissolves intercellular cement
            (e) Kinases—dissolve clots or inhibit their formation
            (f) Collagenase—disintegrates collagen
      b. Cellular destruction—some microbes damage tissues and cause disease by direct mechanical injury to the cells, particularly intracellular parasites (e.g., viruses and rickettsiae)
      c. Capsules—increase virulence apparently by making microbes possessing them less vulnerable to destruction by phagocytosis

REVIEW OF PHYSICAL PRINCIPLES RELATED TO PREOPERATIVE AND POSTOPERATIVE CARE
Electricity
Static Electricity
A. Substances can be charged by friction, whereby a negatively charged object picks up positive charges, which it discharges via a spark when touching an object that is a good conductor
B. Applications
   1. Removing blankets and sheets from a bed will build up electric charges through the hands that should be discharged by touching a grounded object before touching others
   2. Wool, silk, nylon, and Dacron may set off sparks caused by static electric charges and should not be used around combustible gases or monitoring equipment
   3. Electric equipment and operating room tables should be grounded to allow static charges to drain off, thus preventing sparks

Current Electricity
A. Direct current (DC)—flow of electric charge in one direction only (e.g., the electric system of an automobile)
B. Alternating current (AC)—electric charge moves first in one direction and then in the opposite direction, with the voltages and currents alternating back and forth (e.g., the outlets in homes and hospitals)
C. Concept of electric energy and work
   1. Potential energy of the electric field is called electric potential and is measured in volts (V)

2. Rate of flow of electric current is measured in amperes (amp); 1 amp is a current flow of 1 coulomb/second; a coulomb is 6.25 billion electrons
3. Ohm's law—electric potential (volts), rate of flow of electric charge (amperes), and resistance are related; the rate of flow of electricity between 2 points is directly proportional to the impressed voltage and inversely proportional to the resistance between the 2 points; thus the rate of flow of electricity can be increased by either increasing the voltage or decreasing the resistance
   a. Dry fingers or hands touching an ungrounded or faulty electric source can result in a definite shock; the source touched with wet fingers or while standing in water can result in enough electric energy to be fatal
   b. As little as 0.05 amp can be fatal, and 0.1 amp is practically always fatal since the electric currents upset the natural electric rhythms of the heart and can result in fibrillation and also stop the breathing center from working
   c. The shock obtained via alternating current is not caused by electrons pouring from the socket into the body but by the powerful vibrations of electrons and ions already inside the body, which are energized via the electric field that is flowing from the outlet

Power
A. Power represents the quantity of energy used per unit of time and is expressed in watts (W)
B. The kilowatt (kW) is 1000 W; power companies compute the number of kilowatt hours of power used for billing purposes; a kilowatt hour is the quantity of electric power consumed in 1 hour at a rate of 1 kW per hour

Application
A. Electronic cardiac pacemakers—battery-operated devices supplement or replace defective electric stimulation in the human heart and thus help to maintain the individual's heartbeat at a selected rate
B. Electrosurgery—an extremely high-frequency device called an oscillator is utilized to generate high temperatures in a small area to coagulate or desiccate tissue, thus preventing bleeding during surgery; electric cutting (using the oscillator) vibrates the tissues apart and simultaneously cauterizes the small blood vessels, thus preventing bleeding
C. Electronic thermometers—in these devices, temperature changes in a crystal alter the resistance of the crystal to electric flow; changes in an individual's temperature also alter the resistance of the crystal,

allowing a certain amount of current to flow through and the amount to be read on a scale calibrated for temperature readings; these thermometers give readings more accurate than mercury thermometers in about 5 to 7 seconds
D. Electrocardiograms—these devices measure and record the electric activity of the heart as this activity is carried to the surface of the body by the ions of the body fluids; this information provides an electric picture of the heart's activity

Heat
A. Temperature measures the intensity of heat
   1. The 3 common measures of temperature are
      a. Celsius or centigrade
      b. Fahrenheit
      c. Absolute or Kelvin
   2. Conversions
      If
      T_f = Temperature in Fahrenheit degrees
      T_c = Temperature in Celsius degrees
      T_k = Temperature in absolute (Kelvin) degrees
      then
      $T_f = (\%_5\, T_c) + 32$
      $T_c = (T_f - 32) \times \%_9$
      $T_k = T_c + 273°$
B. The unit which expresses the quantity of thermal energy or the amount of heat that could be produced in a body is the calorie
C. The British Thermal Unit (BTU) is defined as the quantity of heat required to change the temperature of 1 lb of water 1° F
D. Specific heat is the quantity of heat required to raise the temperature of a substance 1° C
E. Water has a high specific heat, which means that a relatively large quantity of energy must be added to water to bring about small temperature changes; e.g., a hot water bottle stays hot for a long time because water possesses a great deal of thermal energy
F. Heat is used to kill all living organisms on medical instruments and other materials; dry heat at a temperature of 170° C (338° F) for 30 minutes is considered sufficient for sterilization; dry heat sterilization has an advantage over steam sterilization in that no damage is done to the fine cutting edges of surgical instruments or to ground glass surfaces

Change of State
A. Evaporation—molecules of a liquid become molecules of gas; since the most energetic molecules leave the surface of a liquid during evaporation, the

average kinetic energy and temperature of the remaining liquid molecules are lower; thus evaporation causes cooling

1. Rubbing alcohol applied to the skin will rapidly evaporate, cooling the body
2. Sweating is an important physiologic process because evaporation helps to control body temperature

B. Boiling—evaporation occurring beneath the surface of a liquid; the gas bubbles so formed are buoyed to the liquid's surface and escape into the atmosphere; this evaporation can be speeded up by (1) adding heat to the liquid molecules so that they possess enough energy to burst out from the surface of the liquid or (2) reducing the atmospheric pressure above the liquid

1. Autoclave—by increasing the pressure inside the autoclave (which is like a giant pressure cooker), higher water temperatures can be reached and bacteria and their spores can be readily destroyed by the steam generated; thus the autoclave sterilizes materials placed in it for specified lengths of time
2. Distillation (all chemical and drug solutions are made in distilled water)—purifying water by boiling and collecting the vapor; impurities are left behind during water evaporation

REVIEW OF PHARMACOLOGY RELATED TO PREOPERATIVE AND POSTOPERATIVE CARE
Drugs that Produce Anesthesia

A. Inhalation anesthetics
1. General implications for nurses
   a. Obtain an accurate history of allergies and other medical problems that could alter a patient's response to the drugs used during surgery
   b. Be aware of the stages of anesthesia
      (1) Stage I—euphoria, gradual loss of consciousness
      (2) Stage II—hyperexcitement (thrashing of extremities), hyperactivity of reflexes (eyelids, swallowing), dilation of pupils
      (3) Stage III—depression of corneal reflex and pupillary response to light, voluntary control absent, muscle tone decreased
      (4) Stage IV—medullary paralysis, death
   c. In the operating room be aware of flammable agents and use grounded equipment
   d. Observe the patient for side effects
      (1) Excitement and restlessness
      (2) Nausea and vomiting
      (3) Respiratory distress

2. Actions—in general, balanced anesthesia includes use of several drugs and provides control of pain, consciousness, and muscle relaxation
3. Examples
   a. Cyclopropane, trimethylene
   b. Enflurane (Ethrane)
   c. Ether, diethyl ether
   d. Ethyl chloride
   e. Ethylene
   f. Fluroxene (Fluoromar)
   g. Halothane (Fluothane)
   h. Methoxyflurane (Penthrane)
   i. Nitrous oxide, nitrogen monoxide
   j. Trichloroethylene (Trilene)
   k. Vinyl ether (Vinethene)

B. Intravenous barbiturates as anesthetics
1. General implications for nurses
   a. Obtain a detailed health history to reduce the possibility of untoward effects
   b. Carefully monitor vital signs postoperatively
   c. Observe the patient for adverse effects
      (1) Respiratory depression
      (2) Hypotension and tachycardia
      (3) Laryngospasm
2. Action—high lipoid affinity provides prompt effect on cerebral tissue and rapid induction with ultrashort action
3. Examples
   a. Methohexital sodium (Brevital)
   b. Thiamylal sodium (Surital)
   c. Thiopental sodium (Pentothal)

C. Intravenous and intramuscular nonbarbiturates as anesthetics
1. General implications for nurses
   a. Decrease stimulation, since psychic disturbances may occur when the patient emerges from anesthesia
   b. Observe the patient for adverse effects
      (1) Respiratory failure
      (2) Increased blood pressure
      (3) Rigidity
2. Action—these drugs induce a cataleptic state (patient appears to be awake but dissociated from the environment); pain response aborted; amnesia for the procedure
3. Example—ketamine hydrochloride (Ketaject)

D. Local anesthetics
1. General implications for nurses
   a. Observe the patient for side effects
      (1) Allergic reactions
      (2) Cardiac arrest
      (3) Convulsions
      (4) Hypotension

b. Be aware of sites of administration
  (1) Surface (topical)
  (2) Infiltration (local)—solution injected in limited area where nerve fibers have no sheath and weak solution blocks nerve endings
  (3) Field block—solution injected close to nerves around area to be anesthetized
  (4) Nerve block—solution injected at perineural site distant from desired anesthesia site; stronger solutions are required to allow filtration through the nerve sheath
  (5) Peridural (epidural, extradural, caudal)—solution is injected at a site blocking the paravertebral and peridural sections of spinal nerves controlling sensory stimuli at the manipulation site
  (6) Spinal (intrathecal, subarachnoid)—solution is injected into the spinal subarachnoid space to anesthetize nerve roots emerging from the spinal cord; hypobaric solutions (drug diluted with distilled water) gravitate caudad, and hyperbaric solutions (drug diluted with dextrose) gravitate cephalad

2. Action—there is a decrease in the permeability of the nerve membrane to the influx of sodium ions required for depolarization of the neuron

3. Examples
  a. Local anesthetics used topically
    (1) Benoxinate hydrochloride (Drosacaine)
    (2) Benzocaine
    (3) Butacaine sulfate (Butyn)
    (4) Butyl aminobenzoate (Butesin)
    (5) Cocaine
    (6) Cyclomethycaine (Surfacaine)
    (7) Dibucaine (Nupercaine); also used for spinal anesthesia
    (8) Dimethisoquin hydrochloride (Quotane)
    (9) Diperodon hydrochloride (Diothane)
    (10) Dyclonine hydrochloride (Dyclone)
    (11) Hexylcaine hydrochloride (Cyclaine); also used for nerve block
    (12) Lidocaine hydrochloride (Xylocaine); also used for nerve block
    (13) Phenacaine hydrochloride (Holocaine)
    (14) Piperocaine hydrochloride (Metycaine)
    (15) Pramoxine hydrochloride (Tronothane)
    (16) Proparacaine hydrochloride (Ophthetic, Ophthaine)
    (17) Tetracaine hydrochloride (Tetracel, Anacel, Pontocaine); also used for nerve block

  b. Local anesthetics used primarily for nerve block
    (1) Bupivacaine hydrochloride (Marcaine)
    (2) Chloroprocaine hydrochloride (Nesacaine, Nesacaine-CE)
    (3) Mepivacaine hydrochloride (Carbocaine)
    (4) Prilocaine hydrochloride (Citanest)
    (5) Procaine hydrochloride (Novocain)
    (6) Propoxycaine hydrochloride (Blockain)

Drugs that Produce Sedation and Sleep

1. General implications for nurses
  a. Check with the pharmacist for drug compatibility if the patient is receiving other medications
  b. Observe the patient for adverse effects specific to each medication

2. Barbiturate sedatives
  a. Action—depression of the central nervous system, starting with the diencephalon
  b. Examples
    (1) Hexobarbital (Sombucaps, Sombulex)
    (2) Pentobarbital sodium (Nembutal)
    (3) Secobarbital (Seconal)
    (4) Amobarbital (Amytal)
    (5) Aprobarbital (Alurate)
    (6) Butabarbital sodium (Bubartal, Butisol)
    (7) Probarbital calcium (Ipral)
    (8) Talbutal (Lotusate)
    (9) Barbital (Neuronidia)
    (10) Phenobarbital (Luminal)
  c. Adverse effects
    (1) Drowsiness
    (2) Photosensitivity
    (3) Hypotension

3. Trichloroacetic acid
  a. Action—induction of a natural sleep by depressing the central nervous system
  b. Examples
    (1) Chloral betaine (Beta-Chlor)
    (2) Chloral hydrate (Felsules, Lorinal, Noctec, Somnos)
    (3) Petrichloral (Periclor)
  c. Adverse effects
    (1) Gastric irritation
    (2) Diarrhea

4. Phenothiazine derivatives
  a. Action—relaxation of skeletal muscles; depression of the central and autonomic nervous systems
  b. Examples
    (1) Methotrimeprazine hydrochloride (Levoprome)
    (2) Promazine hydrochloride (Sparine)
    (3) Propiomazine hydrochloride (Largon)

c. Adverse effects
  (1) Hypotension
  (2) Dry mouth
  (3) Pseudoparkinsonian symptoms
  (4) Agranulocytosis

5. Other sedatives and hypnotics
  a. Action—generally depression of the central nervous system and skeletal muscle relaxation
  b. Specific drugs and their adverse effects
    (1) Ethchlorvynol (Placidyl)—morning drowsiness, blurring vision, transient hypotension
    (2) Ethinamate (Valmid)—morning drowsiness
    (3) Flurazepam hydrochloride (Dalmane)—dizziness, tachycardia, gastrointestinal disturbances
    (4) Methaqualone (Quaalude, Sopor)—morning drowsiness, gastrointestinal disturbances
    (5) Methyprylon (Noludar)—morning drowsiness, gastrointestinal disturbances
    (6) Sodium bromide, used primarily for daytime sedation—gastric irritation; generalized rash; tremulousness of hands, lips, and tongue; impaired mental processes; auditory and visual hallucinations; or coma with long-term use of excessive levels of the drug
    (7) Glutethimide (Doriden)
      (a) Adverse effects—morning drowsiness, transient hypotension, and, infrequently, pharyngeal and laryngeal reflex depression
      (b) Drug interactions—acts synergistically with oral anticoagulants to decrease their effectiveness

Drugs that Control Pain

A. Nonnarcotic agents
  1. General implications for nurses
    a. Observe for side effects of each drug
    b. Explain the importance of maintaining a therapeutic dosage when discharged
    c. Observe for toxicity characterized by central nervous system stimulation, excitement, delirium
  2. Salicylates
    a. Action
      (1) Unclear but involves many mechanisms
      (2) Antipyretic activity—lowers hypothalamic "thermostat" and dissipates heat by vasodilation and diaphoresis
      (3) Antiinflammatory
    b. Examples
      (1) Acetylsalicylic acid (aspirin) (A.S.A., Asteric, Ecotrin)
      (2) Carbaspirin calcium (Calurin)

(3) Choline salicylate (Arthropan)
(4) Salicylamide (Amid-Sal, Liquiprin, Raspberin, Salamide, Salicim, Salrin)
(5) Sodium salicylate
  c. Adverse effects
    (1) Gastric irritation
    (2) Visual disturbances
    (3) Decreased clotting time
    (4) Tinnitus
  3. Nonsalicylates
    a. Action—similar to salicylates; used for patients with salicylate allergy or gastric ulcers or those receiving anticoagulants
    b. Examples
      (1) Acetaminophen (Apamide, Febrolin, Fendon, Lyteca, Nebs, Tempra, Tylenol); also has muscle relaxant properties
      (2) Acetophenetidin (used as component of preparations to allow lower dosage because higher dosage causes agranulocytosis, anemia, hepatotoxicity, and methemoglobinemia)
      (3) Dipyrone (Dimethone, Narone, Nartate, Novaldin, Pydirone, Pyrilgin)
      (4) Mefenamic acid (Ponstel); also has antiinflammatory properties
    c. Adverse effects
      (1) Vertigo
      (2) Skin rash
      (3) Depression of leukocyte and erythrocyte production
  4. Propoxyphene hydrochloride (Darvon)
    a. Action—functions as an analgesic without antiinflammatory effects
    b. Adverse effects
      (1) Constipation
      (2) Skin rash
      (3) Psychic dependence
  5. Carbamazepine (Tegretol)
    a. Actions
      (1) Controls trigeminal neuralgia by decreasing synaptic transmission in the nerve nucleus
      (2) Has sedative, anticholinergic, and muscle relaxant properties
    b. Adverse effects
      (1) Dry mouth
      (2) Weakness
      (3) Lethargy

B. Narcotic analgesics
  1. General implications for nurses
    a. Request the physician to rewrite orders for narcotics q. 24 h.

b. Observe for respiratory depression prior to and following administration of narcotics

c. Utilize nursing judgment in evaluating patient needs for narcotic analgesics

d. Evaluate effectiveness of medication

2. Actions

a. Raise the pain threshold and interfere with pain perception centers

b. Have antitussive and sedative actions

3. Examples

a. Codeine sulfate

b. Hydromorphone hydrochloride (Dilaudid)

c. Levorphanol tartrate (Levo-Dromoran)

d. Meperidine hydrochloride (Demerol)

e. Morphine sulfate

f. Oxycodone (used in Percodan)

g. Oxymorphone hydrochloride (Numorphan)

h. Pantopium (Pantopon)

i. Pentazocine hydrochloride (Talwin)

4. Adverse effects

a. Decreased gastric motility

b. Euphoria

c. Urine retention

d. Repiratory depression

e. Hypotension

RELATED PROCEDURES
Intravenous (IV) Therapy

A. Purpose

1. Replace fluid and electrolyte loss

2. Provide route for other medications

3. Maintain nutrition when the patient is unable to tolerate feedings (see hyperalimentation procedure under gastrointestinal disorders)

B. Nursing responsibilities

1. Explain procedure to the patient

2. Assist the patient with care, since mobility will be limited

3. Check solution for clarity and correct type

4. Assist qualified person in starting the IV

5. Regulate flow rate

Per minute drop rate =

$$\frac{\text{Milliliters to be infused} \times \text{Drop factor}}{\text{Number of hours} \times 60 \text{ minutes}}$$

6. Monitor intake and output

7. Observe for signs of complications

a. Infiltration—pain, swelling, coldness, and decreased flow of IV

b. Phlebitis—pain, redness, and heat at site

c. Air embolisms are rare, since the tubing does not contain sufficient air to cause an embolus to form

d. Circulatory overload—dyspnea, cough, frothy sputum, rales evident on auscultation

8. Change tubing and site at intervals specified by agency or if infiltration or phlebitis occurs

C. Physical principle involved—gravity

Blood Transfusion

A. Purpose

1. Restore blood volume after hemorrhage

2. Maintain hemoglobin levels in severe anemias

3. Replace specific blood components

B. Nursing responsibilities

1. Check that blood or blood components have been typed and cross matched, indicating that the blood of the donor and recipient are compatible

2. Blood must never be administered straight from the refrigerator

3. A baseline of the patient's temperature, blood pressure, pulse, and respirations should be determined prior to administration

4. An IV with normal saline and a blood administration set containing a filter are used to start the infusion; solutions containing glucose may cause the blood to clot in the tubing and should not be used

5. Before starting the infusion, it is advisable for 2 nurses to verify the blood type, Rh factor, patient and blood numbers, and expiration date

6. The container should be inverted gently to suspend the red cells within the plasma

7. Observe for signs of hemolytic reaction, which generally occur early in the transfusion (within the first 10 to 15 minutes)

a. Shivering

b. Headache

c. Lower back pain

d. Increased pulse and respiratory rate

e. Hemoglobinuria

f. Oliguria

g. Hypotension

8. Observe for signs of febrile reaction, which usually occur within 30 minutes

a. Shaking

b. Headache

c. Elevated temperature

d. Back pain

e. Confusion

f. Hematemesis

9. Observe for allergic reaction

a. Hives

b. Wheezing

c. Pruritus

d. Joint pain

10. If any reaction occurs
    a. Stop infusion immediately
    b. Notify the physician
    c. Maintain patency of the IV with normal saline
    d. Send blood to the laboratory
    e. Monitor vital signs frequently
    f. Send a urine specimen to the laboratory if a hemolyic reaction is suspected
C. Physical principle involved—gravity

GENERAL NURSING CARE
Preoperative Care

A. Prior to day of surgery
    1. Allow the patient time to ask questions about procedures and surgery
    2. Explain all procedures to the patient and give reasons and objectives for them
    3. Determine the patient's level of understanding of operative procedure to ascertain whether signature on permit represents informed consent
    4. Allow and encourage the patient to ventilate feelings about diagnosis and surgery
    5. Tell the patient what to expect in the operating room, recovery, and/or intensive care units if indicated
    6. Inform the patient if the plan is to return him or her to other than the present room
    7. Provide a spiritual counselor if desired by the patient or family
    8. Consider needs of the family when discussing surgery
    9. Teach the patient the activities that will be instituted after surgery (e.g., deep breathing, coughing, turning)
    10. Teach the patient physical exercises that will be used to promote circulation after surgery (e.g., isometric leg exercises, ambulation routines)
    11. Inform the patient to expect some discomfort after surgery and teach the importance of requesting medication for pain
    12. Make certain that history, physical examination results, recent laboratory tests, and chest x-ray report are entered on the chart
    13. Inform all members of the medical team, especially the anesthesiologist, of the patient's allergies and other health problems and prominently mark the chart
    14. Carry out ordered preoperative preparation (e.g., shave, Betadine, pHisoHex washes, enemas, douches)
    15. Remove nail polish from fingers and toes
    16. Administer prescribed sleeping medication
    17. Inform the patient not to take anything by mouth after midnight, remove fluid, and place obvious signs at bedside
B. Day of surgery
    1. In the morning, check the patient's vital signs and assess overall physical status; record and report any deviations to physician
    2. Have the patient void
    3. See that any drainage tubes (catheter or Levin tube) which were ordered are inserted
    4. Make certain that name identification band is on the patient's wrist
    5. Have the patient remove dentures and other prosthetic devices: store any valuables
    6. Administer prescribed preoperative medication
    7. Put side rails up after administering medications
    8. Transfer the patient to a stretcher when operating room calls; fasten the stretcher strap in place before transporting
    9. Consider needs of the family on the day of surgery

Postoperative Care

A. Be aware of surgical stresses
    1. Depression of the central nervous system from general or regional anesthesia
    2. An interruption in the integrity of the skin
    3. Depressed respiratory functioning
    4. Alterations in circulation and fluid and electrolyte balance
    5. Depression of gastrointestinal and urinary functioning
    6. Emotional trauma
    7. Change in body image
B. Minimize postoperative complications
    1. Maintain a patent airway by keeping the artificial airway in place until gag reflex returns, suctioning trachea as needed, keeping head extended and turned to the side, and observing the rate and character of respirations
    2. Assess the patient's physical status—note and record level of consciousness, vital signs, color and temperature of skin, condition of surgical site, presence and functioning of intravenous and drainage tubes, and return of sensorimotor functioning; report significant changes
    3. Protect the patient from injury by keeping under close observation, keeping side rails in place, positioning the patient to prevent excessive pressure on body parts or on tubing, controlling restlessness and preventing the patient from pulling on tubes or dressing, and making certain that all equipment is in safe working condition and properly used

4. Turn the patient frequently and encourage deep breathing and coughing to prevent the development of atelectasis or hypostatic pneumonia
5. Perform or encourage range of motion and isometric exercises and early ambulation to prevent phlebitis, paralytic ileus, and circulatory stasis
6. Maintain patency of tubing (catheter, gastric tubes, T-tube, chest tubes, etc.) to promote drainage and maintain decompression to reduce pressure on suture line
7. Monitor the patient's overall physical status, vital signs, dressing, and drainage to observe for early signs of hemorrhage and to prevent excessive blood loss and shock
8. Use surgical aseptic technique when changing dressings or as necessary when irrigating tubing to prevent infection
9. Monitor intake and output to prevent dehydration, fluid and electrolyte imbalance, and urinary suppression or retention
10. Observe for abdominal distention to prevent discomfort and intestinal obstruction
11. Give medication for pain as ordered to prevent discomfort and restlessness
12. Regulate IV therapy to prevent circulatory overload
13. Support or encourage the patient to support and splint the incisional site when coughing, moving, or turning to prevent tension on suture line
14. Position the patient as required by type of surgery to prevent misalignment and prevent the accumulation of fluid or the blocking of drainage tubes

C. Immediate care in the recovery room
1. Monitor vital signs
2. Reorient the patient to time, place, and situation
3. Call the patient by name
4. Answer questions as honestly and simply as possible and avoid complicated, involved explanations
5. Medicate for pain and restlessness
6. Expect and accept repetitious questions and give the patient necessary reassurance
7. Maintain patency of all tubing and attach to appropriate drainage as ordered
8. Maintain patency of airway; observe for return of gag reflex

D. Consider postoperative nutritional needs
1. Initial IV therapy for water and electrolytes, but oral intake needed as soon as possible for adequate nutrition
2. Hyperalimentation—parenteral nutrition of high nutrient density; solutions of amino acids, glucose, electrolytes, minerals, vitamins; usually inserted into larger veins (inferior or superior vena cava) to avoid thrombosis in peripheral veins; used in cases of major tissue trauma, injury, or extensive surgery
3. Gradually increase oral intake as permitted
   a. Liquid diets
      (1) Clear liquid—clear broth, bouillon, juices, plain gelatin, fruit-flavored water ices, ginger ale, coffee, tea
      (2) Full liquid—may add milk and items made with milk, such as cream soups, milk drinks, sherbet, ice cream, puddings, custard
   b. Soft diet—may add all soft cooked foods, such as refined cereals, pasta, rice, white bread and crackers, eggs, cheese, meat, potatoes, cooked whole vegetables, cooked fruits, few soft ripe plain fruits without membranes or skins, simple desserts
   c. Light diet—same as soft with few additional whole cooked foods, light raw foods such as fruit; mainly avoid heavily seasoned or fried foods
   d. Full (or general) diet—full, well-balanced diet of all foods as desired and tolerated, including a wide variety for interest and flavor
4. Provide for special nutritional needs
   a. Protein—increased need caused by protein losses and the catabolism of recovery and tissue healing; a period of negative nitrogen balance initially
   b. Calories—adequate amount to supply energy and spare protein for tissue building
   c. Water—adequate fluid therapy to prevent dehydration caused by large fluid losses
   d. Minerals—replacement of deficiencies and ensurance of continued adequacy essential to maintain electrolyte balance; zinc needed for wound healing in deficient individuals
   e. Vitamins—C especially needed for tissue synthesis and wound healing; B complex essential in energy production and tissue building

Controlling Infection
NURSING RESPONSIBILITIES TO PREVENT CROSS-CONTAMINATION

A. Recognize that microorganisms can be transferred directly by fomites and insects and indirectly by airborne particles
B. Use medical aseptic techniques

1. Handwashing before and after patient care, after handling excreta, etc.
2. Bacteriostatic chemicals—antiseptics and disinfectants
   a. To inhibit or destroy pathogens
   b. In concurrent and terminal disinfections of contaminated articles
3. Barriers such as gowns, gloves, and masks to protect personnel when caring for persons with infections
4. Correct disposal of contaminated materials (e.g., linens, tissues, dressings, secretions, excretions)

C. Use surgical aseptic techniques
1. Sterilize by autoclaving, boiling, etc. to destroy all microorganisms
2. Barriers such as gowns, gloves, and masks to protect the patient against microbiologic hazards in the environment
3. Sterile equipment and technique when caring for wounds, irrigating sterile cavities, giving injections, and inserting instruments or devices into body cavities or areas that are normally sterile

DRUGS THAT CONTROL INFECTION
Definition of Terms

A. Antibiotic—a metabolic product of an organism used to destroy another organism
B. Bactericidal effect—capable of destroying bacteria at low concentrations (e.g., disrupt building of cell membrane or wall, allow leak of cytoplasm)
C. Bacteriostatic effect—slows reproduction of bacteria; natural physiologic mechanisms are required for phagocytic abolition of the bacteria
D. Superinfection—emergence of microorganism growth (e.g., yeast and fungi) when natural protective flora is destroyed by antiinfective drug
E. Bacterial resistance—a natural characteristic of an organism or one acquired by mutation preventing destruction by a drug to which it was previously susceptible

General Implications for Nurses Administering Antiinfective Drugs

A. Knowledge of why the patient is receiving specific antiinfective medication
1. Check culture and sensitivity reports
2. Observe for inflammatory response, including elevated temperature and WBC count
B. Be aware that certain foods and other medications may affect the action of the antiinfective
C. Prevent superinfection by providing yogurt or Bacid capsules

D. Administer antibiotics at equal intervals during the day
E. Increase fluid intake
F. Observe for common adverse effects such as skin rashes and GI disturbances, as well as the specific effects listed under each classification

Penicillin Preparations

A. Actions
1. Disrupt bacterial cell wall synthesis when new cells are forming by interfering with the synthesis and cross-linkage of mucopeptides in the final stage of cell wall synthesis
2. Broad spectrum of pathogen susceptibility except to *Staphylococcus aureus*
B. Examples
1. Amoxicillin (Amoxil, Larocin)
2. Ampicillin (Omnipen, Penbritin, Polycillin, Principen)
3. Carbenicillin disodium (Geopen, Pyopen)
4. Methicillin sodium (Staphcillin)
5. Nafcillin sodium (Unipen)
6. Oxacillin sodium (Bactocill, Prostaphlin)
7. Penicillin G potassium (Dramicillin, Pedacillin, Pentids, Pfizerpen)
8. Penicillin G procaine (Crysticillin A.S., Diurnal-Penicillin, Duracillin A.S., Pentids-P, Wycillin)
9. Penicillin V (Pen-Vee, V-Cillin)
C. Adverse effects
1. Allergic reactions
   a. Range from skin rash to anaphylactic shock
   b. Penicillinase (Neutrapen) is used to inactivate circulating penicillin by its enzymatic action
2. Superinfection (e.g., *Candida* or *Pseudomonas* species in vagina or respiratory and intestinal tracts)

Cephalosporins

A. Actions
1. Disrupt synthesis of bacterial cell wall by inactivating transpeptidase required for cross-linkage of peptidoglycan chains
2. Minor structural difference from penicillin allows therapy for penicillin-sensitized patients
3. Broad spectrum limited by sensitivity to action of cephalosporinase of some gram-negative rods (*Enterobacter, Pseudomonas*)
B. Examples
1. Cefazolin sodium (Ancef, Kefzol)
2. Cephacetrile (Celospor)
3. Cephalexin monohydrate (Keflex)

4. Cephaloglycin (Kafocin)
5. Cephaloridine (Loridine)
6. Cephalothin sodium (Keflin)
7. Cephradine (Velosef, Anspor)

C. Adverse effects
1. Allergic reactions (minor rashes, urticaria, fever, eosinophilia)
2. Superinfections
3. Diarrhea
4. Nephrotoxicity with large doses

D. Special considerations—metabolites cause a false positive reaction for glycosuria in tests with Clinitest and Fehling's and Benedict's solutions

Erythromycins and Similar Drugs

A. Actions
1. Compete for receptor sites on the ribosome unit to inhibit mRNA synthesis of protein required for reproduction
2. Excretion route is in the bile through the intestine (90%), which allows use with compromised renal function

B. Examples
1. Clindamycin hydrochloride (Cleocin)
2. Erythromycin (E-Mycin, Erythrocin, Ilotycin)
3. Erythromycin ethylsuccinate (Erythrocin Ethylsuccinate, Pediamycin)
4. Lincomycin hydrochloride monohydrate (Linocin)

C. Adverse effects
1. Nausea and vomiting
2. Diarrhea
3. Abdominal pain
4. Black tongue

Tetracyclines

A. Actions
1. Block tRNA attachment to ribosomes to inhibit protein synthesis
2. Provide broad-spectrum effect

B. Examples
1. Chlortetracycline hydrochloride (Aureomycin)
2. Demeclocycline (Declomycin)
3. Doxycycline hyclate (Vibramycin Hyclate)
4. Oxytetracycline (Terramycin)
5. Tetracycline (Achromycin, Panmycin, Sumycin, Tratracyn)

C. Adverse effects
1. Gastroenteritis—caused by superinfection
2. Hepatotoxicity—lethargy, anorexia, jaundice, fatty necrosis
3. Phototoxicity
4. Nephrotoxicity

5. Hyperuricemia
6. Enamel hypoplasia, dental caries, and bone defects in children under 8 years of age and in fetus after the fourth month of gestation

D. Other considerations
1. Drugs delay blood coagulation and potentiate effect of oral anticoagulants
2. Oral drug forms insoluble mixture with iron and the calcium, magnesium, and aluminum salts of foods and drugs; e.g., absorption of the drug is erratic when milk and antacids are taken concurrently
3. Oral sodium bicarbonate decreases dissolution of capsules that require acid media in stomach
4. Parenteral drugs contain ascorbic acid, causing false positive test with Benedict's solution and Clinitest and false negative test with Clinistix and Tes-Tape

Aminoglycosides

A. Actions
1. Disrupt protein synthesis by providing substitute for essential nucleotide required by mRNA
2. Have broad-spectrum effect but are used only in the treatment of serious infections

B. Examples
1. Gentamicin sulfate (Garamycin)
2. Kanamycin sulfate (Kantrex)
3. Neomycin sulfate (Mycifradin, Neobiotic)
4. Streptomycin sulfate (Strycin)
5. Amikacin sulfate (Amiken)
6. Tobramycin sulfate (Nebcin)

C. Adverse effects
1. Ototoxicity (tinnitus, vertigo, hearing loss)
2. Rapid emergence of resistant bacteria
3. Nausea and vomiting
4. Nephrotoxicity
5. Blood dyscrasias

Polymycin Group

A. Actions
1. Detergent effect on bacterial cell membrane increases permeability, which disrupts intracellular osmotic gradient
2. Oral forms of both drug groups are used to suppress bacterial growth in the intestine (decrease ammonia production or "sterilize bowel")

B. Examples
1. Colistimethate sodium (Coly-Mycin M)
2. Colistin sulfate (Coly-Mycin S)
3. Polymyxin B sulfate (Aerosporin)

C. Adverse effects
1. Circumoral or lingual paresthesias
2. Nephrotoxicity

D. Other considerations
1. Potentiation of neuromuscular blocking agents, general anesthetics, or parenterally administered magnesium
2. Oral forms suppress the intestinal bacteria that synthesize vitamin K, decreasing the available vitamin and potentiating the action of oral anticoagulants

Chloramphenicol

A. Actions
1. Substitutes for essential amino acid phenylalanine, which prevents mRNA activity
2. Used in severe drug-resistant infections
B. Examples
1. Amphicol
2. Chloromycetin
3. Mychel
4. Novochlor
C. Adverse effects
1. Aplastic anemia
2. Leukopenia
3. Thrombocytopenia
4. Headache
5. Confusion
6. Peripheral neuropathy
7. Optic neuritis
8. GI disturbances
9. Gray baby syndrome (abdominal distention, pallid cyanosis, vasomotor collapse, ashen gray color, death)
10. Interference with metabolism of phenytoin, oral antidiabetic agents, and dicumarol, leading to cumulative effects of these drugs

Amantadine Hydrochloride

A. Actions
1. Prophylaxis when exposure to viral infection (e.g., A_2 influenza virus) has occurred
2. Preventing entrance of virus into host cells
B. Adverse effects
1. Insomnia
2. Dizziness
3. Tremor
4. Psychosis
5. Orthostatic hypotension
6. Constipation
7. Urinary retention

Sulfonamides

A. Actions
1. Substitute a false metabolite for paraaminobenzoic acid required in the synthesis of folic acid by bacteria

2. Plasma protein binding maintains tissue levels by liberating drug when tissue levels are low
3. Tenacious plasma protein binding may hold drug until it reaches renal sites, producing high levels in tubular urine
4. Many forms require alkalinization of urine and high fluid intake to maintain urine volume and decrease incidence of nephron crystals
5. Recycling of drug in nephron delays excretion and maintains blood levels of drug
   a. Tubule cells excrete drug into tubular urine after removal from plasma protein binding sites
   b. Tubule cells also reabsorb the drug from tubule urine, and it returns to tissue and liver sites to be metabolized
   c. Alkalinization of urine slows recycling and increases excretion rate
B. Examples
1. Phthalylsulfathiazole (Cremothalidine, Rothalid, Sulfathalidine)
2. Succinylsulfathiazole (Rolsul, Sulfasuxidine)
3. Sulfasalazine (Azulfidine)
4. Sulfadiazine
5. Sulfamethizole (Thiosulfil)
6. Sulfamethoxazole (Gantanol)
7. Sulfaphenazole (Sulfabid)
8. Sulfisomidine (Elkosin)
9. Sulfisoxazole (Gantrisin, SK-Soxazole, Soizole, Sosol, Soxomide, Sulfisocon, Unisulf)
C. Adverse effects
1. Anorexia
2. Nausea and vomiting caused by gastric irritation and action at vomiting centers in medulla
3. Malaise
4. Blood dyscrasias (leukopenia, thrombocytopenia, erythrocytopenia)
5. Fever
6. Headache
7. Stomatitis
8. Conjunctivitis
9. Hepatotoxicity

Kidney-Specific Drugs

A. Nalidixic acid (NegGram)
1. Action—urinary bactericidal that provides high concentration in nephron
2. Adverse effects
   a. Nausea and vomiting
   b. Rash, urticaria
   c. Dizziness
   d. Diplopia
   e. Headache
3. Causes false-positive results with Clinitest

B. Nitrofurantoin (Cyantin, Furadantin, Furalan, Macrodantin, Trantoin)
   1. Actions
      a. Acts as a diffusible acid when tubular urine is acidic
      b. Provides a high concentration of drug in nephrons for antibacterial action
   2. Adverse effects
      a. Nausea and vomiting
      b. Skin rashes
      c. Hemolytic anemia
C. Methenamines
   1. Action—exert antibacterial activity by liberating ammonia and formaldehyde by hydrolysis in acid urine
   2. Examples
      a. Methenamine (Uritone)
      b. Methenamine hippurate (Hiprex)
      c. Methenamine mandelate (Mandelamine)
   3. Adverse effects
      a. Nausea and vomiting
      b. Pruritus
      c. Rash
D. Sulfa drugs specific for urinary tract infections
   1. Action and adverse effects same as for other sulfa drugs
   2. Examples
      a. Sulfisoxazole (Gantrisin)
      b. Sulfamethoxazole (Gantanol)

Sulfones that Control *Mycobacterium leprae* (Hansen's Disease)

A. Actions
   1. Deprive bacteria of the nucleotide required for folic acid synthesis and growth
   2. Slow elimination and wide tissue distribution permit daily administration; mucosal lesions improve in 3 to 6 months; nerve tenderness decreases in 6 to 9 months; however, skin lesions require 1 to 3 years for clearance of bacilli
B. Examples
   1. Acedapsone (repository form with few adverse effects)
   2. Acetosulfone sodium (Promacetin)
   3. Clofazimine (Lamprene)—a red compound that colors the skin, conjunctiva, urine, sputum, and sweat red-brown
   4. Dapsone (Avlosulfon)
   5. Sulfoxone sodium (Diasone)
   6. Thiazolsulfone (Promizole)
C. Adverse effects
   1. Hemolytic anemia at start of therapy
   2. GI disturbances

   3. Serum sickness–like symptoms and exacerbation of lesions

Drugs that Control *Mycobacterium tuberculosis*

A. General considerations
   1. Primary triad of drugs for therapy includes isoniazid, streptomycin sulfate, and aminosalicylic acid or ethambutol
   2. Bacterial resistance to single drugs develops rapidly, and combination decreases resistance and adverse effects
B. Isoniazid (INH, Hyzyd, Niconyl, Nydrazid)
   1. Actions
      a. Interferes with synthesis of the lipoprotein cell wall of *Mycobacterium*
      b. Competes for the enzyme required in the synthesis of pyridoxine; the result is a vitamin B_6 deficiency, which causes neurologic symptoms (hyperreflexia, paresthesia of extremities, vertigo) unless this vitamin is supplied during therapy
      c. Used for prophylaxis of 1 year's duration for individuals who change from a negative to a positive reaction to the tuberculin test and to individuals living with a newly diagnosed tubercular patient
   2. Adverse effects
      a. Hepatotoxicity
      b. Bone marrow depression
      c. Skin rash
      d. Exacerbation of rheumatoid arthritis
   3. May cause false positive reactions with Clinitest
C. Paraaminosalicylic acid preparations
   1. Action—interfere with bacterial synthesis of folic acid by providing a substitute nucleotide
   2. Examples
      a. Calcium aminosalicylate (Teebacin Calcium)
      b. Paraaminosalicylic acid (P.A.S.)
      c. Potassium aminosalicylate (Teebacin Kalium, Paskalium)
      d. Sodium aminosalicylate (Parasal Sodium, Pasdium)
   3. Adverse effects
      a. Gastric irritation
      b. Abdominal pain
      c. Nausea, vomiting, and diarrhea
      d. Blood dyscrasias
D. Streptomycin sulfate (see amino glycosides)
E. Drugs used as substitutes for streptomycin sulfate
   1. Examples
      a. Capreomycin sulfate (Capastat)
      b. Cycloserine (Seromycin)

c. Rifampin (Rifadin, Rimactane)

d. Viomycin sulfate (Viocin)

2. Other considerations

a. Dosage spacing (2 to 3 times per week) after initial intensive therapy decreases incidence of neurotoxicity to these drugs

b. Drug interactions with rifampin—absorption delayed by aminosalicylates (drugs administered on a schedule allowing 8 to 12 hours between them); inhibits activity of oral anticoagulants; phenobarbital interferes with rifampin activity when used concomitantly

F. Second line drugs used in therapy

1. Actions

a. Inhibit cell metabolism

b. Prevent multiplication of cells

2. Examples

a. Ethambutol hydrochloride (Myambutol)

b. Ethionamide (Trecator S.C.)

c. Pyrazinamide (PZA)

Antifungals

A. Griseofulvin, micronized (Fulvicin-U/F, Grifulvin V, Grisactin)

1. Action—acts as an analog of purine and is incorporated into new epithelial cells during synthesis of nucleic acids

2. Adverse effects

a. Peripheral neuritis

b. Vertigo

c. Fever

d. Arthralgia

e. Nausea

f. Diarrhea

g. Headache

B. Nystatin (Mycostatin, Nilstat)

1. Action—binds tenaciously to cell wall sterols and causes a detergent effect that increases permeability of membrane and causes cell to rupture

2. Adverse effects

a. Nausea

b. Vomiting

C. Amphotericin B (Fungizone)

1. Action—detergent-like effect on cell wall that increases permeability of membrane and causes the cell to rupture

2. Adverse effects

a. Paresthesia and muscle weakness (caused by drug effect on normal cells containing sterols)

b. Chills

c. Hyperpyrexia

d. Nephrotoxicity

e. Nausea and vomiting

f. Flushed skin

g. Generalized pain

h. Convulsions

Antiparasitics

A. Metronidazol (Flagyl)

1. Actions

a. Trichomonacidal and amebicidal

b. Used in the treatment of trichomoniasis, intestinal amebiasis, and amebic liver abscess

2. Adverse effects

a. Nausea and vomiting

b. Diarrhea

c. Abdominal cramps

d. Metallic taste

e. If taken with alcohol—nausea, vomiting, headache, and hypotension

B. Emetine hydrochloride

1. Actions

a. Causes degeneration of the nucleus and reticulation of the ameba cytoplasm

b. Used in the treatment of acute amebic dysentery, amebic hepatitis, and abscess

2. Adverse effects

a. Nausea and vomiting

b. Dizziness

c. Tachycardia

d. Muscular weakness

e. Dyspnea

f. Precordial pain

g. Local myositis at injection site

C. Antimalarial drugs

1. Definition of terms

a. Causal prophylaxis—drugs used to intercede at primary tissue sites to eradicate *Plasmodium* before it begins reproduction cycles

b. Radical cure—drugs used to destroy tissue parasites

c. Suppressive prophylaxis and suppressive cure—drugs used to interrupt the blood cycle phase

d. Clinical cure—drugs provide relief of symptoms in an acute exacerbation of malaria

2. Primaquine phosphate

a. Actions

(1) Primary drug for radical cure of *Plasmodium vivax;* also has a gametocytocide action in 3 days

(2) Control requires 14 days; therapy is continued for 8 weeks

   b. Adverse effects
     (1) Leukopenia
     (2) Agranulocytosis
     (3) Intravascular hemolysis
     (4) Visual disturbances
     (5) Nausea and vomiting
3. Chloroquine phosphate (Aralen Phosphate, Roquine) and hydroxychloroquine sulfate (Plaquenil)
   a. Actions
     (1) Inhibit oxygen uptake and interfere with nucleic acid synthesis in plasmodia
     (2) Modify the gametocytes of *P. vivax* to prevent completion of the reproductive cycle
     (3) Used with primaquine phosphate for suppressive prophylaxis of *P. vivax* for individuals traveling to endemic areas
   b. Adverse effects
     (1) Blood dyscrasias
     (2) Dizziness
     (3) Convulsions
     (4) Visual disturbances
     (5) Ototoxicity
     (6) GI distress
4. Amodiaquine hydrochloride (Camoquin, Flavoquin)
   a. Actions
     (1) Used with chloroquine hydrochloride for clinical cure of *P. vivax* or *P. falciparum*
     (2) Rapid-acting schizonticide, providing negative peripheral blood samples in 48 to 72 hours; afebrile in 24 to 48 hours; continuation of therapy provides suppressive cure of *P. falciparum*
   b. Adverse effects
     (1) Blood dyscrasias
     (2) Headache
     (3) Fatigue
     (4) Psychosis
     (5) Visual disturbances
     (6) Ototoxicity
     (7) Nausea and vomiting
5. Chloroguanide hydrochloride (Paludrine) and pyrimethamine (Daraprim)
   a. Actions
     (1) Used for suppressive prophylaxis
     (2) Folic acid antagonist; prevents nucleic acid synthesis by plasmodia; sterilizing effect that inhibits gametocyte development in mosquito breeder of *P. falciparum* and *P. vivax*
     (3) Slow acting; therapy continued 4 weeks after last exposure

   b. Adverse effects
     (1) Blood dyscrasias
     (2) Headache
     (3) Convulsions
     (4) Visual disturbances
     (5) Ototoxicity
     (6) GI disturbances
6. Quinine sulfate
   a. Actions
     (1) Schizonticidal and gametocidal
     (2) Used for radical cure and for suppression
   b. Adverse effects
     (1) Blood dyscrasias (hemolytic anemia, thrombocytopenia, agranulocytosis)
     (2) Severe headache
     (3) Convulsions
     (4) Hypothermia
     (5) Hypotension
     (6) Visual disturbances
     (7) GI distress
     (8) Renal damage

Antineoplastic Drugs
GENERAL INFORMATION

A. Drugs act primarily on malignant cells during reproduction of proteins
B. One drug or a combination of drugs may be used to increase specificity of action and decrease drug tolerance
C. Administration routes, delivering drug to involved organs
   1. Isolation or regional perfusion that requires extracorporeal perfusion
   2. Intraarterial infusion at organ site that allows uptake of drug before it enters the venous route
   3. Intracavity instillation
D. Antineoplastic drugs have a low therapeutic index (T.I.), and evidence of cytotoxic effects occurs in normal tissues
E. General adverse effects—anorexia, nausea, vomiting, lassitude, hyperuricemia (caused by rapid breakdown of tumor tissue), epithelial tissue lesions (stomatitis, abdominal cramps, diarrhea), bone marrow depression (bleeding, infections), alopecia

IMPLICATIONS FOR NURSES

A. Protect the patient from communicable diseases and use strict asepsis
B. Observe the patient for adverse effects of each antineoplastic drug

C. Provide emotional support
D. Allow the patient to ventilate feelings
E. Help set realistic goals

DRUGS USED
Hormones in Chemotherapy

A. Actions
 1. Change hormonal balance and slow growth rate of certain tumors
 2. Especially useful in treatment of neoplasms involving the reproductive organs
B. Examples
 1. Estrogen (Premarin, Diethylstilbestrol, Feminone, Lynoral)
 2. Androgen (Drolban, Halotestin, Teslac, Oreton)
 3. Progesterone (Delalutin, Depo Provera, Megace)
C. Adverse effects
 1. Emergence of characteristics of the opposite sex
 2. Edema
 3. Changes in libido
 4. Irritability
 5. Uterine bleeding

Antimetabolites

A. Action—interfere with production of purine precursors (guanine, adenine) required for DNA or RNA synthesis; pyrimidine precursors (cytosine, thymine) required for DNA synthesis or the precursors (cystosine, uracil) required for RNA synthesis; or the folic acid conversion required for DNA or RNA protein construction
B. Analogs used to interfere in cell reproduction
 1. Purine antagonist (adenine analog)
  a. Azathioprine (Imuran)—action as a sulfhydryl enzyme inhibitor makes it useful as an immunosuppressive drug
  b. Mercaptopurine (Purinethol)
 2. Purine antagonist (guanine analog)—Thioguanine
 3. Pyrimidine antagonist (thymine analog)
  a. Fluorouracil (also uracil analog)
  b. Floxuridine (also uracil analog)
  c. Hydroxyurea (Hydrea)
 4. Pyrimidine antagonist (cytosine analog)—cytarabine (Cytosar)
 5. Folic acid antagonist—methotrexate
C. Adverse effects
 1. Liver dysfunction
 2. Intractable vomiting
 3. Leukopenia
 4. Alopecia

Alkylating Agents

A. Action—cause chromatin disruptive effects similar to those of x rays by transferring their side chains to molecules in the cell and reacting selectively with phosphate groups of DNA
B. Examples
 1. Busulfan (Myleran)
 2. Carmustine
 3. Chlorambucil (Leukeran)
 4. Cyclophosphamide (Cytoxan, Endoxan)
 5. Mechlorethamine hydrochloride (Caryolysine, Mustargen)
 6. Melphalan (Alkeran)
 7. Pipobroman (Vercyte)
 8. Thiophosphoramide (Thiotepa)
 9. Uracil mustard
C. Adverse effects
 1. Persistent vomiting
 2. Ataxia
 3. Convulsions

Plant Alkaloids

A. Action—disorganize the mitotic spindle to decrease cell reproduction
B. Examples
 1. Vinblastine sulfate (Velban)
 2. Vincristine sulfate (Oncovin)
C. Adverse effects
 1. Constipation
 2. Peripheral neuropathy
 3. Ataxia
 4. Muscle weakness
 5. Paresthesia

Antineoplastic Antibiotics

A. Action—By binding to DNA, slow RNA production and interfere with cell building (are highly toxic and not useful as antiinfectives)
B. Examples
 1. Dactinomycin (Cosmegen)
 2. Daunomycin
 3. Mithramycin (Mithracin)
 4. Mitomycin (mutamycin)
 5. Bleomycin sulfate (Blenoxane)
 6. Doxorubicin hydrochloride (Adriamycin)
C. Adverse effects
 1. Irritation of vein on administration
 2. Leukopenia
 3. Alopecia
 4. Nausea and vomiting
 5. Cardiac irritability and arrest

Radioactive Agents

A. Action—Destroy neoplasms by irradiation
B. Examples
 1. Gold (^{198}Au) used for pleural effusions and ascites secondary to cancer
 2. Sodium iodide (^{131}I) avidly taken up by thyroid cells
 3. Sodium phosphate (^{32}P) reduces erythrocyte count (e.g., in polycythemia vera)
C. Adverse effects
 1. Radiation sickness
 2. Low-grade fever
 3. Skin rash

Cancer Immunotherapy

A. Actions
 1. Nonspecific immunotherapy involves the introduction of noncancerous antigens into the body to stimulate the production of lymphocytes and antibodies
 2. Passive immunotherapy involves the transfer of antibodies from an individual who has been cured of cancer to someone with that same cancer
 3. Active specific immunotherapy involves injection of tumor cells intradermally to stimulate the patient's immune system
B. Examples of nonspecific immunotherapy
 1. BCG (bacillus of Calmette-Guérin)
 2. *Corynebacterium parvulum*
C. Adverse effects
 1. Fever
 2. Chills
 3. Malaise
 4. Enlarged lymph nodes
 5. Local abscess formation

Common Combinations of Chemotherapeutic Agents

A. MOPP
 1. Mechlorethamine (nitrogen mustard)
 2. Vincristine (Oncovin)
 3. Procarbazine (Matulane)
 4. Prednisone
B. COP
 1. Cyclophosphamide (Cytoxan)
 2. Vincristine (Oncovin)
 3. Prednisone
C. MAC
 1. Methotrexate
 2. Dactinomycin (Actinomycin D)
 3. Cyclophosphamide (Cytoxan)
D. POMP
 1. 6-Mercaptopurine (Purinethol)
 2. Vincristine (Oncovin)
 3. Methotrexate
 4. Prednisone
E. COMFU-P
 1. Cyclophosphamide (Cytoxan)
 2. Vincristine (Oncovin)
 3. Methotrexate
 4. 5-Fluorouracil (5-FU)
 5. Prednisone
F. CODFU
 1. Cyclophosphamide (Cytoxan)
 2. Vincristine (Oncovin)
 3. Dactinomycin (Actinomycin D)
 4. 5-Fluorouracil (5-FU)

Maintenance of Fluid, Electrolyte, and Acid-Base Balance

FLUID AND ELECTROLYTE BALANCE
Basic Concepts

A. Total volume of fluid and total amount of electrolytes in body normally remain relatively constant
B. Volume of blood plasma, interstitial fluid, and intracellular fluid and the concentration of electrolytes in each remain relatively constant
C. Fluid balance and electrolyte balance are interdependent
D. Intake must equal output
E. Fluid and electrolyte balance maintained primarily by mechanisms that adjust output to intake; secondarily by mechanisms that adjust intake to output
F. Fluid balance is also maintained by a physical mechanism that controls movement of water between fluid compartments (osmosis)
G. The average adult male (68 kg) (150 lb) contains about 40 L of water, comprising 60% of his body weight; 25 L intracellular, 15 to 17 L extracellular
H. Extracellular fluid divided among
 1. Interstitial fluid—10 to 12 L
 2. Plasma—3 L
 3. Small fluid compartments—1 L (e.g., cerebrospinal fluid, aqueous humor, serous and synovial fluid, lymphatic channels)
 4. Gastrointestinal tract—1 L at any given time for all gastrointestinal organs
I. All body fluids are related and mix well with each other: plasma becomes interstitial fluid as it filters across the capillary wall; interstitial fluid can return to the capillary by osmosis or enter lymphatic channels, becoming lymph; interstitial fluid and intracel-

Table 2-1. Average concentrations of major ions in extracellular and intracellular fluids (usually expressed in milliosmols per liter [mOsm/L] of H_2O)

Ion	Intracellular fluid	Extracellular fluid	
		Plasma	Interstitial
Na^+	10	144.0	137.0
K^+	141	5.0	4.7
Cl^-	4	107.0	112.7
HCO_3^-	10	27.0	28.3
Ca^{++}	0	2.5	2.4
Mg^{++}	31	1.5	1.4
$SO_4^=$	1	0.5	0.5
Phosphates ($H_2PO_4^-$; $HPO_4^=$)	11	2.0	2.0
Proteins	4	1.2	0.2

lular fluid are in osmotic equilibrium across the cell membranes, regulated by the sodium ion (Na^+) concentration of interstitial fluid and the potassium ion (K^+) concentration of intracellular fluid

1. Mechanism of fluid flow between plasma and interstitial fluid involves several forces
   a. Blood hydrostatic pressure
   b. Blood osmotic pressure
   c. Interstitial fluid hydrostatic pressure
   d. Interstitial fluid osmotic pressure
2. Blood hydrostatic pressure, interstitial fluid osmotic pressure, and interstitial fluid hydrostatic pressure (normally a negative value) tend to move fluid out of the blood in the capillaries and into the interstitial fluid
3. Blood osmotic pressure moves fluid back into the capillary blood from the interstitial fluid
4. Starling's law of the capillaries states that equal amounts of water move back and forth between blood and interstitial fluid only when the blood hydrostatic pressure plus the interstitial fluid hydrostatic pressure plus the interstitial fluid *osmotic* pressure equals the blood osmotic pressure; under these conditions fluid balance exists between the blood and interstitial fluid
   a. Blood gains liquid from interstitial fluid whenever the blood hydrostatic pressure plus the interstitial fluid hydrostatic pressure plus the interstitial fluid osmotic pressure is less than the blood osmotic pressure
   b. Blood loses liquid to interstitial fluid whenever blood osmotic pressure is less than blood hydrostatic pressure plus interstitial fluid hydrostatic pressure plus interstitial fluid osmotic pressure
J. Chemically, extracellular fluid and intracellular fluid are strikingly different: sodium is the main cation of extracellular fluid; potassium is the main ca-

tion of intracellular fluid; chloride is the main anion of extracellular fluid; phosphate is the main anion of intracellular fluid; protein concentration is much higher in intracellular fluid than in interstitial fluid (see Table 2-1)

K. Chemically, plasma and interstitial fluid are almost identical except that plasma contains slightly more electrolytes, considerably more proteins, somewhat more sodium, and fewer chloride ions that interstitial fluid (see Table 2-1)

Major Ions (Electrolytes)

A. Cations (+)
   1. Sodium (Na^+)
      a. Most abundant cation in extracellular fluid
      b. Sodium pump in most body cells pumps sodium out of intracellular fluid
      c. Regulates cell size by osmotically drawing water from the cells to balance flow of water into the cells due to osmotically active intracellular proteins
      d. Action potential of nervous and muscle fibers requires sodium; sodium is basic to the body's communication system
      e. Helps to regulate acid-base balance by exchanging hydrogen ions for sodium ions in the kidney tubules; excess hydrogen ions (acid) are excreted
   2. Potassium (K^+)
      a. Most abundant cation of intracellular fluid
      b. Potassium pump brings potassium into cells of the body
      c. Resting polarization and repolarization of nerve and muscle fibers depend on potassium
         (1) If potassium concentration of extracellular fluid rises above normal (hyperkalemia), the force of the contracting heart weakens; with extremely high concentrations the heart will not contract

(2) If potassium concentration of extracellular fluid drops below normal (hypokalemia), the resting polarization in nerve and muscle fibers increases, resulting in weakness and eventual paralysis
3. Calcium (Ca^{++})
  a. Forms salts with phosphates, carbonate, and fluoride in bones and teeth to make them hard
  b. Required for correct functioning of nerves and muscles
    (1) If calcium concentrations rise above normal levels (hypercalcemia), nervous system becomes depressed and sluggish
    (2) If calcium concentrations fall below normal levels (hypocalcemia), nervous system becomes extremely excitable, resulting in cramps and tetany
  c. Calcium is required for blood clotting, acting as a cofactor in the formation of prothrombin activator and thrombin
4. Magnesium (Mg^{++})
  a. Cofactor for many enzymes involved in energy metabolism
  b. Normal constituent of bone
B. Anions (−)
1. Chloride (Cl^-)
  a. Most abundant anion in extracellular fluid
  b. In great part balances sodium
  c. Major component of gastric secretions
2. Bicarbonate (HCO_3^-)
  a. Part of bicarbonate buffer system
  b. Reacts with a strong acid to form carbonic acid and a basic salt, thus limiting the drop in pH
3. Phosphate ($H_2PO_4^-$ and $HPO_4^=$)
  a. Part of phosphate buffer system
  b. Functions in cellular energy metabolism: phosphate + ADP → ATP (the energy currency of the cell)
  c. Combines with calcium ions in bone, providing hardness
  d. Involved in structure of genetic material, DNA and RNA

Major Avenues by which Water Enters and Leaves the Body

A. Water enters the body through digestive tract both in liquids (drinking) and in foods (preformed water)
B. Water is formed in the body by metabolism of foods (oxidative water)
C. Water leaves the body via kidneys (as urine), intestines (with feces), and lungs and skin (insensible water losses)

Mechanisms that Maintain Total Fluid Volume

A. Osmoreceptor system
1. Regulates water output volume to balance fluid intake volume
2. Most important mechanism for regulation of water output, since other fluid losses through the skin, lungs, and gastrointestinal system have no feedback mechanism relative to water loss
3. Cells in the hypothalamus synthesize ADH, which is then stored in the posterior pituitary prior to release into the circulation
4. Osmoreceptors respond to dehydration by increasing the frequency of nerve impulses to the posterior pituitary, resulting in an increase in the amounts of ADH released; this increases water reabsorption in the kidney tubules and decreases urinary output
5. Osmoreceptors respond to overhydration by decreasing nerve impulses to the posterior pituitary, which decreases the release of ADH, resulting in an increase in urinary output
B. Interaction of the circulatory system
1. Regulation of blood volume (extracellular fluid volume)
2. Increased fluid intake increases the blood volume
3. Increased blood volume results in an increase in cardiac output, blood pressure, and therefore glomerular filtration
4. Increased glomerular filtration results in an increase in urinary output and a decrease in blood volume
C. Regulation of fluid intake—thirst mechanism
1. Dehydration of cells in the thirst center of the hypothalamus gives rise to thirst sensation
2. Thirst sensations are also induced by dryness of the oral mucosa
3. Fluid intake stretches the stomach and moistens the mouth and throat; these sensations cancel thirst sensation prior to the actual hydration of body fluids
D. Various factors such as hyperventilation, hypoventilation, vomiting, diarrhea, circulatory failure may alter the volume of fluid lost

Mechanisms that Maintain Electrolyte Concentrations

A. Aldosterone feedback mechanism
1. Adrenal cortex secretes the steroid hormone aldosterone when extracellular fluid sodium concentrations decrease or potassium concentrations increase

2. Aldosterone stimulates kidney tubules to reabsorb sodium; potassium reabsorption decreases as sodium reabsorption increases; sodium is salvaged while potassium is excreted
3. This mechanism helps preserve normal sodium and potassium concentrations in extracellular fluid
4. Secondary effects of aldosterone
   a. Chloride conserved with sodium
   b. Water conserved, since it is reabsorbed by osmosis as tubules reabsorb salt
B. Parathyroid regulation of calcium
   1. Parathyroid glands secrete parathormone when extracellular fluid calcium concentrations decrease
   2. Parathormone stimulates the release of calcium from bone, calcium reabsorption in the small intestine (vitamin D required), and calcium reabsorption in kidney tubules
   3. Increased extracellular fluid calcium concentrations result in decreased secretion of parathormone and gradual loss of excess calcium

ACID-BASE BALANCE
Basic Concepts

A. Healthy survival depends on the body's maintaining a state of acid-base balance; more specifically, healthy survival depends on the maintenance of a relatively constant, slightly alkaline pH of blood and other fluids
B. When the body is in a state of acid-base balance, it maintains a stable hydrogen ion concentration in body fluids; specifically, blood pH remains relatively constant between 7.35 and 7.45
C. The body has 3 devices or mechanisms for maintaining acid-base balance; named in order of the speed with which they act, they are the buffer mechanism, the respiratory mechanism, and the renal or urinary mechanisms
D. A state of uncompensated acidosis exists if blood pH decreases below 7.35
E. A state of uncompensated alkalosis exists if blood pH increases above 7.45
F. The pH of body fluids shifts from the ideal of 7.35 to 7.45 for several reasons
   1. Glucose, utilized by almost all body cells, is oxidized; as a result energy, water, and carbon dioxide are produced; the CO_2 combines with the water to produce carbonic acid (H_2CO_3)
   2. Metabolism of sulfur amino acids results in formation of sulfuric acid
   3. Metabolism of phospholipids and phosphoproteins results in formation of phosphoric acid

4. Muscle metabolism under anaerobic conditions produces lactic acid
5. Rapid weight loss results in extra fat metabolism, producing ketone bodies that include alpha keto acids
6. The acid produced by the normal mechanisms just mentioned requires neutralization to avoid acidosis, coma, and death

Buffer Mechanisms for Maintaining Acid-Base Balance

A. The buffer mechanism consists of chemicals called buffers, which are present in the blood and other body fluids and which combine with relatively strong acids or bases to convert them to weaker acids or bases; hence, buffers function to prevent marked changes in blood pH when either acids or bases enter the blood
B. A buffer is often referred to as a buffer pair because it consists of not 1 but 2 substances; the chief buffer pair in the blood consists of the weak acid, carbonic acid (H_2CO_3), and its basic salts, collectively called base bicarbonate ($B \cdot HCO_3$); sodium bicarbonate ($NaHCO_3$) is by far the most abundant base bicarbonate present in blood plasma
C. When the body is in a state of acid-base balance, blood contains 27 mEq base bicarbonate per liter and 1.35 mEq carbonic acid per liter; usually this is written as a ratio, referred to as the base bicarbonate/carbonic acid ratio:

$$\frac{27 \text{ mEq B} \cdot \text{HCO}_3}{1.35 \text{ mEq H}_2\text{CO}_3} = \frac{20}{1}$$

D. Whenever the base bicarbonate/carbonic acid ratio of blood equals 20/1, blood pH equals 7.4
E. Base bicarbonate buffers nonvolatile acids that are stronger than carbonic acid; it reacts with them to convert them to carbonic acid and a basic salt
F. Some facts about the changes in capillary blood produced by the buffering of blood by base bicarbonate
   1. Buffering does not prevent blood pH from decreasing, but it does prevent it from decreasing as markedly as it would without buffering
   2. Buffering removes some sodium bicarbonate from blood and adds some carbonic acid to it; this necessarily decreases the base bicarbonate/carbonic acid ratio, which in turn necessarily decreases the pH of blood as it flows through capillaries (from its arterial level of about 7.4 to its venous level of about 7.38)
   3. Anything that decreases the blood's base bicarbonate/carbonic acid ratio necessarily decreases

blood pH and thus tends to produce acidosis; the corollary is also true: anything that increases the base bicarbonate/carbonic acid ratio necessarily increases blood pH and thus tends to produce alkalosis

G. Other buffer systems in body fluids
   1. Protein buffer
      a. Most plentiful; three fourths of all chemical buffering power lies in proteins of the body fluids
      b. Provides support to other buffering systems such as bicarbonate buffer and phosphate buffer
   2. Phosphate buffer system
      a. One sixth as concentrated as bicarbonate buffer in extracellular fluid
      b. More important in intracellular fluids, where its concentration is considerably higher
      c. Helps to buffer pH of urine in kidney tubules
   3. Hemoglobin buffer system—buffers intracellular fluid of the erythrocyte

H. Bicarbonate buffer is the most important buffer in human body fluids because its components, base bicarbonate and carbonic acid, are actively and constantly regulated by the action of the respiratory and urinary systems

Respiratory Mechanism for Controlling Acid-Base Balance

A. Respiratory system controls acid-base balance by controlling rate of carbon dioxide (CO_2) exhalation from lungs; during normal body metabolism CO_2 is produced, which reacts with water to form carbonic acid, resulting in a decrease in pH (as acidity increases, pH decreases); when the respiratory system blows CO_2 out of the body, carbonic acid breaks down into CO_2 and water, resulting in an increase in pH (as acidity decreases, pH increases)

B. Respiratory acidosis
   1. Conditions impairing the ability of the respiratory system to blow off CO_2 will result in a buildup of CO_2 in the body; excess CO_2 combines with water to form carbonic acid and hydrogen ions, resulting in a decrease in pH
   2. Signs of respiratory acidosis include dyspnea, irritability, tachycardia, and cyanosis
   3. Common causes include emphysema, pneumonia, asthmatic attack, atelectasis, pneumothorax, drug overdose

C. Respiratory alkalosis
   1. Less frequently, hyperventilation blows off too much CO_2 from the body, causing an excessive breakdown of carbonic acid, resulting in an increase of pH

   2. Signs of respiratory alkalosis include deep or deep and rapid breathing, light-headedness, tetany, convulsions, and unconsciousness
   3. Common causes include hysteria, prolonged crying, and mechanical ventilation

Renal Mechanism for Maintaining Acid-Base Balance

A. The renal mechanism is the most effective device the body has for maintaining acid-base balance; unless it operates adequately, acid-base balance cannot be maintained

B. The renal mechanism for maintaining acid-base balance makes the urine more acidic and the blood more alkaline; this neutralizes the constant production of acid products from cells; the mechanism consists of 2 functions performed by the distal renal tubule cells, both of which remove hydrogen ions from blood to urine and in exchange reabsorb sodium ions from tubular urine to blood
   1. Distal tubule cells secrete hydrogen ions and reabsorb sodium ions (Fig. 1)
   2. Distal tubule cells form ammonia, which combines with hydrogen ions they have secreted to form ammonium ions (NH_4^+), which are excreted in the urine in exchange for sodium ions, which are reabsorbed into the blood (Fig. 2)

C. The distal tubule functions produce the following results
   1. They increase blood's sodium bicarbonate content and decrease its carbonic acid content, thereby increasing the base bicarbonate/carbonic acid ratio and blood pH
   2. They acidify urine (decrease urine pH)

D. Metabolic acidosis
   1. Excess acid, other than carbonic acid, which is a respiratory acid, accumulates in the body beyond the body's ability to neutralize it
   2. Signs of metabolic acidosis include weakness, malaise, headache, disorientation, deep rapid breathing, fruity odor to breath, coma
   3. Common causes include diabetes mellitus, salicylate poisoning, severe diarrhea, vomiting of intestinal contents, infection

E. Metabolic alkalosis
   1. Excess base bicarbonate in the body
   2. Signs of metabolic alkalosis include muscle hypertoxicity, tetany, confusion, shallow slow respirations, convulsions, coma
   3. Common causes include vomiting of stomach contents or prolonged gastric suction, excessive ingestion of alkaline drugs, potent diuretics

Fig. 1. Acidification of urine and conservation of base by the distal renal tubular excretion of hydrogen ions (H^+) from the urine and the reabsorption of sodium ions (Na^+) into the blood in exchange for the H^+ excreted into it. (From Anthony, C.P., and Thibodeau, G.A.: Textbook of anatomy and physiology, ed. 11, St. Louis, 1983, The C.V. Mosby Co.)

Fig. 2. Acidification of urine by the tubular excretion of ammonia (NH_3). An acid (glutamine) leaves the blood, enters a tubule cell, and is deaminized to form ammonia. The ammonia is excreted into the urine, where it combines with hydrogen to form the ammonium ion (NH_4^+). In exchange for NH_4^+ the tubule cell reabsorbs Na^+. (From Anthony, C.P., and Thibodeau, G.A.: Textbook of anatomy and physiology, ed. 11, St. Louis, 1983, The C.V. Mosby Co.)

F. Compensation
1. In respiratory acidosis the urinary system excretes increased hydrogen ions to compensate for the respiratory system's inability to blow off CO_2
2. In respiratory alkalosis the urinary system may decrease excretion of hydrogen ions to compensate and maintain the body's pH in the normal range
3. In metabolic acidosis the respiratory system compensates by hyperventilation in an attempt to blow off CO_2 and raise the pH
4. In metabolic alkalosis the respiratory system compensates by decreasing the rate and depth of breathing in an attempt to retain CO_2 and decrease the pH

CHEMICAL PRINCIPLES RELATED TO FLUID AND ELECTROLYTES
Ionization
Ion
A. When an atom loses or gains an electron (electrons), it is no longer a neutral atom but a charged particle—an ion
B. The charge on this particle depends on whether electrons are lost ($+$) or gained ($-$) and the number of electrons lost or gained
C. An electron is a negative particle; the loss of 1 electron makes ion positive (less negative) by 1; with loss of 2 electrons, ion is 2^+, etc.
D. The gain of 1 electron makes ion negative by 1; with 2 electrons gained, the ion is 2^-, etc.

Ionization and Water
A. When certain compounds are placed in water, the polar water molecules dissociate the molecules of the compound into ions—a process called ionization
B. A substance that will ionize when placed in water is called an electrolyte
C. A substance that will ionize in water (an electrolyte) will allow the passage of an electric current through its solution
D. Acids, bases, and salts ionize in water and conduct an electric current

Factors Affecting Strength of Electrolytes
A. Amount of electrolyte present in solution
B. How well the electrolyte dissociates in solution—degree of ionization
1. Weak electrolytes are substances that dissociate into ions to only a slight degree
2. Strong electrolytes are substances that dissociate into ions to a larger degree

Bases, Acids, and Salts
Bases
A. Definition—a base is a substance that usually adds a hydroxyl ion (OH^-) to any solution in which it is placed,

$$\text{in water} \\ \downarrow \\ NaOH \rightarrow Na^+ + OH^-$$

B. Properties of a base
1. Bitter taste
2. Slippery feeling
3. Electrolyte in water
4. Reacts with indicators, giving a base color
   a. Methyl orange—yellow
   b. Litmus—blue
   c. Phenolphthalein—red
5. Reacts with acids to form water and a salt (neutralization)
6. Reacts with certain metals to release hydrogen gas
7. Combines with organic acids (fatty acids) to form soaps
8. In high concentration destroys organic material; corrosive
C. Names and formulas of common bases
1. Calcium hydroxide ($Ca(OH)_2$)—water solution, called lime water
2. Sodium hydroxide ($NaOH$)—caustic soda
3. Potassium hydroxide (KOH)—soap making
4. Ammonium hydroxide (NH_4OH)—household cleaner
5. Magnesium hydroxide ($Mg(OH)_2$)—water solution marketed under trade name Milk of Magnesia—antacid, mild laxative
6. Aluminum hydroxide ($Al(OH)_3$)—component of antacid pills

Acids
A. Definition—an acid is ordinarily thought of as a substance that liberates an H^+ (hydrogen ion) to a solution in which it is placed

$$\text{in water} \\ \downarrow \\ H_2CO_3 \rightarrow H^+ + HCO_3^-$$

B. Properties of an acid
1. Sour taste
2. Reacts with indicators, giving an acid color
   a. Methyl orange—red
   b. Litmus—red
   c. Phenolphthalein—colorless
3. Combines with certain metals, releasing hydrogen gas
4. Reacts with bases to form water and a salt (neutralization)

5. Reacts with carbonates to give carbon dioxide gas
6. Acts as an electrolyte in water
7. In high concentration destroys organic materials—corrosive

C. Names and formulas of common acids
1. Hydrochloric acid (HCl)—secreted by the parietal cells of the stomach; transforms pepsinogen into pepsin, which is a protein-digesting enzyme of gastric juice
2. Nitric acid (HNO_3)—used in test for proteins
3. Sulfuric acid (H_2SO_4)—in storage batteries
4. Carbonic acid (H_2CO_3)
   a. One form in which CO_2 is transported in the blood
   b. Part of the bicarbonate buffer system, which is the most important buffer system regulating the pH of body fluids
5. Boric acid (H_3BO_3)—mild antiseptic
6. Acetic acid (CH_3COOH)—vinegar
7. Lactic acid ($CH_3CHOHCOOH$)—builds up in muscle tissue during exercise; most lactic acid is then transported to the liver via the circulatory system where it is completely oxidized into CO_2, water, and energy (as ATP)

General Considerations Concerning Acids and Bases
A. Weak acids produce few hydrogen ions in solution, whereas strong acids produce many
B. Weak bases produce few hydroxyl ions in solution, whereas strong bases produce many
C. Strong acids and bases can cause serious damage to human tissue
D. Acids and bases can be used to neutralize each other—therefore, in the event of acid or base burn, flood with water and add the opposite chemical in weak, diluted form

Salts
A. Definition—the compound (besides water) formed when an acid is neutralized by a base is a salt; e.g.,

$$HCl + KOH \rightarrow H_2O + KCl$$
Acid　　Base　　　Water　　Salt

B. Properties of a salt
1. Crystalline in nature
2. Ionic even in the dry crystal
3. Electrolyte in solution
4. "Salty" taste
C. Names and formulas of common salts
1. Sodium chloride (NaCl)—salt of intercellular and extracellular spaces
2. Calcium phosphate ($Ca_3(PO_4)_2$)—bone and tooth formation
3. Potassium chloride (KCl)—salt of intracellular spaces

4. Calcium carbonate ($CaCO_3$)—limestone
5. Barium sulfate ($BaSO_4$)—when taken internally, outlines internal structures for x-ray studies
6. Silver nitrate ($AgNO_3$)—antiseptic
7. Iron (II) sulfate ($FeSO_4$)—treatment of anemia
8. Sodium bicarbonate ($NaHCO_3$)—antacid
9. Calcium sulfate ($CaSO_4$)—hydrated form is plaster of paris (casts for broken bones)
10. Magnesium sulfate ($MgSO_4$)—Epsom salt

Hydrogen Ion Concentration (pH)
A. The *p* in pH comes from the French word *puissance,* meaning power
B. The *H* in pH stands for *hydrogen*
C. Thus pH denotes the power or strength of hydrogen (ions) in a solution
D. A neutral solution has the same amount of acid-reacting ions, H^+ (actually H_3O^+), as basic-reacting ions, OH^-
E. An acid-reacting solution has more H^+ than OH^-
F. A basic-reacting solution has more OH^- than H^+
G. pH is used to represent these conditions
1. A neutral solution has a pH of 7.00
2. An acid solution would have a pH in the range from 0 to 6.99; the lower the pH, the more acid the solution
3. A basic solution would have a pH in the range from 7.01 to 14.00; the higher the pH, the more basic the solution
4. The pH of the extracellular (vascular and interstitial) fluid is in the narrow range of 7.35 to 7.45; fluctuations in pH of 0.4 unit above or below this range can result in body distress; a prolonged blood pH of 7 or less or 7.8 or more can result in death
5. Certain body fluids have a pH different from 7.4; gastric juice has a pH of 1 or 2 caused by the presence of hydrochloric acid; bile is basic; urine may be acidic or basic

Circulatory System
REVIEW OF ANATOMY AND PHYSIOLOGY OF THE CIRCULATORY SYSTEM
Functions
A. Primary function—provides communication between widely separated body parts through transportation of hormones, nutrients, wastes, respiratory gases, vitamins, minerals, enzymes, water, leukocytes, antibodies, and buffers
B. Secondary functions—contributes directly or indirectly to all the body's metabolic functions: tissue

perfusion with oxygen and nutrients, water balance, immunity, enzymatic reactions, and pH and temperature regulation

Structures

Blood

A. Blood components
1. Serum—plasma with fewer or no coagulating proteins
2. Plasma
   a. Water—3 L in average adult; constitutes 90% of plasma
   b. Ions—see fluid and electrolytes and Table 2-2
   c. Proteins—all act as buffers; fractionated and separated from each other by electrophoretic and ultracentrifugation techniques
      (1) Albumin
         (a) Largest component of plasma proteins
         (b) Principally responsible for plasma colloid osmotic pressure (COP)

Table 2-2. Plasma constituents

Constituent	Normal concentration range
Water	Approximately 90% by volume
Ions	
Sodium (Na^+)	135 to 145 mEq/L
Potassium (K^+)	4.0 to 5.5 mEq/L
Calcium (Ca^{++})	4.5 to 5.0 mEq/L
Magnesium (Mg^{++})	1.5 to 2.5 mEq/L
Chloride (Cl^-)	100 to 106 mEq/L
Bicarbonate (HCO_3^-)	23 to 28 mEq/L
Phosphate ($H_2PO_4^-$; $HPO_4^=$)	1.5 to 2.5 mEq/L
Plasma proteins	
Albumin	3.5 to 5.5 g/100 ml
Globulins (alpha, beta, and gamma)	1.5 to 3.6 g/100 ml
Glucose	70 to 110 mg/100 ml
Nitrogenous substances	
Blood urea nitrogen (BUN)	5 to 25 mg/100 ml
Uric acid	2 to 8 mg/100 ml
Creatinine	0.7 to 1.5 mg/100 ml
Amino acids	0.1 to 3.0 mg/100 ml
Bilirubin	0.0 to 1.5 mg/100 ml
Lipids	
Cholesterol	150 to 300 mg/100 ml
Fatty acids	200 to 400 mg/100 ml
Triglycerides	15 to 25 mg/100 ml
Other constituents	
Respiratory gases (O_2 and CO_2)	Variable concentrations
Hormones	
Vitamins	
Enzymes	

(c) Reversibly combines with and transports certain lipids, bilirubin, thyroxin, and certain drugs, such as barbiturates
(2) Alpha and beta globulins
   (a) Help establish COP
   (b) Transport certain vitamins, iron, copper, and cortisol
   (c) Hemostasis (prothrombin and fibrinogen are in this blood fraction)
(3) Gamma globulins—antibodies
d. Glucose—prime oxidative metabolite of body cells
3. Formed elements
   a. Erythrocytes
      (1) Shape—pliable biconcave disc that maximizes surface area proportional to volume for ease of diffusion of respiratory gases
      (2) Number—males: 4.5 to 6.2 × 10^6/mm³; females: 4.0 to 5.5 × 10^6/mm³
      (3) Formation—erythropoiesis
         (a) Location—red marrow of vertebrae, sternum, ribs, iliac crests, clavicles, scapulae, and skull
         (b) Maturation process—mature erythrocytes are mainly sacs of hemoglobin without a nucleus, mitochondria, ribosomes, endoplasmic reticula, or Golgi bodies; process requires folic acid and vitamin B_{12}; vitamin B_{12} plus intrinsic factor from the parietal cells of the stomach form hemopoietic factor, which stimulates erythrocyte formation (see pernicious anemia)
         (c) Under conditions of low O_2 tension, liver and kidneys secrete proteins into blood that combine to form erythropoietin, which stimulates erythrocyte production
      (4) Principal component is hemoglobin
         (a) Conjugated protein—globulin plus 4 molecules of heme
         (b) Formed within the erythrocyte utilizing copper, cobalt, iron, nickel, and vitamin B_6
         (c) Functions to bind O_2 through iron in heme and CO_2 through globulin portion; can carry both simultaneously
      (5) Erythrocytes live for about 120 days; old or deteriorated ones are removed by reticuloendothelial cells of the liver, spleen, and bone marrow; 3.5 × 10^6 die

and are replaced daily; heme is converted to bilirubin, which is excreted from the liver as part of the bile
  b. Leukocytes
    (1) Types
      (a) Granulocytes (polymorphonuclear)—originate in red marrow and consist of neutrophils (50% to 70% of total), eosinophils (1% to 4% of the total), and basophils (0% to 1% of the total)
      (b) Agranulocytes (mononuclear)—originate in red marrow and lymphatic tissue and consist of monocytes (3% to 8% of the total), which become macrophages in tissue spaces, and lymphocytes (25% to 40% of the total)
    (2) Functions
      (a) Phagocytosis of bacteria by neutrophils and macrophages; phagocytosis of antibody-antigen complexes by eosinophils
      (b) Antibody synthesis—B lymphocytes produce antibodies; they also become plasma cells, which produce most circulatory antibodies
      (c) Destruction of transplanted tissues and cancer cells by T lymphocytes, which form in lymphoid tissue and mature in the thymus
    (3) Leukocytes live for a few hours or days; some T lymphocytes live for many years and provide long-term immunity
  c. Thrombocytes—anucleate cellular fragments associated with hemostasis
    (1) Origin—fragmentation of megakaryocytes in bone marrow
    (2) Number—150,000 to 500,000/mm^3
    (3) Function in blood coagulation
      (a) Adhere to each other and to damaged areas of circulatory system to limit or prevent blood loss
      (b) Release chemicals that constrict damaged blood vessels
B. Physical properties of blood
  1. Volume
    a. Male: 5 to 6 L; female: 4.5 to 5.5 L
    b. Hematocrit: percent blood volume occupied by red cells (normal range: 36% to 45%)
  2. Specific gravity (sp gr)—normal range: 1.05 to 1.06
  3. Viscosity—about 5.5 times as viscous as pure water

C. Blood groups
  1. Names—indicate type antigens on or in red cell membrane (e.g., type A blood means that red cells have A antigens, type O that red cells have no antigens)
  2. Every person's blood belongs to one of the 4 blood groups—type A, type B, type AB, or type O—and is either Rh positive or Rh negative
  3. Plasma—normally contains no antibodies against antigens present on its own red cells but does contain antibodies against other A or B antigens not present on its red cells (e.g., type A plasma does not contain antibodies against A antigen but does contain antibodies against B antigen)
  4. Blood does not normally contain anti-Rh antibodies; Rh-positive blood never contains them; Rh-negative blood will contain anti-Rh antibodies if the individual has been transfused with Rh-positive blood or has carried an Rh-positive fetus
  5. The potential danger in transfusing blood is that the donor's blood may be agglutinated (clumped) by the recipient's antibodies
D. Hemostasis—arrest of bleeding
  1. Vasoconstriction—reflex spasm in cut or ruptured vessel's smooth muscles
  2. Aggregation of platelets—adhere to damaged blood vessel walls forming plugs
  3. Blood coagulation (clotting)—blood becomes gel as soluble fibrinogen is converted to insoluble fibrin; process brought about by at least a dozen different chemical clotting factors operating in sequence after mechanism is triggered
    a. Extrinsic clotting mechanism—trigger for mechanism is blood contacting damaged tissue
    b. Intrinsic clotting mechanism—trigger for mechanism is release of chemicals (platelet factors) from platelets aggregated at either the site of a wound or at a rough spot on blood vessel wall
  4. Some facts about the blood proteins essential for clotting
    a. Liver cells synthesize prothrombin, fibrinogen, and other clotting factors; adequate amounts of vitamin K must be present in blood for the liver to make normal amounts of prothrombin, Stuart factor (X), factor VIII, and Christmas factor (IX) (PTC)
    b. Normal blood prothrombin content—10 to 15 mg/100 ml of plasma
    c. Normal blood fibrinogen content—350 mg/100 ml of plasma

d. Both prothrombin and fibrinogen are soluble proteins normally present in blood in adequate amounts for clotting to occur at the normal rapid rate

e. Fibrin is an insoluble protein formed from the soluble protein fibrinogen, in the presence of the enzyme thrombin; fibrin appears as a tangled mass of threads having a jelly-like texture; blood cells become enmeshed in these threads, and red cells give the clot its red color

5. Clinical applications

a. Hemophilia—hereditary sex-linked disease characterized by defect in clotting ability of blood caused by lack of a blood protein essential for clotting (factor VIII)

b. Thrombosis—partial or complete occlusion of a blood vessel, caused by presence of a stationary clot (thrombus)

c. Embolism—partial or complete occlusion of a blood vessel by a moving clot (embolus)

d. Atherosclerosis—plaques of lipoid material deposited in endothelium act as rough spots, causing platelet disintegration and thrombus formation

Heart

A. Location—in pericardial cavity within the mediastinum with apex on diaphragm and pointing to left (apical beat may be counted by placing stethoscope in fifth intercostal space on line with left midclavicular point); two thirds of bulk of heart lies to left of midline of body, one third to right

B. Covering—pericardium

1. Structure

a. Fibrous pericardium—loose-fitting, inextensible sac around heart

b. Serous pericardium—consists of 2 layers

(1) Parietal layer—lines inner surface of fibrous pericardium

(2) Visceral layer (epicardium)—adheres to outer surface of the heart; pericardial space, lying between the parietal and visceral layers, contains a few drops of lubricating pericardial fluid

2. Function—protects heart against friction and erosion by providing well-lubricated, smooth sac in which the heart beats

C. Structure of heart

1. Heart wall

a. Myocardium—composed of cardiac muscle cells

b. Endocardium—delicate endothelial lining of myocardium

c. Cardiac skeleton—continuous dense connective tissue regions at the heart's base and in the interventricular septum serving as points of origin and insertion for cardiac muscle fibers and as supports for the heart's valves

2. Cavities

a. Upper 2 called atria

b. Lower 2 called ventricles

3. Valves and openings

a. Openings between atria and ventricles known as atrioventricular orifices

(1) Guarded by cuspid valves

(a) Tricuspid on right

(b) Mitral (bicuspid) on left

(2) Valves consist of 3 parts

(a) Flaps or cusps

(b) Chordae tendineae

(c) Papillary muscles

b. Opening from right ventricle into pulmonary artery guarded by the pulmonary semilunar valve

c. Opening from left ventricle into the aorta guarded by the aortic semilunar valve

4. Blood supply to myocardium (heart muscle)

a. By way of only 2 small vessels: the right and left coronary arteries, the first branches of the aorta

b. Both coronary arteries send branches to both sides of the heart

c. Right coronary branches supply right side of heart mainly but also carry some blood to the left ventricle

d. Left coronary branches supply left side of heart mainly but also carry some blood to the right ventricle

e. Most abundant blood supply goes to the myocardium of the left ventricle

f. Greatest flow of blood into myocardium occurs when heart relaxes due to decreased arterial compression

g. Relatively few anastomoses (branches from one artery to another artery) exist between the larger branches of the coronary arteries (poor collateral circulation); hence, if one of these vessels becomes occluded, little or no blood can reach the myocardial cells supplied by that vessel; deprived of an adequate blood supply, the cells soon die (myocardial infarction)

5. Nerve supply to heart

a. Sympathetic fibers (in cardiac nerves) and parasympathetic fibers (in the vagus nerve) form the cardiac plexuses

b. Fibers from the cardiac plexuses terminate mainly in the sinoatrial node

c. Sympathetic impulses tend to accelerate and strengthen heartbeat

d. Parasympathetic (vagal) impulses slow the heartbeat

6. Conduction system of heart

a. Sinoatrial (SA) node—a cluster of cells located in the right atrial wall near the opening of the superior vena cava

b. Atrioventricular (AV) node—a small mass of special conducting cells located in the base of the right atrium at the top of the interventricular septum

c. AV bundle of His—special conducting fibers that originate in the AV node and extend by 2 branches down the 2 sides of the interventricular septum (right and left bundle branches)

d. Purkinje fibers—special conducting fibers that extend from the AV bundles throughout the wall of the ventricles

e. Normally a nerve impulse begins its course through the heart in the heart's own pacemaker, the SA node; it quickly spreads through both atria, via special conducting fibers, to the AV node; after a short delay at this node, the impulse is conducted by 2 branches of the AV bundle of His down both sides of the interventricular septum; from there, the impulse travels over Purkinje fibers to the lateral walls of the ventricles

f. Impulse conduction through the heart generates electric currents that spread through surrounding tissues to the skin, from which visible records of conduction can be made with the electrocardiograph or oscillograph; conduction from the SA node through the atria causes atrial contraction and gives rise to the so-called P wave of the electrocardiogram; conduction from the AV node down the bundle of His and out the Purkinje fibers causes ventricular contraction and gives rise to the QRS wave; ventricular repolarization is associated with the T wave

g. Refractory period—particularly long (¼ second) to ensure against extra beats arising as electrical energy flows around the surface of the heart; only SA node depolarizations, occurring after a refractory period, produce the next beat

D. Physiology of heart

1. Function—to pump varying amounts of blood through the vessels as the needs of cells change

2. Cardiac cycle

a. Consists of systole (contraction) and diastole (relaxation) of atria and of ventricles; atria contract, and as they relax ventricles contract

b. Time required—about ⅘ second from one cardiac cycle; so 70 to 80 cycles or heartbeats per minute

3. Auscultatory events (heart sounds)—first sound (I), "lub," occurs at the beginning of ventricular systole due to closing of the atrioventricular valves (tricuspid and mitral); second sound (II), "dub," occurs at the end of ventricular systole due to closing of the semilunar valves

Blood Vessels

A. Kinds

1. Arteries—vessels that carry blood away from the heart (all arteries except pulmonary artery carry oxygenated blood); arteries branch into smaller and smaller vessels called arterioles, which branch into microscopic vessels, the capillaries

2. Veins—vessels that carry blood toward the heart (all veins except the pulmonary veins carry deoxygenated blood); veins branch into venules, which collect blood from capillaries; veins in cranial cavity formed by dura mater called sinuses

3. Capillaries—microscopic vessels that carry blood from arterioles to venules; capillaries unite to form small veins or venules, which, in turn, unite to form veins; exchange of substances between blood and interstitial fluid occurs in capillaries

B. Structure of blood vessels

1. Arteries

a. Lining (tunica intima) of endothelium

b. Middle coat (tunica media) of smooth muscle, elastic, and fibrous tissues; this coat permits constriction and dilation

c. Outer coat (tunica adventitia or externa) of fibrous tissue; its firmness makes arteries stand open instead of collapsing when cut

2. Veins

a. Same 3 coats, but thinner and fewer elastic fibers

b. Veins collapse when cut

c. Semilunar valves present in most veins over 2 mm in diameter

3. Capillaries

a. Only lining coat present (intima)

b. Wall only 1 cell thick

C. Fetal circulation—structures that are essential for fetal circulation but that normally cease to exist after birth
   1. Umbilical arteries—2 extensions of hypogastric arteries (internal iliacs) carry fetal blood to placenta
   2. Placenta—attached to uterine wall
   3. Umbilical vein—extends from placenta back to fetus' body; returns oxygenated blood from placental to fetal circulation; 2 umbilical arteries and 1 umbilical vein constitute umbilical cord
   4. Ductus venosus—small vessel that connects umbilical vein with inferior vena cava in fetus
   5. Foramen ovale—opening in fetal heart septum between right and left atria
   6. Ductus arteriosus—small vessel connecting pulmonary artery with descending thoracic aorta
   7. Only 2 fetal blood vessels carry oxygenated blood—umbilical vein and ductus venosus; as soon as blood enters inferior vena cava from ductus venosus it becomes mixed with venous blood

Physiology of Circulation

A. Definitions
   1. Circulation—blood flow through circuit of vessels
   2. Systemic circulation—blood flow from left ventricle into aorta, other arteries, arterioles, capillaries, venules, and veins to right atrium of heart
   3. Pulmonary circulation—blood flow from right ventricle to pulmonary artery to lung arterioles, capillaries, and venules, to pulmonary veins, to left atrium
   4. Hepatic portal circulation—blood flow from capillaries, venules, and veins of stomach, intestines, spleen, pancreas, and gallbladder into portal vein, liver sinusoids, to hepatic veins, to inferior vena cava
   5. Cardiac output (CO)—volume of blood pumped per minute by either left or right ventricle; average for male at rest: 5 L/minute; cardiac output is the stroke volume (systolic discharge) times heart rate; CO increases if heart rate increases or if stroke volume increases, as by sympathetic stimulation

B. Regulation of cardiac output
   1. Starling's law of the heart—within physiologic limits the heart, when stretched by an increased returning volume of blood, contracts more strongly and pumps out the extra returned blood; heart pumps in proportion to peripheral demand
   2. Autoregulation—volume of blood returning to heart and subsequently pumped by the heart is determined by the tissues; precapillary sphincters, which precede every capillary bed of the body, relax and permit more blood flow when O_2 tension falls; they constrict and restrict flow when O_2 tension rises
   3. Venous return—sum of all volumes of blood flowing through all capillary beds of the body; initiates Starling's law of the heart
   4. Nervous and hormonal influences on heart—physiologic limit on heart's ability to increase output as venous return increases; maximum at about 15 L/minute; sympathetic stimulation and epinephrine raise upper limit of cardiac output to 25 to 30 L/minute in normal individuals and to 35 L/minute in athletes; parasympathetic stimulation decreases heart rate and stroke volume
   5. Neural influence on veins—venous constriction due to sympathetic stimulation milks blood toward heart, increasing venous return and cardiac output

C. Principles of circulation
   1. Blood circulates because a blood pressure gradient exists in the vessels; like all fluids, blood moves from regions where its pressure is greater to regions where the pressure is less; because blood pressure is highest in the left ventricle and aorta, successively lower in arteries, arterioles, capillaries, venules, veins, and lowest in the central veins (venae cavae and right atrium), blood flows through the circulatory system in this order
   2. Normal range of systolic blood pressure is 100 to 139 mm Hg; consistent readings in 140s and 150s are borderline high; readings 160 and above are high; difference between systolic and diastolic pressures is the pulse pressure, normally between 30 and 40 mm Hg
   3. Blood pressure normally remains relatively constant over a wide range of activities due to
      a. Neural regulation—maintains blood pressure on a minute-by-minute basis; increase in arterial pressure stimulates baroreceptors in aorta and carotid sinus, which leads to increased parasympathetic impulses to heart via vagus nerve, which slow the heart rate; a decrease in arterial pressure inhibits baroreceptors in the aorta and carotid sinus and thereby leads to decreased parasympathetic impulses and increased sympathetic impulses to the heart, which in turn cause a faster heart rate

b. Intrinsic circulatory regulation—maintains blood pressure on an hour-to-hour basis; increased blood pressure raises the hydrostatic pressure of plasma, leading to increased filtration of plasma from circulatory system to interstitial spaces, this results in reduced venous return, decreased cardiac output, and decreased blood pressure

c. Kidney regulation—provides long-term day-to-day regulation of blood pressure; increased blood pressure drives more blood through the kidneys, which in turn make and excrete more urine; as a result venous return, cardiac output, and blood pressure all decrease

4. Blood flow through the capillary bed—plasma filters through capillary wall at arterial end of capillary bed and becomes interstitial fluid; fluid flows over cells in capillary bed, and diffusion of nutrients and wastes occurs between fluid and cells; about half the interstitial fluid filters back into venous end of capillary bed, becoming plasma again; remaining half of interstitial fluid enters lymphatic channels along with leaked plasma proteins and returns to venous system

5. Regulation of blood flow in the circulatory system—rate of flow in liters per minute is directly proportional to blood pressure gradient and diameter of blood vessels; as pressure gradient and vessel diameter increase, flow rate increases; rate of flow is inversely proportional to blood vessel length and blood viscosity; as vessel length and blood viscosity increase, flow rate decreases; peripheral resistance refers to the combined effects of blood vessel radius and length and blood viscosity

6. Under nonpathologic conditions blood pressure remains relatively constant; since vessel length and blood viscosity are constant, the rate of flow depends almost entirely on blood vessel radius (constriction and dilation)

a. Sympathetic discharge constricts muscular arteries and arterioles leading to the viscera, kidneys, and skin and dilates those leading to skeletal muscles

b. Postural reflexes (baroreceptor system)—arterioles are constricted when one suddenly stands after sitting or lying down; this raises blood pressure and ensures adequate perfusion of brain cells with oxygen and nutrients

c. Sympathetic discharge constricts blood reservoirs, such as the veins, and propels blood toward the heart

D. Pulse
1. Definition—alternate expansion and elastic recoil of blood vessel
2. Cause—variations in pressure within vessel caused by intermittent injections of blood from heart into aorta with each ventricular contraction; pulse can be felt because of elasticity of arterial walls
3. Pulse can be felt wherever artery lies near surface and over firm background such as bone; some of those most easily palpated are
   a. Radial artery—at wrist
   b. Temporal artery—in front of ear, or above and to outer side of eye
   c. Common carotid artery—along anterior edge of sternocleidomastoid muscle, at level of lower margin of thyroid cartilage
   d. Facial artery—at lower margin of lower jaw bone, on line with corners of mouth, in groove in mandible about one third of way forward from angle of bone
   e. Brachial artery—at bend of the elbow, along the inner margin of the biceps muscle
   f. Posterior tibial artery—behind the medial malleolus (inner "ankle bone")
   g. Dorsalis pedis—on anterior surface of the foot, just below the bend of the ankle
4. Venous pulse—in large veins only; produced by changes in venous pressure brought about by alternate contraction and relaxation of the atria rather than the ventricles, as in arterial pulse

Lymphatic System

Lymph Vessels

A. Structure—lymph capillaries similar to blood capillaries in structure; larger lymphatics similar to veins but are thinner walled, have more valves, and have lymph nodes in certain places along their course

B. Names—largest lymphatic known as thoracic duct; drains lymph from entire body, except upper right quadrant, into the left subclavian vein (where it joins the internal jugular); right lymphatic ducts drain lymph from the upper right quadrant into the right subclavian vein

C. Functions
1. Lymphatics return fluid and proteins to blood from interstitial fluid; about 60% of fluid filtered out of blood capillaries returns to circulation via lymphatics rather than by osmosis into venous ends of capillaries; about 50% of total blood proteins leak out of capillaries per day; the only way these large molecules can return to blood is via lymphatics

2. Adequate lymph return is essential for maintaining homeostasis of blood proteins and therefore of blood volume
3. Interference with the return of proteins to the blood results in edema caused by the loss of protein and changes in colloid osmotic pressure

Lymph Nodes

A. Structure—lymphatic tissue, separated into compartments by fibrous partitions; afferent lymphatic vessels enter each node; 1 (usually) efferent vessel drains lymph out of node
B. Location—usually in clusters; some of more important groups, from nursing viewpoint, follow
   1. Submental and submaxillary groups in floor of mouth; lymph from nose, lips, and teeth drains through these nodes
   2. Superficial cervical nodes in neck, along sternocleidomastoid muscle; lymph from head and neck drains through these nodes
   3. Superficial cubital nodes at bend of elbow; lymph from hand and forearm drains through these nodes
   4. Axillary nodes in armpit; lymph from arm and upper part of the chest wall, including the breast, drains through these nodes (may be removed during mastectomy for carcinoma)
   5. Inguinal nodes in groin; lymph from the leg and external genitals drains through these nodes
C. Functions
   1. Help defend the body against injurious substances (notably, bacteria and tumor cells) by filtering them out of lymph and thereby preventing their entrance into bloodstream; leukocytes in lymph nodes destroy many of these substances by phagocytosis and antibody action
   2. Lymphatic tissue of lymph nodes carries on the process of hemopoiesis; specifically, it forms T and B lymphocytes

Lymph

A. Definition—fluid in lymphatics
B. Source—interstitial fluid that has entered the lymphatic capillaries
   1. Interstitial fluid is the fluid in the microscopic tissue spaces
   2. Interstitial fluid is formed by plasma filtering out of the blood capillaries into the tissue spaces

Spleen

A. Location—left hypochondrium, above and behind cardiac portion of the stomach
B. Structure—lymphatic tissue, similar to lymph nodes; size varies, contains numerous spaces filled with venous blood
C. Functions

1. Defense—phagocytosis of particles such as microbes, red cell fragments, and platelets by reticuloendothelial cells of spleen (reticuloendothelial system—phagocytic cells, located mainly in the liver, spleen, bone marrow, and lymph nodes; also, macrophages of connective tissue and microglia in the brain and cord); antibody formation by plasma cells of spleen
2. Hemopoiesis—lymphatic tissue of the spleen, like that of the lymph nodes, forms lymphocytes and possibly monocytes
3. Spleen serves as blood reservoir; sympathetic stimulation causes constriction of its capsule, squeezing out an estimated 200 ml of blood into general circulation within 1 minute

REVIEW OF PHYSICAL PRINCIPLES RELATED TO THE CIRCULATORY SYSTEM
Principles of Mechanics
Newton's Laws of Motion

A. First law: A body remains at rest or in uniform motion in a straight line unless forces act on it to make it change its state of rest or uniform motion; in other words, bodies continue to do whatever they are doing unless some force acts on them
   EXAMPLE: The heart produces the force that propels the blood through the vessels; without such a force the blood would not flow
B. Second law: If a body is accelerated, the greater the force applied to it, the greater the acceleration; the greater the mass of the body, the more force needed to produce a desired acceleration
   EXAMPLE: In polycythemia the greater cell mass of each unit volume of blood requires greater force of cardiac contraction to produce a desired rate of blood flow
C. Third law: For every action there is an equal and opposite reaction
   EXAMPLE: As blood flows through an artery, it exerts an action force on the walls of the artery; the walls of the artery exert a reaction force on the blood, which helps to provide the pressure to keep the blood flowing

Law of Gravitation

Any 2 objects in the universe are attracted to each other with a force equal to the product of the masses of the 2 objects divided by the square of the distance between them (e.g., the greater the mass of the bodies, the greater the gravitational force; the closer they are together, the greater the gravitational force)
EXAMPLE: When a person is standing, blood tends to pool in the lower extremities, resulting in bulging of veins in lower parts of the body and requiring greater

pumping force from the heart to overcome such pooling; orthostatic hypotension and recovery by the baroreceptor reflex are a direct result of gravitational forces; the evolutionary development of valves in the venous system (particularly in the legs) is due to gravitational forces

Momentum

A. Basic concept—an object's momentum is dependent on its mass and the velocity at which it is moving

EXAMPLE: A 112.5 kg (250 lb) person in a heavy motorized wheelchair moving down a corridor at 3 mph (4.8 kph) has greater momentum than a 45 kg (100 lb) person in a light wheelchair rolling along at 5 mph (8 kph)

B. Changes in momentum—an object's momentum can be changed by applying a force to the object for a certain length of time; the greater the force applied and/or the longer the time that the force is applied, the greater is the change in momentum of the object

EXAMPLE: During exercise, the contracting heart imparts great momentum to the blood because the force of contraction of the myocardium is great, and the duration of contraction of the myocardium is relatively long

Energy

A. Basic concept—a property that enables a body to perform work

EXAMPLE: The heart possesses energy because it is capable of doing the work of circulating the blood

B. Work—the product of the force exerted and the distance through which the force moves

EXAMPLE: The heart exerts a force that moves the blood a certain distance

C. Laws concerning energy
1. First law of thermodynamics (law of conservation of energy)—energy cannot be created or destroyed but may be transformed from one form into another

EXAMPLE: The potential energy of the ATP molecule is transformed into the kinetic energy of cardiac muscle contraction during the cardiac cycle

2. Second law of thermodynamics—all systems in the universe have a natural tendency to become disorderly or randomized; the energy of the system continually becomes more spread out and dilute

a. Molecules tend to move from areas where they are in high concentration to areas where they are in low concentration; this is usually stated as the law of diffusion

EXAMPLES
(1) The diffusion of oxygen and carbon dioxide between the air sacs and capillaries of the lungs
(2) The diffusion of water through the membrane systems of cells (osmosis)

b. Heat always flows from a hot body into a colder one

EXAMPLES
(1) Some of the chemical energy stored in muscles is transformed into heat when muscles contract; this heat flows from the hot body (the muscles) into cooler bodies (the surrounding tissues, including blood) and helps to maintain the human body temperature of 37° C (98.6° F)
(2) When the human body is too hot, vasodilation occurs in the skin and heat radiates from the body into the cooler surrounding air

Efficiency

Efficiency—never total, since friction that occurs when two surfaces rub together produces resistance and heat; the greater the efficiency, the less heat produced; friction causes mechanical devices eventually to be worn away

EXAMPLE: If friction did not operate, the human heart would only have to beat once in a lifetime, since the initial force would propel the blood indefinitely through the blood vessels; friction continuously slows blood flow, and consequently the adult heart beats an average of 72 times each minute

Principles of Physical Properties of Matter

Solids

Concept of elasticity—because of external or internal stresses, solids may change their shape or size

EXAMPLE: Heart and blood vessels constantly change shape as blood pressure and degree of neural stimulation undergo change

Liquids

A. Hydrostatic pressure—force per unit area caused by the weight of the fluid on matter submerged in the fluid

EXAMPLE: The weight of blood in a capillary exerts a hydrostatic force that helps to filter the blood through the capillary wall, forming interstitial fluid

B. Pascal's principle—when pressure is applied to a fluid in a closed, nonflexible container, it is transmitted undiminished throughout all parts of the fluid and acts in all directions

EXAMPLES: In the circulatory system the pressure exerted as a result of the contracting ventricles is transmitted throughout the blood vessels of the circulatory system; this pressure is responsible for blood flow

1. Pressure—fluid always flows from regions of higher pressure to those of lower pressure; the pressure in the human circulatory system is highest in the ventricles during systole, decreases throughout the length of the circulatory system, and is lowest in the atria; the normal pressure of blood in the circulatory system varies with age and disease
2. Lumen of the tube—the flow of fluid through a tube is directly proportional to the radius of the tube; e.g., the degree of constriction of the arterioles for the most part determines the quantity of blood entering the capillary beds and returning to the heart
3. Length of the tube—the longer the tube, the less fluid flow there is through it in a unit of time; when blood circulation to the skin is greatly increased, the heart must increase its output to maintain normal circulation, since many more miles of tubing (capillaries) have been added to the system
4. Viscosity—the molecular components of a fluid exert forces of attraction on each other; as the fluid flows along, an internal friction, caused by the molecular attractions of the fluid's components, tends to impede it; this internal resistance to fluid flow is viscosity
   a. Anemia—because of a reduced number of erythrocytes, the viscosity of the blood is decreased; therefore blood returns to the heart more rapidly, increasing cardiac output, which may overwork the heart during periods of increased exercise
   b. Polycythemia—an increased number of erythrocytes in the blood increases its viscosity; blood flows more sluggishly and the blood pressure increases to compensate
C. Capillarity—when a small-diameter tube is dipped into water or other fluid, the water will rise in the tube because of adhesion of the water molecules to the components of the glass; surface tension then causes the film of water to contract and pull itself up the tube; the water continues to rise until its weight balances the adhesive force; this rise of the fluid level in a tube is called capillarity or capillary action
   EXAMPLE: Capillarity draws blood into a capillary tube when a technician takes a small blood sample for various analyses

Gases

Gases are carried in the circulatory system by combining with other molecules

Principles of Acoustics

Basic concept—sound is a mechanical vibration that cannot occur in a vacuum; it is propagated best through solids and through liquids better than gases; it travels in waves from a vibrating source such as human vocal cords, a loudspeaker, or a dropped object

EXAMPLES

1. A very faint heartbeat can be heard only with a stethoscope or by placing the ear on the chest; even strong heartbeats cannot be heard distinctly with just the ears
2. The sound vibrations (waves) pass readily through the tissue of the human body to the surface of the skin where the stethoscope can pick them up
3. Ultrasonic fetal heart monitors can detect the fetal heart beat as early as the twelfth week of gestation
4. Echocardiography—a sound wave–constructed picture of the heart helps in the identification of cardiac diseases

Principles of Electricity

Electric Force

A. The atoms composing all matter represent an almost perfect balance of protons and electrons; the attraction of a positive proton for a negative electron (opposite charges attracting) is the electric force that also makes like charges repel each other
B. Electric forces hold atoms and molecules together and thus hold solid matter together; electric forces also provide the source for all chemical energy; the molecular rearrangements associated with cellular metabolism derive their energy from electric forces between enzymes, substrates, and cofactors

Conductors and Insulators

A. Conductors are good transferrers of electric fields and the energy they contain; copper and aluminum are good conductors and are commonly used for all electric wiring, including the electrodes for cardiac monitoring
B. Insulators—rubber and most nonmetals are good insulators, as is the connective tissue separating the atria and ventricles of the heart and electrically insulating these regions; consequently the only way electrical energy can flow from the AV node to the ventricles is through the heart's specialized conducting system (bundle of His) in the interventricular septum
C. Water as a conductor—distilled water is a poor conductor, although tap water contains enough charged

particles (ions) to make it a fairly good electric conductor; the ions (electrolytes) of body fluids make them excellent conductors of electrical energy

Application of Electricity
A. Electronic devices used in health care
1. Electronic cardiac pacemakers—battery-operated devices supplement or replace defective electric stimulation in the human heart and thus help maintain the individual's heartbeat at a selected rate
2. Defibrillator—electronic device that delivers electrical energy through electrodes strategically placed on an individual whose heart is in atrial or ventricular fibrillation; the use of such a device is based on the premise that the sustaining mechanism of the fibrillation process is different from the initiating mechanism; thus, if the initiating mechanism is no longer present and the sustaining mechanism is terminated by the defibrillating electric current, sinus rhythm will ensue
B. Applications to the human body—the contraction of all types of muscle is preceded by depolarization of the muscle fibers; ions carry the electric charges
   EXAMPLE: Electrocardiograms measure and record the electric activity of the heart as this activity is carried to the surface of the body by the ions of the body fluids; this information provides an electric picture of the heart's activity

Principles of Light (Electromagnetic Waves)

Basic concept—emission of high-frequency electromagnetic waves due to excitation of the innermost orbital electrons of atoms; to excite the innermost orbital electron, considerable energy must be expended
EXAMPLE: Angiography—observation of motion picture x-ray images

REVIEW OF CHEMICAL PRINCIPLES RELATED TO THE CIRCULATORY SYSTEM
Water
General Information
A. Chemical combination of oxygen and hydrogen
B. Most abundant compound
C. Essential to life
D. Sixty percent of the average adult human body weight is water; percentage may be as high as 80% in infants and as low as 40% to 50% in the elderly
Physical Properties
A. Colorless, tasteless, odorless liquid
B. Exists chiefly as ice at low temperatures, liquid at moderate temperatures, and gas at elevated temperatures

1. Water changes from liquid to solid at the freezing point (0° C [32° F])
2. Water changes from liquid to gas at the boiling point (100° C [212° F])
3. These transition points in the physical states of water are the basis of the Celsius and Fahrenheit temperature scales
4. Conversion from one temperature scale to the other is accomplished by using the formula

$$°C = \frac{5}{9} (°F - 32)$$

Chemical Properties
A. Water molecule a dipolar structure; because of this molecular shape, it is an excellent solvent for ionic or slightly ionic substances
B. Water a stable compound; it dissociates very slightly to H^+ and OH^- under normal conditions
C. Electrolysis can dissociate water into its components, hydrogen and oxygen
D. Many chemical reactions need water as a solvent before they can occur
E. Process of splitting a substance with the addition of water called hydrolysis, which is the basis for the digestion of food
F. Crystals formed with water in their molecule are called hydrates
Importance
A. Necessary for life; universal solvent
B. Essential for many chemical reactions
C. Needed for digestion (hydrolysis) of food
D. Forms large percentage of plant and animal tissue
E. Necessary for circulation of blood; plasma is a water solution
F. Necessary for elimination; urine, sweat, feces contain water
G. Lubricating fluid at joints (synovial fluid) contains water
H. Water has a great capacity for absorbing heat or giving off absorbed heat; useful in ice packs, hydrotherapy, and hot compresses
Water as a Standard
A. Thermometer scales—the freezing and boiling points of water are used to standardize Celsius and Fahrenheit scales
B. Specific gravity—compares the density of a volume of water to the density of the same volume of another substance
C. Weight—1 g is the weight of 1 ml of water at 4° C
D. Calorie—the heat needed to raise 1 g of water 1° C
E. pH—water acts as neutrality point on acid-base scale

Body Regulation of Water Content

A. The osmoreceptors of the hypothalamus influence the neurohypophysis in its release of ADH (antidiuretic hormone or vasopressin); working through the kidney tubules, this hormone regulates water reabsorption from urine

B. The thirst center of the hypothalamus detects body dehydration and produces the sensation of thirst

Proteins

A. Polymers of alpha amino acids connected by peptide bonds

B. Characteristics of proteins
1. Protein molecules are very large
2. Proteins form colloid particles in solution
3. Synthesis of proteins occurs in ribosomes of cell according to specific genetic patterns under direction of the nucleic acids DNA and RNA
4. Structure patterns of proteins are extremely specific; proteins differ from species to species, individual to individual, and organ to organ; this presents a problem in transplant operations
5. Proteins are the tissue builders of the body

C. Classification of proteins
1. Simple proteins—give amino acids on hydrolysis
   a. Albumins—water soluble, coagulated by heat (lactalbumin [milk], serum albumin [blood], egg white); albumin is most important in the development of the plasma colloid osmotic pressure, which helps control (through osmosis) the flow of water between the plasma and interstitial fluid; during a condition such as starvation, a fall in the albumin level of the blood results in a fall in the plasma colloid osmotic pressure; this leads to edema because less fluid is being drawn by osmosis into the capillaries from the interstitial spaces
   b. Globulins—insoluble in water, soluble in dilute salt solutions, coagulated by heat (e.g., lactoglobulin [milk], serum globulin [blood], gamma serum globulin [forms antibodies of blood])

Enzymes

A. Organic catalysts that enter into reactions and are reformed at end of reaction

B. Needed in minute amounts

C. Protein in nature and inactivated by all factors that denature proteins (e.g., high temperature, changes in pH)

D. Substrate is the substance acted on by an enzyme; e.g., carbon dioxide and water are the substrate for the enzyme carbonic anhydrase, found in the erythrocyte, which catalyzes the conversion of CO_2 and H_2O into carbonic acid

E. Enzymes usually have ending "ase" added on to name of substrate or to action of enzyme (e.g., sucrase—enzyme hydrolyzing sucrose; lactic acid dehydrogenase—enzyme removing hydrogen from lactic acid)

F. Enzymes, being proteins, are usually quite specific in action
1. One enzyme will usually catalyze only 1 reaction—substrate specificity
2. Enzyme activity will be high at temperature specific for the enzyme and low at other temperatures—temperature specificity
3. Enzyme activity will be high at the pH specific for the enzyme and low at the other pH values—pH specificity

G. Certain inorganic ions act to speed up or slow down enzyme activity—enzyme activators and enzyme inhibitors

H. Enzymes acting within cells are called intracellular enzymes; e.g., the enzymes that bring about the breakdown of glucose and other sugars and the synthesis of carbohydrates, proteins, and nucleic acids all function within cells and are intracellular enzymes

I. Enzymes acting outside cells are called extracellular enzymes; e.g., the digestive enzymes that are found in the mouth, stomach, and small intestine all function outside cells and are extracellular enzymes

J. Some enzymes exist in 2 parts
1. Apoenzyme—protein part of enzyme (inactive)
2. Coenzyme—nonprotein part of enzyme (inactive)
3. Holoenzyme—the apoenzyme and the coenzyme together (active molecule)

Solutions

Basic Concepts

A. Substances that dissolve in other substances form solutions

B. A solution can be classified as a homogeneous mixture

C. Solids, liquids, and gases can be dissolved in other solids, liquids, and gases
1. Substance dissolved is called the solute
2. Substance in which the solute is dissolved is called the solvent
3. Common solution is one in which a solid, liquid, or gas is dissolved in a liquid; e.g., blood is mainly a liquid (water) containing dissolved ions, sugars, amino acids, and respiratory gases

Factors Affecting Solubility
A. Chemical and physical nature of the solvent
B. Chemical and physical nature of the solute
C. Amount of solvent versus amount of solute
D. Temperature—warming aids some solutes (solids) to dissolve; cooling aids others (gases) to dissolve
E. Presence or absence of mixing; mixing usually speeds solution reaction
F. Pressure—especially when one of the components is a gas

Types of Solutions
A. Dilute—small amount of solute in a relatively large amount of solvent
B. Concentrated—large amount of solute in a relatively small amount of solvent
C. Unsaturated—holding less solute than is possible for it to dissolve at a certain temperature and pressure
D. Saturated—holding all the solute it can dissolve at a certain temperature and pressure
E. Supersaturated—unique case of a solution holding more solute than it normally should for a particular temperature and pressure
  1. Very unstable condition
  2. Excess solute easily precipitates from solution
F. Percent solution—grams of solute per gram of solution
G. Molar solution (M)—number of gram-molecular weights of solute per liter of solution
H. Normal solution (N)—number of gram-equivalent weights of solute per liter of solution
I. Molal solution—gram-molecular weight of solute in 1000 g of solvent

Osmosis
A. Process of selective diffusion
B. More concentrated solution is separated from a less concentrated solution by a membrane that is permeable only to the solvent—a semipermeable membrane
C. Solvent moves more rapidly from the dilute solution into the concentrated solution than in the reverse direction
D. Pressure forcing the solvent aross the membrane is called osmotic pressure
E. Isotonic solutions—when the osmotic pressures of 2 liquids are equal, the flow of solvent is equalized and the 2 solutions are said to be isotonic to each other
  1. Physiologic saline—0.89% NaCl in distilled water—is isotonic to blood and body tissues
  2. Five percent dextrose in water is isotonic to blood and body tissues
  3. When isotonic solutions are administered intravenously, the blood cells remain intact

F. Hypertonic solutions—when one solution has less osmotic pressure (is more concentrated) than another, it draws fluid from the other and is said to be hypertonic to it
G. Hypotonic solutions—when one solution has more osmotic pressure (is more dilute) than another, it forces fluid into the other and is said to be hypotonic to it
H. Both hypertonic and hypotonic types of solution are destructive to body cells and should not be used in intravenous injections
I. Osmosis constantly occurs as part of the normal physiology of human beings
  1. Capillary membrane—the colloid osmotic pressure of the plasma draws fluid from the tissue spaces back into the capillaries; edema results when disease states upset the normal colloid osmotic pressure (e.g., starvation, kidney disease)
  2. Plasma membranes—water freely flows from interstitial fluid into intracellular fluid and vice versa, depending on the relative concentration of water in these 2 fluid compartments

Size of the Particle of Solute Determines the Type of Solution
A. Atomic, ionic, and most molecular-sized particles are extremely small—submicroscopic
  1. Particles are freely dispersed by solvent
  2. Particles are kept in solution by movement and attraction of solvent molecules
  3. Substances of this class are called crystalloids
  4. Crystalloids form true solutions
    a. Clear in appearance—particles cannot be seen
    b. Solute stays in solution as long as the solvent is not removed by evaporation or other means
    c. Solute accompanies solvent as it passes through filters and most membranes; e.g, the ions Na^+, K^+, Cl^-, HCO_3^- dissolved in plasma are in true solution
B. Large particles of matter do not form solutions in the real sense of the term
  1. Solute particles easily settle out of solvent
  2. Solute particles can be seen by naked eye or with microscope when suspended in solvent
  3. Solute can be removed by ordinary filtration
  4. Substances of this class are called coarse suspensions; e.g., the erythrocytes are suspended in plasma and can be seen microscopically and removed by fine filters or centrifugation
C. The colloid particle
  1. Intermediate in size between the crystalloid and the coarse suspensoid
  2. Particle much larger than the crystalloid particle

although smaller than particle of coarse suspensoid; diameter of colloid around 0.0000001 to 0.00001 mm

3. Solutions of colloids
   a. Solute particles dispersed by solvent
   b. Solution—clear, cloudy, or opalescent
   c. Show bright path of reflected light passed through the solution—Tyndall effect
   d. More stable than coarse suspensoids, less stable than true solutions
   e. With time, colloid particles will settle out
   f. Affect osmotic pressure less than do crystalloids
   g. Most of the proteins in plasma are dispersed as colloid particles
   h. Blood is classified as a colloid and a suspension
4. Colloid particles will pass through ordinary filters but will be held back by most membranes
5. Colloid particles carry electric charges on their surfaces—not to be confused with ionic charges
6. Importance of colloid suspensions
   a. Proteins, fats, and many carbohydrates form molecules in the colloid size range
   b. These form colloid solutions in the cells and body fluids
   c. Protoplasm of cell itself is a colloid

Buffers

A. A poorly ionized acid or base, plus a salt formed from that acid or base, acts as a buffer in solution; e.g., a typical buffer of the blood is carbonic acid (H_2CO_3) plus its salt, sodium bicarbonate (Na-HCO_3)
B. A buffer allows the addition of acid ions (H_3O^+) and basic ions (OH^-) without a change occurring in the pH of the solution to which the addition is made
C. The body regulates its pH through buffer systems; during normal metabolism, it builds up CO_2, which forms carbonic acid with water; the subsequent ionization of carbonic acid would tend to lower the body fluid pH; but through increased rate and depth of breathing, the excess CO_2 is expelled from the body; thus the circulatory and respiratory systems interact with buffer systems to help regulate the body's pH
D. Blood buffers
   1. Proteins, amino acids, bicarbonates, and phosphates all act to prevent changes in the pH of blood
   2. Blood buffers are necessary to prevent changes in the pH of blood that are incompatible with life

Radioactive Elements

A. Certain elements (e.g., radium) have atoms whose nuclei are naturally unstable and are constantly breaking down at a set rate
B. In the breakdown process these elements emit high-energy particles and rays that can penetrate other materials—radioactive rays
   1. Alpha particle—fast-moving helium nucleus
      a. Weight—4 atomic weight units (awu)
      b. Charge—2^+
      c. Penetration—slight
   2. Beta particle—fast-moving electron
      a. Weight—practically 0 awu
      b. Charge—1^-
      c. Penetration—moderate
   3. Gamma ray—penetrating ray, similar to light ray
      a. Weight—none
      b. Charge—none
      c. Penetration—high
C. Uses of radioactivity
   1. Leukemia, polycythemia, and bone cancer treatments with radioactive phosphorus (^{32}P); radiophosphorus has also been useful in localizing breast tumors because of the uptake of the ^{32}P into the rapidly growing, cancerous tissue
   2. Studies on red cells (erythrocytes) and hemoglobin formation with radioactive iron (^{59}Fe) and radioactive chromium (^{51}Cr)

REVIEW OF MICROBIOLOGIC PRINCIPLES RELATED TO THE CIRCULATORY SYSTEM
Major Pathogens

A. *Streptococcus pyogenes*—gram-positive streptococcus; the most virulent strain (Group A beta hemolytic) causes scarlet fever, septic sore throat, tonsillitis, cellulitis, puerperal fever, erysipelas, rheumatic fever, and glomerulonephritis
B. *Streptococcus viridans*—gram-positive streptococcus; distinguishable from *S. pyogenes* by its alpha hemolysis (rather than beta) of red cells; the most common cause of subacute bacterial endocarditis

Resistance

A. Nonspecific resistance—that directed against all invading microbes; varies considerably from one species to another and even among individuals of same species
   1. Body surface barriers
      a. Intact skin and mucosa
      b. Cilia and secretion of mucus
   2. Antimicrobial secretions
      a. Oil of skin—contains fatty acids effective against many bacteria and fungi

b. Tears—contain lysozyme, a bactericidal (gram-positive) enzyme

c. Gastric juice—contains highly bactericidal hydrochloric acid

d. Vaginal secretions—low pH acts to inhibit microbial growth

3. Internal antimicrobial agents

a. Interferon—antiviral substance produced within the cells in response to a viral attack; it inhibits viral growth and multiplication

b. Properdin—protein agent in blood that destroys certain gram-negative bacteria and viruses

c. Lysozyme—ubiquitous; destroys mainly gram-positive bacteria

4. Phagocytosis—part of the role of the reticuloendothelial system

a. Phagocytes—cells in the blood that ingest and destroy microbes

(1) Microphages—polymorphonuclear leukocytes, of which the neutrophils are the most active; in the inflammatory response they pass through the intact capillary wall (diapedesis) into the intercellular area

(2) Macrophages

(a) Fixed (sessile) macrophages—phagocytes lining the capillary endothelium and sinuses of the liver (Kupffer cells), spleen, bone marrow, lymph nodes, and other organs where they remove microbes from the blood

(b) Wandering macrophages (histiocytes)—blood monocytes that enter the tissues (via diapedesis) and devour intercellular debris, including debilitated microphages

B. Specific resistance—that directed against a specific pathogen (foreign protein) or its toxin

1. Antigen—any substance, including allergens, that stimulates the production of antibodies when introduced into the body; typically, antigens are foreign proteins, the most potent being microbial cells and their products

a. Plasma cells—antibody-producing cells that arise from B lymphocytes in the presence of antigens; a specific antigen provokes the production of a specific antibody (homologous antibody), which is considered to be ineffective against any other antigen

b. Memory cells—large population of antibodies that develop on first encounter with an antigen; they become somewhat dormant un-

til stimulated by subsequent encounters with the antigen; this phenomenon explains the dramatic rise in antibody titer following a booster shot of a vaccine (anamnestic reaction)

2. Antibody—immune substance produced by plasma cells; antibodies are gamma globulin molecules and are commonly referred to as immunoglobulin (Ig)

a. Chemical structure—made up of 4 polypeptide chains in 2 pairs

b. Classification—there are 5 major classes of antibodies

(1) Immunoglobulin G (IgG) antibodies—most important class, making up more than 80% of the total immunoglobulins; only immunoglobulin that passes the placental barrier, providing natural passive immunity to the newborn

(2) Immunoglobulin A (IgA) antibodies—present in blood, mucus, and human milk secretions; play an important role against respiratory pathogens

(3) Immunoglobulin M (IgM) antibodies—first antibodies to be detected after an injection of antigen; bactericidal for gram-negative bacteria under specific conditions

(4) Immunoglobulin D (IgD) antibodies—present in small numbers in normal individuals; specific immunologic role presently under investigation

(5) Immunoglobulin E (IgE) antibodies—responsible for hypersensitivity and allergies; these antibodies exist tightly bound to the surface of mast cells (large basophilic connective tissue cells)

(a) Upon introduction of their homologous antigens (allergens), they cause the mast cells to release histamine and other pharmacologic agents

(b) Release of histamine and other pharmacologic agents causes the symptoms of hypersensitivity reactions

(c) This process explains the relief of symptoms by the administration of antihistamines

3. Antigen-antibody reactions

a. Agglutination—clumping together of cells and specific antigens by homologous antibodies called agglutinins

b. Cytolysis—disruption or dissolution of cells (lysis) by homologous antibodies called cytolysins or lysins

c. Opsonification—rendering of bacteria and other cells susceptible to phagocytosis by homologous antibodies called opsonins

d. Neutralization (viral)—rendering of viruses noninfective by homologous antibodies called neutralizing antibodies

e. Neutralization (toxin)—chemical neutralization of a toxin by homologous antibodies called antitoxins

f. Precipitation—formation of an insoluble complex (precipitate) in the reaction between a soluble antigen and its homologous antibodies called precipitins

4. Complement-fixation—group of blood serum proteins needed in certain antigen-antibody reactions; both the complement and the antibody must be present for a reaction to occur

Immunity

A. Species immunity—certain species are naturally immune to specific microorganisms; e.g., humans are immune to distemper, dogs are immune to measles

B. Active immunity—antibodies formed in the body
1. Natural active immunity—antibodies formed by the individual during the course of the disease; in some instances the antibodies provide lifelong immunity (e.g., measles, chickenpox, yellow fever, smallpox)
2. Artificial active immunity—use of a vaccine or toxoid to stimulate the formation of homologous antibodies; revaccination (booster shots) is often needed to sustain antibody titer (anamnestic effect)
   a. Killed vaccines—antigenic preparations containing microbes grown in the laboratory separated from growth medium and killed by heat or a chemical agent; usually injected subcutaneously; less often given by intramuscular or oral routes (e.g., pertussis vaccine, typhoid vaccine)
   b. Live vaccines—antigenic preparations containing microbes weakened (attenuated) by drying, continued and prolonged passage through culture media or animals (to induce mutations), or by other means; typically such vaccines are more antigenic than killed preparations; (e.g., oral [Sabin] poliomyelitis vaccine, measles vaccine)
   c. Toxoids—antigenic preparations composed of inactivated bacterial toxins (generally an exotoxin treated with formaldehyde) (e.g., tetanus toxoids, diphtheria toxoids)

C. Passive immunity—antibodies acquired from an outside source
1. Natural passive immunity—passage of preformed antibodies from the mother through the placenta or colostrum to the baby; therefore during the first few weeks of life the newborn is immune to certain diseases to which the mother has active immunity
2. Artificial passive immunity—injection of antisera derived from immunized animals or humans; antisera (antiserums) provide immediate and often complete protection in susceptible exposed persons and also are of value in treatment (e.g., diphtheria antitoxin, tetanus antitoxin); individuals may be hypersensitive to certain sera such as horse serum, and pretesting for hypersensitivity must be carried out before administration

PHARMACOLOGY RELATED TO CIRCULATORY SYSTEM DISORDERS

A. Cardiac glycosides
1. General implications for nurses
   a. Check apical pulse for 1 minute before administration; if pulse is below 60 or above 120 beats per minute, the dose should be withheld and the physician notified
   b. Observe for signs of digitalis toxicity, which include nausea and vomiting, visual disturbances, bigeminal rhythm, and muscle weakness
   c. Increase potassium in diet because digitalis toxicity is more common if the patient is hypokalemic
   d. Inform the patient regarding the above factors
   e. Observe the patient for adverse effects
      (1) Most frequent—nausea, vomiting, headache, drowsiness, insomnia, vertigo, confusion are all attributable to drug action at central nervous system sites; oral forms also cause nausea and vomiting by irritation of gastric mucosa
      (2) Bradycardia attributable to drug-induced slowing of the sinoatrial (SA) node firing; arrhythmias are first evidence of toxicity in one third of patients; premature nodal or ventricular impulses are varying degrees of heart block caused by drug action that slows transmission of impulses through the atrioventricular (AV) node

(3) Xanthopsia (yellow vision) caused by drug effect on visual cones

(4) Gynecomastia (mammary enlargement) in males resulting from estrogen-like steroid portion of digitalis glycosides

2. Action

  a. Positive inotropic effect (increased force of contraction) achieved by increasing permeability of muscle membranes to the calcium and sodium ions required for contraction of muscle fibrils

  b. Negative chronotropic effect (decreased rate of contraction) achieved by an action mediated through the vagus nerve (X); slows firing of the SA node and impulse transmission by the AV node

3. Examples of drugs

  a. Digitalis

  b. Digitoxin (Crystodigin, Digitaline)

  c. Digoxin (Lanoxin)

  d. Gitalin (Gitaligin)

  e. Lanatoside C (Cedilanid)

  f. Ouabain

4. Digitalization

  a. Provides an initial loading dose for acute effect on the heart

  b. After desired effect is achieved, the dosage is lowered to maintenance level, replacing drug metabolized and excreted each day

B. Antiarrhythmic drugs

1. General implications for nurses

  a. Observe for variations in cardiac rhythm

  b. If medication given intravenously, maintain the patient on a monitor

  c. Observe for specific adverse effects of each drug

  d. Inform the patient regarding drug action, specific side effects, and the need for continued medical supervision

2. Quinidine preparations

  a. Actions

    (1) Control atrial arrhythmias by prolonging the effective refractory period and slowing depolarization

    (2) Have a mild depressant effect on the hepatic enzyme system, which synthesizes coagulation factors; therefore concomitant use with oral anticoagulants may cause excessive hypoprothrombinemia with bleeding

    (3) Have anticholinergic properties; thus excessive cholinergic blocking (dryness of mouth, constipation) may result with concomitant use of belladonna alkaloids or other drugs possessing anticholinergic properties (phenothiazines, antihistamines, tricyclic antidepressants, procainamide hydrochloride)

  b. Examples

    (1) Quinidine gluconate (Quinaglute)

    (2) Quinidine hydrochloride

    (3) Quinidine polygalacturonate (Cardiaquin)

    (4) Quinidine sulfate (Quinidex, Quinora)

  c. Adverse effects

    (1) Heart block caused by drug depression of AV node and ventricular conduction tissue

    (2) Accelerated AV conduction or ventricular tachycardia occurring with initial dose is caused by vagolytic action (may be lessened by digitalis administration)

    (3) Vasodilation with syncope and hypotension caused by depressant effect on all muscle tissue may occur with high dosage or IV use

    (4) Gastric irritation with nausea, vomiting, and diarrhea may occur with oral use

3. Lidocaine hydrochloride

  a. Action—controls ventricular irritability by shortening the refractory period and suppresses ectopic foci

  b. Adverse effects

    (1) Drowsiness

    (2) Nervousness

    (3) Blurred vision

    (4) Nausea

    (5) Tremors

    (6) Hypotension

    (7) Generalized paresthesias

    (8) Convulsions

    (9) Respiratory arrest

4. Procainamide hydrochloride (Pronestyl)

  a. Actions

    (1) Controls ventricular and atrial arrhythmias by prolonging the refractory period of the heart and slowing the conduction of cardiac impulses

    (2) Has some anticholinergic effects

  b. Adverse effects

    (1) Hypotension

    (2) Bradycardia

    (3) Decreased motility of the gastrointestinal tract (paralytic ileus)

5. Phenytoin (Dilantin)
   a. Action—controls atrial or ventricular arrhythmias by reducing automaticity without decreasing conduction
   b. Adverse effects
      (1) Lack of coordination
      (2) Dizziness
      (3) Nausea
      (4) Vomiting
      (5) Nystagmus
      (6) Megaloblastic anemia
      (7) High alkalinity requires infusion in large veins at a maximum rate of 50 mg/min
6. Disopyramide phosphate (Norpace)
   a. Actions
      (1) Exerts antiarrhythmic effect by decreasing the rate of diastolic depolarization
      (2) Primarily used to treat ventricular arrhythmias
   b. Adverse effects
      (1) Contraindicated in the presence of cardiogenic shock or heart block
      (2) Urinary retention
      (3) Constipation
      (4) Dry mouth
      (5) Hypotension
      (6) Diarrhea
      (7) Nausea
7. Propranolol hydrochloride (Inderal)
   a. Actions
      (1) Used effectively in the treatment of supraventricular arrhythmias and is currently used for therapy of angina pectoris and hypertension
      (2) Has a negative inotropic effect by depressing cardiac response to sympathetic nervous system stimuli via blocking action at beta receptors
         (a) Some vasodilation of coronary arteries occurs
         (b) Reduces inotropic and chronotropic effects of exercise; the patient may be light-headed, weak, and fatigued after exercise
   b. Adverse effects
      (1) Bradycardia
      (2) Cardiac arrest
      (3) AV block
      (4) Nausea, vomiting, and diarrhea
      (5) Visual disturbances and hallucinations
C. Drugs that increase the heart rate
   1. General implications for nurses
      a. Monitor vital signs frequently

b. Awareness of drug effect on preexisting conditions
   c. Observe for adverse effects, such as tachycardia and those specific to each drug
2. Atropine sulfate
   a. Actions
      (1) Suppresses parasympathetic nervous system control at SA and AV nodes
      (2) Administer IV by bolus to increase the heart rate in severe bradycardia
   b. Adverse effects
      (1) Decreased bladder emptying
      (2) Decreased glandular secretions
      (3) Depression of gastrointestinal motility
3. Isoproterenol hydrochloride (Isuprel)
   a. Actions
      (1) Stimulates beta-adrenergic receptors of sympathetic nervous system, thereby also improving tissue perfusion
      (2) Used in cardiogenic shock and Adams-Stokes and carotid sinus syndromes
   b. Adverse effects
      (1) Hypotension
      (2) Tachycardia and palpitation
      (3) Flushing of skin
      (4) Headache
      (5) Anxiety and restlessness
4. Epinephrine hydrochloride
   a. Actions
      (1) Via the sympathetic nervous system, stimulates the rate and force of cardiac contraction; used in cardiogenic shock and heart block
      (2) Reduces blood flow to the abdominal viscera
      (3) Bronchodilation
   b. Examples
      (1) Adrenaline
      (2) Vaponefrin
   c. Adverse effects
      (1) Palpitation, cardiac arrhythmias
      (2) Throbbing headache
      (3) Urinary retention
D. Drugs that dilate the coronary arteries—nitrates
   1. General implications for nurses
      a. Instruct the patient to take sublingual medication only when sitting or lying down because of postural hypotension
      b. Instruct the patient to store medication correctly
      c. Observe for adverse effects
         (1) Facial blushing
         (2) Hypotension, which may be sudden if drug is taken with alcohol

      (3) Vertigo, fainting

      (4) Headache

  2. Actions

    a. Decrease the resistance of the smooth muscle of large-capacity vessels (veins, venules) and high-resistance vessels; this decreases cardiac work and myocardial oxygen requirements

    b. Decrease the incidence of anginal attacks and improve work tolerance

    c. Decrease the central venous pressure (CVP), left ventricle end-diastolic pressure, and pulmonary wedge pressure; this lowers blood pressure, causing a reflexive increase in heart rate

    d. Increase blood flow through the coronary arteries and collateral channels with increased blood flow to ischemic areas of the heart

  3. Examples

    a. Nitrates for sublingual use

      (1) Erythrityl tetranitrate (Cardilate)

      (2) Isosorbide dinitrate (Isordil, Sorbitrate)

      (3) Nitroglycerin

        (a) Effect in 1 to 2 minutes; repeat dose in 5 minutes if pain persists

        (b) When taken 3 minutes before activity known to cause anginal pain, pain-free exercise tolerance increases

        (c) Tablets deteriorate rapidly in heat, light, moisture (potency loss by sublimation)

        (d) Sublingual use causes slight stinging, burning, tingling under the tongue; absence of these signs can indicate deterioration of the drug

    b. Nitrates for oral use

      (1) Erythrityl tetranitrate (Cardilate)

      (2) Mannitol hexanitrate (Nitranitol)

      (3) Pentaerythritol tetranitrate (Peritrate)

      (4) Trolnitrate phosphate (Metamine)

      (5) Isosorbide dinitrate (Sorbitrate, Iso-Bid, Isordil)

    c. Nitrates for topical use

      (1) Nitro-Bid ointment

      (2) Nitrol ointment

      (3) Nitrong ointment

E. Drugs that dilate the peripheral blood vessels

  1. General implications for nurses

    a. Observe for common side effects, such as postural hypotension, weakness, and dizziness, as well as those specific to drugs

    b. Monitor blood pressure in standing and prone positions

    c. Inform the patient and family of the side effects and necessity of continued medical supervision

  2. Rauwolfia alkaloids

    a. Actions

      (1) Inhibit the stimulation of vascular smooth muscles

      (2) Cross the blood-brain barrier and act on the medullary vasomotor centers and central nervous tissue to cause a sedative effect

    b. Examples

      (1) Reserpine (Rau-Sed, Reserpoid, Sandril, Serpasil)

      (2) Syrosingopine (Singoserp)

      (3) Deserpidine (Harmonyl)

      (4) *Rauwolfia serpentina* (Raudixin, Rautina, Wolfina)

      (5) Rescinnamine (Moderil)

    c. Adverse effects

      (1) Bizarre dreams, drowsiness

      (2) Nasal congestion

      (3) Bradycardia, lethargy

  3. Guanethidine sulfate (Ismelin)

    a. Action—depresses activity of the sympathetic nervous system

    b. Adverse effects

      (1) Persistent diarrhea

      (2) Hypotension

      (3) Bradycardia

      (4) Dizziness and weakness

      (5) Inhibits ejaculation

  4. Methyldopa (Aldomet)

    a. Action—depletes norepinephrine at peripheral and central sites

    b. Adverse effects

      (1) Bradycardia

      (2) Dizziness, drowsiness

      (3) Orthostatic hypotension

      (4) Diarrhea

  5. Hydralazine hydrochloride

    a. Actions

      (1) Relaxes smooth muscles of arteries, causing vasodilation and a lowering of blood pressure

      (2) Increases cardiac output

    b. Examples

      (1) Apresoline

      (2) Dralzine

    c. Adverse effects

      (1) Postural hypotension

      (2) Tachycardia

      (3) Numbness and tingling of extremities

(4) Localized edema
(5) GI disturbances
6. Sodium nitroprusside (Nipride)
  a. Actions
    (1) Causes peripheral dilation to lower blood pressure in a hypertensive crisis
    (2) Must be administered by continuous IV infusion and must be protected from heat, light, and moisture
  b. Adverse effects
    (1) Sweating, muscular twitching and apprehension associated with rapid reduction of blood pressure
    (2) Skin rash
    (3) Psychosis, if toxic levels are reached
7. Diazoxide (Hyperstat IV)
  a. Action—dilates peripheral arterioles, producing an immediate fall in blood pressure
  b. Adverse effects
    (1) Hyperglycemia
    (2) Marked sodium and water retention
    (3) Transient tachycardia
    (4) GI disturbances
8. Clonidine hydrochloride (Catapres)
  a. Actions
    (1) Decreases cardiac output
    (2) Reduces peripheral resistance
  b. Adverse effects
    (1) Orthostatic hypotension
    (2) Dry mouth
    (3) Sedation
    (4) Rapid rise in blood pressure if therapy is discontinued abruptly
9. Prazosin hydrochloride (Minipress)
  a. Actions
    (1) Smooth muscle relaxant
    (2) Relaxation of peripheral arterioles results in decreased peripheral resistance
  b. Adverse effects
    (1) Dizziness, drowsiness
    (2) Weakness
    (3) Palpitation and syncope
    (4) Vertigo
10. Cyclandelate (Cyclospasmol)
  a. Action—smooth muscle relaxant, causing decreased peripheral resistance
  b. Adverse effects
    (1) Flushing
    (2) Tachycardia
    (3) Nausea
11. Isoxsuprine hydrochloride (Vasodilan)
  a. Actions

    (1) Vasodilator due to smooth muscle relaxation
    (2) Uterine relaxant
  b. Averse effects
    (1) Palpitation, tachycardia
    (2) Dizziness, weakness
F. Drugs that decrease circulating blood volume (diuretics)
  1. General implications for nurses
    a. Assess intake and output
    b. Weigh the patient daily under standard conditions
    c. Observe for signs of electrolyte imbalance and weakness, as well as specific adverse effects of drugs
    d. Administer in morning
    e. Encourage foods high in potassium if indicated
  2. Thiazides
    a. Actions
      (1) Decrease the circulating blood volume, counteract the sodium-retaining effects of antihypertensives, and improve blood flow from the capillaries
      (2) Interfere with sodium ion transport at ascending limb of Henle's loop and inhibit carbonic anhydrase activity at distal tubule sites
    b. Examples
      (1) Chlorothiazide (Diuril)
      (2) Chlorthalidone (Hygroton)
      (3) Hydrochlorothiazide (Esidrix, Hydro-Diuril, Oretic)
      (4) Methyclothiazide (Enduron)
    c. Adverse effects
      (1) Hypokalemia caused by the rapid exchange of potassium ions for sodium ions at collecting tubules
      (2) Initial diuresis may cause weakness, fatigue, dizziness
      (3) Drug-induced hyperglycemia may convert a prediabetic to a diabetic state
      (4) Headache, dizziness, vertigo, paresthesias
      (5) GI irritation
      (6) Long-term therapy may induce symptoms of gout secondary to increased uric acid reabsorption and asymptomatic hyperuricemia
  3. Potassium-sparing drugs
    a. Action—interfere with aldosterone-induced reabsorption of sodium ions at distal nephron sites to increase sodium chloride excretion

and decrease potassium ion loss (potassium sparing)
   b. Examples
      (1) Spironolactone (Aldactone)
      (2) Triamterene (Dyrenium)
   c. Adverse effects
      (1) Hyponatremia, tissue dehydration
      (2) Mild headache
      (3) Mild acidosis resulting from decreased excretion of ammonium
      (4) Long-term use causes low serum sodium ion concentrations that stimulate aldosterone secretion
4. Mercurial diuretics
   a. Actions
      (1) Block sulfhydryl-containing enzymes that control tubule transport systems for sodium ions in the nephron by release of mercurial ions in tubule cells
      (2) Act chiefly at proximal and distal tubule sites for active transport; also affect the passive transport of chloride and water
   b. Examples
      (1) Mercaptomerin sodium (Thiomerin)
      (2) Mersalyl with theophylline (Salyrgan-Theophylline)
   c. Adverse effects
      (1) Hypokalemic alkalosis caused by potassium and hydrogen ion exchange for sodium ions at collecting tubules (which increases output of potassium and hydrogen ions with prolonged therapy)
      (2) Destruction of tubule cells with excess use
      (3) Hypersensitivity reactions (e.g., pruritus, skin rash, GI disturbances, stomatitis, vertigo, headache)
5. Other potent diuretics
   a. Actions
      (1) Interfere with active transport of sodium ions in ascending limb of Henle's loop
      (2) Action at proximal tubule sites inhibits sodium chloride and water reabsorption
   b. Examples
      (1) Ethacrynic acid (Edecrin)
      (2) Furosemide (Lasix)
      (3) Metolazone (Zaroxolyn)
   c. Adverse effects
      (1) Hypokalemia and alkalosis (drugs exchange sodium ions at collecting tubules, causing loss of potassium and hydrogen ions)
      (2) Hyperuricemia with long-term oral use

      (3) Elevated blood urea nitrogen
      (4) Ototoxicity (rare)
G. Drugs that constrict peripheral blood vessels
   1. General implications for nurses
      a. Careful monitoring of blood pressure at frequent intervals
      b. Infiltration may cause local vasoconstriction and tissue necrosis
      c. Titrate IV with blood pressure to prevent hypertension
      d. Observe for hypertensive headache and abdominal distress, as well as adverse effects listed under specific drugs
   2. Alpha-adrenergic stimulators
      a. Actions
         (1) Alpha receptors cause constriction that elevates the blood pressure
         (2) Increase arterial constriction, which increases the work load of the left ventricle and may reflexively slow cardiac rate, causing reduced cardiac output and less effective blood flow
         (3) Venous alpha receptors cause constriction that improves blood flow toward the heart
      b. Examples
         (1) Hydroxyamphetamine hydrobromide (Paredrine)
         (2) Methoxamine hydrochloride (Vasoxyl)
         (3) Phenylephrine hydrochloride (Neo-Synephrine)
         (4) Levarterenol bitartrate (Levophed); also has a positive inotropic and chronotropic effect on the heart
         (5) Mephentermine sulfate (Wyamine); also stimulates cardiac beta receptors
         (6) Metaraminol bitartrate (Aramine); also stimulates cardiac beta receptors
      c. Adverse effects
         (1) Constriction of resistance vessels without action on capacitance vessels may increase venous pooling and reduce venous return to the heart
         (2) Adrenergic stimulation inhibits intestinal motility, and gaseous distention or constipation may occur with prolonged administration
   3. Vasopressin (Pitressin)
      a. Action—musculotropic effect that constricts small vessels when infused by a route delivering the drug to bleeding sites
      b. Adverse effects
         (1) Tremors
         (2) Diaphoresis

      (3) Pounding in head
      (4) Urticaria
      (5) Abdominal cramps
H. Plasma volume expanders
  1. General implications for nurses
    a. Must be administered slowly to prevent circulatory overload
    b. Observe for signs of pulmonary edema caused by circulatory overload, as well as specific adverse effects
    c. Monitor intake and output
  2. Osmotic agents
    a. Action—cause movement of fluid from interstitial spaces into bloodstream
    b. Examples
      (1) Dextran 40 (Rheomacrodex)
      (2) Dextran 70 (Macrodex)
      (3) Dextran (Expandex)
    c. Adverse effects
      (1) Anaphylactic reaction
      (2) Pulmonary edema
  3. Albumin preparations
    a. Actions
      (1) Expand blood volume
      (2) May provide clotting factors (except plasma protein fraction)
      (3) Decrease the hematocrit
    b. Examples
      (1) Normal human serum albumin
      (2) Normal human serum albumin (salt-poor)
      (3) Plasma protein fraction
    c. Adverse effects
      (1) Rash
      (2) Nausea and vomiting
      (3) Increased salivation
      (4) Hepatitis
I. Drugs that prevent intravascular clot formation (anticoagulants)
  1. General nursing implications
    a. Observe for signs of bleeding, such as hemoptysis and hematuria, and other adverse effects specific to the drug
    b. Check appropriate laboratory tests
    c. Have antidote available—vitamin K for warfarin sodium (Coumadin) and protamine sulfate for heparin
    d. Teach the patient
      (1) Signs of bleeding
      (2) To use an electric razor
      (3) To carry a medical alert card
      (4) Effects of diet and other medications on therapy

  2. Oral anticoagulants
    a. Actions
      (1) Interfere with synthesis of prothrombin by the liver
      (2) Cause an increased prothrombin time
      (3) Effects are counteracted by vitamin K
    b. Examples
      (1) Dicumarol
      (2) Warfarin sodium (Coumadin, Panwarfin)
  3. Heparin sodium
    a. Action—must be administered parenterally and inhibits conversion of prothrombin to thrombin
    b. Examples
      (1) Depo-Heparin
      (2) Lipohep
      (3) Meparin
      (4) Panheprin
    c. Adverse effects
      (1) Chills, fever, pruritus
      (2) Asthmalike reactions
      (3) Local irritation and hematoma from IM or SC injections
J. Drugs that affect red blood cell building
  1. General implications for nurses
    a. Use Z-track procedure for IM administration
    b. Inform the patient about the side effects of hematinics; adverse effects of vitamin replacement are rare
    c. Mouth care to prevent staining of teeth
  2. Vitamin replacements
    a. Action—provide components for protein framework of cells by supplying cofactors for DNA synthesis of nucleotides
    b. Examples
      (1) Vitamin B_{12} replacement
        (a) Cyanocobalamin
        (b) Hydroxocobalamin
        (c) Vitamin B_{12} with intrinsic factor concentrate
        (d) Liver injection
      (2) Tetrahydrofolic acid
        (a) Folate sodium
        (b) Folic acid (Folvite)
        (c) Leucovorin calcium
  3. Hematinics
    a. Action—provide a component of hemoglobin for erythroblasts
    b. Examples
      (1) Oral iron sources
        (a) Ferrocholinate (Chel-Iron, Ferrolip)
        (b) Ferrous fumarate (Ircon, Toleron)
        (c) Ferrous gluconate

(d) Ferrous lactate (Ferro Drops)

(e) Ferrous sulfate

(2) Parenteral iron sources

(a) Iron-dextran injection (Imferon)

(b) Iron sorbitex (Jectofer)

   c. Adverse effects

(1) Injectable preparation causes tissue staining

(2) Fever

(3) Urticaria

(4) Nausea and vomiting

(5) Black stools

RELATED DIAGNOSTIC PROCEDURES
Angiography

A. Definition—an x-ray examination using contrast dye to visualize the patency of an artery

B. Nursing responsibilities

1. Inform the patient of the risks involved in this procedure (allergic reaction, embolus, cardiac arrhythmia)

2. Administer mild sedative as ordered prior to procedure

3. Observe the patient for complications

4. Postprocedure care involves checking the injection site for bleeding and inflammation, assessing circulatory status of the extremities, and enforcing bed rest

Bone Marrow Aspiration

A. Definition—puncture to collect tissue from the bone marrow

1. Sites used include the sternum, vertebral body, iliac crest, or the tibia in infants

2. Performed to study the cells involved in blood production

B. Nursing responsibilities

1. Obtain informed consent

2. Attempt to allay anxiety of the patient

3. Assist the physician in maintaining a sterile field and positioning the patient

4. Send the specimen to the laboratory in a proper container with appropriate label

Cardiac Catheterization

A. Definition—introduction of a catheter into the heart via a peripheral vessel

1. Injection of contrast material for visualization of chambers, coronary circulation, and great vessels

2. Withdrawal of blood samples to evaluate cardiac function

3. Measurement of pressures within chambers and blood vessels (e.g., pulmonary wedge pressure)

B. Nursing responsibilities

1. Obtain an informed consent; the patient should be aware of the purpose of and the complications possible with this procedure as well as the sensations experienced (e.g., urge to cough, nausea, heat)

2. Allow time for verbalization of fears

3. Keep the patient n.p.o. for 6 to 8 hours prior to the procedure

4. Determine the presence of allergies, particularly to iodine

5. Administer sedatives as ordered prior to the procedure

6. After catheterization

a. Monitor vital signs frequently; cardiac arrhythmias are more common during the procedure but may occur afterward also

b. Assess the puncture site for bleeding (sandbags or ice packs may be ordered if the femoral artery is used)

c. Assess the involved extremity for signs of ischemia (e.g., absence of peripheral pulses, changes in sensation, color, and temperature)

d. Maintain bed rest for the prescribed number of hours

Exercise Stress Testing

A. Definition—assessment of cardiac function by ECG, blood pressure, and pulse rate during sustained exercise

1. Common aerobic activities involved include walking on a treadmill or riding a stationary bicycle

2. Cardiac workload is increased by either constant level of activity or graduating levels of difficulty to evaluate ability of the coronary circulation to supply adequate amounts of oxygen to the heart muscle when maximum heart rates are approached (depression of ST segment of ECG is one indication of myocardial hypoxia)

B. Nursing responsibilities

1. Obtain an informed consent

2. Attempt to allay anxiety of the patient

3. Instruct the patient to have only a light meal several hours prior to the test and to avoid stimulants and depressants

4. Ensure that the patient does not smoke (nicotine causes vasoconstriction)

5. Ask the patient to report dizziness, chest pain, dyspnea, fatigue, or nausea if experienced during the test

6. Continually observe the patient, the vital signs, and the ECG during the test

7. Ensure ready access to emergency cardiac drugs and equipment (e.g., defibrillator)
8. Observe the patient after the test and reinforce any medical instructions as required

RELATED EMERGENCY AND CRITICAL CARE PROCEDURES
Cardiac Monitoring
A. Definition
   1. Electric observation of the conductivity patterns of the heart by the use of skin electrodes and a monitoring device; the heart's electric activity is conducted to the surface of the skin by the salty fluids bathing the cells and tissues
   2. Utilized in heart disease, during surgery and intrusive procedures, or when danger of arrhythmias (cardiac irregularities in rhythm) is apparent
   3. P, Q, R, S, and T segments are parts of the normal electrocardiogram (ECG); P wave represents atrial depolarization, QRS waves (QRS complex) ventricular depolarization, and T wave ventricular repolarization
B. Nursing responsibilities
   1. Explain the procedure to patient and attempt to allay anxiety
   2. Prepare the skin on the chest for electrode attachment
      a. Cleanse area with alcohol swab to remove dirt and oils
      b. Shave the area to improve skin-electrode contact
   3. Place electrodes on the skin and attach to the monitor cable as indicated
      a. Right arm (on chest)
      b. Left arm (on chest)
      c. Center (or ground)
   4. Turn on the monitor scope and set the machine's sensitivity when a clear picture is obtained
   5. Observe the monitor for changes in rate and rhythm
   6. Set the alarm and readout attachment (if available) so an electric printout will be made if there is a change in cardiac activity
   7. If arrhythmia occurs, act appropriately
      a. Emergency arrhythmias require immediate intervention
      b. If the arrhythmia is nonemergency, document its occurrence with a rhythm strip and notify the physician
   8. Life-threatening arrhythmias require immediate intervention
      a. Ventricular fibrillation—repetitive rapid stimulation from ectopic ventricular foci to which the ventricles are unable to respond; ventricular contraction is replaced by uncoordinated twitching; circulation ceases, and death ensues
         (1) Defibrillate immediately
         (2) Inject lidocaine
         (3) Institute cardiopulmonary resuscitation
         (4) Document the arrhythmia and notify the physician
      b. Ventricular tachycardia—series of three or more bizarre premature ventricular beats that occur in a regular rhythm; this electric activity results in decreased cardiac output and may rapidly convert to ventricular fibrillation
         (1) Use lidocaine intravenously to convert rhythm
         (2) Be prepared to administer defibrillation and cardiopulmonary resuscitation
         (3) Document the arrhythmia and notify the physician
      c. Premature ventricular contractions (PVCs) of greater than 5 per minute—originate in the ventricles and occur before the next expected sinus beat; they can be life threatening when they occur close to the T wave, since cardiac repolarization is interfered with and ventricular fibrillation may ensue
         (1) Administer lidocaine intravenously
         (2) Document the arrhythmia and notify the physician
         (3) Long-term institution of oral antiarrhythmics may be indicated
      d. Complete heart block—occurs when there is no electric communication between the atria and ventricles and each beats independently; this activity will not provide long-term adequate circulation, and syncope, congestive failure, or cardic arrest may ensue
         (1) Document the arrhythmia and notify the physician
         (2) Use of intravenous isoproterenol is generally indicated
         (3) Prepare for pacemaker insertion (see procedure)
      e. Asystole (cardiac standstill)—occurs when there is no cardiac activity, demonstrated on the ECG tracing as a flat line; this terminates in death unless intervention is begun immediately
         (1) Institute cardiopulmonary resuscitation

(2) Document the arrhythmia and notify the physician

(3) Cardiac stimulants may be given via IV or intracardiac route

(4) Pacemaker insertion may be indicated (see procedure)

Cardiac Pacemaker Insertion

A. Definition—artificial pacemakers replace natural electric stimulation of the heart and are indicated in the treatment of

1. Complete heart block—impulses generated from the SA node of the heart do not reach the ventricles; the atria and ventricles beat independently of each other

2. Second-degree AV (atrioventricular) block—there is intermittent failure of impulse to reach the ventricles

3. Adams-Stokes syndrome—a sudden drop in ventricular rate that causes syncope and temporary loss of consciousness

B. Pacemakers—involve the insertion of an electrode catheter into the right ventricle, which transmits the impulses generated by the pacing unit

1. Demand pacemakers are most frequently used; the pacemaker will stimulate the ventricles to contract only if the patient's ventricular rate falls below the rate set on the pacemaker

2. Fixed-rate pacemakers stimulate the heart a specific amount of times per minute regardless of the patient's rhythm

3. Pacemakers may be temporary and worn externally or permanent and surgically placed under the skin

C. Nursing responsibilities

1. Explain the procedure to the patient

2. Observe the cardiac monitor before, during, and after the procedure to verify pacemaker capture, and observe for arrhythmias

3. Have emergency medications (e.g., lidocaine, atropine sulfate, isoproterenol) available, as well as a defibrillator

4. Teach the patient how to take pulse, to keep a diary of pulse, and to notify the physician immediately if the rate falls below that set on the pacemaker

5. Teach the patient to remain under a physician's supervision, since batteries must be replaced approximately every 2 years; pacemaker function may be checked by special telephone devices

6. Encourage the patient to wear a bracelet or carry a medical alert card

Swan-Ganz Catheter Procedure

A. Definition—catheter used to measure pulmonary capillary wedge pressure, pulmonary artery pressure, and right atrial pressure

1. The double-lumen catheter with a balloon tip is inserted into the brachial vein and advanced through the superior vena cava, into the right atrium and ventricle, and into the pulmonary artery; the catheter is guided further until, when the balloon is inflated, it is wedged in the distal arterial branch

2. This catheter functions to yield information on the patient's circulatory status, left ventricular pumping action, and vascular tone

B. Nursing responsibilities

1. Obtain informed consent for procedure

2. Assist the physician in inserting the catheter using surgical aseptic technique

3. Observe the insertion site for inflammation

4. Observe the line for patency and air bubbles

5. Take readings with transducer at the level of the patient's sternal notch

6. Change the dressing as ordered using surgical asepsis

7. Notify the physician if the waveform changes or pressure readings are altered

8. Normal readings

a. Pulmonary capillary wedge pressure: 5 to 13 mm Hg

b. Pulmonary artery pressure
(1) Systolic: 16 to 30 mm Hg
(2) Diastolic: 0 to 7 mm Hg

c. Right atrial pressure: 5 mm Hg

9. Keep emergency medications and a defibrillator available

Central Venous Pressure (CVP) Monitoring

A. Definition

1. CVP is the right atrial pressure, which is normally 2 to 8 mm Hg

2. A catheter is passed from the subclavian vein into the superior vena cava or right atrium

B. Nursing responsibilities

1. Obtain informed consent

2. Assist the physician with insertion of the catheter using surgical aseptic technique

3. Obtain chest x-ray film after insertion to ascertain the position of the catheter

4. Take readings as ordered

a. Place the patient in a supine position

b. Place the stopcock of the manometer at the midaxillary line (which is approximately the

level of the right atrium) and fill with fluid from line
   c. Allow fluid to enter the catheter by placing the stopcock in "off" position toward the IV bottle
   d. If the patient is on a respirator, remove it during readings
 5. Record and report changes in CVP readings; often these readings are used to regulate the rate of administration of IVs (high readings are present in congestive heart failure, low readings in hypovolemia)

Cardiopulmonary Resuscitation (CPR)

A. Definition—institution of artificial ventilation and circulation with rescue breathing and external cardiac compression
B. Nursing responsibilities
 1. Ascertain the absence of spontaneous respiration and carotid pulse
 2. Place the victim on a firm surface
 3. Ventilate the lungs
   a. Straighten the airway
     (1) Head tilt maneuver
     (2) Chin tilt maneuver
     (3) Jaw thrust maneuver
   b. Pinch the nostrils
   c. Form a seal with the mouth
   d. Ventilate four times quickly
 4. Place heel of hand over lower half of body of sternum, interlock hands and compress the chest 3.8 to 5 cm (1½ to 2 inches for an adult)
 5. Maintain the ventilation/compression ratio
   a. One rescuer: 2 breaths after every 15 compressions (rate, 80 per minute)
   b. Two rescuers: 1 breath after every 5 compressions (rate, 60 per minute)
 6. Terminate CPR as indicated
   a. Return of cardiac rhythm and spontaneous respirations
   b. Lack of response suggestive of permanent, irreversible brain damage

MAJOR DISEASES
Hypertension

A. Etiology and pathophysiology
 1. Hypertension increases the risk of coronary artery disease, heart failure, myocardial infarction, cerebral vascular accidents (CVAs), and renal failure
 2. Essential hypertension
   a. Anxiety and other stresses are believed to play a role in releasing a pressor from kidneys that causes chronic vasoconstriction, thereby raising blood pressure
   b. Individuals with essential hypertension have difficulty handling hostile feelings, are less assertive, and have more obsessive-compulsive traits than do nonhypertensive individuals
   c. Onset is generally between 25 and 55 years of age
 3. Renal hypertension
   a. Narrowing of the lumen of a renal artery as a result of atherosclerosis, causes release of renin
   b. Renin sets off series of reactions, which cause sodium retention and subsequent rise in blood pressure
   c. Onset is generally after 50 years of age
 4. Malignant hypertension results from sustained hypertension of any form, which causes necrosis of the arterioles and proliferative changes of the renal arteries leading to renal failure, CVA, and heart failure, if untreated
 5. Hypertensive crisis may also be caused by endocrine disorders (pheochromocytoma), increased intracranial pressure, and encephalopathy
B. Signs and symptoms
 1. Subjective
   a. Headache (occipital area)
   b. Lightheadedness
   c. Tinnitus
   d. Easy fatigue
   e. Visual disturbances
 2. Objective
   a. Blood pressure greater than 140/90 mm Hg in person younger than 50 years of age; World Health Organization defines hypertension as greater than 160/95 mm Hg
   b. Retinal changes
   c. Possible hematuria
   d. Epistaxis
   e. Cardiac hypertrophy
C. Treatment
 1. Antihypertensive drugs to decrease peripheral resistance (see drugs that dilate the peripheral blood vessels)
 2. Diuretics to decrease amount of water and sodium retained by the body
 3. Sedatives to control tension
 4. Weight reduction
 5. Smoking discouraged

6. Physical as well as psychologic rest (psychotherapy is often helpful for patients with essential hypertension)
7. Sodium-restricted diet (1 to 3 g daily)
8. A sympathectomy (cutting of sympathetic nerve fibers) may be done to cause dilation of arteries

D. Nursing care
1. Encourage early detection by participation in community screening programs
2. Monitor vital signs with patient in both upright and recumbent positions (orthostatic hypotension is a common adverse effect of antihypertensive drugs)
3. Check weight daily
4. Educate the patient regarding drugs, follow-up care, and diet and activity restrictions (caution:salt substitutes often contain potassium and should not be suggested without physician approval)
5. Reassure and support any expression of emotions
6. If epistaxis occurs, place an ice pack on the back of the neck, which may alleviate it; packing is sometimes required
7. Nursing care related to specific medications should also be included

Arterioatherosclerosis

A. Etiology and pathophysiology
1. Deposition of fatty plaques along inner wall of the artery; most often affects the peripheral arteries, aorta, coronary arteries, and arteries supplying the brain
2. Considered to be a loss of elasticity or "hardening," of the arteries

B. Signs and symptoms (depend on arteries affected)
1. Subjective
   a. Intermittent claudication
   b. Pain, depending on degree circulation is impaired
   c. Forgetfulness
2. Objective
   a. Decreased skin temperature
   b. Pallor
   c. Diminished pulsations
   d. May lead to ulcerations and gangrene
   e. Elevated serum cholesterol and lipids
   f. Objective memory loss on testing

C. Treatment
1. Drugs that cause vasodilation
2. Weight loss
3. Dietary restriction of fat and cholesterol

D. Nursing care

1. Evaluate all pulses, color, and temperature of involved area
2. Discourage positions that hamper circulation (e.g., cross-legged)
3. Teach the patient the hazards of smoking (nicotine causes vasoconstriction)
4. Dietary teaching for family as well as patient
5. Teach importance of warm clothing
6. No vigorous massages of involved area

Angina Pectoris

A. Etiology and pathophysiology
1. Commonly caused by narrowed coronary arteries (coronary artery disease)
2. Patients with aortic stenosis or extremely low pressure may also have impaired coronary artery blood flow
3. Increased metabolic demands due to strenuous exercise, emotional stress, hyperthyroidism, or severe anemia may also precipitate angina pectoris
4. When oxygen supplied by the blood cannot meet the metabolic demands of the muscle, hypoxia occurs
5. Pain is thought to be a result of anaerobic metabolic end products

B. Signs and symptoms
1. Subjective
   a. Chest pain associated with activity; generally subsides after a few minutes of rest
   b. Pain is usually substernal and can be described as "crushing" or "pressure"
   c. Pain may radiate to the left shoulder and arm, jaw, epigastric area, or right shoulder
   d. Palpitation
   e. Faintness
   f. Dyspnea
2. Objective
   a. Diaphoresis
   b. Blood pressure may be elevated
   c. Signs of underlying disease may be evident (cardiac enlargement, valvular disease, arrhythmias)
   d. ECG often indicates a previous infarction

C. Treatment
1. Restricted activity
2. Drugs, such as nitroglycerin, and slower acting vasodilators
3. Weight loss
4. Oxygen therapy during attack
5. Coronary artery bypass surgery if medical regimen not successful
6. Restriction of cholesterol and fat in diet

D. Nursing care
  1. Provide physical and mental rest
  2. Relieve pain by administration of vasodilators
  3. Assess activity tolerance
  4. Discourage smoking
  5. Educate the patient regarding diet, medication, and activity
  6. Provide necessary emotional support due to required alterations in life-style

Myocardial Infarction

A. Etiology and pathophysiology
  1. Acute necrosis of part of the heart muscle caused by interruption of the oxygen supply to the area and resulting in altered functioning and reduced cardiac output
  2. Possible causes include atherosclerosis, thrombus formation, and decreased blood flow
B. Signs and symptoms
  1. Subjective
    a. Sudden, severe, crushing, or viselike pain in the substernal region; may radiate to the arms, neck, and back
    b. Nausea and vomiting
    c. Severe anxiety and dyspnea
    d. Patient's health history, including smoking and drinking habits, obesity, high-cholesterol diet, physical and emotional stresses, chest pain, hypertension
  2. Objective
    a. Signs of shock: cold clammy skin, profuse diaphoresis, decreased blood pressure, rapid thready pulse
    b. Slight elevation of temperature
    c. Blood serum enzyme and isoenzyme levels
      (1) Creatinine phosphokinase (CPK)—elevated on days 1 to 3
      (2) Serum glutamic oxaloacetic transaminase (SGOT)—elevated on days 2 to 4
      (3) Lactic dehydrogenase (LDH)—elevated on day 1, reaching a peak on days 3 to 4, and then gradually subsiding
    d. Complete blood studies, particularly white blood cells and sedimentation rate, to determine presence of inflammatory process
    e. Coagulation studies—prothrombin time (PT) and partial thromboplastin time (PTT)
C. Treatment
  1. Admit the patient to the coronary care unit
  2. Morphine sulfate IV or SC to relieve pain and reduce apprehension
  3. Bed rest with cardiac precautions to reduce demand for oxygen

4. Oxygen as necessary
5. Cardiac monitoring for continued surveillance of the heart's electric activity
6. Frequent monitoring of vital signs, including temperature, pulse (apical and radial), respirations, blood pressure, intake and output
7. One or more of the following medications to prevent or reduce complications: antiarrhythmic agents, digitalis, diuretics, anticoagulants, potassium salts, vasopressors or vasodilators, sedatives, and stool softeners
8. IV fluids at slow rate to keep vein open for administration of medications
9. Clear liquid diet is prescribed initially to decrease oxygen consumption, and then advanced to low sodium
10. Swan-Ganz catheter is used to monitor pressure in pulmonary artery, which reflects function of left ventricle
11. Intraaortic balloon pump that inflates during diastole and deflates during systole may be used to decrease cardiac work load
D. Nursing care
  1. Watch the cardiac monitor and immediately document and report changes in rate, conductivity, and rhythm
  2. Observe the patient for ventricular fibrillation and asystole and take appropriate life-saving actions if they occur (e.g., cardiopulmonary resuscitation, electric defibrillation)
  3. Observe for other variations, such as PVCs close to a T wave, ventricular tachycardia, and atrial fibrillation; if they occur, administer prescribed medications, document the rhythm, and notify the physician
  4. Observe the patient's vital signs every 15 minutes until stable
  5. Closely observe the patient's intake and output
  6. Observe for pulmonary congestion and dependent edema
  7. Observe for pain and restlessness and administer medication as ordered
  8. Watch for cyanosis and dyspnea and administer oxygen as necessary
  9. Recognize that the patient is subject to sensory overload
    a. Orient to the unit and machinery
    b. Allow the patient time to express feelings and fears
10. Provide gradual increase in activity
11. Apply antiembolism stockings

Inflammatory Diseases of the Heart (Pericarditis, Myocarditis, Subacute Bacterial Endocarditis)

A. Etiology and pathophysiology
  1. Pericarditis is an acute or chronic inflammation of the pericardium caused by bacterial or viral invasion, trauma, heart disease, or an autoimmune process
     a. Can result in loss of pericardial elasticity or an accumulation of fluid within the sac
     b. Heart failure or cardiac tamponade (compression of the heart due to a collection of fluid within the pericardial sac) may result
  2. Myocarditis is an inflammation of the myocardium due to pericarditis, systemic infection, or allergic response
     a. The contractility of the heart is impaired due to the inflammatory process
     b. Myocardial ischemia and necrosis are critical complications
  3. Subacute bacterial endocarditis is an inflammation of the inner lining of the heart and valves generally caused by *Streptococcus viridans* or other nonhemolytic streptococci spreading through the blood to the heart from infected teeth, gums, and tonsils; structural damage to the valves may occur in a matter of days, and pump failure will ensue
B. Signs and symptoms
  1. Subjective
     a. Precordial or substernal pain
     b. Shortness of breath
     c. Chills
     d. Fatigue and malaise
  2. Objective
     a. Arrhythmias
     b. Increased cardiac enzymes
     c. Fever
     d. Positive blood cultures
     e. Friction rubs evident on auscultation
C. Treatment
  1. Administer oxygen
  2. Bed rest
  3. Antibiotics to relieve underlying infection
  4. Corticosteroids
  5. Antiarrhythmics
  6. Pericardectomy (surgical removal of scar tissue and the pericardium), if indicated
D. Nursing care
  1. Carefully observe the patient for signs of shock, heart failure, and arrhythmias
  2. Maintain a tranquil environment and help the patient achieve maximum rest
  3. If surgical intervention is undertaken, care for chest tubes and follow the postoperative chest surgery routine (see cardiac surgery)
  4. Explain posthospitalization therapy to the patient to improve compliance (lifelong doses of penicillin prophylactically)

Congestive Heart Failure (CHF)

A. Etiology and pathophysiology
  1. Inability of the heart to meet the demands of the body
  2. Pump failure may be caused by cardiac abnormalities or conditions that place increased demands on the heart
     a. Myocardial infarctions
     b. Valvular defects
     c. Hypertension
     d. Anemia
     e. Hyperthyroidism
     f. Obesity
     g. Circulatory overload
  3. When one side of the heart "fails," there is essentially a buildup of pressure in the vascular system feeding into that side: signs of right-sided failure will be evident in the systemic circulation, those of left-sided failure in the pulmonary system
B. Signs and symptoms
  1. Right-sided failure
     a. Dependent, pitting edema; ankle edema is frequently the first sign of CHF; often subsides at night when legs are elevated
     b. Ascites from increased pressure within the portal system
     c. Respiratory distress if ascites is severe
     d. Fatigue
  2. Left-sided heart failure
     a. Dyspnea from fluid within the lungs
     b. Orthopnea
     c. Frothy, blood-tinged sputum
     d. Fatigue
     e. Apprehension, restlessness
C. Treatment
  1. Morphine sulfate is often given to decrease anxiety and dyspnea
  2. Oxygen is generally administered by mask of cannula; however, if acute left-sided failure exists, the patient may require endotracheal intubation and placement on a ventilator
  3. Digitalis is generally prescribed to increase the efficiency of the heart's pumping action
  4. Diuretics such as furosemide (Lasix) are often

ordered to remove excess fluid, thereby decreasing cardiac work load

5. Potassium supplements are ususally prescribed to prevent digitalis toxicity and hypokalemia
6. Rotating tourniquets (dry phlebotomy) may be used to decrease venous return; generally tourniquets are applied to 3 of the extremities, and every 15 minutes a tourniquet is removed and rotated in a clockwise direction; when the patient is stable, tourniquets are removed one at a time in 15-minute intervals
7. A paracentesis may be performed if ascites exists and is causing respiratory distress
8. Sodium-restricted diet

D. Nursing care
1. Maintain the patient in high Fowler's position
2. Elevate extremities
3. Frequently monitor vital signs
4. Change position frequently
5. Monitor intake and output and daily weight
6. Observe for electrolyte imbalances (hyponatremia, hypokalemia)
7. Provide the patient and family teaching and emotional support
8. Nursing implications for digitalis therapy and diuretics should also be considered

Cardiac Surgery

A. May be used to correct
1. Mitral stenosis or regurgitation
2. Aortic stenosis or insufficiency
3. Coronary occlusion
4. Ventricular aneurysm

B. Preoperative procedures
1. Vital signs and weight
2. Coughing and deep breathing exercises are taught and practiced
3. Inhalation therapy to improve pulmonary function
4. Coagulation studies in addition to routine laboratory tests
5. Chest x-ray examination
6. ECG to assess electric pattern of heart
7. Echocardiography, which uses sound, is especially helpful in evaluating valvular defects
8. Cardiac catheterization (see related diagnostic procedures)

C. Types of procedures—open or closed heart surgery (when extracorporeal circulation or the heart-lung machine is used, it is called open heart surgery; hypothermia may be used in either open or closed heart surgery to decrease the metabolic demands of the body)

1. Mitral commissurotomy or valvotomy involves splitting the joined portions of the mitral valve that are present in mitral stenosis
2. Mitral valve replacement is done for mitral insufficiency, which occurs when the mitral valve does not close properly to block the reflux of blood from the ventricle into the atrium during systole (regurgitation)
3. Coronary bypass surgery is done when severe arteriosclerotic disease causes angina pectoris; a segment of a vessel (often the saphenous vein) is anastomosed, bypassing the diseased portion of a coronary artery
4. Aneurysmectomy is done to correct a ventricular aneurysm (which occurs in approximately 10% to 30% of patients with myocardial infarction; i.e., a weakened ventricular wall balloons out, causing decreased cardiac efficiency)

D. Postoperative nursing care
1. Monitor cardiac functioning
2. Evaluate vital signs, including peripheral pulses and neurologic signs
3. Utilize rectal probe to monitor temperature
4. Maintain airway; the patient will have an endotracheal tube in place postoperatively and require mechanical ventilation; suction as necessary
5. Monitor intake and output
6. Assess state of hydration by frequent checks on central venous pressure (CVP) readings, electrolytes, specific gravity, and observation of the patient
7. Care for chest tubes
   a. Milk the tubing to maintain patency
   b. Avoid kinked tubing
   c. Drainage should not be more than 200 ml/hour
8. Maintain a Foley catheter in place; in addition to output, monitor specific gravity
9. Assess pain (nature, site, duration, type) and provide relief
10. Encourage coughing and deep breathing; change position frequently
11. Evaluate arterial blood gases
12. Administer parenteral therapy, including electrolytes and blood
13. Plan with the patient and family for meeting both short- and long-term goals
14. Provide relief of anxiety and fear by staying with the patient and explaining procedures; encourage verbalization of feelings; provide emotional support

E. Complications

1. Hemorrhage that can lead to hypovolemia
   a. Decreased blood pressure, increased pulse rate
   b. Restlessness, apprehension
   c. Lowered CVP readings
   d. Pallor
2. Cardiac tamponade caused by collection of fluid or blood within pericardium
   a. Decreased arterial pressure
   b. Elevated CVP
   c. Rapid, thready pulse
   d. Diminished output
3. Congestive heart failure
   a. Dyspnea
   b. Elevated CVP
   c. Tachycardia
   d. Edema
4. Myocardial infarction
5. Renal failure
6. Embolism
7. Psychosis resulting from an inability to cope with anxiety associated with cardiac surgery

Thrombophlebitis and Emboli

A. Etiology and pathophysiology
   1. Thrombophlebitis is the inflammation of a vein and is associated with clot formation (thrombus)
   2. An embolus is a clot or solid particle carried by the bloodstream that may interfere with circulation to vital organs
   3. Risk factors thought to contribute to this disorder include immobilization, venous stasis, trauma to vessels, and pregnancy
   4. Surgical procedures involving the pelvic area increase the risk of phlebitis because of the vascularity of the area and subsequent vascular impairment
B. Signs and symptoms
   1. Subjective
      a. Pain on dorsiflexion of affected extremity (Homans' sign)
      b. Sometimes no signs are present until embolus is released and lodges in a vessel supplying a vital organ
   2. Objective
      a. Swollen limb with hard veins that are sensitive to pressure
      b. Redness and warmth of area along the vein
      c. If emboli are released, pulse may be lost in area and severe pain may persist
C. Treatment
   1. Bed rest with elastic stockings to promote venous return

2. Warm moist heat to promote vasodilation; however, some believe this may dislodge the clot, and ice packs are ordered
3. Elevation of extremity to reduce edema
4. Anticoagulants to prevent recurrence of deep vein involvement
5. Vasodilators to prevent vascular spasm
6. Amputation of an extremity when vascular supply is severely impaired; may also be indicated for a neoplasm or following trauma
   a. Below-the-knee amputation provides the patient with a more natural gait, since knee movement is maintained
   b. Above-the-knee amputation limits the patient's movement, since prosthesis contains knee joint
   c. A guillotine amputation, in which the wound is left open and skin traction is applied, is performed when the area is infected, gangrenous, or extensively traumatized or if the patient is a poor surgical risk
   d. A flap-type amputation is less prone to infection, since the skin covers the area and healing occurs within 2 weeks; may be above or below the knee
D. Nursing care
   1. Associated with medical management
      a. Observe the patient frequently for signs of vascular impairment (e.g., pallor, cyanosis, coolness, diminished pulses)
      b. Assist the patient in understanding the rationale for prolonged bed rest and minimal activity
      c. Apply antiembolitic stockings and remove for 15 minutes every 8 hours
      d. Observe and record vital signs, including peripheral pulses
      e. Instruct the patient to avoid tight and constricting clothing, cigarette smoking, or maintaining one position for long periods
      f. Observe for signs of embolism (e.g., sudden pain, cyanosis, hemoptysis, shock)
   2. Associated with amputation
      a. Observe the patient for bleeding
      b. Keep tourniquet at bedside
      c. Allow the patient to express emotional reactions to procedure
      d. Elevate the stump for 24 to 48 hours
      e. Keep the patient's extremities close to the body to prevent abduction deformity
      f. Encourage the patient to move the stump
      g. Place the patient with a lower extremity amputation in a prone position twice daily to stretch the flexor muscles

h. Start range-of-motion exercises to the stump after about 10 days

i. Encourage the patient not to sit in any position for prolonged periods, since this inactivity can cause hip flexion contractures

j. Provide and teach good care of the stump
   (1) Stump shrinkage (a change in size and shape of stump) is caused by reduction of subcutaneous fat by pressure of constrictive bandage and socket of prosthesis as well as disuse atrophy occurring in the involved muscles; maximum shrinkage usually takes a minimum of 1 to 1½ years and sometimes longer
   (2) Keep the stump clean: wash with mild soap but do not soak; use clean bandages and socks
   (3) Physical preparation for a prosthesis
       (a) Apply compression bandage to prevent edema and promote stump shrinkage
       (b) Massage the stump to soften the scar, decrease tenderness, and improve vascularity
       (c) Teach and encourage the patient to do stump-conditioning exercises to harden the stump (push stump against pillow and then progress to harder surfaces)

k. With the physical therapist, assist the patient with a lower extremity amputation to learn crutch walking

l. For patients fitted with a prosthesis immediately after surgery, ambulation instruction is begun on the first postoperative day

m. Explain and discuss the phantom limb phenomenon with the patient
   (1) Phantom limb—physiologic reaction of the nerves in the stump causing an unpleasant feeling that the limb is still there; this response may or may not be precipitated by a psychologic overlay
   (2) Phantom limb pain—when the unpleasant feelings become painful or disagreeable
   (3) Characteristics of phantom limb—sensations may be constant or intermittent, and of varying severity
   (4) Approaches that may help relieve phantom limb—have the patient look at the stump or close eyes and put the stump through range of motion as if the full limb were still there; if the patient con-

tinues to have severe pain of long duration, the medical therapy may include
   (a) Injecting the nerve endings in the stump with alcohol to give temporary relief
   (b) Surgical revision of the stump

n. Consider the special needs related to an upper extremity amputation
   (1) Mastery of an upper extremity prosthesis is more complex than that of a lower extremity prosthesis
   (2) The patient must do bilateral shoulder exercises to prepare for fitting the prosthesis
   (3) The artificial arm cannot be used above the head or behind the back because of the harnessing
   (4) There is no artificial hand that can duplicate all the fine movements of the fingers and thumb of the normal hand, although the development of electronic limbs does not negate this possibility for the future
   (5) There is a loss of sensory feedback; therefore the patient must use visual control at all times (a blind person could not adequately use a functional prosthesis)

Varicose Veins

A. Etiology and pathophysiology
   1. The veins in the lower trunk and extremities become dilated, congested, and tortuous due to weakness of valves or loss of elasticity of vessel walls
   2. A positive Trendelenburg test is diagnostic of varicose veins: the patient lies down with legs elevated until veins empty completely; the patient then stands, and observation of filling of veins is made; a normal vein fills from below, whereas a varicose vein fills from above

B. Treatment
   1. Surgical intervention involves ligation of the vein above the varicosity and removal of the involved vein; the great saphenous vein may be ligated near the femoral junction
   2. Postoperative early ambulation is essential to prevent formation of thrombi

C. Nursing care
   1. Elevate the foot of the bed for first 24 hours
   2. Observe vital signs and incisions for indications of hemorrhage
   3. Assist the patient with ambulation
   4. Administer analgesics as ordered

Peripheral Vascular Disorders

A. Etiology and pathophysiology
   1. Buerger's disease (thromboangiitis obliterans)
      a. Peripheral circulation impaired by inflammatory occlusions of the peripheral arteries
      b. Thromboses of both arteries and veins may occur
      c. Incidence is highest in young adult males who smoke
   2. Raynaud's disease
      a. Spasms of digital arteries thought to be caused by abnormal response of the sympathetic nervous system to cold or emotional stress
      b. Primarily occurs in young females
      c. Rarely leads to gangrene
   3. Atherosclerosis is a contributing factor
B. Signs and symptoms
   1. Subjective
      a. Paresthesia
      b. Aching pain
   2. Objective
      a. Pallor or cyanosis
      b. Gangrenous ulcers (more common in Buerger's disease)
      c. Diminished pulses in Buerger's disease
C. Treatment
   1. Vasodilators may be given
   2. Sympathectomy to sever the sympathetic ganglia supplying the area; there is local vasodilation with improved circulation
      a. Lumbar sympathectomy deprives the leg and foot of innervation
      b. Cervicothoracic sympathectomy relieves vasospasm in the arms and hands
   3. Femoropopliteal bypass grafting
      a. Saphenous vein grafting from femoral artery to the area below the obstruction
      b. Polyester fiber grafts in aortic iliac obstructions
   4. Amputation if vascular supply is severely impaired
D. Nursing care
   1. Associated with medical management
      a. Instruct the patient not to smoke or wear constrictive garments
      b. Extremities should be kept warm; instruct the patient to wear gloves when exposed to cold
      c. Protect from injury since there is decreased wound healing ability; lubricants may be applied to keep skin supple
      d. Assess color, temperature, pulses, and sensation of involved extremities
   2. Associated with sympathectomy
      a. Monitor vital signs frequently, since shock can occur
      b. Change position gradually, since dizziness may be a problem
      c. Apply elastic bandages if ordered
   3. Associated with femoropopliteal bypass grafting
      a. Assess circulation of involved extremity by checking pulses, color, temperature, and neurologic function
      b. Observe blood pressure frequently, since hypotension increases the possibility of thrombus formation
      c. Observe for signs of hemorrhage, including pain, change in skin color, and alteration of vital signs
      d. Ambulate patient as ordered; sitting should be avoided in femoropopliteal bypass surgery
   4. Associated with amputation (see thrombophlebitis and emboli)

Aneurysms

A. Etiology and pathophysiology
   1. Distention at the site of a weakness in the arterial wall
      a. Saccular aneurysm—pouchlike projection at one side of the artery
      b. Fusiform aneurysm—entire circumference of the artery wall is dilated
      c. Mycotic aneurysm—tiny weaknesses in the arterial wall that result from infection
      d. Dissecting aneurysm—tear in the inner lining of an arteriosclerotic aorta wall cause blood to form a hematoma between layers of the artery, and actually compress the lumen of the artery
   2. Causes
      a. Congenital weakness
      b. Atherosclerosis (most common cause of both thoracic and abdominal aortic aneurysms)
      c. Syphilis
      d. Trauma
   3. Represent surgical emergency if ruptured
B. Signs and symptoms
   1. Thoracic aortic aneurysm
      a. Subjective
         (1) May be asymptomatic
         (2) Pain resulting from pressure against the nerves or vertebrae
         (3) Dyspnea
         (4) Dysphagia
      b. Objective
         (1) Hoarseness, aphonia from impingement of laryngeal nerve
         (2) Cough

  (3) Unequal pulses and arterial pressure in upper extremities
  (4) Trachea may be displaced from midline due to adhesions between trachea and aneurysm
2. Abdominal aortic aneurysm
  a. Subjective
    (1) May be asymptomatic
    (2) Lower back or abdominal pain (severe if aneurysm leaking)
    (3) Sensory changes in the lower extremities if aneurysm ruptures
  b. Objective
    (1) Hypertension
    (2) Pulsating abdominal mass
    (3) Mottling of the lower extremities if aneurysm ruptures
    (4) Increased abdominal girth if aneurysm ruptures
3. Dissecting aortic aneurysm
  a. Subjective
    (1) Restlessness and anxiety
    (2) Severe pain
  b. Objective
    (1) Diminished pulses
    (2) Signs of shock
C. Treatment
  1. Resection of the aneurysm and use of a Teflon or Dacron graft
  2. Surgical procedures involving the aorta would necessitate use of a heart-lung device (cardiopulmonary bypass)
  3. Medical treatment is aimed at decreasing cardiac output and blood pressure through the use of drugs
D. Postoperative nursing care
  1. Monitor the vital signs and pulses of all extremities, including the posterior tibial and dorsalis pedis
  2. Monitor central venous pressure (CVP) frequently
  3. Record intake and output, since renal failure may occur after surgery
  4. Administer narcotics as ordered to alleviate pain
  5. Apply abdominal binders to provide support when the patient is coughing, deep breathing, and ambulating
  6. Prevent flexion of hip and knees to eliminate pressure on the arterial wall
  7. Apply elastic stockings and encourage dorsiflexion of the foot to help decrease the risk of thrombophlebitis
  8. Maintain patency of the nasogastric tube if present

Shock
A. Etiology and pathophysiology
  1. Hypovolemic—occurs when there is a loss of fluid resulting in inadequate tissue perfusion; caused by
    a. Excessive bleeding
    b. Excessive diarrhea or vomiting
    c. Fluid loss from fistulas or burns
  2. Cardiogenic—occurs when pump failure causes inadequate tissue perfusion; caused by
    a. Congestive heart failure
    b. Myocardial infarction
    c. Cardiac tamponade
  3. Neurogenic—caused by rapid vasodilation and subsequent pooling of blood within the peripheral vessels; caused by
    a. Spinal anesthesia
    b. Emotional tension
    c. Drugs that inhibit the sympathetic nervous system
  4. Anaphylactic—due to an allergic reaction that causes a release of histamine and subsequent vasodilation
  5. Septic—similar to anaphylaxis and is the body's reaction to bacterial toxins (generally gram-negative infections), which results in the leakage of plasma into tissues
B. Signs and symptoms
  1. Subjective
    a. Apprehension
    b. Restlessness
    c. Paresis of extremities
  2. Objective
    a. Weak, rapid, thready pulse
    b. Diaphoresis
    c. Cold, clammy skin
    d. Decreased blood pressure
    e. Decreased urine output
    f. Pallor
    g. Progressive loss of consciousness
    h. Lowered CVP readings
C. Treatment
  1. Aimed at correcting the underlying cause
  2. Fluid and blood replacement
  3. Oxygen therapy
  4. Vasoconstricting drugs to increase blood pressure
  5. Cardiac monitoring
  6. Cardiotonics, such as digitalis preparations, for cardiogenic shock
  7. Antihistamines for anaphylactic shock
  8. Antibiotics for septic shock based on blood cultures

9. Elevation of lower extremities to ensure circulation to vital organs
10. Intraaortic balloon pump may be used to aid the failing heart

D. Nursing care
1. Keep the patient warm
2. Check vital signs and CVP frequently
3. Monitor urine output and specific gravity
4. Allay anxiety
5. Carefully observe all responses to therapy

Anemia

A. Iron deficiency anemia
1. Etiology and pathophysiology
   a. Poor dietary habits leading to inadequate intake of iron
   b. Iron is essential for the formation of hemoglobin and erythrocytes needed to carry oxygen to cells
2. Signs and symptoms
   a. Subjective
      (1) Fatigue
      (2) Headache
      (3) Paresthesias
   b. Objective
      (1) Ankle edema
      (2) Dry, pale mucous membranes
      (3) Pearly white sclera
      (4) Decreased hemoglobin and erythrocytes
      (5) Increased iron binding capacity
3. Treatment
   a. Improve diet; include ascorbic acid, which stimulates iron uptake
   b. Iron supplements
4. Nursing care
   a. Diet teaching
   b. Teach the patient about the side effects of medications

B. Pernicious anemia
1. Etiology and pathophysiology
   a. Lack of intrinsic factor in the stomach prevents the absorption of vitamin B_{12} in the lower portion of the ileum
   b. Subsequent reduced number of erythrocytes formed, leading to anemia
2. Signs and symptoms
   a. Subjective
      (1) Weakness
      (2) Sore mouth
      (3) Paresthesias
      (4) Dyspnea
   b. Objective
      (1) Pallor
      (2) Beefy red tongue
      (3) Positive Romberg test (loss of balance when eyes close)
      (4) Gastric analysis—no intrinsic factor
      (5) Schilling test—urine test for B_{12} absorption
3. Treatment—lifetime cyanocobalamin (B_{12}) injections
4. Nursing care
   a. Explain disease process and the need for continued treatment
   b. Teach family member(s) how to give IM injections or make referral to visiting nurse

C. Aplastic anemia (hypoplastic anemia)
1. Etiology and pathophysiology
   a. Bone marrow is depressed or destroyed by a chemical or drug
   b. Leukopenia, thrombocytopenia, and decreased erythrocytes
2. Signs and symptoms
   a. Subjective
      (1) Headache
      (2) Weakness
      (3) Anorexia
      (4) Dyspnea
   b. Objective
      (1) Fever
      (2) Bleeding from mucous membranes
      (3) Decreased leukocytes, erythrocytes, and platelets
3. Treatment
   a. Identify and eliminate causative agent
   b. Blood transfusions
   c. Maintenance of fluid and electrolyte balance
4. Nursing care
   a. Support the patient and family in understanding illness
   b. Prevent infection by reverse isolation

Blood Dyscrasias

A. Thrombocytopenic purpura
1. Etiology and pathophysiology—bleeding disorder of unknown origin (possibly autoimmune) in which there is a reduction of platelets
2. Signs and symptoms
   a. Subjective
      (1) History of epistaxis
      (2) History of gum bleeding
   b. Objective
      (1) Low platelet count
      (2) Ecchymotic areas
      (3) Hemorrhagic petechiae

3. Treatment
   a. Corticosteroids
   b. Immunosuppressive agents
   c. Splenectomy
   d. Platelet transfusions
4. Nursing care
   a. Prevent injury and bruises
   b. Encourage patient to adhere to medical regimen
   c. Teach the side effects of medications, particularly proness to infection
   d. Provide postoperative care related to splenectomy
B. Polycythemia vera
   1. Etiology and pathophysiology—disorder of unknown origin that results in an increased number of erythrocytes, leukocytes, and platelets
   2. Signs and symptoms
      a. Subjective
         (1) Headache
         (2) Weakness
         (3) Itching
      b. Objective
         (1) Increased hemoglobin
         (2) Purple-red complexion
         (3) Dyspnea
         (4) Bleeding from mucous membranes
   3. Treatment
      a. Phlebotomy several times yearly
      b. Diet low in iron
      c. Radioactive phosphorus; busulfan (Myleran)
   4. Nursing care
      a. Discuss diet with the patient and family
      b. Supportive care and prevention of hemorrhage
      c. Assist with phlebotomy
C. Agranulocytosis
   1. Etiology and pathophysiology
      a. Results in a decreased number of leukocytes
      b. Thought to arise from physical agents (e.g., heavy metals) and cytotoxic drugs
   2. Signs and symptoms
      a. Subjective
         (1) Fatigue
         (2) Malaise
      b. Objective
         (1) High fever
         (2) Necrotic ulcers of mucosa
         (3) Rapid weak pulse
   3. Treatment
      a. Removal of causative agent
      b. Transfusions
      c. Antibiotics

4. Nursing care
   a. Prevent infection and observe for signs of infection
   b. Careful oral hygiene
   c. Bed rest
   d. High-vitamin diet
D. Disseminated intravascular coagulation (DIC)
   1. Etiology and pathophysiology
      a. Body's response to injury or disease in which microthrombi obstruct the blood supply of organs
      b. Complicated by hemorrhage at various sites throughout the body
   2. Signs and symptoms
      a. Subjective
         (1) Restlessness
         (2) Anxiety
      b. Objective
         (1) Laboratory tests indicate low fibrinogen and prolonged prothrombin and partial thromboplastin times
         (2) Hemorrhage, both subcutaneous and internal
   3. Treatment
      a. Goal is to relieve the underlying cause
      b. Heparin to prevent the formation of thrombi
      c. Transfusion of blood products
   4. Nursing care
      a. Observe for bleeding
      b. Minimize skin punctures
      c. Prevent injury
      d. Provide emotional support

Leukemia

A. Etiology and pathophysiology
   1. Incidence highest in children ages 3 to 4; declines until age 35, at which point there is a steady increase
   2. Etiology unknown, although exposure to certain toxic substances such as radiation seems to increase the incidence
   3. In general, an uncontrolled proliferation of white blood cells
   4. Classified according to the type of white cell affected
      a. Acute lymphocytic leukemia
         (1) Primarily occurs in children
         (2) Most favorable prognosis with chemotherapy
         (3) Results from abnormal leukocytes in blood-forming tissue
      b. Acute myelogenous leukemia

(1) Occurs throughout life cycle

(2) Prognosis is poor with or without chemotherapy

(3) Results from inability of leukocytes to mature; those that do are abnormal

c. Chronic myelogenous leukemia

(1) Occurs after the second decade

(2) Prognosis is poor

(3) Results from abnormal production of granulocytic cells

d. Chronic lymphocytic leukemia

(1) Occurs after age 35

(2) Life expectancy some 4 to 5 years

(3) Results from increased production of leukocytes and lymphocytes and proliferation of cells within the bone marrow, spleen, and liver

B. Signs and symptoms

1. Subjective

a. Malaise

b. Bone pain

2. Objective

a. Anemia

b. Thrombocytopenia

c. Elevated leukocytes

d. Decreased platelets

e. Petechiae

f. Gingival bleeding

C. Treatment

1. Chemotherapy

2. Transfusions of whole blood or blood fractions

3. Analgesics

4. Bone marrow transplant

D. Nursing care

1. Discuss the importance of follow-up care with the patient and/or family

2. Emotional support for patient and family

3. Specific nursing responsibilities related to particular chemotherapeutic therapy, transfusion, or diagnostic tests

Infectious Mononucleosis

A. Etiology and pathophysiology

1. Acute infectious disease of the lymphatic system due to Epstein-Barr (EB) herpesvirus

2. Transmitted by respiratory droplets

3. Incubation period is uncertain; probably 28 to 42 days

4. Incidence highest between ages 15 and 35

5. Complications include hepatitis, ruptured spleen, pericarditis, and meningoencephalitis

B. Signs and symptoms

1. Subjective

a. Sore throat

b. Malaise

c. Stiff neck

d. Nausea

2. Objective

a. Elevated temperature

b. Enlarged, tender lymph nodes (generally, posterior cervical nodes involved first)

c. Splenomegaly in approximately 50% of patients

d. Elevated lymphocyte and monocyte counts

e. Positive heterophile antibody agglutination test

C. Treatment

1. Generally directed toward symptoms (recovery is approximately 3 weeks)

2. A.S.A.; steroids if severely ill

3. If spleen ruptures, splenectomy and blood transfusions

D. Nursing care

1. Provide rest

2. Administer A.S.A. as indicated

3. Assess for signs of complications; the spleen should not be palpated once the diagnosis is made

4. Increase fluid intake

Hodgkin's Disease

A. Etiology and pathophysiology

1. Cause unknown

2. Higher incidence in females and young adults

3. Proliferation of malignant cells (Reed-Sternberg cells) within lymph nodes

4. All tissues may eventually be involved, but chiefly lymph nodes, spleen, liver, tonsils, and bone marrow

5. Classification by staging and the presence or absence of systemic symptoms

B. Signs and symptoms

1. Subjective

a. Dyspnea and dysphagia due to pressure from enlarged nodes

b. Pruritus

c. Anorexia

2. Objective

a. Enlarged lymph nodes (generally cervical nodes are involved first)

b. Diagnosis confirmed by histologic examination of a lymph node

c. Progressive anemia

d. Elevated temperature

　　　e. Enlarged spleen and liver may occur
　　　f. Pressure from enlarged lymph nodes may cause symptoms of edema and obstructive jaundice
　　　g. Thrombocytopenia if spleen and bone marrow involved
C. Treatment
　1. Radiotherapy
　　　a. Vital organs must be shielded
　　　b. Potential side effects
　　　　(1) Nausea
　　　　(2) Skin rashes
　　　　(3) Dry mouth
　　　　(4) Dysphagia
　2. Surgical intervention
　　　a. Excision of node for biopsy
　　　b. Excision of masses to relieve pressure on other organs
　　　c. Laparotomy or laparoscopy for determination of stage
　3. Chemotherapy
　　　a. Nitrogen mustard
　　　b. Thiophosphoramide (Thiotepa)
　　　c. Chlorambucil
　　　d. Vincristine
　　　e. Doxorubicin (Adriamycin)
　　　f. Prednisone
D. Nursing care
　1. Provide emotional support for the patient and family
　2. Protect from infection
　3. Monitor temperature
　4. Observe for signs of anemia; provide adequate rest
　5. Examine sclera and skin for signs of jaundice
　6. Provide diet as tolerated; observe for anorexia and nausea

Lymphosarcoma

A. Etiology and pathophysiology
　1. Malignant tumors of the lymph nodes and lymphatic tissue
　2. Gastrointestinal tract, tonsils, spleen, and liver frequently involved
　3. Cause unknown; incidence is increased in patients who have immunologic disorders
B. Signs and symptoms
　1. Subjective
　　　a. Malaise
　　　b. Lethargy
　2. Objective
　　　a. Painless lymphadenopathy

　　　b. Fever
　　　c. Diaphoresis
　　　d. Weight loss
　　　e. Decreased resistance to disease
C. Treatment similar to that for Hodgkin's disease
D. Nursing care similar to that for Hodgkin's disease

Respiratory System

REVIEW OF ANATOMY AND PHYSIOLOGY OF THE RESPIRATORY SYSTEM
Functions

A. To make possible exchange of gases between blood and air
B. To make possible cellular respiration

Organs

Nose

A. Structure
　1. Portions
　　　a. Internal—in skull, above roof of mouth
　　　b. External—protruding from face
　2. Cavities
　　　a. Divisions—right and left
　　　b. Meati—superior, middle, and lower; named for turbinates located above each meatus
　　　c. Openings
　　　　(1) To exterior—anterior nares
　　　　(2) To nasopharynx—posterior nares
　　　d. Conchae (turbinates)
　　　　(1) Superior and middle processes of ethmoid bone; inferior conchae, separate bones
　　　　(2) Conchae partition each nasal cavity into 3 passageways or meati
　　　e. Floor—formed by palatine bones and maxillae; these also act as roof of mouth
　3. Lining—ciliated mucosa
　4. Sinuses draining into the nose (paranasal sinuses)
　　　a. Frontal
　　　b. Maxillary (antrum of Highmore)
　　　c. Sphenoidal
　　　d. Ethmoidal
B. Functions
　1. Serves as passageway for incoming and outgoing air, filtering, warming, moistening, and chemically examining it
　2. Organ of smell (olfactory receptors located in the nasal mucosa)
　3. Aids in phonation

Pharynx

A. Structure—composed of muscle with mucous lining
1. Divisions
   a. Nasopharynx—behind the nose
   b. Oropharynx—behind the mouth
   c. Laryngopharynx—behind the larynx
2. Openings
   a. In the nasopharynx—4 openings: 2 auditory (eustachian) tubes and 2 posterior nares
   b. In the oropharynx—1 opening: fauces, archway into mouth
   c. In the laryngopharynx—2 openings: into esophagus and into larynx
3. Organs in the pharynx
   a. In nasopharynx—nasopharyngeal tonsils (adenoids)
   b. In oropharynx—palatine and lingual tonsils
B. Functions
1. Serves as a passage way and entrance to the respiratory and digestive tracts
2. Aids in phonation
3. Tonsils function to destroy incoming bacteria and detoxify certain foreign proteins

Larynx

A. Location—at upper end of the trachea, just below the pharynx
B. Structure
1. Cartilages—9 pieces arranged in a boxlike formation; thyroid cartilage is the largest (called the "Adam's apple"); epiglottis (the "lid" cartilage); cricoid (the "signet ring" cartilage)
2. Vocal cords
   a. False cords—folds of mucous lining
   b. True cords—fibroelastic bands stretched across the hollow interior of the larynx; the paired vocal cords (folds) and the posterior arytenoid cartilages make up the glottis; the slit between the vocal cords, through which air enters and leaves the lower respiratory passages, is the rima glottidis
3. Lining—ciliated mucosa
C. Functions
1. Voice production—during expiration, air passing through the larynx causes the vocal cords to vibrate; short, tense cords produce a high pitch; long, relaxed cords, a low pitch
2. Serves as part of the passageway for air and as the entrance to the lower respiratory tract

Trachea

A. Structure
1. Walls—smooth muscle; contain C-shaped rings of cartilage at intervals; these keep the tube open at all times but do not constrict the esophagus, which is directly behind the trachea
2. Lining—ciliated mucosa
3. Extent—from the larynx to the bronchi; 10 to 11 cm (about 4½ inches) long
B. Function—furnishes open passageway for air going to and from lungs

Lungs

A. Structure
1. Size—large enough to fill pleural divisions of thoracic cavity
2. Shape—cone, base downward
3. Location—in pleural divisions of thorax; extend from slightly above clavicle to diaphragm; base of each lung rests on diaphragm
4. Divisions
   a. Lobes—3 in the right lung, 2 in the left
   b. Root—consists of the primary bronchus and pulmonary artery and veins bound together by connective tissue
   c. Hilum—vertical slit on medial surface of the lung, through which root structures enter the lung
   d. Apex—pointed upper part of the lung
   e. Base—broad, inferior surface of the lung
5. Bronchial tree—consists of the following
   a. Bronchi—right and left, formed by branching of the trachea; right bronchus slightly larger and more vertical than left; each primary bronchus branches, on entering the lung, into 10 segmental bronchi in each lung; primary and segmental bronchi all contain C-shaped cartilaginous rings
   b. Bronchioles—small branches off the secondary bronchi; distinguished by lack of C-shaped cartilage and a duct diameter of about 1 mm
   c. Terminal bronchioles—last ones possessing a ciliated mucosa
   d. Respiratory bronchioles—composed of cuboidal nonciliated cells
   e. Alveolar ducts—microscopic branches off bronchioles composed of a thin squamous epithelium
   f. Alveoli—microscopic sacs composed of single layer of extremely thin squamous epithelial cells; each alveolar duct terminates in cluster of alveoli, often likened to a bunch of grapes; each alveolus enveloped by network of lung capillaries
6. Covering of lung—visceral layer of pleura

B. Function—place where air and blood can come in close enough contact for rapid diffusion of gases to occur
1. Bronchi, bronchioles, alveolar ducts—lower part of airway through which air moves into and out of alveoli
2. Alveoli—microscopic sacs in which gases are exchanged rapidly between the air and blood; membranous walls of the millions of alveoli provide a surface area large enough and thin enough to make possible rapid gas exchange
3. Alveolar surfaces coated with group of substances called surfactant; effect is to lower alveolar surface tension to facilitate breathing, since sacs have less tendency to collapse with their walls adhering to each other

Physiology of Respiration

A. Mechanism of inspiration
1. Respiratory muscles contract
2. Thorax increases in size
3. Intrathoracic pressure decreases
4. Lungs increase in size
5. Intrapulmonic pressure decreases
6. Air rushes from positive pressure in the atmosphere to negative pressure in the alveoli
7. Inspiration is completed
B. Mechanism of expiration
1. Respiratory muscles relax
2. Thorax decreases in size
3. Intrathoracic pressure increases
4. Lungs decrease in size
5. Intrapulmonic pressure increases
6. Air expelled from higher pressure in the lung to lower pressure in the atmosphere
7. Expiration is completed
C. Neural control
1. Alveolar stretch receptors respond to inspiration (lung inflation) by sending inhibitory impulses to inspiratory neurons in brainstem; this is the Hering-Breuer inflation reflex, and it prevents lung overdistension
2. During expiration (lung deflation) the stretch receptors no longer inhibit inspiratory neurons, and inspiration may begin again; this is the Hering-Breuer deflation reflex
D. Chemical control
1. Blood pH—decrease in pH—stimulates respiration by direct stimulation of neurons of respiratory center and indirectly by stimulation of carotid and aortic chemoreceptors
2. Blood PCO_2—increase in arterial PCO_2 results in

decrease in pH and mimics effects in no. 1 above
3. Stimulation of respiratory center neurons or chemoreceptors results in hyperventilation; hypoventilation occurs when the arterial pH rises or the arterial PCO_2 falls
E. Amount of air exchanged in breathing
1. Directly related to gas pressure gradient between atmosphere and alveoli and inversely related to resistance opposing air flow; the greater the difference between atmospheric pressure and alveolar pressure, the greater the amount of air exchanged in breathing; the greater the resistance opposing air flow to or from the lungs, the less air exchanged
2. Measured by apparatus called a spirometer
3. Tidal air—average amount expired after normal inspiration; approximately 500 ml
4. Expiratory reserve volume (ERV)—largest additional volume of air that can be forcibly expired after a normal inspiration and expiration; normal ERV 1000 to 1200 ml
5. Inspiratory reserve volume (IRV)—largest additional volume of air that can be forcibly inspired after a normal inspiration; normal IRV 3000 to 3300 ml
6. Residual air—that which cannot be forcibly expired from lungs; about 1200 ml
7. Minimal air—that which can never be removed from alveoli if they have been inflated even once, even though lungs are subjected to atmospheric pressure that squeezes part of residual air out
8. Vital capacity—approximate capacity of lungs as measured by amount of air that can be forcibly expired after forcible inspiration; varies with size of thoracic cavity, which is determined by various factors (e.g., size of rib cage, posture, volume of blood and interstitial fluid in the lungs, size of the heart)
9. Maximal expiratory flow rate—an individual should be able to exhale 70% of his vital capacity in the first second and empty more than 90% in 3 seconds; asthma and emphysema prevent such normal, forced expiratory rates; measurable with a spirometer
F. Diffusion of gases between air and blood occurs across alveolar-capillary membranes (i.e., in lungs between air in alveoli and venous blood in lung capillaries)
1. Direction of diffusion
   a. Oxygen—net diffusion toward lower oxygen

Fig. 3. Mechanism of oxygen diffusion.

Fig. 4. Mechanism of carbon dioxide diffusion.

pressure gradient (i.e., from alveolar air to blood)

   b. Carbon dioxide—net diffusion toward lower carbon dioxide pressure gradient (i.e., from blood to alveolar air)

  2. Mechanism of oxygen diffusion (Fig. 3)

  3. Mechanism of carbon dioxide diffusion (Fig. 4)

G. How blood transports oxygen

  1. As solute—about 0.5 ml of oxygen is dissolved in 100 ml of blood; produces the blood P_{O_2} (pressure of oxygen in the blood)

  2. As oxyhemoglobin—each gram of hemoglobin can combine with 1.34 ml of oxygen; hence, with normal hemglobin content (e.g., 15 g per 100 ml of blood) and 100% oxygen saturation, about 20 ml (15×1.34) of oxygen is transported as oxyhemoglobin

  3. Various factors influence rate at which oxygen associates with hemoglobin to form oxyhemoglobin, including

   a. Increasing pressure of oxygen in the blood

   b. Decreasing pressure of carbon dioxide in the blood

  4. Various factors influence the rate at which oxygen dissociates from hemoglobin, including

   a. Decreasing pressure of oxygen in the blood

   b. Increasing pressure of carbon dioxide in the blood

   c. Increased blood temperature

H. How blood transports carbon dioxide

  1. As solute—small amount dissolves in plasma

  2. As bicarbonate ion—more than half of carbon dioxide in blood is present in the plasma as bicarbonate ion (HCO_3^-) formed by ionization of carbonic acid

  3. As carbhemoglobin—less than one third of carbon dioxide is transported in combination with hemoglobin

I. Diffusion of gases between arterial blood and tissues occurs in tissue capillaries

  1. Oxygen—net diffusion of dissolved oxygen out of the blood into the tissues because of lower P_{O_2} there (perhaps 30 mm Hg, compared to arterial P_{O_2} of 100 mm Hg); diffusion of dissolved oxygen out of the blood lowers blood P_{O_2} from arterial to venous level (from 100 to 40 mm Hg); decreasing P_{O_2} as the blood moves through tissue capillaries causes oxygen to dissociate from hemoglobin, thereby releasing more oxygen for diffusion out of the blood to the tissue cells

  2. Carbon dioxide—net diffusion of carbon dioxide into the blood because of lower P_{CO_2} there (40 mm Hg compared with probably over 50 mm Hg in tissues); diffusion of carbon dioxide into tissue capillaries increases blood P_{CO_2} from arterial to venous level (from 40 to 46 mm Hg); increasing P_{CO_2} like decreasing P_{O_2} tends to accelerate oxygen dissociation from hemoglobin

REVIEW OF PHYSICAL PRINCIPLES RELATED TO THE RESPIRATORY SYSTEM
Principles of Mechanics

Law of Gravitation
EXAMPLES
1. Postural drainage—positioning the patient so the throat is below level of the lungs to help drain fluid from the lungs
2. Rocking beds—abdominal viscera alternately push against and then away from the diaphragm, thus aiding in respiration
3. Position of the head postoperatively—head is placed on one side; thus, the force of gravity pulls the tongue down, breathing remains unobstructed and allows for drainage in case of vomiting
4. Use of chest tubes to restore negative pressure to intrapleural space

Momentum
EXAMPLES
1. During a cough or a sneeze, the abdominal and intercostal muscles apply a large force on the air in the lungs; the sudden opening of the vocal cords and epiglottis results in the explosive propulsion of air from the lungs; in this case momentum of the air stream is great, not because of the mass of the particles (since the molecules of gasses in air are light), but because of their high velocity
2. When a person speaks, the vocal cords vibrate and in turn produce vibrations in the air molecules surrounding them; the momentum in these vibrating molecules is transferred from air molecule to air molecule all the way to the ear of the listener, where the vibrations are converted into nerve impulses that the brain interprets as sound

Energy
EXAMPLES
1. Epithelial cells of the human respiratory tract possess energy because their cilia beat back and forth and thus do the work of pushing mucus and foreign matter up toward the throat
2. Every living cell in the body possesses energy because it does work to maintain certain water and electrolyte concentrations within itself
3. The cilia exert a force that moves them through a certain distance in the fluid surrounding them
4. The cell membranes exert a force that moves ions a certain distance through the membrane
5. Second law of thermodynamics

Principles of Physical Properties of Matter

Solids
Concept of elasticity
EXAMPLE: The elastic recoil of the lungs during quiet respiration provides the entire force necessary to effect expiration

Liquids
Surface tension—molecules of a liquid exert forces of attraction on one another; at the surface of the liquid the molecules are attracted by other molecules at the bottom and sides, but not at the top since air is there; this results in a force of contraction at the liquid surface called surface tension
EXAMPLE: The alveoli and respiratory passages of the human lungs have a mixture of surface tension–reducing substances collectively called surfactant that reduce surface tension and the pull that the water molecules would ordinarily have on each other if these surface active agents were absent; breathing is therefore much easier because of this agent

Gases
The molecules composing gases are so far apart that they do not exert any cohesive forces on each other; consequently, the gas will expand to fill any container and will exert pressure on the container because of elastic rebound of the gas molecules with the walls of the container
A. Boyle's law—at constant temperature the pressure exerted by a gas is inversely proportional to its volume; as the volume of a gas is decreased, its pressure increases, and as the volume is increased, the pressure decreases
   1. Respiration—contraction and downward movements of the dome-shaped diaphragm increase the volume of the thoracic cavity containing the lungs; since the volume of air in the lungs is increased, the pressure exerted by the air is decreased; air now flows from the area of higher pressure outside the body to the area of lower pressure inside the lungs; conversely, during expiration, the upward movement of the diaphragm and the elastic recoil of the lungs themselves decrease the volume of air in the thoracic cavity and lungs as air flows out
   2. Pneumothorax—opening that connects the outside air with the intrapleural space; result is that air flows into the intrapleural space; this eliminates the pressure gradient between the thoracic cavity and the atmosphere, and the lungs cannot inflate
   3. Intermittent positive pressure breathing (IPPB) apparatus—special valve is operated by the individual's own respirations; on inspiration, one

part of the valve opens and oxygen or a mixture of gases is forcefully pushed under greater than atmospheric pressure (positive pressure) into the lungs through a special mouthpiece or face mask

B. Dalton's law—pressure exerted (in millimeters of mercury [mm Hg]) by a gas in a mixture of gases is proportional to its percentage in the mixture; e.g., partial pressure of oxygen (O_2) in alveoli is 104 mm Hg; partial pressure of O_2 in pulmonary artery and alveolar capillaries is 40 mm Hg; therefore O_2 diffuses from alveoli air sacs into capillaries

C. Henry's law—quantity of gas dissolving in a liquid is proportional to the partial pressure of the gas at a given temperature; i.e., a person overcome by smoke inhalation or who has some obstruction to normal breathing can benefit from inhalation of either pure O_2 or a mixture of gases having a higher partial pressure of O_2 than is found in air

D. Bernoulli's principle—moving air exerts less pressure than motionless air

Principles of Light

A. X rays use high-frequency electromagnetic waves
   EXAMPLE: The chest x-ray examination permits observation of a variety of lung disorders, such as pneumonia, tumors, and tuberculosis

B. Total internal reflection—at a certain critical angle, light between two media is not refracted (bent) through the media but is reflected back into the first medium
   EXAMPLE: Fiberoptics allows illumination and visualization of trachea and bronchi (bronchoscopy); the image picked up by the lens internally reflects along fiberoptic tubing (even if bent) until it reaches the eye of the observer

REVIEW OF CHEMICAL PRINCIPLES RELATED TO THE RESPIRATORY SYSTEM

(Same as cardiovascular)

REVIEW OF MICROORGANISMS RELATED TO THE RESPIRATORY SYSTEM

A. Bacterial pathogens
   1. *Bordetella pertussis*—small, gram-negative coccobacillus; causes pertussis or whooping cough
   2. *Streptococcus pneumoniae*—gram-positive, encapsulated diplococcus; on the basis of the antigenic nature of the capsule there are about 100 types, the most important being Types I, II, and III; causes pneumococcal pneumonia (most commonly lobar) and often responsible for sinusitis, otitis media, and meningitis
   3. *Haemophilus influenzae*—small gram-negative,

highly pleomorphic bacillus; causes acute meningitis and upper respiratory tract infections
   4. *Klebsiella pneumoniae* (Friedländer's bacillus)—gram-negative, encapsulated, non-spore-forming bacillus; causes pneumonia and urinary tract infections
   5. *Mycobacterium tuberculosis* (tubercle bacillus)—acid-fast actinomycete (thin, waxy rods, often bent, nonmotile, non-spore forming); causes tuberculosis

B. Rickettsial pathogen
   Coxiella burnetii—only species of rickettsiae not associated with a vector; causes Q fever, an infection clinically similar to primary atypical pneumonia

C. Viral pathogens
   1. DNA viruses
      Adenoviruses—spherical, 70 to 80 nm in diameter; cause acute respiratory tract disease, adenitis, pharyngitis, and other respiratory tract infections as well as conjunctivitis
   2. RNA viruses
      a. Coronaviruses—enveloped pleomorphic viruses; frequently associated with a mild upper respiratory tract infection
      b. Picornaviruses—spherical and 20 to 30 nm in diameter; cause poliomyelitis, Coxsackie disease, common cold, and various diseases of animals
      c. Reoviruses—double-stranded RNA virus involved in mild respiratory tract infections of humans

D. Fungal pathogen
   Histoplasma capsulatum—dimorphic fungus producing characteristic spores (chlamydospores) in infected tissue; causes histoplasmosis (a primary lung infection)

PHARMACOLOGY RELATED TO RESPIRATORY SYSTEM DISORDERS

A. Bronchodilators
   1. General implications for nurses
      a. Administer via correct route (oral, rectal, parenteral, inhalation)
      b. Monitor vital signs for changes
      c. Observe for signs of adequate oxygenation such as warmth and color
      d. Teach the patient the action and side effects of therapy
      e. Observe for side effects
         (1) Dizziness, nervousness
         (2) Gastric irritation
         (3) Palpitations

2. Theophylline derivatives
   a. Actions
      (1) Directly on bronchial smooth muscle, decreasing spasm and relaxing smooth muscle of the vasculature
      (2) Direct stimulatory effect on myocardium increases cardiac output, which improves blood flow to kidneys
      (3) Directly on renal tubules, providing a diuretic effect by increasing excretion of sodium and chloride ions
   b. Examples
      (1) Aminophylline
      (2) Dyphylline (Dilor, Neothylline)
      (3) Oxtriphylline (Choledyl)
      (4) Theophylline (Aqualin, Elixophyllin)
3. Sympathetic amines
   a. Actions
      (1) Act at beta-adrenergic receptors in bronchus to relax smooth muscle and increase respiratory volume
      (2) Inhalants have a local action causing vasoconstriction that reduces congestion or edema
      (3) With large doses the myocardium is stimulated, which results in an increased cardiac output
   b. Examples
      (1) Epinephrine hydrochloride (Adrenalin, Epifrin)
      (2) Epinephrine, aqueous (Sus-Phrine)
      (3) Ethylnorepinephrine hydrochloride (Bronkephrine)
      (4) Ephedrine sulfate
      (5) Pseudoephedrine hydrochloride (Sudafed)
      (6) Metaproterenol sulfate (Alupent, Metaprel)
      (7) Terbutaline sulfate (Brethine)
      (8) Aminophylline
      (9) Isoproterenol hydrochloride (Isuprel)
B. Mucolytic agents and expectorants
   1. General implications for nurses
      a. Observe for respiratory distress
      b. Have mechanical suction apparatus available in the event the patient is unable to cough up secretions
      c. Wash the patient's face after administration, since stickiness is common
      d. Administer drugs diluted as ordered; do not directly follow expectorants with other fluid intake
      e. Observe the patient for adverse effects

(1) Nausea
(2) Skin eruptions
(3) Jitteriness
      f. Increase fluid intake to loosen secretions
      g. Encourage coughing and deep breathing
   2. Mucolytic agents
      a. Action—raise osmolality of bronchial glandular secretions, causing fluid to dilute the secretions
      b. Examples
         (1) Calcium iodide
         (2) Glyceryl guaiacolate (Robitussin)
         (3) Iodinated glycerol (Organidin)
         (4) Potassium iodide (SSKI, Pima Syrup)
   3. Expectorants
      a. Action—increase production of thinner, less viscid secretions that protect bronchial tissues
      b. Examples
         (1) Acetylcysteine (Mucomyst)
         (2) Glyceryl guaiacolate (Guaifenesin, Robitussin)
         (3) Terpin hydrate elixer
C. Antitussives
   1. General implications for nurses
      a. Explain side effects to the patient
      b. Advise the patient not to take liquids for 15 minutes after administration
      c. Provide adequate fluids and put the patient in a semi-Fowler or high Fowler position to support respiratory processes
      d. Observe for adverse effects
         (1) Hypersensitivity
         (2) Nausea
         (3) Drowsiness
   2. Narcotic antitussives
      a. Actions
         (1) Suppress cough reflex by acting on the medullary control center
         (2) Usually employed when cough is not productive
      b. Examples
         (1) Hydrocodone bitartrate (Codone, Dicodid)
         (2) Levopropoxyphene napsylate (Novrad)
         (3) Noscapine (Nectadon)
   3. Nonnarcotic antitussives
      a. Action—inhibit cough reflex at afferent endings of the vagus nerve and at medullary transmission sites
      b. Examples
         (1) Benzonatate (Tessalon)
         (2) Dextromethorphan hydrobromide (Romilar, Sucrets)

4. Antihistaminic cough suppressants
   a. Action—prevent histamine-induced edema, causing irritation of cough-sensitive nerve endings in tracheobronchial structures
   b. Examples
      (1) Chlophedianol hydrochloride (Ulo)
      (2) Diphenhydramine hydrochloride (Benadryl)
D. Drugs that antagonize the effects of narcotics
   1. General implications for nurses
      a. Carefully monitor vital signs, especially respirations
      b. Prepare for emergency resuscitative measures
      c. Be alert to withdrawal symptoms
      d. Observe for adverse effects
         (1) Respiratory depression when drug used alone
         (2) Lethargy, dizziness
         (3) Nausea and vomiting
         (4) Miosis (constriction of pupils)
   2. Actions
      a. Compete with narcotics for receptors at the respiratory center
      b. Lower threshold for carbon dioxide stimulation of respiration (increase respiratory rate and tidal volume, which decreases blood CO_2 level)
   3. Examples
      a. Levallorphan tartrate (Lorfan)
      b. Nalorphine hydrochloride (Nalline)
      c. Naloxone hydrochloride (Narcan)
E. Drugs that have an antihistaminic effect
   1. General implications for nurses
      a. Caution the patient regarding operating machinery and driving while taking this medication
      b. Advise the patient to report side effects to the physician
      c. If given IM, inject deep to prevent irritation to tissue
      d. Observe for adverse effects
         (1) Inability to concentrate
         (2) Insomnia
         (3) Ataxia
         (4) Tremors
         (5) Headache
         (6) Nausea, anorexia
         (7) Diarrhea
   2. Actions
      a. Interfere with histaminic effect by competing for extravascular receptors at arteriole sites

   b. Block histamine-induced irritation of nerve endings, causing itching or burning, dilation of arterioles, and constriction of venules, which leads to transudation of fluid into the tissues
   c. Prevent progression but have no effect on existing problems
   d. Also have an antiemetic, anticholinergic, and central nervous system depressant effect
3. Examples
   a. Brompheniramine maleate (Dimetane)
   b. Chlorpheniramine maleate (Chlor-Trimeton, Histaspan, Teldrin)
   c. Cyproheptadine hydrochloride (Periactin)
   d. Methdilazine hydrochloride (Tacaryl)
   e. Chlorothen citrate (Tagathen)
   f. Methapyrilene hydrochloride (Histadyl)
   g. Pyrilamine maleate
   h. Tripelennamine citrate (Pyribenzamine)
   i. Carbinoxamine maleate (Clistin)
   j. Diphenhydramine hydrochloride (Benadryl)
   k. Doxylamine succinate (Decapryn)
   l. Hydroxyzine hydrochloride (Atarax)
   m. Hydroxyzine pamoate (Vistaril)

RELATED DIAGNOSTIC PROCEDURES
Bronchoscopy

A. Definition
   1. Visualization of the tracheobronchial tree via a scope advanced through the mouth into the bronchi
   2. Procedure may be performed to remove foreign body, to remove secretions, or to obtain specimens of tissue or mucus for further study
B. Nursing responsibilities
   1. Obtain an informed consent
   2. Maintain the patient n.p.o. prior to procedure and remove dentures and jewelry
   3. Administer ordered preprocedure medications to produce sedation and decrease anxiety
   4. Postprocedure responsibilities
      a. Monitor vital signs until stable
      b. Do not allow the patient to drink until the gag reflex returns
      c. Inform patient to expect some hemoptysis after the procedure
      d. Observe the patient for signs of hemorrhage and/or respiratory distress

Pulmonary Function Tests

A. Definition
   1. Series of tests used to detect problems in the performance capabilities of the pulmonary system

2. A spirometer is used to measure amounts of gas exchanged between the patient and the atmosphere; nose clips are used to allow only mouth breathing and prevent air leakage
3. Measurement studies include
   a. Tidal volume—amount of air inhaled or exhaled during one respiration
   b. Vital capacity—volume of air that can be forcefully exhaled after a maximum inspiration
   c. Total lung capacity—volume of air in the lungs following a maximum inspiration
B. Nursing responsibilities
   1. Explain procedure to the patient to allay anxiety and promote compliance at time of test
   2. Notify the respiratory therapist of all medications that the patient is receiving which affect respiratory function

Thoracentesis

A. Definition
   1. Surgical aseptic procedure in which the chest wall is punctured with a trocar to remove fluid or air; this is done for diagnostic purposes or to alleviate respiratory embarrassment
   2. No more than 1000 ml of fluid should be removed at a time; fluid withdrawn should be sent to the laboratory for culture and sensitivity tests
   3. Complications include pneumothorax from trauma to the lung and pulmonary edema as a result of sudden fluid shifts
B. Nursing responsibilities
   1. Obtain an informed consent
   2. Explain procedure to the patient
   3. Ensure that chest x-ray examination is done prior to and after the procedure
   4. Assist and support the patient in the sitting position
   5. Set up a sterile field for the physician
   6. Assess pulse and respirations prior to, during, and after the procedure
   7. Inform the patient not to cough during the procedure to prevent trauma to the lungs
   8. After the procedure, label and send specimens for laboratory tests
   9. Note and record the amount, color, and clarity of the fluid withdrawn
   10. Place the patient on opposite side for approximately 1 hour to prevent leakage of fluid through the thoracentesis site
   11. Observe the patient for coughing, bloody sputum, and rapid pulse rate and report their occurrence immediately

Sputum Studies

A. Definition—analysis of sputum for pathogenic bacteria or tumor cells
   1. Culture and sensitivity—identification of bacteria and appropriate antibiotic therapy; the specimen should be obtained prior to institution of antibiotic therapy
   2. Acid-fast bacteria (AFB)—staining technique to identify bacilli as acid fast, generally indicative of *Mycobacterium tuberculosis*
   3. Cytology—microscopic examination of pulmonary epithelial cells that have sloughed off into the sputum; performed when malignancy is suspected
B. Nursing responsibilities
   1. Collect in the early morning before the patient has eaten or drunk, or after aerosol treatment
   2. Have the patient rinse his mouth with water to decrease contamination of specimen with oropharyngeal microorganisms
   3. Instruct the patient to take several deep breaths and cough deeply to raise sputum and expectorate into a sterile specimen container; care must be taken to avoid touching the inside of the container
   4. Transport the specimen to the laboratory promptly
   5. Offer oral hygiene after collection to eliminate foul taste of sputum

Arterial Blood Gases

A. Definition—measurement of arterial pH, partial pressures of oxygen and carbon dioxide, bicarbonate ion, and oxygen saturation (see acid-base balance)
B. Nursing responsibilities
   1. Explain procedure to the patient
   2. Obtain a heparinized syringe or vacuum container tube
   3. Notify the laboratory to calibrate equipment
   4. Aseptically obtain approximately 3 ml of arterial blood; most common sites include the radial, brachial, and femoral arteries
   5. Avoid introducing room air into the syringe, for this can alter results
   6. Apply pressure over the arterial site for 5 minutes to prevent bleeding
   7. Place the specimen in ice to decrease the metabolic rate of blood cells and subsequent alteration of values; transport promptly to the laboratory

RELATED EMERGENCY AND CRITICAL CARE PROCEDURES
Administration of Oxygen

A. Definition
  1. Administration of supplemental oxygen when the patient's respiratory system is compromised and tissue hypoxia is threatened
  2. May be accomplished via a catheter, cannula, mask, or tent
B. Nursing responsibilities
  1. Explain the procedure to the patient and family
  2. Attach "no smoking" signs to door of room and instruct the patient and visitors to adhere to this rule, since oxygen supports combustion
  3. Assess the patient's color (nail beds, general appearance) and vital signs prior to and during therapy
  4. Ascertain if the patient has chronic lung disease before administering high concentrations of oxygen
  5. Attach appropriate apparatus to the oxygen source and fill the humidification cannister with water to prevent drying of mucous membranes

Management of Airway Obstruction

A. Suctioning of airway
  1. Definition
    a. Mechanical aspiration of mucous secretions from the tracheobronchial tree by application of negative pressure
    b. Utilized to maintain a patent airway, obtain a sputum specimen, or stimulate coughing
    c. May be nasotracheal, oropharyngeal, or through an endotracheal or tracheostomy tube
  2. Nursing responsibilities
    a. Maintain surgical asepsis
    b. Assess proper functioning of the equipment
    c. Lubricate the suction catheter with sterile water
    d. Insert the catheter
      (1) If tracheal suction is being utilized, insert approximately 4 inches
      (2) If nasotracheal suction is being utilized, insert until the cough reflex is induced
    e. Apply no suction while the catheter is being inserted
    f. Rotate and withdraw the catheter while suction is applied; suction should not exceed 10 to 15 seconds
    g. Clear the catheter with sterile solution and encourage the patient to breathe deeply
    h. If deeper suction is required, ask the patient to turn his head to the side to permit entry of the suction catheter into the opposite bronchus
B. Abdominal thrust (Heimlich maneuver)
  1. Definition—short abrupt pressure against the abdomen (halfway between the umbilicus and xyphoid) to raise intrarespiratory pressure, which will dislodge an obstruction such as a bolus of food or a foreign body
  2. Symtoms of obstruction
    a. Partial—noisy respiration, dyspnea, lightheadedness, dizziness, flushing of face, bulging of eyes, repeated coughing
    b. Total—cessation of breathing, inability to speak or cough, extension of head, facial cyanosis, bulging of eyes, panic, unconsciousness
  3. Nursing responsibilities
    a. Partial obstruction: allow the individual's expulsive cough to dislodge the obstruction; do not perform back slaps or abdominal thrusts; assess for signs of total obstruction
    b. Total obstruction: open the individual's mouth and remove the obstruction if possible; give four sharp blows between the scapulas (some experts believe abdominal thrusts should be initiated first); standing behind the victim, encircle arms around the victim's hypochondrium and thrust upward and inward against the diaphragm; alternate four abdominal thrusts with four backslaps until the obstruction is dislodged
    c. Remove any foreign bodies coughed up into the mouth
    d. Assess for signs of injury to the liver or spleen; there is a higher risk of this when abdominal thrusts are performed with the victim in a recumbent position

Tracheostomy Care

A. Definition—removal of dried secretions from the cannula to maintain a patent airway, prevent infection, and prevent irritation
B. Nursing responsiblities
  1. Tracheostomy care should be done at least every 8 hours
  2. Suction to remove secretions from the lumen of the tube (see procedure for suctioning of airways)
  3. If an inner cannula is present
    a. Remove and place in a container of hydrogen peroxide and rinse with normal saline, using surgical aseptic technique

b. Remove dried secretions within the cannula, using a sterile pipe cleaner or brush

c. Drain excess saline before reinserting the tube, which is then locked in place

4. Clean the area around the stoma with peroxide and saline, using aseptic technique; apply antiseptic ointment if ordered

5. Change the tracheostomy string or tape, being careful not to dislodge the cannula

6. Place a tracheostomy dressing or fenestrated 4 × 4 inch (unfilled) dressing below the stoma to absorb expelled secretions

7. Humidify inhaled air mechanically or by the use of a moistened 4 × 4 inch dressing over the tracheostomy, since air is bypassing normal humidification process in the nasopharynx

Mechanical Ventilation

A. Definition—use of a mechanical device to instill a mixture of air and oxygen into the lungs using positive pressure

B. Types of ventilators
1. Volume control—delivers a preset tidal volume at various pressures
2. Pressure control—delivers preset pressure at various volumes

C. Types of ventilation
1. Controlled—the patient receives a specified volume at a specific pressure with no triggering of the machine by the patient; the nurse may have to administer drugs such as curare or morphine to decrease the patient's own respiratory response
2. Assisted—the patient triggers the machine so that the rate may vary; however, if the patient has periods of apnea, the machine will take over initiation of respirations

D. Nursing responsibilities
1. Keep the respirator at settings as ordered and notify the respiratory therapy department and the physician if distress occurs
2. Maintain a sealed system between the respirator and the patient so that volume to be delivered is kept constant and air is not lost around the tubing; this is accomplished by inflating the cuff of the endotracheal tube or tracheostomy tube to the minimum occlusive volume
3. Perform suction frequently, since humidified oxygen helps to liquefy secretions that must be removed
4. Observe the patient for signs of respiratory insufficiency, such as tachypnea, cyanosis, and changes in sensorium

5. Ascertain blood gases as ordered to determine effectiveness of ventilation
6. Establish a means of communication, since patient will be unable to speak while on a ventilator

Chest Tubes

A. Definition
1. Use of tubes and suction to return negative pressure to the intrapleural space
2. To drain air from the intrapleural space, the chest tube is placed in the second or third intercostal space; to drain blood or fluid, the catheter would be placed at a lower site, usually the eighth or ninth intercostal space
3. One-bottle underwater system—allows air or fluid to drain from the pleural cavity by gravity via a glass rod, which extends approximately 2 cm below the surface of the water within the collection bottle
4. Two-bottle drainage system—involves 1 bottle that acts as a collection chamber and provides the water seal while a second bottle can be connected to a suction apparatus; the bubbling of water within the second bottle indicates that the desired suction is maintained
5. Three-bottle system—includes 1 bottle that serves to collect drainage, 1 that acts as the water-seal chamber, and 1 that controls suction
6. Pleurevac—commercially prepared plastic unit designed for closed chest suction; it combines the features of the other systems and may or may not be attached to suction

B. Nursing responsibilities
1. Ensure that the tubing is not kinked; tape all connections to prevent separation
2. Milk the tubing in the direction of the drainage system to maintain patency
3. Maintain the drainage system below the level of the chest
4. Turn the patient frequently, making sure the chest tubes are not compressed
5. Report drainage on dressing immediately, since this is not a normal occurrence
6. Observe for fluctuation of fluid in glass tube; the level will rise on inhalation and fall on exhalation; if there are no fluctuations, either the lung has expanded fully or the chest tube is clogged
7. Palpate the area around the chest tube insertion site for subcutaneous emphysema or crepitus, which indicates that air is leaking into the subcutaneous tissue

8. Situate the drainage bottles or Pleurevac to avoid breakage
9. Place 2 clamps at the bedside for use if the underwater-seal bottle is broken; clamp the chest tube immediately to prevent air from entering the intrapleural space, which would cause pneumothorax to occur or extend
10. Encourage coughing and deep breathing every 2 hours, splinting the area as needed
11. When the physician removes the chest tube, instruct the patient to exhale or strain (Valsalva maneuver) as the tube is withdrawn; apply a gauze dressing immediately and firmly secure with tape to make an airtight dressing
12. Encourage movement of the arm on the affected side

MAJOR DISEASES
Pulmonary Embolism and Infarction

A. Etiology and pathophysiology
   1. Postoperative patients, as well as those confined to bed, are prone to venous stasis, which causes peripheral thrombus formation
   2. When an embolus lodges in the pulmonary artery causing hemorrhage and necrosis of lung tissue, it is called a pulmonary infarction
B. Signs and symptoms
   1. Subjective
      a. Severe dyspnea that occurs suddenly
      b. Anxiety
      c. Restlessness
      d. Sharp upper abdominal or thoracic pain
   2. Objective
      a. Violent coughing with hemoptysis
      b. On auscultation, dullness over area of infarction
      c. Increased temperature
C. Treatment
   1. Anticoagulant therapy
   2. Maintenance of blood pressure
   3. Angiography; if the condition is severe, an embolectomy may be indicated
D. Nursing care
   1. Place in the high Fowler position to aid respiration
   2. Monitor vital signs
   3. Administer medications and oxygen as ordered

Pulmonary Edema

A. Etiology and pathophysiology
   1. An acute emergency condition characterized by a rapid accumulation of fluid in the alveolar spaces resulting from increased pressure within the pulmonary system
   2. Possible causes include valvular disease, left ventricular failure, circulatory overload, or congestive heart disease
B. Signs and symptoms
   1. Subjective
      a. History of premonitory symptoms such as shortness of breath, paroxysmal nocturnal dyspnea, wheezing, and orthopnea
      b. Acute anxiety, apprehension, restlessness
   2. Objective
      a. Rapid thready pulse
      b. Pink frothy sputum
      c. Elevated central venous pressure (CVP)
      d. Decreased circulation time
      e. Cyanosis
      f. Wheezing
      g. Stertorous respirations
C. Treatment
   1. Medications aimed at decreasing cardiac work load and improving cardiac output, such as morphine sulfate, digitalis, diuretics, bronchodilators
   2. Oxygen in high concentration or by IPPB as necessary
   3. Phlebotomy to remove approximately 500 ml of blood or the application of rotating tourniquets to reduce the volume of circulating blood
   4. Cardiac monitoring
D. Nursing care
   1. Support the patient in a high Fowler or semi-Fowler position
   2. Observe and record vital signs and monitor cardiac activity and intake and output
   3. Provide a reassuring environment to allay anxiety
   4. Suction as needed to maintain a patent airway
   5. Apply rotating tourniquets when ordered
      a. Tourniquets are generally placed around extremities without completely obliterating the pulse
      b. One touniquet is moved in a clockwise direction every 15 minutes
      c. When the patient is no longer in distress, tourniquets are removed 1 at a time at 15-minute intervals to prevent sudden cardiac overload; legs are rotated off last

Pleural Effusion

A. Etiology and pathophysiology
   1. Collection of fluid in the pleural space
   2. Generally occurs secondary to diseases such as cancer of the lung, tuberculosis, and congestive heart failure

B. Signs and symptoms
   1. Subjective
      a. Pleuritic pain that is sharp and increases on inspiration
      b. Dyspnea
      c. Malaise
   2. Objective
      a. Tachycardia
      b. Elevated temperature
      c. Cough (may be productive or nonproductive depending on cause)
      d. Decreased breath sounds
      e. Chest x-ray examination shows obliteration of the angle between the ribs and diaphragm; may also reveal a mediastinal shift away from the fluid
C. Treatment
   1. Thoracentesis (see procedure)
   2. Treatment of underlying cause
D. Nursing care
   1. Monitor vital signs, particularly temperature and respirations
   2. Auscultate lung fields
   3. Encourage coughing and deep breathing
   4. Increase fluid intake
   5. Place the patient in a high Fowler position for maximum air exchange

Pleurisy

A. Etiology and pathophysiology
   1. Inflammation of the visceral and parietal membranes, which rub together during respiration and cause pain
   2. Caused by chest trauma, tuberculosis, pneumonia, or chest surgery
B. Signs and symptoms
   1. Subjective
      a. Knifelike pain on inspiration
      b. Apprehension
      c. Dyspnea
   2. Objective
      a. Decreased excursion of the involved chest wall
      b. Pleural friction rub discernible on auscultation of chest wall
C. Treatment
   1. Treat the underlying condition
   2. Analgesics for pain
   3. Applications of heat or cold to thoracic area
D. Nursing care
   1. Instruct the patient to lie on the affected side to splint the chest wall and lessen pain on inspiration
   2. Administer medications as ordered

   3. Allay anxiety
   4. Observe for signs of shock or pulmonary emboli

Empyema

A. Etiology and pathophysiology
   1. Collection of pus within the thoracic cavity
   2. May occur following staphylococcal pneumonia, tuberculosis, chest trauma, or surgery
B. Signs and symptoms
   1. Subjective
      a. Unilateral chest pain
      b. Malaise
      c. Anorexia
      d. Dyspnea
   2. Objective
      a. Chest x-ray examination shows pleural exudate
      b. Elevated temperature
      c. Cough
      d. Unequal chest expansion
C. Treatment
   1. Thoracentesis to obtain a specimen of exudate to culture
   2. Chest tubes inserted to drain thoracic cavity
   3. Antibiotics may be instilled through the chest tube or given systemically
   4. If condition is long-standing, the area of inflammation is surgically removed; this is known as decortication
D. Nursing care
   1. Monitor chest tube (see procedure)
   2. Provide emotional support
   3. Administer antibiotics as ordered
   4. Monitor vital signs, particularly temperature and character of respirations

Pneumonia

A. Etiology and pathophysiology
   1. Inflammatory disease usually caused by an infectious agent (bacterial, viral, or fungal) but may also be caused by inhalation of chemicals and aspiration of gastric contents
   2. Pneumonia is commonly spread by respiratory droplets
   3. Pneumococcal pneumonia, the most common type of bacterial pneumonia, occurs in winter and spring; other bacterial pneumonias include *Klebsiella pneumoniae, Haemophilus influenzae,* species of *Pseudomonas, Proteus,* and *Streptococcus,* and *Staphylococcus aureus*
   4. Aspiration pneumonia occurs when gastric contents and the normal flora of the upper respiratory tract are aspirated into the lung
B. Signs and symptoms

1. Subjective
   a. Lassitude
   b. Chest pain that increases on inspiration
   c. Dyspnea
2. Objective
   a. Elevated temperature
   b. Increased WBC
   c. Cough
   d. Chest x-ray examination shows pulmonary infiltration
   e. Sputum production
      (1) Pneumococcal—purulent, rusty sputum
      (2) Staphylococcal—yellow, blood-streaked sputum
      (3) Klebsiella—red gelatinous sputum
      (4) Mycoplasmal—nonproductive that advances to mucoid
C. Treatment
   1. If bacterial pneumonia, culture and sensitivity tests will be done of blood and sputum to determine appropriate antibiotic therapy
   2. Oxygen therapy usually via nasal cannula
   3. Inhalation therapy such as IPPB or the use of incentive spirometer
D. Nursing care
   1. Encourage coughing and deep breathing, splinting the chest as necessary
   2. Observe amount and characteristics of sputum
   3. Collect sputum specimen for culture and sensitivity tests in sterile container; notify the physician if organism is resistant to the antibiotic being given
   4. Increase fluid intake
   5. Monitor vital signs
   6. Observe for signs of respiratory distress, such as labored respirations, cool clammy skin, and cyanosis

Atelectasis

A. Etiology and pathophysiology
   1. Respirations shallow and ineffective, as in postoperative patients
   2. Bronchioles obstructed by secretions, and alveoli distal to the bronchioles collapse; many small bronchioles or a stem of the bronchus may be involved
   3. Causes include compression due to large pleural effusion, empyema, or pneumothorax, obstruction of a bronchus by a tumor, and deficiency of surfactant in an infant
B. Signs and symptoms
   1. Subjective
      a. Restlessness
      b. Anxiety

2. Objective
   a. Rapid shallow respirations
   b. Diminished breath sounds in lower lobes
   c. Productive cough
   d. Temperature elevation
C. Treatment
   1. Oxygen therapy
   2. IPPB
   3. Prophylactic antibiotics
D. Nursing care
   1. Encourage coughing and deep breathing
   2. Monitor respirations closely
   3. Auscultate breath sounds for signs of decreased ventilation
   4. Place in a high Fowler position; turn every 2 hours

Sarcoidosis

A. Etiology and pathophysiology
   1. Characterized by epithelioid cell tubercles, most commonly in the lung
   2. Cause unknown, although 80% have high titers of Epstein-Barr virus
   3. Incidence is highest in blacks and young adults
B. Signs and symptoms
   1. Subjective
      a. Fatigue
      b. Malaise
      c. Dyspnea
   2. Objective
      a. Night sweats
      b. Fever
      c. Weight loss
      d. Cough
      e. Nodules of face
      f. Polyarthritis
      g. Mild anemia
      h. Elevated serum calcium
      i. Kveim test—sarcoid node antigen is injected intradermally and causes local nodular lesion in approximately 1 month
      j. Biopsy of skin, lymph node, or liver
      k. X-ray findings include bilateral hilar and paratracheal adenopathy
C. Treatment
   1. No specific treatment
   2. Corticosteroids to control symptoms
D. Nursing care
   1. Monitor temperature and other vital signs
   2. Increase fluid intake
   3. Provide frequent periods of rest
   4. Provide small nutritious meals, taking into consideration the patient's preferences

Pulmonary Tuberculosis

A. Etiology and pathophysiology
  1. Infection of lungs caused by *Mycobacterium tuberculosis,* an acid-fast bacterium
  2. Causes tubercles, fibrosis, and calcification within the lungs
  3. Tubercle bacillus may be communicated to others by means of droplet formation (inhalation), ingestion, or inoculation
  4. Predisposing factors include debilitating diseases such as alcoholism, cardiovascular disease, diabetes mellitus, and cirrhosis, as well as poor nutrition and crowded living conditions
  5. Chronic, progressive, and reinfection phase is most frequently encountered in adults and involves progression or reactivation of primary lesions after months or years of latency
  6. Swallowing infected sputum may lead to laryngeal, oropharyngeal, and intestinal tuberculosis
B. Signs and symptoms
  1. Subjective
    a. Malaise
    b. Pleuritic pain
    c. Easily fatigued
  2. Objective
    a. Fever
    b. Night sweats
    c. Cough that progressively becomes worse
    d. Hemoptysis
    e. Weight loss
    f. Chest x-ray examination to determine presence of calcified lesions
    g. Analysis of sputum and gastric contents for the presence of acid-fast bacilli
    h. Tuberculin testing
      (1) Examples
        (a) Tine
        (b) Heaf
        (c) Mantoux, which frequently involves the use of purified protein derivative (PPD)
      (2) Determines antibody response to the tubercle bacillus
      (3) Indicates prior exposure to bacillus, which may or may not indicate active disease state (a sudden change from negative to positive requires follow-up testing)
      (4) In each test, either old tuberculin (OT) or PPD is injected intradermally; redness and edema present 48 to 72 hours later indicate a positive finding

C. Treatment
  1. Program of combined antituberculin drugs such as isoniazid, paraaminosalicylic acid, streptomycin, pyrazinamide
  2. Bed rest until symptoms abate or therapeutic regimen is established
  3. Determine whether surgical resection of the involved lobe is necessary if symptoms such as hemorrhage develop or chemotherapy is unsatisfactory
  4. Provide prophylactic therapy to immediate contacts (all cases and follow-up of contacts must be reported to public health agency)
  5. Have the patient begin a high-carbohydrate, high-protein, high-vitamin diet with supplemental vitamin B_6
D. Nursing care
  1. Teach the patient to provide for scheduled rest periods
  2. Teach which foods to include in the diet and which are nutritious between-meal supplements
  3. Teach the importance of maintaining the drug program that has been established without variation
  4. Teach the proper techniques to prevent spread of infection
    a. Frequent hand washing
    b. Cover the mouth when coughing
    c. Proper use and disposal of tissues
    d. Proper cleansing of eating utensils and disposal of food wastes
    e. Isolation when sputum is positive for the organism
  5. Encourage the patient to participate in developing a schedule of activities and therapy and following the schedule once established
  6. Instruct the patient to be alert to the early symptoms of hemorrhage such as hemoptysis and to contact the physician immediately if any occur
  7. Instruct the patient to be alert to the early symptoms of adverse drug reactions (e.g., neuritis, ringing in the ears, ataxia, dermatitis) and to contact the physician immediately if any occur
  8. Encourage the patient to follow prescribed program for productive coughing and deep breathing
  9. Instruct the patient to avoid any medications such as cough syrups without physician's approval
  10. Explain the need and instruct the patient to continue follow-up care and supervision

11. Encourage the patient to express feelings about disease and the many ramifications (stigma, isolation, fear) it creates
12. Expect and accept the patient's expression of hostility and depression
13. Encourage the patient to limit activities until the physician gives approval for gradual increase
14. Help the patient plan a realistic schedule for taking the large number of necessary medications

Chronic Obstructive Pulmonary Disease (COPD)

A. Etiology and pathophysiology
1. Group of diseases that result in an obstruction of airflow; etiology includes air pollution, smoking, chronic respiratory infections, exposure to molds and fungi, and allergic reactions
2. Types
   a. Asthma—obstruction of the bronchioles characterized by attacks that occur suddenly and last from 30 to 60 minutes; an asthmatic attack that is difficult to control is referred to as status asthmaticus
   b. Bronchitis—inflammation of the bronchial walls with hypertrophy of the mucous goblet cells; characterized by a chronic cough
   c. Emphysema—characterized by distended, inelastic, or destroyed alveoli with bronchiolar obstruction and collapse; these alterations greatly impair the diffusion of gases through the alveolocapillary membrane
3. Patients with COPD become accustomed to an elevated residual carbon dioxide level and do not respond to high CO_2 concentrations as the normal respiratory stimulant; they respond instead to a drop in oxygen concentration in the blood

B. Signs and symptoms
1. Subjective
   a. Fatigue and weakness
   b. Headache, impaired sensorium
   c. Dyspnea
2. Objective
   a. Orthopnea, expiratory wheezing, stertorous breathing sounds, cough
   b. Barrel chest, cyanosis, clubbing of fingers
   c. Distention of neck veins
   d. Edema of extremities
   e. Increased P_{CO_2} and decreased P_{O_2} of arterial blood gases
   f. Polycythemia

C. Treatment
1. Antibiotics and cortisone to prevent and reduce inflammation
2. Bronchodilators to reduce muscular spasm
3. Mucolytics and expectorants to liquefy secretions and to facilitate their removal
4. Oxygen at 2 to 3 L even if hypoxia is severe
5. Respiratory therapy program to include IPPB, postural drainage, exercise, and blow bottles
6. High-protein, soft diet

D. Nursing care
1. Advise the elimination of smoking and other external irritants, such as dust, as much as possible
2. Supervise the patient's respiratory exercises, such as pursed lip or diaphragmatic breathing
3. Teach the proper use of nebulizer and other special equipment
4. Carefully observe for symptoms of carbon dioxide intoxication if oxygen is being administered
5. Teach the patient to adjust activities to avoid overexertion
6. Teach the patient to avoid people with respiratory infections
7. Teach the patient to maintain resistance by getting proper rest, eating proper food, dressing properly for existing weather conditions
8. Teach the patient to be alert to early symptoms of infection, hypoxia, hypercapnea, or adverse response to medications
9. Encourage the patient to continue with close medical supervision
10. Encourage the patient to express feelings about disease and therapy
11. Accept the patient's feelings about life-long restrictions in activity
12. Encourage the patient to take an active role in planning therapy
13. Encourage the patient to take medications as ordered
14. Support the patient's efforts to give up smoking by providing diversional activities such as eating hard candies
15. Encourage the family to support the patient's efforts to give up smoking

Silicosis (Black Lung)

A. Etiology and pathophysiology
1. Fibrotic disease of lungs caused by inhalation of inorganic dusts over long periods
2. Common in people whose professions expose

them to free silica, such as miners and sandblasters

   3. Tuberculosis a frequent complication

B. Signs and symptoms

   1. Subjective

     a. Exertional dyspnea

     b. Anxiety

   2 Objective

     a. Frequent respiratory infections

     b. Sputum may be blood streaked

     c. Cough

     d. Chest x-ray examination reveals nodular lesions and enlarged hilar nodes

     e. Biopsy to establish diagnosis

C. Treatment

   1. Relieve cough with antitussives

   2. Prescribe medications for complications such as tuberculosis

   3. Eliminate toxic substances from the environment

D. Nursing care

   1. Assess the patient's ability to meet oxygen needs

   2. Encourage coughing and deep breathing

   3. Involve the patient and family in programs aimed at improved occupational health and safety

Pneumothorax

A. Etiology and pathophysiology

   1. Collapse of a lung caused by disruption of the negative pressure that normally exists within the intrapleural space due to the presence of air in the pleural cavity

   2. Reduces the surface area for gaseous exchange and leads to hypoxia and retention of carbon dioxide (hypercarbia)

   3. Types

     a. Spontaneous—thought to occur when a weakened area of the lung (bleb) ruptures; air then moves from the lung to the intrapleural space causing collapse; highest incidence is in men 20 to 40 years of age

     b. Open—laceration (e.g., a stab wound) through the chest wall into the intrapleural space

     c. Hemothorax—collection of blood within the pleural cavity

     d. Hydrothorax—accumulation of fluid in the pleural cavity

     e. Tension—buildup of pressure as air accumulates within the pleural space; the pressure increase likely to induce a mediastinal shift

   4. Mediastinal shift may occur toward the uninvolved side as a result of increased pressure within the pleural space; this involves the trachea, esophagus, heart, and great vessels

B. Signs and symptoms (depend on extent of collapse)

   1. Subjective

     a. Chest pain, usually described as sharp and increasing on exertion

     b. Dyspnea

   2. Objective

     a. Rapid, shallow respirations (nonsymmetrical)

     b. Breath sounds on the affected side will be diminished or absent

     c. Chest x-ray examination will reveal extent of the pneumothorax

     d. Tachycardia

     e. Hypotension

C. Treatment

   1. Bed rest initially

   2. Analgesics

   3. Negative pressure is returned to the intrapleural space by the insertion of chest tubes attached to underwater drainage

D. Nursing care

   1. Assess respiratory status

     a. Vital signs

     b. Color

     c. Chest motion during respirations

     d. Auscultate the lung fields

   2. Maintain patency of chest tubes (see procedure)

Chest Injuries

A. Etiology and pathophysiology

   1. Penetrating or crushing wounds of the chest wall generally caused by acts of violence (stabbing, gunshot wounds) or motor vehicle accidents

   2. Flail chest—occurs when ribs are fractured in more than one area; the chest wall on the involved side becomes unstable; the portion of lung below the injury moves in the opposite direction to the remainder of the lung, which results in hypoxia

B. Signs and symptoms

   1. Subjective

     a. Dyspnea

     b. Anxiety

   2. Objective

     a. Presence of a wound with a sucking sound on inspiration

     b. Presence of cyanosis and symptoms of mild to profound shock, depending on size of wound

c. Mediastinal shift may occur toward the un-affected side caused by the pressure exerted by a pneumothorax or hemothorax, causing a change in the site of the apical pulse and paradoxical respirations
d. Absence of breath sounds on the affected side

C. Treatment
1. Apply a pressure dressing over the wound
2. Aspiration of the pleural cavity to promote lung expansion
3. Establish a water-seal suction drainage
4. Reduce the oxygen demand by maintaining bed rest and limitation of activity
5. Oxygen as necessary
6. Restore blood volume and treat shock
7. Antibiotics and mild analgesics
8. Respiratory therapy to promote lung expansion
9. Volume-controlled respirator is utilized in cases of severe chest trauma

D. Nursing care
1. Maintain chest tubes if present (see procedure)
2. Observe the respiratory status
3. Encourage the patient to move and cough
4. Teach the patient to self-splint with hands and arms
5. Explain the purpose and functioning of chest tubes and water-seal drainage
6. Administer oxygen and analgesics as ordered and as necessary
7. Encourage the patient to follow directions of respiratory therapists (e.g., blow bottles, IPPB)

Bronchogenic Carcinoma

A. Etiology and pathophysiology
1. Carcinoma of the lungs may be primary or metastatic
2. Etiology unknown, but is much more common in smokers than nonsmokers
3. Incidence highest in men over the age of 40
4. Symptoms may occur after metastasis to other organs such as the ribs, liver, adrenal glands, mediastinal organs, kidneys, and brain

B. Signs and symptoms
1. Subjective
a. Dyspnea
b. Chills
c. Fatigue
d. Chest pain
2. Objective
a. Persistent cough
b. Hemoptysis
c. Unilateral wheeze detected by auscultation

d. Weight loss
e. Clubbing of fingers
f. Pleural effusion
g. "Coin" lesions detected by x-ray examination of the chest
h. Cytologic test of sputum positive

C. Treatment
1. Surgical
a. Lobectomy—removal of 1 lobe of the lung when the lesion is limited to 1 area
b. Wedge section—removal of a small confined lesion; may also be done for biopsy
c. Pneumonectomy—removal of an entire lung
d. Exploratory thoracotomy—opening of the thoracic cavity to confirm diagnosis
e. Thoracoplasty—removal of ribs to reduce the size of the pleural cavity; may be done to prevent complications after resection of lung
2. Radiation therapy may be used as an adjunct therapy or to alleviate symptoms of pain, dyspnea, and hemoptysis
3. Chemotherapy

D. Nursing care
1. Maintain open communication between self, the patient, and the family; refer to community agencies and mental health practitioner as necessary
2. Monitor temperature and vital signs
3. Encourage coughing and deep breathing
4. Change position frequently; semi-Fowler or high Fowler promotes greater lung expansion
5. Specific care based on therapy being used
a. Care of the patient with chest tubes (see procedure)
b. Radiation therapy
(1) Adjust diet to the patient's preference; provide small frequent feedings
(2) Avoid washing off port marks used for radiation therapy
(3) Do not apply powders and ointments that might contain metals
(4) Apply a nonadherent dressing to areas of skin breakdown
c. Chemotherapy (refer to specific drugs)

Cancer of the Larynx

A. Etiology and pathophysiology
1. Most tumors of the larynx (vocal cords, epiglottis, laryngeal cartilages, and ventricle) are squamous cell carcinoma
2. Cigarette smoking and heavy alcohol consumption appear to be related to increased incidence
3. More common in men 50 to 65 years of age

B. Signs and symptoms
 1. Subjective
   a. Sore throat
   b. Dyspnea
   c. Dysphagia
   d. Weakness
 2. Objective
   a. Increasing hoarseness
   b. Weight loss
   c. Enlarged cervical lymph nodes
   d. Foul breath
C. Treatment
 1. Radiation therapy
 2. Chemotherapy (e.g., methotrexate, bleomycin, fluorouracil)
 3. Surgical intervention
   a. Thyrotomy—removal of tumor from the larynx via an incision through the thyroid cartilage
   b. Total laryngectomy—removal of total larynx with construction of a permanent tracheostomy
   c. Radical neck dissection (used when the tumor has metastasized into surrounding tissue and lymph nodes)—removal of larynx, surrounding tissue and muscle, lymph nodes, and glands with a permanent tracheostomy
D. Nursing care of the patient with a total laryngectomy
 1. Provide time to discuss the diagnosis and the ramifications of surgery
 2. Assist and encourage the patient to express feelings
 3. Answer questions as thoroughly and honestly as possible
 4. Arrange for individuals with laryngectomies to visit the patient and discuss the rehabilitative process
 5. Instruct the patient as to the method of communication that will be used postoperatively (e.g., slate board and chalk, pencil and paper, sign language)
 6. Observe for obstruction of airway by mucous plugs, edema, or blood (e.g., air hunger, dyspnea, cyanosis, gurgling)
 7. Observe for signs of hemorrhage (e.g., increased pulse rate, drop in blood pressure, cold clammy skin, appearance of blood on dressing)
 8. Stay with the patient but provide a bell or other system for the patient to signal for help
 9. Provide, at the patient's bedside, suction apparatus and catheters (additional laryngectomy tube and a surgical instrument set with additional hemostats should be immediately available in case the tube becomes dislodged or blocked)
 10. Suction the tracheostomy tube that is left in place for approximately 3 days (see procedure)
 11. Provide humidity to compensate for loss of normal humidification of air in the nasopharynx; later the tracheostomy may be covered with a moistened unfilled gauze pad
 12. Prevent cross infection and contamination of the wound by providing special oral hygiene, cleanliness at tracheal site, avoidance of people with respiratory infections, use of clean equipment
 13. In patients receiving radiation or chemotherapy, observe for signs of adverse reactions
 14. Expect and accept a period of mourning but prevent withdrawal from reality by
   a. Involving the patient in laryngectomy care
   b. Keeping channels of communication open
   c. Supporting the patient's strengths
   d. Encouraging a return to activities of daily living
   e. Allowing the patient time to write responses or use sign language
 15. Encourage the patient to become involved in speech therapy and realistically support efforts and gains
 16. Teach the skills necessary to handle altered body functioning
   a. Method of tracheobronchial suctioning to maintain patency of airway emphasizing pressure, depth, frequency, and safety
   b. Method of changing, cleaning, and securing the laryngectomy tube
   c. Care of skin around the opening
   d. Importance of providing humidified air for inspiration to prevent drying of secretions (can be achieved by use of moist dressing)
 17. Teach the patient to avoid activities that may permit water or irritating substances to enter the trachea, since the usual defensive mechanisms (glottis and cilia) are absent; the patient should avoid showers, swimming, dust, hair spray, and other volatile substances
 18. Teach the patient to avoid wearing clothes with tight collars or constricting necklines
 19. Teach the patient that certain other activities will be interrupted (e.g., sipping through a straw, whistling, blowing the nose)

Adult Respiratory Distress Syndrome (ARDS)

A. Etiology and pathophysiology
   1. Respiratory failure in patients with previously healthy lungs as a complication of conditions such as trauma, aspiration, prolonged mechanical ventilation, severe infection, or open heart surgery
   2. Involves
      a. Pulmonary capillary damage with loss of fluid and interstitial edema
      b. Impaired alveolar gas exchange and tissue hypoxia due to pulmonary edema
      c. Alteration in surfactant production; collapse of alveoli
      d. Atelectasis resulting in labored and inefficient respiration
B. Signs and symptoms
   1. Subjective
      a. Restlessness
      b. Anxiety
      c. Dyspnea
   2. Objective
      a. Increased P_{CO_2} and decreased P_{O_2} arterial blood gases
      b. Tachypnea
      c. Cyanosis
C. Treatment
   1. Relieve the underlying cause
   2. Mechanical ventilation
   3. Positive end expiratory pressure (PEEP)—this setting on a mechanical ventilator maintains positive pressure within the lungs on expiration, which increases the residual capacity, reducing hypoxia
   4. Monitoring arterial blood gases
   5. Corticosteroids may be used
D. Nursing care
   1. Allow frequent rest periods between therapeutic interventions
   2. Provide tranquil supportive environment because sedation is contraindicated due to its depressant effect on respirations
   3. Observe behavioral changes and vital signs, since confusion and hypertension may indicate cerebral hypoxia
   4. Auscultate breath sounds to observe for signs of pneumothorax when the patient is on PEEP (lung tissue that is frail may not withstand increased intrathoracic pressure, and pneumothorax occurs)
   5. Monitor arterial blood gases, as ordered; use a heparinized syringe to obtain specimen
   6. Maintain a patent airway
   7. Care of the patient on mechanical ventilation (see procedure)

Carbon Monoxide Poisoning

A. Etiology and pathophysiology
   1. Caused by inadequately vented combustion devices
   2. Carbon monoxide combines with hemoglobin more readily than does oxygen, causing tissue anoxia
B. Signs and symptoms
   1. Subjective
      a. Headache
      b. Faintness
      c. Vertigo
      d. Tinnitus
   2. Objective
      a. Color may be normal, cyanotic, or flushed, but is usually cherry pink
      b. Paralysis
      c. Loss of consciousness
      d. ECG changes
C. Treatment
   1. Administer artificial respiration
   2. 100% oxygen until carboxyhemoglobin is reduced and respirations are normal
   3. Administer 50% glucose or mannitol
   4. Administer synthetic erythrocytes (Fluosol), which deliver oxygen to cells in the presence of carbon monoxide
D. Nursing care
   1. Remove the individual from the immediate area
   2. Evaluate for cardiopulmonary function
   3. Institute cardiopulmonary resuscitation if necessary and maintain until additional help arrives
   4. Administer oxygen if available
   5. Maintain respirations with assistance if needed
   6. Maintain body temperature
   7. Observe vital signs, with special concern for respirations
   8. Maintain oxygen flow at prescribed levels

Gastrointestinal System

REVIEW OF ANATOMY AND PHYSIOLOGY OF THE GASTROINTESTINAL SYSTEM
Functions

A. Digestion of food, essential preparation for absorption and metabolism
B. Absorption of digested food
C. Elimination of wastes of digestion

Organs

Mouth (Buccal Cavity)

A. Lips
B. Cheeks
C. Hard palate—formed by 2 palatine bones and palatine processes of maxillae
D. Soft palate—formed of muscle in shape of an arch that forms a partition between the mouth and nasopharynx; fauces (archway) or opening from mouth into oropharynx; uvula, conical dependent process; possesses numerous mucus-secreting glands
E. Gums (gingivae)
F. Teeth
   1. Deciduous or "baby teeth"—10 in each jaw (20 in set)
   2. Permanent—16 per jaw (32 in set)
   3. Eruption
     a. Deciduous—first 1 erupts usually at 6 months of age; rest follow at intervals of 1 or more months; however, great individual variation in time of eruption of teeth; deciduous teeth are shed between 6 and 13 years of age
     b. Permanent—usually between 6 years and about 17 years; third molars (wisdom teeth) last to erupt
G. Tongue
   1. Papillae—many rough elevations on surface
   2. Taste buds—specialized receptors of cranial nerves VII (facial) and IX (glossopharyngeal) located in papillae
   3. Frenum (or frenulum)—fold of mucous membrane that helps anchor tongue to floor of mouth
H. Tonsils—lymphatic tissue connected to the surface epithelium by a channel (crypt); produces lymphocytes; defense against infection
I. Salivary glands—produce saliva, a mixture of water, mucin, salts, enzyme (salivary amylase)
   1. Parotid—below and in front of the ear
   2. Submandibular—posterior part of floor of mouth
   3. Sublingual—anterior part of floor of mouth, under tongue

Pharynx

See respiratory system discussion

Esophagus

A. Location and extent
   1. Posterior to trachea; anterior to the vertebral column
   2. Extends from the pharynx through an opening in the diaphragm (hiatus) to the stomach
B. Structure—collapsible muscular tube; about 25 cm (10 inches) long and 0.13 cm (0.05 inch) wide
C. Secretions and functions—secretes mucus; facilitates movement of food

Stomach

A. Size, shape, position
   1. Size—varies in different persons and according to degree of distention
   2. Shape—elongated pouch, with greater curve forming the lower left border
   3. Position—in epigastric and left hypochondriac portions of the abdominal cavity
B. Divisions
   1. Fundus—portion above the esophageal opening
   2. Body—central portion
   3. Pylorus—constricted lower portion
C. Curves
   1. Lesser—upper right border
   2. Greater—lower left border
D. Sphincters
   1. Cardiac—guarding opening of the esophagus into the stomach
   2. Pyloric—guarding opening of the pylorus into the duodenum
E. Glands of the stomach—secrete gastric juice composed of mucus, hydrochloric acid, and enzymes
   1. Simple columnar epithelial cells form the surface of the gastric mucosa; goblet cells secrete mucus
   2. Millions of microscopic gastric glands embedded in gastric mucosa composed of different types of cells; mainly chief cells (zymogen cells) that secrete gastric juice enzymes, and parietal cells that secrete hydrochloric acid and intrinsic factor
F. Functions—food storage and liquefaction (chyme)

Small Intestine

A. Size—approximately 2.5 cm (1 inch) in diameter, 6.1 m (20 feet) in length when relaxed
B. Divisions
   1. Duodenum—joins pylorus of the stomach; about 25 cm (10 inches) in length; C shaped
   2. Jejunum—middle section about 2.4 m (8 feet) in length
   3. Ileum—lower section, about 3.6 m (12 feet) in length; no clear boundary between jejunum and ileum
C. Functions—digestion and absorption
D. Process—mixing movements; peristalsis; secretion of water, ions, and mucus; receives secretions from the liver, gallbladder, and pancreas

Large Intestine

A. Size—approximately 6.3 cm (2½ inches) in diameter, but only 1.5 m (5 or 6 feet) long when relaxed
B. Divisions
   1. Cecum—first 5 to 7.6 cm (2 or 3 inches)
   2. Colon

a. Ascending—extends vertically along the right border of the abdomen up to level of the liver

b. Transverse—extends horizontally across the abdomen, below liver and stomach and above the small intestine

c. Descending—extends vertically down the left side of the abdomen to level of the iliac crest

d. Sigmoid—S-shaped part of large intestine curving downward below the iliac crest to join the rectum; lower part of the sigmoid curve that joins rectum bends toward the left

3. Rectum—last 17.7 or 20.3 cm (7 or 8 inches) of intestines

4. Anus—terminal opening of the alimentary tract

C. Functions—water and sodium ion absorption; temporary storage of fecal matter; defecation

D. Process—weak mixing movements, mass movements, and peristalsis

Vermiform Appendix

A. Size, shape, location—about size and shape of a large angleworm; blind-end tube off the cecum just beyond the ileocecal valve; 7.6 to 10 cm (3 to 4 inches) long; 0.6 cm (¼ inch) in diameter

B. Structure—same coats as compose the intestinal wall

C. Function—part of the immune system; submucosa unique in the large size of its lymphatic nodules

Liver

A. Location and size—occupies most of the right hypochondrium and part of the epigastrium; largest gland in the body

B. Lobes—divided into thousands of lobules by blood vessels and fibrous partitions

1. Right lobe—subdivided into 2 smaller lobes (caudate and quadrate) and right lobe proper

2. Left lobe—single lobe

C. Ducts

1. Hepatic duct—from liver

2. Cystic duct—from gallbladder

3. Common bile duct—formed by union of the hepatic and cystic ducts in a Y formation; drains bile into the duodenum at the hepatopancreatic papilla, surrounded by the sphincter of Oddi

D. Functions—liver is one of the most vital organs because of its role in metabolism of proteins, carbohydrates, and fats

1. Carbohydrate metabolism by liver cells

a. Glycogenesis—conversion of glucose to glycogen for storage

b. Glycogenolysis—conversion of glycogen to glucose and release of glucose into the blood; epinephrine and glucagon accelerate glycogenolysis

c. Gluconeogenesis—formation of glucose from proteins or fats; glucocorticoids (hydrocortisone, corticosterone) have an accelerating effect on gluconeogenesis

2. Fat metabolism by liver cells

a. Ketogenesis—first step in fat catabolism, occurs mainly in liver cells; consists of a series of reactions by which fatty acids are converted to ketone bodies (acetoacetic acid, acetone, beta-hydroxybutyric acid)

b. Fat storage

c. Synthesis of triglycerides, phospholipids, cholesterol, and the B complex factor choline

3. Protein metabolism by liver cells

a. Anabolism—synthesis of various proteins, notably blood proteins (e.g., prothrombin, fibrinogen, albumins, alpha and beta globulins, and clotting factors V, VII, IX, and X)

b. Deamination—first step in protein catabolism; chemical reaction by which amino group is split off from amino acid to form ammonia and a keto acid

c. Urea formation—liver cells convert most of the ammonia formed by deamination to urea

4. Secretes bile, substance important for emulsifying fats prior to digestion and as a vehicle for excretion of cholesterol and bile pigments

5. Detoxifies various substances (e.g., drugs, hormones)

6. Vitamin metabolism—stores vitamins A, D, K, and B_{12}; synthesizes B_3 from tryptophan

Gallbladder

A. Size, shape, location—approximately the size and shape of a small pear; lies on undersurface of the liver

B. Structure—sac made of smooth muscle, lined with mucosa arranged in rugae (expandable longitudinal folds)

C. Functions—concentrates and stores bile

Pancreas

A. Size, shape, location—larger in men than in women, but considerable individual variation; fish shaped, with body, head, and tail; extends from the duodenal curve to the spleen

B. Structure—that of both a duct gland and a ductless gland

1. Pancreatic cells—pour secretion (pancreatic juice) into the duct that runs length of the gland and empties into the duodenum at the hepatopancreatic papilla

Fig. 5. Major insulin effects.

2. Islands of Langerhans (or islet cells)—clusters of cells not connected with pancreatic ducts; 2 main types of cells compose islets (namely, alpha and beta cells); constitute the endocrine glands

C. Functions
 1. Pancreatic cells connected with pancreatic ducts secrete pancreatic juice, enzymes of which help digest all three kinds of foods
 2. Islet cells constitute endocrine gland
    a. Alpha cells secrete the hormone glucagon, which accelerates liver glycogenolysis; hence, tends to increase blood sugar
    b. Beta cells secrete insulin, one of most important metabolic hormones, which exerts a profound influence on the metabolism of carbohydrates, proteins, and fats (Fig. 5)
       (1) Insulin accelerates the active transport of glucose (along with potassium and phosphate ions) through cell membranes; therefore it tends to decrease blood glucose (hypoglycemic effect) and to increase glucose utilization by the cells for either catabolism or anabolism
       (2) Insulin stimulates the production of liver cell glucokinase; therefore it promotes liver glycogenesis, another effect that tends to lower blood glucose
       (3) Insulin inhibits liver cell phosphatase and therefore inhibits liver glycogenolysis

(4) Insulin accelerates the rate of amino acid transfer into cells, so it promotes anabolism of proteins within the cells
(5) Insulin accelerates the rate of fatty acid transfer into cells, promotes fat anabolism (also called fat deposition or lipogenesis), and inhibits fat catabolism

Digestion

A. Definition—all changes that food undergoes in the alimentary canal
B. Purpose—conversion of foods into chemical and physical forms that can be absorbed and metabolized
C. Kinds
 1. Mechanical digestion—all movements of the alimentary tract that
    a. Change physical state of foods from comparatively large solid pieces into minute dissolved particles
    b. Propel food forward along the alimentary tract, finally eliminating digestive wastes from the body
       (1) Deglutition—swallowing
       (2) Peristalsis—wormlike movements that squeeze food downward in the tract
       (3) Mass peristalsis—moving of entire intestinal contents into the sigmoid colon and rectum; usually occurs after a meal
       (4) Defecation—emptying of the rectum, so-called bowel movement

Table 2-3. Absorption of protein, carbohydrate, and fat

Substance	Structures into which absorbed	Circulation
Protein—amino acids	Into blood in intestinal capillaries	Portal vein, liver, hepatic vein, inferior vena cava to heart, etc.
Carbohydrate—monosaccharides (glucose and fructose)	Same as amino acids	Same as amino acids
Fat—glycerol and fatty acids; fatty acids are insoluble and must first combine with bile salts to form water-soluble substance	Chiefly into lymph in intestinal lacteals; some into blood	During absorption while in epithelial cells of intestinal mucosa, glycerol and fatty acids recombine to form microscopic particles of fats (chylomicrons); lymphatics carry them by way of thoracic duct to left subclavian vein, superior vena cava, heart, etc.

c. Churn intestinal contents so all become well mixed with digestive juices and all parts of contents come in contact with the intestinal mucosa to facilitate absorption

2. Chemical digestion—series of hydrolytic processes dependent on specific enzymes; hydrolysis, decomposition of complex compound into 2 or more simple compounds by means of chemical reaction with water

D. Control of digestive gland secretion

1. Secretion of saliva—neural control of this reflex results from parasympathetic impulses to glands, initiated by taste, smell, and sight of food (cephalic phase of digestion)

2. Gastric juice

a. Neural control similar to that of salivary glands

b. Hormonal control—partially digested proteins cause gastric mucosa to release hormone (gastrin) into blood; gastrin stimulates gastric mucosa to secrete juice with high pepsin and hydrochloric acid content

3. Pancreatic juice

a. Hormonal control—hydrochloric acid in chyme entering the duodenum from the stomach causes intestinal mucosa to release a hormone, secretin, into the blood; secretin stimulates pancreatic cells to secrete a juice high in sodium bicarbonate to neutralize hydrochloric acid but low in enzymes; products of protein digestion (e.g., proteoses, peptones, and amino acids) cause the intestinal mucosa to release another hormone, pancreozymin, which stimulates the pancreatic cells to secrete enzymes

b. Neural control—reflex secretion of pancreatic juice results from parasympathetic impulses via the vagus nerve

4. Bile

a. Although bile is secreted continuously, secretin increases amount of bile secreted

b. Presence of fats in the intestine causes the intestinal mucosa to release a hormone, cholecystokinin, into the blood; cholecystokinin stimulates the smooth muscle of the gallbladder to contract, ejecting bile into the duodenum

5. Intestinal juice—control obscure but believed to be both reflexive and hormonal; food in the small intestine causes the mucosa to release hormone (enterocrinin) into blood; enterocrinin stimulates intestinal glands to secrete

Absorption

A. Definition—passage of substances through the intestinal mucosa into the blood or lymph

B. Accomplished mainly through active transport by the intestinal cells; makes it possible for both water and solutes to move through the intestinal mucosa in a direction opposite that expected in osmosis and diffusion

C. Absorption occurs in the duodenum and jejunum of the small intestine; however, absorption of alcohol, certain drugs, and some water occurs in the stomach; most water is absorbed from the large intestine

D. Absorption of protein, carbohydrate, and fat (Table 2-3)

Metabolism

A. Definition—sum of all the chemical reactions in the body

B. Catabolism

1. Consists of a complex series of chemical reactions that take place inside the cells and yield energy, carbon dioxide, and water; about half the energy released from food molecules by ca-

tabolism is put back in storage as unstable, high-energy bonds of ATP molecules; the rest is transformed to heat; the energy in high-energy bonds of ATP can be released as rapidly as needed for cellular work

2. Two processes involved; glycolysis and the Krebs citric acid cycle
3. Purpose—to provide cells continually with utilizable energy

C. Anabolism
1. Synthesis of various compounds from simpler compounds
2. Cellular work that uses some of the energy made available by catabolism

D. Metabolism of carbohydrates
1. Consists of the following processes:
   a. Glucose transport through cell membranes and phosphorylation
      (1) Insulin promotes this transport through cell membranes
      (2) Glucose phosphorylation—conversion of glucose to glucose-6-phosphate, catalyzed by the enzyme glucokinase; insulin increases the activity of glucokinase and promotes glucose phosphorylation, which is essential prior to both glycogenesis and glucose catabolism
   b. Glycogenesis—conversion of glucose to glycogen for storage; occurs mainly in the liver and muscle cells
   c. Glycogenolysis
      (1) In muscle cells glycogen is changed back to glucose-6-phosphate, which is then catabolized in the muscle cells
      (2) In liver cells glycogen is changed back to glucose; an enzyme, glucose phosphatase, is present in the liver cells and catalyzes the final step of glycogenolysis, the changing of glucose-6-phosphate to glucose; glucagon and epinephrine accelerate liver glycogenolysis
   d. Glucose catabolism
      (1) Glycolysis—series of anaerobic reactions that break 1 glucose molecule down into 2 pyruvic acid molecules, with conversion of about 5% of energy stored in glucose to heat and ATP molecules
      (2) Krebs citric acid cycle—series of aerobic chemical reactions by which 2 pyruvic acid molecules (from 1 glucose molecule) are broken down to 6 carbon

dioxide and 6 water molecules, with the release of some energy as heat and some stored again in ATP; citric acid cycle releases about 95%, and glycolysis only about 5%, of the energy stored in glucose; citric acid cycle occurs in the mitochondria of cells

   e. Gluconeogenesis—sequence of chemical reactions carried on in liver cells; process converts protein or fat compounds into glucose
   f. Principles of normal carbohydrate metabolism
      (1) Principle of preferred energy fuel—cells first catabolize glucose, sparing fats and proteins; when their glucose supply becomes inadequate, they next catabolize fats, sparing proteins; and finally, when fats are used up, they catabolize their own cell proteins
      (2) Principle of glycogenesis—glucose in excess of about 120 to 140 mg per 100 ml blood brought to the liver by the portal veins enters the liver cells, where it undergoes glycogenesis and is stored as glycogen
      (3) Principle of glycogenolysis—when blood glucose decreases below the midpoint of normal, liver glycogenolysis accelerates and tends to raise the blood glucose concentration back toward the midpoint of normal
      (4) Principle of gluconeogenesis—when blood glucose decreases below normal or when the amount of glucose entering the cells is unadequate, liver gluconeogenesis accelerates and tends to raise the blood glucose concentration
      (5) Principle of glucose storage as fat—when the blood insulin content is adequate, glucose in excess of the amount used for catabolism and glycogenesis is converted to fat and stored in fat depots

E. Control of metabolism—primarily by hormones
1. Pancreatic hormones
   a. Insulin—exerts predominant control over carbohydrate metabolism but also affects protein and fat metabolism; in general, it accelerates carbohydrate metabolism by the cells, thereby decreasing blood glucose
   b. Glucagon (secreted by the alpha cells of the islands of Langerhans)—accelerates liver glycogenolysis only

2. Anterior pituitary hormones
   a. Growth hormone tends to
      (1) Accelerate protein anabolism; hence promotes growth of skeleton and soft tissues
      (2) Accelerate fat mobilization from adipose cells, which tends to bring about a shift from the use of glucose to the use of fats for catabolism
      (3) Accelerate liver gluconeogenesis from fats, which tends to increase blood glucose
      (4) Stimulate glucagon secretion, which in turn stimulates liver glycogenolysis and glucose release into the blood
   b. ACTH (the adrenocorticotropic hormone)—stimulates the secretion of glucocorticoids by the adrenal cortex
3. Adrenal cortex hormones—glucocorticoids—mainly cortisol and corticosterone, tend to
   a. Accelerate fat mobilization and catabolism, thereby promoting shift to fat catabolism from glucose catabolism whenever the latter is inadequate for energy needs
   b. Accelerate tissue protein mobilization (catabolism)
   c. Accelerate liver gluconeogenesis; presumably a secondary effect; results from protein mobilization and tends to increase blood sugar
4. Adrenal medulla hormones—epinephrine and norepinephrine (catecholamines) tend to accelerate both liver and muscle glycogenolysis, with release of glucose from the liver into the circulation; therefore tend to increase blood sugar
5. Male sex gland hormone—testosterone, secreted by interstitial cells of testes, tends to accelerate protein anabolism

F. Metabolic rate—calories of heat energy produced and expended per hour or per day
   1. Basal metabolic rate (BMR)—calories of heat produced when an individual is awake but resting in a comfortably warm environment 12 to 18 hours after the last meal
      a. Factors determining basal metabolic rates
         (1) Size—BMR is directly related to square meters of surface area of the body; the larger the surface area, the higher the BMR
         (2) Sex—5% to 7% higher in males than in females of the same size and age
         (3) Age—BMR inversely related to age; as age increases, BMR decreases
         (4) Amount of thyroid hormones secreted; thyroid hormones accelerate BMR
         (5) Body temperature—BMR directly related to body temperature; 1° C increase in body temperature above normal is accompanied by about a 13% increase in BMR
         (6) Miscellaneous factors such as sleep (decreases BMR), pregnancy, and emotions (increase BMR)
      b. Measurement
         (1) Determined by measuring the amount of oxygen inspired in a given time
         (2) Reported as normal or as a definite percentage above or below normal
   2. Total metabolic rate—calories of heat energy expended per day; equal to basal metabolic rate plus number of calories of energy used for muscular work, eating and digesting food, and adjusting to cool temperatures
   3. Some principles about the metabolic rate and its relation to body weight
      a. For body weight to remain constant (except for variations in water content) the energy balance must be maintained; body weight remains constant when energy input equals energy output
      b. Whenever the energy input (food intake) is greater than the energy output (total metabolic rate), body weight increases
      c. Whenever energy input (food intake) is less than the energy output (total metabolic rate), body weight decreases

REVIEW OF PHYSICAL PRINCIPLES RELATED TO THE GASTROINTESTINAL SYSTEM
Principles of Mechanics
Law of Motion
EXAMPLE: The greater the force of contraction of the intestinal wall and the more frequent the contractions, the more rapid the propulsion of food and fecal matter through digestive tract; under irritating conditions, rapid powerful peristalsis leads to abdominal cramps and diarrhea
Gravity
EXAMPLE: Colostomy irrigations and enemas
Energy
A. Potential and kinetic energy
   EXAMPLE: The potential energy in glucose (food) molecules is captured in the bonds of the high-energy molecule ATP; such potential energy is released as kinetic energy when ATP powers the

contraction of muscle and the beating of cilia and flagella

B. First law of thermodynamics

EXAMPLE: The energy stored in an ATP molecule exactly equals the energy of work (of muscles, cilia, etc.) and heat energy liberated during the process

C. Second law of thermodynamics

EXAMPLE: The diffusion of nutrients and enzymes in the various digestive juices results in their collisions and chemical interactions because it is the natural tendency of molecules and systems to become more randomized

Principles of Physical Properties of Matter

Solids

EXAMPLE: The elastic properties of the connective and muscular tissues of the stomach permit distention during a meal and the consequent storage and slow digestion and absorption of food over the next several hours

Liquids

A. Pascal's principle

EXAMPLE: The voluntary contraction of muscles of the abdominal wall, such as the external and internal oblique, applies pressure on the fluids of the abdominal cavity, which is transmitted undiminished throughout the abdominopelvic cavity and aids in defecation; chronic constipation with chronic straining during defecation may predispose to hemorrhoids

B. Surface tension

EXAMPLE: Bile salts partly combine with fats and with water; this dual combination lowers the surface tension of the water molecules surrounding large fat droplets, which disperse into thousands of smaller droplets whose greater total surface area promotes more rapid hydrolysis (digestion) by pancreatic lipase

Gases

Boyle's law

EXAMPLES

1. During gastric analysis, the volume of gas in the tube is increased as the barrel of the syringe attached to the tube is pulled out; the result is a flow of gastric contents from the stomach due to the decreased pressure exerted by the gas in the tube as compared with gas pressure in the stomach
2. The same applies during paracentesis
3. During gastric gavage the process is reversed

Heat

A. Body temperature maintained by heat produced as a by-product of biochemical reactions; basal metabolic rate is a measure of heat production under specified conditions

B. The normal metabolism in each of the cells of the human body produces heat; in addition, heat is a by-product of muscular contraction

Light

A. Refraction

EXAMPLE: Total internal reflection in fiberoptics permits viewing of interior walls of stomach and intestines for diagnostic purposes such as endoscopic procedures, gastroscopy, sigmoidoscopy, and proctoscopy

B. X rays

EXAMPLES

1. GI series and barium enemas allow visualization of the soft tissues of the upper and lower gastrointestinal tract; the barium salts coat the inner walls of the alimentary tube and absorb the x rays striking them; as a result, the organ surfaces are outlined
2. Fluoroscopy can be considered the observation of "live" x-ray images; after the x rays pass through the individual, they strike a fluorescent screen that absorbs them and emits visible light; with x-ray–opaque (radiopaque) chemicals the intestinal and biliary tracts can be observed

REVIEW OF CHEMICAL PRINCIPLES RELATED TO THE GASTROINTESTINAL SYSTEM
Oxidation and Reduction

A. Uniting oxygen with a substance results in oxidation

B. Uniting hydrogen with a substance results in reduction

Oxidation-Reduction Reactions in the Body

A. Important in body chemistry as a source of energy through cellular oxidation of foods in cytoplasm and mitochondria; oxidation of nutrients like glucose results in the formation of high-energy ATP molecules and heat—both useful to the body

B. Oxygen is the usual oxidizing agent in cells

C. Some forms of life (anaerobes) can use substances other than oxygen for cellular oxidation (e.g., *Clostridium perfringens* found in gangrenous tissue)

Diffusion and Osmosis

EXAMPLES

1. Diffusion of nutrients and enzymes results in the collisions necessary to promote chemical (metabolic) reactions
2. Absorption of water by osmosis occurs through the mucosa of the GI tract

Active Transport

The movement of molecules against a concentration gradient due to energy (ATP) expenditure

EXAMPLE: The absorption of most simple sugars and amino acids in the small intestine involves active transport processes

Buffers

Pairs of chemical substances that resist changes in pH

EXAMPLE: The sodium bicarbonate part of the bicarbonate buffer system secreted from the pancreas into the duodenum acts as a buffer to prevent acidification of intestinal juices due to the presence of hydrochloric acid from gastric juice

Types of Compounds

Organic Acids

$$\overset{\displaystyle O}{\overset{\displaystyle \|}{}}$$

All organic acids contain the C—OH (carboxyl) group

EXAMPLES

1. Lactic acid—end product of anaerobic muscle metabolism; converted to pyruvic acid and oxidized completely to carbon dioxide and water aerobically
2. Citric acid—one intermediate in the Krebs citric acid cycle; cycle occurs in mitochondria as a major oxidation—reduction pathway for the generation of ATP (potential chemical energy)
3. Salicylic acid—synthesis of aspirin

Amino Acids

A. Amino acids possess 2 functional groups: an amine group and an acid or carboxyl group
B. Amino acids are amphoteric—act as both acids or bases; therefore proteins act as buffers in body fluids
C. Reactions of amino acids
   1. Amino acids are able to act as an acid and as a base (amphoteric character)
   2. Condense via peptide bond to form proteins
D. Essential amino acids cannot be synthesized well enough in the body to maintain health and growth and must be supplied in the food

Carbohydrates

A. Aldehyde or ketone derivatives of single oxidation of polyhydric alcohols, or compounds yielding aldehyde or ketone derivatives on hydrolysis
B. Include simple sugars, starches, celluloses, gums, and resins
C. Widespread in plant and animal tissue
D. Contain carbon, hydrogen, and oxygen; the hydrogen and oxygen are present in approximately the ratio of 2 to 1
E. Synthesis—plants synthesize carbohydrates from carbon dioxide and water with the aid of the green pigment chlorophyll (which acts as an enzyme) and solar energy
F. Classification
   1. By functional group
      a. Carbohydrates having the aldehyde group are called aldoses (e.g., glucose)
      b. Carbohydrates having the ketone group are called ketoses (e.g., fructose)
   2. By complexity of the molecule
      a. Carbohydrate having a single ketose or aldose molecule is called a monosaccharide—a simple sugar (e.g., glucose, fructose)
      b. Carbohydrate formed by combining 2 aldose molecules or an aldose and a ketose molecule is called a disaccharide (e.g., sucrose, lactose, maltose)
      c. Carbohydrate having more than 2 simple sugars joined in a molecule is called a polysaccharide (e.g., starch, glycogen)
G. Tests for glucose in urine
   1. Benedict's test and Clinitest tablets use copper ions in basic medium—show presence of sugar in urine by change in color
   2. Positive reaction gives colors from green (very little sugar) to brick red (more than 2 g sugar/100 ml urine)
   3. Iron ions and silver ions can be used instead of copper to give a test for sugar
   4. Most monosaccharides and disaccharides except sucrose are reducing sugars; therefore sucrose put into urine will not produce a reaction
H. Important carbohydrates
   1. Glycerose and dihydroxyacetone—triose intermediates in cellular metabolism of carbohydrates
   2. Ribose and deoxyribose—pentose constituents in nucleic acids
   3. Glucose (dextrose—hexose monosaccharide; a sugar found abundantly in body fluids, fruits, and vegetables; the pancreatic hormones insulin and glucagon regulate the blood glucose concentration in the normal range of 70 to 105 mg/100 ml blood; glucose is the basic food molecule that is broken down first in glycolysis (in the cytoplasm of cells) and then in the Krebs cycle (in mitochondria); the breakdown of each molecule of glucose results in the release of 38 molecules of ATP, which can be used in almost all cellular energy requiring functions
   4. Fructose (levulose)—ketose monosaccharide;

found in fruits and honey, sweetest sugar known; important intermediate in cellular metabolism of carbohydrates

5. Galactose—hexose monosaccharide; present in brain and nervous tissue
6. Lactose (milk sugar)—disaccharide of glucose and galactose molecules; bacterial fermentation of lactose to lactic acid causes milk to sour
7. Sucrose (cane sugar)—disaccharide of glucose and fructose molecules; nonreducing sugar, common table sugar used in sweetening and baking
8. Maltose—disaccharide of 2 glucose molecules; found in grains and malt
9. Starch—mixed polysaccharide of glucose molecules found in plants
   a. Amylose—straight-chained glucose polymer
   b. Amylopectin—branched-chain glucose polymer
   c. Chief food carbohydrate in human nutrition
   d. Starch polymers react with iodine to form a blue complex; used as a test for starch
      (1) Test becomes colorless as starch is hydrolyzed
      (2) Starch (blue) → amylodextrin (purple) → erythrodextrin (red) → achroodextrin (colorless) → maltose (colorless) → glucose (colorless)
10. Glycogen—polysaccharide polymer of glucose molecules found in human and animal tissue; storage compound in the body; hydrolyzes to glucose, maintaining blood glucose levels
11. Cellulose—polysaccharide polymer of glucose found in plants; not digestible by humans; important in the manufacture of cotton cloth, paper, and cellulose acetate synthetics
12. Inulin—polysaccharide polymer of fructose, used in kidney function test (inulin clearance test)
13. Agar-agar—polysaccharide polymer of galactose used as a solid medium for bacteriologic studies

Lipids

A. Organic substances essentially insoluble in water but soluble in organic solvents (ether, chloroform, acetone, etc.)
B. Fatty acids—important constituents of all lipids (except sterols)
   1. Usually straight-chain carboxylic acids
   2. Naturally occurring fatty acids contain even numbers of carbon atoms
   3. Saturated fatty acids—have no double bonds (points of unsaturation) between their carbon atoms
   4. Unsaturated fatty acids—have 1 or more points of unsaturation between their carbon atoms
   5. Essential fatty acids—cannot be synthesized by the body; must be taken in by diet
C. Classification of lipids
   1. Simple lipids—esters of fatty acids and alcohols
      a. Fats—the alcohol of fats is the trihydric alcohol glycerol
         (1) Solid fats—fats that are solid at room temperature contain long-chain, saturated fatty acids
         (2) Liquid fats (oils)—fats that are liquid at room temperature contain short-chain, unsaturated fatty acids
      b. Waxes—esters of long-chained fatty acids and an alcohol other than glycerol; lanolin, a mixed wax from wool, is used in creams and salves
      c. Reactions of simple lipids
         (1) Hydrolysis—splitting into fatty acid(s) and alcohol by breaking the ester bond is effected by acid, base, or enzyme action
         (2) Saponification—basic hydrolysis; soap is formed from organic salts of a fatty acid and metal ion of base
         (3) Addition—fats containing unsaturated fatty acids will form addition products at points of unsaturation
            (a) Addition of oxygen will cause fat to become rancid; antioxidants slow this reaction in packaged foods
            (b) Unsaturated oils used in paints add oxygen and oils become hard and glossy
            (c) Hydrogenation—liquid fats can form solid fats by adding in hydrogen at double bonds
   2. Compound lipids—fats containing chemical substances other than fatty acids and alcohols
      a. Phospholipids—contain alcohol, fatty acids, phosphoric acid, and a nitrogenous base (or inositol)
         (1) Lecithins—contain the alcohol glycerol, fatty acids, phosphoric acid, and the nitrogenous base choline; are found in brain and nervous tissue; in blood, lecithin serves to render fats soluble in plasma (a lipotropic agent)
         (2) Cephalins—similar in structure to lecithin except base is ethanolamine; important in brain and nerve tissue; help blood-clotting mechanism

(3) Sphingomyelins—made from amino alcohol (sphingosinol), a fatty acid, phosphoric acid, and choline; important in brain and nerve tissue

b. Cardiolipids—made from unsaturated fatty acids, glycerol, and phosphoric acid; found in heart tissue

c. Glycolipids (cerebrosides) structure contains the monosaccharide galactose, amino alcohol (sphingosinol), and a fatty acid; found in brain tissue and the myelin sheaths of nerves

3. Steroids—complex monohydroxy alcohols found in plant and animal tissues—basic structure, the phenanthrine structure plus a cyclopentane ring; characteristic side chains determine specific steroids

a. Cholesterol—a sterol found in human and animal tissue, chiefly in brain and nerve tissue; an important, normal component of membranes; found in blood within a normal range of 150 to 300 mg/100 ml; high blood cholesterol seems associated with coronary thrombosis

b. Ergosterol—a plant sterol that can be converted to vitamin D by ultraviolet light

c. Bile acids—sterols that aid in digestion and absorption of fats

d. Steroid hormones—sex and adrenal gland hormones (glucocorticoids, mineralocorticoids)

e. Vitamin D—steroid helping to control calcium metabolism by regulating calcium uptake from the gastrointestinal tract

Proteins

A. Classification of proteins

1. Simple proteins—give amino acids on hydrolysis

a. Albumins—water soluble, coagulated by heat (e.g., lactalbumin [milk], serum albumin [blood], egg white); albumin is most important in the development of the plasma colloid osmotic pressure, which helps control (through osmosis) the flow of water between the plasma and interstitial fluid; during a condition such as starvation, a fall in the albumin level of the blood leads to a fall in the plasma colloid osmotic pressure; this results in edema because less fluid is drawn by osmosis into the capillaries from the interstitial spaces

b. Globulins—insoluble in water, soluble in dilute salt solutions, coagulated by heat (e.g., lactoglobulin [milk], serum globulin [blood],

gamma serum globulin—forms antibodies of blood)

c. Glutelins—soluble in dilute bases or acids, insoluble in neutral solutions; coagulated by heat (e.g., glutenin [wheat])

d. Albuminoids—soluble in water (e.g., collagen [connective tissue], elastin [ligaments])

e. Histone—water soluble (e.g., globin [hemoglobin])

f. Prolamines—insoluble in water, soluble in 70% to 80% alcohol (e.g., gliadin [wheat], zein [corn])

g. Protamines—water soluble (e.g., protamine [fish spermatozoa])

2. Compound proteins—contain molecules other than amino acids

a. Chromoproteins—proteins containing a colored molecule (e.g., hemoglobin, flavoproteins)

b. Glycoproteins—proteins containing carbohydrate molecule(s) (e.g., mucopolysaccharide of synovial fluid)

c. Lipoproteins—simple proteins combined with lipid substances (e.g., lipovitellin in egg yolk)

d. Nucleoproteins—proteins complexed with nucleic acids (e.g., the DNA [genetic material] found in chromosomes is complexed with proteins); chromosomes are sometimes referred to as nucleoprotein structures

e. Metalloproteins—proteins containing metal ions (e.g., ferritin [iron transport compound of plasma])

f. Phosphoproteins—proteins containing the phosphoric acid radical (e.g., casein of milk)

3. Derived proteins—also called *denatured* proteins; treatment with acids, bases, heat, x-radiation, ultraviolet rays, etc. causes proteins to alter their molecular arrangements

B. Reactions of proteins

1. Amphoteric properties—like the amino acids forming them, proteins can act as an acid or a base in solution; can act as buffers

2. Hydrolysis—acid, base, or enzyme hydrolysis splits the peptide bond; yields proteose → peptones → peptides → amino acids

3. Denaturation—change in structure renders the protein less soluble, leads to coagulation of the protein

a. Heat—protein and heat → coagulated protein (e.g., cooked egg white, cooked meat)

b. Salts of heavy metals—silver, lead, mercury, etc.; taken internally, they are poison because they denature the enzymes of the cells, which are protein in nature

   c. Acetone and alcohol—both harden skin proteins

   d. Inorganic acids and bases—coagulate and hydrolyze proteins

   e. Alkaloids and organic acids—tanning of hides, precipitation of blood proteins for clinical tests

   f. Rays—x rays, infrared rays, ultraviolet rays—long exposure can cause cataracts (precipitation of lens protein in the eye)

  4. Salting out—concentrated salt solutions render soluble proteins insoluble

  5. Color reactions

   a. Xanthoproteic test—protein having a benzene ring (as found in the amino acids tyrosine and phenylalanine) will turn yellow on addition of concentrated nitric acid; heat and a second addition of sodium hydroxide will turn the yellow to orange

   b. Millon test—protein having a phenolic ring (as found in the amino acid tyrosine) will form a red precipitate on addition of a mixture of mercuric and mercurous nitrates

   c. Biuret test—test for the peptide bond; violet appears on addition of a hydroxide and dilute copper sulfate solution; negative for free amino acids (no peptide bond)

   d. Hopkins-Cole test—protein that contains the indole structure (amino acid tryptophan) shows violet on addition of glyoxylic acid and concentrated sulfuric acid

   e. Ninhydrin test—test for free amino acids, ninhydrin reagent gives blue color

Nucleoproteins

A. Specific proteins found in cells, made of large and complex molecules having important functions

B. Composition of nucleoproteins

  1. Hydrolysis of nucleoproteins results in nucleic acids and protein

  2. Hydrolysis of nucleic acid yields

   a. Phosphoric acid—H_3PO_4

   b. Pentose sugars—ribose or deoxyribose

   c. Purine or pyrimidine bases

    (1) Purine bases—adenine, guanine

    (2) Pyrimidine bases—cytosine, uracil, thymine

  3. Combination of a purine or pyrimidine base with either ribose or deoxyribose forms a nucleoside

  4. Addition of phosphoric acid to a nucleoside forms a nucleotide

  5. Polymerization of nucleotide molecules via ester bonds yields a nucleic acid—the shape of DNA is that of a double helix

C. Two main forms of nucleic acid—RNA and DNA (ribonucleic acid and deoxyribonucleic acid)

  1. RNA yields the following on hydrolysis: adenine, guanine, cytosine, uracil, ribose, phosphoric acid

  2. DNA yields the following on hydrolysis: adenine, guanine, cytosine, thymine, deoxyribose, phosphoric acid

D. Role of DNA and RNA in protein synthesis

  1. DNA is found chiefly in the chromatin material of interphase cells and in the chromosomes of cells in mitosis

   a. Portions of DNA molecules are the genes of classic genetics; the genetic code consists of sequences of bases (adenine, guanine, cytosine, and thymine) linearly arranged along the DNA molecule; every 3 bases represent a code for 1 amino acid (a triplet code)

   b. One enormous DNA molecule represents thousands of genes separated from each other by specific triplets (codons) representing periods or commas; i.e., the linear triplet code is punctuated so it can eventually be translated correctly on the ribosome

   c. DNA is also found in mitochondria, chloroplasts, and certain other cellular organelles (like centrioles) and is thought to play some role in their replication and metabolism

  2. RNA is found both inside the nucleus and in the cytoplasm of cells

  3. RNA occurs in three forms: messenger RNA (mRNA), transfer RNA (tRNA), and ribosomal RNA (rRNA)

   a. DNA transcribes its coded message of how to make proteins into mRNA; the function of mRNA is to carry this coded genetic information from the DNA in the nucleus to the ribosome in the cytoplasm where proteins can be synthesized

   b. The transcribed genetic code being carried by mRNA is translated into the synthesis of proteins on the ribosomes; these proteins then serve both structurally and enzymatically in the cell

   c. tRNA molecules each carry an amino acid to the ribosome where protein synthesis is occurring; there is a specific tRNA molecule for each amino acid

   d. rRNA is part of the structure of the ribosome

4. The protein difference between individuals is ultimately determined by differences in the genetic code carried by DNA; the DNA and RNA molecules are presently the only known molecules that store information and can result in the accurate transmission of genetic information from one generation of cell or organism to the next; the cellular mitotic and meiotic processes are elaborate and precise mechanisms for partitioning the genetic material appropriately between daughter cells

E. Other important related compounds
   1. ATP and ADP (adenosine triphosphate and adenosine diphosphate) are energy-storing compounds in cells
   2. NAD (nicotinamide adenine dinucleotide) and NADP (nicotinamide adenine dinucleotide phosphate) are important in hydrogen transport in the metabolism of foods

Enzymes

Hormones involved in regulating the GI tract
A. Gastrin—stimulates flow of gastric juices
B. Enterogastrone—inhibits flow of gastric juices
C. Secretin—stimulates flow of sodium bicarbonate from the pancreas to the duodenum
D. Pancreozymin—stimulates the flow of pancreatic enzymes from the pancreas to the duodenum
E. Cholecystokinin—stimulates contraction of the gallbladder
F. Enterocrinin—stimulates flow of intestinal juice

REVIEW OF MICROORGANISMS RELATED TO THE GASTROINTESTINAL SYSTEM

A. Bacterial pathogens
   1. *Brucella*—three species (*B. abortus, B. suis,* and *B. melitensis*); small, gram-negative, somewhat pleomorphic (variable shape) bacilli, cause brucellosis, an infection primarily of domestic animals (cattle, goats, swine, sheep); humans can acquire it by drinking infected milk
   2. *Escherichia coli*—small, gram-negative bacillus composing the major portion of the normal flora of the large intestine; certain strains are the most common cause of urinary tract infections and infantile diarrhea
   3. *Leptospira icterohaemorrhagiae*—long, tightly coiled spirochete similar in appearance to *Treponema pallidum;* causes infectious jaundice (Weil's disease)
   4. *Shigella*—gram-negative bacillus, similar to *Salmonella; Shigella dysenteriae* and a number of other species cause an illness known as bacillary dysentery or shigellosis

5. *Vibrio cholerae* (formerly *V. comma*)—curved, gram-negative bacillus with a single polar flagellum; causes Asiatic cholera

B. Protozoal pathogens
   1. *Balantidium coli*—ciliated protozoan; causes enteritis
   2. *Entamoeba histolytica*—an ameba; causes amebiasis (amebic dysentery)
   3. *Giardia lamblia*—flagellated protozoan; causes enteritis

C. Parasitic pathogens
   1. Nematodes (roundworms)
      a. *Ancylostoma duodenale* (hookworm)—intestinal parasite similar to *Necator americanus*
      b. *Ascaris lumbricoides* (roundworm)—intestinal parasite resembling the earthworm
      c. *Enterobius vermicularis* (pinworm, seatworm)—small, white parasitic worm found in upper part of the large intestine; the female lays eggs in perianal area, causing irritation
      d. *Necator americanus* (the American hookworm)—intestinal parasite about 1.2 cm (½ inch) long
      e. *Trichuris trichiura* (whipworm)—intestinal parasite about 5 cm (2 inches) long
   2. Cestodes (tapeworm)
      a. *Diphyllobothrium latum* (fish tapeworm)—large tapeworm 6.1 m (about 20 feet) long found in adult form in the intestine of cats, dogs, and humans (vertebrate and aquatic hosts in sequence)
      b. *Echinococcus granulosa* (dog tapeworm)—small tapeworm of dogs; larval stage (hydatid) may develop in humans forming hydatid tumors or cysts in the liver, lungs, kidneys, and other organs
      c. *Hymenolepsis nana* (dwarf tapeworm)—a species about 2.5 cm (1 inch) long, found in adult form in the intestine
      d. *Taenia marginata* (beef tapeworm)—the common tapeworm of humans, a species 3.6 to 7.6 m (12 to 24 feet) long, found in adult form in the human intestine
      e. *Taenia solium* (pork tapeworm)—a species 0.9 to 1.8 m (3 to 6 feet) long found in the adult form in the intestines of humans
   3. Trematodes (flukes)
      a. *Clonorchis sinensis*—one of the most common liver flukes, especially in China and Japan
      b. *Fasciola hepatica*—common liver fluke of

herbivorous animals; occasionally found in the human liver
c. *Fasciolopis buski*—largest of the intestinal flukes
d. *Paragonimus westermani*—lung fluke; found in cysts in the lungs, liver, abdominal cavity, and elsewhere

PHARMACOLOGY RELATED TO GASTROINTESTINAL SYSTEM DISORDERS

A. Antiemetics
  1. General implications for nurses
    a. Observe occurrence and characteristics of vomitus
    b. Eliminate noxious substances from the diet and environment
    c. Provide oral hygiene
    d. Observe the patient for adverse effects
      (1) Drowsiness
      (2) Hypotension
      (3) Dry mouth
      (4) Blurred vision
      (5) Uncoordination
  2. Actions
    a. Diminish the sensitivity of the chemoreceptor trigger zone to irritants (e.g., drugs, radiation therapy)
    b. Those drugs prescribed for motion sickness decrease labyrinthine excitability and the conduction of vestibular-cerebellar stimuli (motion sickness control)
  3. Examples of antiemetics
    a. Promethazine hydrochloride (Fellozine, Ganphen, Phenergan)
    b. Trimethobenzamide hydrochloride (Tigan)
    c. Prochlorperazine (Compazine)
    d. Dimenhydrinate (Dramamine)
    e. Diphenidol hydrochloride (Vontrol)
    f. Hydroxyzine hydrochloride (Atarax, Vistaril)
    g. Meclizine hydrochloride (Bonine)
B. Anorexiants (drugs for appetite suppression)
  1. General implications for nurses
    a. Educate the patient regarding drug misuse
    b. Counsel concerning diet and exercise
    c. Observe for adverse effects
      (1) Constipation
      (2) Blurred vision
      (3) Nausea and vomiting
      (4) Metallic taste
      (5) Tachycardia
      (6) Irritability
  2. Actions

    a. Primary drugs are amphetamines or drugs with comparable action, which act at hypothalamic appetite centers to suppress the desire for food
    b. Amine oxidase inhibition in cerebrocortical and reticular structures; provides elevated mood and increased mental acuity
  3. Examples
    a. Amphetamine sulfate (Benzedrine)
    b. Benzphetamine hydrochloride (Didrex)
    c. Chlorphentermine hydrochloride (Pre-Sate)
    d. Dextroamphetamine sulfate (Dexedrine)
    e. Diethylpropion hydrochloride (Tenuate, Tepanil)
    f. Fenfluramine hydrochloride (Pondimin)
    g. Phenmetrazine hydrochloride (Preludin)
C. Antacids
  1. General implicatons for nurses
    a. Teach the patient about overuse of antacids
    b. Explain need for continued supervision
    c. Attempt to eliminate the source of discomfort
    d. Caution the patient eating a sodium-restricted diet that many of the antacids contain sodium
    e. Observe for adverse effects
      (1) Constipation or diarrhea
      (2) Systemic antacids (sodium bicarbonate) may lead to alkalosis and renal insufficiency
  2. Actions
    a. Provide a protective film on the stomach lining
    b. Lower the gastric acid level, which allows more rapid movement of stomach contents into the duodenum
    c. Drugs containing aluminum, magnesium, and calcium have minimal absorptive tendency
  3. Examples
    a. Aluminum carbonate gel, basic (Basaljel)
    b. Aluminum hydroxide gel (Amphojel)
    c. Aluminum hydroxide with magnesium trisilicate (Gelusil)
    d. Aluminum and magnesium hydroxides (Maalox)
    e. Aluminum phosphate gel (Phosphaljel)
    f. Magaldrate (Riopan)
    g. Sodium bicarbonate (which is absorbed from the intestine and may cause alkalosis)
D. Anticholinergics
  1. General implications for nurses

a. Provide dietary counseling with emphasis on bland foods

b. Observe the patient for adverse effects
   (1) Abdominal distention
   (2) Constipation
   (3) Urinary retention

2. Actions
   a. Decrease production of glandular (salivary, gastric, pancreatic) secretions
   b. Decrease the motility of the digestive tract
   c. Used in the treatment of peptic ulcer

3. Examples
   a. Atropine sulfate
   b. Belladonna leaf, tincture
   c. Isopropamide (Darbid)
   d. Propantheline bromide (Pro-Banthine)
   e. Dicyclomine hydrochloride (Bentyl)

E. Antidiarrheal agents

1. Absorbants
   a. General implications for nurses
      (1) Observe color, characteristics, and frequency of stool
      (2) Observe for signs of electrolyte imbalance
      (3) Assess and eliminate cause of diarrhea
      (4) Give after each loose bowel movement
      (5) Because these drugs are not absorbed, there are minimal side effects
   b. Actions
      (1) Absorb toxic substances as well as nutrients from the digestive tract
      (2) Given after each loose bowel movement; improve consistency of the stool but do not necessarily stop the diarrhea
   c. Examples
      (1) Bismuth subcarbonate
      (2) Kaolin and pectin (Kaopectate)

2. Enteric bacteria replacements
   a. General implications for nurses
      (1) Store in refrigerator
      (2) Contraindicated in children with high fever
      (3) Observe the patient for adverse effects
         (a) Excessive flatulence
         (b) Abdominal cramps
   b. Actions
      (1) Administered when prolonged use of antibiotics has suppressed the natural bacterial flora and overgrowth of pathogenic bacteria has occurred
      (2) Enhance production of lactic acid from carbohydrates in the intestinal lumen; acidity suppresses pathogenic bacterial overgrowth
   c. Examples
      (1) *Lactobacillus acidophilus* (Bacid)
      (2) *Lactobacillus bulgaricus* (Novaflor, Lactinex)

3. Motility suppressants
   a. General implications for nurses
      (1) Warn the patient of the risk of physical dependence with long-term use
      (2) Observe for adverse effects
         (a) Urinary retention
         (b) Tachycardia
         (c) Dry mucous membranes
         (d) Sedation
         (e) Paralytic ileus
         (f) Respiratory depression
   b. Actions
      (1) Increase tone of the intestinal musculature, ileocecal valve, and anal sphincter to slow expulsion of intestinal contents
      (2) Decrease motility so that more water will be absorbed from the large intestine
   c. Examples
      (1) Diphenoxylate hydrochloride (Lomotil)
      (2) Tincture of opium (Paregoric)
      (3) Camphorated opium tincture (0.04% opium content)

F. Cathartics

1. Intestinal lubricants
   a. General implications for nurses
      (1) Do not administer with meals or immediately following meals, since they delay entry of food into the intestines
      (2) Teach the patient regarding overuse of cathartics
      (3) Warn the patient to be aware of side effects of continued use
         (a) Inhibited absorption of fat-soluble vitamins from various foods as well as drug sources
         (b) Anal leaking of oil with continued use
   b. Actions
      (1) Nonabsorbable oils that decrease dehydration of feces
      (2) Lubricate intestinal tract
   c. Examples
      (1) Mineral oil
      (2) Olive oil

2. Fecal softeners

a. General implications for nurses
  (1) Encourage increased roughage and fluid in the diet
  (2) Increase the patient's activity level
  (3) Observe consistency and frequency of stool
b. Actions
  (1) Lower the surface tension of feces in the colon
  (2) Allow water and fats to penetrate feces and ease evacuation of softer stool
c. Examples
  (1) Dioctyl calcium sulfosuccinate (Surfak)
  (2) Dioctyl sodium sulfosuccinate (Colace, Doxinate)
  (3) Peri-Colace

3. Bulk-forming cathartics
  a. General implications for nurses
    (1) Explain to the patient that overuse leads to dependence
    (2) Encourage increased fluid and roughage in diet
    (3) Use with caution for patients taking sodium-restricted diets if the drug contains sodium
    (4) Observe consistency and frequency of stool
  b. Action—increased bulk in the intestinal lumen stimulates propulsive movements by pressure on the mucosal lining
  c. Examples
    (1) Methylcellulose (Cellothyl, Cologel, Hydrolose, Melozets, Methulose, Syncelose)
    (2) Sodium carboxymethylcellulose (Bu-Lax, C.M.C.)
    (3) Psyllium hydrophilic mucilloid (Metamucil, Mucilose)
    (4) Agar

4. Colon irritants
  a. General implications for nurses
    (1) Explain to the patient that prolonged use may lead to dependence
    (2) Observe for adverse effects
      (a) Nausea
      (b) Abdominal cramps
      (c) Diarrhea
    (3) Increase fluid and roughage in the diet
    (4) Observe the consistency and frequency of stool
  b. Action—stimulate peristalsis by reflexive response to irritation caused by the drug's contacting the mucosa of the intestinal lumen

c. Examples
  (1) Cascara sagrada (Peristim)
  (2) Senna (Senokot)
  (3) Castor oil
  (4) Bisacodyl (Dulcolax)

5. Saline cathartics
  a. General implications for nurses
    (1) Instruct the patient to increase bulk in the diet with bran, fresh fruit, cereals, vegetables
    (2) Observe for adverse effects
      (a) Nausea
      (b) Dehydration
      (c) Increased accumulation of sodium ions in the blood
  b. Actions
    (1) Increase osmotic pressure within the intestine, drawing fluid from the blood and bowel wall
    (2) This increases bulk and stimulates peristalsis
    (3) May be used to treat edema
  c. Examples
    (1) Magnesium sulfate (Epsom salts)
    (2) Milk of magnesia
    (3) Magnesium citrate solution
    (4) Effervescent sodium phosphate (Fleet Phospho-Soda)

G. Intestinal antibiotics
  1. General implications for nurses
    a. Know why the drug is being administered
    b. Observe the characteristics of bowel movements
    c. Avoid using drugs that are also ototoxic and nephrotoxic while the patient is receiving the antibiotics
    d. Observe the patient for adverse effects
      (1) Damage to the auditory nerve and kidney
      (2) Nausea, vomiting, diarrhea
      (3) Fungal infections if therapy is prolonged
  2. Actions
    a. Used in the treatment of bacterial diarrhea and as preparation for bowel surgery
    b. Neomycin also used in treatment of hepatic coma, since it suppresses the growth of intestinal flora that will cause a secondary decrease in the blood ammonia level
  3. Examples
    a. Neomycin sulfate
    b. Kanamycin sulfate (Kantrex)

H. Pancreatic enzymes
  1. General implications for nurses

a. Do not crush drugs that are enteric coated (the coating protects against destruction by gastric juices)

b. Administer with meals

c. Provide a balanced diet to prevent indigestion

2. Action—supply digestive enzymes; lipase, protease, amylase

3. Examples

a. Pancrelipase (Cotazym)

b. Pancreatin (Viokase)

RELATED DIAGNOSTIC PROCEDURES
Endoscopy

A. Definition—visualization of the esophagus, stomach, colon, or rectum using a hollow tube with a lighted end

1. Gastroscopy—stomach
2. Esophagoscopy—esophagus
3. Sigmoidoscopy—sigmoid colon
4. Proctoscopy—rectum

B. Nursing responsibilities

1. Obtain an informed consent for the procedure
2. If rectal examination is indicated, administer cleansing enemas prior to the test
3. Restrict diet (n.p.o.) prior to procedure
4. Following the procedure, observe the patient for bleeding, changes in vital signs, or nausea
5. If the throat is anesthetized (as for a gastroscopy or esophagoscopy), check for the return of gag reflex before offering oral fluids

C. Physical principle involved: light refraction

Gastrointestinal (GI) Series

A. Definition—introduction of barium, an opaque medium, into the upper GI tract via the mouth, gastrostomy tube, or nasogastric tube to visualize the area by x-ray methods

B. Nursing responsibilities

1. Explain procedure to the patient
2. Maintain the patient n.p.o. after midnight
3. Inform the patient that the stool will be white or pink for 24 to 72 hours after the procedure
4. Encourage fluids and administer cathartics as ordered

C. Physical principle involved: x rays

Barium Enema

A. Definition—introduction of barium, an opaque medium, into the intestines for the purpose of x-ray visualization for pathologic changes

B. Nursing responsibilities

1. Explain procedure to the patient
2. Prepare the patient for the procedure by

a. Administration of cathartics and/or enemas as ordered to evacuate the bowel

b. Maintaining the patient n.p.o. for 8 to 10 hours prior to the test

3. Inspect stool after the procedure for the presence of barium

4. Administer enemas and/or cathartics as ordered if the stool does not return to normal

C. Physical principle involved: x rays

Gastric Analysis

A. Definition

1. Analysis of stomach contents for the presence of abnormal constituents or lack of normal constituents such as hydrochloric acid, blood, acid-fast bacteria, and lactic acid

2. Acid content is elevated in ulcers, decreased in malignant conditions of the stomach, and absent in pernicious anemia

B. Nursing responsibilities

1. Explain procedure to the patient
2. Maintain the patient n.p.o. prior to the test and have a nasogastric tube passed at time of procedure
3. Administer histamine or caffeine to stimulate hydrochloric acid secretion prior to the procedure if ordered
4. Obtain contents, secure in an appropriate container, and send to laboratory

C. Physical principle involved: Boyle's law

Stool Specimens

A. Definitions

1. Stool for guaiac (occult blood)—specimen or smear of stool on a commercially prepared card is sent to the laboratory for analysis; positive results indicate the presence of blood in the stool and may suggest diverse diseases such as peptic ulcer, gastritis, gastric or colonic carcinoma, colitis, or diverticulitis

2. Stools for O and P (ova and parasites)—must be sent to the laboratory while still warm for microscopic examination

3. Stool culture—specimen or swab of stool is sent in a sterile container for identification of abnormal bacterial growth

B. Nursing responsibilities

1. Explain procedure to the patient
2. Collect specimen in an appropriate container
3. Label the container with the patient's name, identification number, physician and room number
4. Chart that the specimen was sent and any unusual assessment of the stool

RELATED CRITICAL CARE AND GENERAL NURSING PROCEDURES
Enemas

A. Definitions
1. Tap water enema (TWE)—introduction of water into the colon to stimulate evacuation
2. Soapsuds enema (SSE)—introduction of soapy water into the colon to stimulate peristalsis by bowel irritation; contraindicated as a preparation for an endoscopic procedure because it may alter the appearance of the mucosa
3. Harris flush or drip—introduction of water into the colon as tolerated and subsequent repeated drainage of that water through the same tubing to facilitate passage of flatus
4. High colonic irrigation—introduction of water into the upper portion of the colon to facilitate complete fecal evacuation
5. Instillation—introduction of a liquid (usually mineral oil) into the colon to facilitate fecal activity through lubricating effect

B. Nursing responsibilities
1. Explain procedure to the patient
2. Provide privacy
3. Obtain the correct solution
4. Lubricate the tip of a rectal catheter with water-soluble jelly
5. Insert the catheter 10 to 15 cm (4 to 6 inches) into the rectum
6. Allow the solution to enter slowly; keep it no more than 30.5 to 45.7 cm (12 to 18 inches) above the rectum
7. Allow ample time for the patient to expel the enema
8. Observe and record the amount and consistency of returns

C. Physical principle involved: gravity

Irrigation of Nasogastric (Levin) Tube

A. Definition
1. The Levin tube is commonly used for gastric decompression
2. Purposes of insertion of a nasogastric tube include emptying the stomach, obtaining a specimen for diagnostic purposes, or providing a means for nourishment
3. Irrigation is the insertion of fluid (usually normal saline) to maintain patency

B. Nursing responsibilities
1. Check that the order for irrigations has been written by the physician
2. Ascertain the patency of the Levin tube attached to intermittent suction by observing for drain-

age; nausea or abdominal discomfort may indicate that the tube is occluded
3. Assemble equipment: 30-ml syringe or bulb syringe, irrigating solution, and basin for returning fluid
4. Verify placement (see gastric gavage)
5. Instill approximately 30 ml of fluid into the tube
6. Gently withdraw the same volume of fluid as was instilled; if the patient has undergone gastric surgery, the physician will generally order instillations; in this case, irrigation fluid is instilled but not withdrawn; the amount instilled must be subtracted from total gastric output
7. Chart the amount, color, and consistency of drainage

C. Physical principle involved: Boyle's law

Paracentesis

A. Definition—surgical puncture of the peritoneal membrane of the abdominal cavity for the purpose of removing fluid

B. Nursing responsibilities
1. Explain the procedure; obtain consent
2. Have the patient void prior to procedure
3. Assist the patient to a sitting position
4. Observe for signs of shock; sudden fluid shifts can result in hypotension
5. Chart the amount and characteristics of fluid withdrawn
6. Apply a dry sterile dressing to the puncture site
7. Properly label the specimen if required and send to the laboratory

C. Physical principle involved: Boyle's law

Ileostomy Care

A. Definition—physical care of the ileostomy stoma and surrounding skin

B. Nursing responsibilities
1. Protect the skin from irritation, since the feces will be liquid because of the anatomic location of the stoma
2. Explain procedure to the patient and family and encourage self-care
3. Do not irrigate the stoma
4. Affix an appliance with an adequate seal (Karaya) to prevent accidental leakage around the stoma; the appliance is generally worn for 2 to 4 days but emptied every 6 hours

Colostomy Care

A. Definition
1. Instillation of fluid into the lower colon via a stoma on the abdominal wall to stimulate peristalsis and facilitate the expulsion of feces

2. Cleansing the colostomy stoma and collection of feces (stool consistency will depend on location of the ostomy: a colostomy of the sigmoid colon will tend to produce formed stools; a transverse colostomy will produce less formed stools)

B. Nursing responsibilities
1. Secure a physician's order
2. Irrigate the stoma at the same time each day to approximate normal bowel habits
3. Insert a well-lubricated catheter tip into the stoma approximately 7 cm in the direction of the remaining bowel (anatomy of ascending, transverse, and descending colon should be considered); as the solution is allowed to flow, the catheter may be advanced
4. Hold the irrigating container 30.5 to 45.7 cm (12 to 18 inches) above the colostomy; irrigating solution should be 40.5° C (105° F)
5. Clamp tubing or temporarily lower the container if the patient complains of cramping
6. Provide privacy while waiting for fecal returns or permit the patient to ambulate with the collection bag in place to further stimulate peristalsis
7. Cleanse the stoma; if excoriation occurs, a soothing ointment may be ordered
8. Apply a colostomy bag or gauze dressing (if the colostomy is well regulated)
9. Teach the patient to control odor when necessary by placing two aspirin tablets (or commercially available deodorizers) in the colostomy bag or by taking bismuth subcarbonate tablets orally to control odor

C. Physical principle involved: gravity

Gastric Gavage (Tube Feeding)

A. Definition—feeding a prepared liquid formula via a tube passed into the stomach
B. Nursing responsibilities
1. Verify the placement of the tube before feedings
   a. Inject a small amount of air into the tube and, with a stethoscope placed over the epigastric area, listen for the passage of air into the stomach
   b. Aspirate for stomach contents
   c. Place the end of the nasogastric tube in water; presence of bubbling indicates the tube is in the lungs (this method is the least reliable)
2. Place the patient in a sitting position to prevent aspiration
3. Introduce a small amount of water first to verify the patency of the tube; the tube should not be allowed to empty during feeding so that excess air is not forced into the stomach

4. Administer the feeding (which may be the patient's normal foods blenderized) at room or body temperature slowly; observe and question the patient to determine tolerance; the higher the feeding container and the larger the lumen of the feeding tube, the more rapid the flow
5. Administer a small amount of water to clear the tube at the completion of feeding
6. Clamp the tubing and clean the equipment
7. Provide special skin care if the patient has a gastrostomy tube; the skin may become irritated from gastric enzymes; wash and apply a protective ointment as necessary
8. Encourage the patient to chew certain foods that will stimulate gastric secretions while providing psychologic comfort

C. Physical principle involved: Boyle's law

Hyperalimentation (Total Parenteral Nutrition [T.P.N.])

A. Definition
1. High-protein, high-caloric intravenous feeding used for patients with disturbances of ingestion or digestion
2. One liter of the specially prepared solution may provide 70 to 80 g of protein in the form of amino acids, as well as vitamins, electrolytes, and 1000 to 2000 calories

B. Nursing responsibilities
1. Infuse fluid through a large vein such as the subclavian because of the high osmolarity of the solution
2. Ensure proper placement of the tube by chest x-ray examination after insertion of a catheter; accidental pneumothorax can occur during insertion
3. Precisely regulate the fluid infusion rate; an intravenous pump should be used if available
   a. Rapid infusion may result in movement of the fluid from an intravascular compartment; dehydration, circulatory overload, and hyperglycemia can occur
   b. Slow infusion may result in hypoglycemia, since the body adapts to the high osmolarity of this fluid by secreting more insulin; for this reason, hyperalimentation is never terminated abruptly but is gradually discontinued
4. Use aseptic technique when handling the infusion or changing the dressing (in many institutions, only nurses specially trained are allowed to change the dressing because of the high risk of infection)

5. Record daily weights and monitor urinary sugar and acetone levels every 4 to 6 hours
6. Check laboratory reports daily, especially glucose, creatine, BUN, and electrolytes
7. Monitor temperature q. 4 h. since infection is the most common complication of hyperalimentation; if the patient has a temperature elevation, order cultures of blood, urine, and sputum to rule out other sources of infection

MAJOR DISEASES
Stomatitis

A. Etiology and pathophysiology
  1. Inflammation of the buccal mucosa because of disease, trauma, irritants, nutritional deficiencies, or medications
  2. Categories
    a. Aphthous stomatitis—canker sore that can result from chronic cheek biting
    b. Herpes simplex—virus that causes vesicle formation in mouth, on lips, or on nose
    c. Vincent's angina—ulceration of the buccal membrane due to *Borrelia vincentii* (trench mouth)
    d. Thrush—fungal invasion of the mouth by *Candida albicans,* characterized by white patches
B. Signs and symptoms
  1. Subjective
    a. Foul taste in the mouth
    b. Pain in the mouth
  2. Objective
    a. Erythema of the mucous membranes
    b. Changes in salivation
    c. Unpleasant odor to the breath
    d. Bleeding gums in Vincent's angina
    e. White patches in thrush
C. Treatment
  1. Adequate nutrition and hydration
  2. Alkaline mouthwashes
  3. Antifungal agents for thrush
  4. Antibiotics for Vincent's angina
D. Nursing care
  1. Provide mouthwashes every 2 hours
  2. Encourage foods that can be tolerated, such as soft foods, cool drinks, eggnogs
  3. Promote oral hygiene; use soft toothbrush or padded tongue blade

Fracture of the Jaw

A. Etiology and pathophysiology—generally the result of trauma such as motor vehicle accidents or physical combat

B. Signs and symptoms
  1. Subjective
    a. History of trauma to the face
    b. Pain in the face and jaw
  2. Objective
    a. Bloody discharge from the mouth
    b. Swelling of face on the affected side
    c. Difficulty opening or closing the mouth
C. Treatment
  1. Separated fragments of the broken bone are reunited and immobilized by wires and rubber bands; usually placed without surgical incision
  2. Open reduction of the jaw is indicated for severely fractured or displaced bones; interosseous wiring is done
D. Nursing care
  1. Postoperatively control vomiting and reduce the chance of aspiration pneumonia by positioning patient on abdomen
  2. Keep wire cutters at the bedside to release the wires and rubber bands if emesis occurs
  3. Explain diet to the patient and family; no solid foods are permitted; encourage high-protein liquids or blenderized soft foods
  4. Stress the importance of regular oral hygiene and institute it early in the postoperative period

Cancer of the Mouth

A. Etiology and pathophysiology
  1. Primarily in patients who smoke and drink alcohol in large quantities
  2. Cancer of the lip, easily diagnosed; prognosis is very good; incidence highest in pipe smokers
  3. Cancer of the tongue, usually occurs with cancer of the floor of the mouth; metastasis to the neck common
  4. Cancer of the submaxillary glands, highly malignant and grows rapidly
B. Signs and symptoms
  1. Subjective
    a. Pain not an early symptom
    b. Alterations of taste sensation
  2. Objective
    a. Leukoplakia (white patches on mucosa, which are considered precancerous)
    b. Ulcerated areas in the involved structure
C. Treatment
  1. Reconstructive surgery if indicated
  2. Radiation or implantation of radioactive material may arrest growth of tumor
D. Nursing care
  1. Maintain fluid and electrolyte balance

2. Provide for a means of communication
3. If radiation therapy is indicated, relieve dryness of the mouth by frequent mouthwashes and ample fluids
4. Consider time and distance in relation to the radioactive material when giving nursing care

Cancer of the Esophagus

A. Etiology and pathophysiology
   1. Etiology unknown—occurs predominantly in persons with a history of alcohol abuse or hiatus hernia
   2. Tumor may develop anywhere in the esophagus, but most commonly in the middle and lower third
B. Signs and symptoms
   1. Subjective
      a. Dysphagia
      b. Substernal pain
      c. Substernal burning after drinking hot liquids
   2. Objective
      a. Regurgitation
      b. X-ray examination of esophagus reveals irregularities of the lumen
      c. Cytologic examination of cells obtained after esophageal lavage reveals malignant cells
C. Treatment
   1. Surgical removal of the esophagus is the treatment of choice
      a. Esophagogastrostomy—resection of a portion of the esophagus; a portion of the bowel may be grafted between the esophagus and stomach, or the stomach may be brought up to the proximal end of the esophagus
      b. Esophagectomy—removal of part or all of the esophagus, which is replaced by a Dacron graft
      c. Gastrostomy—opening directly into the stomach in which a feeding tube is usually inserted to bypass the esophagus
   2. Radiation and/or chemotherapy may be used prior to or instead of surgery as a palliative measure
D. Nursing care
   1. Support the patient and family emotionally
   2. Formulate realistic goals in planning patient care
   3. Observe for respiratory distress caused by pressure of tumor on the trachea; place in a semi-Fowler or high Fowler position to facilitate respirations
   4. Monitor vital signs, especially respirations
   5. Provide oral care, since dysphagia may result in increased accumulation of saliva in mouth
   6. Maintain nutritional status by providing high-protein liquids along with vitamin and mineral replacements

Hiatal Hernia

A. Etiology and pathophysiology
   1. Portion of the stomach protruding through a hiatus (opening) in the diaphragm into the thoracic cavity
   2. May result from a congenital weakness of the diaphragm or from injury, pregnancy, or obesity
   3. Function of the cardiac sphincter is lost, gastric juices enter the esophagus, and edema and hyperemia may result
B. Signs and symptoms
   1. Subjective
      a. Substernal burning pain
      b. Heartburn after eating, which increases in the recumbent position
      c. Nocturnal dyspnea
   2. Objective
      a. GI series and endoscopy show protrusion of the stomach through the diaphragm
      b. Regurgitation
C. Treatment
   1. Small, frequent, bland feedings
   2. Antacids
   3. Surgical repair (done infrequently)
D. Nursing care
   1. Teach the patient and family about the dietary regimen
   2. Encourage attempts at weight loss
   3. Avoid constricting clothing
   4. Elevate head of the bed after meals
   5. Encourage the patient to eat slowly

Gastritis

A. Etiology and pathophysiology
   1. Inflammation of the stomach; either acute or chronic
   2. May be caused by
      a. Ingestion of irritating chemicals such as aspirin and alcohol
      b. Bacterial or viral infections
      c. Allergic reactions
      d. Chronic uremia, which often leads to chronic gastritis
B. Signs and symptoms
   1. Subjective
      a. Anorexia
      b. Nausea and vomiting
      c. Epigastric fullness
   2. Objective

  a. Diarrhea and cramps if caused by an infection
  b. Dehydration
  c. Hemorrhage if aspirin or other chemicals are involved
C. Treatment
  1. Early treatment aimed at correcting the fluid and electrolyte imbalance; the patient is kept n.p.o. during the acute phase of illness and then progresses to a bland diet
  2. If caused by infection, appropriate antibioics may be given
  3. Other medications that may be prescribed include antispasmodics, anticholinergics, and antacids
D. Nursing care
  1. Observe for signs of dehydration and electrolyte imbalance
  2. Provide adequate fluid intake
  3. Alert the patient to possible causes
  4. Teach the patient the necessary dietary alterations such as omission of coffee, alcohol, and spices and maintaining a bland diet

Peptic Ulcer

A. Etiology and pathophysiology
  1. Ulcerations of the gastrointestinal mucosa and underlying tissues caused by gastric secretions that have a low pH (acid)
  2. Causes include conditions that increase the secretion of hydrochloric acid by the gastric mucosa or that decrease that tissue's resistance to the acid
    a. Zollinger-Ellison syndrome—tumors secreting gastrin, which will stimulate the production of excessive hydrochloric acid
    b. Certain drugs such as aspirin and indomethacin will decrease tissue resistance
    c. Many believe that psychosomatic causes are strongly related to peptic ulcers; a person who is considered a perfectionist may have an increased risk of developing a peptic ulcer
  3. Peptic ulcers may be present in the esophagus, stomach, or duodenum (the most common site)
  4. Complications include pyloric or duodenal obstruction, hemorrhage, and perforation
B. Signs and symptoms
  1. Subjective
    a. Gnawing or burning epigastric pain that occurs 1 to 2 hours after eating and may be relieved by eructation, vomiting, food, or antacids
    b. Nausea
  2. Objective

  a. If bleeding occurs, signs of anemia will be evident; passage of tarry stools (melena) may occur
  b. Vomiting (coffee ground to port wine color if bleeding has occurred)
C. Treatment
  1. Institute measures to neutralize or buffer hydrochloric acid, inhibit acid secretion, and decrease the activity of pepsin and hydrochloric acid such as
    a. Radiation and gastric hypothermia to suppress gastric secretions
    b. Diet regulation through the use of bland foods, and restriction of irritating substances such as nicotine, caffeine, alcohol, spices, and gassy foods
    c. Antacids to reduce acidity
  2. Type and cross match so that blood will be available if gastric hemorrhage occurs
  3. Sedatives, tranquilizers, anticholinergics, and analgesics for pain and restlessness
  4. Antiemetics for nausea and vomiting
  5. Bed rest to reduce physical activity
  6. Encourage the patient to seek counseling or psychotherapy to explore the emotional components of the illness
  7. If hemorrhage occurs, a nasogastric tube is inserted and iced saline lavages may be ordered; irrigations with medications that cause vasoconstriction to control bleeding are also used
  8. Surgical intervention
    a. Vagotomy—cutting of the vagus nerve (X), which innervates the stomach, to decrease the secretion of hydrochloric acid
    b. Bilroth I—removal of the lower portion of the stomach and attachment of the remaining portion to the duodenum
    c. Bilroth II—removal of the antrum and distal portion of the stomach and subsequent anastomosis of remaining section to the jejunum
    d. Antrectomy—removal of the antral portion of the stomach
    e. Gastrectomy—removal of 60% to 80% of the stomach
  9. Common complications of partial or total gastric resection
    a. Dumping syndrome—involves the rapid passage of food from the stomach to the jejunum; the food, being hypertonic (especially if high in carbohydrates), will draw fluid from the circulating blood into the jejunum causing diaphoresis, faintness, and palpitations
    b. Hemorrhage

c. Pneumonia
d. Pernicious anemia
D. Nursing care
1. Allow ample time for the patient to express feelings and concerns
2. Administer and assess effects of sedatives, antacids, anticholinergics, and dietary modifications
3. Encourage hydration to reduce anticholinergic side effects and dilute the hydrochloric acid in the stomach
4. Refrain from administering drugs such as salicylates, phenylbutazone, steroids, and ACTH, which are normally contraindicated
5. Observe for complications such as gastric hemorrhage, perforation, and drug toxicity
6. Postoperative care after gastric resection
a. Monitor vital signs; assess the dressing for drainage
b. Maintain a patent nasogastric tube to the suction apparatus to prevent stress on the suture line
c. Observe the color and amount of nasogastric drainage; excessive bleeding or the presence of bright red blood after 12 hours should be reported immediately
d. Have the patient cough, deep breathe, and change position frequently to prevent the occurrence of pulmonary complications
e. Monitor intake and output
f. Apply an abdominal binder if ordered
g. Apply antiembolism stockings; have the patient ambulate early to prevent vascular complications
h. To prevent dumping syndrome, instruct the patient to
(1) Eat smaller meals at more frequent intervals
(2) Avoid high-carbohydrate intake
(3) Limit the amount of fluid ingested with meals
(4) Lie down or rest after eating
7. Teach drug regimen and signs and symptoms of recurrence
8. Prevent recurrence by teaching patient to modify dietary, working, and living patterns; maintain regularity in activities of daily living; continue medical supervision

Carcinoma of the Stomach

A. Etiology and pathophysiology
1. Often not diagnosed until metastasis occurs; the stomach is able to accommodate to the growth of a tumor, and pain occurs late in the disease
2. May metastasize by direct extension, lymphatics, or blood to the esophagus, spleen, pancreas, liver, or bone
3. Heredity apparently a factor in the development of carcinoma of the stomach, as is the presence of precursors such as ulcerative disease and pernicious anemia
4. Incidence higher in men over 40 years of age; Japan has a 4 times greater rate of cancer of the stomach than does the United States
B. Signs and symptoms
1. Subjective
a. Anorexia
b. Nausea
c. Belching (eructation)
d. Heartburn
2. Objective
a. Weight loss
b. Anemia
c. Positive stools for guaiac (occult blood)
d. Achlorhydria (absence of hydrochloric acid, determined by gastric analysis)
C. Treatment
1. Subtotal or total gastrectomy
2. Radiation
3. Chemotherapy (fluorouracil is often used)
D. Nursing care
1. Offer the patient every opportunity to verbalize fears (i.e., cancer, death, family problems, self-image)
2. Postoperative care the same as nursing care after a gastric resection (see peptic ulcers); in addition, if a total gastrectomy is performed, the chest cavity is usually entered, so the patient will have chest tubes (see pneumothorax for related nursing care)
3. Modify diet to include smaller, more frequent meals
4. If total gastrectomy has been performed, the patient will have a vitamin B_{12} deficiency (see pernicious anemia)
5. Patient may require gavage feedings via nasogastric tube or gastrostomy tube (see procedures)

Cholecystitis

A. Etiology and pathophysiology
1. Inflammation of the gallbladder; usually caused by the presence of stones (cholelithiasis), which are composed of cholesterol, bile pigments, and calcium
2. Diseased gallbladder is unable to contract in response to fatty foods entering the duodenum because of obstruction by calculi or edema

    3. When the common bile duct is completely obstructed, the bile is unable to pass into the duodenum and is absorbed into the blood
    4. Incidence is highest in obese women in the fourth decade

B. Signs and symptoms
    1. Subjective
      a. Indigestion after eating fatty or fried foods
      b. Pain, usually in the right upper quadant of the abdomen, which may radiate to the back
      c. Nausea
    2. Objective
      a. Vomiting
      b. Elevated temperature and WBC
      c. Jaundice in approximately 25% of patients
      d. Diagnostic tests
        (1) Intravenous cholangiogram; patients who are allergic to the dye will complain of sensation of warmth, urticaria, nausea, and vomiting
        (2) Serum bilirubin will be elevated
        (3) Gallbladder series; approximately 6 radiopaque tablets such as Telepaque or Bilopaque are taken with water the evening before so that the gallbladder will be visible on x-ray examination

C. Treatment
    1. Rest
    2. Low-fat diet to avoid stimulating the gallbladder, which constricts to excrete bile with subsequent pain; calories principally from carbohydrate foods in acute phases; if weight loss is indicated, calories may be reduced to 1000 to 1200; postoperatively patients may take fat-restricted diets initially but progress to regular diets
    3. Surgical intervention
      a. Cholecystotomy—incision into the gallbladder for the purpose of drainage
      b. Cholecystectomy—removal of the gallbladder
      c. Choledochotomy—incision into the common bile duct

D. Nursing care
    1. Teach dietary modification to limit fatty foods
    2. Relieve pain both preoperatively and postoperatively
    3. Observe for signs of bleeding (vitamin K is fat soluble and is not absorbed in the absence of bile); administer vitamin K preparations as ordered
    4. Postoperative care
      a. Patients will generally have a nasogastric tube attached to suction to prevent distention
        (1) Maintain patency of the tube
        (2) Assess and measure drainage
      b. Fluid and electrolytes are initially provided by IV route
        (1) Monitor intake and output
        (2) Check IV site for redness, swelling, heat, or pain
      c. Keep the patient in a low Fowler position
      d. Have the patient cough and deep breathe; splint the incision (incision is high and midline, making coughing extremely uncomfortable)
      e. Care of patients with a T tube to bile drainage (if the common bile duct has been explored, a T tube is inserted to maintain patency)
        (1) Secure the drainage bag; avoid kinking of the tube
        (2) Measure drainage at least every shift; drainage during the first day may reach 500 to 1000 ml and then gradually decline
        (3) Apply protective ointments, if ordered, to prevent excoriation
        (4) When the tube is removed, usually in 7 days, observe stool for normal brown color, which indicates bile is again entering the duodenum

Acute Pancreatitis

A. Etiology and pathophysiology
    1. May result from gallstones, alcoholism, carcinoma, or acute trauma to the pancreas or abdomen
    2. Inflammation with or without edema of pancreatic tissues, suppuration, abscess formation, hemorrhage, or necrosis, depending on the severity of the disease and the cause

B. Signs and symptoms
    1. Subjective
      a. Abrupt onset of pain in the central epigastric area that may radiate to shoulder, chest, and back described as aching, burning, stabbing, or pressing
      b. Abdominal tenderness
      c. Nausea
    2. Objective
      a. Elevated temperature
      b. Vomiting
      c. Tachycardia

d. Changes in character of the stools

e. Hypotension

f. Shock

g. Grossly elevated serum amylase and lipase

3. Severity of symptoms depends on the cause of the problem, the amount of fibrous replacement of normal duct tissue, the degree of autodigestion of the organ, the type of associated biliary disease if present, and the amount of interference in blood supply to the pancreas

4. Symptoms may be exaggerated by the development of complications such as pseudocysts, abscesses, pancreatic fistulas, and hyperglycemia

C. Treatment

1. Antacids to neutralize gastric secretions

2. Barbiturates and tranquilizers to reduce emotional tension

3. Narcotics to control pain

4. Cardiotonics to lessen strain on the heart caused by increased metabolic demands and altered circulatory volume

5. Bed rest to decrease metabolic demands and promote healing

6. Nasogastric decompression to control nausea and remove gastric hydrochloric acid

7. Diet regulated according to the patient's condition: nothing by mouth; parenteral administration of fluid, electrolytes, and other nutrients; diet low in fats and proteins, with restriction of stimulants such as caffeine and alcohol

8. Anticholinergics to supress vagal stimulation and decrease gastric motility and duodenal spasm

9. Antibiotics to prevent secondary infections and abscess formation

10. Surgical intervention if the patient fails to respond to medical management, develops persistent jaundice, or bleeds; type of surgery is determined by the cause (e.g., biliary tract surgery, removal of gallstones, drainage of cysts)

D. Nursing care

1. If the patient has a nasogastric tube

a. Administer frequent, thorough mouth care

b. Apply lubricant to the external nares to prevent irritation and eventual breakdown of mucous membranes

c. Observe for electrolyte imbalances (manifested by symptoms such as tetany, irritability, jerking, muscular twitching, mental changes, and psychotic behavior)

d. Observe for signs of adynamic ileus (e.g., nausea and vomiting, abdominal distention)

2. Be alert for hyperglycemic states

3. Monitor vital signs

4. Teach the importance of taking medications containing amylase, lipase, and trypsin in controlling pancreatic insufficiency

5. Encourage the adoption of a life-style that allows for emotional stability, rest, follow-up medical care

6. Use the semi-Fowler position and encourage deep breathing and coughing to promote deeper respiration and prevent respiratory problems

7. Maintain n.p.o. during the acute stage of illness

8. Closely monitor IV feedings until oral feedings can be tolerated

9. Assist in ingestion of small feedings of low-fat, gaseous-free fluids, progressing to diet as tolerated and prescribed

10. Teach the patient and family the importance of dietary discretion, especially the avoidance of alcohol, coffee, spicy foods, and heavy meals, while recognizing religious and cultural factors

11. Help the patient set realistic goals for convalescent period

12. Teach the patient and family about prevention of recurrences and/or control of symptoms (e.g., diet therapy, drug therapy, avoiding foods and substances such as alcohol and caffeine, regular medical supervision, rest requirements)

Cancer of the Pancreas

A. Etiology and pathophysiology

1. Malignant growth from the epithelium of the ductal system producing cells that block the ducts of the pancreas

2. Fibrosis, pancreatitis, and obstruction of the pancreas

3. Lesion tends to metastasize by direct extension to the duodenal wall, splenic flexure of the colon, posterior stomach wall, and common bile duct

4. Cause unknown

B. Signs and symptoms

1. Subjective

a. More common in middle-aged men than women

b. History of chronic pancreatitis, diabetes mellitus, and alcoholism is common

c. Weight loss, anxiety, depression, anorexia, and nausea

d. Severe pain present in most patients

2. Objective
   a. Jaundice
   b. Diarrhea and steatorrhea, along with clay-colored stools and dark urine
   c. Physical examination usually demonstrates presence of a right upper quadrant mass
   d. Decreased serum amylase and lipase levels due to decreased secretion of enzymes
   e. Increased serum bilirubin and alkaline phosphatase levels when biliary ducts are obstructed
C. Treatment
   1. Prepare for surgical intervention by ordering red blood cell and blood volume replacement and medications to correct coagulation problems and nutritional deficiencies
   2. Chemotherapy and radiation when surgery is not possible to provide comfort, or in conjunction with surgery to limit metastasis
   3. Medications to control diabetes if present
   4. Drug therapy such as pancreatic enzymes, bile salts, and vitamin K to correct deficiencies
   5. Analgesics and tranquilizers for pain
   6. Surgery (the treatment of choice, although the postsurgical prognosis is grim): Whipple procedure (removal of the head of the pancreas, the duodenum, a portion of the stomach, and the common bile duct) or a cholecystojejunostomy (creation of an opening between the gallbladder and jejunum)
D. Nursing care
   1. Provide emotional support for the patient and family and set realistic goals in planning care
   2. Administer analgesics as ordered, and as soon as needed, to promote rest and comfort
   3. Use soapless bathing and antipruritic agents to relieve pruritus
   4. Observe the patient for complications such as peritonitis, gastrointestinal obstruction, jaundice, hyperglycemia, and hypotension if patient has undergone surgery
   5. Observe the stools for undigested fat
   6. Frequently monitor the vital signs, observing for wound hemorrhage caused by coagulation deficiency
   7. Administer vitamin K parenterally as ordered
   8. Encourage coughing, turning, and deep breathing
   9. Assist with IPPB therapy as required
   10. Monitor urinary output
   11. Observe for chemotherapeutic and radiation side effects; (e.g., skin irritation, anorexia, nausea, vomiting)
   12. Maintain skin markings of the radiation therapist
   13. Encourage frequent and supplemental feedings as tolerated
   14. Control nausea and vomiting before feedings, if possible
   15. Administer vitamin supplements, bile salts, and pancreatic enzymes, as ordered
   16. Provide oral hygiene and maintain an esthetic environment especially at mealtime

Hepatitis

A. Etiology and pathophysiology
   1. Type A hepatitis (infectious hepatitis)
      a. Caused by Type A hepatitis virus
      b. Transmitted via fecal-oral route, contact with blood or contaminated food (e.g., shellfish)
      c. Incubation period 30 to 40 days
      d. Immune serum antigen (ISG) given after exposure is helpful in preventing disease
      e. Confers immunity on individual
   2. Type B hepatitis (serum hepatitis)
      a. Caused by Type B hepatitis virus
      b. Transmitted by contact with contaminated blood or blood products (e.g., toothbrush, razor, needle)
      c. Incubation period 40 to 180 days
   3. Phases of disease
      a. Prodromal or preicteric
      b. Icteric
      c. Recovery (may take 4 months)
   4. Progression to cirrhosis, hepatic coma, and death may occur, although this is rare
   5. Other causes of hepatitis include chemical agents such as halothane (an anesthetic agent), carbon tetrachloride, gold compounds, and arsenic
B. Signs and symptoms
   1. Prodromal (preicteric) phase
      a. Malaise
      b. Weight loss
      c. Anorexia
      d. Symptoms of upper respiratory tract infection
      e. Intolerance for smoking
   2. Icteric phase
      a. Jaundice
      b. Bile-colored urine that foams when shaken
      c. Acholic (clay-colored) stools
   3. Recovery phase—easy fatiguability
C. Treatment
   1. Rest
   2. Diet therapy

a. High protein—healing of liver tissue vital; daily intake should include 1 qt milk, 2 eggs, 8 oz lean meat, fish, or cheese; total should approximate 75 to 100 g protein

b. High carbohydrate—energy needs, restore glycogen reserves; use daily 4 servings vegetables including potato, 4 servings fruit with frequent juices, 6 to 8 servings bread or cereal; total carbohydrate should be 300 to 400 g

c. Moderate fat—2 to 4 tablespoons butter or fortified margarine, sufficient for making food palatable; a moderate amount of easily digestible foods such as whole milk, cream, butter, margarine, or vegetable oil is beneficial; total fat should be 100 to 150 g daily

d. High calorie—increased energy needs for disease process and tissue regeneration and to spare protein for healing; these food amounts should provide about 2500 to 3000 calories daily

D. Nursing care
1. Encourage quiet activities
2. Attempt to stimulate the appetite
   a. Oral hygiene
   b. Selection of foods based on the patient's preferences
   c. Provide a pleasant, unhurried atmosphere for eating
3. Use special precautions to prevent the spread of infectious hepatitis to others
   a. Special handling of needles
   b. Food and utensils isolated and sterilized; visitors taught how to handle these or to use disposable utensils
   c. Gloves worn when handling the patient's bedpan

Hepatic Cirrhosis

A. Etiology and pathophysiology
1. Irreversible fibrosis and degeneration of the liver
2. Several types of cirrhosis; Laënnec's (alcoholic cirrhosis, nutritional cirrhosis) most common
3. Incidence higher in alcoholics, who are often malnourished, and in those who have had hepatitis
4. Pressure rises in the portal system (which drains blood from the digestive organs), causing stasis and backup in digestive organs
5. As liver failure progresses, there is increased secretion of aldosterone, decreased absorption and utilization of the fat-soluble vitamins (A, D, E, K), and ineffective detoxification of protein wastes

6. Hepatic coma may result from high blood ammonia levels when the liver is unable to convert the ammonia to urea

B. Signs and symptoms
1. Subjective
   a. Nausea
   b. Weakness, fatigue
   c. Anorexia
   d. Abdominal discomfort
2. Objective
   a. Weight loss
   b. Ascites
   c. Esophageal varices as a result of portal hypertension
   d. Hemorrhoids
   e. Edema of extremities
   f. Hematemesis
   g. Hemorrhage due to decreased formation of prothrombin
   h. Jaundice
   i. Delirium caused by rising blood ammonia levels
   j. Elevated liver enzymes (SGOT, SGPT, LDH)
   k. Decreased serum albumin

C. Treatment
1. Rest
2. Restriction of alcohol intake
3. Vitamin therapy—especially A, D, E, and K
4. Diuretics to control ascites and edema
5. Neomycin and lactulose may be prescribed for elevated blood ammonia levels
6. If respiratory distress occurs as a result of ascites, a paracentesis is done; slow removal of fluid from the peritoneal cavity will relieve acute symptoms
7. Surgical intervention for portal hypertension—a portal-caval shunt, in which the circulation from the portal vein bypasses the liver and enters the vena cava, usually decreases portal hypertension
8. Blakemore-Sengstaken tube is utilized in the treatment of bleeding esophageal varices to apply direct pressure to the varices
9. Dietary modification
   a. Cirrhosis
      (1) Protein according to tolerance—with increasing liver damage protein metabolism is hindered; hold to 80 to 100 g as long as tolerated; reduce as necessary
      (2) Continue high carbohydrate–moderate fat as in hepatitis, to supply energy; vitamin supplements, especially B complex
      (3) Low sodium—usually restricted to 500

to 1000 mg daily by eliminating salt and controlling foods processed with salt or sodium-based preservatives; sodium restriction helps to control the increasing ascites

(4) Soft foods—if esophageal varices are present, to prevent danger of rupture and bleeding

(5) Alcohol strictly forbidden, to avoid continued irritation and malnutrition

b. Hepatic coma
(1) Low protein—reduced according to tolerance, 15 to 30 g
(2) High calories and vitamins according to need—about 1500 to 2000 calories, sufficient to prevent tissue catabolism and the liberation of additional nitrogen
(3) Fluid carefully controlled according to output

D. Nursing care
1. Observe the patient for objective signs of disease
2. Observe mental status, which may vary
3. Observe for bleeding
4. Provide special skin care and keep nails trimmed, since pruritus is associated with jaundice
5. Maintain the patient in a semi-Fowler position to prevent ascites from causing dyspnea
6. Monitor intake and output, abdominal girth, and daily weight to assess fluid and electrolyte balance
7. Assist with paracentesis (see procedure)
8. When a Blakemore-Sengstaken tube is in place
   a. Maintain traction once the tube is passed and the gastric balloon is inflated to ensure proper placement
   b. Maintain the esophageal balloon as it has been inflated to 30 to 35 mm Hg
   c. If ordered, deflate the balloon for a few minutes at specific intervals to prevent necrosis
   d. Irrigate with iced saline if ordered
   e. Suction orally as necessary, since the patient is unable to swallow saliva

Carcinoma of the Liver

A. Etiology and pathophysiology
1. May be primary or metastatic carcinoma; primary carcinoma of the liver is rare
2. Generally lethal within a few months

B. Signs and symptoms
1. Subjective
   a. Anorexia
   b. Ache in epigastric area

2. Objective
   a. Weight loss
   b. Anemia

C. Treatment
1. Generally palliative
2. Hepatic lobectomy if the tumor is confined (the liver has extraordinary regenerative capacity)
3. Percutaneous infusions with cytotoxic agents

D. Nursing care
1. Provide comfort
2. Be available to both the patient and family members to discuss their feelings
3. Postoperatively
   a. Maintain fluid and electrolyte balance with IV therapy
   b. Monitor intake and output
   c. Observe for signs of bleeding, hypoglycemia, and other metabolic dysfunctions resulting from impaired liver function
   d. Have the patient cough, deep breathe, and change position frequently to prevent pulmonary and circulatory complications
   e. Because the thoracic cavity may be entered during surgery, also be aware of the care of a patient with chest tubes (see pneumothorax)

Sprue

A. Etiology and pathophysiology
1. Etiology unknown; possible hereditary factor
2. Nontropical sprue similar to celiac disease in children and is characterized by intolerance to gluten, abnormalities in the structure of the small intestines, and malabsorption
3. Tropical sprue is endemic in the Indian subcontinent and the Caribbean and is thought to be due to infection rather than diet
4. Intolerance to gluten results in blunting of the intestinal villi, which reduces absorption surface of the intestinal mucosa

B. Signs and symptoms
1. Subjective
   a. Anorexia
   b. Fatigability
2. Objective
   a. Weight loss
   b. Anemia (macrocytic)
   c. Diarrhea
   d. Steatorrhea
   e. Visualization of the small bowel demonstrates flat, blunt villi
   f. Tetany
   g. Demineralization of the skeletal system

C. Treatment
1. Tropical sprue may respond to a high-protein, normal-fat diet with supplemental vitamin B_{12}, A, D, E, K, folic acid, and iron; in addition, antibiotics such as tetracycline for at least 6 months may be helpful
2. Nontropical sprue may respond to a high-protein, normal-fat, gluten-gliadin–free diet and vitamin supplements of A, D, K, B complex, and folic acid as well as iron and calcium
3. Whenever the disease does not respond to diet, corticosteroids may be used
4. Fluid and electrolyte imbalances must be restored

D. Nursing care
1. Teach the patient and family how to modify the diet to comply with medical management
2. Instruct the family that rice, corn, and soy flours should be used in place of wheat, rye, barley, and oats
3. Advise the patient as to the importance of follow-up care for disease management
4. Provide an opportunity for the patient and family to verbalize feelings about the illness
5. Observe the patient for signs of electrolyte imbalance
6. Record weight on a regular basis

Appendicitis

A. Etiology and pathophysiology
1. Compromised circulation and inflammation of the vermiform appendix
2. Causes include obstruction by a fecalith, foreign body, or kinking
3. Inflammation may be followed by edema, necrosis, and rupture

B. Signs and symptoms
1. Subjective
   a. Anorexia
   b. Nausea
   c. Right lower quadrant pain
   d. Rebound tenderness
2. Objective
   a. Vomiting
   b. Fever
   c. Leukocytosis

C. Treatment
1. Surgical removal of the appendix without delay to decrease the chance of rupture and the risk of peritonitis
2. Prophylactic use of antibiotics postoperatively
3. Fluid and electrolyte maintenance
4. Analgesics for pain

D. Nursing care
1. Provide emotional support, since this condition is unanticipated and the individual needs to ventilate any fear of surgery
2. Monitor fluid and electrolyte balance
3. Assess the patient for signs of infection
4. Encourage early ambulation, if not contraindicated by the patient's condition, to prevent complications
5. Assess the patient's return of bowel function

Regional Enteritis

A. Etiology and pathophysiology
1. Etiology unknown
2. Usually occurs in young adults, but can occur at any age
3. Inflammatory changes involving any part of the alimentary tract but usually demarcated segments of the small bowel
4. Ulceration of the intestinal submucosa accompanied by congestion, thickening of the small bowel, and fissure formations
5. Enlargement of regional lymph nodes
6. Fibrosis and narrowing of the intestinal wall
7. Abscesses and fistulas to the abdominal wall, bladder, and vagina

B. Signs and symptoms
1. Subjective
   a. Pain in the lower right quadrant, cramping, and spasms
   b. Nausea
   c. Exacerbations related to emotional upsets or dietary indiscretions with milk, milk products, and fried foods
2. Objective
   a. Borborygmus (rumbling, gurgling sound in the intestines), flatulence
   b. Weight loss
   c. Fever
   d. Electrolyte disturbance
   e. Diarrhea
   f. Gastrointestinal x-ray series to detect and outline the congested, thickened, fibrosed, and narrowed appearance of the intestinal wall; also abscesses and fistulas, partial bowel obstruction, and ulceration of the mucosa
   g. Proctosigmoidoscopy is performed to exclude other disease, such as ulcerative colitis and diverticulitis
   h. Stools are examined for the presence of blood, fat, protein, parasites, or ova
   i. Fecal fat test is performed to determine fat content, an abnormal amount of which is sig-

nificant in malabsorptive disorders or hyper-motility

    j. D-Xylose tolerance test is performed to determine absorptive ability of upper intestinal tract

C. Treatment

  1. Nothing by mouth in the presence of vomiting

  2. Clear fluid diet progressing to bland low-residue, low-fat diet but increased calories, proteins, vitamins (especially vitamin K), and carbohydrates

  3. Hyperalimentation may be ordered when oral intake is inadequate

  4. Medications such as

    a. Antiemetics

    b. Vitamins and minerals

    c. Anticholinergics

    d. Antidiarrheics

    e. Antiinflammatories

    f. Antiinfectives

  5. Surgery (resection of diseased part) if the patient does not respond to medical therapy or if complications such as obstruction, abscesses, or fistulas occur

D. Nursing care

  1. Monitor intake and output

  2. Offer clear liquids hourly as ordered once the patient ceases to experience nausea and vomiting

  3. Encourage high-calorie, high-protein, high-carbohydrate diet supplemented with vitamins and potassium as ordered

  4. Assist with hyperalimentation therapy if ordered (see procedure)

  5. Offer small, frequent feedings considering patient preference, types of foods allowed, and esthetic factors

  6. Record weight daily

  7. Observe for signs of complications such as elevated temperature, increasing nausea and vomiting, abdominal rigidity

  8. Communicate concern and awareness regarding the patient's discomfort and emotional lability during exacerbations of this chronic illness

  9. Teach the patient

    a. To avoid taking laxatives and salicylates that irritate the intestinal mucosa

    b. How to take antidiarrheics and mucilloid drugs effectively and the observations to make during their use

    c. Skin care if the perineal area is irritated

    d. The importance of seeking help early when exacerbations occur

Crohn's Disease

A. Etiology and pathophysiology

  1. Although the causative mechanisms are unknown, there are various theories involving genetic predisposition, autoimmune reaction, or environmental causes

  2. Cobblestone ulcerations form along the mucosal wall of the terminal ileum, cecum, and ascending colon, which form scar tissue and inhibit food absorption in the area

  3. Ulcerations may perforate through the intestinal wall and form fistulas with adjoining organs

B. Signs and symptoms

  1. Subjective

    a. Severe pain in the right lower quadrant

    b. Malaise

  2. Objective

    a. Moderate fever

    b. Elevated WBC

    c. Mild diarrhea with mucus but *no blood*

    d. Anemia

C. Treatment

  1. High-calorie, high-protein diet

  2. Vitamin supplements, including B_{12}, if a large portion of ileum is involved

  3. Medications such as

    a. Anticholinergics

    b. Analgesics

    c. Intestinal antibiotics

    d. Immunosuppressives

  4. Surgery when fistulas or intestinal obstruction occurs; the involved area of intestine is removed and the ends are anastomosed, if possible; an ostomy is indicated if large areas of intestine are involved

D. Nursing care

  1. Provide an emotionally therapeutic environment in which patient can communicate concerns and stresses resulting from this illness

  2. Plan diet with patient and family, using sample menus to promote compliance

  3. Observe patient for signs of fluid and electrolyte imbalances

Ulcerative Colitis

A. Etiology and pathophysiology

  1. May be caused by emotional stress, an autoimmune response, or a genetic predisposition

  2. Edema of the mucous membrane of the colon leads to bleeding and shallow ulcerations

  3. Abscess formation occurs, and the bowel wall shortens and becomes thin and fragile

  4. Due to the shortening of the intestinal wall,

there is increased flow of contents, which leads to diarrhea
B. Signs and symptoms
  1. Subjective
    a. Weakness, debilitation
    b. Anorexia
    c. Nausea
  2. Objective
    a. Dehydration with poor skin turgor
    b. Passage of bloody, purulent, mucoid, watery stools
    c. Anemia
    d. Low-grade fever
C. Treatment
  1. If tolerated, unrestricted fluid intake; high-protein, high-calorie diet; avoidance of food allergens, especially milk
  2. Medications such as
    a. Antiemetics
    b. Anticholinergics
    c. Corticosteroids
    d. Antibiotics
    e. Sedatives, analgesics, and tranquilizers
    f. Antidiarrheics
  3. Replacement of fluids and electrolytes that are lost because of diarrhea
  4. A temporary ileostomy, a partial colectomy, or a total colectomy with a permanent ileostomy may be performed when (a) no response to medical treatment is evident, (b) course of the disease is downhill, (c) massive hemorrhage or colonic obstruction occurs, or (d) cancer is suspected
D. Nursing care
  1. Serve small frequent feedings of a high-protein, high-calorie, low-residue, bland nature
  2. Teach the patient about importance of diet in controlling and/or minimizing symptoms
  3. Involve the patient in dietary selection, recognizing preferences as much as possible
  4. Initiate accurate administration and recording of fluid, electrolyte, or blood replacements as ordered by the physician
  5. Plan nursing care to allow the patient complete bed rest and the maximum number of rest periods
  6. Institute comfort measures (e.g., a warm powdered bedpan, sheepskin under the buttocks, gentle thorough perineal care) as required
  7. Observe for complications such as rectal hemorrhage, fever, dehydration
  8. Allow the patient and family time to verbalize feelings and participate in care
  9. If an ileostomy is performed, help the patient accept the changes of body image and function involved (see ostomy care)

Intestinal Obstruction
A. Etiology and pathophysiology
  1. Interference with normal peristaltic movement of intestinal contents due to neurologic or mechanical impairments
  2. Causes
    a. Carcinoma of the bowel
    b. Hernias
    c. Adhesions (scar tissue that forms abnormal connections after surgery or inflammation)
    d. Intussusception (telescoping of the bowel on itself)
    e. Volvulus (twisting of the intestines)
    f. Paralytic ileus (interference with neural innervation of the intestines resulting in a decrease in or absence of peristalsis; may be caused by surgical manipulation, electrolyte imbalance, or infection)
B. Signs and symptoms
  1. Subjective
    a. Colicky abdominal pain
    b. Constipation
  2. Objective
    a. Abdominal distention
    b. Vomiting; may contain fecal matter
    c. Decreased or absent bowel sounds
    d. Signs of dehydration and electrolyte imbalance
    e. Flat plate of the abdomen shows the bowel distended with air
C. Treatment
  1. Restriction of oral intake; administration of parenteral fluid and electrolytes
  2. Surgical correction of cause (i.e., hernias, adhesions)
  3. Colostomy, cecostomy, or ileostomy as necessary
  4. Drugs such as pantothenyl alcohol (Ilopan) and neostigmine (Prostigmin) to stimulate the passage of flatus
  5. Gastric decompression by means of a nasogastric, Cantor, or Miller-Abbott tube
D. Nursing care
  1. Assess the patient for dehydration and electrolyte imbalance
  2. Monitor intake and output
  3. Auscultate for bowel sounds; note the passage of flatus
  4. Administer mouth care frequently

5. Measure abdominal girth daily to assess distention
6. Provide special care for the patient with a Miller-Abbott or Cantor tube
   a. Once the lubricated tube is inserted, position the patient first on the right side, to facilitate passage of tube through the pylorus, and then in a semi-Fowler position, to continue the gradual advance into the intestines
   b. Coil and loosely attach extra tubing to the patient's gown to avoid tension against peristaltic action
   c. Irrigate as ordered to maintain patency
   d. Frequently assess placement of the tube; record the level of advancement
   e. Remove the tube gradually because it is being pulled against peristalsis

Cancer of the Small and Large Intestines

A. Etiology and pathophysiology
   1. Cancer of the colon and rectum—can cause a narrowing of the lumen of the bowel, ulcerations, necrosis, or perforation
   2. Predisposing factors include familial polyps, chronic ulcerative colitis, and possibly bowel stasis or ingestion of food additives
   3. Cancer of the colon—more common in males, and incidence increases after 50 years of age
   4. Cancer of the small intestine—usually adenocarcinoma
B. Signs and symptoms
   1. Subjective
      a. Abdominal discomfort
      b. Weakness
   2. Objective
      a. Alterations in usual bowel function (constipation or diarrhea or alternating constipation and diarrhea)
      b. Blood in stool
      c. Distention
      d. Changes in shape of stool (pencil shaped, ribbon)
      e. Weight loss
      f. Secondary anemia
C. Diagnosis and treatment
   1. Diagnostic measures
      a. Digital examination of the rectum to detect any palpable masses
      b. Proctosigmoidoscopy to visualize the bowel directly to determine the presence of abnormalities and to perform a biopsy
      c. Stool examination to test for occult blood
      d. Cytologic examination to detect for malignant cells
      e. Hemoglobin level to detect anemia
      f. Alkaline phosphatase and SGOT levels to detect metastasis to the liver
      g. Serum carcinoembryonic antigen (C.E.A.) measure to screen for carcinoma of the colon
   2. After diagnosis is established, the physician may prepare the patient for surgery by
      a. Prescribing antibiotics to reduce bacteria in the bowel
      b. Typing and cross matching of blood for transfusions to correct the anemia
      c. Ordering vitamin supplements to improve the nutritional status
      d. Inserting a Cantor or Miller-Abbott tube with suction to decompress the colon
   3. Surgical intervention to remove the mass and restore bowel function (e.g., hemicolectomy, resection of the transverse colon, abdominal perineal resection)
   4. Radiation in nonsurgical situations in an attempt to relieve symptoms or postoperatively limit metastases
   5. Chemotherapy orally or parenterally in an attempt to reduce the lesion and limit metastases
   6. Postoperatively
      a. Antibiotic therapy to reduce infection
      b. Parenteral fluids and electrolytes to maintain levels
      c. Cholinergics to stimulate peristalsis
      d. Cantor or Miller-Abbott tube clamped for regular, increasing periods and removed when the patient is able to tolerate clamping and bowel sounds have returned
      e. Sips of water progressing to clear liquid diet and to low-residue diet as tolerated
   7. If colostomy has been performed
      a. Colostomy irrigations as required
      b. Irrigations of perineal incision if present and the application of enzymes such as streptokinase to liquefy protein matter and promote drainage
D. Nursing care
   1. Observe vital signs, increasing abdominal pain, nausea, and vomiting to detect early signs of complications
   2. Monitor patency of the Cantor or Miller-Abbott tube to ensure that accumulated air and fluid are decreased and distention is minimized; instill or irrigate the tube with normal saline as ordered
   3. Note the character of drainage from the decompression tube
   4. Implement measures for mechanical cleansing

and intestinal antisepsis preoperatively (e.g., enemas, colonic irrigations, antibacterial therapy such as neomycin or sulfonamides)

5. Administer chemotherapeutic drugs if ordered and observe for significant side effects such as stomatitis (ulceration of the mouth), dehydration, nausea and vomiting, diarrhea, leukopenia
6. Administer electrolyte and parenteral fluid replacement as ordered in situations of bleeding, vomiting, and/or obstruction
7. Carefully note the patient's tolerance to the introduction of oral fluids and foods while the intestinal tube is clamped
8. Teach the patient and family dietary modifications, including low-residue, non-gas-forming foods, avoidance of stimulants, adequate fluid intake; diet should be as close to the patient's normal as possible
9. Provide colostomy care using medical aseptic technique (see procedure)
10. Recognize that the patient with a colostomy may experience sadness, withdrawal, depression, and suicidal thoughts as a result of body image changes
11. Assess the patient's reaction to the colostomy, recognizing that a great deal will depend on how the patient sees its affecting life-style, physical and emotional status, social and cultural background, and place and role in the family
12. Encourage the patient's involvement in colostomy care as soon as physical and emotional status permits
13. Encourage visiting by family members, stressing the patient's increased need for love and acceptance
14. Recognize that the patient with a cecostomy or colostomy is especially sensitive to gestures, odors, facial expressions, and the amount of attention given
15. Teach the patient and family care of the colostomy, measures to facilitate acceptance and adjustment, resumption of activities, and the need for regular medical supervision
16. Teach the patient that colostomy drainage can be controlled by following a regular irrigation schedule and dietary modifications
17. Arrange for follow-up care with community agencies as required (e.g., Public Health, Home Care Program, Cancer Society, ostomy resource person)

Peritonitis

A. Etiology and pathophysiology
 1. Inflammation of the peritoneum
 2. Generally caused by infection from perforation of GI tract or by chemical stress, as in pancreatitis
B. Signs and symptoms
 1. Subjective
  a. Abdominal pain, rebound tenderness
  b. Malaise
  c. Nausea
 2. Objective
  a. Muscle rigidity over the area
  b. Elevated temperature and WBC
  c. Vomiting
C. Treatment
 1. Bed rest in a semi-Fowler position to drain the area
 2. Nasogastric tube attached to suction and left in place until the patient passes flatus
 3. Fluids and electrolytes replaced parenterally
 4. Antibiotic therapy
 5. Surgery to correct the cause of peritonitis (e.g., appendectomy, incision and drainage of abscesses, closure of a perforation)
D. Nursing care
 1. Maintain the semi-Fowler position to help localize infection in the pelvic area
 2. Assess the patient's temperature, vital signs, and pain
 3. Monitor IV therapy and gastrointestinal decompression
 4. Monitor intake and output
 5. Auscultate for bowel sounds; note the passage of flatus

Hemorrhoids

A. Etiology and pathophysiology
 1. Varicosities of the rectum that can be internal or external
 2. Constipation, prolonged sitting or standing, straining at defecation, and pregnancy increase the risk of developing hemorrhoids
B. Signs and symptoms
 1. Subjective
  a. Anal pain
  b. Pruritus
 2. Objective
  a. Protrusion of varicosities around the anus
  b. Rectal bleeding and mucus discharge
C. Treatment
 1. Low-roughage diet (elimination of raw fruits and vegetables)

2. Use of laxatives and stool softeners to regulate bowel habits
3. Analgesic suppositories and ointments may be prescribed in addition to sitz baths to alleviate discomfort
4. Internal hemorrhoids may be ligated with rubber bands; as necrosis occurs, the tissue sloughs off
5. Hemorrhoidectomy—surgical removal of hemorrhoids

D. Nursing care
1. Administer medication as ordered to relieve discomfort
2. Provide privacy and sufficient time for defecation
3. Educate the patient about the use of roughage, fluids, laxatives, and stool softeners
4. Assist the patient with sitz baths
5. Administer cleansing enemas and prepare the perineal area preoperatively
6. Observe for rectal hemorrhage and urinary retention postoperatively
7. Administer a retention enema on the second or third postoperative day if ordered to stimulate defecation and soften the stool
8. Explain to the patient that postoperatively a small amount of bleeding with a bowel movement is normal

Hernias

A. Etiology and pathophysiology
1. Protrusion of an organ or structure through a weakening in the abdominal wall; may contain fat, intestine, or an organ, such as the bladder
2. Abdominal wall can become weakened due to a congenital or acquired defect
3. If the protruding structure can be manipulated back in place, the hernia is said to be reducible; if it cannot, it is considered incarcerated
4. Strangulation occurs when blood supply to the tissues within the hernia is disrupted; this is an emergency situation, since gangrene occurs
5. Hernias are named according to location
   a. Incisional—due to failure of fascia or muscles to heal postoperatively; intraabdominal pressure causes herniation through the scar tissue
   b. Umbilical—due to failure of the umbilicus to close at birth or to a congenital weakness of the musculature in the area; increased intraabdominal pressure due to obesity, pregnancy, or chronic cough causes herniation through the umbilicus
   c. Femoral—when a loop of intestine herniates through the femoral canal due to a weakness in the femoral ring; more common in women than men; strangulation is a common complication
   d. Inguinal—when a loop of intestine herniates through a weakened abdominal ring (frequently through the spermatic cord) into the inguinal canal; more common in men than women

B. Signs and symptoms
1. Subjective
   a. History of the appearance of swelling after lifting, coughing, or vigorous exercise
   b. Pain (may be due to irritation or strangulation)
   c. Nausea can accompany strangulation
2. Objective
   a. Swelling (lump) in the groin or umbilicus, or near an old surgical incision, that may subside when the patient is in a recumbent position
   b. Vomiting and abdominal distention may develop when strangulation occurs

C. Treatment
1. Manual reduction by gently pushing the mass back into the abdominal cavity
2. When the patient is a poor surgical risk, use of a truss (pad worn next to skin held in place under pressure by a belt)
3. Herniorrhaphy (surgical repair of the defect in the abdominal musculature or fascia)
4. Hernioplasty to prevent recurrence (wire, mesh, or plastic may be inserted to strengthen the abdominal wall)

D. Nursing care
1. Teach the patient using a truss that it should be applied prior to getting out of bed
2. After surgery
   a. Observe the patient for signs of respiratory infection; administer cough suppressants as ordered to prevent stress on the incision
   b. Instruct the patient to self-splint when coughing and turning to provide incisional support
   c. When spinal anesthesia is used, peristalsis is not interfered with and postoperative diet can be normal; when general anesthesia is used, nasogastric decompression may be employed until peristalsis returns
   d. Administer mild cathartics as ordered to prevent straining and increased intraabdominal pressure at defecation
   e. Apply an ice bag and scrotal support with a rolled towel or suspensory if the scrotum is

edematous postoperatively to reduce the edema and pain
  f. Administer medication for pain as ordered when necessary
  g. Instruct the patient to avoid lifting or strenuous exercise on discharge until permitted by the surgeon

Anorexia Nervosa

A. Etiology and pathophysiology
  1. Most common in adolescent through 30-year-old population
  2. More common in females
  3. Aversion to food may result from neurotic concern with obesity
  4. Variety of psychiatric disorders may lead to an emaciated state
B. Signs and symptoms
  1. Subjective
    a. Fatigue or hyperactivity
    b. Globus hystericus (lump in the throat)
    c. Epigastric fullness
    d. Nausea
  2. Objective
    a. Vomiting, usually self-induced
    b. Constipation
    c. Emaciation
    d. Hypotension
    e. Low blood glucose
    f. Anemia
    g. Low BMR
    h. Amenorrhea
C. Treatment
  1. Gradually increase caloric and protein intake
  2. Psychiatric consultation when the individual is receptive
  3. Forced supplements (tube feedings) may be indicated if malnutrition is severe
D. Nursing care
  1. Briefly discuss dietary modification with the individual in a nonthreatening manner; do not focus on eating or weight loss
  2. Develop a therapeutic environment and offer emotional support; develop a trusting relationship

Obesity

A. Etiology and pathophysiology
  1. Occurs when intake of calories exceeds expenditure over a time
  2. Causative factors—overeating, genetic predisposition to certain body types, metabolic imbalances, social and emotional stresses, childhood obesity (resulting in excess numbers of fat cells)

B. Signs and symptoms
  1. Subjective
    a. Malaise
    b. Depression
    c. Fatigue
    d. Dyspnea
  2. Objective
    a. Weight gain that exceeds 20% of ideal weight of the standard height-weight table
    b. Skinfold thickness greater than 0.2 inch measured with skinfold calipers
    c. Tachycardia
    d. Hypertension
C. Treatment
  1. Balanced calorie-restricted diet that may be followed for a more long-term effect (fad dieting should be avoided)
  2. 1 or 2 pound/week loss yields optimal results
  3. Behavior modification program
    a. Food diary (self-monitoring)
    b. Control speed of eating; food should be chewed for a preset length of time
    c. Control the response to hunger stimuli
    d. Reinforce compliance (system of rewards should be established for changes in eating patterns or reduction of pounds)
  4. Support groups
  5. Psychotherapy
D. Nursing care
  1. Provide emotional support
  2. Encourage long-range nutritional counseling
  3. Encourage involvement in an exercise program
  4. Educate regarding the hazards of obesity
  5. Assess for complications (hypertension, diabetes mellitus, respiratory insufficiency)

Food Poisoning

A. *Staphylococcus aureus*
  1. Etiology and pathophysiology
    a. Gram-positive *Staphylococcus* strain that clots plasma (coagulase positive); is the most virulent type and causes a variety of infections
    b. Most food poisoning resulting in GI upset occurs as a result of this bacterium
    c. Organism is found in unrefrigerated creams, mayonnaise, stuffing, meats, and fish
    d. Bacteria usually are transmitted to food on the hands of food handlers
    e. Incubation period is 1 to 6 hours after ingestion of contaminated food, with symptoms lasting 24 to 48 hours
  2. Signs and symptoms
    a. Subjective

(1) Nausea
(2) Malaise
(3) Abdominal cramps and pain
  b. Objective
(1) Diarrhea
(2) Subnormal temperature
(3) Vomiting
3. Treatment
  a. Supply with adequate fluid and electrolytes orally or parenterally
  b. Bed rest
4. Nursing care
  a. Offer fluids in small amounts as tolerated
  b. Teach the patient the importance of eating foods that are properly prepared and stored
B. Botulism
1. Etiology and pathophysiology
  a. *Clostridium botulinum*—large, gram-positive bacillus; an obligate anaerobe; its exotoxin, the most powerful biologic toxic known, is responsible for botulism
  b. Organism causes the most serious, often fatal, form of food poisoning
  c. Toxins found in improperly processed foods (mostly canned foods) that have been infected with the anaerobic bacillus *Clostridium botulinum*
  d. Toxins block neuromuscular transmission in cholinergic nerve fibers by possibly binding with acetylcholine
  e. Incubation period usually 12 to 72 hours after ingestion of contaminated food, but may be as long as 4 to 8 days
2. Signs and symptoms
  a. Subjective
(1) Lassitude and fatigue
(2) Diplopia
(3) Weakness of muscles in the extremities
(4) Dysphasia and dysphagia
  b. Objective
(1) Diminished visual acuity
(2) Loss of pupillary light reflex
(3) Diminished gag reflex
3. Treatment
  a. Keep the patient in a darkened room
  b. IV feedings to prevent aspiration
  c. Tracheostomy and other supportive measures as necessary
  d. Cathartics and cleansing enemas to remove toxins from the body
  e. Trivalent antitoxins as necessary
4. Nursing care
  a. Prevent aspiration pneumonia by proper positioning; keep suction equipment available at the bedside
  b. Carefully observe the patient's neurologic status to determine progression of the disease
  c. Prevent contractures and emboli by the use of range-of-motion exercises
  d. Provide emotional support to the patient and family in an attempt to reduce anxiety
C. Salmonellosis
1. Etiology and pathophysiology
  a. Many species of *Salmonella* cause a local GI infection in which organisms do not enter blood (unlike S. *typhosa* and S. *paratyphi*); such infections are referred to as salmonellosis or salmonella food poisoning
  b. Organisms found in inadequately cooked meats
  c. Multiply in the intestines, causing GI upset and infection
  d. Incubation period usually 10 to 24 hours after ingestion of contaminated food, and symptoms usually last 2 to 3 days
2. Signs and symptoms
  a. Subjective
(1) Nausea
(2) Malaise
(3) Abdominal cramps end pain
  b. Objective
(1) Chills and fever
(2) Vomiting
3. Treatment
  a. Bed rest
  b. Fluid and electrolyte replacement
4. Nursing care
  a. Offer the patient small amounts of fluids as tolerated
  b. Teach the patient the importance of eating foods that have been cooked properly

Genitourinary System

REVIEW OF ANATOMY AND PHYSIOLOGY OF THE GENITOURINARY SYSTEM
Urinary System

Functions
A. Secrete urine
B. Eliminate urine from body (urination, micturition, or voiding) to
1. Excrete various normal and abnormal metabolic wastes
2. Regulate the composition and volume of blood and regulate blood pressure; especially impor-

tant in maintenance of fluid and electrolyte balance and acid-base balance (see section on maintenance of fluid, electrolyte, and acid-base balance)

Organs
Kidneys
A. Gross anatomy
1. Size, shape, and location—about $10 \times 5 \times 2.5$ cm ($4 \times 2 \times 1$ inches); shaped like lima beans; lie against the posterior abdominal wall, behind the peritoneum at the level of the last thoracic and first 3 lumbar vertebrae; right kidney slightly lower than the left
2. External structure
   a. Hilum—concave notch on the mesial surface; blood vessels, nerves, lymphatics, and ureter enter through this notch
   b. Renal capsule—protective fibrous tissue that envelops the kidney
3. Internal structure
   a. Cortex—outer layer of the kidney substance; composed of renal corpuscles convoluted tubules and adjacent parts of loops of Henle
   b. Medulla—inner portion of the kidney; composed of loops of Henle and collecting tubules
   c. Pyramids—triangular wedges of medullary substance that have striped appearance and are composed of collecting tubules
   d. Columns—inward extensions of cortex between the pyramids
   e. Papillae—apices of the pyramids; collecting tubules drain into minor calyces here
   f. Calyces—bell-mouthed cups that drain the papillae; 8 to 12 minor calyces open into 2 or 3 major calyces that form the pelvis
   g. Pelvis—a small funnel tapering into the ureter and formed by union of several calyces
B. Blood flow in the kidney
1. Kidneys receive 20% of cardiac output during rest; reduced to 2% to 4% during physical or emotional stress
2. Abdominal aorta gives rise to the renal artery, which enters the hilum of each kidney; renal artery branches into interlobar arteries which fan out into kidney cortex; smaller arterial branches form afferent arterioles, which enter glomerular capillary beds
3. Efferent arterioles leave the glomerular capillary bed forming the peritubular capillary network which then converges into progressively larger veins until the renal vein leaves the kidney

C. Nephron—anatomic and functional unit of the kidney; approximately one million per kidney
1. Anatomy
   a. Glomerulus—cluster of capillaries invaginated in Bowman's capsule
   b. Bowman's capsule—the funnel-shaped upper end of the urinary tubules
   c. Renal corpuscle—composed of Bowman's capsule and the glomerulus invaginated in it
   d. Proximal convoluted tubule—first portion of kidney tubules
   e. Henle's loop—second portion of kidney tubules
   f. Distal convoluted tubule—third portion of kidney tubules
2. Physiology—nephron functions via principles of filtration, reabsorption, and secretion (Fig. 6)
   a. Glomerulus—urine formation starts with process of filtration; water and solutes (except cellular elements of blood, albumins, fibrinogen, and other blood proteins) filter out of capillaries through glomerular-capsular membrane and into Bowman's capsule
   b. Bowman's capsule—filrate collects here prior to flow to the tubules
   c. Tubular reabsorption and secretion—epithelial lining of tubules reabsorbs substances useful to the body and excretes, dissolved in water, all excess and waste substances; secretes electrolytes essential to acid-base balance
      (1) Proximal tubule
         (a) Reabsorption of glucose and other nutrients (e.g., vitamins and amino acids) from the tubular filtrate to the blood in the peritubular capillaries; mainly by active transport mechanisms in the tubular epithelium
         (b) Reabsorption of electrolytes from the tubule filtrate to blood in the peritubular capillaries; cations (notably sodium) are reabsorbed by active transport, stimulated by aldosterone; anions (notably chlorides and bicarbonate) are reabsorbed by diffusion following cation transport
         (c) Reabsorption of about 80% of the water from the tubular filtrate to the blood in the peritubular capillaries by osmosis as a result of electrolyte reabsorption
      (2) Loop of Henle

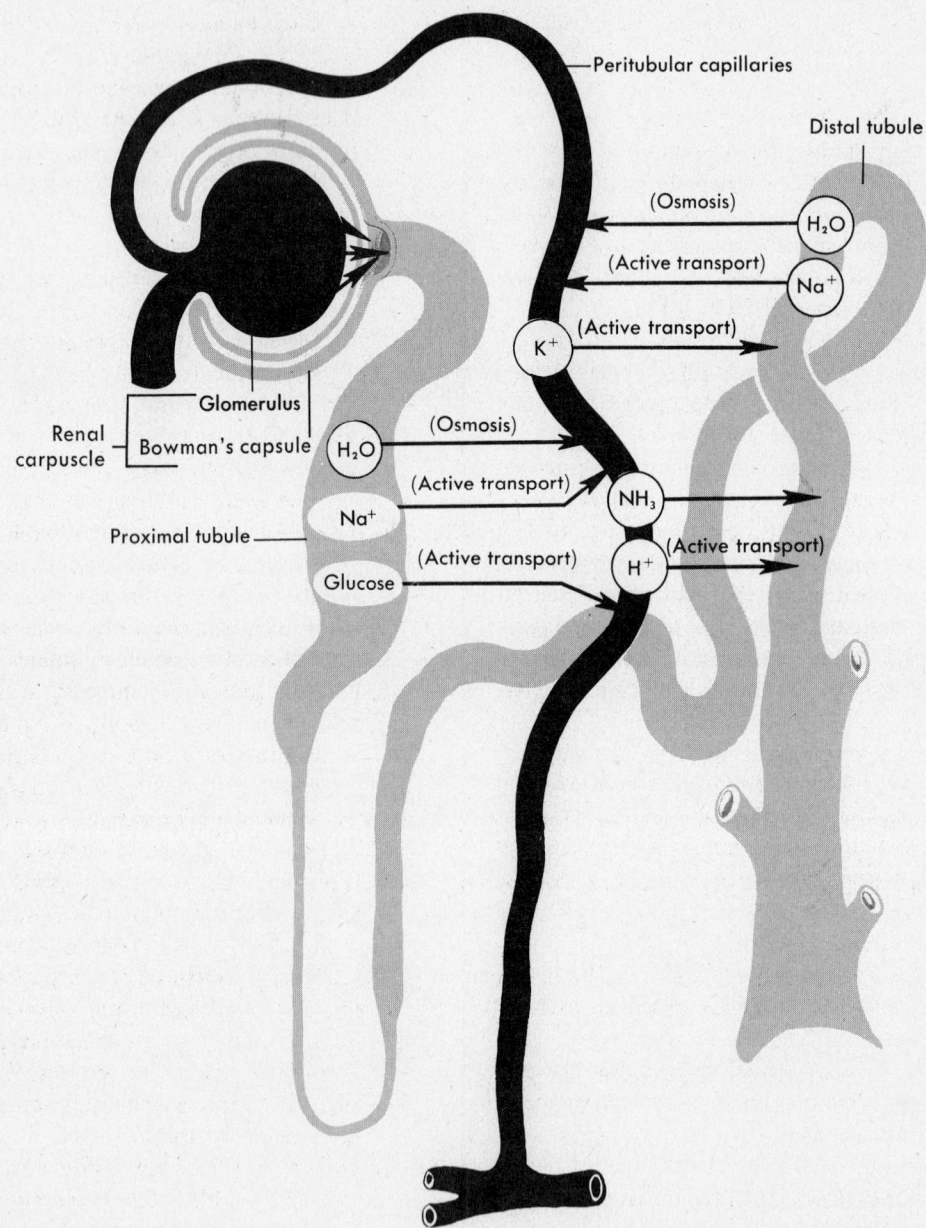

Fig. 6. Diagram showing glomerular filtration, tubular reabsorption, and tubular secretion—the three processes by which the kidneys secrete urine. In the proximal tubule note that water is reabsorbed from the tubular filtrate and moves into the blood by osmosis (a passive transport mechanism) but that sodium and glucose are reabsorbed mainly by active transport mechanisms. Note also that water and sodium are reabsorbed from the distal tubule. Potassium and hydrogen ions (K^+ and H^+) and ammonia (NH_3), by contrast, are secreted into the tubule from the blood. (From Anthony, C.P., and Thibodeau, G.A.: Textbook of anatomy and physiology, ed. 11, St. Louis, 1983, The C.V. Mosby Co.)

    (a) Establishes osmotic conditions that promote water reabsorption

    (b) Actively transports chloride ions from the filtrate, thus passively removing sodium ions with the chloride; sodium chloride excretion results in increased osmotic force and promotes reabsorption of water in the collecting tubules

  (3) Distal tubule

    (a) Reabsorption of electrolytes, particularly sodium, under the influence of the mineralocorticoid aldosterone

    (b) Reabsorption of water into the blood by osmosis; ADH controls the amount of water osmosing out of the distal tubule, whereas amount of electrolytes reabsorbed controls the amount of osmosis out of the proximal tubule

    (c) Secretion of hydrogen, potassium, ammonia, and some other substances from the blood in the peritubular capillaries to the tubular filtrate; accomplished by active transport mechanism

D. Collecting tubules
1. Each collecting tubule receives urine from several nephrons
2. Under ADH influence, final osmotic reabsorption of most of the remaining water in urine occurs

E. Urine composition
1. Water—1.5 L per day average
2. Urea—waste product of protein and amino acid metabolism
3. Uric acid—waste product of muscle metabolism of purines by liver
4. Creatinine—waste product of muscle metabolism
5. Ions (electrolytes)—K^+, Na^+, Ca^{++}, Cl^-
6. Hormones and their breakdown products—presence of chorionic gonadotropin is the basis for a pregnancy test
7. Vitamins—particularly the water-soluble B vitamins and C
8. Drugs secreted in the urine—e.g., aspirin, penicillin, sulfa
9. Other molecules, in low concentrations
10. Abnormal constituents—glucose, albumin, red blood cells, calculi

F. Urine volume is controlled normally by mechanisms that regulate the amount of water reabsorbed by the kidney tubules; only under abnormal conditions does the glomerular filtration rate influence urine volume

1. ADH mechanism—neurons in the hypothalamus (mainly in the supraoptic nucleus) produce the antidiuretic hormone, and the posterior pituitary gland secretes it into the blood; ADH secretion is stimulated by two conditions, an increase in the osmotic pressure of extracellular fluid or a decrease in the volume of extracellular fluid; ADH acts on distal and collecting tubules, causing more water to osmose from the tubular filtrate back into the blood; this increased water reabsorption tends to increase the total volume of body fluid by decreasing the urine volume; ADH has both a water-retaining and an antidiuretic effect
2. Aldosterone mechanism—an increase in aldosterone secretion tends to decrease urine volume by stimulating kidney tubules to reabsorb primarily more sodium and secondarily more water; thus aldosterone tends to produce sodium retention, water retention, and a low urine volume
3. Control by the amount of solutes in tubular filtrate; in general, an increase in tubular solutes causes decreased osmosis of water from proximal tubule back into blood and therefore an increase in urine volume; e.g., in diabetes, excess glucose in the tubule filtrate leads to increased urine volume (polyuria, diuresis)
4. Glomerular filtration rate normally is quite constant at about 125 ml per minute; it does not vary enough to alter volume of urine produced, but in certain pathologic conditions glomerular filtration rate may change markedly and alter urine volume; e.g., in shock the glomerular filtration decreases or even ceases, causing decreased urine volume (oliguria) or urinary suppression (anuria)

G. Control of amount of blood flow through kidneys
1. Reduced renal blood flow results in renal excretion of the hormone renin
2. Renin chemically interacts with blood proteins, producing angiotensin II
3. Angiotensin II causes vasoconstriction and aldosterone secretion, resulting in an increase in blood pressure and renal blood flow

Ureters
A. Location—behind the parietal peritoneum; extend from the kidneys to posterior part of the bladder floor
B. Structure—ureter expands as it enters the kidney to form the renal pelvis; subdivided into calyces, each

of which contains renal papillae; ureter walls composed of smooth muscle with mucosa lining and fibrous outer coat

C. Function—collect urine secreted by the kidney cells and propel it to the bladder by peristaltic waves

Urinary Bladder

A. Location—behind symphysis pubis, below parietal peritoneum

B. Structure—collapsible bag of smooth muscle lined with mucosa arranged in rugae, 3 openings—2 from ureters and 1 into the urethra

C. Functions
1. Reservoir for urine until sufficient amount accumulated for elimination
2. Expulsion of urine from body by way of urethra

Urethra

A. Location
1. Female—behind the symphysis pubis, in front of the vagina
2. Male—extends through the prostate gland, fibrous sheet, and penis

B. Structure—musculomembranous tube lined with mucosa; opening to exterior called urinary meatus

C. Functions
1. Female—passageway for expulsion of urine
2. Male—passageway for expulsion of both urine and semen

Reproductive System

Male Reproductive Organs

Glands

A. Main male sex glands (gonads) are the testes
1. Structure—fibrous capsule covers each testis and sends partitions into interior of gland, dividing it into lobules composed of tiny tubules called seminiferous tubules, embedded in connective tissue containing interstitial cells; ducts emerge from top of gland to enter head of epididymis
2. Location—in the scrotum, 1 testis in each compartment (2 compartments)
3. Functions
   a. Seminiferous tubules carry on spermatogenesis; that is, they form spermatozoa, the male sex cells, or gametes
   b. Interstitial cells secrete testosterone, the main androgen, or male hormone
4. Structure of spermatozoon—consists of a head, middle piece, and whiplike tail that propels sperm; microscopic

B. Accessory glands
1. Seminal vesicles
   a. Location—on posterior surface of the bladder

   b. Structure—convoluted pouches, mucous lining
   c. Function—secrete nutrient-rich fluid estimated to constitute about 30% of semen
2. Prostate gland
   a. Location—encircles urethra just below bladder
   b. Structure—walnut sized gland with ducts opening into urethra
   c. Function—secretes estimated 60% of semen; prostatic secretion is alkaline, which increases sperm motility; prostatic secretion contains abundance of enzyme, acid phosphatase; therefore blood level of this enzyme increases in metastasizing cancer of prostate
3. Bulbourethral glands (Cowper's)
   a. Location—just below prostate gland
   b. Structure—small, pea-shaped structures with duct leading into urethra
   c. Function—secrete alkaline fluid that lubricates urethra prior to ejaculation

Ducts

A. Epididymis
1. Location—lies along top and side of each testis
2. Structure—each epididymis consists of single, tightly coiled tube enclosed in fibrous casing
3. Function—conducts seminal fluid (semen) from testes to vas deferens; secretes small part of semen; stores semen prior to ejaculation, sperm mature during this period

B. Vas deferens (seminal ducts)
1. Location—extend through inguinal canal into abdominal cavity, over top and down posterior surface of bladder to join ducts from seminal vesicles.
2. Structure—pair of tubes or ducts
3. Function—conduct sperm and small amount of fluid from each epididymis to an ejaculatory duct
4. Clinical application—vasectomy is the surgical procedure in which a short section of each vas is cut out and its separated ends tied off; as a result, sperm cannot enter the ejaculatory ducts and be ejaculated; semen from a vasectomized male contains no sperm; hence vasectomy sterilizes a man (makes him infertile); it does not render him impotent; it does, however, slightly decrease the amount of semen ejaculated

C. Ejaculatory ducts—formed by union of each vas with duct from seminal vesicle; pass through prostate gland to terminate in urethra; function—ejaculate semen into urethra

D. Urethra—described under urinary system

Supporting Structures

A. External—scrotum and penis
   1. Scrotum—skin-covered pouch suspended from perineal region; divided into 2 compartments, each containing testis, epididymis, and first part of seminal duct; allows sperm to develop at 2° to 3° below the temperature of rest of body, which is ideal for sperm development
   2. Penis—made up of 3 cylindrical masses of erectile tissue that contain large vascular spaces; filling of these with blood causes erection of penis; 2 larger upper cylinders (corpora cavernosa) and one smaller lower cylinder (corpus cavernosum); the lower cylinder surrounds the urethra; glans penis—a bulging structure at distal end of the penis, over which a double fold of skin, the prepuce or foreskin, fits loosely (removed in circumcision)
B. Internal—spermatic cords are fibrous tubes located in each inguinal canal; serve as casing around each vas deferens and its accompanying blood vessels, lymphatics, and nerves

Female Reproductive Organs
Ovaries—Female Gonads

A. Location—behind and below uterine tubes, anchored to uterus and broad ligaments
B. Size and shape of large almonds
C. Microscopic structure—each ovary of the newborn female consists of several hundred thousand graffian follicles embedded in connective tissues; follicles are epithelial sacs in which ova develop; usually, between the years of menarche and menopause; 1 follicle matures each month, ruptures surface of the ovary, and expels its ovum into the pelvic cavity
D. Functions
   1. Oogenesis—function of a mature ovum in a graafian follicle
   2. Ovulation—expulsion of the ovum from follicle into the pelvic cavity
   3. Secretion of female hormones—maturing follicle secretes estrogens; corpus luteum secretes progesterone and estrogens

Uterine Tubes (Fallopian Tubes, Oviducts)

A. Location—attached to upper, outer angles of uterus
B. Structure—same 3 coats as uterus; distal ends fimbriated and open into pelvic cavity; mucosal lining of tubes and peritoneal lining of pelvis in direct contact here (facilitates spread of infection from tubes to peritoneum)
C. Function—serve as ducts through which ova travel from ovaries to uterus; fertilization normally occurs in tube

Uterus

A. Location—in pelvic cavity between the bladder and rectum
B. Structure
   1. Shape and size—pear-shaped organ approximately the size of a clenched fist
   2. Divisions
      a. Body—upper and main part of the uterus; fundus, the bulging upper surface of the body
      b. Cervix—narrow, lower part of the uterus; projects into the vagina
   3. Walls—composed of smooth muscle (myometrium) lined with mucosa (endometrium)
   4. Cavities
      a. Body cavity—small and triangular with 3 openings into it; 2 from uterine tubes, 1 into cervical canal
      b. Cervical cavity—canal with constricted opening, internal os into body cavity and another, external os, into vagina
C. Position—flexed between body and cervix portions with the body portion lying over the bladder, pointing forward and slightly upward; cervix joins the vagina at right angles; ligaments hold the uterus in position
   1. Broad ligaments (2)—double fold of parietal peritoneum that forms a kind of partition across pelvic cavity, suspending uterus between its folds
   2. Uterosacral ligaments (2)—foldlike extensions of peritoneum from posterior surface of uterus to sacrum, 1 on each side of rectum
   3. Posterior ligament (1)—fold of peritoneum between posterior surface of uterus and rectum; forms deep pouch, cul-de-sac of Douglas (or rectouterine pouch); this pouch is the lowest point in the pelvic cavity and therefore the place where pus accumulates in pelvic inflammations; can be drained by posterior colpotomy (incision at top of the posterior vaginal wall)
   4. Anterior ligament (1)—fold of peritoneum between uterus and bladder; forms shallow cul-de-sac
   5. Round ligaments (2)—fibromuscular cords from upper, outer angles of uterus, through inguinal canals, terminating in labia majora
D. Functions
   1. Menstruation
   2. Pregnancy
   3. Labor

Vagina

A. Location—between rectum and urethra
B. Structure—collapsible, musculomembranous tube, capable of great distention; outlet to exterior protected by fold of mucous membrane called hymen
C. Functions
  1. Receives semen from the male
  2. Constitutes lower part of birth canal
  3. Acts as excretory duct for uterine secretions and menstrual flow

Vulva

Consists of numerous structures that together constitute external genitals

A. Mons veneris—hairy, skin-covered pad of fat over the symphysis pubis
B. Labia majora—hairy, skin-covered lips
C. Labia minora—small lips covered with modified skin
D. Clitoris—small mound of erectile tissue, below junction of two labia minora
E. Urinary meatus—just below clitoris; opening into urethra
F. Vaginal orifice—below urinary meatus; opening into vagina; hymen, fold of mucosa, partially closes orifice
G. Skene's glands—small mucous glands whose ducts open on each side of the urinary meatus
H. Bartholin's glands—2 small, bean-shaped glands; duct from each gland opens on side of the vaginal orifice; both Bartholin's glands and Skene's glands have clinical interest because they frequently become infected (especially by gonococci)

Breasts, or Mammary Glands

A. Location—just under skin, over the pectoralis major muscles
B. Size—depends on deposits of adipose tissue rather than on amount of glandular tissue (which is approximately same in all females)
C. Structure—divided into lobes and lobules that, in turn, are composed of racemose glands; excretory duct leads from each lobe to opening in nipple; circular pigmented area, the areola, borders nipples
D. Function—secrete milk (lactation)
  1. Shedding of placenta causes marked decrease in blood levels of estrogens and progesterone, which, in turn, stimulates anterior pituitary to increase prolactin secretion; high blood level of prolactin stimulates alveoli of breast to secrete milk
  2. Suckling controls lactation in 2 ways; by acting in some way to stimulate anterior pituitary secretion of prolactin and to stimulate posterior pituitary secretion of oxytocin, which stimulates release of milk out of alveoli into ducts from which infant can remove it by suckling (letdown reflex)

Menstrual Cycle

A. Refers mainly to changes in the uterus and ovaries, which recur cyclically from the time of the menarche to the menopause
B. Length of cycle—usually 28 days, although considerable variations occur
C. Hormonal control of menstrual cycle
  1. Menses—brought on by marked decrease in blood levels of progesterone and estrogens at about cycle day 25
  2. Growth of new follicle and ovum—the low blood concentration of estrogens present for a few days before and during the menses stimulates the anterior pituitary gland to secrete follicle-stimulating hormone (FSH); the resulting high blood concentration of FSH stimulates 1 or more primitive graafian follicles and their ova to start growing and also stimulates the follicle cells to secrete estrogens; this leads to a high blood concentration of estrogens, which, in turn, has a negative feedback effect on FSH secretion by the anterior pituitary gland
  3. Endometrial thickening—in the preovulatory phase, is caused by proliferation of endometrial cells stimulated by the increasing concentration of estrogens in blood; the premenstrual phase is caused partly by endometrial cell proliferation and partly by fluid retention caused by increasing progesterone concentration
  4. Ovulation—brought on by high concentrations of luteinizing hormone (LH)
  5. Postovulatory phase—increased secretion of estrogen and progesterone from corpus luteum further prepares the uterine endometrium in event of fertilization and implantation of an ovulated egg
  6. Premenstrual phase—gradual drop in level of estrogens and progesterone, leading to menses
D. Clinical applications
  1. Contraceptive pills contain synthetic preparations of estrogen-like and/or progesterone-like compounds
  2. Most commonly used contraceptive pills prevent pregnancy by preventing ovulation—pituitary secretion of FSH inhibited
E. Progestogen replacement provides the stimulus for desquamation of the uterine lining required for completion of the menstrual cycle or for maintenance of the uterine lining during pregnancy
  1. Drugs

a. Dydrogesterone (Duphaston, Gynorest)
b. Ethisterone
c. Hydroxyprogesterone caproate (Delalutin)
d. Medroxyprogesterone acetate (Depo-Provera, Provera)
e. Norethindrone (Norlutin)
f. Norethindrone acetate (Norlutate)
g. Progesterone (Gesterol, Lipo-Lutin, Proluton)

2. Adverse effects—initial use causes profuse vaginal flow (shedding of accumulatioins of endometrial tissue), spotting, irregular bleeding, nausea, lethargy, jaundice

Development of the Individual

Formation of Gametes

A. The egg and spermatozoon each have 1 set of chromosomes (23); this is in contrast to other cells of the body, which have 2 sets, or 46 chromosomes (23 pairs)
B. The production of ova (eggs) and spermatozoa (sperm) requires a special type of nuclear division (meiosis) in which the chromosome number is reduced from 2 sets (46 chromosomes) to 1 set (23 chromosomes)

Fertilization

A. Spermatozoa are deposited in the vagina
B. Fertilization usually occurs in the uterine tube when the egg is about one third the way down the tube; usually this is about 24 hours after ovulation
C. Sperm must be in the genital tract 4 to 6 hours before they are able to fertilize an egg; during this period the enzyme hyaluronidase is activated; this enzyme is able to dissolve the cement substance (hyaluronic acid) which holds together the cells that surround the ovum
D. Male nucleus enters the cytoplasm of the egg and several events follow:
  1. Fertilization membrane forms around the egg to prevent the entrance of other sperm
  2. Sperm tail is lost and the male nucleus (male pronucleus) moves toward the female nucleus (female pronucleus)
E. Fertilization proper occurs when the male pronucleus unites with the female pronucleus; thus the chromosome number is restored to 2 sets (46 chromosomes)
F. Contraception
  1. Contraceptive pill
  2. IUD (intrauterine device)—placed in the uterus; irritates endometrium or in some other unidentified manner prevents implantation; does not prevent fertilization
  3. Diaphragm with spermicidal jelly—provides physical barrier to movement of sperm flow from the vagina into the uterus; also provides acid conditions unfavorable to sperm
  4. Condom—most widely used method of contraception (cheapest); prevents entering of sperm into female genital tract; only form of contraception providing protection from most venereal disease
  5. Tubal ligation—egg cannot be reached by sperm because fallopian tubes are blocked or severed; fertilization prevented
  6. Vasectomy—sperm cannot be ejected because vas deferens has been blocked or severed

Cleavage

A. In a short time after fertilization the zygote undergoes rapid division to produce a mass of cells (morula) that descends in the uterine tube
B. As it descends it also divides to form a hollow ball referred to as the blastocyst

Implantation

A. The blastocyst implants in the uterine wall
  1. The blastocyst is differentiated into an inner cell mass, a blastocoele (internal cavity)
  2. An outer covering of cells, the trophectoderm, that become trophoderm and will form the fetal portion of the placenta
  3. Implantation occurs 7 to 8 days after fertilization
B. During implantation, cells of trophoderm secrete enzymes that digest the endometrium and allow the embryo to sink below surface; endometrium heals over the implantation site

Embryonic Period

A. First 2 months, after this period it is called a fetus
B. The inner cell mass differentiates into germ layers
  1. Ectoderm—outer layer of skin and mouth cavity and nervous tissue
  2. Mesoderm—connective tissue, including blood and muscle tissue
  3. Endoderm—linings of the alimentary tract, respiratory system, and several glands
C. About the twelfth day after fertilization a fetal membrane, the amnion, forms around the embryo; another membrane, the yolk sac, develops beneath the embryo
  1. Amnion is fluid filled (amniotic fluid) and serves as a fetal shock absorber
  2. Yolk sac serves as an initial embryonic source of erythrocytes
D. Later an allantois develops that will supply the placental blood vessels
E. A chorion surrounds the embryo; this will eventually form the major part of the placenta; fingerlike

projections of the chorion called chorionic villi grow into the endometrium; chorionic villi project into placental blood sinuses; the combination of chorionic villi, placental blood sinuses, and placental blood constitutes the placenta

Umbilical Cord

A. Consists of an outer layer of amnion
B. Contains 2 umbilical arteries and 1 umbilical vein

Fetal Growth

A. Differentiation of cells occurs
B. Development of organs progresses from anterior to posterior in the growing fetus

Hormones

A. During pregnancy the chorion of the placenta secretes a hormone, chorionic gonadotropin, that maintains the corpus luteum; the continuation of progesterone and estrogen secretion from the corpus luteum maintains the pregnancy during the early weeks of development
B. Chorionic gonadotropin reaches a peak in the third month and then drops
C. Estrogen and progesterone increase and continue to be secreted from the placenta during the last 6 months of pregnancy; progesterone acts to inhibit uterine contractions, which might occur due to uterine stretching as the fetus grows
D. In the last month uterine contents shift downward so that the fetus is in contact with the cervix; this contact may induce oxytocin secretion by the posterior pituitary
E. The secretion of oxytocin, which stimulates uterine contractions, coupled with the drop in progesterone brings about labor; uterine contractions increase in frequency and intensity, culminating in fetal expulsion (birth)

Heredity

Chromosomes

A. Humans have 23 pairs of homologous chromosomes
B. In males the sex chromosomes (the X and Y) are not equal in size
C. Homologous chromosomes carry sets of matching genes (alleles) in which 1 may be dominant and the other recessive, or they may have blending expressions

Sex Determination in Humans

A. Genetic females have 2 sets of autosomes (nonsex chromosomes) and 2 X chromosomes, whereas genetic males have 2 sets of autosomes and 1 X chromsome and 1 Y chromosome
B. All eggs produced by females have 1 set of autosomes and 1 X chromosome; spermatozoa produced by a male have a set of autosomes and either an X or a Y chromosome
C. If an X-bearing spermatozoon fertilizes an egg, a female will result; if a Y-bearing spermatozoon fertilizes an egg, a male will result

Genes

A. Sex-linked genes—genes carried on the X chromosome are called sex-linked genes and are always expressed in the male, even though they may be recessive; examples of such genes cause hemophilia and color blindness
B. Multiple genes—many different genes may combine to produce cumulative effects, such as the degree of pigmentation or height
C. Multiple alleles—an example of human traits controlled by multiple alleles are the genes controlling normal blood types; the genes for type O are dominated by the genes for type A or type B; the genes for A and B are both expressed

Genes	Blood type
OO	O
AO	A
AA	A
BO	B
BB	B
AB	AB

D. Following are some other obvious human traits controlled by genes

Dominant	Recessive
Brown eyes	Blue eyes
Normal blood clotting	Hemophilia (sex-linked)
Normal color vision	Color blind (sex-linked)
Normal pigmentation	Albinism
Rh positive (multiple alleles)	Rh negative
Normal red blood cell development	Sickle cell trait

Chromosomal Alterations

A. In rare cases additional sex chromosomes may appear and produce abnormal individuals
  1. X chromosome and no Y chromosome—Turner's syndrome
  2. Two or more X chromosomes and a Y chromosome—Klinefelter's syndrome
B. Translocation of chromosome—a cytogenetic abnormality such as trisomy 21 (Down's syndrome)
C. Mutations
  1. Changes in the DNA are mutations; there may also be chromosomal changes
  2. The frequency of mutations may be increased by certain agents such as ultraviolet radiation, x-ray films, radioactive radiation, and certain chemical substances

REVIEW OF PHYSICAL PRINCIPLES RELATED TO THE GENITOURINARY SYSTEM
Principles of Mechanics
Law of Motion
Newton's law
EXAMPLES
1. Pumping action of the heart supplies hydrostatic force to filter blood in the glomerular capillary bed
2. Contraction of the muscle is responsible for the force of propulsion of semen along and out the male reproductive tract

Momentum
EXAMPLE: During micturition, the walls of the urinary bladder exert a force of prolonged duration that imparts great momentum to the urine being expelled from the body

Energy
EXAMPLE: Chemical energy of ATP is used to actively transport nutrients and electrolytes from glomerular filtrate into the tubular epithelium

Principles of Physical Properties of Matter
Elasticity
EXAMPLES
1. Elastic properties of the bladder permit it to hold several hundred milliliters of urine before micturition
2. Elastic properties of uterine connective tissue partly account for the tremendous increase in size of the uterus during pregnancy

Surface Area
EXAMPLE: The proximal convoluted tubules of the nephron have a brush border consisting of numerous microvilli that have very high surface-to-volume ratio; these tiny cellular extensions greatly increase the surface area of the tubule for reabsorption of materials from the glomerular filtrate

Liquids
Pascal's principle
EXAMPLE: In conditions causing a lack of the micturition reflex, manual pressure over the bladder region will be transmitted to the urine, which results in the opening of the sphincters and the expulsion of urine from the bladder

REVIEW OF CHEMICAL PRINCIPLES RELATED TO THE GENITOURINARY SYSTEM
Urine
A. Water solution of inorganic salts and organic compounds
B. Important in excretion of wastes
C. Analysis yields information of physical condition in health and disease

D. Normal urine
1. Amount—800 to 1800 ml/24 hours
2. Color—light yellow to dark brown, resulting from pigments (urobilin, urochrome, etc.)
3. Odor—aromatic (fresh); food and drugs alter odor
4. Sediment—varies; caused by diet and other normal changes
   a. Few blood cells
   b. Few epithelial cells
   c. Phosphates
   d. Urates
   e. Uric acid crystals
   f. Calcium oxalate
5. Specific gravity (1.005 to 1.025) varies greatly, depending on fluid intake and the quantity of solutes dissolved in the urine; the individual having diabetes insipidus may excrete 5 to 15 L of urine daily; this urine has a very low specific gravity (close to that of pure water); a person with diabetes mellitus may excrete urine of high specific gravity caused by excessive quantities of glucose dissolved in the urine
6. Reaction—usually acid (pH 4.5 to 7.5 is the normal range); alkaline immediately after a meal
7. Proteins—none; protein in the urine is usually associated with a pathologic condition although albumin traces will occasionally appear after heavy exercise or cold showers (these are of no consequence)
8. Sugar—trace to none; the presence of urinary carbohydrate is usually pathologic
9. Ketone bodies—none; ketone bodies in the urine appear in metabolic disorders
10. Indican—none; positive results indicate intestinal obstruction
11. Bile—none; positive results indicate liver or gallbladder dysfunction
12. Blood—trace to none; positive results indicate bleeding in organs of urinary system

Hormones
See endocrine system

REVIEW OF MICROORGANISMS RELATED TO THE GENITOURINARY SYSTEM
A. Bacterial pathogens
1. *Enterobacter aerogenes*—small, gram-negative bacillus (morphologically indistinguishable from *Escherichia coli*); causes urinary tract infections
2. *Haemophilus ducreyi*—morphologically indis-

tinguishable from *H. influenzae* and *H. aegyptius;* causes the venereal ulcer called chancroid (soft chancre)

3. *Neisseria gonorrhoeae*—gram negative diplococcus; causes gonorrhea
4. *Pseudomonas aeruginosa*—gram-negative, motile bacillus; a common secondary invader of wounds, burns, outer ear, and urinary tract; the infection characterized by blue-green pus; may be transmitted by catheters and other hospital instruments
5. *Treponema pallidum*—long, slender, highly motile spirochete; causes syphilis

B. Protozoal pathogen—*Trichomonas vaginalis*—flagellated protozoan; causes trichomonas vaginitis (a venereal disease)

PHARMACOLOGY RELATED TO URINARY SYSTEM DISORDERS

See kidney-specific drugs under section on controlling infection

RELATED DIAGNOSTIC PROCEDURES
Cystoscopy

A. Definition
1. The visualization of the bladder wall through a tube with a fiberoptic end
2. Indicated as a diagnostic measure or as a means to enter the bladder for therapy
B. Nursing responsibilities
1. Obtain an informed consent
2. Maintain the patient n.p.o. before the procedure (which may be done with or without general anesthesia)
3. After the procedure
   a. Maintain the patient in a comfortable state
   b. Observe the patient's urine for blood and clots
   c. Ascertain that the patient has voided through observation and palpation of the bladder

Intravenous Pyelography (IVP)

A. Definition—x-ray examination of the kidneys, ureters, and bladder after the injection of a contrast medium into an antecubital vein
B. Nursing responsibilities
1. Explain procedure to the patient
2. Obtain an informed consent
3. Administer a cathartic as ordered the evening before the test to remove feces and flatus
4. Allow the patient a light supper before the procedure and maintain n.p.o. for 6 to 8 hours prior to the test

Common Urine Tests

A. Definition
1. Urinalysis—microscopic examination of urine for cells, as well as chemical study for pH and specific gravity
2. Culture and sensitivity tests of urine—microscopic examination of urine for bacterial growth and determination of antibiotic appropriate to control growth
B. Nursing responsibilities
1. Explain procedure to the patient
2. Obtain container for the specimen
   a. For urinalysis a urine container is used
   b. For culture a sterile specimen jar is used
3. For urinalysis obtain a freshly voided specimen and place in the container
4. For culture
   a. Cleanse the outer urinary meatus with a bacteriostatic solution
   b. Instruct the patient to void a small amount into a bedpan, urinal, or toilet and then stop the stream
   c. Instruct the patient to continue voiding into a container without contaminating the lid or inside of the container
   d. Seal the container
5. Send the specimen to the laboratory with label indicating contents, patient's name, and date

RELATED GENERAL NURSING PROCEDURES
Urinary Catheterization

A. Definitions
1. Sterile introduction of a catheter through the urethra to the bladder for the purpose of urine collection
2. Intermittent catheterization is performed with a one-lumen catheter, which is removed after the bladder is drained (patients with neurogenic bladder dysfunction may be taught this procedure)
3. Retention catheterization involves use of a catheter with an inflatable balloon around its tip to hold it in place in the bladder (Foley catheter); once inserted, it is attached to a collecting bag and thus the bladder is continually emptied by gravity
B. Nursing responsibilities
1. Explain procedure to the patient
2. Provide privacy
3. Obtain equipment, including a bright light
4. Position the female patient supine with her knees flexed and abducted and the male patient supine with the knees slightly abducted

5. Wash hands, open catheterization tray, and put on sterile gloves
6. Place the sterile fenestrated drape over the external genitalia, exposing the meatus
7. Lubricate tip of the catheter and leave catheter on the sterile tray
8. Saturate cotton pledgets with a suitable cleansing solution
9. Cleanse the urinary meatus
   a. For female patients separate the labia minora with thumb and forefinger and cleanse from anterior to posterior using one pledget for each stroke (keep labia separated)
   b. For male patients hold the penis between thumb and forefinger and cleanse from meatus to shaft using one pledget for each stroke (retract foreskin during this procedure)
10. Insert lubricated catheter into the bladder
    a. For female patients insert approximately 7.5 cm or slightly past the point at which urine returns
    b. For male patients, hold the penis perpendicular to the body and insert catheter 17 to 25 cm or slightly past the point at which urine returns
11. Drain urine (do not exceed 1 L); clamp catheter and notify the physician if drainage is in excess of 1L
    a. Intermittent catherization—remove catheter when bladder is empty
    b. Retention catherization—inflate the balloon with sterile solution or air after the bladder is emptied and the catheter is attached to a sterile closed collection system (to reduce chance of infection)
12. Assist the patient to a comfortable position, remove equipment, and record data on appropriate records

Retention Catheter Care

A. Definition—special care to the urinary meatus and catheter to reduce the likelihood of infection
B. Nursing responsibilities
   1. Explain procedure to the patient
   2. Provide privacy
   3. Gather equipment, wash hands, and don gloves
   4. Perform catheter care at least twice daily
   5. Wash the genital area well with soap and warm water and dry; uncircumcised males should have foreskin retracted to remove sebaceous secretions
   6. Use soap and water to wash encrustations

from catheter (they may harbor microorganisms)
   7. Apply antiseptic solution to the urinary meatus and adjacent catheter (this may vary from institution to institution)
   8. Check drainage tubing at frequent intervals to assess for kinks or clogs
   9. Fasten catheter to the patient's thigh to prevent tension
   10. Keep the drainage bag below bladder level without loops or kinks to ensure gravity drainage
   11. Use a syringe to remove urine if a specimen is needed; use the port site and surgical aseptic technique
   12. Empty the drainage bag at least every 8 hours and record the amount, odor, color, and consistency
   13. Change the drainage bag and catheter according to institutional policy

MAJOR DISEASES
Cystitis

A. Etiology and pathophysiology
   1. Inflammation of the bladder wall usually caused by an ascending bacterial infection (*Escherichia coli* most common)
   2. More common in females due to
      a. Shorter urethra
      b. Childbirth
      c. Anatomic position of the urethra
B. Signs and symptoms
   1. Subjective
      a. Urgency, frequency, burning, and pain on urination
      b. Nocturia
      c. Bearing down on urination
   2. Objective
      a. Pyuria and hematuria
      b. Bacterial growth evident on culture of urine
C. Treatment
   1. Chemotherapeutic and antibiotic agents (e.g., sulfonamides, penicillin, tetracycline)
   2. Antispasmodics to soothe the irritable bladder (e.g., phenazopyridine [Pyridium])
   3. Diet directed toward maintaining an acid urine (e.g., cranberry juice)
   4. Intake of additional fluids to dilute the urine
D. Nursing care
   1. Teach the patient to seek medical attention at the first sign of symptoms
   2. Teach the patient to take medications as directed
   3. Encourage the patient to drink additional fluids

4. Monitor intake and output with attention to character of urine
5. Teach the patient proper perineal care

Renal and Ureteral Calculi

A. Etiology and pathophysiology—formation of stones in the urinary tract; stones may be composed of calcium phosphate, uric acid, or oxalate; they tend to recur and may cause obstruction, infection, and/or hydronephrosis
B. Signs and symptoms
   1. Subjective
      a. Severe pain in kidney area radiating down the flank to the pubic area
      b. Frequency and urgency of urination
      c. History of prior or associated health problems (e.g., gout, parathyroidism, immobility, dehydration, urinary tract infections)
   2. Objective
      a. Diaphoresis, pallor, nausea, vomiting
      b. Hematuria; pyuria may occur if infection is present
C. Treatment
   1. Narcotics for pain
   2. Antispasmodics to reduce the renal colic
   3. Allopurinol or sulfinpyrazone to reduce uric acid excretion
   4. Antibiotics to reduce infection
   5. Monitor intake and output; forced fluids and straining of urine
   6. Diet therapy
      a. Large fluid intake to produce dilute urine
      b. Diet altered according to type of stone
         (1) Calcium stones—low calcium, low phosphate or oxalate according to the calcium compound, acid ash; calcium foods, mainly dairy products, are eliminated; acid ash foods such as meat, egg, and grains are emphasized; alkaline foods such as milk, vegetables, and fruits are controlled
         (2) Uric acid stones—low purine (uric acid is a metabolic product of purines in the body), controlling purine foods such as meat, especially organ meats, meat extractives, and to a lesser extent plant sources (e.g., whole grains and legumes); alkaline ash, since the stone composition is acid
         (3) Cystine stones (rare)—low methionine, since methionine is the essential amino acid from which the nonessential amino acid cystine is formed; controlling pro-

tein foods such as meat, milk, egg, cheese; alkaline ash, since the stone is an acid composition
   7. Surgical intervention if stone is not passed or complications are present (e.g., nephrolithotomy, litholapaxy)
D. Nursing care
   1. Administer medications as ordered
   2. Permit the patient to set own pattern of activity
   3. Plan care to provide the patient with periods of undisturbed rest
   4. Strain all urine
   5. Monitor intake and output
   6. Force fluids
   7. Administer medication as ordered
   8. Encourage the patient to accept medication for pain
   9. Provide as much privacy as possible
   10. Encourage the patient to remain on diet
   11. Teach the patient to read labels on food preparations for the presence of contraindicated additives such as calcium or phosphate

Hydronephrosis (Renal Colic)

A. Etiology and pathophysiology
   1. Obstruction at any point in the urinary system leading to pressure that can damage renal tissue
   2. Due to tumors, trauma, calculi, polycystic disease, congenital abnormalities, lymph enlargement, or nephrotosis (floating kidney)
B. Signs and symptoms
   1. Subjective
      a. Pain, local tenderness
      b. Dull pain in flank region or colicky pain
   2. Objective
      a. Nausea and vomiting
      b. Nocturia
C. Treatment
   1. Treat the underlying cause
   2. Promote urinary drainage with a catheter
   3. Urinary antiseptics
   4. Antispasmodics for colicky spasm
D. Nursing care
   1. Observe for signs of uremia
   2. Medicate as ordered
   3. Maintain patency of drainage tubes

Acute Renal Failure

A. Etiology and pathophysiology
   1. Usually follows direct trauma to the kidneys or overwhelming physiologic stress (e.g., burns,

septicemia, nephotoxic drugs and chemicals, hemolytic blood transfusion reaction, severe shock, renal vascular occlusion)

2. Sudden and almost complete loss of glomerular and/or tubular function
3. Acute renal failure may result in death from acidosis, potassium intoxication, pulmonary edema, or infection
4. May progress from the anuric or oliguric phase through the diuretic phase to the convalescence phase (which can take 6 to 12 months) to recovery of function
5. May progress to chronic renal failure; chronic renal failure may develop as a separate entity and does not have to be a sequela of acute failure

B. Signs and symptoms
1. Subjective
   a. Lethargy and drowsiness than can progress from stupor to coma
   b. Irritability and headache
   c. Circumoral numbness
   d. Tingling extremities
   e. Anorexia
2. Objective
   a. Sudden dramatic drop in urinary output appearing a few hours after the causative event
   b. Oliguria—urinary output less than 400 ml but more than 100 ml/24 hours; anuria—urinary output less than 100 ml/24 hours
   c. Restlessness, twitching, convulsions
   d. Nausea and vomiting
   e. Skin pallor, anemia, and increased bleeding time, which can progress to epistaxis and internal hemorrhage
   f. Ammonia (urine) odor to breath and perspiration, which can progress to uremic frost on skin and pruritus
   g. Generalized edema, hypervolemia, hypertension, and increased venous pressure, which can progress to pulmonary edema and congestive heart failure
   h. In addition, respirations are deep and rapid as a compensatory response to the developing metabolic acidosis
   i. Elevated serum levels of
      (1) BUN
      (2) Creatinine
      (3) Potassium
   j. Decreased serum levels of
      (1) Calcium
      (2) Sodium
      (3) pH
      (4) Carbon dioxide combining power

   k. Anemia
   l. Albumin in urine
   m. Decreased specific gravity

C. Treatment
1. Direct treatment toward correcting the underlying cause of renal failure (e.g., treat shock, eliminate drugs and toxins, treat transfusion reactions, restore integrity of urinary tract)
2. Maintain patient on complete bed rest
3. Diet therapy
   a. Protein low to moderate according to tolerance: 30 to 50 g
   b. Carbohydrate relatively high for energy: 300 to 400 g
   c. Fat relatively moderate: 70 to 90 g
   d. Calories adequate for maintenance and to prevent tissue breakdown: 2000 to 2500 daily
   e. Sodium controlled according to serum levels and excretion tolerance: varying from 400 to 2000 mg
   f. Potassium controlled according to serum levels and excretion capacities: varying from 1300 to 1900 mg
   g. Water controlled according to excretion: about 800 to 1000 ml; careful intake-output records vital
4. Frequent monitoring of vital signs and intake and output
5. Packed cells, electrolytes, and glucose IV as necessary
6. Exchange resins to decrease serum potassium
7. Antibiotics to reduce possibility of infection
8. Peritoneal dialysis or hemodialysis
9. Surgical intervention if kidney transplant is a viable alternative

D. Nursing care
1. Monitor intake and output at frequent intervals
2. Limit fluid intake as ordered
3. Weigh the patient daily
4. Observe for signs of overhydration (e.g., dependent, pitting, sacral, or periorbital edema; rales or dyspnea; headache, distended neck veins, and hypertension)
5. Observe for signs of hyperkalemia and hyponatremia
6. Administer electrolytes as ordered
7. Provide periods of undisturbed rest to conserve energy and oxygen
8. Protect patient from injury caused by bleeding tendency, the possibility of convulsions, and a clouded sensorium
9. Protect patient from cross infection

10. Observe for early signs and symptoms of complications (e.g., hemorrhage, convulsions, cardiac problems, pulmonary edema)
11. Provide special skin care frequently to prevent breakdown and remove uremic frost
12. Monitor vital signs and intake and output at frequent intervals; record and report any deviations immediately
13. Administer antibiotics as ordered
14. Encourage intake of diet as ordered and record amount consumed
15. Allow the patient as much choice as possible in the selection of food while recognizing that little variation is possible
16. Provide mouth care before, after, and between meals
17. Administer dietary and electrolyte supplements as ordered
18. Administer antiemetics to control nausea and antacids to reduce GI irritation

Chronic Renal Failure

A. Etiology and pathophysiology
  1. Chronic renal failure can occur as the result of chronic kidney infections, developmental abnormalities, and vascular disorders
  2. The ongoing deterioration in renal function results in uremia
B. Signs and symptoms
  1. Subjective
    a. Lethargy or drowsiness
    b. Headache
  2. Objective
    a. Vomiting
    b. Mental clouding
    c. Kussmaul respirations
    d. Uremic frost (powdery substance on the skin from urate wastes)
    e. Convulsions, coma, death
C. Treatment
  1. Fluid and salt restrictions
  2. Antihypertensive medications
  3. Peritoneal dialysis—warmed dialyzing solution is introduced via a trocar, which is in the peritoneal cavity; the peritoneal membrane is used as a dialyzing membrane to remove toxic substances, metabolic wastes, and excess fluid
  4. Hemodialysis—the patient is attached (via a surgically created arteriovenous fistula) directly to a machine that pumps his or her blood along a semipermeable membrane; dialyzing solution is on the other side of the membrane, and osmosis of wastes, toxins, and fluid from the patient occurs

5. Diet management
  a. General protein and electrolyte control
  b. The low-protein, essential amino acid diet (modified Giordano-Giovannetti regimen) to sustain patients with uremia and alleviate their difficult symptoms
    (1) Very low protein (20 g); minimal essential amino acids
    (2) Controlled potassium (1500 mg); feed only essential amino acids, causing the body to use its own excess urea nitrogen to synthesize the nonessential amino acids needed for tissue protein production; foods used include 1 egg, 6 oz milk, low-protein bread, 2 to 4 fruits, and 2 to 4 vegetables from special lists to control protein and potassium
D. Nursing care
  1. Monitor intake and output
  2. Provide skin care as needed
  3. Monitor vital signs
  4. When the patient is undergoing dialysis
    a. Explain the procedure and answer questions related to it
    b. Take vital signs and weigh the patient before the procedure is begun
    c. Use surgical asepsis in preparation of the site (abdomen or radial vessels)
    d. Assure the patient that a staff member will be present at all times
    e. If an indwelling catheter is not in place, have the patient void before procedure is started
    f. Once the procedure is instituted by the physician, monitor the patient's response and add dialysate as prescribed
    g. Monitor vital signs every 15 minutes
    h. During peritoneal dialysis keep an accurate flow chart
    i. During hemodialysis watch the site for clotting; check clotting time and administer heparin as prescribed by the physician
    j. During both procedures check tubes for patency
    k. Since both procedures are long, provide back care to promote comfort and diversional activities to help pass the time

Kidney Transplantation

A. Etiology and pathophysiology
  1. Patients with chronic renal failure who have no kidney function are candidates for transplantation
  2. Least risk of rejection of the new kidney occurs if donor and recipient are identical twins

3. At the time of surgery, the patient's own kidney is not removed unless it is infected or enlarged
4. New kidney is placed generally in the iliac fossa retroperitoneally, and the donor's ureter is attached to the bladder to prevent reflux of urine

B. Preoperative care
1. Prepare the patient and family emotionally for the possible outcomes of surgery
2. Explain that, postoperatively, immunosuppressive drugs and dialysis may be indicated as well as isolation to prevent infection
3. Explain routine preoperative and postoperative procedures

C. Postoperative care
1. Maintain patency of the drainage tubes, including the Foley catheter; gross hematuria or clots are *not* expected postoperatively
2. Monitor fluid and electrolyte balance carefully, since no urine output may occur for several days
3. Monitor vital signs, weight, and temperature
4. Observe the patient for signs of rejection
   a. Increased serum creatinine
   b. Decreasing urinary output
   c. Malaise
   d. Fever
   e. Flank pain or tenderness
5. Administer steroids and immunosuppressives as ordered to prevent rejection

Adenocarcinoma of the Kidneys

A. Etiology and pathophysiology
1. Most common cancer affecting the kidneys
2. Common sites of metastasis include lungs, liver, and long bones
3. Incidence higher in males

B. Signs and symptoms
1. Subjective
   a. There may be none until metastasis
   b. Dull back pain
   c. Weakness
2. Objective
   a. Painless hematuria
   b. Enlarged kidney palpable during physical examination
   c. Elevated temperature
   d. Weight loss
   e. Anemia

C. Treatment
1. Nephrectomy
2. Radiation therapy if tumor is sensitive
3. Chemotherapy
4. Hormonal therapy with medroxyprogesterone (Provera)

D. Nursing care
1. Monitor intake and output
2. Increase oral fluid intake
3. Administer analgesics as ordered to alleviate postoperative pain
4. Encourage coughing and deep breathing while splinting the incision
5. Examine dressing and linen under the patient for drainage; a small amount of serosanguineous drainage is expected
6. Maintain integrity of the urinary drainage system; avoid kinking of tubes
7. Observe urine for color, amount, and any abnormal components

Glomerulonephritis

A. Etiology and pathophysiology
1. Involves damage to both kidneys resulting from filtration and trapping of antibody-antigen complexes within the glomeruli
2. As a result, inflammatory and degenerative changes affect all renal tissue
3. Often follows some form of streptococcal infection such as tonsillitis
4. May be acute or chronic in nature; decreases life expectancy if progressive renal damage occurs
5. Complications include hypertensive encephalopathy, heart failure, and infection

B. Signs and symptoms
1. Subjective
   a. Flank pain, costovertebral tenderness
   b. Headache
   c. Malaise
   d. Dyspnea due to salt and fluid retention
   e. Weakness
   f. Visual disturbances
2. Objective
   a. Hematuria
   b. Periorbital and facial edema
   c. Oliguria
   d. Fever
   e. Tachycardia
   f. Urine analysis reveals protein and casts
   g. Elevated plasma BUN and creatinine
   h. Anemia

C. Treatment
1. Antibiotics such as penicillin to treat underlying infection
2. Dietary restriction of sodium, fluids, and protein based on clinical status
3. Diuretics and antihypertensives to control blood pressure

D. Nursing care

1. Monitor intake and output
2. Assess specific gravity of urine
3. Weigh the patient daily
4. Monitor vital signs and temperature
5. Special prophylactic skin care (these patients are prone to skin breakdown)
6. Protect the patient from infection
7. Observe for complications such as renal failure, cardiac failure, and hypertensive encephalopathy
8. Evaluate laboratory results (BUN, creatinine, urinalysis)
9. Encourage continued medical supervision
10. Refer to social service as needed; the long-term nature of the illness may create economic problems for the family

Bladder Tumors

A. Etiology and pathophysiology
  1. Occur most frequently in men over 50 years of age
  2. Smoking, exposure to radiation, schistosomiasis, and exposure over prolonged periods to certain chemicals increase the risk of development of tumor
  3. Common sites of metastasis include lymph nodes, bone, liver, and lungs
B. Signs and symptoms
  1. Subjective
    a. Frequency and urgency of urination
    b. Dysuria
  2. Objective
    a. Direct visualization by cystoscopic examination
    b. Painless hematuria
C. Treatment
  1. Surgical intervention
    a. Resection of tumor
    b. Cystectomy (removal of the bladder); requires urinary diversion
      (1) Ureterosigmoidostomy—ureters are attached to the sigmoid colon, and urine is excreted through the rectum; these patients have constant drainage and are usually troubled by recurrent infection of the urinary tract
      (2) Ileal conduit—section of the ileum is resected and attached to the ureters; one end of this ileal conduit is sutured closed and the other is brought to the skin as an ileostomy to drain urine; technique most widely used to divert urine
      (3) Nephrostomy—catheter is inserted into the kidney through an incision
      (4) Ureterostomy—ureters are implanted in the abdominal wall to drain urine
  2. Radiation therapy
  3. Chemotherapy
D. Nursing care
  1. Allow time for the patient to verbalize fears of surgery, cancer, death, and body image alterations
  2. Preoperatively, in addition to routine care and explanations, prepare the bowel by cleansing with laxatives, antibiotics, and enemas as ordered
  3. Assess the color and amount of urine frequently; maintain patency of drainage system
  4. If the patient has undergone a ureterosigmoidostomy, a drainage tube may be in the rectum for a few days; after removal, encourage the patient to void frequently via the rectum to prevent complications such as reflux and absorption of urine through the intestinal wall
  5. If the patient has an ileal conduit, a urinary drainage bag will be cemented around the stoma to collect urine; encourage self-care; teach the patient to change the appliance by using a mirror
    a. After equipment is collected, remove the collection bag; use water or a commercial solvent to loosen the cement
    b. Hold a rolled gauze pad against the stoma to absorb urine during the procedure
    c. Cleanse the skin around the stoma and under the drainage bag with soap and water; inspect for excoriation
    d. After the skin is dry, apply skin cement to the area around the stoma and to the appliance
    e. Place the appliance over the stoma and secure in place by an adjustable belt
  6. Expect a variety of psychologic manifestations such as anger or depression postoperatively
  7. Arrange visit from a member of an ostomy club
  8. Set realistic goals
  9. Encourage fluids such as cranberry juice to keep the pH of the urine acidic and help prevent infection

Bladder Trauma (Rupture)

A. Etiology and pathophysiology
  1. Traumatic rupture of the bladder occurs following external crushing injury to the area, as in automobile accidents

2. An overdistended bladder at time of trauma increases the risk of this occurrence
B. Signs and symptoms
   1. Subjective
      a. Pain
      b. Anxiety
   2. Objective
      a. Oliguria or anuria
      b. Hematuria
C. Treatment
   1. Exploration of the bladder to aid in diagnosing rupture
   2. Surgical repair of laceration
   3. Insertion of a suprapubic catheter to aid in urinary drainage (a tube inserted directly through the peritoneal cavity into the bladder to drain urine)
D. Nursing care
   1. Observe the vital signs for changes indicative of shock or hemorrhage
   2. Observe the urine for amount and color
   3. Promote rest and analgesia
   4. Maintain patency of catheters

Urethritis

A. Etiology and pathophysiology
   1. Inflammation of the urethra caused by staphylococci, *Escherichia coli, Pseudomonas* species, and streptococci
   2. Although these inflammatory symptoms are similiar to gonorrheal urethritis, sexual contact is not the cause
B. Signs and symptoms
   1. Subjective
      a. Burning on urination
      b. Urgency
      c. Frequency
   2. Objective
      a. Purulent drainage
      b. Bacteria in urine
C. Treatment
   1. Ascertain the causative organism through a culture of urine
   2. Administer antibiotics
   3. Hot sitz baths
   4. Dilation of the urethra and subsequent instillation of antiseptic solution
D. Nursing care
   1. Promote rest and comfort
   2. Encourage fluid intake
   3. Observe urine for clarity and hemorrhage

PHARMACOLOGY RELATED TO REPRODUCTIVE SYSTEM DISORDERS

A. Estrogens
   1. General implications for nurses
      a. Instruct the patient to report unusual vaginal bleeding
      b. Observe for edema and teach the patient to watch for this at home, especially by weighing at least twice per week
      c. If ointments are used, explain how to apply; if vaginal suppositories, explain how to insert
      d. Reassure male patients that feminizing side effects will subside when therapy is completed
      e. Observe the patient for adverse effects
         (1) Purpura
         (2) Thrombophlebitis
         (3) Decreased glucose tolerance
         (4) In males, gynecomastia, loss of libido, testicular atrophy
   2. Actions
      a. Secreted by ovarian follicles in women; trigger the proliferation phase of the menstrual cycle
      b. Regulate menstrual disorders, uterine bleeding, and menopausal problems
      c. May be used for inoperable prostatic cancer, postpartum breast engorgement, and breast cancer
      d. Also used as contraceptives
   3. Examples
      a. Chlorotrianisene (Tace)
      b. Diethylstilbestrol (DES)
      c. Esterified estrogens
      d. Estradiol cypionate
      e. Estradiol valerate
      f. Estrone (Theelin, Menformon)
      g. Ethinyl estradiol (Estinyl)
B. Progesterone and progestins
   1. General implications for nurses
      a. Observe the patient for edema and instruct to observe for this by recording weight and reporting increases
      b. Inform the patient's family that the drugs may result in psychiatric depression
      c. Observe for adverse effects
         (1) Scleral jaundice
         (2) Blurred vision or decreased vision
         (3) Thrombophlebitis
   2. Actions
      a. Progesterone—female ovarian hormone that prepares the uterus for implantation of a fer-

tilized ovum and is essential for the maintenance of pregnancy

    b. Used in the treatment of endometriosis, infertility, dysmenorrhea, and threatened abortion; also in suppression of ovulation

  3. Examples

    a. Hydroxyprogesterone caproate (Delalutin)

    b. Medroxyprogesterone acetate (Provera)

    c. Megestrol acetate (Megace)

    d. Progesterone (Proluton, Progestin, Lipo-Lutin)

C. Androgens

  1. General implications for nurses

    a. Use with a diet that is high in calories and proteins to aid in building body tissues

    b. Watch for signs of virilization in females

    c. Observe the patient for side effects

      (1) Weight gain

      (2) Acne

      (3) Changes in libido

      (4) Hoarseness; deep voice

  2. Actions

    a. Aid in the development of secondary sex characteristics in men and have anabolic properties, which stimulate the building and repair of body tissue

    b. Used in debilitating conditions and to restore hormone levels

  3. Examples

    a. Fluoxymesterone (Halotestin, Ultandren)

    b. Nandrolone phenpropionate (Durabolin)

    c. Norethandrolone (Nilevar)

    d. Testosterones (Testosterone, Oreton, Delatestryl, Andronate)

D. Oral contraceptives

  1. General implications for nurses

    a. Assist the patient in choosing the best method of birth control by providing an accepting atmosphere

    b. Discuss the importance of regular visits to a gynecologist

    c. Observe the patient for adverse effects

      (1) Thrombophlebitis

      (2) Hypertension

      (3) Libido changes

      (4) Hyperglycemia

  2. Actions

    a. Cause thickening of cervical mucus to inhibit sperm travel

    b. Inhibit ovulation

    c. Cause atrophic changes in the endometrium to prevent implantation

  3. Examples

    a. Estrogen and progesterone tablets (Demulen, Enovid, Norlestrin, Ortho-Novum, Ovral, Provest)

    b. Sequential contraceptives were also used but have been removed from the market because of adverse effects

RELATED PROCEDURES
Bilateral Vasectomy

A. Definition

  1. Surgical procedure to produce sterilization in men; often performed on an outpatient basis

  2. Small incision made into the scrotum, and the vas deferens is ligated

B. Nursing responsibilities

  1. Explain possible complications to the patient, such as bruising, edema, mild discomfort

  2. Explain the possibility of residual fertility; sterility is not achieved until semen is sperm free (there will be sperm in semen distal to the point of ligation following a vasectomy)

Tubal Ligation

A. Definition

  1. Surgical procedure to produce sterilization in women; generally performed in the hospital

  2. Laparoscope introduced through a small incision in the abdominal wall; an electric current is passed through forceps grasping the tubes to cause coagulation of the tissue

B. Nursing responsibilities

  1. Observe the incision for signs of swelling or hemorrhage and report to physician

  2. Explain to the patient that effects of the procedure are immediate and that hormonal function is not altered

MAJOR DISEASES
Prostatitis

A. Etiology and pathophysiology

  1. Generally the result of urethritis

  2. Prostate gland becomes swollen and tender

B. Signs and symptoms

  1. Subjective

    a. Difficult urination

    b. Pain

  2. Objective

    a. Fever

    b. Hematuria

C. Treatment

  1. Antibiotics or chemotherapeutics

  2. Application of heat

D. Nursing care

1. Administer antibiotics
2. Apply heat as ordered
   a. Sitz baths
   b. Rectal irrigations
3. Encourage fluids

Cancer of the Prostate

A. Etiology and pathophysiology
   1. Slow, malignant change in the prostate gland
   2. Tends to spread by direct invasion of surrounding tissues and metastases to the bony pelvis and spine
B. Signs and symptoms
   1. Subjective
      a. Frequency and urgency
      b. Difficulty initiating stream
   2. Objective
      a. Decreased force of stream
      b. Urinary retention
      c. Elevated serum acid phosphatase
      d. Enlarged hardened prostate detected by palpation
C. Treatment
   1. Type of surgical intervention depends on the extent of the lesion, the physical condition of the patient, and the patient's full awareness of the outcome (impotency follows radical prostatectomy)
   2. Radical prostatectomy, done by perineal or retropubic approach, removing the seminal vesicles and a portion of the bladder neck
   3. Radiation therapy alone or in conjunction with surgery may be ordered preoperatively or postoperatively to reduce the lesion and limit metastases
   4. Diethylstilbestrol (estrogen) may be ordered to reduce the size of an inoperable lesion or postoperatively to limit metastases
   5. Orchiectomy may be done to limit production of testosterone
D. Nursing care
   1. Similar to care of the patient who has undergone a prostatectomy for benign prostatic hypertrophy
   2. Explain to the patient that development of secondary female sexual characteristics will occur as a result of the medication and not the surgery
   3. Allow time and opportunity for the patient to express feelings about impotence
   4. Support the patient's male image
   5. Explain the situation to the patient's family and include them in planning
   6. Assist the patient and family in dealing with the diagnosis of cancer

Epididymitis

A. Etiology and pathophysiology
   1. Acute or chronic inflammation of the epididymis
   2. Occurs as a sequela of urinary tract infections, venereal disease, prostatitis
B. Signs and symptoms
   1. Subjective
      a. Chills
      b. Scrotal pain
      c. Groin pain
   2. Objective
      a. Fever
      b. Edema
      c. Elevated WBC
      d. Pyuria and bacteriuria
C. Treatment
   1. Medication to control pain, fever, and infection
   2. Scrotal support to facilitate drainage
   3. Notification of the state department of health if venereal disease is present
D. Nursing care
   1. Maintain the patient in a restful state
   2. Explain to the patient the importance of good hygiene practices
   3. Encourage fluid intake
   4. Ascertain contacts if due to venereal disease
   5. Teach the patient to protect himself from contracting most venereal disease by use of a condom

Benign Prostatic Hypertrophy

A. Etiology and pathophysiology
   1. Slow enlargement of the prostate gland common in men over 40 years of age
   2. Constriction of urethra and subsequent interference in urination
B. Signs and symptoms
   1. Subjective
      a. Frequency and urgency
      b. Difficulty initiating stream
   2. Objective
      a. Decreased force of stream
      b. Nocturia
      c. Total urinary retention
C. Treatment
   1. Reestablish emptying of the bladder by ordering a hot bath to induce voiding or by inserting an indwelling catheter or a cystotomy tube
   2. Urinary antiseptics and medications for reduction of pain and anxiety
   3. Have the patient prepared for surgical removal of the prostate by means of a suprapubic, transurethral, perineal, or retropubic prostatectomy

4. Postoperatively maintain drainage, force fluids, medicate for pain, administer antibiotics and stool softeners

D. Nursing care
   1. Observe for or initiate measures to maintain patency of the catheter
   2. Irrigate the catheter as ordered
   3. Encourage increased fluid intake (2400 to 3000 ml/day)
   4. Use sterile technique when necessary (e.g., insertion of the urinary catheter, irrigations, dressing changes)
   5. Maintain integrity of the closed drainage systems
   6. Administer antiseptics, bacteriostatics, and antibiotics as ordered
   7. In acute urinary retention, decompress the bladder slowly via a Foley catheter (not more than 800 to 1200 ml at a time) to prevent shock and hematuria
   8. Observe for signs of hemorrhage (e.g., change in vital signs, nature of drainage, pain, symptoms of shock, frank bleeding)
   9. Avoid postoperative complications by encouraging the patient to deep breathe and cough and to exercise muscles in lower extremities
   10. Teach the patient preoperatively what can be expected postoperatively (e.g., presence of catheters, bloody drainage, bladder spasms, pain)
   11. Accept and encourage the patient to express concerns about sexual functioning
   12. Provide the patient as much privacy as possible
   13. Administer medication for pain as ordered

Cancer of the Cervix

A. Etiology and pathophysiology
   1. Slow, malignant change in the tissue forming the neck of the uterus
   2. Most common form of genital tract malignancy in women
   3. High cure rate when diagnosed early
   4. Tends to spread by direct invasion of surrounding tissues and metastases to the lungs, bones, and liver

B. Signs and symptoms
   1. Subjective
      a. Back pain
      b. Leg pain
   2. Objective
      a. Spotting after intercourse
      b. Vaginal discharge
      c. Lengthening of the menstrual period
      d. Papanicolaou cytologic finding of Class V is considered conclusive of cervical cancer; Papanicolaou cytologic findings of Class I, II, III, or IV require further studies before a conclusive diagnosis can be determined

C. Treatment
   1. Type of surgical intervention depends on the extent of lesion and the physical condition of the patient
   2. Hysterosalpingo-oophorectomy (panhysterectomy) to remove the uterus, fallopian tubes, and ovaries; in advanced lesions the parametrial tissue and lymph nodes may also be removed
   3. Simple hysterectomy when preservation of ovarian function is desirable
   4. Radiation therapy alone or in conjunction with surgery may be ordered to reduce the lesion and limit metastases

D. Nursing care
   1. Assist the patient and family in dealing with the diagnosis of cancer
   2. Allow and encourage the patient to express feelings and concerns about change in self-image and sexual functioning
   3. Support the patient's feminine image
   4. If she is receiving or is to receive internal radiation therapy
      a. Explain the side effects that may occur and the procedures involved, especially the need for isolation during treatment
      b. Instruct her in maintaining proper positioning (supine and side-lying)
      c. Inspect the implant for proper position
      d. Provide low-residue diet and prevent bowel and urinary distention to avoid displacement of radioactive substance and irradiation of adjacent tissues
      e. Explain to the patient and family that visitors and staff will be limited in the amount of time they can spend in the room to avoid their overexposure to radiation
   5. If surgical intervention is used
      a. Maintain patency of the urinary catheter that was inserted prior to surgery to decompress the bladder and reduce stress on the operative site
      b. Observe for reestablishment of bowel sounds
      c. Maintain accurate intake and output
      d. Following removal of the urinary catheter, note the amount of output and pattern of voiding; catheterize for residual urine if ordered and whenever necessary for urinary retention
      e. For additional nursing responsibilities, see postoperative care

Vaginitis

A. Etiology and pathophysiology
1. Trichomoniasis—overgrowth of *Trichomonas vaginalis,* which normally is present in the vagina
2. Candidiasis (moniliasis)—caused by *Candida albicans,* a fungus; incidence is high in patients with diabetes mellitus and those receiving antibiotic therapy because of change in normal flora
3. Atrophic vaginitis—common in the postmenopausal period because atrophied vaginal mucosa is prone to infection

B. Signs and symptoms
1. Subjective
   a. Pruritus, burning
   b. Dyspareunia (pain with intercourse)
2. Objective
   a. Vaginal discharge
      (1) Malodorous, thin yellow discharge (trichomoniasis)
      (2) White "cheesy" discharge (moniliasis)
   b. Vaginal smear can indicate *Trichomonas vaginalis, Candida albicans,* or other microorganisms

C. Treatment
1. Douches (acetic acid may be added)
2. Antifungal preparations for candidiasis
   a. Nystatin (Mycostatin) vaginal suppositories
   b. Propionic acid gel inserted vaginally
   c. Gentian violet applied to vaginal mucosa and cervix
3. Antiprotozoan preparations for trichomoniasis
   a. Metronidazole (Flagyl) tablets taken orally
   b. Furazolidone-nifuroxime (Tricofuron) vaginal suppositories
4. Estrogen therapy prescribed for atrophic vaginitis

D. Nursing care
1. Advise the patient to have sexual partner use a condom during coitus until vaginitis is resolved
2. Explain to the patient that frequent douching will alter the normal pH environment of the vagina, predisposing to vaginitis
3. Instruct the patient to use tampons to prevent discharge from irritating vulvar area
4. Administer a douche if ordered
   a. Explain procedure to the patient; provide privacy
   b. Assemble equipment, including douche can, tip, bedpan, gloves, waterproof pads, and solution at 45° C (110° F) (30 ml of vinegar may be added to a liter of solution for acetic solution; alkaline solutions should never be utilized)
   c. Assist the patient onto a bedpan while maintaining privacy
   d. Wearing gloves, separate the labia and insert the tip into the vagina
   e. Rotate the douche tip gently so the solution reaches all vaginal folds
   f. When all solution is used, instruct the patient to bear down to expel as much remaining solution as possible; solution returns during the entire procedure
   g. Dry the perineal area gently
   h. Resterilize nondisposable equipment

Endometriosis

A. Etiology and pathophysiology
1. Growth of endometrial cells in areas outside the uterus
2. Generally affects young nulliparous women
3. Endometrial cells are stimulated by the ovarian hormones; will cause bleeding during the normal menstrual cycle
4. Adhesions are common and may result in sterility
5. Adenomyosis is a similar condition affecting women 40 to 50 years old in which the endometrial cells invade the muscles of the uterus

B. Signs and symptoms
1. Subjective
   a. Lower abdominal pain beginning 2 to 7 days prior to menstruation, becoming progressively worse, and then diminishing as the menstrual flow decreases
   b. Dyspareunia
   c. Pain associated with defecation
2. Objective
   a. Abnormal uterine bleeding (metrorrhagia, menorrhagia)
   b. Infertility

C. Treatment
1. Hormone therapy to suppress ovulation; young married women are advised not to delay pregnancy if children are desired
2. Surgical intervention
   a. Resection of lesions
   b. Oophorectomy, salpingectomy, and total hysterectomy if the condition is severe

D. Nursing care
1. Provide the patient as much privacy as possible
2. Explain procedures to the patient
3. Ascertain the patient's understanding of risks of sterility
4. Provide the patient time to talk about feelings
5. Administer analgesics as ordered

6. Observe for hemorrhage (e.g., check for signs of shock, vaginal bleeding); check vaginal packing
7. Check the patient's output; make certain that the patient is emptying her bladder
8. Routine preoperative and postoperative care if surgery is necessary

Pelvic Inflammatory Disease (PID)

A. Etiology and pathophysiology
1. Occurs within the female pelvic cavity; can affect the fallopian tubes (salpingitis), ovaries (oophoritis), peritoneum, surrounding connective tissue, and pelvic veins
2. May be acute or chronic, bilateral or unilateral
3. Caused by the introduction of bacteria (usually through the cervical opening) such as gonococci, streptococci, or tubercle bacilli that are transported by the blood from the lungs
4. If untreated, can lead to adhesions and sterility
B. Signs and symptoms
1. Subjective
   a. Severe cramping pain in lower abdomen
   b. Nausea
   c. Malaise
   d. Dysmenorrhea, dypareunia
2. Objective
   a. Temperature elevation
   b. Foul-smelling, purulent vaginal discharge
   c. Elevated WBC
   d. Cultures of vaginal discharge reveal causative organism
C. Treatment
1. Medication to control pain and fever
2. Specific antibiotics depending on the organism identified
3. Identify and notify sexual contacts and the state department of health if venereal disease is present
D. Nursing care
1. Maintain the patient on bed rest in a semi-Fowler position to localize the infection and prevent the formation of abscesses within the abdominal cavity
2. Apply heat if ordered to the abdomen or via a douche to improve circulation
3. Observe and record the amount and character of vaginal discharge
4. Change perineal pads frequently using gloves; tampons should not be used
5. Explain safety measures to prevent reinfection of the patient or others; during the acute phase the patient should abstain from intercourse

6. Provide psychologic support because of the social aspects of venereal disease

Vaginal Fistula

A. Etiology and pathophysiology
1. Abnormal opening between two organs
2. May be congenital or occur as a result of carcinoma or radiation therapy
3. Types
   a. Rectovaginal—opening between the rectum and vagina
   b. Vesicovaginal fistula—opening between the bladder and vagina
   c. Ureterovaginal fistula—opening between a ureter and the vagina
B. Signs and symptoms
1. Subjective
   a. Burning sensation
   b. Frequency of urination (if secondary urinary tract infection)
2. Objective
   a. Discharge of urine, feces, or flatus from the vagina
   b. Excoriation of vaginal mucosa
   c. Odor
C. Treatment
1. Dietary modification including high-protein, low-residue diet with vitamin supplement
2. Enemas, bladder irrigations, and douches using antibiotic solutions
3. Fistulas may be repaired surgically
D. Nursing care
1. Provide psychologic support, since the patient may be embarrassed by odor and drainage and become withdrawn
2. Provide privacy during any treatments
3. Change pads frequently; sitz baths and irrigations to maintain cleanliness of area
4. Observe drainage and perineum for signs of inflammation
5. Assess urine for signs of infection; maintain patency of drainage tubes
6. Monitor temperature as an indication of secondary infection

Cystocele and Rectocele

A. Etiology and pathophysiology
1. Cystocele—herniation of the bladder into the vagina
2. Rectocele—herniation of the rectum into the vagina
3. Both conditions may be present at the same time and are generally associated with relaxation or injury of the pelvic muscles during childbirth

B. Signs and symptoms
 1. Subjective
   a. Feeling of fullness in vagina
   b. Constant urge to defecate
   c. Dysuria
 2. Objective
   a. Soft reducible mass evident during vaginal examination that increases when patient is asked to bear down
   b. Stress incontinence
   c. Residual urine (60 ml or more after voiding)
C. Treatment
 1. Anterior colporrhaphy to correct a cystocele
 2. Posterior colporrhaphy to correct a rectocele
D. Nursing care
 1. Encourage voiding every 4 hours to prevent strain on the suture line from a distended bladder (no more than 150 ml should accumulate)
 2. If the patient has difficulty voiding, insert a Foley catheter if ordered
 3. After each bowel movement and voiding, cleanse the perineum with warm normal saline and sterile cotton balls; always cleanse away from the vagina and toward the anus
 4. Administer douches if ordered; include patient instruction
 5. Apply heat lamp, anesthetic spray, or ice packs if ordered to relieve discomfort
 6. Limit diet to liquids for first 5 days to avoid defecation and prevent strain on the suture line
 7. Administer medications to decrease GI motility if ordered
 8. Administer cathartics and an oil-retention enema using a thin rectal tube if prescribed

Prolapsed Uterus

A. Etiology and pathophysiology
 1. As a result of weakness of the pelvic floor, the uterus descends into the vagina; most often associated with childbirth
 2. If severe, the entire uterus may protrude outside the vaginal orifice; in this case, the vagina is actually inverted; referred to as procidentia
 3. Ulcerations in procidentia increase risk of cancer
B. Signs and symptoms
 1. Subjective
   a. Heaviness within the pelvis
   b. Low back pain
   c. Incontinence
 2. Objective
   a. Mass in the lower vagina or outside the orifice
   b. Elongated cervix
   c. Urinary retention

C. Treatment
 1. Vaginal pessary to maintain the uterus in correct position
 2. Surgical intervention
   a. Suspension of the uterus and correction of retroversion
   b. Hysterectomy (if postmenopausal)
D. Nursing care
 1. Encourage the patient to seek medical assistance if there is a prolapsed uterus
 2. If procidentia is present, observe for ulcerations; apply warm saline compresses or protective ointment to prevent ulceration
 3. Explain to the patient that if pessary is used, it must be taken out by the physician frequently and cleaned
 4. Observe the color, amount, and frequency of urination
 5. See section on cancer of the cervix for postoperative care

Carcinoma of the Breast

A. Etiology and pathophysiology
 1. Frequently begins as a hard, nontender, relatively fixed nodule found most often in the upper outer quadrant of the breast
 2. Metastasis by direct extension to the surrounding tissue and via lymph and blood to the axillary nodes, lungs, bone, brain, and liver
 3. Incidence increases with age and is influenced by heredity and the number of menstrual cycles a woman has had; multiparas and women with early menopause have a lower incidence, as do Japanese women
 4. Paget's carcinoma is a type of breast cancer that invades the nipple and milk ducts
B. Signs and symptoms
 1. Subjective
   a. Lesion generally *non*tender
   b. Malaise in later stages
 2. Objective
   a. Dimpling of skin by lesion
   b. Inversion and discharge from nipple
   c. Changes in color of breast over lesion; in late stages skin has orange peel appearance
   d. Enlarged axillary lymph nodes
   e. Positive findings in following tests
     (1) Mammography—x-ray examination of the breast—when there is an increased risk of developing breast cancer
     (2) Thermography—heat-sensing device to evaluate abnormal circulatory signs
     (3) Xerography—special x-ray plate sub-

jected to an electric charge—to image all breast tissue

    (4) Biopsy for microscopic evaluation

        (a) Aspiration of tissue by syringe

        (b) Excised tissue may be sent to the laboratory for a frozen section from which thin slices are examined

    (5) Estrogen receptor assay—if positive, indicates need for alteration of the hormonal environment by surgical or chemical means

    (6) Elevated carcinoembryonic antigen (CEA) in serum, plasma, or cerebrospinal fluid—indicative of progression of cancer, particularly of the breast, ovaries, and gastrointestinal tract; also used in detecting cancer of the prostate

C. Treatment

  1. Type of surgical and medical intervention depends on the extent of the lesion and the physical condition of the patient

  2. Surgical intervention

    a. Lumpectomy—removal of the lump and a fourth to a third of the breast (only for early, minute, peripheral lesions)

    b. Simple mastectomy—removal of the breast only

    c. Radical mastectomy—removal of the breast, pectoral muscles, pectoral fascia, and nodes (pectoral, subclavicular, apical, and axillary); this procedure may be modified

    d. Oophorectomy, adrenalectomy, and/or hypophysectomy to control metastases through alteration of the endocrine environment; most successful if normal numbers of estrogen receptor sites are maintained as determined by estrogen receptor assay

  3. Radiation therapy alone or in conjunction with surgery preoperatively or postoperatively to reduce the lesion and limit metastases

  4. Corticosteroids, androgens, and antiestrogens (tamoxifen citrate) may be given to alter hormonal environment

  5. Chemotherapy

    a. Alkylating agents

      (1) Cyclophosphamide (Cytoxan)

      (2) Chlorambucil (Leukeran)

      (3) Triethylenethiophosphoramide (Thiotepa)

    b. Antimetabolites

      (1) 5-fluorouracil (5-FU, Fluorouracil)

      (2) Methotrexate (Amethopterin, MTX)

    c. Other drugs

      (1) Adriamycin (Doxorubicin)

      (2) Vincristine (Oncovin)

D. Nursing care

  1. Encourage and instruct the patient concerning monthly breast self-examination

    a. Inspect while sitting with hands at sides and then overhead for retraction of the nipple, dimpling of skin, color change, and asymmetry

    b. Palpate the axillary and supraclavicular nodes

    c. Palpate the breast tissue using a circular pattern when lying down with the arms abducted

    d. Do after each menstrual cycle because premenstrual hormones can cause harmless nodules that will disappear after menses; if postmenopausal, do on the same date each month

  2. Assist the patient and family to cope with the diagnosis of cancer and altered body image by encouraging them to talk with staff and each other

  3. Administer medication for pain as ordered

  4. Listen to and accept the patient's anger and depression and do not attempt to minimize it

  5. Help the patient identify feelings and encourage discussion of them

  6. Support the patient's feminine image

  7. If the patient is receiving cobalt therapy or antineoplastic drugs, inform, explain, and assist her to accept the side effects that may occur (e.g., nausea, vomiting, hair loss, anorexia, diarrhea, stomatitis, malaise, itching)

  8. If surgery is performed

    a. Observe for hemorrhage by checking all areas of the dressing, the drainage unit, and vital signs

    b. Maintain functioning of portable vacuum drainage unit by ensuring patency of tube, emptying when necessary, and supporting to avoid tension at site of insertion

    c. Encourage good posture and provide assistance with ambulation until the patient adjusts to her altered balance

    d. Prevent or reduce lymphedema by elevating and supporting the patient's hand above her elbow and the elbow above her shoulder

    e. Instruct the patient who has undergone a radical mastectomy to avoid carrying heavy articles with the affected arm and to avoid cuts or bruises, having blood drawn, injections, or blood pressure readings in the affected arm because of impaired lymphatic drainage

f. Encourage active exercises of the affected arm, beginning gradually the day after surgery if approved by the physician
   (1) Wall hand climbing
   (2) Brushing hair
   (3) Turning rope
g. Instruct the patient as to the types of prostheses and where to obtain them; cotton covered by gauze may be used to fill a patient's bra until she is seen by a professional fitter
h. Use agencies such as Reach for Recovery to help the patient with physical and emotional readjustment
9. If the patient is receiving radiation therapy
   a. Observe for signs of radiation burns (erythema, desquamation)
   b. Avoid removal of skin markings drawn by the radiologist
   c. Instruct her to use only ointments or emollients prescribed by the physician

SEXUALLY TRANSMITTED DISEASES (VENEREAL DISEASES)

A. Etiology and pathophysiology
1. As a result of changing sexual habits, incidence of these diseases has increased and infections of the rectum and pharynx are common
2. Examples
   a. Syphilis, caused by the spirochete *Treponema pallidum*
   b. Gonorrhea, caused by the bacterium *Neisseria gonorrhoeae*
   c. Herpesvirus type 2 may also cause genital infections
3. During childbirth, infant may acquire gonococcal ophthalmia neonatorum; 1% silver nitrate solution or another ophthalmic antimicrobial is instilled into the infant's eyes at birth to prevent blindness
4. Organisms are inactivated easily if exposed to dryness, refrigeration, or other harsh environments
B. Signs and symptoms
1. Syphilis
   a. Primary (10 days to 3 months)
      (1) Chancre on genitalia, mouth, or anus
      (2) Serous drainage from chancre
      (3) Enlarged lymph nodes
      (4) Positive tests for syphilis (VDRL, Kolmer, or Wasserman can be used)
   b. Secondary (2 weeks to 6 months after the chancre heals)

(1) Skin lesions on palms and soles
(2) Erosions of oral mucous membrane
(3) Condylomata lata (wartlike growths) on the genitalia
(4) Alopecia
(5) Enlarged lymph nodes
   c. Latent
      (1) May remain asymptomatic for life
      (2) Positive laboratory tests for syphilis
   d. Tertiary (affects approximately one fourth of cases)
      (1) Gummas (granulomas) attack almost any organ and cause cardiovascular syphilis (aortitis and thoracic aortic aneurysms) and neurosyphilis (personality changes, ataxia, strokes, and blindness)
      (2) During this stage it is rare for an individual to infect another; however, a fetus can be infected
2. Gonorrhea
   a. Males
      (1) Symptoms begin within a few days after exposure
      (2) Discharge from the penis, initially clear mucus progressing to purulent drainage
      (3) Dysuria
      (4) Urethral smear positive for gonococcus
      (5) If untreated, complications such as sterility, urethral stricture, prostatitis, and epididymitis
   b. Females
      (1) Purulent yellow vaginal discharge
      (2) Dysuria, urgency
      (3) Endocervical smear positive for gonococcus
      (4) May be asymptomatic
3. Herpes genitalia
   a. Subjective
      (1) Anorexia
      (2) Genital pain
      (3) Dysuria
   b. Objective
      (1) Vesicles and papules on genitalia
      (2) Leukorrhea
      (3) Vaginal bleeding
      (4) Cultures reveal herpesvirus type 2
      (5) Increased risk of neonatal death and spontaneous abortion
      (6) Possible carcinogen
C. Treatment
1. Identification of patient contacts; report all cases to the state health department

2. Antibiotics (in particular, penicillin) used to cure syphilis and gonorrhea; herpes genitalia is treated only by supportive therapy
3. Abstention from sexual contact until determined to be noninfectious

D. Nursing care
   1. Provide a supportive nonjudgmental environment
   2. Encourage the use of early screening and educational program such as V.D. clinics, "hot lines," and workshops
   3. Explain to the patient that careful cleansing of the genitals as well as the use of condoms helps prevent the transmission of most venereal disease
   4. Teach about the diseases and their transmission
   5. Encourage fluids
   6. Assess any genital discharge for color, amount, and consistency

Endocrine System

REVIEW OF ANATOMY AND PHYSIOLOGY OF THE ENDOCRINE SYSTEM
Functions

Endocrine glands secrete products called hormones, which are chemical messengers that deliver stimulatory or inhibitory signals to target cells (Table 2-4)

Glands

Thyroid Gland

A. Anatomy
   1. Soft, red-brown mass having right and left pear-shaped lobes joined by a narrow isthmus
   2. Extends from sides of cricoid and thyroid cartilages to sixth tracheal cartilage
   3. Half of glands observed have a pyramidal lobe extending upward from the isthmus

B. Actions of thyroid hormones (Table 2-5)
   1. Accelerate cellular reactions in most body cells
      a. Increase BMR
      b. Accelerate growth
      c. Alter the metabolic rate of over 100 enzyme systems by profound stimulatory effect on cellular protein synthesis
   2. Bind to nuclear and cytoplasmic receptor sites
      a. Intranuclear chromatin protein binds thyroid hormones; this stimulates cellular protein synthesis and influences growth, development, and cell differentiation
      b. Mitochondrial membranes bind thyroid hormones, which regulate energy metabolism

C. Metabolism (inactivation) of thyroid hormones
   1. Liver the principal organ regulating blood concentration of thyroid hormones; thyroxine and tril-iodothyronine deaminated, deiodinated, and conjugated; conjugates excreted in the bile
   2. Skeletal muscle, kidney, liver, and heart tissues deiodinate thyroid hormones; this mechanism of hormone inactivation not as important as conjugation in liver

Parathyroid Glands

A. Anatomy—generally 4 small yellow glands (but may be 2 to 12); 0.6 cm (¼ inch) in diameter at their widest part; usually embedded in the capsule of the posterior part of the thyroid (but may be behind the pharynx or in the thorax with the thymus)

B. Actions of parathyroid hormones
   1. Parathormone—major sites of action are skeleton, kidneys, and intestine
      a. Bone tissue releases Ca^{++} into blood (requires active form of vitamin D)
         (1) Osteoclastic osteolysis stimulated
         (2) Osteocytic osteolysis stimulated
         (3) Enhanced rate of maturation of precursor cells into osteoclasts and osteoblasts
         (4) Inhibition of osteoblastic collagen synthesis
      b. Kidney tubule reabsorption of Ca^{++} and Mg^{++} is enhanced, which helps prevent further decreases in serum Ca^{++} levels; excretion of K^+, P^{+++}, and HCO_3^- also is enhanced; that of H^+ and NH_4^+ is decreased
      c. Parathormone, through adenylate cyclase activation, stimulates kidney's production of the enzyme that converts 25-dihydroxycholecalciferol into 1,25-hydroxycholecalciferol, which is the active form of vitamin D that works with parathormone in bone to mobilize Ca^{++}
      d. The intestinal mucosa increases its absorption of Ca^{++} and P^{+++}, with subsequent release into the blood
   2. Calcitonin
      a. Decreases loss of Ca^{++} from bone through inhibition of osteocytic and osteoclastic osteolysis (cAMP mechanism)
         (1) Action opposite that of parathormone
         (2) Some bone cells respond specifically to calcitonin; others to parathormone
      b. Decreases loss of Ca^{++} from bone and promotes hypocalcemia; this effect offsets postprandial hypercalcemia

Table 2-4. Location and hormones of endocrine glands

Endocrine gland	Location	Hormones
Pituitary Anterior (adenohypophysis)	Cranial cavity, in sella turcica of sphenoid bone	Growth hormone (GH, somatotropin, somatropic hormone, STH)* Thyrotropin (thyroid-stimulating hormone, or TSH) Adrenocorticotropic hormone (ACTH, corticotropin)* Follicle-stimulating hormone (FSH) Luteinizing hormone (LH) in female; interstitial cell-stimulating hormone (ICSH) in male Prolactin (lactogenic hormone, luteotropin) Melanocyte-stimulating hormone (MSH) Alpha and beta lipotropins
Posterior (neurohypophysis)	In sella turcica of sphenoid bone	Antidiuretic hormone (ADH, vasopressin)† Oxytocin†
Pineal	Midbrain	Melatonin
Thyroid	Overlies thyroid cartilage below the larynx	Thyroid hormones (thyroxine and triiodothyronine) Calcitonin
Parathyroids	Usually 4 beads on posterior wall of the thyroid	Parathormone Calcitonin
Thymus	Root of neck and anterior thorax	Thymosin‡
Adrenals	Situated on medial anterior surface of each kidney	
Cortex		Glucocorticoids (mainly cortisol and corticosterone) Mineralocorticoids (mainly aldosterone) Sex hormones (small amounts of androgens and estrogens)
Medulla		Epinephrine (mainly) Norepinephrine
Pancreas (islets of Langerhans)	Retroperitoneal in abdominal cavity	Insulin (secreted by beta cells) Glucagon (secreted by alpha cells) Somatostatin Pancreatic polypeptide

Ovaries
  Graafian follicles
  Corpus luteum
	Pelvic cavity (female)	Estrogens (estradiol, estrone)
		Progesterone

Testes Interstitial cells of testes	Scrotum (male)	Testosterone

*Also present in placenta along with estrogens and progesterone.
†ADH and oxytocin are synthesized in the hypothalamus but are secreted by the posterior pituitary gland. Synthesis occurs in cell bodies of neurons of the supraoptic and paraventricular nuclei. From here they migrate down the neurons' axons into the posterior pituitary gland, which secretes them into the blood.
‡One of several active thymic hormones

Table 2-5. Functions of thyroid and parathyroid hormones

Hormones	Functions	Hypofunction effects	Hyperfunction effects
Thyroid hormones Thyroxine Triiodothyronine Thyrocalcitonin	Stimulate metabolic rate; therefore essential for normal physical and mental development Inhibit anterior pituitary secretion of TSH Quickly decreases blood calcium concentration if it increases about 20% above normal level; presumably accelerates calcium movement from blood into bone	Cretinism, if occurs early in life; myxedema, if occurs in older children or adults	Hyperthyroidism
Parathyroid hormone (parathormone)	Increases blood calcium concentration by accelerating following three processes: 1. Breakdown of bone with release of calcium into blood 2. Calcium absorption from intestine into blood 3. Kidney tubule reabsorption of calcium from tubular urine into blood, thereby decreasing calcium loss in urine Decreases blood phosphate concentration by slowing its reabsorption by kidney tubules and thereby increasing phosphate loss in urine	Decreased blood calcium (hypocalcemia), which causes increased neural excitability and tetany Increased blood phosphorus (hyperphosphatemia)	Increased blood calcium (hypercalcemia), which causes decreased neural excitability and muscle weakness Bone "softening"—decalcification Hypophosphatemia

Table 2-6. Sex hormones (ovarian and testicular)

Hormones	Functions
Estrogens (secreted by graafian follicle and corpus luteum) Estradiol Estrone Estriol	Stimulate proliferation of epithelial cells of female reproductive organs (e.g., thickening of endometrium, breast development) Stimulate uterine contractions Accelerate protein anabolism (including bone matrix synthesis) so promote growth; but also promote epiphyseal closure so limit height Mildly accelerate sodium and water reabsorption by kidney tubules; increase water content of uterus High blood estrogen concentration inhibits anterior pituitary secretion of FSH and prolactin but stimulates its secretion of LH Low blood estrogen concentration after delivery of baby stimulates anterior pituitary secretion of prolactin
Progesterone (secreted by corpus luteum and placenta)	Name "progesterone" indicates hormone's general function, "favoring pregnancy" Stimulates secretion by endometrial glands, thereby preparing endometrium for implantation of fertilized ovum Inhibits uterine contractions, thereby favoring retention of implanted embryo Promotes development of alveoli (secreting cells) of estrogen-primed breasts; necessary for lactation Protein-catabolic and salt- and water-retaining effects similar to those of corticoids but milder; increases water content of endometrium
Testosterone (secreted by interstitial cells of testes)	Growth and development of male reproductive organs; promotes "maleness" Marked stimulating effect on protein anabolism, including synthesis of bone matrix and muscular development, hence, promotes growth; however, it also tends to limit height by promoting epiphyseal closure Mild acceleration of kidney tubule reabsorption of sodium chloride and water Inhibits secretion of ICSH by anterior pituitary

Testes

A. Anatomy—see genitourinary system

B. Actions of testicular (androgenic) hormones
1. Major androgenic action in target tissues is stimulation of protein synthesis through enhancement of nuclear DNA and RNA
2. Increased protein synthesis manifests itself as increased tissue growth, particularly in younger individuals; at puberty, rise in androgen level induces growth of long bones, muscular development, enlargement of the external genitalia, increased sex drive, laryngeal growth, and growth of body hair
3. Androgens influence fetal brain development through contributing to establishment of neural pathways that help to regulate adult brain functions and behavior

C. Metabolism of androgens
1. Liver the major site for androgen metabolism: testosterone and other androgenic steroids are enzymatically converted into other less androgenic steroids and then conjugated with glucuronic acid or sulfate
2. The generally biologically inactive conjugates are excreted in bile and urine

Ovaries

A. Anatomy—see genitourinary system

B. Actions of ovarian hormones
1. Estrogens
a. Enter target cells, bind cycloplasmic receptors, and enter nucleus; estrogen receptor complex regulates mRNA synthesis with overall effect of stimulating cellular RNA and protein synthesis
b. Stimulate uterine and liver lipid metabolism
c. Stimulate long bone calcification
d. Play a major role in the ovulatory-menstrual cycle
e. Increased protein and lipid synthesis are manifested in the reproductive system as uterine growth
f. Participate also in growth of pubic and axillary hair, pelvic enlargement, subcutaneous lipid distribution, growth of mammary glands, and maturation of skin (increased glandular activity)
2. Progesterone
a. Increases mucus secretory activity of endometrium; such action required for implantation of young embryo
b. Promotes growth of breasts
c. Keeps uterine smooth muscle quiescent during pregnancy

d. Inhibits oxytocin release by neurohypophysis (otherwise released in response to vaginal distention)

C. Metabolism of estrogens and progesterone
1. Liver conjugates estrogens with glucuronic and sulfuric acids; the conjugates are excreted chiefly in the urine
2. Conversion of estradiol to the less active estrone in the liver; placenta also carries out this conversion
3. Liver converts progesterone, synthesized from cholesterol in corpus luteum, placenta, and adrenals, to pregnanediol, which is then conjugated with glucuronic acid or sulfate; conjugates are excreted in urine

Adrenal Glands

A. Anatomy
1. Wedge-shaped, flattened, yellowish structure positioned like a cap at the kidney's superior border
2. Actually two closely associated structures—inner adrenal medulla and outer adrenal cortex; medulla and cortex each produce hormones with distinct effects on distant target structures
3. Medulla produces two catecholamines, D-epinephrine and D-norepinephrine, in approximate ratio of 80% to 20% respectively
4. Cortex secretes three steroid hormones in relatively large amounts: aldosterone (a mineralcorticoid), cortisol (known as hydrocortisone), and corticosterone (both glucocorticoids); also small amounts of several androgenic steroids; adrenocortical secretion is circadian, with higher levels produced during daytime; aldosterone secretion increases as sodium ions (Na^+) decrease or potassium ions (K^+) increase

B. Actions of adrenal hormones
1. Epinephrine and norepinephine
a. Stimulate liver and skeletal muscle to break down glycogen
b. Increase oxygen utilization and increase carbon dioxide production
c. Increase blood concentration of free fatty acids through stimulation of lipolysis in adipose tissue
d. Cause constriction of nearly all blood vessels of body, thereby greatly increasing total peripheral resistance and arterial pressure
e. Increase heart rate and force of contraction and thereby raise cardiac output
f. Epinephrine significantly dilates bronchial smooth muscle

Table 2-7. Functions of adrenal cortex hormones

Hormones	Functions	Hypofunctions effects (e.g., in Addison's disease)	Hyperfunction effects (e.g., in Cushing's syndrome)
Glucocorticoids, mainly cortisol (hydrocortisone) and corticosterone	In general, a normal blood concentration of glucocorticoids promotes normal metabolism of all three kinds of foods and a high blood concentration produces various stress responses		
	Accelerates mobilization and catabolism of fats; i.e., causes shift from usual utilization of carbohydrates for energy to fat utilization		
	Accelerates tissue protein mobilization and catabolism (tissue proteins hydrolyzed to amino acids, which enter blood and are carried to liver for deamination and gluconeogenesis)		Muscle atrophy and weakness; osteoporosis
	Accelerates liver gluconeogenesis (i.e., formation of glucose from mobilized proteins [hyperglycemic effect])		Hyperglycemia
	Causes atrophy of lymphatic tissues, notably thymus and lymph nodes		Lymphocytopenia
	Decreases antibody formaton (immunosuppressive, antiallergic effect)		Decreased immunity Decreased allergy
	Slows the proliferation of fibroblasts characteristic of inflammation (antiinflammatory effect)		Spread of infections; slower wound healing
	Mild acceleration of sodium and water reabsorption and potassium excretion by kidney tubules		High blood sodium (hypernatremia); sodium retention; also water retention; low blood potassium (hypokalemia)
	Decreases ACTH secretion		
Mineralcorticoids, mainly aldosterone	Marked acceleration of sodium and water reabsorption by kidney tubules	Low blood sodium (hyponatremia); dehydration	High blood sodium (hypernatremia); water retention, edema
	Marked acceleration of potassium excretion by kidney tubules	High blood potassium (hyperkalemia)	Low blood potassium (hypokalemia)

g. Inhibit contractions of gastrointestinal and uterine smooth muscle
2. Glucocorticoids and mineralcorticoids (Table 2-7)
C. Metabolism of adrenocortical steroids
1. Liver the major organ metabolizing adrenal steroids
2. Conjugation of steroids with glucuronic acid or sulfate produces inactive products primarily excreted in urine
3. In liver disease, adrenal steroids increase in blood due to decreased inactivation

Pancreas
A. Anatomy (see gastrointestinal system)
B. Actions of pancreatic hormones
1. Regulate glucose homeostasis through action of insulin and glucagon; also secrete somatostatin and pancreatic polypeptide
2. Insulin stimulates intracellular macromolecular syntheses, such as glycogen synthesis, protein synthesis, and lipogenesis
3. Insulin stimulates cellular uptake of Na^+ and K^+ (latter are significant in the treatment of diabetic coma with insulin); glucose also requires K^+ supplement to offset hypokalemia
4. Glucagon induces liver glycogenolysis similar to that produced by epinephrine, but glucagon functions at lower concentration and also does not raise blood pressure; antagonizes the glycogen synthesis stimulated by insulin
5. Glucagon inhibits hepatic protein synthesis; this makes amino acids available for gluconeogenesis and also increases urea production
6. Glucagon stimulates hepatic ketogenesis and release of glycerol and fatty acids from adipose tissue
7. Primary target organs are muscle, liver, and adipose cells, but other tissues also affected

8. Somatostatin inhibits release of both insulin and glucagon
9. Pancreatic polypeptide increases pancreatic and gastric secretions; secreted into blood after a protein-rich meal; secretion inhibited by somatostatin

Thymus
A. Anatomy
1. Soft, pink mass extending from lower border of thyroid to the fourth costal cartilages; great variation in size; 2 asymmetric lobes
2. Large at birth; decreases in size after puberty; hardly visible beyond middle age
B. Actions of thymic hormones
1. Regulate immunologic processes, possibly through regulation of the numbers and types of lymphoid cells; decrease in immune response; with aging, parallels thymus involution and decreasing blood concentrations of thymic hormones
2. Just after birth the thymus produces specific lymphocytes that migrate to peripheral regions (e.g., lymph nodes, spleen) to provide immunologic potential
3. Thymus synthesizes hormones that regulate the rate of development of lymphoid cells, particularly T cells

Pineal Gland
A. Anatomy
1. A firm, reddish, conical structure lying in the midbrain between the superior colliculi and attached by a short stalk to the roof of the third ventricle
2. Composed of cords of pinealocytes (or chief cells) separated by connective tissue; septa continuous with the pia mater covering the organ; cells accumulate calcareous granules (brain sand) by age 18 clearly visible at x-ray examination
B. Actions of pineal hormone
1. Secretes melatonin
2. Melatonin may regulate diurnal fluctuations of hypothalamic-hypophyseal hormones

Pituitary Gland
A. Anatomy
1. Rounded body 1.2 cm (½ inch) in diameter extending downward from the floor of the brain's third ventricle by a stalk (infundibulum); supported and protected by the sella turcica of the sphenoid bone; located near the optic chiasm
2. Composed of an anterior lobe (adenohypophysis) and a posterior lobe (neurohypophysis)
B. Actions of pituitary hormones (Tables 2-8 and 2-9)

PHARMACOLOGY RELATED TO ENDOCRINE SYSTEM DISORDERS
A. Drugs that affect glucose assimilation
1. General implications for nurses
   a. Administer all forms of insulin subcutaneously
   b. Use only regular insulin for intravenous administration
   c. When mixing insulins, draw regular insulin into the syringe first
   d. Rotate sites of administration
   e. Observe the patient for adverse effects of each medication
2. Insulin
   a. Action and types (Table 2-10)
      (1) Enables all tissues to utilize carbohydrates
      (2) Aids in metabolism of fat and protein
   b. Adverse effects
      (1) Irritability
      (2) Confusion
      (3) Convulsions
      (4) Tachycardia
      (5) Tremor
      (6) Moist skin
      (7) Headache
      (8) Hunger
3. Oral hypoglycemic agents
   a. Action—stimulates pancreatic beta cells to produce insulin in adults with residual functioning cells
   b. Examples
      (1) Acetohexamide (Dymelor)
      (2) Chlorpropamide (Diabinese)
      (3) Tolazamide (Tolinase)
      (4) Tolbutamide (Orinase)
      (5) Phenformin hydrochloride (DBI)
   c. Adverse effects
      (1) Skin reactions
      (2) Jaundice
      (3) Pruritus
      (4) Possible arteriosclerotic disease
4. Insulin antagonist
   a. Actions
      (1) Mobilizes glucose, which is stored in the liver
      (2) Stimulates gluconeogenesis from fats
   b. Example—glucagon
   c. Adverse effects
      (1) Nausea and vomiting
      (2) Circulatory collapse
B. Drugs that affect the thyroid gland
1. General implications for nurses

Table 2-8. Functions of anterior pituitary hormones

Hormones	Functions	Hyposecretion effects	Hypersecretion effects
Growth hormone (GH)	Promotes protein anabolism (hence essential for normal growth)	Dwarfism (well-formed type) if it occurs before skeletal growth is completed	Giantism if it occurs before skeletal growth is completed
	Promotes fat mobilization and catabolism (i.e., causes shift from carbohydrate catabolism to fat catabolism)	Simmonds' disease after skeletal maturity	Acromegaly (if occurs after skeletal maturity)
	Slows carbohydrate metabolism; has antiinsulin, hyperglycemic, diabetogenic effect (promotes glucagon secretion)		Hyperglycemia; chronic excess GH may cause diabetes mellitus
Thyroid-stimulating hormone (TSH)	Stimulates synthesis and secretion of thyroid hormones	Hypothyroidism: cretinism in early life, myxedema in adults	Hyperthyroidism (exophthalmic goiter, various other names)
Adrenocorticotropic hormone (ACTH)	Stimulates adrenal cortex growth and secretion of glucocorticoids; slight mineralocorticoid stimulation	Atrophy of adrenal cortex and hyposecretion (e.g., Addison's disease)	Hypertrophy of adrenal cortex and hypersecretion (Cushing's syndrome)
		Increased skin pigmentation	
Follicle-stimulating hormone (FSH)	Stimulates primary graafian follicle to start growing and to develop to maturity	Failure of follicle and ovum to grow and mature; sterility	
	Stimulates follicle cells to secrete estrogens		
	In male, FSH stimulates development of seminiferous tubules and spermatogenesis by them		
Luteinizing hormone (LH)	Essential for bringing about complete maturation of follicle and ovum		
	Required for ovulation		
	Causes formation of corpus luteum in ruptured follicle following ovulation; hence the name luteinizing hormone		
	Stimulates corpus luteum to secrete progesterone		
	In males LH is called interstitial cell–stimulating hormone (ICSH) because it stimulates interstitial cells of testes to secrete testosterone		
Prolactin	Promotes breast development during pregnancy	Failure to lactate	
	Initiates milk secretion after delivery of baby		
	Stimulates progesterone secretion by corpus luteum		
Alpha and beta lipoproteins	Cause release of lipid from adipose cells		

Table 2-9. Functions of posterior pituitary hormones

Hormones	Functions	Hyposecretion effects	Hypersecretion effects
Antidiuretic hormone (ADH); vasopressin	Increases water reabsorption by kidney's distal and collecting tubules, thereby producing antidiuresis (less urine volume; name based on this effect) Stimulates vasoconstriction; raises blood pressure	Diuresis (polyuria); diabetes inspidisus	Antidiuresis (oliguria)
Oxytocin	Stimulates powerful contractions by pregnant uterus Stimulates milk ejection from alveoli (milk-secreting cells) of lactating breasts into ducts; essential before milk can be removed by suckling		
Coherin	Regulates peristaltic rhythmicity in intestinal smooth muscle		
Melanocyte-stimulating hormone (MSH)	Stimulates synthesis and dispersion of melanin in skin, causing darkening		

Table 2-10. Types of insulin

Insulin	Action		
	Onset (hr)	Peak (hr)	Duration (hr)
Rapid acting			
Insulin injection (regular insulin)	½ to 1	2 to 6	5 to 8
Prompt insulin zinc suspension (Semilente)	½ to 1	3 to 9	12 to 16
Intermediate acting			
Globin zinc insulin injection	1 to 4	6 to 16	16 to 24
Insulin zinc suspension (Lente)	1 to 4	7 to 12	24 to 30
Isophane insulin suspension (NPH)	1 to 2	7 to 12	24 to 30
Long acting			
Extended insulin zinc suspension (Ultralente)	4 to 8	10 to 30	34 to 46
Protamine zinc insulin suspension (PZI)	1 to 8	12 to 24	30 to 36

    a. Anticipate that treatment is started in small doses and increased slowly

    b. Teach the patient the importance of medical follow-up

    c. Observe the patient for changes in weight, increased mental alertness and improved condition of skin and hair

  2. Thyroid hormone substitutes

    a. Actions

      (1) Regulate the rate of metabolism in most cells

      (2) Aid in growth and development of bones and teeth

      (3) Affect protein, fat, and carbohydrate metabolism

    b. Examples

      (1) Levothyroxine sodium (Synthroid)

      (2) Liothyronine sodium (Cytomel)

      (3) Thyroglobulin (Proloid)

      (4) Thyroid (Thyrolar)

    c. Adverse effects

      (1) Hyperactivity

      (2) Accelerated metabolism

  3. Antithyroid drugs

    a. Inhibit oxidation of iodides to prevent their combination with tyrosine in formation of thyroxine

    b. Examples

      (1) Methylthiouracil (Methiacil, Muracil)

      (2) Propylthiouracil (Propacil)

      (3) Methimazole (Tapazole)

    c. Adverse effects

      (1) Hypothyroidism in fetus

      (2) Urticaria

      (3) Agranulocytosis

  4. Strong iodine solution

a. Actions
   (1) Makes the thyroid gland less vascular by producing involution of an enlarged gland
   (2) Used preoperatively to decrease the risk of hemorrhage
b. Example—Lugol's solution
c. Adverse effects
   (1) Laryngeal edema
   (2) Hypersecretion of glands
   (3) Discoloration of teeth (administer diluted through a straw)

C. Adrenocorticosteroids
1. General implications for nurses
   a. Avoid infections
   b. Check patient for signs of other illnesses, since symptoms may be masked
   c. Monitor vital signs and weight
   d. Instruct the patient to carry a card indicating the medication prescribed
   e. Report symptoms of gastric distress
   f. Administer with antacids or milk
2. Actions
   a. Play an important role in most of the metabolic processes in the body
   b. Antiinflammatory effect aids the individual in coping with stress
   c. Alterations in the metabolism of protein, fat, and carbohydrates, as well as in fluid and electrolyte balance
3. Examples
   a. Betamethasone valerate (Valisone)
   b. Corticotropin (ACTH, Cortigel)
   c. Dexamethasone (Decadron, Hexadrol)
   d. Fludrocortisone acetate (Florinef Acetate)
   e. Hydrocortisone (Cortef, Hydrocortone)
   f. Hydrocortisone succinate (Solu-Cortef)
   g. Methylprednisolone sodium succinate (Solu-Medrol)
   h. Prednisone
4. Adverse effects
   a. Cushinglike symptoms
   b. Osteoporosis
   c. Hypertension
   d. Peptic ulcer
   e. Cataracts
   f. Delayed wound healing
   g. Eurphoria, psychosis

D. Antidiuretic hormones from the posterior pituitary
1. General implications for nurses
   a. Observe the patient for signs of dehydration
   b. Monitor intake and output
   c. If drug is administered to improve bladder or bowel tone, observe for continence or the passage of flatus
2. Actions
   a. In general, used in the treatment of diabetes insipidus since they promote water reabsorption by the distal renal tubules
   b. Vasopressin also causes vasoconstriction and increased muscle tone of the bladder, GI tract, uterus, and blood vessels
3. Examples
   a. Lypressin (Diapid)—intranasal administration
   b. Vasopressin (Pitressin)
   c. Vasopressin tannate (Pitressin Tannate)
4. Adverse effects
   a. Increased intestinal activity
   b. Hyponatremia
   c. Pallor
   d. Water intoxication

MAJOR DISEASES
Hyperpituitarism

A. Etiology and pathophysiology
1. May be due to overactivity of gland or the result of an adenoma
2. Characterized by an excessive concentration of pituitary hormones in the blood, overactivity, and changes in the anterior lobe of the pituitary gland
3. Two classifications
   a. Giantism—generalized increase in size, especially in children; involves the long bones
   b. Acromegaly—occurs after epiphyseal closing, with subsequent enlargement of cartilage, bone, and soft tissues of body
B. Signs and symptoms
1. Subjective
   a. Headaches
   b. Depression
   c. Weakness
2. Objective
   a. Increased soft tissue and bone thickness
   b. Facial features become coarse and heavy, with enlargement of lower jaw, lips, and tongue
   c. Enlarged hands and feet
   d. Increased somatotropin serum levels
   e. X-ray examination of long bones, skull (sella turcica area), and jaw demonstrates change in structure
   f. Amenorrhea
   g. Glycosuria

h. Diabetes and hyperthyroidism may also occur

C. Treatment
1. Medications to relieve symptoms of other endocrine imbalances resulting from pituitary hyperfunctioning
2. Surgical intervention (hypophysectomy) or irradiation of the pituitary

D. Nursing care
1. Help the patient accept the altered body image that is irreversible
2. Assist family to understand what the patient is experiencing
3. Help the patient recognize that medical supervision will be required for duration of life
4. Help the patient to understand the basis for the change in sexual functioning
5. Assist the patient in expressing feelings
6. If the patient has undergone a hypophysectomy
   a. Encourage the following of an established medical regimen
   b. Protect from stress situations
   c. Protect from infection
   d. Follow and maintain an established schedule for hormone replacement
   e. Follow nursing care for the patient undergoing intracranial surgery

Hypopituitarism (Simmonds' Disease)

A. Etiology and pathophysiology
1. Total absence of pituitary hormones
2. Occurs when there is destruction of the anterior lobe of the gland by trauma, tumor, or hemorrhage

B. Signs and symptoms
1. Subjective
   a. Lethargy
   b. Loss of strength
   c. Decreased tolerance for cold
2. Objective
   a. Decreased temperature
   b. Decreased blood pressure
   c. Emaciation
   d. Diminished axillary and pubic hair

C. Treatment
1. Replace hormones
2. If tumor is present, surgical intervention is indicated

D. Nursing care
1. Discuss the importance of adhering to medical regimen on a long-term basis
2. Allow the patient ample time to verbalize feelings regarding the long-term nature of the disease

Diabetes Insipidus

A. Etiology and pathophysiology
1. Etiology unknown; but may occur as a result of head trauma or surgical ablation or irradiation of the pituitary gland or an adenoma
2. Occurs when there is a deficiency of vasopressin (ADH), which is secreted by posterior pituitary

B. Signs and symptoms
1. Subjective
   a. Polydipsia
   b. Craving for cold water
2. Objective
   a. Polyuria (5 to 25 L/24 hr)
   b. Dilute urine; specific gravity 1.001 to 1.005
   c. Signs of dehydration (poor skin turgor, dry mucous membranes, elevated temperature)

C. Treatment
1. Administer vasopressin (Pitressin Tannate), antidiuretic hormone
2. Determine the underlying cause and attempt to treat it

D. Nursing care
1. Weigh the patient daily
2. Carefully monitor intake and output
3. Replace fluid by mouth or parenterally
4. Check results of the serum electrolyte evaluation
5. Monitor specific gravity of urine

Hypothyroidism

A. Etiology and pathophysiology
1. Absence or decreased production of thyroid hormone
2. Classified according to the time of life in which it occurs
   a. Cretinism—hypothyroidism in infants and young children
   b. Hypothyroidism without myxedema—mild degree of thyroid failure in older children and adults
   c. Hypothyroidism with myxedema—severe degree of thyroid failure in older individuals

B. Signs and symptoms
1. Subjective
   a. Dull mental processes
   b. Apathy
   c. Lethargy
   d. Intolerance to cold
2. Objective
   a. Stolid masklike facies
   b. Increase in weight
   c. Constipation
   d. Subnormal temperature and pulse
   e. Dry brittle hair

   f. Thickened skin

   g. Enlarged tongue; drooling

   h. Decreased BMR

   i. Decreased thyroxine (T_4) and radioactive iodine uptake

C. Treatment
1. Administer thyroid hormones
2. Maintain vital functions

D. Nursing care
1. Explain to the patient and family the importance of continued use of medication
2. Have patience with a lethargic patient
3. Teach the patient and family to be alert for signs of complications: angina pectoris—chest pain, feeling of indigestion; cardiac failure—dyspnea, palpitations; myxedema coma—weakness, syncope, slow pulse rate, subnormal temperature, slow respirations, lethargy
4. Teach the patient to seek medical supervision on a regular basis and when any signs of illness develop
5. Help the patient and family recognize that patient's inability to adapt to cold temperature requires the use of additional protection and modification of outdoor activity in cold weather
6. Teach the patient to avoid constipation by the use of adequate hydration and roughage in the diet

Hyperthyroidism (Graves' Disease)

A. Etiology and pathophysiology
1. Excessive concentration of thyroid hormones in the blood
2. Overactivity and changes in the thyroid gland may be present
3. May occur at periods of high physiologic and psychologic stress, although considered by some to be an autoimmune reaction
4. The gland may also enlarge (goiter) due to decreased iodine intake; no increase in secretion of thyroid is present

B. Signs and symptoms
1. Subjective
   a. Polyphagia
   b. Emotional lability and apprehension
   c. Heat intolerance
2. Objective
   a. Weight loss
   b. Increased systolic blood pressure and pulse
   c. Tremors
   d. Hyperhidrosis
   e. Increased respiratory rate
   f. Exophthalmos

   g. Increased BMR

   h. Increased radioactive thyroid uptake

   i. Increased triiodothyronine (T_3), thyroxine (T_4), and protein-bound iodine (PBI)

   j. Loose stools

C. Treatment
1. Antithyroid medications such as propylthiouracil and methimazole (Tapazole) to block the synthesis of thyroid hormone
2. Antithyroid medications such as iodine to reduce the vascularity of the thyroid gland
3. Radioactive iodine to destroy thyroid gland cells, thereby decreasing the production of thyroid hormone (atomic cocktail)
4. Medications to relieve the symptoms related to the increased metabolic rate (e.g., digitalis, propranolol [Inderal], phenobarbital)
5. Well-balanced, high-calorie diet with vitamin supplements
6. Surgical intervention involves a subtotal or total thyroidectomy

D. Nursing care
1. Assign the patient a private room with the means for temperature control when possible
2. Provide for periods of uninterrupted rest
3. Administer medications to promote sleep
4. Use nursing measures such as warm milk, warm bath, and back rub to establish a climate for rest
5. Protect the patient from stress-producing visitors
6. Provide diet high in calories, vitamins, carbohydrates, and proteins with supplementary feedings between meals and at bedtime
7. Understand that the patient is upset by lability of mood and exaggerated response to environmental stimuli; take time to explain disease processes involved
8. If the patient has undergone thyroid surgery
   a. Observe for signs of respiratory distress and laryngeal stridor caused by tracheal edema (keep tracheotomy set available)
   b. Provide humidity with cold steam nebulizer to keep secretions moist
   c. Keep the bed in a semi-Fowler position without pillows and teach patient to support head
   d. Use a soft cervical collar if ordered to prevent unnecessary neck movement
   e. Observe dressings at the operative site and back of the neck and shoulders for signs of hemorrhage
   f. Observe for signs of thyroid storm; may result from manipulation of the gland during surgery, which releases thyroid hormone into bloodstream

(1) High fever
(2) Tachycardia
(3) Irritability, delirium
(4) Coma
g. Symptomatic treatment is indicated if thyroid storm occurs
h. Observe for signs of tetany, which can occur after accidental trauma or removal of the parathyroid glands
(1) Numbness of extremities
(2) Spasm of the glottis
i. If tetany occurs, give calcium gluconate IV

Hyperparathyroidism
A. Etiology and pathophysiology
1. Hyperfunction of the parathyroid glands; usually caused by adenoma; hypertrophy and hyperplasia of the glands may also be responsible
2. As a result the kidneys excrete excess calcium and phosphorus
3. If dietary intake is not enough to meet calcium levels demanded by high levels of parathormone, demineralization of the bone occurs
B. Signs and symptoms
1. Subjective
a. Apathy
b. Fatigue
c. Muscular weakness
d. Anorexia
e. Emotional irritability
f. Deep bone pain (if demineralization occurs)
g. Constipation
2. Objective
a. Bone cysts, pathologic fractures
b. Renal calculi composed of calcium
c. Pyelonephritis, renal damage, uremia
d. Vomiting
e. Elevated serum calcium
f. Decreased serum phosphorus
g. Cardiac arrhythmias
C. Treatment
1. Surgical excision of a parathyroid tumor
2. Increased fluid intake
3. Activity encouraged
4. Calcium intake restricted
D. Nursing care
1. Observe the patient for signs of skeletal (deep bone pain, deformities) and renal (lower back pain, hematuria) involvement
2. Strain the urine, observing for stones
3. Encourage fluid intake, especially fluids like cranberry juice that acidify the urine

4. Assist the patient in ambulating to help prevent demineralization
5. Monitor intake and output
6. Encourage foods such as prune juice and roughage to combat constipation
7. Instruct the patient to limit intake of foods high in calcium, especially milk products
8. Provide cardiac monitoring if hypercalcemia is severe
9. If surgery is performed, postoperative care is the same as for patients undergoing thyroid surgery (see hyperthyroidism)

Hypoparathyroidism
A. Etiology and pathophysiology
1. Parathyroid glands may not secrete a sufficient amount of parathormone after thyroid surgery, parathyroid surgery, or x-ray therapy of the neck; idiopathic hypoparathyroidism rare
2. As levels of parathormone drop, the serum calcium also drops, causing signs of tetany; a concomittant rise in serum phosphate occurs
B. Signs and symptoms
1. Subjective
a. Photophobia
b. Diplopia
c. Muscle cramps
d. Irritability
e. Dyspnea
2. Objective
a. Trousseau's sign (carpopedal spasm)
b. Chvostek's sign (contraction of the facial muscle in response to tapping near the angle of the jaw)
c. Decreased serum calcium
d. Elevated serum phosphate
e. Stridor, wheezing from laryngeal spasm
f. Convulsions
g. Cataracts if the disease is chronic
h. X-ray examination reveals increased bone density
i. Cardiac arrhythmias
C. Treatment
1. Calcium chloride or calcium gluconate given IV for emergency treatment
2. Calcium salts administered orally (calcium carbonate, calcium gluconate)
3. Dihydrotachysterol to increase absorption of calcium from the GI tract
4. Calciferol (vitamin D) to help raise serum calcium levels
5. Parathormone injections
6. High-calcium, low-phosphate diet

D. Nursing care
1. Observe respiratory status and have emergency equipment available to perform a tracheostomy
2. Observe seizure precautions
3. Monitor serum calcium and phosphate levels
4. Check vital signs frequently if a history of cardiac problems is present; place on a monitor
5. Provide a calm environment free of harsh stimuli
6. Provide dietary instruction including elimination of milk, cheese, and egg yolks because of high phosphorus content

Diabetes Mellitus

A. Etiology and pathophysiology
1. Occurs when there is insufficient supply of insulin; may be due to
   a. Failure in body's production
   b. Blockage of insulin supply
   c. Autoimmune response wherein the insulin may bind to an immune serum globulin fraction, preventing utilization
2. Incidence increases with obesity, aging, and familial predisposition
3. Type I—insulin-dependent diabetes mellitus (IDDM), formerly called juvenile type; has a rapid onset and requires insulin administration
4. Type II—non-insulin-dependent diabetes mellitus (NIDDM), formerly called adult onset type; has a gradual onset and sometimes can be controlled by diet
5. Body does not have adequate insulin to convert glucose to glycogen
   a. Glucose level in the blood remains high
   b. Body attempts to rid itself of excess glucose by excreting some via the kidneys
   c. Osmotic force is created within the kidneys due to glucose excretion, and body fluid is lost
   d. Body is unable to utilize carbohydrates properly, and fat is oxidized as a compensatory mechanism; oxidation of fats gives off ketone bodies
B. Signs and symptoms
1. Subjective
   a. Polydipsia
   b. Polyphagia
   c. Fatigue
   d. Blurred vision from retinopathy
   e. Peripheral neuropathy
2. Objective
   a. Polyuria
   b. Weight loss
   c. Hyperglycemia
   d. Glycosuria
   e. Peripheral vascular changes and gangrene
C. Treatment
1. Attempt to manage mild uncomplicated diabetes by the use of diet, considering individual nutritional needs, maintenance of ideal weight, calories, and situational adaptations; a planned follow-up program according to need
   a. Characteristics of diet
      (1) Calories as needed to maintain ideal weight
      (2) Protein—optimum normal age group needs; usually 65 to 85 g for average adult
      (3) Carbohydrate—adequate for need but not excessive; usually about 100 to 250 g for an adult
      (4) Fat—moderation is the guideline; substitution of vegetable fats for some of the animal fats; usually about 70 to 100 g for adult
      (5) Dietary ratio—carbohydrate to protein to fat usually about 2:1:1
      (6) Distribution—fairly even distribution of food throughout the day in 3 meals, with snacks added between as needed from the day's total food allowances according to need and therapy with insulin or oral hypoglycemics
   b. Basic tools for planning diet—food exchange groups, using the exchange system of dietary control
2. Insulin administration
   a. Adjusted after considering the patient's physical and emotional stresses, selecting a specific type of insulin depending on the condition and needs of the patient (see pharmacology section for discussion of insulin)
   b. Somogyi effect—insulin-induced hypoglycemia
      (1) Epinephrine is released and the blood sugar level is low
      (2) Glucagon is released by alpha cells of the pancreas
      (3) These reactions cause mobilization of the liver's stored glucose and iatrogenically induce hyperglycemia
      (4) Somogyi phenomenon is treated by gradually lowering insulin dosage while monitoring blood glucose, particularly during the night (when hypoglycemia is most likely to occur)

c. Insulin pump
   (1) External device worn on a belt or harness, connected to the patient's subcutaneous tissue via an 18-gauge needle
   (2) Usual site of needle placement is the abdomen; needle is changed q. 48 h.
   (3) Regular insulin is pumped at a continual rate with a bolus (extra preset amount) prior to meals
3. Oral hypoglycemics for certain patients; however, these patients must have some functioning beta cells in the islets of Langerhans; more commonly prescribed for adults with late developing mild diabetes (see pharmacology section)

D. Nursing care
1. Assist the patient to accept the diagnosis
2. Encourage the patient to express feelings about illness and the necessary changes in life-style and self-image
3. Assist the patient and family in understanding the disease process
4. Help the patient with the administration of medication until self-administration is both physically and psychologically possible
5. Assist the patient to recognize the need for continuing health supervision
6. Assist the patient in recognizing the need for activities and diet that promote and maintain health
7. Patient teaching should include
   a. Testing urine for sugar and acetone and interpreting results; inaccurate readings may be obtained when the patient is taking cephalosporins, aspirin, and ascorbic acid
   b. Selection of correct testing method based on the patient's medication
   c. Avoidance of infection
   d. Proper care of the legs, feet, and toenails
   e. Method of administration of insulin—using sterile technique, rotating injection sites, measuring dosage, types and strengths of insulin, peak action periods
   f. Proper use of dietary chart and how to make substitutions
8. Encourage the patient to continue medical supervision and follow-up care, including visits to an eye care specialist and podiatrist
9. Teach the patient and the family the signs of impending hypoglycemia (headache, nervousness, diaphoresis, rapid thready pulse, slurred speech)
10. Teach the patient and family the signs of impending diabetic coma (restlessness; hot, dry, flushed skin; thirst; rapid pulse; nausea; fruity odor to breath)
11. For the patient with an insulin pump
   a. Allow time to adjust psychologically
   b. Teach the following:
     (1) Technique of inserting the needle and filling the syringe; use of aseptic methods
     (2) When to remove the pump (e.g., before showering or sexual relations)
     (3) How to test capillary blood glucose levels to monitor insulin dosage at home

Diabetic Coma (Ketoacidosis)

A. Etiology and pathophysiology
1. Occurs when there is insufficient insulin available, a systemic infection, diarrhea and vomiting, overindulgence in eating, emotional stress, injury, surgery, or pregnancy
2. Lack of insulin results in alterations of metabolism; proteins and fats are utilized; dehydration and electrolyte imbalance occur; and ketone bodies appear in the urine

B. Signs and symptoms
1. Subjective
   a. Thirst
   b. Anorexia
   c. Drowsiness
   d. Headache
2. Objective
   a. Vomiting
   b. Flushed appearance
   c. Lowered blood pressure
   d. Coma
   e. Sweet odor to breath
   f. Kussmaul breathing due to acidosis: very deep respirations as the body attempts to blow off CO_2
   g. Hyperglycemia
   h. Glycosuria and ketonuria

C. Treatment
1. Insert IV to provide direct access to the circulatory system and a Foley catheter to obtain urine samples at frequent intervals
2. Administer rapid-acting insulin
3. Replace lost fluids and electrolytes, using blood studies to determine dosage
4. Cardiac monitoring may be indicated if circulatory collapse is imminent
5. Establish cause of acidosis and treat appropriately

D. Nursing care
1. Stress adherence to dietary and therapeutic regimen to prevent occurrence

2. Administer insulin as ordered
3. Keep accurate records of urine tests, vital signs, and fluid balance
4. Teach the patient regarding dietary habits, prevention of infection, and signs of ketoacidosis

Hypoglycemia, or Insulin Shock

A. Etiology and pathophysiology
   1. May result when a diabetic patient receiving insulin therapy omits a meal, makes an error in insulin dosage, or vomits a meal; the majority of attacks occur in morning or late afternoon
   2. Occurs when blood sugar falls below 60 mg/100 ml
B. Signs and symptoms
   1. Subjective
      a. Muscular weakness
      b. Diplopia
      c. Faintness
      d. Numbness and tingling in fingers, tongue, lips
   2. Objective
      a. Diaphoresis
      b. Trembling
      c. Tachycardia
      d. Disorientation
C. Treatment
   1. Oral glucose administration if the patient is alert
   2. Administration of glucagon parenterally to stimulate glucogenolysis
   3. Insertion of an IV line for access to a vein in an emergency
   4. Administration of 50% dextrose
D. Nursing care
   1. Administer medications as ordered
   2. Keep accurate record of intake and output, vital signs, and fractional urine tests
   3. If ordered, give patient protein or fat feeding after an easily absorbed carbohydrate meal is given

Primary Aldosteronism (Conn's Syndrome)

A. Etiology and pathophysiology
   1. Aldosterone, a mineralocorticoid, causes the kidneys to retain sodium and excrete potassium
   2. Hypersecretion of aldosterone is usually caused by an adenoma of the adrenal cortex but may also be caused by hyperplasia or carcinoma
   3. The disease is more common in females
B. Signs and symptoms
   1. Subjective
      a. Muscle weakness

      b. Polydipsia, polyuria
      c. Paresthesia
   2. Objective
      a. Hypertension
      b. Hypokalemia
      c. Hypernatremia
      d. Elevated urinary aldosterone levels
      e. Renal damage
         (1) Proteinuria
         (2) Alkaline urine
         (3) Decreased specific gravity of urine
         (4) Pyelonephritis
C. Treatment
   1. Surgical removal of the tumor
   2. Temporary management with spironolactone
   3. Occasionally a bilateral adrenalectomy involving lifelong corticosteroid therapy is necessary
D. Nursing care
   1. Monitor vital signs
   2. Observe for signs of electrolyte imbalance
   3. Provide fluids to meet excessive thirst
   4. Encourage continued medical supervision
   5. Monitor intake and output and specific gravity of urine
   6. If bilateral adrenalectomy is performed
      a. Administer steroids with milk or antacid
      b. Protect the patient from infection
      c. Explain drug and side effects to patient
      d. Instruct the patient to carry medical alert identification card
   7. Provide dietary instruction; include foods high in potassium such as orange juice and bananas while avoiding or limiting intake of foods that contain sodium

Cushing's Syndrome

A. Etiology and pathophysiology
   1. Results from excess secretion of adrenocortical hormones
   2. Caused by hyperplasia or by a tumor of the adrenal cortex; however, the primary lesion may occur in the pituitary gland, causing excess production of ACTH
   3. Administration of excess glucocorticoids or ACTH will also cause Cushing's syndrome
B. Signs and symptoms
   1. Subjective
      a. Weakness
      b. Decreased libido
      c. Mood swings to psychosis
   2. Objective
      a. Obese trunk with relatively thin arms and legs

b. Hypertension
c. Moon face
d. Buffalo hump
e. Acne
f. Increased susceptibility to infections
g. Hirsutism
h. Ecchymotic areas
i. Purple striae on the breast and abdomen
j. Amenorrhea
k. Hyperglycemia
l. Hypokalemia
m. Elevated 17-hydroxysteroids
n. Osteoporosis may be evident on x-ray examination
C. Treatment (aimed at correcting cause)
1. Reduce dosage of externally administered corticoids
2. If lesion on pituitary is causing hypersecretion of ACTH, a hypophysectomy or irradiation of the pituitary may be done
3. Surgical excision of adrenal tumors (adrenalectomy)
4. Potassium supplements
5. High-protein diet with sodium restriction
D. Nursing care
1. Monitor vital signs
2. Protect the patient from exposure to infections
3. Collect 24-hour urine specimens for diagnostic purposes (17-ketosteroids and 17-hydroxysteroids)
4. Encourage ventilation of feelings by the patient and spouse, since changes in body image and sex drives can alter marital support
5. Attempt to minimize stress in the environment by measures such as limiting visitors and explaining procedures carefully
6. Monitor sugar and acetone

Addison's Disease

A. Etiology and pathophysiology
1. Hyposecretion of adrenocortical hormones
2. Generally caused by destruction of the cortex or by idiopathic atrophy
B. Signs and symptoms
1. Subjective
a. Weakness
b. Easy fatigue
c. Nausea
2. Objective
a. Increased bronze pigmentation of skin
b. Vomiting
c. Diarrhea
d. Hypotension
e. Hypoglycemia
f. Small heart
g. Increased plasma ACTH
h. Decreased 17-ketosteroids and 17-hydroxysteroids in 24-hour urines
i. Hyponatremia
C. Treatment
1. Replacement of hormones
a. Glucocorticoids to correct metabolic imbalance
b. Mineralocorticoids to correct electrolyte imbalance and hypotension
2. High-carbohydrate, high-protein diet
3. Special diagnostic tests to determine whether disease is caused by primary adrenocortical insufficiency or is secondary to pituitary insufficiency
a. Eight-hour IV ACTH test to measure urinary steroid output after administration of ACTH; if output fails to rise, the problem is primary adrenocortical insufficiency (Addison's); if output rises slowly (normal response is rapid rise), the problem is secondary to pituitary insufficiency
b. Plasma cortisol ACTH test to measure plasma cortisol level before and 30 minutes after administration of ACTH; if level fails to rise, the problem is primary adrenocortical insufficiency (Addison's); if level rises (which is also the normal response), the problem is secondary to pituitary insufficiency
c. Thorn test to measure eosinophil count before and after administration of ACTH; if count remains the same, the problem is primary adrenocortical insufficiency (Addison's)
D. Nursing care
1. Administer steroids as ordered
2. Administer steroids with milk or an antacid to limit ulcerogenic factor of the drug
3. Put the patient in a quiet room to prevent contact with patients having infectious diseases
4. Limit the number of visitors
5. Monitor vital signs 4 times a day; be alert for elevation in temperature (infection, dehydration), alterations in pulse rate (hyperkalemia), and alterations in blood pressure
6. Observe for signs of sodium and potassium imbalance
7. Monitor intake and output and weigh daily
8. Encourage adequate diet and fluid intake
9. Administer antiemetics to prevent fluid and electrolyte loss by vomiting

Pheochromocytoma

A. Etiology and pathophysiology
  1. Tumor of the adrenal medulla; usually benign
  2. Causes increased secretion of epinephrine and norepinephrine
  3. Heredity believed to be involved in the development of the tumor
B. Signs and symptoms
  1. Subjective
    a. Headache
    b. Visual disturbances
    c. Nausea
  2. Objective
    a. Hypertension and orthostatic hypotension
    b. Tachycardia
    c. Diaphoresis
    d. Increased BMR
    e. Increased urinary catecholamines
    f. Hyperglycemia
C. Treatment
  1. Surgical removal of the tumor
  2. Antihypertensive and antiarrhythmic drugs
D. Nursing care
  1. Monitor blood pressure frequently in both upright and horizontal positions
  2. Administer parenteral fluids and blood as ordered preoperatively and postoperatively to maintain blood volume
  3. Collect a 24-hour urine specimen to evaluate urinary catecholamines
  4. If bilateral adrenalectomy is performed, instruct the patient regarding maintenance doses of steroids
  5. Emphasize the importance of continued medical supervision and screening for other family members

Neuromusculoskeletal Systems

REVIEW OF ANATOMY AND PHYSIOLOGY OF THE NEUROMUSCULOSKELETAL SYSTEMS
Nervous System

Cells

Neurons (nerve cells) are basic structural and functional unit; about 10 billion in the human brain
A. General properties and functions
  1. Irritability—response to stimulus
  2. Conductivity—conduct electrical energy (nerve impulse); basis for body's rapid communication and integration network
  3. Types
    a. Sensory (afferent) neurons—transmit impulses to spinal cord or brain
    b. Motoneurons (motor or efferent neurons)—transmit impulses away from brain or spinal cord toward or to muscles or glands
      (1) Somatic motoneurons—transmit impulses from the cord or brainstem to skeletal muscle
      (2) Visceral or autonomic motoneurons—transmit impulses from the cord or brainstem to smooth muscle, cardiac muscle, or glands
    c. Interneurons (internuncial or intercalated neurons)—transmit impulses from sensory neurons to motoneurons
  4. Neurons cannot be replaced if lost; but neuronal contents are constantly being replenished; a system of axonal flow distributes neural components to all regions from the cell body, where most synthesis occurs
B. Structure—well suited to transmitting impulses over distances
  1. Cell body contains a nucleus and other cytoplasmic organelles
  2. Axon and dendrites—cellular extensions; single axon or dendrite referred to as a nerve fiber
    a. Axon—one per neuron; carries impulse away from cell body; longer and thinner than dendrites; travels only at end where it communicates with other neurons, muscles, or glands; may be over 1 m (39 inches) in length and may communicate with 1000 other neurons
    b. Dendrites—delicate cellular extensions carry impulses toward cell body; several per neuron; each repeatedly branches, forming complex, bushlike network around cell body; increases surface area for reception by neuron of incoming electric signals; dendrite of sensory neurons exceptional in being extremely long, extending to periphery from ganglia near brain and spinal cord
  3. Supportive coverings and sheaths
    a. Myelin—multiple, dense layers of membrane wrapped around an axon or dendrite; gaps in myelin every millimeter or so along the fiber are called nodes of Ranvier; myelinated nerve fibers transmit nerve impulses more rapidly than nonmyelinated fibers of same diameter
    b. Neurilemma—sheath of cells (Schwann cells) forming an envelope around axons and some dendrites

(1) Responsible for effective regeneration of a nerve fiber after injury in the peripheral nervous system; the neurilemma forms a cellular tube down which the regenerating fiber travels

(2) Forms the myelin sheath

4. Neuronal cell membrane—similar in lipid content to cell membranes of all other body cells; however, specific proteins embedded in and attached to the surface of the lipid provide special characteristics; membrane proteins can be grouped into five classes

a. Pumps—actively transport ions (notably Na^+ and K^+) between intracellular and interstitial fluid; establish ionic conditions for resting potential and nerve impulse

b. Channels—provide selective pathways for diffusion of specific ions, as in neuronal depolarization and repolarization; channels open and close (gating mechanisms) in response to voltage changes and chemicals

c. Receptors—depolarization and repolarization; channels provide specific binding sites for various naturally occurring transmitters and drugs

d. Enzymes—catalyze chemical reactions on the membrane surface

e. Structural proteins—interconnect cells to form tissues and organs; hold cell parts together

5. Synapse—point of contact between 1 neuron and another

a. Typical neuron may have between 1000 and 10,000 synapses

b. Most often occurs between axon of 1 cell and dendrite of another, also commonly between axon and the cell body of another

c. Physical gap (synaptic cleft; separates the terminal axonal branches and dendrite or cell body of the next neuron

d. At the synapse, the axon terminals enlarge to form a terminal button, which is the information-delivering part of the synapse; some synapses are excitatory and others inhibitory

6. Neuroglia takes up most of the space in the nervous system not occupied by neurons; it supports, defends, and nourishes neurons; chief source of CNS tumors; unlike neurons, neuroglia retains the ability to divide; astrocytes, a type of neuroglial cell, provide framework of cells and fibers that suspend neurons and help provide the blood-brain barrier

Nerve Impulse

A. General considerations

1. Wave of electrical energy that flows over the surface of neurons and permits communication and integration between distant body regions

2. The larger the nerve fiber and the thicker the myelin sheath, the greater the velocity of the nerve impulse

3. Based on concentration differences between ions in the intracellular fluid of neuron and surrounding interstitial fluid

4. Ionic differences depend on ion pumps—most often studied is called sodium pump

a. Requires ATP to work

b. Pumps 3 sodium ions out of the cell in exchange for 2 potassium ions taken into the cell

c. Due to action of the sodium pump, intracellular fluid is about 10 times richer in potassium ions than is interstitial fluid, and interstitial fluid is about 10 times richer in sodium ions than is intracellular fluid

B. Impulse generation

1. Resting potential—after the sodium pump establishes ionic gradients, some potassium diffuses out of cell through permanently open potassium channels; such potassium flow results in an excess of positive charge on the membrane's outer surface and a deficit of positive charge on the membrane's inner surface; the result is a voltage difference of 70 millivolts (mV) with the cell interior being negative; this is the resting potential

2. Action potential—change in voltage across the neuronal membrane activates (opens) specific sodium ion channels in the membrane, allowing sodium ions to enter the cell and reverse the membrane's charge (inside becomes positive and outside becomes negative); as depolarization proceeds, the sodium channel closes and a voltage-gated potassium channel opens so that repolarization occurs with the voltage difference returning to the resting potential

3. Nerve impulse—action potential, composed of depolarization and repolarization, propagates itself down the axon or dendrite and is known as the nerve impulse

C. Basic route of impulse conduction—reflex arc

1. Description—impulse conduction

a. Starts in receptors

b. Continues over reflex arc(s)

c. Terminates in effectors (muscles and glands)

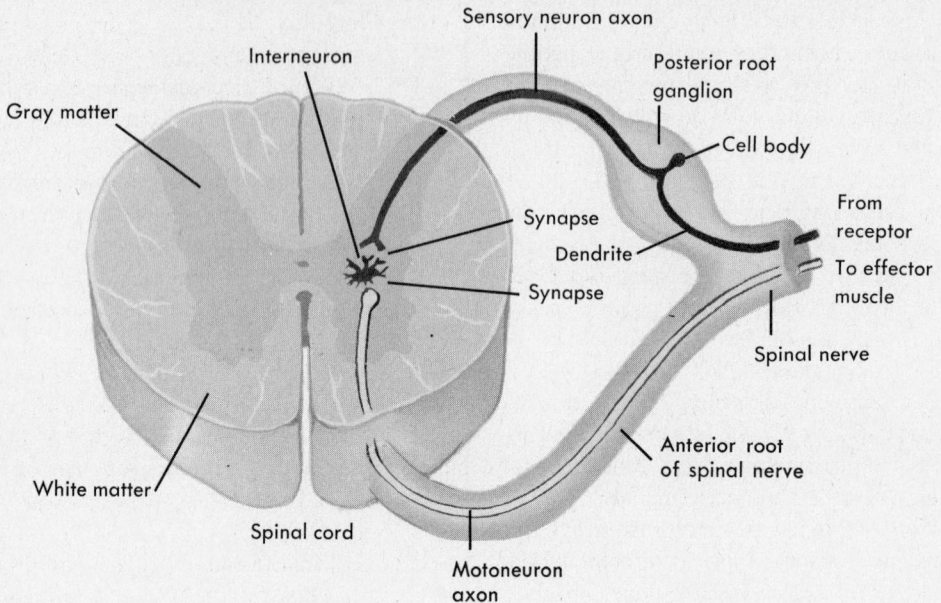

Fig. 7. Three-neuron ipsilateral reflex arc, consisting of an afferent (sensory) neuron, an interneuron, and an efferent (motor) neuron (motoneuron). Note the presence of two synapses in this arc: (1) between sensory neuron axon terminals and interneuron dendrites and (2) between interneuron axon terminals and motoneuron dendrites and cell bodies (located in the anterior gray matter). Nerve impulses traversing such arcs produce many spinal reflexes (e.g., withdrawing the hand from a hot object). (From Anthony, C.P., and Thibodeau, G.A.: Textbook of anatomy and physiology, ed. 11, St. Louis, 1983, The C.V. Mosby Co.)

d. Results in a reflex—response by muscles or glands in which the impulse terminates; a reflex, therefore, is either contraction of muscle or secretion by gland

e. Not all impulses result in reflexes; many are inhibited at some point along the reflex arc

2. Types of reflex arcs

a. Two-neuron (monosynaptic) reflex arc—simplest arc possible; consists of at least 1 sensory neuron, 1 synapse, and 1 motor neuron (motoneuron); synapse is a region of contact between axon terminals of one neuron and dendrites or the cell body of another neuron

b. Three-neuron arc (Fig. 7)—consists of at least 1 sensory neuron, 1 synapse, 1 interneuron, 1 synapse, and 1 motoneuron

c. Complex multisynaptic neural pathways also exist; many not yet clearly mapped

D. Conduction across synapses

1. Given synapse can transmit only 1 type of transmitter substance

2. There are 30 different types of neurotransmitters, including

a. Monoamines (norepinephrine, dopamine, serotonin, acetylcholine); axons that release acetylcholine are called cholinergic; those that release norepinephrine are called adrenergic

b. Amino acids (gamma-aminobutyric acid [GABA], glutamic acid, glycine, taurine); GABA is the most common inhibitory transmitter in the brain

c. Neuropeptides (hormone-releasing hormones, enkephalins, and endorphins); some influence hormone levels and some influence perception and integration of pain and emotional experience

d. Prostaglandins—high levels in brain tissue; some inhibit and some excite; may moderate the action of other transmitters by influencing the neuronal membrane

3. Overall response of the neuron—sum or average of excitatory and inhibitory inputs determines whether the cell will fire and the rate at which it will fire; the neuron is seen to be an evaluator of signals, not just a passive transmitter; the result of its evaluation is its individual rate of impulse transmission

Organs of Nervous System

A. Central nervous system (CNS)—spinal cord and brain

B. Peripheral nervous system (PNS)—nerves and ganglia

C. Definitions
1. White matter—bundles of myelinated nerve fibers
2. Gray matter—clusters of mainly neuronal cell bodies
3. Nerves—bundles of myelinated nerve fibers located outside the CNS
4. Tracts—bundles of myelinated nerve fibers located within the CNS
5. Ganglia (singular: ganglion)—microscopic structures consisting of neuron cell bodies; mainly located outside the CNS

Spinal Cord

A. Location—in the spinal cavity, from the foramen magnum to the first lumbar vertebra

B. Structure
1. Deep groove (anterior median fissure) and more shallow groove (posterior median sulcus) incompletely divide the cord into right and left symmetric halves
2. Inner core of the cord consists of gray matter shaped like a 3-dimensional H
3. Long columns of white matter surround the cord's inner core of gray matter; namely, right and left anterior, lateral, and posterior columns; composed of numerous sensory and motor tracts (Fig. 8)

C. Functions
1. Sensory tracts conduct impulses up cord to brain; motor tracts conduct impulses down cord from brain
2. Gray matter of cord contains reflex centers for all spinal cord reflexes

Brain

A. General considerations
1. Most active of all body organs in energy consumption; has large blood supply and high oxygen consumption, which increases even further during dreaming stage of sleep
2. Unlike other cells of body, neurons can only utilize glucose for energy metabolism; therefore hypoglycemia can seriously alter brain function and lead to coma
3. Brain cells protected by the blood-brain barrier, a selective filtration system that isolates the brain from substances in the general circulation; barrier is based on the relative impermeability of blood vessels in the brain and the tight wrapping of neuroglial cells around the neurons and blood vessels of the brain; only selected brain regions designed to monitor the chemical composition of blood are not protected by the blood-brain barrier
4. Ease of drug entry into the brain depends on size and fat solubility; the smaller the molecule and the greater the fat solubility, the more easily the drug enters brain tissue
5. Overall function of the brain and spinal cord is to channel sensory input to a variety of neural structures whose analysis culminates in the convergence of impulses on various motor neurons, which effect movements of all types of muscles and activity of glands

B. Regions of brain and their functions
1. Basic tissue types
   a. Gray matter—aggregations of neuron cell bodies
   b. White matter—composed primarily of tracts of fibers (axons) interconnecting neurons in different regions of the CNS
2. Basic cellular types in the CNS
   a. Association (intercolated) neurons—about 99.9% of all the neurons in the CNS
   b. Motor neurons—several million found in the CNS
3. Gross anatomic regions
   a. Hindbrain (brainstem)—lowermost brain division; formed by enlargement of the spinal cord as it enters the cranial cavity
      (1) Medulla—lowest portion of the hindbrain
         (a) Consists mainly of white matter (sensory and motor tracts); also contains reticular formation (mixture of gray and white matter); some important reflex centers located in reticular formation: cardiac, vasomotor, respiratory, and swallowing centers
         (b) Functions—contains centers for vital heart, blood vessel diameter (blood pressure), and respiratory reflexes; also centers for vomiting, coughing, swallowing, etc.; conducts impulses between the cord and brain (both sensory and motor)
      (2) Pons
         (a) Part of the brain located just above the medulla; consists mainly of white matter (sensory and motor tracts) interspersed with gray matter (reflex centers)

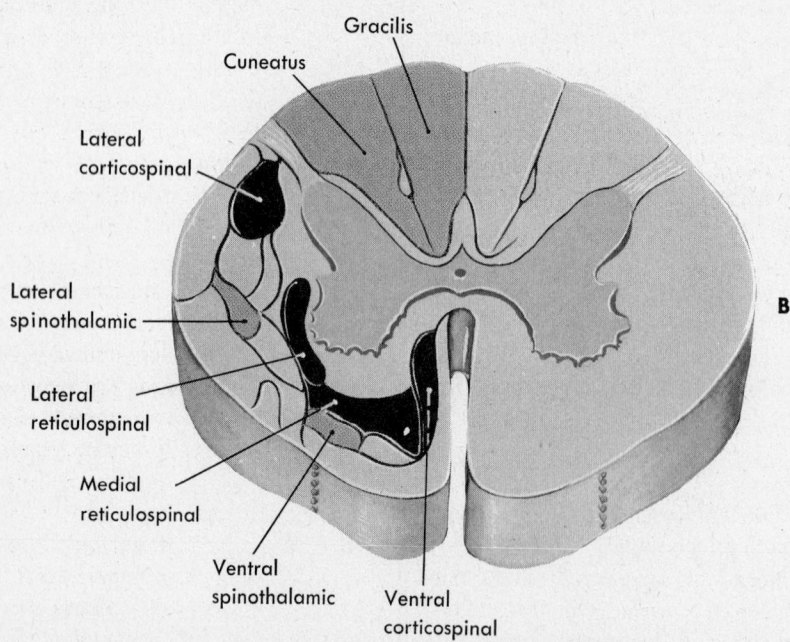

Fig. 8. A, Distribution of gray matter (horns) and white matter (columns) in a section of the spinal cord at the thoracic level. **B,** Location in the spinal cord of some major projection tracts. Black areas are descending motor tracts. Shaded areas are ascending sensory tracts. (From Anthony, C.P., and Kolthoff, N.J.: Textbook of anatomy and physiology, ed. 9, St. Louis, 1975, The C.V. Mosby Co.)

(b) Conducts impulses between the cord and various parts of the brain and contains reflex centers for cranial nerves V, VI, VII, and VIII (trigeminal, abducent, facial, and acoustic)

b. Cerebellum—dorsal appendage of the hindbrain
   (1) Structure—second largest part of the human brain; surface marked with sulci (grooves) and very slightly raised, slender convolutions; internal white matter forms pattern suggestive of veins of a leaf
   (2) Functions
       (a) Cerebellum exerts synergic control over the skeletal muscles; this means that impulses conducted by cerebellar neurons regulate and modulate output of the somatomotor region of the neocortex, which results in coordination of skeletal muscle contractions to produce smooth, steady, and precise movements
       (b) Because it coordinates skeletal muscle contractions, the cerebellum plays an essential part in producing normal postures and maintaining equilibrium

c. Midbrain—part of the brain located between the pons, which lies below it, and the diencephalon and cerebrum, which lie above it; consists mainly of white matter (cerebral peduncles) with scattered bits of gray matter
   (1) Superior and inferior colliculi (corpora quadrigemina)—integrate and analyze sensory input from the ears, eyes, and various regions of the cerebral cortex; put out motor information to lower motor system
   (2) Reflex centers for cranial nerves III (oculomotor) and IV (trochlear)—pupillary reflexes and eye movements
   (3) Pineal body—precise function unknown; may be part of endocrine system, helping to regulate secretion of gonadotropins from the hypophysis cerebri

d. Forebrain
   (1) Optic vesicles—develop into the retinas connected to base of the forebrain by their stalks, the optic nerves
   (2) Diencephalon—unpaired division of the forebrain; cerebral hemispheres diverge from this structure

(a) Thalamus—mass of gray matter in each cerebral hemisphere
    [1] Processes incoming sensory information prior to distribution to the somatosensory cortex; crudely translates sensory impulses into sensations but does not localize them on a body region
    [2] Ventral nucleus of the thalamus processes motor information from the cerebral cortex and cerebellum and projects its analysis back to the motor cortex
    [3] Contributes to the concentrating ability by filtering out distracting sensory input
    [4] Contributes to emotional component of sensations (pleasant or unpleasant)

(b) Hypothalamus—gray matter that forms floor of third ventricle and lower part of its lateral walls
    [1] Contains many higher autonomic reflex centers; these centers integrate autonomic functions by sending impulses to each other and to the lower autonomic centers; they form a crucial part of the neural path by which emotions and other cerebral functions can alter vital, automatic functions such as the heartbeat, blood pressure, peristalsis, and secretion by glands and thereby produce psychosomatic diseases; neural path for psychosomatic disease—impulses from the cerebral cortex to autonomic centers in the hypothalamus, to lower autonomic centers in the brainstem and cord, to visceral effectors (e.g., heart, smooth muscle, glands)
    [2] Helps control the anterior pituitary gland; certain neurons in the hypothalamus secrete neuropeptides into the pituitary portal veins, which transport them to the anterior pituitary gland where they influence secretion of various important hormones; e.g., TRH and LH-RH regulate

the pituitary secretions of TSH and gonadotropic hormones respectively

[3] Neurons in the supraoptic nucleus of the hypothalamus synthesize ADH and oxytocin; from the cell bodies of these neurons, ADH and oxytocin are transmitted down their axons into the posterior pituitary gland, from which they are released into the blood; in short, hypothalamic neurons make ADH and oxytocin, but the posterior pituitary gland secretes them

[4] Certain hypothalamic neurons serve as an appetite center and others function as a satiety center; together these centers regulate appetite and food intake

[5] Certain hypothalamic neurons serve as heat-regulating centers by relaying impulses to lower autonomic centers for vasoconstriction, vasodilation, and sweating, and to somatic centers for shivering

[6] Maintains waking state; constitutes part of the arousal or alerting neural pathway

(c) Corpus callosum—mass of white matter (nerve tracts) that interconnects the two cerebral hemispheres

(d) Optic chiasm—the point of crossing over (decussation [X, Latin *decem*]) of optic nerve fibers from the nasal half of each retina to the opposite side where they join optic nerve fibers from the lateral half of the other eye's retina to form the optic tracts

(3) Paired cerebral hemispheres (telencephalon)—longitudinal fissure divides the cerebrum into 2 hemispheres connected only by the corpus callosum; each cerebral hemisphere divided by fissures into 4 major lobes: frontal, parietal, temporal, occipital; also contains deeper regions of gray matter and fiber tracts

(a) Cerebral cortex is outer layer of gray matter forming folds (convolutions) composed of hills (gyri) and valleys (sulci)

(b) Frontal lobes
antenor + posterior

[1] Abstract thinking, sense of humor, and uniqueness of personality

[2] Contraction of skeletal muscles and synchronization of muscular movements

[3] Exert control over hypothalamus; influence basic biorhythms

[4] Control muscular movements necessary for speech; found only in 1 cerebral hemisphere

(c) Parietal lobes
[1] Translate nerve impulses into sensations (e.g., touch, temperature)
[2] Interpret sensations; provide appreciation of size, shape, texture, and weight
[3] Sense of taste

(d) Temporal lobes
[1] Translate nerve impulses into sensations of sound and interpret sounds
[2] Sense of smell
[3] Control behavior patterns

(e) Occipital area
[1] Translates nerve impulse into sights and interprets sights
[2] Provides appreciation of size, shape, and color

(f) Angular gyrus—analysis and integration of sights, sounds, and somatic sensations

(g) Amygdala—controls patterns of emotional behavior

(h) Corpus striatum—helps regulate muscle contraction and emotional reactions

(i) Cerebral tracts—bundles of axons compose the white matter in the interior of the cerebrum; ascending projection tracts transmit impulses toward the cerebral cortex; descending projection tracts transmit impulses from cerebral cortex; commissural tracts transmit from 1 hemisphere to the other; association tracts transmit from 1 convolution to another in the same hemisphere

4. Brain and spinal cord coverings
   a. Bony—vertebrae around the cord; cranial bones around the brain

b. Membranous—called meninges; consist of 3 layers
  (1) Dura mater—white fibrous tissue, outer layer
  (2) Arachnoid membrane—cobwebby middle layer
  (3) Pia mater—innermost layer; adheres to outer surface of the cord and brain; contains blood vessels
5. Cord and brain fluid spaces
  a. Subarachnoid space around the cord and extending beyond the cord into the fourth and fifth lumbar vertebrae
  b. Subarachnoid space around the brain
  c. Central canal inside the cord
  d. Ventricles and cerebral aqueduct inside the brain; 4 cavities
    (1) First and second (lateral) ventricles—large cavities, one in each cerebral hemisphere
    (2) Third ventricle—vertical slit in the cerebrum beneath the corpus callosum and longitudinal fissure
    (3) Fourth ventricle—diamond-shaped space between the cerebellum and medulla and pons; expansion of the central canal of the cord
6. Formation and circulation of the cerebrospinal fluid (CSF)
  a. Formed by plasma filtering from the network of capillaries (choroid plexus) in each ventricle; active transport of plasma also involved
  b. Circulates from the lateral ventricles to the third ventricle, cerebral aqueduct, fourth ventricle, central canal of the cord, and the subarachnoid space of the cord and brain; returns to blood via venous sinuses of the brain

Cranial Nerves—12 Pairs
See Table 2-11

Table 2-11. Distribution and function of cranial nerve pairs

Name and number	Distribution	Function
Olfactory (I)	Nasal mucosa, high up along the septum especially	Sense of smell (sensory only)
Optic (II)	Retina of eyeball	Vision (sensory only)
Oculomotor (III)	Extrinsic muscles of eyeball, except superior oblique and external rectus; also intrinsic eye muscles (iris and ciliary)	Eye movements; constriction of pupil and bulging of lens, which together produce accommodation for near vision
Trochlear (IV), smallest cranial nerve	Superior oblique muscle of eye	Eye movements
Trigeminal (V) (or trifacial), largest cranial nerve	Sensory fibers to skin and mucosa of head and to teeth; muscles of mastication (sensory and motor fibers)	Sensation in head and face; chewing movements
Abducent (VI)	External rectus muscle of eye	Abduction of eye
Facial (VII)	Muscles of facial expression; taste buds of anterior two thirds of tongue; motor fibers to submaxillary and sublingual salivary glands	Facial expressions; taste; secretion of saliva
Acoustic (VIII) (vestibulocochlear)	Inner ear	Hearing and equilibrium (sensory only)
Glossopharyngeal (IX)	Posterior third of tongue; mucosa and muscles of pharynx; parotid gland; carotid sinus and body	Taste and other sensations of tongue; secretion of saliva; swallowing movements; function in reflex arcs for control of blood pressure and respiration
Vagus (X) (or pneumogastric)	Mucosa and muscles of pharynx, larynx, trachea, bronchi, esophagus; thoracic and abdominal viscera	Sensations and movements of organs supplied; for example, slows heart, increases peristalsis and gastric and pancreatic secretion; voice production
Spinal accessory (XI)	Certain neck and shoulder muscles (muscles of larynx, sternocleidomastoid, trapezius)	Shoulder movements; turns head; voice production; muscle sense
Hypoglossal (XII)	Tongue muscles	Tongue movements, as in talking; muscle sense

Note: The first letters of the words in the following sentence are the first letters of the names of the cranial nerves, and many generations of anatomy students have used it as an aid to memorizing the names: "On Old Olympus' Towering Tops, A Finn And German Viewed Some Hops." (There are several slightly different versions of this mnemonic.)

Spinal Nerves—31 Pairs

A. Each nerve attaches to the cord by 2 short roots, anterior and posterior; the posterior roots are marked by a swelling, the spinal ganglion

B. Branches of the spinal nerves form plexuses or intricate networks of fibers (e.g., brachial plexus), from which nerves emerge to supply various parts of the skin, mucosa, and skeletal muscles

C. All spinal nerves are mixed nerves composed of both sensory dendrites and motor axons; they function in both sensations and movements

D. Nerve consists of bundles of nerve fibers (axons and dendrites) supported by connective tissue

Sensorineural Pathways—Conduction

A. Sensory pathways to the cerebral cortex from the periphery consist of relays of at least 3 neurons, which are identified by Roman numerals
  1. Sensory neuron I—conducts from the periphery to the cord or to the brainstem
  2. Sensory neuron II—conducts from the cord or brainstem to the thalamus
  3. Sensory neuron III—conducts from the thalamus to the somatosensory area of the cerebral cortex

B. Crude awareness of sensations occurs when impulses reach the thalamus

C. Full consciousness of sensations with accurate localization and discrimination of fine details occurs when impulses reach the cerebral cortex

D. Most sensory neuron II axons decussate; so one side of the brain registers most of the sensations for the opposite side of the body

E. Principle of divergence applies to the sensorineural pathways; each sensory neuron synapses with many neurons, and therefore impulses may diverge from any sensory neuron and be conducted to many brain regions, including the cerebellum, reticular formation, and also more directly the motor neurons

F. Impulses that produce pain and an awareness of temperature are conducted up the cord to the thalamus by the lateral spinothalamic tracts

G. Impulses that produce touch and pressure sensations are conducted up the cord to the thalamus by the following 2 pathways:
  1. Impulses that result in discriminating touch and pressure sensations (e.g., stereognosis, precise localization, vibratory sense) are conducted by the tracts of the posterior white columns of the cord to the medulla and from there are transferred to the thalamus
  2. Impulses that result in crude touch and pressure sensations are conducted up the cord to the thalamus by fibers of the ventral spinothalamic tracts

H. Sensory impulses that result in conscious proprioception or kinesthesia (sense of position or movement of body parts) are conducted over the same pathway as are impulses that result in discriminating touch and pressure sensations

I. Sensory impulses, in addition, are also conducted to the cerebral cortex via complex multineuron pathways known as the reticular activating system; spinoreticular tracts relay sensory impulses up the cord to the brainstem reticular gray matter, and from there other neurons relay them to the hypothalamus, thalamus, and probably other parts of the brain, then finally to the cerebral cortex; conduction by the reticular activating system is essential for producing and maintaining consciousness; presumably, general anesthetics produce unconsciousness by inhibiting conduction by the reticular activating system; conversely, amphetamines and norepinephrine are thought to produce wakefulness by stimulating the reticular activating system

Motoneural Pathways to Skeletal Muscles

A. Principle of the final common path—the final common path for impulse conduction to skeletal muscles consists of anterior horn neurons (i.e., motoneurons whose dendrites and cell bodies lie in the anterior gray columns of the cord and whose axons extend out through the anterior roots of spinal nerves and their branches to terminate in skeletal muscles); besides being referred to as the final common path and as anterior horn cells, these neurons are also called lower motoneurons, somatic motoneurons, and lower motor system

B. Principle of convergence—axons of many neurons converge on (i.e., synapse with) each anterior horn motoneuron

C. Motor pathways from the cerebral cortex to anterior horn cells are classified according to the route by which the fibers enter the cord
  1. Pyramidal tracts (corticospinal tracts)—axons of neurons whose dendrites and cell bodies lie in the cerebral cortex; axons descend from cortex through internal capsule, pyramids of medulla, and spinal cord; a few of these axons synapse with anterior horn cells, but most of them synapse with internuncial neurons that synapse with anterior horn cells; conduction by pyramidal tracts is necessary for willed movements to occur; hence 1 cause of paralysis is interruption of pyramidal tract conduction
  2. Extrapyramidal tracts—all tracts that conduct between the motor cortex and the anterior horn cells, except the pyramidal tracts; upper extrapyramidal tracts relay impulses between the cor-

tex, basal ganglia, thalamus, and brainstem; reticulospinal tracts (the main lower extrapyramidal tracts) relay impulses from the brainstem to the anterior horn cells in the cord; impulse conduction via extrapyramidal tracts is essential for producing large, automatic movements (e.g., walking, swimming) and for producing facial expressions and movements that characterize many emotions

D. Motor conduction pathway from the primary motor area of the cerebral cortex to skeletal muscles via pyramidal tracts consists of a 2-neuron relay; an upper motoneuron conducts impulses from cerebrum to cord and a lower motoneuron (anterior horn cell) conducts from cord to skeletal muscle (Fig. 9)

E. Motor conduction pathway from the cerebral cortex via the extrapyramidal tracts consists of complex multineuron relays; several upper motoneurons re-

Fig. 9. Crossed pyramidal (lateral corticospinal) tracts, the main motor tracts of the body. Axons that compose the pyramidal tracts come from neuron cell bodies in the cerebral cortex. After they descend through the internal capsule of the cerebrum and the white matter of the brainstem, about three fourths of the fibers decussate—cross over from one side to the other—in the medulla, as shown here. Then they continue downward in the lateral corticospinal tract on the opposite side of the cord. Each lateral corticospinal tract, therefore, conducts motor impulses from one side of the brain to skeletal muscles on the opposite side of the body. (From Anthony, C.P., and Thibodeau, G.A.: Textbook of anatomy and physiology, ed. 11, St. Louis, 1983, The C.V. Mosby Co.)

lay impulses through the basal ganglia, thalamus, and brain stem down the cord to the lower moto-neuron

F. Motor pathways from the cerebral cortex to anterior horn cells classified according to their influence on anterior horn cells as follows:
   1. Facilitatory tracts—conduct impulses that have a facilitating or stimulating effect on anterior horn cells; main facilitatory tracts are the pyramidal tracts and the facilitatory reticulospinal tracts
   2. Inhibitory tracts—conduct impulses that have an inhibiting effect on anterior horn cells; main inhibitory tracts are the inhibitory reticulospinal tracts; interruption of inhibitory reticulospinal tracts results in spasticity and rigidity

G. Ratio of facilitatory and inhibitory impulses impinging on anterior horn cells determines their activity (whether they are facilitated, stimulated, or inhibited)

Autonomic Nervous System

A. Definition—Division of the nervous system that conducts impulses from the brainstem or cord out to visceral effectors: cardiac muscle, smooth muscle, and glandular tissue

B. Divisions—consists of 2 divisions: the sympathetic (thoracolumbar) system and the parasympathetic (craniosacral) system
   1. Sympathetic system
      a. Sympathetic ganglia—2 chains of 21 or 22 ganglia located immediately in front of the spinal column, 1 chain to the right, 1 to the left
      b. Collateral ganglia—located a short distance from the cord (e.g., celiac ganglia [solar plexus], superior and inferior mesenteric ganglia)
      c. Sympathetic nerves—(e.g., splanchnic nerves, cardiac nerves)
   2. Parasympathetic system
      a. Parasympathetic ganglia—located some distance from the spinal column, in or near the visceral effectors (e.g., ciliary ganglion in posterior part of the orbit, near the iris and ciliary muscle)
      b. Parasympathetic nerves—(e.g., vagus nerve, called the great parasympathetic nerve of the body)

C. Neurons
   1. Preganglionic sympathetic neurons—dendrites and cell bodies lie in the lateral gray columns of thoracic and lumbar segments of the cord; their axons conduct from the cord to the sympathetic ganglia or the collateral ganglia; see D,3 below
   2. Postganglionic sympathetic neurons—dendrites and cell bodies lie in the sympathetic ganglia or the collateral ganglia; their axons conduct to visceral effectors
   3. Preganglionic parasympathetic neurons—dendrites and cell bodies of some of these neurons lie in gray matter of the brain stem; others exit at sacral segments of the cord; conduct impulses from the brain stem or cord to the parasympathetic ganglia; see D,3 below
   4. Postganglionic parasympathetic neurons—dendrites and cell bodies lie in the parasympathetic ganglia; their axons conduct to visceral effectors; see D,3 below

D. Some principles about the autonomic nervous system
   1. Dual autonomic innervation—both sympathetic and parasympathetic fibers supply most visceral effectors
   2. Single autonomic innervation—only sympathetic fibers supply sweat glands and probably the smooth muscles of hairs and of most blood vessels; preganglionic sympathetic fibers terminate in adrenal medulla (not postganglionic fibers as in other glands)
   3. Autonomic chemical transmitters—all preganglionic axons are cholinergic fibers, as are most (or perhaps all) parasympathetic postganglionic axons and a few sympathetic postganglionic axons (to sweat glands, external genitalia, and smooth muscle in walls of blood vessels located in skeletal muscles); sympathetic postganglionic axons are the only adrenergic (i.e., norepinephrine-releasing) fibers; but, as just mentioned, a few of them are cholinergic
   4. Autonomic antagonism and summation—sympathetic and parasympathetic impulses tend to produce opposite effects; the algebraic sum of 2 opposing tendencies determines the response made by dually innervated visceral effectors (Table 2-12)
   5. Principle of parasympathetic dominance of the digestive tract—normally, parasympathetic impulses to digestive tract glands and smooth muscle dominate over sympathetic impulses to these effectors; the dominance of parasympathetic impulses promotes digestive gland secretion, peristalsis, and defecation
   6. Principle of sympathetic dominance in stress situations—under conditions of stress, sympathetic impulses to the visceral effectors usually increase greatly and dominate over parasympathetic impulses; however, in some individuals

Table 2-12. Autonomic functions

Visceral effector	Effect of sympathetic stimulation (neurotransmitter, norepinephrine unless otherwise stated)	Effect of parasympathetic stimulation (neurotransmitter, acetylcholine)
Heart	Increased rate and strength of heartbeat (beta receptors)	Decreased rate and strength of heartbeat
Smooth muscle of blood vessels		
Skin blood vessels	Constriction (alpha receptors)	No parasympathetic fibers
Skeletal muscel blood vessels	Dilation (beta receptors)	No parasympathetic fibers
Coronary blood vessels	Dilation (beta receptors)	No parasympathetic fibers
Abdominal blood vessels	Constriction (alpha receptors)	No parasympathetic fibers
Blood vessels of external genitals	Ejaculation (contraction of smooth muscle in male ducts, e.g., epididymis and vas deferens)	Dilation of blood vessels causing erection in male
Smooth muscle of hollow organs and sphincters		
Bronchi	Dilation (beta receptors)	Constriction
Digestive tract, except sphincters	Decreased peristalsis (beta receptors)	Increased peristalsis
Sphincters of digestive tract	Contraction (alpha receptors)	Relaxation
Urinary bladder	Relaxation (beta receptors)	Contraction
Urinary sphincters	Contraction (alpha receptors)	Relaxation
Eye		
Iris	Contraction of radial muscle; dilated pupil	Contraction of circular muscle; constricted pupil
Ciliary	Relaxation; accommodates for far vision	Contraction; accommodates for near vision
Hairs (pilomotor muscles)	Contraction produces goose pimples, or piloerection (alpha receptors)	No parasympathetic fibers
Glands		
Sweat	Increased sweat (neurotransmitter, acetylcholine)	No parasympathetic fibers
Digestive (salivary, gastric, etc.)	Decreased secretion of saliva; not known for others	Increased secretion of saliva
Pancreas, including islets	Decreased secretion	Increased secretion of pancreatic juice and insulin
Liver	Increased glycogenolysis (beta receptors); increases blood sugar level	No parasympathetic fibers
Adrenal medulla*	Increased epinephrine secretion	No parasympathetic fibers

From Anthony, C.P., and Thibodeau, G.A.: Textbook of anatomy and physiology, ed. 11, St. Louis, 1983, The C.V. Mosby Co.
*Sympathetic preganglionic axons terminate in contact with secreting cells of the adrenal medulla. Thus the adrenal medulla functions (to quote a descriptive phrase) as a "giant sympathetic postganglionic neuron."

under stress, parasympathetic impulses via the vagus nerve to glands and smooth muscle of the stomach greatly increase, causing increased hydrochloric acid secretion and increased gastric motility; this can eventually cause peptic ulcer, a condition that may aptly be called the great parasympathetic stress disease

7. In general, when the sympathetic system dominates control of visceral effectors, it causes them to function in ways that enable the body to expend maximum energy as is necessary in strenuous exercise and other types of stress; see Table 2-12 for sympathetic effects on specific effectors

8. Principle of nonautonomy—the autonomic nervous system is neither anatomically nor physiologically independent of rest of the nervous system; all parts of nervous system work together as a single functional unit; i.e., dendrites and cells of all preganglionic neurons in gray matter of the brainstem or cord (lower autonomic centers) are influenced by impulses conducted to them from higher autonomic centers, notably the hypothalamus

9. Importance of autonomic nervous system—plays a major role in maintaining physiologic balance; under usual conditions, autonomic impulses regulate activities of the visceral effectors so they maintain or quickly restore this balance; under highly stressful conditions, problems may occur

Sense Organs

Millions of receptors distributed widely throughout the skin and mucosa; muscles, tendons, joints, and viscera are sense organs of body (Table 2-13)

A. General considerations
 1. Receptors monitor internal and external environment
 2. Stimuli are interpreted and converted to nerve impulses, which are conducted through sensory neurons to the brain
 3. Receptors' degrees of depolarization depend on the strength of the stimulus; the variable degree of depolarization is called the generator potential
 4. Generator potential determines the frequency of nerve impulses sent to the CNS by afferent nerve fibers attached to receptors
 5. Most receptors display sensory adaptation—steady and prolonged stimulus results in a steady decrease in strength of generator potential

B. Types of receptors
 1. Exteroceptors of skin and mucosa—consist of receptors for spinal or cranial nerve branches; different types of receptors for different sensations such as heat, cold, pain, touch, and pressure
 2. Proprioceptors of muscles, tendons, and joints—stretching of muscles or tendons during movements initiates stretch reflexes
 3. Visceroceptors—pressoreceptors (baroreceptors) respond to stretch in walls of the aorta and carotid arteries, providing the brain with information on blood pressure; oxygen chemoreceptors in the aortic and carotid bodies monitor O_2 levels; carbon dioxide chemoreceptors in the respiratory center (in medulla) help control the rate and depth of respirations
 4. Taste
  a. Taste buds consist of groups of receptor cells bundled together with sensory hairs protruding from a pore in the taste bud and connected to the facial and glossopharyngeal nerves (VII and IX)
  b. Respond to chemicals—sweet at tongue tip; sour and salt at tip and sides; bitter at back; receptors for bitter most sensitive
  c. Olfaction intimately involved in the sense of taste

5. Olfaction
 a. Receptors in epithelium of the nasal mucosa
 b. Odors sensed as chemicals interact with receptor sites on sensory hairs of olfactory cells
 c. Olfactory neural pathways utilize cranial nerve I

6. Sight
 a. Coats of the eyeball
  (1) Outer—sclera proper and cornea
  (2) Middle—choroid proper, ciliary body, suspensory ligament holding lens, and iris
  (3) Inner—retina
 b. Cavities and humors of the eyeball
  (1) Anterior cavity with an anterior and posterior chamber; both contain aqueous humor
  (2) Posterior cavity has no divisions; contains vitreous humor
 c. Muscles of the eye (Table 2-14)
 d. Refractory media of the eye
  (1) Cornea
  (2) Aqueous humor
  (3) Crystalline lens (has greatest refractive power)
  (4) Vitreous humor
 e. Accessory structures of the eye
  (1) Eyebrows and lashes
  (2) Eyelids or palpebrae—lined with mucous membrane (conjunctiva) that continues over surface of eyeball; corners of eyes, where upper and lower lids join, called inner and outer canthi
  (3) Lacrimal apparatus—lacrimal glands, ducts, sacs, and nasolacrimal ducts
 f. Physiology of vision
  (1) Formation of an image on the retina, accomplished by
   (a) Refraction—bending of light rays as they pass through the eye
   (b) Accommodation—bulging of the lens for viewing near objects
   (c) Constriction of pupils—occurs simultaneously with accommodation and in bright light
   (d) Convergence of the eyes for near objects so light rays from the object may fall on corresponding points of 2 retinas; necessary for single binocular vision

Table 2-13. Receptors

Kinds	Locations	Stimulated by	Functions
Exteroceptors	Skin, mucosa, ear, eye	Changes in external environment (e.g., pressure, heat, cold, light waves, sound waves)	Initiate reflexes Initiate sensations of many kinds (e.g., pressure, heat, cold, pain, vision, hearing)
Visceroceptors (interoceptors)	Viscera	Changes in internal environment (e.g., pressure, chemical)	Initiate reflexes Initiate sensations of many kinds (e.g., hunger, sex, nausea, pressure)
Proprioceptors	Muscles, tendons, joints, semicircular canals of inner ear	Pressure changes	Initiate reflexes Initiate muscle sense, or sense of position and movement of parts; also called kinesthesia

Table 2-14. Eye muscles

Location	Kind of muscle	Names	Functions
Extrinsic—attached to outside of eyeball and to bones of orbit	Skeletal (voluntary, striated)	Superior rectus Inferior rectus Lateral rectus Medial rectus Superior oblique Inferior oblique	Move eyeball in various directions
Intrinsic—within eyeball	Visceral (involuntary, smooth)	Iris Ciliary muscle	Regulate size of pupil Control shape of lens, making possible accommodation for near and far objects

(2) Stimulation of the retina—dim light causes breakdown of the chemical rhodopsin present in rods, thereby initiating impulse conduction by the rods; bright light causes breakdown of chemicals in the cones; rods considered receptors for night vision, cones receptors for daylight and color vision

(3) Most cones concentrated in small region of the retina called fovea centralis; provides sharpest color vision

(4) Conduction to visual area in occipital lobe of cerebral cortex by fibers of optic nerves and optic tracts

7. Hearing
    a. External ear—consists of the auricle (or pinna), external acoustic meatus (ear opening), and external auditory canal
    b. Middle ear—separated from the external ear by the tympanic membrane; middle ear contains auditory ossicles (malleus, incus, stapes) and openings from the auditory (eustachian) tubes, mastoid cells, external ear, and internal ear; auditory tube is collapsible and lined with mucosa and extends from the nasopharynx to the middle ear; equalizes pressure on both sides of eardrum, as when tubes open during yawning, swallowing, or sucking
    c. Inner ear (or labyrinth)—composed of a bony labyrinth that has a membranous labyrinth inside it; parts of the inner ear
    (1) Bony vestibule—contains the membranous utricle and saccule, each of which, in turn, contains a sense organ called the macula; vestibular nerve (branch of eighth cranial [acoustic or vestibulocochlear] nerve) supplies the maculae acusticae; these sense organs give information about equilibrium, position of the head, and acceleration and deceleration
    (2) Bony semicircular canals—contain the membranous semicircular canals in which are located the crista ampullaris, the sense organ for sensations of equilibrium and head movements; vestibular nerve supplies the crista as well as the macula
    (3) Bony cochlea—contains the membranous cochlear duct in which is located

the organ of Corti, the hearing sense organ; cochlear nerve (branch of eighth cranial nerve) supplies the organ of Corti
  d. Physiology of hearing
    (1) Sound waves moving through the air enter the ear canal and move down it to strike against the tympanic membrane, causing it to vibrate
    (2) Vibrations of the tympanic membrane move the malleus, whose handle is attached to the membrane
    (3) Movement of the malleus moves the incus, to which the head of the malleus attaches
    (4) Incus attaches to the stapes; so, as the incus moves, it moves the stapes against the oval window, into which it fits; as the stapes presses inwardly on the perilymph around the cochlear duct, it starts a ripple in the perilymph
    (5) Movement of the perilymph is transmitted to the endolymph inside the cochlear duct and stimulates the organ of Corti, which projects into the endolymph
    (6) Cochlear nerve conducts impulses from the organ of Corti to the brain; hearing occurs when impulses reach the auditory area in the temporal lobe of the cerebral cortex

Muscular System

A. Functions
  1. Movement
  2. Posture
  3. Heat production—metabolism in muscle cells produces relatively large share of body heat
B. Types of muscles and neural control
  1. Striated—controlled by voluntary nervous system via somatic motoneurons in spinal and some cranial nerves
  2. Smooth—controlled by autonomic nervous system via autonomic motoneurons in autonomic, spinal, and some cranial nerves; not under voluntary control (with rare exceptions)
  3. Cardiac—control is identical to that of smooth muscle
C. Anatomy of skeletal muscle as a whole
  1. Typically spindle shaped; composed of long muscle cells referred to as muscle fibers; invested by coating of fibrous connective tissue (fascia), which binds muscle to surrounding tissues

  2. Arranged in bundles or fasciculi; each muscle contains several fasciculi
  3. Contains rich blood supply; numerous capillary beds provide nutrients to and remove wastes from muscle
  4. Characteristics of individual skeletal muscle fibers
    a. Generally long and spindle shaped
    b. Multinucleate; called a syncytium
    c. Cell membrane called sarcolemma; endoplasmic reticulum called sarcoplasmic reticulum; mitochondria may be referred to as sarcosomes
    d. Contain myofibrils specialized for contraction; composed of two types of protein myofilaments, actin and myosin
D. Neuromuscular junction
  1. Axon terminal forms junction with the sarcolemma of muscle fiber; tiny synaptic cleft separates the presynaptic membrane (axon) from postsynaptic membrane (sarcolemma)
  2. Axon terminals contain tiny sacs, synaptic vesicles; these contain the neurotransmitter acetylcholine
  3. When a nerve impulse reaches the axon terminal, acetylcholine is released from synaptic vesicles into synaptic cleft; acetylcholine diffuses across synaptic cleft and attaches to receptor sites on sarcolemma; receptor sites are attached to channels in the membrane; when acetylcholine binds to the receptor site, a channel opens and sodium and potassium ions flow down their concentration gradients; the sarcolemma is depolarized, and electrical energy flows into the muscle fiber
  4. The enzyme cholinesterase, found in the synaptic cleft, inactivates acetylcholine; additional stimulation of muscle requires release of more acetylcholine
E. Muscle fiber contraction
  1. Electrical energy flows deep into muscle fiber along transverse intracellular tubules associated with sarcoplasmic reticulum
  2. Calcium ions released by flow of electrical energy inactivate troponin, which normally blocks the interaction between actin and myosin
  3. Myosin releases and uses energy from ATP to cause action to slide along myosin filaments (contraction); cessation of impulses leaves actin and myosin in a relaxed unassociated phase
  4. Energy for contraction—immediate energy is ATP; creatine phosphate, a high-energy mole-

cule stored in abundance in muscle, replenishes supply of ATP as needed; the ultimate source of energy is glucose and fatty acids oxidized aerobically to carbon dioxide and water, with the release of energy

5. Anaerobic breakdown of glucose during prolonged and vigorous muscle contraction results in lactic acid buildup associated with fatigue and an aching feeling; this oxygen debt is paid off during rest, when oxygen is plentiful

F. Basic principles of skeletal muscle action

1. Skeletal muscles contract only if stimulated; a skeletal muscle and its motor nerve function as a physiologic (motor unit) unit; either is useless without the other's functioning; for this reason anything that prevents impulse conduction to a skeletal muscle paralyzes the muscle

2. Most skeletal muscles attach to at least 2 bones; as a muscle contracts and pulls on its bones, it mobilizes the bone that moves most easily; the bone that moves is called the muscle's insertion bone, and that which remains stationary is its origin bone

3. Bones serve as levers, and joints as fulcrums of these levers; a muscle's contraction exerts a pulling force on its insertion bone at the point where it inserts, pulling that point nearer the muscle's origin bone

4. Skeletal muscles almost always act in groups rather than singly; members of groups are classified as follows:

   a. Prime movers—muscle or muscles whose contraction actually produces the movement
   b. Synergists—muscles that contract at the same time as the prime mover, helping it produce the movement or stabilizing the part (i.e., holding it steady) so the prime mover can produce a more effective movement
   c. Antagonists—muscles that relax while the prime mover is contracting (exception: antagonist contracts at the same time as the prime mover when a part needs to be held rigid, as the knee joint does in standing); antagonists are usually located directly opposite the bones they move; e.g., muscle that flexes the lower arm lies on anterior surface of the upper arm bone, whereas that which extends the lower arm lies on posterior surface of the upper arm

5. Body of a muscle usually does not lie over the part moved by the muscle; instead it lies above or below, or anterior or posterior to, the part;

thus the body of a muscle that moves the lower arm will not be located in the lower arm but in the upper arm; e.g., biceps and triceps brachii muscles

6. Contraction of a skeletal muscle either shortens the muscle, producing movement, or increases the tension (tone) in the muscle; contractions are classified according to whether they produce movement or increase muscle tone as follows:

   a. Tonic contractions—produce muscle tone; do not shorten the muscle so do not produce movements; only a few fibers contract at one time, and this produces a moderate degree of muscle tone; in the healthy, awake body all muscles exhibit tone
   b. Isometric contractions—increase the degree of muscle tone; do not shorten the muscle so do not produce movements; daily repetition of isometric contractions gradually increases muscle strength
   c. Isotonic contractions—the muscle shortens, thereby producing movement; all movements are the result of isotonic contractions

G. Origins, insertions, and functions of main skeletal muscles grouped according to functions (Table 2-15)

H. Weak places in abdominal wall where hernias may occur

1. Inguinal rings—right and left internal, right and left external
2. Femoral rings—right and left
3. Umbilicus

I. Metabolism of skeletal muscle

1. Hypertrophy is physical enlargement of the muscle due to the addition of more myofibrils to muscle fibers, making them swell; muscle fibers do not divide to produce new fibers

2. Atrophy is reduction in size of muscle due to decrease in number of myofibrils in muscle fiber

3. Treppe (staircase phenomenon)—when a muscle has contracted a few times, subsequent contractions are more powerful; may be related to the release of increased quantities of calcium ions from sarcoplasmic reticulum after the first few contractions

4. Shivering—rapid, repeating, involuntary skeletal muscle contractions; caused by hypothalamic temperature regulating center; makes use of inefficiency of muscle contraction (i.e., most of the energy of ATP is converted to heat; a smaller part goes into the mechanical motion of contraction)

Table 2-15. Origins, insertions, and functions of main skeletal muscles

Part of body moved	Movement	Muscle	Origin	Insertion
Upper arm	Flexion	Pectoralis major	Clavicle (medial half) Sternum Costal cartilages of true ribs	Humerus (greater tubercle)
	Extension	Latissimus dorsi	Vertebrae (lower thoracic, lumbar, and sacral) Ilium (crest) Lumbodorsal fascia	Humerus (intertubercular groove)
	Abduction	Deltoid	Clavicle Scapula (spine and acromion)	Humerus (lateral side on deltoid tubercle)
	Adduction	Latissimus dorsi contracting with pectoralis major	See above (Latissimus dorsi) See above (Pectoralis major)	Humerus (greater tubercle) Humerus (intertubercular groove)
Shoulder	Shrugging, elevating	Trapezius	Occipital bone Vertebrae (cervical and thoracic)	Scapula (spine and acromion) Clavicle
	Lowering	Pectoralis minor Serratus anterior	Ribs (second to fifth) Ribs (upper 8 or 9)	Scapula (coracoid) Scapula (anterior surface)
Lower arm	Flexion			
	With forearm supinated	Biceps brachii	Scapula (supraglenoid tuberosity) Scapula (coracoid)	Radius (tubercle at proximal end)
	With forearm pronated	Brachialis	Humerus (distal half, anterior surface)	Ulna (front of cornoid process)
	With forearm semi-supinated or semi-pronated	Brachioradialis	Humerus (above lateral epicondyle)	Radius (styloid process)
	Extension	Triceps brachii	Scapula (infraglenoid tuberosity) Humerus (posterior surface—lateral head above radial groove; medial head, below)	Ulna (olecranon process)
Thigh	Flexion	Iliopsoas (iliacus and psoas major)	Ilium (iliac fossa) Vertebrae (bodies of twelfth thoracic to fifth lumbar)	Femur (small trochanter)
		Rectus femoris	Ilium and anterior inferior iliac spine	Tibia (by way of patellar tendon)
	Extension	Gluteus maximus	Ilium (crest and posterior surface) Sacrum and coccyx (posterior surface)	Femur (gluteal tuberosity) Iliotibial tract
		Hamstring group (see below)	Ischium (tuberosity) Femur (linea aspera)	Fibula (head of) Tibia (lateral condyle, medial condyle, and medial surface)
	Abduction	Gluteus medius and minimus	Ilium (lateral surface)	Femur (greater trochanter)
		Tensor fasciae latae	Ilium (anterior part of crest)	Iliotibial tract
	Adduction	Adductor group Brevis Longus Magnus	Pubic bone	Femur (linea aspera)
Lower leg	Flexion	Hamstring group Biceps femoris Semitendinosus Semimembranosus	Ischium (tuberosity) Femur (linea aspera)	Fibula (head of) Tibia (lateral condyle, medial condyle, and medial surface)
		Gastrocnemius	Femur (condyles)	Tarsal bone (calcaneus by way of tendo calcaneus)

Table 2-15. Origins, insertions, and functions of main skeletal muscles—cont'd

Part of body moved	Movement	Muscle	Origin	Insertion
Lower leg—cont'd	Extension	Quadriceps femoris group Rectus femoris Vastus lateralis Vastus medialis Vastus intermedius	Ilium (anterior inferior spine) Femur (linea aspera and anterior surface)	Tibia (by way of patellar tendon)
Foot	Flexion (dorsiflexion)	Tibialis anterior	Tibia (lateral condyle)	First cuneiform tarsal Base of first metatarsal
	Extension (plantar flexion)	Gastrocnemius	Femur (condyles)	Calcaneus (by way of tendo calcaneus)
		Soleus	Tibia	Same as gastrocnemius, but underneath
Head	Flexion	Sternocleidomastoid	Sternum Clavicle	Temporal bone (mastoid process)
	Extension	Trapezius	Vertebrae (cervical) Scapula (spine and acromion) Clavicle	Occiput
Abdominal wall	Compress abdominal cavity; therefore assists in straining, defecation, forced expiration, childbirth, posture, etc.	External oblique	Ribs (lower 8)	Innominate bone (iliac crest and pubis by way of inguinal ligament) Linea alba
		Internal oblique	Innominate bone (iliac crest, inguinal ligament) Lumbodorsal fascia	Ribs (lower 3) Pubic bone Linea alba
		Transversus	Ribs (lower 6) Innominate bone (iliac crest, inguinal ligament) Lumbodorsal fascia	Pubic bone Linea alba
		Rectus abdominis	Innominate bone (pubic bone and symphysis pubis)	Ribs (costal cartilage of fifth, sixth, seventh)
Chest wall	Elevate ribs, thereby enlarging anteroposterior and anterolateral dimensions of chest and causing inspiration	External intercostals	Ribs (lower border of all but twelfth)	Ribs (upper border of rib below origin)
	Depress ribs	Internal intercostals	Ribs (inner surface, upper border of all except first)	Ribs (lower border of rib above origin)
	Pull floor of thorax downward, thereby enlarging vertical dimension of chest and causing inspiration	Diaphragm	Lower circumference of rib cage	Central tendon of diaphragm
Trunk	Flexion	Iliopsoas	Femur (small trochanter)	Ilium Vertebrae (bodies of twelfth thoracic to fifth lumbar)
	Extension	Sacrospinalis Iliocostalis (lateral) Longissimus (medial)	Vertebrae (posterior surface of sacrum, spinous processes of lumbar, and last 2 thoracic) Ilium (posterior part of crest)	Ribs (lower 6) Vertebrae (transverse processes of thoracic) Ribs Vertebrae (spines of thoracic)
		Quadratus lumborum	Ilium (posterior part of crest) Vertebrae (lower 3 lumbar)	Ribs (twelfth) Vertebrae (transverse processes of first 4 lumbar)

5. Rigor mortis—ATP must combine with myosin to effect release of actin from myosin, which permits relaxation; after death, ATP is depleted from muscle fibers, and actin and myosin strongly associate, producing rigor mortis; subsequent bacterial decomposition of muscle proteins brings about relaxation; body enters rigor state about 24 hours after death and comes out of rigor about 24 hours later

J. Bursae
  1. Definition—small sacs lined with synovial membrane and containing synovial fluid
  2. Locations—wherever pressure is exerted over moving parts
     a. Between skin and bone
     b. Between tendons and bone
     c. Between muscles or ligaments and bone
  3. Names of bursae that frequently become inflamed (bursitis)
     a. Subacromial—between the acromion and the capsule of the shoulder joint
     b. Olecranon—between the olecranon process of the ulna and the skin; inflammation called student's elbow
     c. Prepatellar—between the patella and the skin; inflammation called housemaid's knee
  4. Function—act as cushions, relieving pressure between moving parts

K. Tendon sheaths
  1. Definition and location—tube-shaped structures that enclose certain tendons, notably those of wrist and ankle; made of connective tissue lined with synovial membrane
  2. Function—facilitate gliding movements of tendon

Skeletal System

A. Functions
  1. Furnishes supporting framework
  2. Affords protection for the viscera, brain, and hemopoietic system
  3. Provides levers for the muscles to pull on to produce movements
  4. Hemopoiesis by red bone marrow—formation of all kinds of blood cells; note that some lymphocytes and monocytes are formed in lymphatic tissue
  5. Mineral storage—calcium, phosphorus (in the form of phosphates), and sodium are stored in bone

B. Nature of bone substance
  1. Organic matter—makes up about 33% of bone by weight

  a. Cells
     (1) Osteoblasts—bone-producing cells
     (2) Osteoclasts—bone-dissolving cells
     (3) Osteocytes—former osteoblasts embedded in and maintaining bone substance
  b. Collagen—collagen fibers make up about 97% of organic matter of bone; give bone tough and somewhat flexible quality; responsible for high tensile strength of bone
  c. Polysaccharides—part of ground substance of bone consists of polysaccharides such as hyaluronic acid and sialic acid
  d. Protein—polysaccharide complexes such as chondroitin sulfate are part of ground substance of bone
  2. Inorganic matter—makes up about 67% of bone by weight
     a. Apatite salts—apatite, a complex ion composed of calcium and phosphates, forms hydroxyapatite, carbonate apatite, and fluoride apatite; makes bone hard and is responsible for the high compressional strength of bone
     b. Magnesium and sodium ions are part of bone matrix
     c. Certain radioactive isotopes accumulate in bone (e.g., strontium 90, calcium 45, phosphorus 32, plutonium 259); may increase likelihood of bone tumors and leukemia

C. Bone formation
  1. Intramembranous ossification—fibrous membranes composing certain parts of fetal skeleton, such as skull bones and lower jaw, are converted to bone
  2. Endochondral ossification—conversion of cartilage bone models into actual bone in fetus; most of fetal skeletal system ossifies by endochondral ossification
  3. Ossification—end result of either intramembranous or endochondral ossification is the same, cancellous (spongy) bone; the denser type of bone substance, compact bone, forms later in development through conversion of selected regions of cancellous bone into compact bone
     a. Distribution of cancellous and compact bone
        (1) Outer surface of all bones, except at joints, composed of compact bone
        (2) Interior of short, flat, and irregular bones (all bones except long bones) composed of cancellous bone; epiphyses of long bones composed of cancellous bone in their interior
        (3) Diaphyses of long bones hollow; walls of diaphysis composed of compact bone

b. Ossification process
   (1) Formation of bone matrix (the intercellular substance of bone), made up of collagen fibers and a cementlike ground substance composed of polysaccharides and protein-polysaccharide complexes; osteoblasts (bone-forming cells) synthesize collagen and cement substance from proteins provided by the diet; vitamin C promotes the formation of bone matrix; exercise and estrogens act to stimulate osteoblasts to form bone matrix
   (2) Calcification of bone matrix—calcium salts deposited in the bone matrix; vitamin D promotes calcification by stimulating calcium uptake in small intestine

c. Bone growth
   (1) In length—by continual thickening of epiphyseal cartilage followed by ossification; as long as bone growth continues, epiphyseal cartilage grows faster than it can be replaced by bone; therefore line of cartilage persists between diaphysis and epiphyses and can be seen on x-ray film; during adolescence cartilage is completely transformed into bone, at which time bone growth is complete
   (2) In diameter—osteoclasts destroy bone surrounding the medullary cavity, thereby enlarging the cavity; at the same time, osteoblasts add new bone around outer surface of the bone; bones may thicken throughout life, depending on the stresses placed on the bone; the more prolonged the stress (walking, running, weight lifting), the thicker the bones become (within physiologic limits)

D. Structure of long bones (Fig. 10)

E. Names and numbers of bones (Table 2-16)

F. Joints
  1. Synarthrotic—generally nonmovable joints; also called fibrous joints—no joint cavity or capsule; joining bones held together by fibrous tissue
    a. Sutures—bind skull bones together
    b. Syndesmoses—bind tibia and fibula; also the diaphyses of the radius and ulna
  2. Amphiarthrotic—slightly movable joints; also called cartilaginous joints—no joint cavity or capsule; joining bones held together by cartilage and ligaments
    a. Symphyses—disc of cartilage between bones, as between vertebrae or at the pubic symphysis

Fig. 10. Diagram to show the structure of a long bone as seen in longitudinal section. (From Anthony, C.P., and Kolthoff, N.J.: Textbook of anatomy and physiology, ed. 9, St. Louis, 1975, The C.V. Mosby Co.)

    b. Synchondroses—costal cartilages bind ribs to the sternum
  3. Diarthrotic—freely movable joints; the joint cavity or space between articular surfaces of two bones is lined by a thin layer of hyaline cartilage covering the articular surfaces of the joining bones; the bones are held together by a fibrous capsule lined with synovial membrane and ligaments; may be ball and socket (as in hip), hinge (as in elbow), condyloid (as at wrist), pivot, gliding, or saddle
    a. Kinds of movement possible at diarthrotic joints
      (1) Flexion—bending one bone on another; (e.g., bending forearm on upper arm)
      (2) Extension—stretching one bone away from another (e.g., straightening lower arm out from a flexed position)
      (3) Abduction—moving bone away from body's midline (e.g., moving arms straight out from sides)

Table 2-16. Bones of the body

Part of body	Name of bone	Number	Description
1. Axial skeleton			
a. Skull*			
(1) Cranium	1. Frontal	1	1. Forehead bone
	2. Parietal	2	2. Bulging bones that form top sides of cranium
	3. Temporal	2	3. Form lower sides of cranium and part of cranial floor
	4. Occipital	1	4. Forms posterior part of cranial floor and walls
	5. Sphenoid	1	5. Forms mid portion of cranial floor
	6. Ethmoid	1	6. Composes part of anterior portion of cranial floor; lies anterior to sphenoid, posterior to nasal bones
(2) Face	1. Nasal	2	1. Form upper part of bridge of nose
	2. Maxillary	2	2. Upper jaw bones
	3. Zygomatic (malar)	2	3. Cheek bones
	4. Mandible	1	4. Lower jaw bone
	5. Lacrimal	2	5. Fingernail-shaped bones posterior and lateral to nasal bones, in medial wall of orbit
	6. Palatine	2	6. Form posterior part of hard palate
	7. Inferior conchae (turbinates)	2	7. Thin scroll of bone along inner surface of side wall of nasal cavity
	8. Vomer	1	8. Lower, posterior part of nasal septum
(3) Ear ossicles	1. Malleus (hammer)	2	Tiny bones in middle ear cavity in temporal bone; resemble, respectively, miniature hammer, anvil, and stirrup
	2. Incus (anvil)	2	
	3. Stapes (stirrup)	2	
b. Hyoid bone		1	U-shaped bone in neck between mandible and upper part of larynx; only bone in body that forms no joints with any other bones
c. Vertebral column	1. Cervical vertebrae	7	1. Upper 7 vertebrae
	2. Thoracic vertebrae	12	2. Next 12 vertebrae; ribs attached to these
	3. Lumbar vertebrae	5	3. Next 5 vertebrae, located in "small" of back
	4. Sacrum	1	4. In embryo, 5 separate vertebrae, but fused in adult into 1 wedge-shaped bone
	5. Coccyx	1	5. In embryo, 4 or 5 separate vertebrae, but fused in adult into 1 bone
d. Ribs and sternum	1. True ribs	7 pairs	1. Upper 7 pairs fastened to sternum by costal cartilages
	2. False ribs	5 pairs	2. Do not attach to sternum directly; upper 3 pairs of false ribs attached by means of costal cartilage of seventh ribs; last 2 pairs not attached at all and therefore called "floating" ribs
	3. Sternum	1	3. Breast bone
2. Appendicular skeleton			
a. Upper extremities	1. Clavicle	2	1. Collar bone; shoulder girdle fastened to axial skeleton by articulation of clavicle with sternum
	2. Scapula	2	2. Shoulder blade
	3. Humerus	2	3. Long bone of upper arm
	4. Radius	2	4. Thumb side of forearm
	5. Ulna	2	5. Little finger side of forearm
	6. Carpals	16	6. Wrist bones; arranged in 2 rows at proximal end of hand
	7. Metacarpals	10	7. Long bones; form framework of palm of hand
	8. Phalanges	28	8. Miniature long bones of fingers; 3 in each finger, 2 in each thumb
b. Lower extremities	1. Os coxae, or pelvic bone	2	1. Large hip bones; lower extremities attached to axial skeleton by articulation of pelvic bones with sacrum
	2. Femur	2	2. Thigh bone
	3. Patella	2	3. Kneecap
	4. Tibia	2	4. Shin bone
	5. Fibula	2	5. Long, slender bone of lateral side of lower leg
	6. Tarsals	14	6. "Ankle" bones; form heel and proximal end of foot
	7. Metatarsals	10	7. Long bones of feet
	8. Phalanges	28	8. Miniature long bones of toes
	TOTAL	206†	

*Paranasal sinuses—holes in frontal, sphenoidal, maxillary, and ethmoid bones reduce weight of skull, serve as resonating chambers in speech, produce mucus, and often become inflamed due to allergic responses and viral or bacterial infection.

†Sesamoid bones (rounded bones found in various tendons) have not been counted except for patellae, which are largest sesamoid bones; number of these bones varies greatly between individuals. Wormian bones (small islets of bone in some cranial sutures) have not been counted because of variability of

(4) Adduction—moving bone back toward the body's midline (e.g., bringing arms back to sides of body from an outstretched, or abducted, position)

(5) Rotation—pivoting bone on its axis (e.g., partial rotation such as turning the head from side to side)

(6) Circumduction—describing surface of a cone with the moving part (e.g., moving arm around so the hand describes a circle)

(7) Supination—forearm movement turning the palm forward

(8) Pronation—forearm movement turning the back of the hand forward

(9) Inversion—ankle movement turning the sole of the foot inward

(10) Eversion—ankle movement turning the sole outward

(11) Protraction—moving a part, such as the lower jaw, forward

(12) Retraction—pulling a part back; opposite of protraction

(13) Plantar flexion—pointing the toes (as a ballerina) away from the body

(14) Dorsiflexion—pointing toes toward the body

G. Differences between male and female skeletons
1. Male skeleton larger and heavier than female skeleton
2. Male pelvis deep and funnel shaped with narrow pubic arch; female pelvis shallow, broad, and flaring with wider pubic arch

H. Age changes in skeleton
1. From infancy to adulthood, not only do bones grow but their relative sizes change as well; the head becomes proportionately smaller, the pelvis relatively larger, the legs proportionately longer, etc.
2. From young adulthood to old age, bone margins and projections change gradually; bone piles up along them (marginal lipping and spurs), thereby restricting movement; such continuing growth is due, in part, to stimulation of somatotrophic hormone

I. Repair of skeleton
1. When bone is fractured, connective tissue called a callus grows into and around the broken region
2. Macrophages reabsorb dead and damaged cells
3. Osteoclasts dissolve bone fragments
4. Osteoblasts produce new bone substance and fuse bone together
5. Final bone shape slowly remodeled; the complete process takes several months; much slower than epithelial tissue, which has a higher metabolic rate and richer blood supply

REVIEW OF PHYSICAL PRINCIPLES RELATED TO THE NEUROMUSCULOSKELETAL SYSTEMS
Principles of Mechanics

A. Applications of energy laws—machines
Apart from friction, the work output of a machine is equal to the work input to the machine; the first law of thermodynamics indicates that energy cannot be created or destroyed; a machine can multiply force, that is, provide a mechanical advantage, but at the expense of distance
1. Lever—rigid bar that moves about a fixed point known as the fulcrum; a small force is applied through a large distance and the other end of the lever exerts a large force over a small distance; the musculoskeletal system operates through lever systems
   a. First-class lever—fulcrum between resistance and effort (e.g., scissors, hemostat, bending head backward or forward)
   b. Second-class levers—resistance between fulcrum and effort (e.g., wheelbarrow, oxygen tank carrier)
   c. Third-class lever—effort between resistance and fulcrum (e.g., forceps, bending over and using your back muscles to lift an object with your hips acting as the fulcrum; swinging the arm when using a tennis racquet)
2. Pulleys—can multiply force at the expense of distance; the use of a number of pulleys together, as in a block and tackle, provides a mechanical advantage equal to the number of ropes excluding the pull rope; thus a block and tackle with 2 ropes gives a mechanical advantage of 2; a 100-lb weight can be lifted by application of a force of 50 lb (e.g., traction, lifting heavy objects like engines; pulleys used to change direction of a force); used in traction to apply tension in back injuries

B. Center of gravity
1. Position in a body where all the weight is considered to be located; sphere, such as a rubber ball, has its center of gravity in its center
2. Object is stable (will not topple over) as long as a line dropped from its center of gravity to the ground is within the base of the object; in a human the center of gravity is in the pelvic cavity, and for upright balance the line drawn from this point to the ground must fall somewhere between the legs

a. When lifting a patient, the back should be kept straight to keep torque at a minimum; in addition, when bending over, the body's center of gravity shifts from a stable position between the legs to an unstable position outside the legs; the back muscles must then work even harder to prevent the body from toppling over

b. When walking and carrying a load, the load should be carried as close to the body (center of gravity) as possible to maintain balance and to avoid strain

Principles of Physical Properties of Matter

A. Pascal's principle—when pressure is applied to a fluid in a closed, nonflexible container, it is transmitted undiminished throughout all parts of the fluid and acts in all directions

EXAMPLE: Cerebrospinal fluid—abnormal increase of pressure on this fluid is transmitted to all parts of the central nervous system containing the fluid

1. Brain tumor—mass of tissue displaces fluid and increases the pressure of the cerebrospinal fluid

2. Hydrocephalus—blockage in the canal of Sylvius or overactivity of the choroid plexuses results in a tremendous collection of fluid and increased pressure

B. Electromagnetic radiation

1. X ray

EXAMPLE: Pneumoencephalogram—ventricles of the brain can be imaged radiographically if the cerebrospinal fluid of the ventricles is temporarily replaced by air; as x rays pass through the brain, the ventricles are outlined; the picture obtained is called a pneumoencephalogram

2. Radiation hazards—individuals working with x rays should leave the room, stand behind a lead shield, or wear a lead apron when activating the x-ray machine, since there is some scattering of radiation in all directions even though the x-ray beam is aimed at a particular area; film badges (photographic film) should be worn when working near sources of radiation to provide a record of the individual's overall exposure to the radiation

C. Sound—mechanical vibration; cannot occur in a vacuum; propagated best through solids, and through liquids better than gases; travels in waves from vibrating source such as vocal cords, loudspeaker, or dropped object

1. Properties of waves

a. Transverse waves—particles of the medium vibrate at right angles to the direction of the wave (e.g., waves on the surface of liquids and all electromagnetic waves [light, infrared, and ultraviolet])

b. Longitudinal waves—particles of the medium vibrate back and forth along the same direction as the wave (e.g., sound waves)

c. Frequency—number of complete vibrations (or waves) generated or moving along per second; referred to as cycles per second or as a hertz (Hz)

d. Passage of a wave through a medium (gas, liquid, solid, or plasma) is actually the passage of a disturbance in the medium, not a flowing of the medium itself; the wave represents sequential vibration or swinging of the molecules of the medium from the vibrating source to the ears

e. Refraction of sound waves—sound travels faster in warm air than in cool air; in warm air the average kinetic energy of the air molecules is higher than in cool air and the wave can be propagated more quickly

f. Reflection of sound waves—many solid objects reflect sound waves from their surfaces resulting in an echo; a reverberation is a series of echoes

g. Energy of sound waves—all waves possess energy but to differing degrees; ultraviolet waves and gamma radiation possess high energy, whereas sound waves possess little energy; the structure of the ear reflects the need to amplify the relatively weak energy of sound waves into more energetic waves capable of stimulating the liquid-filled organ of hearing, the cochlea in the inner ear

h. Velocity of sound—frequency of the wave multiplied by the length of the wave; the velocity of sound waves varies with the nature and temperature of the medium; since light travels much faster than sound, lightning is seen before thunder is heard

2. Interpretation of sounds

a. Loudness—neurologic or pyschologic interpretation of intensity; although the exact relationship is complex, one could say that the greater the intensity of the sound waves stimulating the organ of Corti the greater will be the frequency of nerve impulses reaching the auditory centers of the brain and the louder the sound seems to be

(1) Noise level is measured in decibels (dB); a normal conversation is about 65 dB,

amplified rock music about 120 dB, and the sound of a nearby jet airplane about 140 dB; the decibel scale is logarithmic so that 120 dB is 1 million times more intense than 60 dB

(2) Excessive noise can result in hearing loss at certain frequencies of sound; noise levels of about 85 dB and over can damage the organ of Corti; damage increases with the length and intensity of noise and is irreversible

(3) Doppler effect—when a vibrating source and a receiver of sound move toward each other, the pitch or frequency of the sound produced by the source becomes higher; as the vibrating source and the receiver move away from each other, the frequency of the sound becomes lower

(4) Speech audiometry—this technique detects the threshold of hearing of actual speech for individuals by presenting groups of 2-syllable words at successively lower levels until the person fails to hear; these data are presented as a speech reception threshold (SRT) in decibels; phonetically balanced single-syllable words can also be presented; these words represent a frequency of sounds of speech that approximates a typical conversation; the percentage of words repeated correctly is the Davis Social Adequacy Index (SAI); a score of 94% to 100% is considered normal

b. Pitch—corresponds to frequency; the higher the frequency, the higher the pitch of the sound

(1) Humans can potentially hear sounds whose frequencies range from 16 to 20,000 Hz; with increasing age, the upper range decreases slightly, which presents no problem in hearing speech, since speech falls in the range of 85 to 1050 Hz

(2) Audiometers are capable of electronically producing sounds at a variety of frequencies as well as intensities and are used to measure hearing loss

c. Quality—people have different and distinct qualities or timbres to their voices; similarly, the sounds of different musical instruments are easily recognized; a musical sound or a voice rarely represents a pure tone but usually many frequencies occurring simultaneously

d. Ultrasonic sound—vibrational frequencies exceeding the upper level of human hearing (20,000 Hz)

(1) Can be used in cleaning metal parts; the high-frequency vibrations shake the solution and produce bubbles that help in the cleaning process; ultrasonic cleaners are available for hospital use in cleaning syringes and needles

(2) Low-intensity ultrasonic waves have been used to treat arthritis and bursitis, to break kidney stones, and to help dissolve scars

(3) Ultrasonic dental drills can quickly drill into teeth without the pain associated with tooth vibrations, which stimulate the nerve of the tooth

(4) Sonograms are pictures of the body derived through differential reflection or transmission of sound waves

e. Deafness—condition wherein sound vibrations are not transmitted to the brain for interpretation

(1) Perforation or tear of the tympanic membrane

(2) Inflexibility of the 3 middle ear bones or ossicles; vibrations are thus only poorly transmitted to the oval window

(3) Otosclerosis—abnormal bone formation over the oval window immobilizes the stapes

(a) Surgery can remove the abnormal bony tissue in the early stages of the disease

(b) In later stages the stapes may be removed and a prosthesis implanted

(c) If the oval window is ossified, a new opening in the cochlea is made to replace the oval window (fenestration)

(d) Bone-conduction hearing aids can essentially bypass the middle ear

(4) Deafness caused by auditory nerve damage; the nerve cannot be regenerated nor can hearing be helped by hearing aids

f. Hearing aids—electronic devices that amplify sounds and assist partially deaf persons to hear; a miniature microphone picks up the sound, sends it to an amplifier and then to a miniature loudspeaker fitted in or behind the ear

(1) Air-conduction type sends an amplified sound wave into the ear, thus utilizing the person's own middle ear

(2) Bone-conduction type bypasses the middle ear and transmits amplified vibrations to the skull bones, which in turn produce vibrations in the inner ear

D. Light
1. Basic concepts
   a. Visible light is a type of electromagnetic radiation; all electromagnetic radiation consists of moving electric and magnetic energy fields that come into existence because of the vibrations of electrically charged particles
   b. All types of electromagnetic radiation have the same electric and magnetic nature and travel at the same constant velocity: 186,000 miles per second (speed of light)
   c. Electromagnetic spectrum varies from extremely long AM and FM radio waves measured in miles to very short gamma and cosmic rays measured in millimeters
   d. Product of the frequency of vibration and the wavelength is constant (the velocity of light); the lower the frequency of vibration of the wave, the longer will be the wavelength, and the higher the frequency, the shorter the wavelength
   e. The higher the frequency (or the shorter the wavelength) of electromagnetic radiation, the greater will be the energy content of the radiation
2. Wavelengths of electromagnetic radiation
   a. Wavelengths are measured in either millimicrons or Angstrom units
      (1) A millimicron is one thousandth of a micron; a micron is one millionth of a meter (39 inches)
      (2) An Angstrom unit is one tenth of a millimicron
   b. Wavelengths of visible light possess just the right amount of vibrational energy to excite the photoreceptor cells (rods and cones) of the retina
   c. Different wavelengths of light are bent or refracted to slightly different degrees and appear to the eyes and brain as different colors; this principle of dispersion is responsible for a rainbow
   d. Emission of light—atoms can be excited by absorbing energy that causes orbiting electrons to jump to higher energy levels within the atom; as the electrons fall back to their lower (more stable) energy levels (deexcitation), the energy of excitation is released and may appear as visible light (e.g., advertising signs, mercury vapor street lamps)

(1) Characteristic pattern of wavelengths of light (a discontinuous spectrum) is emitted from every element in the vapor state; this pattern is best seen by means of a spectroscope
(2) Fluorescence—property of absorbing radiation of one frequency and emitting radiation of a lower frequency and energy; a substance is said to be fluorescent if it emits visible light when energized or bombarded with ultraviolet (UV) light; high-intensity fluorescent light bulbs have been used to treat jaundice in newborn infants; the excess bilirubin in the blood, which is responsible for the jaundice, is oxidized by exposure to the bright light as blood passes through the vessels of the thin skin
(3) Phosphorescence—atoms of a phosphorescent substance become deexcited a relatively long time after being excited; the phosphorescent atoms in the dial of a luminous clock are excited during the day by the visible light striking them; the dial then glows throughout the night as billions of excited atoms gradually become deexcited, releasing their energy as visible light

3. Laser
   a. Acronym for light amplification by stimulated emission of radiation; a laser produces coherent light, which means that the light waves are all of the same frequency, are all in phase with each other (peak with peak, trough with trough), and are all traveling in the same direction; in coherent light, millions of light waves becomes additive and form a single, concentrated beam of light that travels in a straight line without spreading out and that can be precisely focused on minute areas
   b. As coherent light leaves the laser (ruby crystal), it can be utilized for a variety of purposes
      (1) Eye surgery—energy in the coherent light produced by a laser is used to fuse minute areas of the retina to the surrounding choroid coat; an ophthalmoscope is used to focus the coherent light precisely on specific, tiny areas of the retina; a detached retina can thus be reattached, and the fusion points are so tiny that there is no apparent loss of light-sensitive retinal tissue; the machine used

in this type of surgery is called a photo-coagulator and uses a ruby laser

(2) Cancer therapy—laser has been used in the selective treatment of pigmented skin cancers, which apparently absorb the light more readily than do surrounding, less pigmented, normal tissues

4. Color
   a. Perception of color is the result of the translation and interpretation of certain nerve impulses in the brain that come from the retina; the frequency of light determines the color that is seen; the lowest frequency stimulating the retina is red, the highest is violet, in between are all the colors of nature
   b. Objects may appear to be colored because they emit electromagnetic radiation that falls within the visible range; may also appear colored not because they emit light, but because of selective reflection
   c. Color mixing
      (1) Red, green, and blue are the additive primaries; any color in the spectrum can be obtained with the proper blend of these 3; equal amounts of the 3 produce white light
      (2) Magenta, yellow, and cyan (turquoise) are the subtractive primaries; any color in the spectrum can be obtained using the proper blend of these 3; they are sometimes loosely called red, yellow, and blue
      (3) Complementary colors are any 2 colors that, when added together, produce white: red and cyan, magenta and green, and yellow and blue
   d. Perception of color is believed to depend on the cones of the retina, which are located most densely at the part of the retina called the fovea centralis; one type of cone detects red, another detects green, and another blue; it is generally thought that the brain blends nerve impulses from these three types of cones to produce our perception of all the colors of nature
      (1) Faulty color vision is thought to be caused by cones that are either missing or not functioning properly; red-green color blindness is the most common type and is a genetically inherited trait that causes individuals to see red and green objects as shades of gray; more men are affected than women, since the trait appears to be sex linked

(2) Color and emotion—even though red light has a lower frequency and therefore less energy than a quantum of blue light, the human mind generally associates red with warmth, excitement, and mental stimulation, and blue with coolness and calmness; for many individuals the color of an object or a room determines to a great extent whether they will keep and use the object or stay in the room; thus color has a physical basis in the electromagnetic radiation but involves complex interpretation by the human mind

5. Reflection and refraction
   a. General principles
      (1) Source of light—sun the primary outdoor source; incandescent and fluorescent bulbs are indoor sources
      (2) Most objects visible because they reflect light emitted from various sources
      (3) Pane of glass is transparent if it allows light to pass through it in straight lines
      (4) Thin cloth window shade or a piece of paper is translucent if it allows light to pass through it in a diffused manner so objects cannot be seen; in hospitals, shades or blinds diffuse light and cut down on harsh glare
      (5) Heavy pair of curtains is opaque if light cannot pass through it
      (6) Light traveling in any single medium travels in straight lines; each straight line called a ray
   b. Reflection
      (1) When light strikes a surface off which it can reflect, the angle of incidence equals the angle of reflection as measured from the normal (a line perpendicular to the plane of the reflecting surface)
         (a) When successive elevations of any surface are less than about one fourth the wavelength of the incident light, the light reflected from the surface travels mainly in one direction and the surface is polished
         (b) Light reflected from rougher surfaces travels in many directions and is diffusely reflected; it is easier to read a page of text printed on paper that provides a more diffuse than polished reflection, since glare is eliminated
         (c) The word *ambulance* is often printed backward on the front of these ve-

hicles so that motorists seeing the lettering via reflected light through their rearview mirrors will be able to read the lettering correctly

(2) Virtual images—as light reflects off a mirror, the angles of incidence and reflection are equal; the reflected rays of light appear to come from a point behind the mirror; because the light rays do not actually come from this point, the image is referred to as a virtual image as opposed to a real image; the virtual image of a mirror is as far behind the mirror as the object is in front of the mirror

c. Refraction

(1) Refraction—bending of an oblique ray of light as it travels from one transparent medium into another; refraction is caused by the change in average velocity of light as it passes through the medium

(2) Index of refraction—average speed of light varies in different, transparent media; the average speed of light in water is only 75% of its average speed in a vacuum; the average speed in a diamond is 41% of its average speed in a vacuum; the index of refraction is a measure of how much the average speed of light differs from its speed in a vacuum; index of refraction equals the speed of light in a vacuum divided by its speed in a medium; the higher the index of refraction, the slower the average speed of light through the medium

EXAMPLES

1. Thermometer or syringe half immersed in a beaker of water appears to be bent at the point of immersion

2. Object in water appears to be nearer the surface than it actually is; thus it seems larger because it is magnified

3. Mirage—average speed of light is slightly greater in hot air than in cool air; on a hot paved road or a desert the light reflected from an object is refracted upward, away from the hot surface and may then produce an upside-down virtual image to an individual some distance away; the wet shimmering look of a hot road is refracted light from the sky reaching a motorist's eye after passing through hot air layers

4. Total internal reflection—at a certain critical angle, light between 2 media is not refracted (or bent) but is reflected back into the first medium

   a. This phenomenon permits viewing of the interior walls of the stomach, intestines, and blood vessels

   b. Dentist's flashlight will "curve" the light (via total internal reflection) to the appropriate part of an individual's mouth

   c. Total internal reflection via the paired prisms in a pair of binoculars permits higher magnifications in a short optic tube

6. Diffraction

Bending of light or any type of electromagnetic wave around corners; the longer the wavelength of electromagnetic radiation, the larger the object that it can be bent around

EXAMPLES

1. AM radio waves, some of which are over 3 miles long, easily bend around objects, thereby allowing AM broadcasts to come in clearly even in cities having many tall buildings and mountainous regions

2. FM radio waves, which are from 9 to 12 feet long, cannot easily bend around large objects; consequently, a specific location in a city or suburban area with large obstructing objects can determine the quality of the reception of FM broadcasts

3. Some spectrophotometers used in certain laboratory analyses of blood and urine rely on diffraction gradings to disperse white light into its component wavelengths and to utilize these specific wavelengths in the analytic procedure

4. X-ray diffraction—because of their very short wavelengths, x rays diffract around the atoms in large molecules and produce diffraction patterns on photographic plates; analyses of these patterns can reveal the details of the arrangement of the atoms in a molecule; used in DNA analysis

7. Polarization

Certain naturally occurring crystals, like tourmaline and herapathite, absorb light waves striking them in all planes but one; the light transmitted through and emerging from the crystal vibrates in only one plane; this is called plane-polarized light

EXAMPLES
1. Polaroid filters contain a material, like herapathite or certain synthetic molecules, that will permit only light vibrating in a single plane to pass through; when used in sunglasses, they cut down on glare and eye strain; much of the light reflected from nonmetallic surfaces, such as water, glass, or roadways, is already polarized because these surfaces tend to absorb light waves perpendicular to their surfaces and to reflect light waves parallel to their surfaces; when this polarized light strikes the Polaroid filters in the sunglasses, many of the light waves are absorbed; thus fewer waves are transmitted and the harsh glare is reduced
2. Polarizing filters for cameras cut down on glare in photographs and also have the effect of deepending the blue color of the sky
3. Polarizing microscopes are used in research laboratories to analyze the molecular structure of many substances

8. Lenses
   a. Refraction of light through transparent glass (or quartz or fluorite) lenses is of great practical importance; magnification of objects is possible using simple lenses as well as groups of lenses arranged in telescopes and microscopes; the principal axis of a lens is the line joining the 2 points that represent the centers of curvature of the curved surfaces of a given lens
   b. Convex lenses (converging or positive lenses) converge light rays passing through them; concave lenses (diverging or negative lenses) diverge light rays passing through them
   c. When light rays parallel with the principal axis pass through a converging lens, they converge on the focal point; light rays not parallel with the principal axis converge in a series of points above and below the focal point, making up the focal plane
      (1) Converging lens will magnify an object (acting as a simple magnifying glass) if it is held inside the focal point of the lens; the image is enlarged, right side up and virtual; this means that the image only appears to exist but has no physical reality
      (2) When an object is placed outside the fo-

cal point of a converging lens, a real, inverted image is obtained that can be focused on a screen; whenever a real image is formed, the object and image are on opposite sides of the lens

EXAMPLES
1. Motion pictures utilize converging lenses, and the movie screen is the plane where light rays are converged; slide projectors also operate under the same principle
2. In cameras the film is flattened out and placed in the focal plane of the camera's lens; in popular single-lens reflex (SLR) cameras a mirror diverts the light to a prism, which erects the image, allowing the viewer to see exactly what will be focused on the film; when the shutter button is pushed and the mirror flips out of the way, light is focused on and exposes the photographic film
3. Diverging lenses used alone produce smaller, virtual images; they are used on some cameras (not SLR cameras) as "finders," since the virtual image seen approximates the proportions of the photograph; whenever a virtual image is formed, the object and the image are on the same side of the lens
4. Lens defects—distortions in an image produced by a given lens are called aberrations; combining a number of lenses as a system can usually minimize aberrations; this is the reason that microscopes and telescopes employ compound lenses in their construction
   a. Spherical aberration—unsharp (uncrisp) images are formed because light refracted from the outer edges of the lens is focused at a point slightly different from the point at which light refracted from more central areas of the lens is focused
      (1) In cameras and microscopes this is corrected by using more than one lens and also by using diaphragms to cover the outer regions of the lens
      (2) In the human eye the iris is generally contracted to varying degrees and acts, in effect, like a diaphragm to block light from being refracted through the outer regions of the lens

b. Chromatic aberration—each wavelength of visible light refracts through lenses at different angles; thus each wavelength (color) of white light is brought to focus at a slightly different point; the result of this is that objects take on colors that they do not possess; this is corrected in cameras, microscopes, and telescopes by using combinations of simple lenses made of different types of glass called achromatic lenses; in the human eye, vision is sharpest when the pupil is the smallest; cutting down on light moving through the periphery of the lens minimizes chromatic as well as spherical aberration

c. Astigmatism—human eye astigmatism is a type of abberration caused by the surface of the cornea possessing irregular curves; since the cornea in addition to the lens is important in refracting (focusing) light on the retina, the result of astigmatism is blurred vision, which can be corrected by using lenses that have variable curvature to compensate for the irregular curvature of the cornea

5. Focusing—camera focuses on objects at varying distances by changing the distance between the lens and the film; the human eye focuses on objects at varying distances by changing the degree of curvature of the lens; this ability of the human eye to change the focal length of the lens is called accommodation; whereas the cornea, aqueous humor, and vitreous humor all help to focus light on the retina, only the crystalline lens is able to accommodate; the muscle responsible for accommodation is the ciliary body; when the ciliary body contracts, the suspensory ligaments loosen and the lens rounds out and is in position for focusing on near objects; when the ciliary body relaxes, the suspensory ligaments pull the lens into a flattened position, which allows for focusing on distant objects; the limit for accommodation is represented by the near point; objects closer to the eye than the near point (about 15 cm [6 inches] from the surface of a normal eye) cannot be clearly focused on the retina

a. Emmetropia—normal refractive state of the eye

b. Ametropia—any abnormality in refractive ability of the eye
   (1) Myopia—eye focuses light anterior to the retina (somewhere in the vitreous humor); from this abnormal focal point, light rays diverge and produce a blurred image on the retina; however, if objects are held about 2.5 cm (1 inch) from the eye, they will focus on the retina; for this reason, myopia is also called near-sightedness; glasses containing diverting lenses correct this condition
   (2) Hyperopia—eye focuses light posterior to the retina; thus a circle of not-yet-converged light strikes the retina, producing a blurred image; hyperopia is also called far-sightedness and can be corrected using glasses containing converging lenses

c. Contact lenses—thin lenses that are molded to the shape of the outer surface of the cornea; this can correct near-sightedness, far-sightedness, and astigmatism; the lens is applied to the surface of the eye using a saline solution that helps adhere the lens to the eye's surface

6. Eye examination with the ophthalmoscope and the retinoscope
   a. Ophthalmoscope—permits visualization of the interior of the eye; thus the examiner can study a patient's vision with this instrument; light shone into an eye with normal refractive ability will be focused on the retina and reflected back to the examiner's eye; persons with myopia or hyperopia will not converge the light on the retina, and the examiner will not clearly see the eye's interior; then by using lenses of varying refractive abilities the examiner can compensate for the person's abnormal refraction, study the interior of the eye, and determine the state of vision
   b. Retinoscope—permits diagnosis and evaluation of the refractive state of the eye; a beam of light shone into the

eye is reflected from the retina as it leaves the pupil; by observing its distribution as it leaves the pupil, the examiner can determine the refractive error in the eye

7. Binocular vision—visual fields of the 2 human eyes overlap; while each eye sees some areas of the environment that the other eye cannot see, both eyes also see large areas in common; the human brain interprets these overlapping fields in terms of depth; the environment appears in 3 dimensions, as opposed to the visual effect of a movie projected on a flat screen; the blind spot of the right eye can be seen by the left eye and vice versa; therefore no gaps in the field of vision exist

REVIEW OF CHEMICAL PRINCIPLES RELATED TO THE NEUROMUSCULOSKELETAL SYSTEMS
Amines

A. Organic compounds containing an amino group (NH_2) that can be considered derivatives of ammonia
B. Reactions of the amines
1. Basic, in water solution
2. Like a base with acids, forming complex ions
C. Important amines
1. Monoamines such as norepinephrine, dopamine, serotonin, acetylcholine, and histamine serve as transmitter chemicals in the nervous system
2. Amino acids such as gamma-aminobutyric acid (GABA) and glycine act as inhibitors; glutamic acid has an excitatory influence on the nervous system

Lipids

Phospholipids, lecithin, cephalins, and sphingomyelins are important components of nerve membranes and sheaths

Proteins

Actin, myosin, and troponin are important in muscle contraction

Group I A Alkali Metals

A. Sodium—in the extracellular fluid these ions are responsible for action potentials of nervous and muscular tissues; after some stimulus, it is the diffusion of Na^+ from the interstitial fluid into the intracellular fluid of neurons and muscle fibers that brings about depolarization; thus sodium ions are basic to

the functioning of the body's communication system, the nervous system, and all muscular movements
B. Potassium
1. Resting polarization of neurons, all types of muscle fibers (i.e., smooth, cardiac, striated), and most cells of the body is caused by the continual diffusion of K^+ from the intracellular fluid to the interstitial fluid; similarly, repolarization of neurons and muscle fibers is caused by the outward diffusion of K^+ to the interstitial fluid from the intracellular fluid
2. Several important cellular enzymes functioning in glucose and amino acid metabolism require K^+ as a cofactor

Group II A Alkali Earth Metals

A. Magnesium
1. Activator for many enzymes
2. Present in bones
B. Calcium
1. Gives hardness to bones and teeth by forming phosphate, carbonate, and fluoride salts
2. Important in muscle contraction; ATP must combine with CA^{++} before its energy can be used to slide actin and myosin filaments together
3. Extracellular Ca^{++} concentration must be precisely regulated (through the parathyroid glands) for normal body functioning; hypocalcemia can result in tetany; hypercalcemia can result in depression of the nervous system
C. Strontium
1. May substitute for calcium in body
2. Radioactive isotope (strontium 90) can be a health hazard, forming pockets of radiation in tissues

Group VII A Halogens

Fluorine—prevents tooth decay when added to water supply

Group I B

A. Silver—filling for teeth, surgical mending of bone, photography
B. Gold—filling for teeth

REVIEW OF MICROORGANISMS RELATED TO THE NEUROMUSCULOSKELETAL SYSTEMS

A. Bacterial pathogens
1. *Clostridium tetani*—large, gram-positive, motile bacillus forming large terminal spores; like all clostridia, it is an obligate anaerobe; causes tetanus (lockjaw)

2. *Haemophilus aegyptius* (Koch-Weeks bacillus)—indistinguishable morphologically from *Haemophilus influenzae;* causes a common conjunctivitis called pinkeye
3. *Neisseria meningitidis*—gram-negative diplococcus; causes epidemic (meningococcic) meningitis
B. DNA viruses—herpetoviruses; spherical and 150 to 200 nm in diameter; cause herpes simplex, varicella (chickenpox), herpes zoster (shingles), infectious mononucleosis, and cytomegalic inclusion disease
C. RNA viruses—togaviruses; spherical and 40 to 60 nm in diameter; mostly borne by mosquitoes and ticks; cause eastern equine encephalomyelitis, western equine encephalomyelitis, Venezuelan equine encephalomyelitis, and a number of other infections
D. Fungal pathogen—*Cryptococcus neoformans*—pathogenic yeast with a characteristic large capsule around the cell; causes cryptococcosis (torulosis, European blastomycosis), a serious infection involving the lungs and central nervous system
E. Protozoa—*Trypanosoma*—flagellated ribbonlike protozoa; *T. gambiense* and *T. rhodesience* cause African sleeping sickness (transmitted by tsetse flies) and *T. cruzi* causes South American trypanosomiasis or Chagas' disease (transmitted by reduviid bugs)
F. Worm—*Trichinella spiralis*—one of smallest parasitic nematodes (about 1.5 mm in length), causes trichinosis (muscle infestation with trichina)

PHARMACOLOGY RELATED TO DISORDERS OF THE NEUROMUSCULOSKELETAL SYSTEMS

A. Anticonvulsant drugs
1. General implications for nurses
   a. Teach the patient regarding maintaining therapeutic blood level of drug as well as continued medical supervision
   b. Instruct the family about treatment and how to care for the patient during a seizure
   c. Suggest a medical alert card or other form of identification be carried by the patient
   d. If seizure occurs
      (1) Maintain airway
      (2) Protect the patient from injury
      (3) Observe the type and duration of seizure
   e. Observe for adverse effects
      (1) Dizziness, drowsiness
      (2) Nausea and vomiting
      (3) Hydantoins (phenytoin and mephenytoin) cause

(a) Respiratory and cardiovascular depression
(b) Ataxia
(c) Gingivitis and hyperplasia of the gums
(d) Hirsutism
(e) Inhibition of the action of corticosteroids, digitalis, and folic acid
   f. Anticoagulants potentiate the action of phenytoin
   g. Depression of cardiac and respiratory centers can be caused by magnesium sulfate 50% and diazepam
2. Actions
   a. Modify bioelectric activity at subcortical and cortical sites
   b. Raise the threshold response to stimuli precipitating seizure control
3. Examples
   a. Grand mal seizure control
      (1) Carbamazepine (Tegretol)—also used for control of psychomotor seizure and trigeminal neuralgia
      (2) Phenytoin (Dihycon, Di-Lan, Dilantin)—also used for psychomotor seizure control
      (3) Magnesium sulfate 50%
      (4) Mephobarbital (Mebaral)
      (5) Mephenytoin (Mesantoin)
      (6) Primidone (Mysoline)—also used for psychomotor seizure control
      (7) Diazepam (Valium)—given intravenously in instances of status epilepticus
   b. Petit mal seizure control
      (1) Ethosuximide (Zarontin)
      (2) Methsuximide (Celontin)
      (3) Paramethadione (Paradione)
      (4) Trimethadione (Tridione)
B. Osmotic diuretics for increased intracranial pressure (mannitol)
1. General implications for nurses
   a. Observe the patient for signs of increased intracranial pressure (e.g., decreasing pulse rate, increasing blood pressure, unequal pupils, change in level of consciousness)
   b. Monitor intake and output
   c. Mannitol contraindicated in patients with congestive heart failure or impaired renal function
   d. Generally the head of the bed should be elevated
   e. Observe for adverse effects
      (1) Headache

(2) Nausea

(3) Chills

(4) Hyponatremia and hypochloremia

2. Actions

    a. Increase osmotic pressure within the glomeruli, causing more fluid to be excreted in the urine

    b. Used to reduce cerebral edema and intraocular pressure

C. Drugs to increase calcium ion balance

1. General implications for nurses

    a. Observe the patient for signs of tetany and hypercalcemia

    b. Increase fluid intake

    c. Check the patient's electrolytes

    d. Increase amounts of calcium and vitamin D in the diet

    e. Recognize that parathyroid hormone may be given to increase osteoclastic activity, which would raise serum calcium

2. Actions

    a. Vitamin D improves the absorption of calcium from the intestines

    b. Observe the patient for adverse effects

        (1) Nausea and vomiting

        (2) Constipation

        (3) Possible renal calculi

        (4) Muscle flaccidity

3. Examples

    a. Calcium ion replacement

        (1) Calcium chloride

        (2) Calcium gluconate

        (3) Calcium carbonate (Os-Cal)

    b. Vitamin D replacement

        (1) Dihydrotachysterol (Hytakerol)

        (2) Calciferol

D. Antiparkinsonism drugs

1. General implications for nurses

    a. Understand that treatment controls symptoms but is not a cure

    b. Provide emotional support

    c. Eliminate vitamin B_6 from diet if L-dopa is prescribed

    d. Observe the patient for adverse effects

        (1) Levodopa and amantadine hydrochloride

           (a) Orthostatic hypotension

           (b) Ataxia

           (c) Depression, psychic disturbances

        (2) Anticholinergic drugs (ethopropazine, benztropine mesylate, and trihexyphenidyl)

           (a) Dry mouth

           (b) Blurred vision

2. Actions

    a. Anticholinergic drugs act at central sites to inhibit cerebral motor impulses and to block efferent impulses that cause rigidity of the musculature

    b. Supplies or causes the release of dopamine required for norepinephrine synthesis and maintenance of the neurohormonal balance at subcortical, cortical, and reticular sites that control motor function

3. Examples

    a. Levodopa (Dopar, Larodopa)

    b. Amantadine hydrochloride (Symmetrel)

    c. Ethopropazine hydrochloride (Parsidol)

    d. Benztropine mesylate (Cogentin)

    e. Trihexyphenidyl hydrochloride (Artane, Tremin)

E. Cholinesterase inhibitors

1. General implications for nurses

    a. Observe the patient closely, because dosage is adjusted according to needs

    b. Be aware of signs of drug toxicity, which can mimic myasthenia gravis

    c. Observe the patient for adverse effects

        (1) Intestinal colic, diarrhea

        (2) Excess salivary secretion

        (3) Weak rapid pulse

        (4) Acute toxicity—pulmonary edema and respiratory failure

    d. Atropine sulfate may be given for treatment of overdose

2. Actions

    a. Prevent enzymatic breakdown of acetylcholine at nerve endings, which allows accumulation of the neurotransmitter

    b. Improves strength of contraction in all muscles, but a primary concern is maintaining the contractile strength of respiratory muscles

3. Examples

    a. Neostigmine bromide (Prostigmin Bromide)—also used for stimulation of smooth muscle contraction in the abdominal viscera (uterus, bladder)

    b. Ambenonium chloride (Mytelase)

    c. Pyridostigmine bromide (Mestinon Bromide)

    d. Edrophonium chloride (Tensilon)—because of its short-lived action, this drug is primarily used for diagnostic purposes

F. Skeletal muscle relaxants

1. General implications for nurses

    a. Caution the patient to avoid activity requiring mental alertness

    b. Avoid giving to patients with a history of liver disease, since it may cause jaundice

    c. Provide for safety because of depression of CNS

    d. Advise the patient not to take other CNS depressants

  2. Actions

    a. Cause a relaxation of voluntary muscles by depressing the central nervous system

    b. Decrease effects of muscle spasms, trauma, arthritis, etc.

  3. Examples

    a. Carisoprodol (Rela, Soma)

    b. Chlormezanone (Trancopal)

    c. Chlorphenesin carbamate (Maolate)

    d. Chlorzoxazone (Paraflex)

    e. Mephenesin (Mephson, Romeph, Tolax, Tolserol)

    f. Metaxalone (Skelaxin)

    g. Methocarbamol (Robaxin)

    h. Parafon Forte (which contains both chlorzoxazone and acetaminophen)

    i. Diazepam (Valium)

G. Drugs used in the treatment of arthritis

  1. General implications for nurses

    a. Teach the patient the serious nature of side effects, especially blood dyscrasias

    b. Encourage the patient to remain under medical supervision even when relief of pain occurs

    c. Observe for diminishing signs of inflammation

    d. Administer with milk, meals, or antacids

    e. Alters effects of other drugs, especially anticoagulants

    f. Observe the patient for adverse effects

      (1) Salicylates

        (a) Tinnitus, dizziness

        (b) Gastric irritation

        (c) Prolonged bleeding time

      (2) Gold compounds

        (a) Pruritus

        (b) Stomatitis

        (c) Albuminuria, hematuria

        (d) Thrombocytopenia, agranulocytosis

      (3) Phenylbutazone

        (a) Edema

        (b) Gastric distress

        (c) Vertigo

        (d) Hepatitis

        (e) Psychosis

        (f) Leukopenia, thrombocytopenia, agranulocytosis

      (4) Indomethacin

        (a) Peptic ulcer

        (b) Light-headedness

        (c) Skin rashes

        (d) Bone marrow depression

      (5) Ibuprofen

        (a) Gastric irritation

        (b) Dizziness

        (c) Skin rash

  2. Actions

    a. Analgesia thought to be caused by action at peripheral nerve endings; therefore these drugs are effective in the treatment of musculoskeletal pain but not visceral pain

    b. Interfere with the normal inflammatory process

  3. Examples

    a. Salicylates (aspirin, sodium salicylate)

    b. Gold compounds (usually given with salicylates)

    c. Phenylbutazone (Butazolidin, Butazolidin Alka)

    d. Indomethacin (Indocin)

    e. Steroids

    f. Ibuprofen (Motrin)

H. Drugs used in the treatment of gout

  1. General implications for nurses

    a. Administer antiinflammatory drugs, such as corticosteroids and indomethacin, in addition to drugs that will lower serum uric acid during acute phase

    b. Increase fluids to discourage the formation of renal calculi

    c. Encourage weight reduction

    d. Monitor serum urate levels to determine effectiveness of treatment

    e. Observe for adverse effects

      (1) Nausea, vomiting

      (2) Blood dyscrasias

      (3) Liver damage

  2. Actions and examples

    a. Colchicine thought to decrease urate crystal deposits by inhibiting lactic acid production by leukocytes

    b. Probenecid (Benemid) prevents the formation of tophi by inhibiting the reabsorption of urate by the kidneys

    c. Allopurinol (Zyloprim) actually blocks the formation of uric acid within the body

I. Drugs that affect the eyes

  1. General implications for nurses

    a. Observe for adverse effects (see specific drug)

b. Minimize side effects by administering drugs at bedtime

c. Stress the need for medical supervision while on medications

2. Ophthalmic cholinergics (miotics)
   a. Actions
      (1) Used in the treatment of glaucoma
      (2) Constrict the pupil, pull the iris away from the filtration angle, and improve outflow of aqueous humor
   b. Examples
      (1) Timolol maleate (Timoptic)
      (2) Pilocarpine hydrochloride (or nitrate)
      (3) Carbachol
      (4) Methacholine chloride (Mecholyl)
      (5) Physostigmine
      (6) Neostigmine bromide (Prostigmin)
      (7) Demecarium (Humorsol)
      (8) Isoflurophate (Floropryl)
      (9) Echothiophate (Phospholine)
   c. Adverse effects
      (1) Twitching of eyelids
      (2) Brow ache
      (3) Headache
      (4) Conjunctival pain
      (5) Contact dermatitis

3. Anticholinergic drugs
   a. Actions
      (1) Paralyze accommodation (cycloplegia)
      (2) Dilate the pupil (mydriasis) by relaxing the ciliary muscle and the sphincter muscle of the iris
      (3) Facilitate examination of the interior of the eye
   b. Examples
      (1) Atropine
      (2) Scopolamine
      (3) Homatropine hydrobromide
      (4) Cyclopentolate (Cyclogyl)
      (5) Eucatropine
      (6) Tropicamide (Mydriacyl)
   c. Adverse effects
      (1) Dry mouth and skin
      (2) Flushing
      (3) Fever
      (4) Rash
      (5) Tachycardia
      (6) Ataxia

4. Mydriatics
   a. Action—dilate pupil (mydriasis) by causing contraction of dilator muscle of the iris with minimal effect on ciliary muscle, which lessens effect on accommodation

b. Examples
   (1) Tropicamide (Mydriacil)
   (2) Phenylephrine hydrochloride (Neo-Synephrine)
   (3) Hydroxyamphetamine (Paredrine)
c. Adverse effects
   (1) Brow ache
   (2) Headache
   (3) Blurred vision
   (4) Tachycardia
   (5) Hypertension

5. Carbonic anhydrase inhibitors
   a. Action—decrease inflow of aqueous humor in control of intraocular pressure (administered orally or parenterally)
   b. Examples
      (1) Acetazolamide (Diamox)
      (2) Dichlorphenamide (Daranide, Oratrol)
      (3) Ethoxzolamide (Cardrase, Ethamide)
      (4) Methazolamide (Neptazane)
   c. Adverse effects
      (1) Diuresis
      (2) Paresthesia
      (3) Nausea, vomiting
      (4) Depression
      (5) Confusion
      (6) Destruction of the angle

6. Osmotic agents
   a. Actions
      (1) Reduce volume of intraocular fluids
      (2) Administered systemically to decrease blood osmolality, which mobilizes fluid from the eye
   b. Examples
      (1) Glycerin (Glyrol, Osmoglyn)
      (2) Urea (Urevert, Ureaphil)
      (3) Mannitol (Osmitrol)
   c. Adverse effects
      (1) Headache
      (2) Nausea
      (3) Vomiting

RELATED DIAGNOSTIC PROCEDURES
Lumbar Puncture

A. Definition—involves the introduction of a needle into the subarachnoid space, usually between L_3 and L_4 or L_4 and L_5, to prevent injury to the spinal cord above this level

B. Purposes
   1. Withdrawal of spinal fluid for diagnostic purposes or to reduce spinal pressure (normal is 70 to 200 mm H_2O)
   2. Measurement of spinal pressure (Queckenstedt

test involves compression of the jugular veins; normally pressure will rise; but if blockage exists, pressure will not change)
3. Injection of air or dye for diagnostic x-ray examination
4. Injection of medication such as anesthetics
C. Nursing responsibilities
1. Explain procedure to the patient and obtain a signed consent
2. Set up a sterile field
3. Assist the patient into a position that will enlarge the opening between the vertebrae
   a. Lying on side with feet drawn up and head lowered to chest; back near edge of mattress
   b. Sitting over side of bed, leaning on overbed table, feet supported on a stool
4. Observe the patient for signs of shock, such as tachycardia, diaphoresis, and pallor
5. After procedure assist the patient into a recumbent position; the patient should remain recumbent up to 24 hours, depending on the physician's orders
6. Label specimens and send to laboratory
7. Note color and amount of spinal fluid, as well as the patient's condition, and record
8. Administer fluids unless contraindicated

Bárány's Caloric Test

A. Definition
1. Used to assess vestibular labyrinthine function
2. Warm or cold water is instilled rapidly into the auditory canal, causing motion of the endolymph within the semicircular canals and normally resulting in vertigo, nystagmus, and nausea
3. Eyes deviate toward the stimulated ear if cold water is used and away if warm water is used
B. Nursing responsibilities
1. Explain procedure to the patient
2. Assemble equipment for the procedure
3. Assist the physician and support the patient during irrigation
4. Observe and record reaction of the patient

Neurologic Assessment

A. Definition—systematic evaluation of the cranial nerves, motor and sensory functioning, and mental status to detect neurologic abnormalities
1. Critical aspects of a complete neurologic assessment are generally extracted and compose a "Neuro checklist," which is used when the nature of the situation does not warrant complete evaluation

2. See review of anatomy and physiology of the neuromusculoskeletal systems
B. Nursing responsibilities
1. Perform assessment as dictated by the patient's needs
   a. Cranial nerves
      (1) Olfactory (I): ability to identify familiar odors such as mint or alcohol with eyes closed and one nostril occluded at a time
      (2) Optic (II): visual acuity measured by use of Snellen chart or by gross estimation with reading material; gross comparison of visual fields with those of examiner; color perception
      (3) Oculomotor (III), trochlear (IV), and abducent (VI): ability of the pupils to react equally to light and to accommodate to varying distances; normal range of extraocular movement (EOM) evaluated by asking the patient to follow a finger or object with the eyes; should also include assessment for nystagmus (jerking motion of eyes) particularly when eyes are directed laterally
      (4) Trigeminal (V): sensations of the face evaluated by lightly stroking cotton across forehead, chin, and cheeks while the patient's eyes are closed; ability to clench the teeth (jaw closure)
      (5) Facial (VII): symmetry of the facial muscles as the patient speaks or is asked to make faces
      (6) Acoustic or vestibulocochlear (VIII): hearing acuity determined by a watch tick or whispered numbers; Weber test may be performed by holding the stem of a vibrating tuning fork at midline of the skull (should be heard equally in both ears)
      (7) Glossopharyngeal (IX) and vagus (X): uvula should hang in midline; swallow and gag reflexes should be intact
      (8) Spinal accessory (XI): symmetrical ability to turn the head or shrug the shoulders against counterforce of the examiner's hands
      (9) Hypoglossal (XII): ability to protrude the tongue without deviation to left or right, and without tremors
   b. Motor function (including cerebellar function)
      (1) Balance
         (a) Observation of gait

(b) Romberg test: positive if the patient fails to maintain an upright position with feet together when the eyes are closed

(2) Coordination: ability to touch the finger to the nose when arms are extended or to perform similar tasks smoothly

(3) Muscle strength: evaluated by having the patient move major muscle groups against opposition supplied by the examiner

c. Sensory function: bilateral testing of the response to light touch with cotton, superficial pinprick, vibration of a tuning fork

d. Mental status or cerebral functioning

(1) Level of consciousness: determined by the response to stimuli (e.g., verbal or physical); a patient may be in any state, ranging from alert to comatose

(2) Orientation to person, place, and time: determined by general conversation and direct questioning

(3) Judgment, memory, and ability to perform simple calculations

(4) Appropriateness of behavior and mood

e. Reflexes

(1) Deep tendon (biceps, triceps, patellar, Achilles reflexes) with a reflex hammer; classification from 0 (absent) to 4+ (signifying hyperactive)

(2) Plantar: plantar flexion of the foot when the sole is stroked firmly with a hard object such as a tongue blade; abnormal adult response (dorsiflexion of the foot and fanning of the toes) is described as a positive Babinski and is indicative of corticospinal tract disease

2. Accurately record findings

3. Report any deviations that warrant immediate treatment

4. Explain and reassure the patient when the examination must be repeated frequently (e.g., after head trauma)

Computerized Axial Tomography (CAT Scan)*

A. Definition

1. Cross-sectional visualization of the brain determined by computer analysis of relative tissue density as an x-ray beam passes through

---

*Now called "computed tomography" (CT).

2. Provides valuable information about location and extent of tumors, infarcted areas, atrophy, and vascular lesions

3. May be done with or without intravenous injection of dye for contrast enhancement

B. Nursing responsibilities

1. Explain procedure to the patient; inform the patient that it will be necessary to lie still and that the equipment is complex but will cause no pain or discomfort

2. If the facility is small, arrange transportation to a larger facility that has the required equipment

3. Evaluate the patient for possible allergy to iodine, a component of the contrast material

4. Withhold food for approximately 4 hours prior to testing; dye may cause nausea in sensitive patients

5. Remove wigs, clips, and pins prior to the test

6. No special care is required after the procedure

Electroencephalography (EEG)

A. Definition

1. Measurement and recording of electrical activity of the brain in the form of waves

2. Provides information about seizure disorders, local tumors, infections of the central nervous system, and chemical toxicity

3. May be done at the bedside with portable equipment but generally is done in a special room to decrease distractions and interference

4. The patient may be asked to hyperventilate, or flashing lights may be utilized to trigger any abnormal wave pattern

B. Nursing responsibilities

1. Explain procedure to the patient; common misconceptions include fear of receiving electrical shock and fear that personal thoughts will be revealed

2. Provide the patient with a normal meal to avoid hypoglycemia; stimulants such as coffee or tea and depressants are withheld because of their effect on the EEG

3. Shampoo hair after the test to remove collodion, the conducting jelly

Electromyography

A. Definition

1. Measurement and recording of the electrical activity of specific muscles into which needle electrodes have been inserted

2. In addition to providing information about primary muscle disease, it helps differentiate be-

tween motor symptoms that are secondary to neurologic disturbances
B. Nursing responsibilities
1. Explain procedure to the patient
2. No special preparation or postprocedure care is required

Pneumoencephalography
A. Definition
1. Visualization of the ventricles and subarachnoid space of the brain by means of air contrast
2. Air is injected into the cerebrospinal fluid usually at L4 or L5 and rises to the brain
3. X-ray pictures of the brain are taken with the patient in a variety of positions to allow the air to disperse to the required spaces
B. Nursing responsibilities
1. Explain procedure to the patient and obtain a signed consent
2. Withhold fluid and food prior to the procedure
3. Remove dentures
4. Remove hair decorations; comb the hair back to prevent interference with the procedure
5. After the procedure
a. Observe the patient for neurologic signs
b. Observe for signs of shock, such as tachycardia
c. Keep the patient in a recumbent position for 24 hours
d. Encourage fluids

Cerebral Angiography
A. Definition—visualization of the cerebral vasculature with a contrast dye and x-ray projection
B. Nursing responsibilities (see angiography under related diagnostic procedures of the circulatory system)

Myelography
A. Definition—visualization of the spinal canal after it has been injected with radiopaque dye
B. Nursing responsibilities
1. Explain procedure to the patient and obtain a signed consent
2. Maintain the n.p.o. status prior to the test
3. Remove dentures and metal objects
4. Administer a sedative as ordered prior to the procedure
5. After the procedure
a. Observe for neurologic signs
b. Keep the patient in a recumbent position for 24 hours
c. Encourage fluid intake

RELATED GENERAL NURSING PROCEDURES
Care of the Unconscious Patient
A. Observe for changes in vital signs and neurologic status
B. Keep the patient's head slightly elevated to reduce venous pressure within the cranial cavity
C. Do the following as needed:
1. Maintain the airway by suctioning as necessary; use an airway or endotracheal tube
2. Provide sterile tracheostomy care as well as frequent oral hygiene
3. Position the patient to prevent pressure areas from forming decubiti
4. Maintain adequate fluid balance
5. Evaluate the patient's level of consciousness at frequent intervals
6. If the patient's eyes remain open, protect the corneas with moistened pads, mineral oil, or ointment as ordered
7. Protect the patient during seizures

Transfer of Patients
A. Definitions
1. Methods of moving a patient from one surface to another (e.g., bed to wheelchair, wheelchair to commode)
2. Weight-bearing transfers—by patients who have at least one stable lower extremity (e.g., hemiplegics, patients who have undergone a unilateral lower extremity amputation, patients with a fractured hip)
3. Non-weight-bearing transfers—by patients who do not have a stable lower extremity (e.g., paraplegics not wearing braces, patients with double lower extremity amputations)
B. Nursing responsibilities
1. Assess the patient's abilities (e.g., sitting tolerance, balance, weight-bearing potential, strength, motivation, understanding of principles of transfer)
2. Identify need for and selection of assistive devices (e.g., slide board, trapeze, wheelchair with a removable arm, hydraulic lift)
3. Select most appropriate transfer method and teach and assist the patient with this new technique
4. Provide for patient safety (e.g., encourage use of low-heeled shoes, lock wheelchair brakes during transfer, remove hazards [scatter rugs, slippery floors, stepstools], ensure adequate assistance)
5. Communicate individualized transfer techniques

by instructing the patient and family and informing the entire health team

6. Consider the patient's abilities and disabilities when deciding appropriate transfer technique and need for assistive devices (e.g., hemiplegia—place the wheelchair on the side opposite the affected extremities; paraplegia—may use trapeze, slide board, or wheelchair with removable arm)

7. Maintain correct proximity and visual relationship of wheelchair to the bed (e.g., paraplegia—place the wheelchair lateral or perpendicular to the bed; hemiplegia—place the wheelchair at a 30-degree angle to the bed on the unaffected side)

Use of Assist Devices for Passive Positioning

A. Devices and their purposes
1. Stryker or Foster frames—allow for horizontal turning of the patient
2. CircOlectric bed—allows for vertical turning of the patient; the patient can be placed in a variety of positions (Trendelenburg, prone, standing, supine); one nurse can turn the patient, with the electric motor providing the power; attachments permit application of traction and other accessories
3. Purposes
   a. Hyperextension
   b. Immobilization
   c. Correction of deformities
   d. Facilitation of turning
   e. Relief of pressure
   f. Promotion of body functions (circulation, respiration, elimination)
B. Nursing responsibilities
1. Turn the patient all in one piece
2. Since frames are narrow, for safety purposes do not permit the patient to sit up, roll over, or reach out to the side; do not place extremely obese and disoriented patients on a frame
3. Since only the prone and supine and, on the CircOlectric bed, vertical positions can be used, strict attention must be paid to prevention of decubiti
4. Before releasing pivot pins, secure all bolts and straps to ensure patient safety
5. When turning the CircOlectric bed, do so slowly so that the patient's cerebral circulation can adjust to the new position; observe for signs of hypotension

Walking with a Cane

A. Purposes
1. Improve stability of the patient with a lower limb disability
2. Maintain balance
3. Prevent further injury
4. Provide security while developing confidence in ambulating
5. Relieve pressure on weight-bearing joints
6. Assist in increasing speed of ambulation with less fatigue
7. Provide for greater mobility and independence
B. Nursing responsibilities
1. Ascertain that the patient is able to bear weight on the affected extremity
2. Ensure that the patient is able to use the upper extremity opposite the affected lower extremity
3. Measure to determine the length of cane required
   a. Highest point should be about level with the great trochanter
   b. Handpiece should allow 30 degrees of flexion at the elbow with the wrist held in extension
4. Explain the proper techniques in using a cane
   a. Hold in the hand opposite the affected extremity
   b. Advance the cane and the affected extremity simultaneously, and then the unaffected leg
   c. Keep the cane close to the body
   d. When climbing, step up with the unaffected extremity and then place the cane and the affected lower extremity on the step; when descending, reverse the procedure
5. Observe the patient for incorrect use of the cane
   a. Leaning the body over the cane
   b. Shortening the stride on the unaffected side
   c. Inability to develop a normal walking pattern
   d. Persistence of the abnormal gait pattern after the cane is no longer needed

Locomotion on Wheels

The patient is propelled or propels himself on wheels or casters in a sitting position

A. Purposes
1. Support the body
2. Decrease cardiac workload
3. Promote independence and stimulate activities
4. Provide mobility for those who cannot ambulate or those who can ambulate but whose ambulation is unsteady, unsafe, or too strenuous
B. Nursing responsibilities
1. Instruct the patient that prolonged sitting in one

position can cause flexion contractures of the hips and knees and ischial decubiti (encourage the patient to change body positions and to use padded cushions and exercises such as push-ups every hour to relieve pressure)
  2. Ensure that specific devices necessary for patient safety (e.g., wheel brakes, arm locks, seat belts, swing foot rests) are in operating condition
  3. Alert the wheelchair-bound patient to the accessories that meet the patient's specific needs (e.g., removable arms, lap boards, knobs on the handrims, extra long leg panels, battery or motor propulsion)

Crutch Walking

A. Purposes
  1. Support body weight, assist weak muscles, and provide joint stability
  2. Relieve pain
  3. Prevent further injury and provide for improvement of function
  4. Allow for greater patient independence
B. Nursing responsibilities
  1. Ensure proper fit of crutches by measuring the distance from the anterior fold of the axilla to a point 15 cm (6 inches) out from the heel
     a. Axillary bars must be 5 cm (2 inches) below the axillae and may or may not be padded
     b. Hand bars should allow almost complete extension of the arm with the elbow flexed about 30 degrees when the patient places weight on the hands
     c. Rubber crutch tips should be in good condition, about 5.1 to 7.6 cm (2 to 3 inches) in height, with a circumference of 3.8 to 4.4 cm (1½ to 1¾ inches)
  2. Assist the patient in use of proper technique, depending on ability to bear weight and to take steps with either one or both of the lower extremities
     a. Four-point alternate crutch gait
        (1) Right crutch, left foot, left crutch, right foot
        (2) Equal but partial weight bearing on each limb
        (3) Slow but stable gait; there are always 3 points of support on the floor
        (4) The patient must be able to manipulate both extremities and get one foot ahead of the other (e.g., persons with polio, arthritis, cerebral palsy)
     b. Two-point alternate crutch gait
        (1) Right crutch and left foot simultaneously

        (2) There are always 2 points of support on the floor
        (3) This is a more rapid version of the 4-point gait and requires more balance and strength (e.g., a bilateral amputee)
     c. Three-point gait
        (1) Advance both crutches and the weaker lower extremity simultaneously, then the stronger lower extremity
        (2) Fairly rapid gait, but requires more balance and strength in the arms and the good lower extremity
        (3) Used when one leg can support the whole body weight and the other cannot take full weight-bearing (e.g., a patient with a fractured hip)
     d. Swing crutch gaits
        (1) Swing-to gait
           (a) Place both crutches forward, lift and swing the body *up* to the crutches, then place crutches in front of the body and continue
           (b) There are always 2 points of support on the floor
           (c) This technique is indicated for any patient with adequate power in the upper arms
        (2) Swing-through gait
           (a) Place both crutches forward, lift and swing the body *through* the crutches, then place crutches in front of the body and continue
           (b) Very difficult gait, because as the patient swings through the crutches it necessitates rolling the pelvis forward and arching the back to get the center of gravity in front of the hips
           (c) Indicated for the patient who has power in the trunk and upper extremities, excellent balance, self-confidence, and a dash of daring (e.g., a bilateral amputee, a paraplegic with braces)
     e. Tripod crutch gaits
        (1) Tripod alternate gait
           (a) Right crutch, left crutch, drag the body and legs forward
           (b) The patient constantly maintains a tripod position—both crutches are held fairly widespread out front while both feet are held together in the back
           (c) Necessary for the individual who

cannot place one extremity ahead of the other (e.g., a person with flaccid paralysis from poliomyelitis, one with spinal cord injuries)

(2) Tripod simultaneous gait

(a) Place both crutches forward, drag the body and legs forward

(b) Because the tripod must have a large base, the patient's body must be inclined forward sufficiently to keep the center of gravity in front of the hips

3. Observe the patient for incorrect use of crutches
   a. Using the body in poor mechanical fashion
   b. Hiking hips with abduction gait (common in amputees)
   c. Lifting crutches while still bearing down on them
   d. Walking on ball of foot with foot turned outward and flexion at hip or knee level
   e. Hunching shoulders (crutches usually too long) or stooping with shoulders (crutches usually too short)
   f. Looking downward while ambulating
   g. Bearing weight under arms should be avoided to prevent injury to the nerves in the brachial plexus; damage to these nerves can cause paralysis and is known as crutch palsy

Ambulation with a Walker

A. Purposes
   1. Maintain balance
   2. Provide additional support because of wide area of contact with floor
   3. Allow for some ambulatory independence
B. Nursing responsibilities
   1. Assist the patient in selecting a walker
      a. Device should not be used unless the patient will never be able to ambulate with a cane or crutches
      b. Measurements for a walker are the same as for a cane
      c. The patient must have strong elbow extensors and shoulder depressors and partial strength in the hands and wrist muscles
      d. The patient needs maximum support to ensure security and enhance confidence
      e. Device is ordinarily limited to the home because it cannot be used on steps
   2. Assist the patient in ambulating with the walker
      a. Lift the device off the floor and place forward a short distance, then advance between the walker

b. Two-wheeled walkers—raise back legs of the device off the floor, roll walker forward, then advance to it
c. Four-wheeled walkers—push device forward on floor and then walk to it

3. Observe the patient for incorrect use of the walker
   a. Keeping arms rigid and swinging through to counterbalance the position of the lower extremity
   b. Tending to lean forward with abnormal flexion at the hips
   c. Tending to step forward with the good leg and shuffle the affected leg up to the bar

Ambulation with Braces or Splints

A. Purposes
   1. Support and protect weakened muscles
   2. Prevent and correct anatomic deformities
   3. Aid in controlling involuntary muscle movements
   4. Immobilize and protect a diseased or injured joint
   5. Provide for improvement of function
B. Nursing responsibilities
   1. Keep equipment in good repair (e.g., oil joints, replace straps when worn, wash with saddle soap)
   2. Provide adequate shoes (e.g., keep in good repair, heels low and wide, high top to hold the heel in the shoe)
   3. Examine the skin daily for evidence of breakdown at pressure points
   4. Check alignment of the braces (e.g., leg braces—joints should coincide with body joints; back brace—upright bars in center of back, brace should grip the pelvis and trocanter firmly, lacing should begin from the bottom)

Ear Irrigations

A. Definition
   1. Introduction of fluid into the external auditory canal
   2. Usually done for cleansing purposes but can be used to apply antiseptic solutions
B. Nursing responsibilities
   1. Explain procedure to the patient
   2. Assemble equipment: irrigating solution, sterile irrigating syringe, cotton balls, cotton-tipped applicators, towel
   3. Assist the patient to sitting position with the head tilted to affected side to facilitate drainage
   4. Gently pull up and back on the external ear of

an adult, down and forward on a child, to straighten the canal

5. Direct solution into the canal without exerting excessive force; collect returns in a basin
6. Dry the outer ear and have patient lie on the affected side
7. Record the procedure, type of drainage, etc.

Instillation of Eye Medications

A. Purpose—to provide therapeutic effect of medication ordered
B. Nursing responsibilities
1. Explain procedure to the patient
2. Position the patient with the head slightly backward
3. Pull lower eyelid down and place ointment or solution in the center of the cul-de-sac of the eye that is to be medicated (check order: O.D.— right eye, O.U.—both eyes, O.S.—left eye)
4. Allow the patient to close the eyes gently and instruct that they should not be rubbed
5. Record administration of medication appropriately

MAJOR DISEASES
Migraine Headache

A. Etiology and pathophysiology
1. Caused by constriction and then dilation of the cerebral arteries
2. Individuals who have migraines are frequently described as perfectionists, inflexible, and ambitious
3. Incidence higher in females
B. Signs and symptoms
1. Subjective
a. Severe throbbing pain, often in temporal or supraorbital area, that lasts several hours to a day
b. Fatigue and irritability may precede headache
c. Nausea
d. Visual disturbances
2. Objective
a. Pallor
b. Vomiting
C. Treatment
1. Methysergide maleate (Sansert) to prevent attacks; should not be continued for more than 6 to 12 months consecutively; then, should be omitted for a few months before it is resumed
2. Ergotamine tartrate (Glynergen) or ergotamine with caffeine (Cafergot) to relieve migraines

3. Elimination of factors (physical, psychologic, environmental) that precipitate illness
D. Nursing care
1. Assist the patient in identifying situations that seem to precipitate attacks
2. Suport the patient in modification of life-style and development of insight
3. Provide a dark, quiet environment when migraine begins
4. If the patient is nauseated
a. Administer an antiemetic if ordered
b. Offer small, frequent sips of fluid as tolerated
c. Assist with mouth care

Head Injuries

A. Etiology and pathophysiology
1. Result from trauma, frequently seen after motor vehicle accidents
2. Fractures
a. Linear—simple break in the bone
b. Depressed—break that results in fragments of bone penetrating the brain tissue
3. Hemorrhages
a. Epidural—hematoma forms between the dura and the skull; may result from a laceration of the middle meningeal artery
b. Subdural—hematoma forms between the dura and arachnoid layers; generally follows venous damage
4. Concussion—temporary disruption of synaptic activity
5. Contusions—bruising of brain tissue, with slight bleeding of small cerebral vessels into surroundng tissues
B. Signs and symptoms
1. Subjective
a. Lethargy
b. Indifference to surroundings
2. Objective
a. Signs of increased intracranial pressure (see brain surgery)
b. Lack of orientation to time and place
c. Paresthesia
d. Labored respirations
e. Positive Babinski sign (stroking bottom of the foot causes dorsiflexion of the foot)
f. Coma
g. Dilation and fixation of pupils
C. Treatment
1. Control seizures with anticonvulsants
2. Maintain adequate fluid and electrolyte balance

3. Surgical intervention in cases of depressed skull fractures or hematomas
D. Nursing care
1. Observe the patient for signs of increased intracranial pressure (see brain surgery); institute neural checks every 15 minutes for several hours, progressing to every hour and then every 4 hours
2. Maintain airway
3. If the patient is unconscious, see care of the unconscious patient
4. If surgery is indicated, see care of the patient undergoing brain surgery
5. Institute seizure precautions; administer anticonvulsants if ordered

Brain Tumor

A. Etiology and pathophysiology
1. Either benign or malignant; they require intervention, since the skull can not accommodate the increasing size of the tumor, and intracranial pressure rises
2. Classified according to tissue of origin
   a. Meningioma—occurs outside the brain from the covering meninges
   b. Acoustic neuroma and optic nerve spongioblastoma polare—occur from the cranial nerves
   c. Gliomas—originate in brain tissue
   d. Hemangioblastomas—occur from within blood vessels
B. Signs and symptoms
1. Subjective
   a. Headache that increases with stooping
   b. Lethargy
2. Objective
   a. Vomiting
   b. Papilledema (noted on ophthalmoscopy)
   c. Abnormal brain waves on the EEG
3. Symptoms may vary depending on location of tumor
   a. Frontal lobe—personality changes, focal seizures, blurred vision, hemiparesis or aphasia
   b. Temporal lobe—seizures, headache, papilledema, aphasia
   c. Parietal lobe—jacksonian convulsions, visual loss
   d. Occipital region—focal seizures, visual hallucinations
   e. Cerebellar region—loss of coordination, papilledema
C. Treatment

1. Radiation therapy or chemotherapy for inaccessible tumors
2. Brain surgery for complete removal of the lesion if location and extension into surrounding tissues permit
3. Steroids, anticonvulsives, and osmotic diuretics to control symptoms
D. Nursing care
1. Give emotional support to the patient undergoing palliative procedures
2. Maintain the patient as comfortably as possible with analgesics and antiemetics as ordered
3. If the patient is to undergo brain surgery
   a. Obtain consent for surgery and removal of hair (save the hair)
   b. After surgery keep the patient's head elevated 30 cm (12 inches) to aid drainage
   c. Observe for return of cough and swallowing reflexes
   d. Assess the patient's level of consciousness and neurologic status for changes
   e. Utilize hypothermia as ordered if the patient is febrile; fever increases metabolic needs of the brain
   f. Observe dressings for CSF leakage or hemorrhage
   g. Maintain accurate intake and output records
   h. Observe for signs of increased intracranial pressure
      (1) Restlessness
      (2) Weakness or paralysis
      (3) Increased blood pressure
      (4) Decreased pulse
      (5) Pupillary dilation

Brain Abscess

A. Etiology and pathophysiology
1. Occurs when there is an infection in another region of the body that spreads to the brain or after a penetrating head wound
2. Results from invasion of the brain: formation and collection of exudate within the brain tissue
B. Signs and symptoms
1. Subjective
   a. Malaise
   b. Headache
   c. Anorexia
2. Objective
   a. Fever
   b. Vomiting
   c. Weight loss
C. Treatment

1. Large doses of antibiotics
2. In severe cases, a craniotomy may be performed to allow removal of the abscess
D. Nursing care
   1. Observe the patient for changes in vital signs or neurologic responses
   2. See care of the patient undergoing brain surgery

Cerebral Aneurysm

A. Etiology and pathophysiology
   1. Sac formed by dilation of the walls of an artery within the cranial cavity
   2. May be the result of a congenital weakness in the vessel, trauma, or arteriosclerosis
   3. Symptoms occur when the aneurysm compresses nearby nerves or when it ruptures
B. Signs and symptoms
   1. Subjective
      a. Unilateral headache
      b. Pain in the eye
      c. Diplopia
      d. Tinnitus
   2. Objective
      a. Rigidity of the back of the neck and spine
      b. Ptosis of the eyelid
      c. Hemiparesis
C. Treatment
   1. Attempt to keep the patient hypotensive, usually with rauwolfia alkaloids
   2. If there is a stalk connecting the aneurysm, clips may be inserted surgically to cut off blood supply to the aneurysm permanently
D. Nursing care
   1. See care of the patient undergoing brain surgery
   2. See care of the patient with a cerebral hemorrhage

Cerebral Hemorrhage

A. Etiology and pathophysiology
   1. Result of arteriosclerosis, trauma, hemorrhagic disorder, brain tumor, or ruptured aneurysms
   2. May occur in various areas of the brain
      a. Subarachnoid hemorrhage—generally from a congenital aneurysm near the circle of Willis
      b. Intracerebral hemorrhage—generally occurs because of hypertension, although may result from various disorders; the bleeding is usually located in the basal ganglia
      c. Subdural hemorrhage—generally involves a bridging vein, and therefore more time may pass before a hematoma is formed
B. Signs and symptoms

1. Subjective
   a. Headache
   b. Dizziness
2. Objective
   a. Convulsions
   b. Hemiplegia
   c. Unconsciousness
   d. Right-sided hemiplegia usually accompanied by aphasia
C. Treatment
   1. Complete bed rest
   2. Steroids, stool softeners, anticonvulsants, analgesics, aminocaproic acid (Amicar) by continuous IV drip to inhibit fibrinolysis
   3. Surgical intervention if indicated
   4. See care of the unconscious patient

Cerebral Vascular Accident (CVA or Stroke)

A. Etiology and pathophysiology
   1. Term applied to destruction (infarction) of brain cells caused by a reduction in the oxygen supply
   2. Caused by a sudden or gradual interruption in the blood supply following an intracerebral hemorrhage, blockage of vessels by thrombi or emboli, or vascular insufficiency
   3. Symptoms depend on the area of the brain involved and extent of damage
   4. Conditions that predispose to a CVA include cerebral arteriosclerosis, syphilis, dehydration, trauma, and hypertension
   5. Transient ischemic attacks (TIA) may also occur without causing permanent damage; these usually last only a few minutes
   6. Incidence increases with age
B. Signs and symptoms
   1. Subjective
      a. Syncope
      b. Changes in level of consciousness
      c. Transient paresthesias
      d. Headache
      e. Mood swings
   2. Objective
      a. Convulsions
      b. Nuchal rigidity (if caused by subarachnoid or intracerebral hemorrhage)
      c. Hemiplegia on side opposite the lesion
      d. Aphasia—brain unable to fulfill its communicative functions because of damage to its input, integrative, or output centers; a disturbance of language function that may involve impairment of the ability to read, write, speak, or interpret messages

(1) Expressive aphasia—difficulty making thoughts known to others; speaking and writing is most affected

(2) Receptive aphasia—difficulty understanding what others are trying to communicate; interpretation of speech and reading is most affected

(3) Expressive-receptive aphasia—equal difficulty with speaking, writing, interpreting speech, and reading

e. Alterations in reflexes
f. Functional disorders of the bladder and bowel
g. CSF is bloody if cerebral or subarachnoid hemorrhage is present
h. Abnormal EEG
i. Cerebral angiography may reveal vascular abnormalities such as aneurysms, narrowing, or occlusions
j. If increased intracranial pressure exists, as with hemorrhage, elevated blood pressure and bounding pulse

C. Treatment
1. Complete bed rest with sedation as needed
2. Maintenance of nutrition by the parenteral route or nasogastric feedings if the patient is unable to swallow
3. Anticoagulant therapy
4. Antihypertensive agents if indicated
5. Surgical intervention
   a. To relieve pressure and control bleeding if hemorrhage is present
   b. Carotid endarterectomy to improve cerebral blood flow when carotid arteries are narrowed by arteriosclerotic patches may be done on a patient in stable condition

D. Nursing care
1. Assess the patient's respiratory functioning (vital signs, type and rate of respirations, color, blood gases, etc.)
2. Observe for level of consciousness
3. Monitor vital signs
4. Observe for signs of increasing intracranial pressure
5. Assess swallowing and gag reflexes
6. Maintain patency of the airway by positioning, suctioning, and inserting an artificial airway
7. Provide for drainage and expansion of lungs by placing patient in a low semi-Fowler position with the head turned to the side
8. Provide oxygen as necessary
9. Provide frequent oral hygiene
10. Encourage the patient to breathe deeply and cough; administer intermittent positive pressure if necessary
11. Provide elastic stockings for both legs
12. Provide for frequent nursing observations, since the patient may be unable to signal for assistance
13. Prevent decubiti
    a. Provide special care to the back and bony prominences; keep the patient clean and dry
    b. Relieve pressure by use of mechanical and supportive devices
    c. Turn the patient every 2 hours
    d. Provide adequate hydration to maintain skin turgor
14. Prevent muscle atrophy and contractures
    a. Provide for active and passive range of motion and other exercises
    b. Use footboards and other devices to prevent footdrop, flexion of fingers, abduction of hips, adduction of shoulders and arms
15. Encourage the aphasic patient to communicate
    a. Be aware of own reactions to the speech difficulty
    b. Evaluate extent of the patient's ability to understand and express self at a simple level
    c. Include the health team, especially the speech therapist, in planning patient care
    d. Involve the family as much as possible
    e. Convey to the patient that there is a problem with communication, not with intelligence
    f. Try to eliminate anxiety and tension related to communication attempts (e.g., be consistent, give the patient time to respond, employ a calm, accepting, and deliberate manner)
    g. Help the patient set attainable goals
    h. Stimulate the patient's communication without pushing to point of frustration
    i. Keep distractions at a minimum, since they interfere with the reception and integration of messages (e.g., one-to-one conversations rather than group conversations, shut off the radio when speaking)
    j. Speak slowly, clearly, and in short sentences and do not raise voice
    k. Use alternate means of communication (e.g., gestures, writing, picture board)
    l. Involve the patient in social interactions (e.g., encourage socialization, do not anticipate all needs, ask questions and expect

answers, do not ignore the patient in group conversations)

m. Make a definite transition between tasks to prevent or reduce confusion

n. Be alert for clues and gestures when speech is garbled (e.g., continue to listen, nod, and make occasional neutral statements, let the patient know when you cannot understand)

o. Provide for periodic reevaluation to demonstrate to the patient and health team the effect and nature of progress

16. Attempt to prevent fecal impaction and/or urinary tract problems

a. Provide adequate fluid intake

b. Provide a diet with enough roughage for sufficient quantity of bowel content and proper consistency for evacuation

c. Avoid preoccupation with elimination

d. Avoid the overt encouragement of incontinence (e.g., through the routine use of diapers, Chux, and other depersonalizing devices)

e. Stimulate normal elimination by exercise and activity

f. Help the patient develop regular bowel and bladder patterns

g. Respect the individual (e.g., provide for privacy, individuality of routine, avoidance of delay); encourage the patient to make decisions

h. Utilize physical and psychologic techniques to stimulate elimination (e.g., running water, place the patient's hands in warm water, place the patient in as normal a position as possible for elimination)

i. Create an environment that keeps sensory monotony to a minimum (e.g., orient to time and place, use a radio and television selectively, increase the patient's social contacts, provide visual stimuli, extend environment beyond the patient's room)

j. Provide for self-esteem (e.g., encourage the patient to wear own clothes, do self-care activities, make decisions)

k. Accept and explore the patient's feelings of fear, anger, and depression; a disabled person has few avenues by which to express anger; incontinence is often used in this manner

17. Keep the side rails in place or use safety straps

18. Provide the patient with tube feedings if swallowing and gag reflexes are depressed or absent

19. Provide food in a form that is easily swallowed

20. Assist the patient with feeding (e.g., use a padded spoon handle; feed on the unaffected side of mouth; feed in as close to a sitting position as possible)

21. Provide realistic encouragement and praise

22. Accept the patient's mood swings and emotional outbursts

23. Assist the patient and family to set realistic goals

24. Help the patient to adjust to change in body image and altered self-concept

Epilepsy (Convulsive Disorders)

A. Etiology and pathophysiology

1. Abnormal discharge of electric impulses by the nerve cells in the brain from idiopathic or secondary causes resulting in the typical manifestation of seizures

2. Onset of idiopathic epilepsy generally before age 30

3. Other conditions associated with seizures include brain tumor, CVA, hypoglycemia, and head trauma

4. Types of seizures

a. Generalized motor seizures (grand mal)—aura, loss of consciousness, tonic and clonic movements, interruption of respirations, loss of bladder and bowel control

b. Petit mal seizures—brief transient loss of consciousness with or without minor motor movements of eyes, head, or extremities

c. Jacksonian seizures (focal-motor seizures)—disturbed sensations and interrupted motor functioning, beginning in a somewhat localized area of the body and progressing to other parts of the body; the areas affected by the seizure usually reflect the area of the brain involved

d. Psychomotor seizures—characterized by a transient clouding of consciousness, behavioral alterations, and changes in affect and perception; may become violent and engage in antisocial activity

e. Status epilepticus—continuous convulsion that may completely exhaust the patient and lead to death

B. Signs and symptoms (grand mal seizures)

1. Subjective

a. Aura or warning sensation such as seeing spots or feeling dizzy often precedes a grand mal seizure

b. Loss of consciousness during seizure
c. Lethargy often follows return to consciousness
d. Dyspnea
2. Objective
a. Pupils become fixed and dilated
b. Often the patient cries out as seizure begins or as air is exhaled forcefully
c. Tonic and clonic movement of the muscles
d. Incontinence
e. Abnormal EEG
C. Treatment
1. Anticonvulsant therapy continued throughout life
a. Phenytoin sodium (Dilantin), mephenytoin (Mesantoin) and primidone (Mysoline) often used to control grand mal seizures
b. Trimethadione (Tridione), phensuximide (Milontin), and ethosuximide (Zarontin) to control petit mal seizures
c. Diazepam (Valium) given IV to treat status epilepticus
2. Sedatives (e.g., phenobarbital) used to reduce emotional stress
D. Nursing care
1. Assist the patient to identify the aura
2. Help the patient prepare and provide some protection before the seizure develops
3. Provide protection for the patient during and after the seizure by maintaining and protecting from injury; a tongue blade should not be forced into a patient's mouth when teeth are firmly clenched, since this may cause the tongue to occlude the airway or may loosen teeth
4. Encourage the patient to carry and wear a medical alert tag
5. Encourage the patient to take medications even when seizure free
6. Help the patient plan a schedule that provides for adequate rest and a reduction of stress
7. Instruct the patient to refrain from excessive use of alcohol, since it is contraindicated with the medications
8. Observe and teach the patient and family to observe the aura, initial point of seizure, type of seizure, level of consciousness, loss of control of bladder and bowel, progression of seizure, and postseizure condition
9. Encourage the patient to express feelings about illness and the necessary changes in life-style and self-image
10. Assist the patient and family to accept the diagnosis and develop some understanding of the disease process
11. Help the patient understand that medication must be taken continuously for the remainder of life
12. Refer the patient for job counseling as needed
13. Encourage the patient and family to attend meetings of the local epilepsy association
14. Refer the patient for genetic counseling if appropriate (age of patient, cause of seizures)

Mononeuritis and Polyneuritis

A. Etiology and pathophysiology
1. May involve only one nerve (mononeuritis) or several nerves (polyneuritis)
2. Mononeuritis occurs when there is trauma to the trunk of a nerve, such as from pressure of a tumor, dislocation of a joint, or infection; the nerve involved near the area of injury becomes part of the scar tissue or callus of bone
3. Polyneuritis occurs when there is a deficiency of thiamine (e.g. in alcoholism) and subsequent disturbances in metabolism of nerve tissue
B. Signs and symptoms
1. Subjective
a. Pain which increases after any body movement that stretches nerve involved
b. Burning pain along the injured nerve in mononeuritis
2. Objective
a. Swelling over the affected nerve in mononeuritis
b. Paresis or paralysis of the affected limb in polyneuritis
C. Treatment
1. Mononeuritis
a. Sympathetic nerve block
b. Physical therapy
c. Analgesics
2. Polyneuritis
a. Thiamine replacement
b. Bed rest
c. Analgesics
D. Nursing care
1. Administer pain medications as ordered
2. Provide emotional support for the patient during the course of hospitalization

Bell's Palsy

A. Etiology and pathophysiology
1. Paralysis that occurs on one side of the face as a result of an inflamed seventh cranial (facial) nerve; generally lasts only 2 to 8 weeks but may last longer in older patients

2. May follow trauma or exposure to the elements
3. Most common between ages 20 and 50 years
B. Signs and symptoms
  1. Subjective
    a. Facial pain
    b. Difficulty eating
  2. Objective
    a. Distortion of face
    b. Speech difficulty
    c. Diminished blink reflex
    d. Increased lacrimation
C. Treatment
  1. Prednisone therapy
  2. Heat, massage, and electric stimulation are used to maintain circulation and muscle tone
  3. Prevention of corneal irritation with eyedrops and the use of a protective eye shield
D. Nursing care
  1. Explain to the patient in most cases recovery occurs within 2 to 8 weeks
  2. Assess blink reflex and the patient's ability to close the eye
  3. Keep the face warm
  4. Teach the patient to massage the face gently and perform simple exercises such as blowing
  5. Encourage ventilation of feelings, since self-image will be affected

Trigeminal Neuralgia (Tic Douloureux)

A. Etiology and pathophysiology
  1. Disorder of the fifth cranial (trigeminal) nerve characterized by excruciating knifelike pain along the branches of the nerve
  2. Etiology unknown
  3. Incidence higher in women of middle and older age
B. Signs and symptoms
  1. Subjective
    a. Burning or knifelike pain lasting 1 to 15 minutes, usually over the lip or chin and in teeth
    b. Pain precipitated by stimulation of trigger zones during activities such as brushing hair and eating or when sitting in a cold draft
  2. Objective
    a. Sudden closure of an eye
    b. Twitching of the mouth
C. Treatment
  1. Carbamazepine (Tegretal) to relieve and prevent pain
  2. Antiepileptic drugs
  3. Injection of alcohol into the ganglion to relieve pain for several months or years until nerve regenerates

4. Surgical intervention involves sectioning the sensory root of the nerve, which will cause loss of all sensation in the area supplied by the nerve
D. Nursing care
  1. Prevent factors that can trigger an attack
    a. Avoid foods that are too hot or cold
    b. Use cotton pads to gently wash the patient's face
    c. Avoid jarring the bed
    d. Keep the room free of drafts
  2. Provide teaching to patients who have had surgery
    a. Inspection of the eye for foreign bodies, which the patient will not be able to feel, should be done several times a day
    b. Warm normal saline irrigation of the affected eye 2 or 3 times a day is helpful in preventing a corneal infection
    c. Dental checkups every 6 months, since dental caries will not produce pain

Paralysis Agitans (Parkinson's Disease)

A. Etiology and pathophysiology
  1. Progressive disorder in which there is a destruction of nerve cells in the basal ganglia of the brain, which results in a generalized degeneration of muscular function
  2. Suspected causes include neuromuscular imbalance (dopamine and acetylcholine), unknown virus, cerebral vascular disease, and chemical or physical trauma
B. Signs and symptoms
  1. Subjective
    a. Mild diffuse muscular pain
    b. Feelings of stiffness and rigidity, particularly of large joints
    c. Defects in judgment and emotional lability may be present, but intelligence is usually not impaired
    d. Sensitivity to heat
  2. Objective
    a. Increased difficulty in performing usual activities such as writing, dressing, and eating
    b. Generalized tremor commonly accompanied by "pill-rolling" movements of the thumb against the fingers; tremors usually reduced by intentional movements
    c. Various disorders of locomotion (e.g., bent posture, difficulty in rising from a sitting position, shuffling propulsive gait, loss of rhythmic arm swing when walking)
    d. Masklike facial expression with unblinking eyes

e. Low-pitched, slow, poorly modulated, poorly articulated speech
f. Drooling because of difficulty in swallowing saliva
g. Various autonomic symptoms (e.g., lacrimation, constipation, incontinence, decreased sexual capacity, excessive perspiration)

C. Treatment
1. Medical regimen is palliative rather than curative
2. Levodopa may be utilized to alleviate dopamine deficiency and decrease dyskinesia and rigidity
3. Anticholinergic agents that counteract the action of acetylcholine in the central nervous system
4. Medications to relieve related symptoms (e.g., antispasmodics, antihistamines, analgesics, sedatives)
5. Physiotherapy to reduce rigidity of muscles and prevent contractures
6. Surgical intervention using alcohol, freezing (cryosurgery), electric cautery, ultrasound, etc. to destroy the globus pallidus (to relieve rigidity), and/or the thalamus (to relieve tremor) portions of the brain

D. Nursing care
1. Provide a safe environment
2. Teach the patient or family to cut food into small bite-size pieces to prevent choking
3. Teach the patient activities to limit postural deformities (e.g., use firm mattress without a pillow, periodically lie prone, keep head and neck as erect as possible, consciously think about posture when walking)
4. Teach the patient activities to maintain gait as normal as possible (e.g., clasp hands behind the back when walking, exercise with stationary bicycle, use low-heeled shoes)
5. Teach and encourage daily physical therapy to limit rigidity and prevent contractures (e.g., warms baths, passive and active exercises)
6. Attempt to administer care when the patient is able to accept it emotionally and avoid rushing the patient, since he or she is unable to function under pressure
7. Encourage the patient to continue taking medications even though results may be minimal
8. Limit foods high in pyridoxine (vitamin B_6), since it decreases the effectiveness of L-dopa (e.g., dried beans, dry milk, salmon, tuna, pork, beef liver, kidneys)
9. Encourage small intake of alcohol, since it promotes relaxation and reduces rigidity

10. Encourage the intake of a well-balanced diet in small frequent amounts prepared so it is easily masticated
11. Encourage an adequate intake of roughage and fluids to avoid constipation
12. Suction when necessary to maintain an adequate airway (usually advanced stages)
13. Administer medications as ordered

Multiple Sclerosis, Disseminated Sclerosis

A. Etiology and pathophysiology
1. Chronic, debilitating, progressive disease with periods of remission and exacerbation characterized by randomly scattered patches of demyelination in the brain stem, cerebrum, cerebellum, and spinal cord
2. Cause unknown
3. Onset in early adult life

B. Signs and symptoms
1. Subjective
   a. Paresthesia
   b. Altered position sense
   c. Dysphagia
   d. Ataxia
   e. Weakness
   f. Diplopia
   g. Inappropriate emotional affect (euphoria occurs in later stages)
2. Objective
   a. Nystagmus
   b. Intention tremors
   c. Slurred speech
   d. Spastic paralysis
   e. Increased deep tendon reflexes
   f. Pallor of optic discs evident on examination with ophthalmoscope
   g. Increased gamma globulin levels in the CSF

C. Treatment
1. Generally palliative
2. Corticosteroids
3. Physiotherapy, rehabilitation, and psychotherapy

D. Nursing care
1. Encourage the patient to use supportive devices to maintain ambulation
2. Provide active and passive range of motion and other exercises
3. Teach the patient to use assistive devices in carrying out activities of daily living
4. Assist the family to understand why the patient should be permitted and encouraged to be active

5. Assist the patient and family to plan and implement a bowel and bladder regimen
6. Explain the disease process to both the patient and the family in understandable terms
7. Do not encourage false hopes during periods of remission
8. Spend time listening to both the patient and the family and encourage them to ventilate feelings
9. Attempt to refer the patient and family to the National Multiple Sclerosis Society
10. Encourage the patient to seek counseling and rehabilitation
11. Explain to the patient and family that mood swings and emotional alterations are part of the disease process
12. Help the patient reestablish a realistic self-image
13. Teach the patient to compensate for problems with gait (walk with feet farther apart to broaden base of support, use low-heeled shoes) and provide assistive devices when necessary (tripod cane, walker, wheelchair)
14. Teach the patient to compensate for loss of sensation by using a thermometer to test water temperature, avoiding constricting stockings, using protective clothing in cold weather, changing position frequently
15. Teach the patient to compensate for difficulty in swallowing by taking small bites, chewing well, using a straw with liquids using foods of more solid consistency
16. If the patient is immobilized
    a. Provide special skin care to prevent the formation of decubiti
    b. Provide special attention to joints and attempt to prevent dysfunctional contractures

Myasthenia Gravis

A. Etiology and pathophysiology
1. Neuromuscular disorder in which there is a disturbance in the transmission of impulses at the myoneural junction
2. Dysfunction thought to be caused by rapid breakdown or insufficient supply of acetylcholine at the junction
3. Highest incidence in young adult females
4. Myasthenic crisis refers to the sudden inability to swallow or maintain respirations due to weakness of the muscles of respiration
B. Signs and symptoms
1. Subjective
    a. Extreme muscle weakness, which becomes progressively worse as the muscle is used but disappears with rest
    b. Dysphagia (difficulty chewing)
    c. Diplopia
    d. Dysarthria (difficulty speaking)
2. Objective
    a. Ptosis of the lid
    b. Weak voice
    c. Myasthenic smile (snarling, nasal smile)
    d. Strabismus
    e. Diagnostic measures include administration of neostigmine (Prostigmin) subcutaneously or IV administration of edrophonium (Tensilon) to provide spontaneous relief of symptoms; edrophonium is also used to distinguish myasthenic crisis from toxic effects of neostigmine and similar drugs
C. Treatment
1. Specific medications that block the action of cholinesterase at the myoneural junction
    a. Neostigmine (Prostigmin)
    b. Pyridostigmine bromide (Mestinon)
    c. Ambenonium chloride (Mytelase)
2. X-ray therapy of the thymus may cause partial remission
3. Corticosteroids or ACTH
4. Tracheostomy with mechanical ventilation is often necessary in myasthenic crisis
D. Nursing care
1. Administer medications on strict time schedule to prevent onset of symptoms; instruct the patient and family to do the same
2. Observe for signs of dyspnea, dysphagia, and dysarthria, which may indicate myasthenic crisis
3. Have an emergency tracheostomy set at bedside
4. Plan activity to avoid fatigue based on the individual's tolerance
5. Instruct the patient to avoid people with upper respiratory tract infections, since pneumonia may develop as a result of fatigued respiratory muscles
6. Encourage the patient to carry a medical alert card or identification stating condition
7. Do not administer morphine to patients receiving anticholinesterases, since these drugs potentiate the effects of morphine and may cause respiratory depression
8. Provide emotional support and close contact with the patient to allay anxiety
9. Administer tube feedings when necessary if the

patient has difficulty swallowing so that aspiration will not occur

10. In severe instances anticipate all needs, since the patient is too weak to turn, drink, or even request assistance

Guillain-Barré Syndrome

A. Etiology and pathophysiology
   1. Cause unknown; thought to be linked to swine flu–like virus
   2. Changes in the motor cells of the spinal cord and medulla with areas of demyelination
   3. Most common in young adults
B. Signs and symptoms
   1. Subjective
      a. Generalized weakness
      b. Paresthesia
   2. Objective
      a. Paralysis begins in lower extremities; ascends within the body, usually 24 to 27 hours
      b. Respiratory paralysis
      c. Hypertension, tachycardia, and low-grade fever
C. Treatment
   1. Steroids
   2. Support vital functions (similar to that for poliomyelitis)
D. Nursing care
   1. Observe vital signs and vital capacity
   2. Suction, provide fluid replacement therapy, and monitor functioning of the respirator as required
   3. Provide emotional support to the patient and family because of the severity and lengthy convalescent period

Amyotrophic Lateral Sclerosis (ALS)

A. Etiology and pathophysiology
   1. Cause unknown
   2. Progressive degenerative process involving the spinal, corticobulbar, and lower motor neurons, with subsequent atrophic and spastic changes in the cranial as well as the spinal muscles
   3. Occurs more frequently in men than in women
B. Signs and symptoms
   1. Subjective
      a. Muscular weakness
      b. Malaise
   2. Objective
      a. Irregular spasmodic twitching in small muscle groups (fasciculations)
      b. Difficulty in chewing, swallowing, speaking
      c. Outbursts of laughter or crying

C. Treatment
   1. Physiotherapy may be helpful in relieving spasticity
   2. Support respiratory functions
D. Nursing care
   1. Provide emotional support for the patient and family
   2. Encourage range-of-motion exercises
   3. Explain the importance of maintaining good nutrition and preventing infection

Poliomyelitis

A. Etiology and pathophysiology
   1. Invasion of the lymph system by the poliovirus through the pharynx, with eventual spread to the lymph nodes, circulatory system, and nervous system
   2. Virus causes inflammation and necrosis of the cells, with resultant paralysis
   3. When it occurs in spinal cord, the anterior horn cells are affected; bulbar poliomyelitis involves the cranial nerves, and encephalitic poliomyelitis the cerebrum
   4. Incubation period 5 to 12 days
B. Signs and symptoms
   1. Subjective
      a. Fatigue
      b. Headache
      c. Muscular pain, especially in head and back
   2. Objective
      a. Flaccid paralysis
      b. Absent deep tendon reflexes
      c. Increased spinal fluid pressure
      d. Poliovirus in stool, throat secretions, blood, or spinal fluid
      e. Fever
      f. Respiratory paralysis may occur
C. Treatment
   1. Strict bed rest
   2. Support vital functions
      a. Tracheostomy
      b. Fluid replacement
      c. Urinary drainage
   3. Antibiotics
D. Nursing care
   1. Stress the importance of immunizations as a way to prevent disease
   2. Carefully observe vital signs and vital capacity
   3. Maintain body alignment
   4. Allow the patient time to verbalize feelings; realize that paralysis may make this impossible, which can be frustrating for the patient

Huntington's Chorea

A. Etiology and pathophysiology
 1. Inherited disorder, considered autosomal dominant
 2. Progressive atrophy of the basal ganglia and some portions of the cerebral cortex
 3. Appears during the middle adult years
B. Signs and symptoms
 1. Subjective
   a. Memory loss
   b. Disorientation
   c. Eventual dementia
 2. Objective
   a. Uncontrolled jerky movements of the extremities or trunk
   b. Disorganized gait
   c. Uncontrolled periods of anger
   d. Hesitant or explosive patterns of speech
   e. Grimacing facial movements
C. Treatment
 1. Control of jerky movements with haloperidol, fluphenazine, or L-dopa
 2. Symptoms are treated as they occur
D. Nursing care
 1. Provide emotional support for patient and family
 2. Provide for safety
 3. Utilize community agencies to provide situational support

Rheumatoid Arthritis

A. Etiology and pathophysiology
 1. Chronic disease characterized by inflammatory changes in the body's connective tissue particularly areas that have a cavity and easily moving surfaces
 2. Cause unknown, although theories include autoimmunity, heredity, and psychosomatic factors
B. Signs and symptoms
 1. Subjective
   a. Fatigue
   b. Malaise
   c. Joint pain
   d. Muscle stiffness after periods of inactivity
   e. Paresthesia
 2. Objective
   a. Anemia
   b. Weight loss
   c. Joint deformity as demonstrated by x-ray examination
   d. Subcutaneous nodules
   e. Elevated sedimentation rate
   f. Presence of rheumatoid factors in serum through latex fixation test

C. Treatment
 1. Corticosteroids, antiinflammatories, analgesics, immunosuppressive drugs
 2. Physiotherapy to minimize deformities
 3. Surgical intervention to remove severely damaged joints (e.g., hip replacement)
 4. Paraffin dips of affected extremity for relief of joint pain by providing uniform heat
D. Nursing care
 1. Administer analgesics and other medications as ordered
 2. Teach the patient to take medications as ordered
 3. Apply heat and cold as ordered; heat paraffin to 52° to 54° C (125° to 129° F)
 4. Promote rest and position to ease joint pains
 5. Provide for range-of-motion exercises up to the point of pain, recognizing that some discomfort is always present
 6. Encourage the patient to verbalize feelings
 7. Set realistic goals, focusing on strengths
 8. Encourage use of supportive devices to help patient conserve energy and maintain independence
 9. For nursing care of the patient following hip replacement see fractured hip

Osteoarthritis

A. Etiology and pathophysiology
 1. Etiology is unknown, but predisposing factors include obesity, aging, and joint trauma
 2. A degeneration and atrophy of the cartilages and calcification of the ligaments
B. Signs and symptoms
 1. Subjective
   a. Pain after exercise
   b. Stiffness of joints
 2. Objective
   a. Heberden's nodes symmetrically occurring on fingers (bony extensions)
   b. Decreased range of motion
C. Treatment
 1. Weight reduction in instances of obesity
 2. Local heat to affected joints
 3. Medications to reduce symptoms, such as analgesics, antiinflammatory agents, and steroids
 4. Exercise of affected extremities
 5. Surgical intervention
   a. Synovectomy—removal of the enlarged synovial membrane before bone and cartilage destruction occurs
   b. Arthrodesis—fusion of a joint performed when the joint surfaces are severely dam-

aged; this leaves the patient with no range of motion of the affected joint
  - c. Reconstructive surgery—replacement of a badly damaged joint with a prosthetic device (see hip replacement)
- D. Nursing care
  1. Assist patient in activities that require using affected joints; allow for rest periods
  2. Attempt to relieve the patient's discomfort by the use of medications or the application of heat as ordered
  3. Allow patient ample time to verbalize feelings regarding limited motion and changes in lifestyle

Gouty Arthritis (Gout)

- A. Etiology and pathophysiology
  1. Disorder in purine metabolism that leads to high levels of uric acid in the blood and the deposition of uric acid crystals (tophi) in tissues, especially joints; followed by an inflammatory response
  2. Incidence highest in males; a familial tendency has been demonstrated
  3. Renal urate lithiasis (kidney stones) may result from precipitation of uric acid in the presence of a low urinary pH
- B. Signs and symptoms
  1. Subjective
     - a. Sudden onset of asymmetric joint pain usually in the metatarsophalangeal joint of the great toe
     - b. Local pruritus
     - c. Malaise
     - d. Headache
     - e. Anorexia
  2. Objective
     - a. Elevated serum uric acid
     - b. Signs of inflammation of joint including swelling, heat, and redness
     - c. Tophi in outer ear, hands, and feet
- C. Treatment
  1. Administration of antiinflammatory and uricosuric agents (see pharmacology)
  2. Alkaline-ash diet to increase the pH of urine to discourage precipitation of uric acid and enhance the action of drugs such as probenicid (Benemid)
  3. Elimination of foods high in purines
  4. Weight loss is encouraged if indicated
- D. Nursing care
  1. Assess joint pain, motion, and appearance

  2. Administer antiinflammatory agents such as phenylbutazone (Butazolidin), oxyphenbutazone (Tandearil), or indomethacin (Indocin) with antacids or milk to help prevent peptic ulcers; observe therapeutic response
  3. Carefully align joints so they are slightly flexed during acute stage; encourage regular exercise, which is important for long-term management
  4. Use a bed cradle during the acute phase to keep pressure of sheets off joints
  5. Increase fluid intake to 2000 to 3000 ml daily to prevent formation of calculi
  6. Instruct the patient to avoid foods such as brains, kidneys, liver, and sweetbreads that have a high purine content
  7. Provide education regarding drug therapy and avoidance of excess alcohol intake

Osteomyelitis

- A. Etiology and pathophysiology
  1. Occurs as the result of bacterial invasion of the bone by *Staphylococcus aureus,* streptococcal organisms, *Escherichia coli,* or *Salmonella* organisms
  2. Infection of the bone results from trauma or systemic infection and involves the entire bone and surrounding soft tissue
- B. Signs and symptoms
  1. Subjective
     - a. Pain and tenderness of the bone
     - b. Malaise
     - c. Difficulty in weight-bearing
  2. Objective
     - a. Fever
     - b. Swelling over the affected bone
     - c. Signs of sepsis
- C. Treatment
  1. Antibiotic therapy
  2. Incision and drainage of a bone abscess
  3. Sequestrectomy—surgical removal of the dead infected bone and cartilage
- D. Nursing care
  1. Administer pain medications and antibiotics as ordered
  2. Use surgical aseptic technique when changing dressings
  3. Maintain good body alignment and promote comfort
  4. Utilize room deodorizer if a foul odor is apparent
  5. Allow the patient ample time to express feelings about long-term hospitalization

Osteoporosis

A. Etiology and pathophysiology
  1. Decrease in bone substance so the bone can no longer maintain the skeletal structure
  2. Most commonly affects the vertebrae, pelvis and femur
  3. Related factors include menopause, aging, inactivity, insufficient calcium intake or absorption, hyperparathyroidism, acromegaly, Cushing's syndrome, and hyperthyroidism
B. Signs and symptoms
  1. Subjective
     a. Backache
     b. Difficulty maintaining balance
  2. Objective
     a. Decreased height resulting from compression of the vertebrae
     b. X-ray examination reveals a demineralization of bone and compression of the vertebrae
C. Treatment
  1. Planned program of exercise
  2. Estrogen therapy to decrease bone reabsorption
  3. High-protein, high-calcium diet with vitamin D supplement
  4. Support for the spine (e.g., corset, Taylor brace)
  5. Treatment of underlying disorder vital to halt the process
D. Nursing care
  1. Encourage active exercise and assist with passive exercises
  2. Instruct the patient about proper body mechanics
  3. Provide a diet that includes meats and milk products
  4. Consider safety factors associated with instability; a cane or walker may be necessary for ambulation
  5. Provide rest periods to prevent fatigue
  6. Encourage fluids in acute osteoporosis to discourage the formation of renal calculi

Osteogenic Sarcoma

A. Etiology and pathophysiology
  1. Malignant bone tumor that usually begins in the long bones, especially around the knee
  2. Metastasis to the lungs common and occurs early; prognosis is poor
  3. Highest incidence between 20 and 30 years of age
B. Signs and symptoms
  1. Subjective
     a. Pain
     b. Limited motion
     c. Malaise
  2. Objective
     a. Local swelling
     b. Weight loss
     c. Anemia
     d. Elevated serum alkaline phosphatase
     e. Fever
     f. Microscopic evaluation of biopsy reveals neoplastic cells
C. Treatment
  1. Amputation of limb or resection of tumor
  2. Chemotherapy
  3. Radiation
D. Nursing care
  1. Be available for the patient and family to discuss fears, concerns, and treatment
  2. Provide high-protein, high-calorie meals based on the patient's preference
  3. Administer special nursing care following surgery (see amputations)
  4. Administer analgesics and antiemetics as needed
  5. Provide special care if the patient is receiving radiation therapy
     a. Observe the skin for breakdown
     b. Do not wash off port marks
     c. Avoid use of powders and ointments that contain metals

Multiple Myeloma

A. Etiology and pathophysiology
  1. Cause unknown, although genetic and viral factors are being closely considered
  2. Malignant overgrowth of plasma cells and malignant tumor growth in bone and bone marrow
  3. Occurs primarily in middle-aged men
B. Signs and symptoms
  1. Subjective
     a. Bone pain
     b. Progressive weakness
     c. Low back pain
  2. Objective
     a. Anemia
     b. Cachexia
     c. Idiopathic bone fractures
     d. Macroglobulinemia
     e. Platelet deficiency with resultant bleeding tendency
     f. Punched-out appearance of the bones at x-ray examination
     g. Presence of Bence Jones protein in urine
C. Treatment
  1. Chemotherapeutic agents, especially melphalan (Alkeran)
  2. Radiation therapy

3. Analgesics and narcotics for pain
4. Supportive therapy such as transfusions as indicated
D. Nursing care
  1. Carefully ambulate the patient to prevent pneumonia and reduce pathologic fractures
  2. Allow the patient ample time to express feelings about the disease and related therapies
  3. Allow the patient to participate in planning nursing care to aid in self-esteem and promote a feeling of self-control

Intractable Pain

A. Etiology and pathophysiology
  1. Pain not relieved by conventional treatment
  2. Causes include cancer, neuralgia, tic douloureux, and ischemia
B. Signs and symptoms
  1. Subjective
    a. Pain
    b. Fatigue
    c. Irritability
  2. Objective
    a. Evidence of a related disease process
    b. Pallor
C. Treatment
  1. Surgical intervention
    a. Rhizotomy—posterior spinal nerve root is resected between the ganglion and the cord, resulting in permanent loss of sensation; the anterior root may be cut to alleviate painful muscle spasm
    b. Cordotomy—to alleviate intractable pain in the trunk or lower extremities; the transmission of pain and temperature sensation is interrupted by creation of a lesion in the ascending tracts, percutaneously using an electrode or surgically via laminectomy
    c. Sympathectomy—to control pain of vascular disturbances and phantom limb pain (see procedures related to gastrointestinal disorders)
  2. Acupuncture therapy
  3. Biofeedback helps the patient develop control over anxiety and physiologic function
  4. Electronic stimulation may alter the electric potential of the nerve to prevent complete depolarization or block the transmission of pain sensations to the brain
    a. Percutaneous stimulator—electrodes applied over the painful area or along the nerve pathway
    b. Dorsal column stimulator and peripheral nerve implant—involve direct attachment of an electrode to the sensory nerve; a transmitter attached to the electrode is carried by the patient so electric stimulation can be administered as needed
D. Nursing care
  1. Assess pain, including location, duration, type, and severity
  2. Eliminate factors from the environment that seem to intensify pain
  3. Support the patient and family, since the patient frequently will withdraw
  4. Educate the patient and family about treatments available and the potential side effects
  5. Provide postoperative care
    a. Nursing care for a patient undergoing a cordotomy or rhizotomy or implantation of a dorsal column stimulator (see ruptured nucleus pulposus)
    b. Neurologically assess the extremities for movement, sensation, and skin temperature
    c. Carefully inspect skin, since the patient will not feel pain of ulceration
    d. Instruct the patient to avoid extreme environmental conditions and the use of heating pads and to check the temperature of bath water, since temperature sensitivity is absent

Ruptured Nucleus Pulposus ("Slipped Disc," Herniation of an Intervertebral Disc)

A. Etiology and pathophysiology
  1. Involves protrusion of the nucleus pulposus into the spinal canal with subsequent compression of the cord or nerve roots; usually occurs as a result of trauma
  2. Most common site is lumbosacral area (between L4 and L5), but herniation can also occur in the cervical region (between C5 and C6 or C6 and C7)
B. Signs and symptoms
  1. Subjective
    a. Lumbosacral disc
     (1) Acute pain in lower back, radiating across the buttock and down the leg (sciatic pain)
     (2) Pain when raising the unflexed leg on the affected side (Lasègue's sign)
     (3) Weakness of the foot
    b. Cervical disc
     (1) Neck pain that may radiate down arm to the hand
     (2) Weakness of the affected upper extremity

   2. Objective
     a. Straightening of the normal lumbar curve with scoliosis away from the affected side (lumbosacral disc)
     b. Atrophy of the biceps and triceps may be present (cervical disc)
     c. Elevated CSF protein
     d. Myelogram shows impingement on the spinal cord
     e. Electromyography (EMG) can help localize the site of a herniated disc

C. Treatment
   1. Bed rest with traction to the lower extremities (lumbosacral disc) or cervical traction (cervical disc)
   2. Back brace or support; cervical collar
   3. Local application of heat
   4. Muscle relaxant
   5. Surgical intervention
     a. Laminectomy—excision of the ruptured portion of the nucleus pulposus through an opening created by removal of part of the vertebra
     b. Spinal fusion—if 3 or more discs are involved, the affected vertebrae are permanently fused to stabilize the spine.

D. Nursing care
   1. Administer analgesics and other medications as ordered
   2. Use a firm mattress and bed board under the patient
   3. Make certain that traction and/or braces are correctly applied and maintained and that weights hang freely
   4. Use the fracture bedpan to avoid lifting of hips
   5. Give frequent and extensive back care to relax muscles and promote circulation
   6. Support the patient's body alignment at all times
   7. Use log-rolling method to turn the patient (instruct the patient to fold arms across the chest, bend the knee on the side opposite the direction of the turn, and then roll over)
   8. Increase fluid intake and roughage in the diet to prevent constipation; use stool softeners to prevent straining
   9. Keep the patient flat for 24 hours and encourage fluids to limit headache after a myelogram is done
   10. Provide special care for the patient undergoing a laminectomy
     a. Explain to the patient that pain may persist postoperatively for some time because of edema
     b. Place the bedside table, phone, and call bell within reach to prevent twisting
     c. Observe the dressing for hemorrhage and leakage of spinal fluid; notify the physician immediately if either occurs
     d. Observe for inadequate ventilation, especially in patients who have undergone a cervical laminectomy
     e. Assess the patient for changes in neurologic functioning
   11. Allow the patient to be dependent, but foster independence
   12. Encourage the patient to express feelings about altered functioning and self-image
   13. Encourage the patient to verbalize fears about the present condition and future disability
   14. Teach the patient to use proper body mechanics to prevent subsequent injury

Fractures

A. Etiology and pathophysiology
   1. Breaks in the continuity of bone, usually accompanied by localized tissue reponse and muscle spasm
   2. Cause usually trauma, but pathologic fractures may occur as a result of osteoporosis, multiple myeloma, or bone tumors, which weaken bone structure
   3. Types
     a. Complete fracture—bone completely separated into 2 parts; may be transverse or spiral
     b. Incomplete fracture—only part of the bone broken
     c. Comminuted fracture—bone broken into several fragments
     d. Greenstick fracture—splintering on one side of the bone, with bending of the other side; occurs only in pliable bones, usually in children
     e. Simple (or closed) fracture—bone broken but no break in the skin
     f. Compound (or open) fracture—break in the skin at the time of fracture with or without protrusion of the bone
   4. Stages of healing include formation of a hematoma followed by cellular proliferation and callus formation by the osteoblasts; finally ossification and remodeling of the callus

B. Signs and symptoms
   1. Subjective
     a. Pain aggravated by motion
     b. Tenderness
   2. Objective

a. Loss of motion
b. Edema
c. Crepitus (grating sound heard when fractured limb is moved)
d. Ecchymosis
e. X-ray examination reveals break in continuity of bone

C. Treatment
1. Traction may be used to reduce the fracture or to maintain alignment of bone fragments until healing occurs
   a. Skin traction—weights attached to adhesive, which is applied to the skin
      (1) Buck's extension—exerts a straight pull on a limb; often used temporarily to immobilize the leg when a patient fractures a hip
      (2) Bryant's traction—both lower limbs extended vertically; used to align fractured femurs in young children
      (3) Russell traction—lower leg is supported in a hammock, which is attached to rope and pulleys on a Balkan frame; used to treat fractures of the femur (the foot of the bed is usually elevated for countertraction)
   b. Skeletal traction applied to the bone
      (1) Steinmann pin or Kirschner wire may be inserted through the bone and skin; weights are then attached to a spreader, which is attached to both ends of the pin or wire (this may be used in conjunction with a cast)
      (2) Crutchfield tongs are inserted into the skull and weights are attached to immobilize the patient with a cervical fracture in a position of hyperextension
2. Surgical intervention to align the bone (open reduction), often with plates and screws to hold fracture in alignment
3. Manipulation to reduce fracture (closed reduction)
4. Application of cast to maintain alignment and immobilize limb

D. Nursing care
1. Provide emergency nursing care
   a. Evaluate the patient's general physical condition
   b. Treat for shock
   c. Splint suspected fractures before moving the patient; consider all suspected fractures to be fractures until x-ray films are available
   d. Cover open wound with sterile dressing if available

2. Observe for signs of emboli (fat or blood clot)—severe chest pain, dyspnea, pallor, diaphoresis
3. Provide special care to a patient with a cast
   a. Observe for signs of circulatory impairment—change in skin temperature or color, numbness or tingling, unrelieved pain, decrease in pedal pulse, prolonged blanching of toes after compression
   b. Protect the cast from damage until dry by elevating it on a pillow; handle with palms of hands only
   c. Promote drying of the cast by leaving it uncovered; a hair dryer or light may be used, with care to prevent burning
   d. Maintain bed rest until the cast is dry and ambulation is permitted
   e. Observe the patient for signs of hemorrhage and measure extent of drainage on cast when present
   f. Observe for irritation caused by rough cast edges, and pad as necessary for comfort and to prevent soiling
   g. Observe for swelling and notify the physician if necessary
   h. Administer analgesics judiciously and report unrelieved pain
   i. Observe for signs of infection (e.g., elevated temperature, odor from cast, swelling)
4. Provide special care to a patient in traction
   a. Check that weights are hanging freely and that the affected limb is not resting against the bed; countertraction may be necessary to prevent this by raising the foot of the bed (Russell traction and Buck's extension) or head of the bed (cervical traction)
   b. Maintain the patient in proper alignment
   c. Observe for foot-drop in patients with Russell traction or Buck's extension, since this may be indicative of nerve damage
   d. Observe for signs of thrombophlebitis; this is a more common complication of Russell traction because there is pressure on the popliteal space in addition to the stress of immobility
   e. Provide careful skin care
   f. Observe skin for irritation and observe site of insertion of skeletal traction for signs of infection
   g. Use aseptic technique when cleansing the site of insertion of skeletal traction (frequently an antiseptic ointment is also ordered)
5. Encourage high-protein, high-vitamin diet to

promote healing; high-calcium diet is not recommended for the patient confined to prolonged bed rest, since decalcification of the bone will continue until activity is restored, and a high calcium intake could lead to formation of renal calculi

6. Encourage fluids to help prevent complications of constipation, renal calculi, and urinary tract infection
7. Teach patient isometric exercises to promote muscle tone.
8. Teach patient appropriate crutch-walking technique; nonweight-bearing (3-point swing-through); weight-bearing (4-point) progressing to use of cane (see procedures)

Fractured Hip

A. Etiology and pathophysiology
   1. Fractures of the head or neck of the femur (intracapsular fracture) or trochanteric area (extracapsular fracture)
   2. Incidence highest in elderly females due to osteoporosis
B. Signs and symptoms
   1. Subjective
      a. Pain
      b. Changes in sensation
   2. Objective
      a. Affected leg appears shorter
      b. External rotation of the affected limb
      c. X-ray examination reveals lack of continuity of the bone
C. Treatment
   1. Buck's extension or Russell traction as a temporary measure to relieve the pain of muscle spasm or if surgery is contraindicated
   2. Closed reduction with a hip spica cast in fractures of the intertrochanteric region
   3. Open reduction and internal fixation
      a. Austin Moore prosthesis
      b. Thompson prosthesis
      c. Smith-Petersen nail
      d. Jewett nail
D. Nursing care
   1. See nursing care of the patient with a fracture
   2. Encourage the use of a trapeze to facilitate movement
   3. Use the fracture pan for elimination
   4. Postoperative care
      a. Inspect dressing and linen for bleeding
      b. Use a trochanter roll to prevent external rotation of legs
      c. Do not turn the patient on the operated side unless specifically ordered

d. Use pillows or abductor pillow to maintain the legs in slight abduction; after hip replacement it prevents dislodging of the prosthesis
      e. Encourage quadriceps setting exercises
      f. Assist the patient to ambulate—first using a walker, progressing to 3-point crutch walking, and then to total weight-bearing using a cane to provide stability
      g. Avoid flexing the hips of a patient with a total-hip replacement; assist to a lounge chair position when permitted to sit

Spinal Cord Injury

A. Etiology and pathophysiology
   1. Sudden impingements on the spinal cord as a result of trauma
   2. Fractures of the vertebrae can cut, compress, or completely sever the spinal cord if the patient is not positioned and moved correctly at the scene of an accident; the symptoms depend on the location (lumbar, thoracic, cervical) and extent of the damage (complete transection, partial transection, compression) and may be temporary or permanent; the sensation and mobility of areas that are supplied by nerves below the level of the lesion are lost
B. Signs and symptoms
   1. Subjective
      a. Loss of sensation below the level of the injury
      b. Inability to move
   2. Objective
      a. Early symptoms of spinal shock
         (1) Absence of reflexes below the level of the lesion
         (2) Flaccid paralysis (immobility accompanied by weak, soft, flabby muscles) below the level of injury
         (3) Hypotonia caused by disruption of neural impulses results in bowel and bladder distention
         (4) Inability to perspire in affected parts
         (5) Hypotension
      b. Later symptoms of spinal cord injury
         (1) Reflex hyperexcitability (spastic paralysis)—muscles below the site of injury become spastic and hyperreflexic
         (2) State of diminished reflex excitability (flaccid paralysis) below the site of injury follows the state of reflex hyperexcitability in all instances of total cord damage and may occur in some instances of partial cord damage

(3) In total cord damage, since both upper and lower motoneurons are destroyed, the symptoms depend totally on the location of the injury; loss of motor and sensory function present at this time is usually permanent
   (a) Sacral region—paralysis (usually flaccid type) of the lower extremities (paraplegia) accompanied by atonic (autonomous) bladder and bowel with impairment of sphincter control
   (b) Lumbar region—paralysis of the lower extremities that may extend to the pelvic region (usually flaccid type) accompanied by a spastic (automatic) bladder and loss of bladder and anal sphincter control
   (c) Thoracic region—same symptoms as in the lumbar region except extends to the trunk below level of the diaphragm
   (d) Cervical region—same symptoms as in the thoracic region except extends from the neck down and includes paralysis of all extremities (quadriplegia); if injury is above C4, respirations are depressed
(4) In partial cord damage either the upper or the lower motoneurons, or both, may be destroyed; therefore the symptoms depend not only on the location but also on the type of neurons involved; destruction of lower motoneurons will result in atrophy and flaccid paralysis of the involved muscles, whereas destruction of upper motoneurons causes spasticity

C. Treatment
   1. Neurologic assessment
   2. Maintain vertebral alignment by use of the following:
      a. Bed rest with supportive devices (bed board, sand bags, etc.)
      b. Bed rest with total immobilization (see procedures)—Stryker frame, CircOlectric bed
      c. Traction (skeletal or skin traction)—e.g., Crutchfield tongs, Buck's extension
      d. Corsets, braces, and other devices when mobility is permitted
   3. Surgery to reduce pain or pressure and/or stabilize the spine (e.g., laminectomy, spinal fusion)
   4. Mechanical ventilation as needed
   5. Temperature control via hypothermia or tepid baths
   6. Extensive rehabilitation therapy
D. Nursing care
   1. Maintain frequent observation of the patient's respiratory and neurologic functioning
   2. Maintain spinal alignment at all times; when turning the patient, use the log-rolling method and make certain enough help is available to move the patient as a single unit
   3. Check safety locks on Stryker frames and CircOlectric beds before turning patient
   4. Maintain surgical asepsis for the patient with Crutchfield tongs or spinal surgery
   5. Provide special skin care to back and bony prominences
   6. Maintain body parts in a functional position; prevent dysfunctional contractures
   7. Institute active and passive range-of-motion exercises as soon as approved by physician
   8. Provide the patient with simple explanations
   9. Encourage the patient to verbalize and accept that hostility will surface
   10. Stay with the patient when possible to provide assurance
   11. Allow the patient to be independent when possible
   12. Include the patient in decision-making process
   13. Help the patient to adjust to changes in body image and altered self-concept
   14. Accept periods of depression that occur
   15. Allow the patient time to reorganize life-style
   16. Set realistic short-term goals so the patient can achieve some success
   17. Test the temperature of bath water to avoid burns; teach the patient to test water temperature in any water-related activity
   18. Avoid bumps and bruises when involved in activities; utilize techniques to prevent pressure and examine skin for signs of pressure from positioning, braces, or splints
   19. Use a footboard to stimulate pressure sensation and proprioception
   20. Provide an opportunity for the patient to touch, grasp, and manipulate objects of different sizes, weights, and textures to stimulate tactile sensation
   21. Encourage the patient to be aware of all body segments: look at both extremities, comb both sides of the hair, shave both sides of the chin, put make-up on both sides of the face
   22. Protect the affected limbs by proper positioning during transfer; use a sling when indicated

23. Teach the patient to use the unaffected extremities to manipulate, move, and stabilize the affected ones
24. Attempt to reestablish a scheduled pattern of bowel function
    a. Understand what the individual's bowel functioning means to the patient and family
    b. Involve the patient, family, and entire health team in the development of a plan of care
    c. Review the patient's bowel habits prior to illness as well as the current pattern of elimination
    d. Supply a diet adequate in bulk, roughage, and bowel-stimulating properties
    e. Encourage sufficient fluid intake—2000 to 3000 ml per day
    f. Encourage the patient to be as active as possible to develop the tone and strength of the muscles that can be used
    g. Establish a specific and definite time for the bowel movement; regularity is the most important aspect of bowel reeducation
       (1) Exact time depends on the patient's schedule
       (2) Depends on the patient's past pattern
       (3) Consider scheduling evacuation after a meal to utilize the gastrocolic reflex (peristaltic wave in the colon induced by entrance of food into a fasting stomach)
    h. Determine if the patient is aware of the need to defecate (e.g., feeling of fullness or pressure in the rectum, flatus, borborygmus)
    i. Provide privacy for the patient during toileting activities
    j. Encourage the patient to assume a position most near the physiologic position for defecation (sitting the patient up frequently assists in preparing for this)
    k. Utilize assistive measures to induce defecation by
       (1) Teaching the patient to bear down and contract abdominal muscles (the Valsalva maneuver should be avoided by people with cardiac problems)
       (2) Teaching the patient to lean forward to increase intraabdominal pressure by compressing the abdomen against the thighs
       (3) Digital stimulation

       (4) Using suppository if necessary
       (5) Using enemas only as a last resort
    l. Provide for adaptation of equipment as necessary (e.g., elevated toilet seat, grab bars, padded backrest)
    m. Teach the family the bowel training program
25. Attempt to reestablish bladder function
    a. Determine the type of bladder problem
       (1) Neurogenic bladder—any disturbance in bladder functioning caused by a lesion of the nervous system
       (2) Spastic bladder (reflex or autonomous)—disorder caused by a lesion of the spinal cord above the bladder reflex center, in the conus medullaris; there is a loss of conscious sensation and cerebral motor control; the bladder empties automatically when the detrusor muscle is sufficiently stretched (about 500 ml)
       (3) Flaccid bladder (atonic, nonreflex, or autonomous)—disorder caused by a lesion of the spinal cord at the level of the sacral conus or below; the bladder continues to fill, becomes distended, and periodically overflows; the bladder muscle does not contract forcefully and therefore does not empty except with a conscious effort
    b. Understand what the individual's bladder functioning means to the patient and family
    c. Involve the patient, family, and entire health team in the development of a plan of care
    d. Review the patient's bladder habits prior to illness as well as the current pattern of elimination
    e. Encourage activity
    f. Encourage sufficient fluid intake
       (1) 3000 to 5000 ml per 24-hour period
       (2) Glass of water with each attempt to void
       (3) Reduce the amount of fluid as the day progresses and restrict fluid after 6 P.M. to limit the amount of urine in the bladder during the night
    g. Provide for privacy during toileting activities
    h. Encourage the patient to assume as normal a position as possible for voiding
    i. Establish a voiding schedule

(1) Begin trial voiding at the time the patient is most often incontinent
(2) Attempt voiding every 2 hours all day and 2 to 3 times during the night
(3) Time intervals between voiding should be shorter in the morning than later in the day
(4) As the patient's ability to maintain control improves, lengthen the time between attempts at voiding
(5) Time of intervals is not as important as regularity
j. Determine whether the patient is aware of need or act of urination (e.g., fullness or pressure, flushing, chilling, goose pimples, cold sweats)
k. Utilize assistive measures to induce urination by teaching the patient to
(1) Use the Credé maneuver—manual expression of the urine from the bladder with moderate external pressure, downward and backward, from the umbilicus to over the suprapubic area
(2) Bend forward to increase intraabdominal pressure
(3) Stimulate "trigger points"—areas that, for the individual, will instigate urination (e.g., stroke the thigh, pull pubic hair, touch meatus)
l. Record intake, output, voiding times, and times of incontinence
m. Provide for adaptive equipment as necessary (e.g., elevated toilet seats, commode, urinals, drainage systems)
n. Teach the family the bladder training program

Anterior Segment Disorders of the Eye

A. Etiology and pathophysiology
  1. Conjunctivitis—inflammation of the conjunctiva; can result from invasion by organisms, allergens, or irritants
  2. Blepharitis—inflammation of the lid margins; classified as staphylococcal or seborrheic
  3. Keratitis—inflammation of the cornea due to invasion of an organism
  4. Uveitis—an inflammation of the iris, ciliary body, and/or the choroid
  5. Pterygium—segment of thickened conjunctiva that can extend over the cornea
  6. Trachoma—viral infection of the lids and conjunctiva that can result in corneal ulceration and blindness

7. Chalazion—sterile cyst of the meibomian gland that causes inflammation of the lid; the cyst remains when the inflammation subsides
8. Hordeolum—infection of a follicle of the eyelash commonly caused by staphyloccocal organisms
B. Signs and symptoms
  1. Subjective
    a. Photophobia (keratitis, uveitis)
    b. Blurred vision (keratitis, uveitis, trachoma)
    c. Pain (keratitis, uveitis)
    d. Burning and itching of eyes (conjunctivitis, blepharitis, hordeolum)
  2. Objective
    a. Scaling and crust formation of lids (conjunctivitis, blepharitis, keratitis, uveitis)
    b. Swelling and redness (conjunctivitis, blepharitis, keratitis, uveitis, hordeolum)
    c. Tearing (keratitis)
    d. Ciliary injection (uveitis)
    e. Purulent drainage (conjunctivitis)
C. Treatment
  1. Conjunctivitis, blepharitis, hordeolum
    a. Antibiotic ointments
    b. Warm compresses
  2. Keratitis
    a. Culture analysis to determine causative organism
    b. Topical steroids and antibiotics
    c. If the cornea is badly damaged, corneal transplant
  3. Uveitis
    a. Mydriatics to keep the iris at rest
    b. Topical steroids and antibiotics
    c. Dark glasses
  4. Pterygium—surgical removal
  5. Trachoma—oral antibiotics, usually tetracycline, for 3 to 5 weeks
  6. Chalazion—usually surgical excision of cyst
D. Nursing care
  1. Instruct the patient on proper care of the eyes (hand washing, avoidance of rubbing)
  2. Administer antibiotic ointment and instruct patient in its use
  3. Apply soaks as ordered
  4. Prepare the patient for surgery, if indicated
  5. If the patient has undergone a corneal transplant (keratoplasty)
    a. Maintain bed rest for 1 or 2 days with the eyes bandaged
    b. Explain to the patient the importance of avoiding the Valsalva maneuver during healing

c. Explain to the patient that healing may take up to 6 months because the circulatory supply of the cornea is decreased

Tumors of the Eye

A. Etiology and pathophysiology
   1. May be benign or malignant; can form in or metastasize to the eye
   2. Retinoblastoma a congenital malignant neoplasm found in children; spreads easily by extension to the brain
   3. Melanoma common in the iris and choroid; grows slowly but metastasizes to the liver and lungs
B. Signs and symptoms
   1. Subjective
      a. Headache
      b. Visual complaints
   2. Objective
      a. Increased injection of the conjunctiva
      b. Decreased vision
      c. In retinoblastoma, white pupillary reflex, strabismus, retinal detachment
C. Treatment
   1. Chemotherapy
   2. Radiation therapy
   3. Enucleation (surgical removal of the eye)
D. Nursing care
   1. Support the patient and family as they attempt to cope with the diagnosis
   2. Observe the patient for side effects of medical therapy and attempt to limit their effects
   3. If the patient has undergone an enucleation, care involves
      a. Maintaining pressure dressings on the eye for 1 or 2 days to minimize hemorrhage
      b. Watching for signs of meningitis, which occurs as a complication, including headache or pain on the operative side
      c. Explaining that monocularity results in the loss of depth perception, and activities that require this should be avoided
      d. Explaining that the artificial eye may be inserted when healing is complete, usually 6 to 8 weeks; support adaptation to changes in body image

Cataract

A. Etiology and pathophysiology
   1. Opacity of the crystalline lens or its capsule
   2. Results from injury, exposure to heat, heredity, aging, or congenital factors that cause a diminution of sight

B. Signs and symptoms
   1. Subjective
      a. Distortion of vision (e.g., haziness, cloudiness, diplopia)
      b. Photophobia
   2. Objective
      a. Progressive loss of vision
      b. Usual black pupil appears clouded, progressing to milky white appearance
C. Treatment
   1. Corrective lenses until the cataract matures enough for removal
   2. Surgical intervention to remove the opaque lens
      a. Preoperative preparation with mydriatics and ophthalmic antibiotics
      b. Antiemetics, analgesics, and stool softeners postoperatively
      c. Corrective lenses (contact lenses or glasses)
         (1) Contacts fitted approximately 3 months postoperatively
         (2) Temporary eyeglasses given soon after discharge, with the final prescription several weeks later
   3. Insertion of a lens implant sometimes at the time of surgery
D. Nursing care
   1. Instruct the patient to prevent pressure on eyes by
      a. Not touching or rubbing the eyes
      b. Not closing the eyes tightly
      c. Avoiding coughing, sneezing, or bending from the waist (teach the patient to open the mouth when coughing)
      d. Lying on the back or the nonoperated side
      e. Avoiding rapid head movements
      f. Avoiding straining at stool
   2. Instruct the patient to request prescribed analgesics and antiemetics as required
   3. Administer stool softeners
   4. Provide side rails to help in turning and preventing falls
   5. Assist the patient with ambulation because of distortions in depth perception and extremely blurred vision
   6. Provide an easily accessible call bell
   7. Reduce the amount of light and encourage the use of sunglasses when the eye patch is removed
   8. Provide a quiet environment to promote rest
   9. Avoid substances that might precipitate coughing or sneezing (e.g., pepper, talcum powder)
   10. Observe for signs of increased intraocular pressure (e.g., pain, restlessness, increased pulse rate)

11. Observe for signs of infection (e.g., pain, changes in vital signs)
12. Encourage deep breathing
13. Explain to the patient that depth perception will be altered but assure patient that the corrective lenses will help to compensate for this distortion

Angle Closure Glaucoma

A. Etiology and pathophysiology
1. Condition in which the pressure within the eyeball is higher than normal
2. Closed angle of the drainage system of the canal of Schlemm prevents aqueous from reaching the lymph drainage spaces called the trabecular meshwork

B. Signs and symptoms
1. Subjective
   a. Nausea
   b. Halos around lights
   c. Malaise
2. Objective
   a. Gradual loss of peripheral vision
   b. Increased intraocular pressure (24 to 32 mm Hg) as measured with a tonometer
   c. Steamy cornea
   d. Conjunctival injection

C. Treatment
1. Lowering the intraocular pressure with miotics or carbonic anhydrase inhibitors
2. Surgical intervention to facilitate drainage of the aqueous humor is called an iridectomy; a surgical incision is made through the cornea to remove a portion of the iris to facilitate aqueous drainage

D. Nursing care
1. Explain the importance of continued use of eye medications as ordered
2. Explain the need for continued medical supervision for observation of intraocular pressure to ensure control of the disorder
3. Teach the patient to avoid exertion, stooping, heavy lifting, or wearing constricting clothing, since these increase intraocular pressure

Detached Retina

A. Etiology and pathophysiology
1. May result from trauma, the aging process, or cataract surgery; also seen in cases of myopia
2. Retina separates from the choroid, and vitreous humor seeps behind the retina

B. Signs and symptoms
1. Subjective
   a. Flashes of light
   b. Floaters
   c. Sensation of a veil in the line of sight
2. Objective
   a. Retinal separation noted on ophthalmoscopy
   b. Assessment of visual loss

C. Treatment
1. Bed rest, with the area of detachment in a dependent position to promote healing
2. Tranquilizers to promote rest and reduce anxiety
3. Surgical intervention
   a. Cryosurgery—supercooled probe causes retinal scarring and healing of area
   b. Photocoagulation—laser beam through the pupil produces a retinal burn, which causes scarring of the involved area
   c. Scleral buckling—shortening of the sclera to force the choroid closer to the retina

D. Nursing care
1. Keep the patient on bed rest in position as ordered
2. Provide the patient with a call bell and answer promptly
3. Observe for signs of hemorrhage postoperatively (severe pain, restlessness)
4. Diminish lights in the room
5. Explain to the patient that return to a sedentary occupation may occur in approximately 3 weeks and to a more active job in 6 to 8 weeks

Chronic Otitis Media

A. Etiology and pathophysiology
1. Chronic inflammatory disease of the middle ear; usually begins in childhood
2. Related to perforation of the eardrum; may be associated with mastoiditis

B. Signs and symptoms
1. Subjective
   a. Hearing loss
   b. Feeling of fullness within the ear
2. Objective
   a. Drainage from the ear that may be foul smelling
   b. Perforation of the eardrum apparent during examination with an otoscope
   c. Presence of cholesteatoma (epidermal inclusion cyst)

C. Treatment
1. Systemic antibiotics
2. Antibiotic eardrops
3. Gentle irrigations to cleanse the ear
4. Treatment of upper respiratory tract infections

D. Nursing care
  1. Instill antibiotics as prescribed
  2. Instruct the patient to report headache or stiff neck immediately, since this may indicate complications of meningitis

Mastoiditis

A. Etiology and pathophysiology
  1. Disease of the mastoid process; may be acute or chronic
  2. Generally occurs secondary to otitis media
  3. Disruption of the intercellular construction of the bone; suppurative mastoiditis
B. Signs and symptoms
  1. Subjective
    a. Tenderness over the mastoid process
    b. Headache and ear pain
  2. Objective
    a. Drainage from the ear
    b. Elevated temperature
C. Treatment
  1. Antibiotics—eardrops or systemic
  2. Cleansing of the ear
  3. Surgical intervention
    a. Mastoidectomy (radical or modified)
    b. Tympanoplasty
D. Nursing care
  1. Instruct the patient to seek treatment for any ear infections
  2. Care of the patient undergoing mastoidectomy
    a. Cleanse the postauricular area preoperatively
    b. Postoperatively reinforce the dressing over drain site from the mastoid
    c. Observe the patient for facial paralysis and report, since this may indicate damage to facial nerve
    d. Utilize safety precautions such as side rails to prevent injury to the patient who is experiencing vertigo

Otosclerosis

A. Etiology and pathophysiology
  1. Fixation of the stapes, preventing transmission of auditory vibrations to the inner ear (conduction deafness)
  2. Cause unknown, but incidence higher in females; heredity a factor
B. Signs and symptoms
  1. Subjective
    a. Loss of hearing reported by the patient
    b. Ringing or buzzing in the ears
  2. Objective

    a. Use of a tuning fork shows bone conduction better than air conduction (Rinne test)
    b. Presence of spongy bone in the labyrinth
C. Treatment
  1. Hearing aids to amplify sound
  2. Stapedectomy—removal of the diseased portion of the stapes, and replacement with a prosthetic implant to conduct vibrations from the middle to inner ear
D. Nursing care
  1. Position the patient postoperatively according to the physician's preference
    a. Lying on the operated side facilitates drainage
    b. Lying on the nonoperated side helps prevent displacement of the graft
  2. Instruct the patient to alter position gradually to prevent vertigo
  3. Question the patient about pain, headache, vertigo, or unusual sensations in ear and report
  4. Instruct the patient to avoid sneezing and blowing nose, swimming, showers, and flying until permitted by the physician; if the patient must sneeze, instruct to keep the mouth open to equalize pressure in the ear
  5. Explain to the patient that because of edema from surgery and the presence of packing, hearing will be diminished but will improve

Ménière's Disease

A. Etiology and pathophysiology
  1. Chronic disease of the inner ear causing severe vertigo
  2. Cause unknown, but follows infections of the middle ear or trauma
  3. Incidence highest in males between the ages of 40 and 60 years
B. Signs and symptoms
  1. Subjective
    a. Vertigo
    b. Nausea
    c. Headache
    d. Sensitivity to loud sounds
    e. Sensory hearing loss, usually unilateral
    f. Tinnitus
  2. Objective
    a. Vomiting
    b. Diaphoresis
    c. Nystagmus during attacks
    d. Bárány's caloric test (reveals diminished or absent response)
    e. Weber test and auditory testing document hearing loss

C. Treatment
1. Diuretics
2. Antihistamines
3. Surgical destruction of the labyrinth or vestibular nerve, which will cause deafness in that ear
4. Salt-free diet combined with administration of ammonium chloride
D. Nursing care
1. Support the patient emotionally
2. To prevent the onset of symptoms, encourage the patient not to move rapidly
3. Protect from injury during attack; use side rails; encourage the patient to lie down during an attack
4. Instruct the patient to pull off the road if driving when an attack occurs
5. Postoperative care for the patient with a total labyrinthectomy
   a. Bed rest may be necessary because of severe vertigo
   b. Instruct the patient to avoid sudden movements
   c. Explain that Bell's palsy may occur postoperatively but will subside within a few months
6. Instruct the patient to avoid foods such as salted meats and fish, cheese, condensed milk, carrots, and spinach

Integumentary System
REVIEW OF ANATOMY AND PHYSIOLOGY OF THE INTEGUMENTARY SYSTEM
Functions

A. Prevents loss of body fluids
B. Protects deeper tissues from pathogenic organisms, noxious chemicals, and short wavelength ultraviolet radiation
C. Helps regulate body temperature
D. Provides location for sensory reception of touch, pressure, temperature, pain, wetness, tickle, etc.
E. Assists in vitamin D synthesis
F. Plays a minor excretory role

Anatomy

A. Epidermis—contains no blood or lymphatic vessels; cells nourished by diffusion from underlying dermal papillae
1. Layers from the dermis outward
   a. Stratum germinativum—cell layers undergoing mitosis; gradually pushed to surface to replace those exfoliated
   b. Stratum granulosum—granule-filled cells in several layers; contain keratohyalin, intermediate in keratin formation; most free nerve endings of epidermis are here; contains epidermal pigment
   c. Stratum lucidum—translucent layers; nails are outgrowths of this layer
   d. Stratum corneum—upper horny layer of flat, dead cells that exfoliate rapidly, taking bacterial flora with them; responsible for variations in skin thickness
2. Melanocytes of the lower epidermis produce melanin, which colors skin
3. Exceptional epidermal regions
   a. Conjunctiva—epidermis so thin it is transparent
   b. Lips—epidermis very thin and highly vascular, which accounts for redness
B. Dermis
1. Extremely vascular fabric of collagen and elastic fibers woven to provide strength and flexibility
2. Upper papillary layer joined to epidermis by upward projecting papillae; vascular loops in papillae nourish overlying epidermis; contain abundant touch receptors; double-row papillae in finger pads and palms and soles give great strength against shearing stress, provide fingerprint pattern as unique arrangement of ridges projected to epidermal surface, and allow hands and feet to grip surfaces
3. Deeper reticular layer contains loose arrangement of connective tissue gradually merging with subcutaneous fatty layer (superficial fascia)
4. Skin stretched beyond certain limits (e.g., during pregnancy) may rupture dermal collagen and elastic fibers; consequent scar tissue repair produces striae gravidarum
C. Glands
1. Eccrine—tubular coiled glands deep in dermis; duct rises straight through dermis and spirals through epidermis, opening in sweat pore on crest of skin ridges; secretes clear fluid
2. Apocrine—scent glands; very large branched tubular glands found in the axillary, mammary, and genital areas that produce an originally odorless secretion rapidly metabolized by bacteria to produce typical body odors
3. Ceruminous—wax glands in external auditory canal; large branched glands frequently opening into hair sheaths along with sebaceous glands
4. Sebaceous—small saclike glands lacking innervation, usually forming close to hairs and open-

ing into upper portion of hair follicle; form independent of hairs at corners of mouth and in
eyelids as meibomian glands; absent on palms
and soles, accounting for wrinkling of these
areas after lengthy immersion in water
5. Mammary—milk-secreting, compound tubular
alveolar glands developing to full extent only
during pregnancy
D. Hair
1. Long strands of tightly compacted and cemented, dead and keratinized cells sheathed in
hair follicles (tubes of epidermal cells plunged
obliquely into dermis surrounded by dermal connective tissue sheath)
2. About the same number of follicles in males and
females; hormones stimulate differential growth
3. Determines appearance; round (straight hair);
ribbon shaped (kinky hair); alternately round
and oval (wavy hair)
4. Arrector pili (smooth muscle) attached at one
end to connective sheath in middle of the hair
follicle and at other end to the dermal papillary
region of the dermis; on contraction, elevates
hair and surrounding skin but depresses skin
overlying the dermal papillary attachment point;
result is "gooseflesh"; such contraction also
stimulates sebaceous gland secretion

Tissue Repair

A. Inflammation
1. Vascular changes—initially there is vasoconstriction (5 to 10 minutes); vessel walls lined
with leukocytes (margination); then vasodilation
with increased blood flow and increased vessel
permeability (effects of histamine from mast
cells, kinins, and prostaglandins); lymphatics
become plugged with fibrin to wall off damaged
area
2. Polymorphonuclear and mononuclear leukocytes
leave the vessels (diapedesis) and phagocytize
foreign substances
3. Chronic inflammation—longer-lived mononuclear leukocytes (macrophages) predominate,
and fibroblasts deposit a wall of collagen around
each group of macrophages and foreign substances; stage of granuloma formation
B. Fibroplasia
1. Epithelization—epithelial cells of the epidermis
begin to cover tissue defect through migration of
basal cells across wound defect with continued
mitosis in intact epithelium

2. Deep in the wound, fibroblasts synthesize collagen and ground substance; process begins about
fourth or fifth day and continues for 2 to 4
weeks
3. Capillaries regenerate by endothelial budding;
tissue becomes red
4. Fibrin plugs are lysed
C. Scar maturation
1. Collagen fibers rearranged into a stronger, more
organized pattern
2. Scar remodels, sometimes for months and years
due to collagen turnover; if collagen synthesis
exceeds breakdown, a hypertrophic scar or ke-
loid forms; if collagen breakdown exceeds synthesis, scar gradually softens and fades
3. Wound contracture—contraction of wound margins begins about 5 days after injury; caused by
fibroblast migration into the wound along the
lines of fibrin strands initially deposited in the
wound; assists in closing the defect but may also
result in contractures that can be debilitating

REVIEW OF PHYSICAL PRINCIPLES RELATED TO THE INTEGUMENTARY SYSTEM
Principles of Mechanics

Friction—epidermal ridges resulting from upthrusting
dermal papillae provide palms of hands, fingers, and
soles of feet with friction surfaces for grasping and
walking

Principles of Physical Properties of Matter

Elasticity—molecular structure of elastin, a protein,
permits stretching of skin under tension and the ability
to snap back to its original shape when tension is relieved; less elastic properties of collagen give skin its
strength to resist tearing and shearing forces

Principles of Heat

A. Radiation—heat brought to the dermis by blood radiates through the epidermis; allows for elimination
of excess heat
B. Evaporation—sweat evaporating cools the body surface and acts to drain heat from the body interior

Principle of Light

Radiation absorption
A. Ultraviolet absorption by melanin protects the skin
and underlying structures from damage
B. Quantity and degree of dispersed melanin, which
absorbs visible light wavelengths differently, produces different skin colors

REVIEW OF CHEMICAL PRINCIPLES RELATED TO THE INTEGUMENTARY SYSTEM
Solutions (Solubility)

A. Fat-soluble substances have a greater tendency to penetrate skin than do water-soluble substances
   EXAMPLE: Oleoresins of poison ivy, fat-soluble vitamins (A, D, E), and insecticides are absorbed, whereas water is repelled
B. Fat-soluble (oily) substances secreted by the Meibomian glands (modified sebaceous glands) of the eyelids, which are not capable of mixing with water; act as barriers to prevent tears from constantly flooding over lower eyelid

Water

Dehydration of epidermal cells leaves water-insoluble keratin impregnated in surface and corneum providing a water-resistant protective barrier

PHARMACOLOGY RELATED TO DISORDERS OF THE INTEGUMENTARY SYSTEM

A. Antibiotics and antifungals
   1. General implications for nurses
      a. Assess the lesion, including size, location, color, configuration, drainage, and any accompanying sensation such as pain or pruritus
      b. Thoroughly cleanse the area before application of ointment, cream, or lotion
      c. Recognize that topical antiinfectives begin to act quickly after application but systemic absorption is minimal
      d. Observe the skin after application of anti-infective; if no improvement is noted, notify physician
      e. Obtain and check results of culture and sensitivity tests on drainage
      f. Observe for side effects
         (1) Erythema
         (2) Drying
         (3) Pruritus
         (4) Swelling
         (5) Vesicle formation
   2. Actions
      a. Antibiotics generally interfere with one of the following cellular functions:
         (1) Cell wall synthesis
         (2) Protein synthesis
         (3) Membrane permeability
      b. Antifungal agents usually act by altering the permeability of the cell membrane
      c. May be an ointment, lotion, cream, or powder

   3. Examples
      a. Antibiotic preparations
         (1) Bacitracin (ototoxicity and nephrotoxicity have been reported as side effects)
         (2) Neomycin
         (3) Chloramphenicol (Chloromycetin)
         (4) Clotrimazole (Lotrimin)
         (5) Polysporin
         (6) Nitrofurazone (Furacin)
         (7) Silver sulfadiazine (Silvadene) (see drugs used in the treatment of burns)
      b. Antifungal preparations
         (1) Gentian violet
         (2) Nystatin (Mycostatin); may cause ototoxicity and nephrotoxicity with prolonged use
         (3) Potassium permanganate solution
B. Pediculicides and scabicides
   1. General implications for nurses
      a. Inspect skin, particularly the scalp, for scabies and pediculosis before and after treatment
      b. Use gown, gloves, and cap to prevent spread of parasitic arthropods
      c. Keep linen of an infected patient separate and sterilize to prevent reinfection
      d. Observe for irritation
      e. Assess source of infection; provide patient and family education
      f. Avoid contact with the eyes and mucous membranes
   2. Actions
      a. Exact mechanism for destruction of parasitic arthropods unknown
      b. May be absorbed through skin and mucous membranes; are then metabolized by the liver and excreted in the feces and urine
   3. Examples
      a. Gamma benzene hexachloride (Gexane, Kwell)
      b. Benzyl benzoate lotion (Benylate, Albacide, Scabanca)
C. Topical drugs used in the treatment of burns
   1. General implications for nurses
      a. Adhere to strict surgical asepsis
      b. Observe burns and the patient's general condition
      c. See nursing care of burns
      d. Observe for side effects listed with each drug
   2. Action—antiinfective agents act on bacterial cell wall or alter cellular function to produce bactericidal effects

3. Examples
   a. Silver sulfadiazine (Silvadene)
      (1) Apply to a thickness of 1/16 inch
      (2) Cleanse burns and debride prior to application
      (3) Because hemolysis can occur in patients with deficiency of glucose-6-phosphate dehydrogenase, monitor G-6-PD level before initiation of treatment
      (4) Observe for other adverse effects
          (a) Rash
          (b) Pruritus
   b. Mafenide acetate (Sulfamylon)
      (1) Cleanse and debride prior to application
      (2) May cause burning sensation when first applied
      (3) Observe the patient for acidosis, since medication acts as carbonic anhydrase inhibitor; if the patient becomes dyspneic, ointment should be removed
   c. Silver nitrate 0.5% solution
      (1) Apply dressings soaked in $AgNO_3$ and keep moist
      (2) Causes brown/black discoloration of anything it comes in contact with
      (3) May cause electrolyte imbalance if used on large area over long period because it is hypotonic; electrolyte levels should be evaluated frequently; observe for signs of electrolyte disturbance such as a change in behavior

D. Antipruritics
   1. General implications for nurses
      a. Assess the lesion, including location and size
      b. Question the patient regarding relief obtained from treatment
      c. Advise medical follow-up, since these medications provide only temporary relief of symptoms
      d. Observe for local irritation
      e. Discourage the patient from scratching; keep nails well trimmed
   2. Actions
      a. Tars act as irritants, promoting circulation and decreasing inflammatory exudates
      b. Local anesthetics block the conduction of nerve impulses
      c. Antiinflammatory agents decrease inflammation
   3. Examples
      a. Benzocaine (Anbesol, Dermoplast, Solarcaine)
      b. Lidocaine hydrochloride (Xylocaine jelly, ointment, or spray)
      c. Phenol
      d. Tars
      e. Calamine

E. Antiinflammatory agents
   1. General implications for nurses
      a. Assess lesions for color, location, size, etc.
      b. Protect the skin from scratching or rubbing
      c. Use appropriate topical agent
         (1) Use lotions in areas such as the axillae and groin
         (2) Use creams if the lesion is draining
         (3) Use ointments on dry lesions
      d. Avoid contact with eyes
      e. Cleanse the skin before application
      f. Utilize occlusive dressings if ordered
      g. Observe for signs of sensitivity
         (1) Contact dermatitis
         (2) Irritation
         (3) Burning
         (4) Itching
         (5) Folliculitis
         (6) Adrenal insufficiency may occur if absorbed systemically
   2. Actions
      a. Reduce signs of inflammation; vasoconstriction decreases swelling and pruritus
      b. Absorbtion through skin is increased if a large area of skin is involved or if occlusive dressings are used
   3. Examples
      a. Betamethasone (Celestone)
      b. Betamethasone valerate (Valisone, Celestoderm)
      c. Fluocinolone acetonide (Fluonid, Synalar)
      d. Fluocinonide (Lidex)
      e. Flurandrenolone (Cordran, Drenison)
      f. Hydrocortisone (Acticort, Cortril, Hytone)
      g. Triamcinolone acetonide (Aristocort, Kenalog, Triamalone)

RELATED PROCEDURES
Skin Grafts
A. Definition
   1. Covering of denuded tissue with skin to prevent infection and loss of body fluids, promote healing, and prevent contractures
   2. Applied between the fifth and twenty-first day, depending on extent of the burn
   3. Types of skin grafts
      a. Xenografts—skin from animals, usually pigs (porcine xenograft)

b. Homografts—skin from another person

c. Autografts—skin from another part of the patient's body

   (1) Mesh graft—machine used to mesh skin obtained from a donor site so it can be stretched to cover a larger area of burn

   (2) Postage stamp graft—earlier method of accomplishing the same goal as a mesh graft; a small amount of skin is used to cover a larger area; the donor skin is cut into small pieces and applied to the burn

   (3) Sheet grafting—large strips of skin placed over the burn as close together as possible

B. Nursing responsibilities

1. Explain procedure to the patient; obtain a written consent

2. Prepare the donor site carefully

3. Postoperatively keep donor sites (which are covered with a nonadherent dressing and wrapped in an absorbent gauze) dry using a heating lamp or hair dryer as ordered; remove absorbent gauze as ordered; nonadherent dressing will separate as healing occurs

4. Grafts are generally left with a light pressure dressing for approximately 3 days; after the graft has "taken," roll cotton-tipped applicators gently over the graft to remove underlying exudate; allowed to remain, exudate could promote infection, which could prevent the graft from adhering

5. Observe for foul-smelling drainage, temperature elevation, and other signs of infection

MAJOR DISEASES
Primary Skin Lesions

A. Macule—flat circumscribed area from 1 to several centimeters in size, without elevation (freckle, flat pigmented moles)

B. Papule—raised circumscribed area less than 1 cm in size (acne)

C. Nodule—raised solid mass that extends into the dermis and is 1 to 2 cm in size (pigmented nevi)

D. Tumor—solid raised mass that extends into the dermis and is over 2 cm in size (dermatofibroma)

E. Wheal—flattened collection of fluid 1 mm to several centimeters in size (mosquito bites)

F. Vesicle—raised collection of fluid less than 1 cm in size (chickenpox, herpes simplex)

G. Bulla—fluid-filled vesicle over 1 cm in size (second-degree burn, pemphigus)

H. Pustule—vesicle or bulla filled with pus, 1 mm to 1 cm in size (acne vulgaris)

I. Cyst—mass of fluid-filled tissue that extends to the subcutaneous tissues or dermis, over 1 cm in size (epidermoid cyst)

Burns

A. Etiology and pathophysiology

1. Thermal, radiation, and chemical burns—cause cell destruction and result in depletion of fluid and electrolytes

2. Extent of the fluid and electrolyte loss directly related to extent and degree of the burn

   a. First degree (also known as partial thickness)—erythema, edema, and pain; fluid loss slight, especially if less than 15% of body surface is involved

   b. Second degree (also known as deep dermal)—erythema, pain, vesicles, with oozing; fluid loss slight to moderate, especially if less than 15% of the body surface is involved

   c. Third degree (also known as full thickness)—charred or pearly white, dry skin, absence of pain; fluid loss usually severe, especially if more than 2% of the body surface is involved

3. Classification of second- and third-degree burns

   a. Minor burns—no involvement of hands, face, or genitalia; total burn area does not exceed 15%, and third-degree burns do not exceed 2% of body area

   b. Major burns—involvement of 15% to 30% of body; but third-degree burns do not exceed 10% of body area

   c. Critical burns—involvement exceeds 30% of body surface; this classification is also used if the patient has a preexisting chronic health problem, is under 18 months or over 50 years of age, or has additional injuries

4. Pulmonary injury should be suspected if 2 of the following factors are present and expected if 3 or all 4 are present:

   a. Hair in nostrils singed

   b. The patient was trapped in a closed space

   c. Face, nose, and lips burned

   d. Initial blood sample contains carboxyhemoglobin

5. Extent of trauma can be estimated by rule of nines or other burn area chart

6. Curling's ulcer may occur after a burn

   a. The patient may complain of gastric discomfort, or there may be profuse bleeding

   b. Usually occurs by end of the first week after a burn

    c. Treatment essentially the same as for a gastric ulcer; however, mortality following surgical repair is high because of the patient's debilitated state

B. Signs and symptoms
  1. Subjective
    a. Extreme anxiety
    b. Restlessness
    c. Pain, severity depending on the type of burn
    d. Paresthesia
    e. Disorientation
  2. Objective
    a. Changes in appearance of skin indicate degree of burn (see etiology and pathophysiology)
    b. Hematuria; blood hemolysis with subsequent rise in plasma hemoglobin may occur with third-degree burns
    c. Elevated hematocrit as a result of fluid loss
    d. Electrolyte imbalance
    e. Presence of symptoms of hypovolemic shock caused by circulatory failure resulting from seepage of water, plasma, proteins, and electrolytes into burned area
    f. Presence of symptoms of neurogenic shock (symptoms similar to hypovolemic shock) caused by the fright, terror, hysteria, and pain involved in the situation
    g. Disorientation and confusion may be present

C. Treatment
  1. Tetanus toxoid immediately
  2. IV replacement therapy at a rate of 250 ml per hour to achieve an intake of between 6000 and 7000 ml for the first 24 hours (half of total IV solutions will be an electrolyte solution such as Ringer's lactate and half will be plasma or plasma substitute)
  3. Reduction of total IV solutions during second 24 hours depending on the patient's urinary output, blood work, and central venous pressure
  4. Foley catheter; monitor the urinary output and specific gravity hourly to observe kidney functioning and determine fluid replacement
  5. Insert a central venous pressure (CVP) line and take an hourly reading to monitor circulating fluid volume
  6. Vital signs monitored every 15 minutes
  7. Serum electrolytes and blood gases to observe for levels and assist in deciding replacement therapy
  8. IPPB and continuous oxygen to assist with respirations

  9. Tracheostomy if laryngeal edema occurs
  10. Reverse isolation
  11. Permit the patient nothing by mouth except mineral water for first 24 to 48 hours; allow clear liquids as tolerated after 2 days; then place the patient on high-protein, high-carbohydrate, high-fat, high-vitamin diet as tolerated
  12. Daily Hubbard tank baths after the fifth day; use antibiotic ointment and Kling dressing
  13. Intervene surgically to perform debridement and skin grafting (see procedures), promote healing, and limit contractures
  14. Mechanical debridement (wet to dry dressings) or enzymatic debridement (e.g., Travase ointment) may be used
  15. IV and topical antibiotics to limit infection (Keflin and penicillin intravenously; Sulfamylon ointment; gentamicin; silver nitrate solution; and silver sulfadiazine)
  16. Narcotics to reduce pain and sedatives to decrease anxiety, given IV or orally due to decreased muscle absorption

D. Nursing care
  1. Observe vital signs, central venous pressure, intake and output, and specific gravity as ordered; notify the physician if deviations occur or if output falls below 30 ml or rises above 50 ml per hour
  2. Maintain patency of the Foley catheter to ascertain the correct information regarding fluid balance
  3. Make certain that blood electrolyte and gas tests are performed and results are available
  4. Administer fluid and electrolytes as ordered
  5. Observe the patient for signs of electrolyte imbalance (calcium, potassium, and sodium) and metabolic acidosis
  6. Observe for signs of tracheal edema (dyspnea, stridor)
  7. Elevate head of the bed
  8. Encourage the patient to cough and deep breathe
  9. Maintain reverse isolation to prevent infection of burned areas
  10. Use sterile technique (irrigating drainage tubes, dressings, and bed linens)
  11. Administer tetanus toxoid as ordered
  12. Administer IV and topical antibiotics as ordered
  13. Observe for signs of infection (rising temperature and white blood cell count, odor)
  14. Support the joints and extremities in a functional position

15. Support the patient while turning
16. Keep room temperature as constant as possible
17. Observe for symptoms of Curling's (stress) ulcer
18. Give small, frequent high-protein, high-carbohydrate, high-fat, high-vitamin feedings
19. Give medication for pain as ordered and particularly before dressing change
20. Expect the patient to express negative feelings about burns, and accept it
21. Explain need for staff wearing gowns and masks
22. Give realistic reassurance

Acne Vulgaris

A. Etiology and pathophysiology
   1. Hormonal activity produces hyperkeratosis of the follicular orifices, leading to blockage of secretions and the subsequent formation of fatty plugs known as blackheads (comedones)
   2. When a blackhead (comedo) forms, the sebaceous gland involved becomes hypertrophic and infected
   3. Cysts and nodules form, leaving scars
   4. Most common among adolescents
B. Signs and symptoms
   1. Subjective
      a. Pain when sebaceous glands become infected
      b. Depression
   2. Objective
      a. Blackheads on skin (open comedones)
      b. Whiteheads on skin (closed comedones)
C. Treatment
   1. Mechanical removal with a comedo extractor
   2. Abrasive cleaners, astringents, and bacteriostatic creams
   3. Ultraviolet light as a peeling agent
   4. Cryotherapy to produce desquamation of skin
   5. Oral administration of antibiotics such as tetracycline
   6. Intralesional injections of corticosteroids
   7. Dermabrasion to improve the scars but not to cure the condition
      a. Instrument that functions at a high speed with a cylinder of wire or sandpaper at its end
      b. Epidermis and some dermis are removed at high points of the scars so they do not appear as deep
      c. Local anesthesia for treatment of small areas; general is indicated for large areas
D. Nursing care
   1. Promote good hygienic care when instructing the patient how to wash areas and apply topical medications
   2. Discuss the use of water-base cosmetics to prevent clogging of pores
   3. Instruct the patient on how to take medications
   4. Emphasize the importance of diet, especially vitamin A, and increased fluid intake
   5. Postoperative care following dermabrasion
      a. Apply ointment to lubricate skin and remove crust from area
      b. Observe serum draining from the area and report copious amounts of drainage to the surgeon
      c. Explain to the patient that the feeling of being sunburned is normal after dermabrasion

Contact Dermatitis

A. Etiology and pathophysiology
   1. Results from contact with a substance that reacts with the protein in the skin to form an antigen in a sensitized patient
   2. Antigen causes proliferation of lymphocytes, and the interaction of these factors causes eczematous changes
   3. Common causes—poison ivy, hair dye containing paraphenylenediamine, benzocaine, soaps, cements, insecticides, rubber compounds
B. Signs and symptoms
   1. Subjective
      a. Discomfort
      b. Pruritus
   2. Objective
      a. Erythema at the point of contact
      b. Vesicles and papules
      c. Edema
      d. Thickening of the skin and scaling
C. Treatment
   1. Identification of the allergen through patch testing; a suspected allergen is applied to the unbroken skin; the skin is observed for erythema, papules, and vesicles in 24 to 48 hours
   2. Antihistamines, antipruritics
   3. Topical corticosteroids
D. Nursing care
   1. Instruct the patient to avoid situations or substances that involve the identified allergen
   2. Cool environment, provide tepid baths, and trim finger nails to help control injury from scratching
   3. Provide diversional activities
   4. If topical corticosteroids are ordered, apply occlusive plastic dressings (Saran Wrap) over the ointment or lotion as ordered

Psoriasis

A. Etiology and pathophysiology
1. Inflammatory disease that may be acute or chronic
2. Genetic predisposition is thought to be a factor
3. Uncommon in blacks
4. Injury to the skin and psychologic stress appear to be factors in flare-ups

B. Signs and symptoms
1. Subjective
   a. Mild pruritus (severe if in skin folds)
   b. If psoriatic arthritis is present, joint pain and stiffness
2. Objective
   a. Bright red, well-demarcated plaque covered with silvery scales, usually on knees, elbows, and scalp
   b. Stippling and thickening of the nails
   c. Inflammatory changes of the joints if psoriatic arthritis is present
   d. Uric acid levels may be elevated

C. Treatment
1. Exposure to solar or ultraviolet irradiation
2. Application of coal tar ointment or antiinflammatory topical agents
3. Systemic corticosteroid therapy may be used in severe cases
4. Methotrexate may also be used for severe psoriasis
5. Exposure to black light combined with oral administration of methoxsalen useful in treatment of intractable cases

D. Nursing care
1. Encourage the patient to ventilate feelings about changes in body image; show acceptance
2. Assess lesions and the response to therapy
3. Determine factors linked to flare-ups; the patient may need help coping with stressful situations
4. Instruct the patient to use a soft brush to remove scales when bathing
5. If occlusive dressings are ordered with topical ointment, Saran Wrap, plastic bags, or rubber gloves may be used

Pemphigus

A. Etiology and pathophysiology
1. Potentially fatal skin disease
2. Occurs only in adults
3. Cause unknown

B. Signs and symptoms
1. Subjective
   a. Debilitation
   b. Malaise
   c. Pain associated with lesions
2. Objective
   a. Bullae on normal skin and mucosa
   b. Separation of epidermis caused by rubbing skin (Nikolsky's sign)
   c. Acantholysis (changes in intercellular connections of the epidermis) evident on microscopic examination
   d. Leukocytosis, eosinophilia
   e. Foul-smelling discharge

C. Treatment
1. Oral corticosteroids
2. Antibiotics for secondary infections
3. Topical treatment for relief of symptoms
   a. Potassium permanganate baths
   b. Oatmeal baths

D. Nursing care
1. Administer steroids with antacid or milk to prevent gastric irritation (see drugs)
2. Monitor intake and output (NaCl and fluid are lost through the skin)
3. Test urinary sugar and acetone levels, since the patient is receiving large doses of corticosteroids
4. Protect the patient from infection
5. Watch for signs of infection such as elevated temperature and WBC
6. Provide oral hygiene and increased fluid intake to soothe oral lesions
7. Encourage ventilation of feelings; patients are often discouraged and depressed

Cancer of the Skin

A. Etiology and pathophysiology
1. Most common cancer; however, early detection and slow progression make the cure rate high
2. Exposure to the sun, irritating chemicals, and chronic friction implicated; more common in persons with fair complexions
3. Types
   a. Basal cell carcinoma—generally located on the face and appears as a waxy nodule that may have telangiectasias visible; the most common type of skin cancer, but metastasis is rare
   b. Squamous cell carcinoma—develops rapidly and may metastasize through local lymph nodes; may develop secondarily to precancerous lesions such as keratosis and leukoplakia and is found most frequently on upper extremities and face, which are exposed to the sun; it appears as a small red nodular lesion
   c. Malignant melanoma—most serious type and arises from the pigment producing melanocytes; the color of the lesion may vary

greatly (white, flesh, gray, brown, blue, black); changes in size, color, sensation, or characteristics of a mole suggest the possibility of malignant melanoma; metastasis via blood can be extensive

B. Signs and symptoms
  1. Subjective
    a. Pruritus may or may not be present
    b. Localized soreness
  2. Objective
    a. Change in color, size, or shape of preexisting lesion
    b. Oozing, bleeding, or crusting
    c. Biopsy of tumor reveals type of cancer
    d. Lymphadenopathy if metastasis has occurred

C. Treatment
  1. Surgical excision of the lesion and surrounding tissue
  2. Chemosurgery, which involves the use of zinc chloride to fix the cells before they are dissected
  3. Cryosurgery utilizing liquid nitrogen to destroy the tumor cells by freezing
  4. Radiation (malignant melanoma does not respond well to this mode of treatment)
  5. Chemotherapy
  6. Nonspecific immunostimulants such as BCG vaccine

D. Nursing care
  1. Assess skin lesions
  2. Instruct the patient to examine moles for changes and have those subject to chronic irritation (bra or belt line) removed
  3. Encourage limitation of exposure to sun
  4. Emphasize continued medical supervision
  5. Use surgical aseptic technique when caring for surgical site
  6. Encourage verbalization; maintain a therapeutic environment
  7. Provide care to the patient receiving radiation
    a. Observe skin for local reaction
    b. Avoid use of ointments or powders containing metals
  8. Care related to specific chemotherapeutic agents (see pharmacology)

Herpes Zoster (Shingles)

A. Etiology and pathophysiology
  1. Acute viral infection of nerve structures caused by the varicella-zoster virus
  2. Inflammation occurs along the pathway of one or more peripheral sensory nerves
  3. Occurs in patients who have not had chickenpox and are exposed to an affected individual
  4. May frequently occur in patients with other debilitating illness; (e.g., tuberculosis, Hodgkin's disease)

B. Signs and symptoms
  1. Subjective
    a. Malaise
    b. Headache
    c. Pain
    d. Paresthesias
  2. Objective
    a. Painful, pruritic vesicles arranged along the pathway of the involved nerves
    b. Stains made from lesion exudate isolate the organism

C. Treatment
  1. Medications for pain, relaxation, itching, and preventing secondary infection
  2. Control of pain by blocking the nerve through injection of drugs such as lidocaine or applying medication such as triamcinolone (Kenalog)
  3. Antiinflammatory drugs such as systemic steroids or Kenalog ointment to decrease inflammation

D. Nursing care
  1. Administer analgesics and other medications as ordered
  2. Reduce itching and protect lesions from air by the application of salves, ointments, lotions, and sterile dressings as ordered
  3. Protect from pressure by use of air mattress, bed cradle, and light loose clothing (avoid synthetic and woolen materials and use cotton fabrics)
  4. Use aseptic technique when caring for a patient with open lesions
  5. Administer antibiotics as ordered
  6. Encourage the patient to avoid scratching and to use gloves at night to limit the possibility of accidental scratching
  7. Assist the patient in understanding the basis for the rash and the itch
  8. Allay fears that may be based on old wives' tales about shingles
  9. Encourage the patient to express feelings

Systemic Lupus Erythematosus (SLE)

A. Etiology and pathophysiology
  1. Origin unknown; affects the connective tissue and is thought to be due to a defect in the body's immunologic mechanisms or to genetic predisposition
  2. Fibrinoid deposits in blood vessels, among collagen fibers, and on organs
  3. Necrosis of the glomerular capillaries, inflam-

mation of cerebral and ocular blood vessels, necrosis of lymph nodes, vasculitis of the GI tract and pleura, and degeneration of the basal layer of skin

B. Signs and symptoms
   1. Subjective
      a. Malaise
      b. Photosensitivity
      c. Joint pain
   2. Objective
      a. Fever
      b. Butterfly erythema on the face
      c. Erythema of palms
      d. Positive LE prep
C. Treatment
   1. Corticosteroids and analgesics to reduce pain and inflammation
   2. Supportive therapy as major organs become affected (heart, kidneys, CNS, GI tract)
D. Nursing care
   1. Administer medications and observe for side effects
   2. Help the patient and family cope with severity of the disease as well as its poor prognosis

Polyarteritis Nodosa

A. Etiology and pathophysiology
   1. Cause unknown; occurs primarily in women in midlife
   2. Collagen disease that causes inflammation and necrosis of small and medium-sized arteries
   3. When healing of the arteries occurs, there is a thickening of the walls with subsequent circulatory impairment
   4. Common areas involved are the kidneys, heart, liver, and GI tract
B. Signs and symptoms
   1. Subjective
      a. Malaise
      b. Weakness
      c. Severe abdominal pain, muscle aches
   2. Objective
      a. Weight loss
      b. Low-grade fever
      c. Bloody diarrhea
      d. Proteinuria if kidneys are affected
      e. Positive rheumatoid factor (RF) and elevated sedimentation rate
C. Treatment
   1. Corticosteroids and analgesics to control pain and inflammation
   2. Balanced diet to combat weight loss

D. Nursing care
   1. Provide relief of symptomatic pain
   2. Provide emotional support for both the patient and the family because of the poor prognosis

Progressive Systemic Sclerosis (Scleroderma)

A. Etiology and pathophysiology
   1. Thought to be caused by an autoimmune defect; occurs in women more frequently than in men
   2. Systemic disease that causes fibrotic changes in connective tissue throughout the body
   3. May involve the skin, synovial membranes, esophagus, heart, lungs, kidneys, or GI tract
B. Signs and symptoms
   1. Subjective
      a. Articular pain
      b. Muscle weakness
   2. Objective
      a. Masklike hard skin that eventually adheres to underlying structures
      b. Telangiectases on the lips, fingers, face, and tongue
      c. Dysphagia
      d. Restriction of body motion as the disease progresses
      e. Positive LE prep, elevated gamma globulin levels, false-positive test for syphilis
C. Treatment
   1. Corticosteroids
   2. Salicylates or analgesics for joint pain
   3. Physical therapy
   4. Skin care to prevent decubitus formation
D. Nursing care
   1. Support the patient and family emotionally; there is no cure at present
   2. Administer medications as ordered
   3. Encourage the patient to exercise actively
   4. Observe vital signs, urinary output, and vital capacity for changes in function of vital organs

INFECTIOUS DISEASES
Acquired Immune Deficiency Syndrome (AIDS)

A. Etiology and pathophysiology
   1. Etiology unclear; some evidence that it is caused by a virus
   2. Incidence highest among young male homosexuals; IV drug users and individuals requiring frequent transfusions (hemophiliacs) also at risk
   3. Both humoral and cellular immunity suppressed, making individuals susceptible to opportunistic

organisms such as *Pneumocystis carinii* and cancer such as Kaposi's sarcoma
  4. Mortality rates estimated at 40% to 70%
 B. Signs and symptoms
   1. Subjective
    a. General malaise
   2. Objective
    a. Persistent fever
    b. Night sweats
    c. Enlarged lymph nodes
    d. Leukopenia
    e. Macular-papular lesions on body or mucous membranes
 C. Treatment
   1. Kaposi's sarcoma—antineoplastics
   2. Opportunistic infections—antimicrobial agents such as sulfamethoxazole
   3. Other therapies are under investigation
 D. Nursing care
   1. Protect the patient from secondary infection; carefully assess for early signs
   2. Provide emotional support in light of the patient's developmental level and life-style and the presence of potentially fatal illness
   3. Maintain both "enteric" and "blood and needle" precautions to protect staff and visitors

Gas Gangrene

 A. Etiology and pathophysiology
   1. Caused by an anaerobic gram-positive clostridium *(Clostridium perfringens, C. novyi)* that enters through a deep wound
   2. Usually occurs 2 to 5 days after injury
   3. Bacilli colonize in muscle tissue surrounding the wound
 B. Signs and symptoms
   1. Subjective
    a. Pain
    b. Apprehension
    c. Anorexia
   2. Objective
    a. Bronzed or blackened wound tissue
    b. Crepitus
    c. Sweetish-smelling exudate
    d. Necrosis of muscle tissues
    e. Presence of clostridia on culture
    f. Pallor
    g. Diarrhea
    h. Vomiting
    i. Temperature elevation (may be slight)
    j. Anemia
 C. Treatment

   1. Multiple incisions for decompression and drainage
   2. Extirpation and debridement of involved tissue with copious irrigations
   3. Penicillin G, tetracycline, chloramphenicol, or erythromycin, depending on drug sensitivity
   4. Amputation
   5. Hyperbaric oxygenation
   6. Whole blood, packed erythrocytes, or plasma transfusions to combat hemolysis and profound anemia
   7. Antitoxin therapy may be started
 D. Nursing care
   1. Prevent infection whenever the wound is near the rectum, since the organism is found in feces
   2. Utilize wound and skin precautions in caring for the patient
   3. Monitor fluid and electrolyte balance
   4. Check cardiovascular status frequently to determine complications

Hansen's Disease (Leprosy)

 A. Etiology and pathophysiology
   1. Thought to be transmitted by direct contact with the acid-fast bacillus *Mycobacterium leprae*
   2. Bacillus causes lesions of the peripheral nervous system that extend to and destroy nearby skin tissues
 B. Signs and symptoms
   1. Subjective—loss of sensation
   2. Objective—painless, colorless, or red-brown macules and papules, nodules, sores, and ulcers
 C. Treatment
   1. Sulfone drugs
   2. Reconstructive surgery
 D. Nursing care
   1. Provide emotional support for the patient and the family, allowing ample time for verbalization of feelings
   2. Maintain mobility of the patient with decreased use of painful extremities
   3. Encourage case-finding examinations of all family members and friends; assure them that the disease has a very low incidence of communicability

Malaria

 A. Etiology and pathophysiology
   1. Caused by a protozoon *(Plasmodium falciparum, P. vivax, P. ovale, P. malariae)* that enters during a bite by an infected *Anopheles* mosquito, through the use of dirty needles, or by a transfusion from an infected donor

2. When the parasite enters the bloodstream, it invades the red blood cells; destruction of red blood cells, blockage of capillaries, and irreversible damage to the spleen and liver may follow
3. Rare complication is "blackwater fever"; name derived from the fact that there is intravascular hemolysis and hemoglobinuria

B. Signs and symptoms
  1. Subjective
     a. Malaise
     b. Headache
     c. Muscle aches
     d. Chills
     e. Thirst
  2. Objective
     a. High fever
     b. Anemia
     c. Enlarged spleen
     d. Dehydration
     e. Renal failure

C. Treatment
  1. Antimalarial drugs (see chemoprophylaxis under nursing care)
  2. Aspirin

D. Nursing care
  1. Monitor fluid and electrolyte balance
  2. Utilize needle and blood precautions; prevent mosquito bites
  3. Use therapeutic measures such as sponges to decrease the fever; maintain hydration
  4. Maintain bed rest until the fever and other symptoms have ceased
  5. Assist with dialysis and monitor blood transfusions as needed when blackwater fever is present
  6. Teach preventive measures
     a. Avoiding stagnant pools
     b. Initiating chemoprophylaxis 1 week prior to visiting infested areas and regularly while in the area: pyrimethamine, proguanil hydrochloride, chloroquine diphosphate, or amodiaquine dihydrochloride

Rabies

A. Etiology and pathophysiology
  1. Caused by a virus found in the saliva of an infected animal and usually spread by bite; the animal can be a carrier and not be ill with the disease
  2. Incubation period 30 to 50 days in bites of the upper parts of the body, 4 months in bites of the lower parts
  3. Bites are usually unprovoked; suspected animals are observed for 10 days
  4. Negri bodies (round objects) found in the brain tissue of infected animals
  5. Virus affects the CNS; may cause punctate hemorrhages and neuronal destruction

B. Signs and symptoms
  1. Subjective
     a. Anxiety
     b. Depression, malaise, lethargy
     c. Irritability
     d. Headaches
     e. Stiff neck
     f. Anorexia, nausea
     g. Photophobia
     h. Respiratory difficulty such as wheezing, hyperventilation, and dyspnea
     i. Thirst
     j. Paresthesia or pain near the bite or in the bitten extremity
  2. Objective
     a. Severe difficulty swallowing
     b. Excessive salivation
     c. Choking
     d. Aerophobia
     e. Apnea
     f. Paralysis
     g. Coma
     h. Cardiac arrhythmias

C. Treatment
  1. Cleansing of the wound with aqueous benzalkonium chloride
  2. Tracheostomy if respiratory embarrassment severe
  3. Human rabies globulin; dose given in the buttock; wound is bathed with the drug
  4. Duck embryo rabies vaccine (DEV) is also used; a total of 23 doses is administered subcutaneously
  5. Sedative or anesthetics as necessary; phenytoin (Dilantin) used for seizures

D. Nursing care
  1. Maintain strict isolation technique
  2. Monitor blood gases, fluid and electrolyte balance, and electrocardiograms
  3. Keep the room dark and quiet to prevent agitation
  4. Monitor the tracheostomy and the need for suctioning
  5. Prevent drafts, which may result in spasms
  6. Allow the family and patient to verbalize their feelings

Rocky Mountain Spotted Fever

A. Etiology and pathophysiology
1. Contamination of an individual by a tick infected with *Rickettsia rickettsii* (through bite or contamination by a crushed tick on the fingers or in the eye); there may or may not be a history of tickbite
2. Sudden onset, with an incubation period of 3 to 17 days
3. Organism attacks endothelial cells and extends into the vessel walls, causing thrombi, inflammation, and necrosis

B. Signs and symptoms
1. Subjective
   a. Malaise
   b. Insomnia
   c. Headache
   d. Anorexia
   e. Photophobia
   f. Joint and muscle discomfort
2. Objective
   a. Fever
   b. Rash (rose-colored macules)
   c. Subcutaneous hemorrhage
   d. Necrosis
   e. Enlarged spleen
   f. Hearing loss
   g. Hypotension
   h. Circulatory collapse

C. Treatment
1. Prompt recognition and treatment vital
2. Tetracycline or chloramphenicol therapy continued until the patient is afebrile for 3 to 5 days
3. Treatment of symptoms and complications as they develop

D. Nursing care
1. Assure the family that the patient's disturbed emotional responses are associated with the disease
2. Monitor symptoms to determine progression of the disease
3. Assess the cardiovascular status to determine developing circulatory collapse
4. Reassure the patient that hearing loss will last only several weeks
5. Teach prevention such as wearing tick repellents and checking pants legs and animals for the presence of ticks
6. Teach all individuals to kill ticks with a tweezer to prevent contamination of fingers

Tetanus (Lockjaw)

A. Etiology and pathophysiology
1. Caused by the anaerobic bacillus *Clostridium tetani,* which is transmitted through an open wound
2. Symptoms from 2 days to 3 weeks after exposure to the bacillus
3. Toxins from the bacillus invade the nervous tissue, and the motor and sensory nerves become hypersensitive, resulting in prolonged contractions and respiratory failure

B. Signs and symptoms
1. Subjective
   a. Irritability
   b. Restlessness
2. Objective
   a. Muscle rigidity
   b. Local or general spastic contractions of the voluntary muscles
   c. Trismus (spasm of the masticatory muscles)
   d. Spasms of the respiratory tract
   e. Convulsions

C. Treatment
1. TIG (tetanus immune globulin)
2. Maintain adequate pulmonary ventilation
3. Debridement of the wound to allow exposure to air
4. Control of muscle spasms
5. Penicillin G to limit secondary infection
6. Maintain fluid balance and nutrition
7. Diazepam and barbiturates to sedate the patient and limit spasms
8. Once symptoms develop, specific therapy is ineffective; therefore institution of supportive therapy is necessary until toxins are reduced by time

D. Nursing care
1. Prevent the disease through immunization programs
2. Maintain a quiet environment to decrease stimuli, which may result in convulsions
3. Frequently assess respiratory status; administer oxygen as needed
4. Frequently suction the airway to maintain patency and promote ventilation; keep an endotracheal tube and tracheostomy set at the bedside
5. Allow the patient and family to verbalize fears and feelings

Typhoid Fever

A. Etiology and pathophysiology
1. Caused by the bacterium *Salmonella typhi,* which can be carried in human feces and transmitted through sewage, flies, and shellfish

2. Incubation period 3 to 20 days
3. Bacterium invades the GI tract and localizes in lymph tissue of the intestinal wall (Peyer's patches); these areas may become thrombosed and tissue sloughs off, leaving ulcers
4. Hemorrhage, peritonitis, perforation, and hepatitis are serious complications
B. Signs and symptoms
1. Subjective
   a. Headaches
   b. Drowsiness
2. Objective
   a. Fever
   b. Bradycardia
   c. Rose-colored papules on the abdomen
   d. Enlarged spleen
   e. Enlarged liver
   f. Delirium
   g. Constipation during the early stage; diarrhea during the late stage
C. Treatment
1. Chloramphenicol or sulfamethoxazole and trimethoprim
2. Corticosteroids the first 4 to 5 days of treatment
D. Nursing care
1. Encourage a diet high in calories
2. Employ methods to decrease the fever
3. Monitor fluid and electrolytes to prevent imbalance
4. Maintain enteric precautions and isolation technique
5. Utilize enemas and mild laxatives as ordered to limit constipation
6. Educate the public to prevent disease through proper sewage treatment
7. Encourage vaccination programs with booster injections every 3 years in endemic areas
8. Allow the patient and family ample time to verbalize emotional reactions and concerns resulting from the illness

EMERGENCY NURSING CARE

A. Assessing potentially life-threatening conditions
1. Airway—see CPR
2. Breathing
3. Circulation
4. Other indications of emergencies: shock, altered consciousness, uncontrolled bleeding, chest pains, spinal injuries
B. Establishing priority of needs

1. Triage—system of patient evaluation to establish priorities and assign appropriate treatment or personnel
2. Determination of priority
   a. Emergency situations: greatest risk receives priority
   b. Major disasters: classification based on principles to benefit the largest number; those requiring highly specialized care may be given minimal or no care
C. Offering psychologic support
1. Establish and maintain open communication with the patient and family to mediate feelings of "loss of control"
2. Allow contact between the client and family as soon as feasible
D. Caring for specific emergency situations
1. Circulatory
   a. See specific disease: myocardial infarction, hypertensive crisis, shock, asystole
   b. See related emergency and critical care procedures
   c. Uncontrolled hemorrhaging
      (1) Stop the bleeding by direct pressure, application of a pressure dressing or ice to constrict vessels, elevation of the involved extremity, or (rarely) tourniquet application
      (2) Treat for shock
2. Respiratory
   a. See specific disease: pneumothorax, pulmonary edema, pulmonary embolism, carbon monoxide poisoning, COPD, ARDS
   b. See related emergency and critical care procedures
   c. Near drowning
      (1) Assessment
         (a) Possible airway obstruction from bronchospasm
         (b) Evaluation of arterial blood gases for hypoxia, hypercarbia, and acidosis
         (c) Possible pulmonary edema
            [1] *Salt water:* high osmotic pressure of aspirated water draws additional fluid into alveolar spaces from the vascular bed
            [2] *Fresh water:* removes surfactant, leading to alveolar collapse
      (2) Management
         (a) Establish an airway and ventilate

with 100% oxygen and positive pressure
  (b) Correct the acidosis
  (c) Insert a nasogastric tube to prevent aspiration of gastric contents
  (d) Treat pulmonary edema, hypothermia if present
3. Gastrointestinal
  See specific diseases: perforated peptic ulcer, appendicitis, intestinal obstruction, bleeding esophageal varices associated with cirrhosis
4. Genitourinary
  See specific disease: bladder trauma
5. Endocrine
  See specific diseases: hypoglycemia, ketoacidosis, thyroid storm
6. Neuromusculoskeletal
  See specific diseases: fractures, spinal cord injury, head injury, cerebral vascular accident, myasthenic crisis
7. Integumentary
  See specific disease: burns
8. Poisoning
  See pediatric nursing: poisoning
9. Thermal trauma
  a. Heat stroke
    (1) Risk factors: advanced age, strenuous exercise in heat, medications such as anticholinergics that interfere with sweating
    (2) Signs and symptoms
      (a) Hot, dry, flushed skin progressing to pallor in the late stages of circulatory collapse
      (b) Elevation of body temperature above 40.5° C (105° F)
      (c) Complaints of dizziness, nausea, and headaches
      (d) Convulsions
      (e) Altered level of consciousness
    (3) Management
      (a) Rapidly reduce temperature: hypothermia blanket, cold-water baths and enemas
      (b) Administer oxygen to meet increased metabolic demands
      (c) Institute seizure precautions
  b. Hypothermia
    (1) Risk factors: exposure to cold; submersion in cold water; age (elderly and very young)

    (2) Signs and symptoms
      (a) Local (frostbite): pallor, paresthesia, pain to absence of sensation of involved body part
      (b) Systemic: core temperature less than 34.4° C (94° F), weak and irregular pulse, decreased level of consciousness
    (3) Management
      (a) Monitor core temperature with an esophageal or rectal probe
      (b) Continually assess cardiac status, arterial blood gases, electrolytes, glucose, and BUN
      (c) Rewarm: to prevent cardiovascular collapse, core rewarming with heated oxygen and/or irrigations must precede surface rewarming
      (d) Correct fluid and electrolyte imbalances

Medical-Surgical Nursing Review Questions

1 A nursing hypothesis is a nurse's:
1. Actual intervention
2. Prescription
3. Evaluation of data
4. Evaluation of care

2 Where primary nursing is practiced, the nurse who plans for and delegates care with full authority to see that the plan is followed is the:
1. Clinical specialist
2. Head nurse
3. Nurse clinician
4. Primary nurse

3 The following is an example of primary health care by the nurse:
1. Correction of dietary deficiencies
2. Assisting in immunization programs
3. Prevention of disabilities
4. Rehabilitation

4 An objective method for data collection includes:
1. Direct observation of the patient
2. Speaking with the patient's family
3. The patient's description of the illness
4. Collection of specimens

5 The determining factor in the revision of a nursing care plan is the:
1. Correctness of the original hypothesis
2. Method for providing care
3. Available time
4. Effectiveness of implementation

6 Which of the following best defines the term ''nursing process''? Nursing process is the:
1. Activities a nurse employs to identify a nursing problem
2. Process the nurse uses to determine nursing goals
3. Steps the nurse employs in planning and giving nursing care
4. Implementation of nursing care by the nurse

7 To begin the nursing process, the nurse must first:
1. State the patient's nursing needs
2. Identify goals for nursing care
3. Obtain information about the patient
4. Evaluate the effectiveness of nursing actions

8 The effectiveness of nurse-patient communication is validated by:
1. Health team conferences
2. Medical assessments
3. Patient feedback
4. Patient's physiologic adaptations

Situation: A small urban community in the western area of the country is flattened by a severe, widespread tornado. Questions 9 through 13 refer to this situation.

9 Immediately after the storm has passed the rescue team with which you are working is searching for injured people. You split up to search, and you find a man lying next to a broken natural gas main. He is not breathing and is bleeding heavily from a wound on the foot. Your first step would be to:
1. Remove him from the immediate vicinity
2. Apply surface pressure to the foot wound
3. Start rescue breathing immediately
4. Treat him for shock

10 You find a young boy under the wreckage of a frame house. He is conscious, breathing satisfactorily, and lying on his back. He complains of pain in his back and is unable to move his legs. First you would:
1. Gently raise him to a sitting position to see if the pain either diminishes or increases in intensity
2. Leave him lying on his back, give him instructions not to move, and seek additional help
3. Roll him on his abdomen, place a pad under his head, and cover him
4. Gently lift him onto a flat piece of lumber and, using any available transportation, rush him to medical help

11 You find another injured person, obviously in shock. You would keep him lying on his back and:
1. Elevate the head higher than the rest of the body; give stimulants in small sips
2. Surround the body with hot water bottles or chemical heating pads if available
3. After evaluation, allow the patient to walk around if injuries permit
4. Raise the legs higher than the rest of the body, prevent chilling, and give fluids if possible

12 When a disaster occurs, you may have to treat the mass hysteria first. The person or persons to be cared for immediately would be those in:
1. Depression
2. Euphoria
3. Panic
4. Comatose state

13 In any disaster concerning a number of people the function that contributes most to saving of lives is sorting, or triage. Assume that you are the nurse who has to determine this priority of patient needs. The patients who need immediate care are those with:
1. Second-degree burns of 10% of the body
2. Severe lacerations involving open fractures of major bones
3. Closed fractures of major bones
4. Significant penetrating or perforating abdominal wounds

14 A disease produced when a *Clostridium* organism enters wounds and produces a toxin causing crepitus is:
1. Tetanus
2. Gas gangrene
3. Botulism
4. Anthrax

15 The major benefit in using tetanus antitoxin is that it:
1. Stimulates plasma cells directly
2. Provides high titer of antibodies
3. Provides immediate active immunity
4. Stimulates long-lasting passive immunity

16 Antibodies are also produced by:
1. Plasma cells
2. Eosinophils
3. Lymphocytes
4. Erythrocytes

Situation: Mrs. Hollens, age 30 and a chemist, is the mother of 2 young children. For the past few months she has noticed that she tires easily, has painless swelling of the lymph nodes, and has been running a low-grade fever with excessive diaphoresis at night. She also has anorexia with loss of weight. She does not recall having had any serious illness except that once during the winter she experienced what she believed was a viral infection. On her admission to the hospital the physician ordered a complete medical examination for Mrs. Hollens. On the basis of diagnostic tests, Mrs. Hollens is said to have Hodgkin's disease. Questions 17 through 21 refer to this situation.

17 The lymph nodes usually affected first are the:
1. Inguinal
2. Axillary
3. Cervical
4. Mediastinal

18 The highest incidence of Hodgkin's disease is in:
1. Children
2. Young adults
3. Middle-aged persons
4. Elderly persons

19 Which of the following would you expect Mrs. Hollens to develop as a result of whole-body irradiation? Increased:
1. Red blood cell production
2. Susceptibility to infection
3. Tendency for pathologic fractures
4. Blood viscosity

20 Whole-body irradiation injures or destroys bone marrow, making it unable to function normally. As a result, which of the following would you expect to develop?
1. Decreased number of erythrocytes
2. Decreased susceptibility to infections
3. Increased tendency for bones to break
4. Increased blood viscosity

21 The apparent paradox of radiation being a known cancer-inducing agent as well as a widely used therapy for cancer is clarified when one considers the:
1. Extent of the body irradiated
2. Nutritional environment of the cells
3. Dosage of radiation utilized
4. Physical condition of the patient

Situation: Mrs. Johnson, a 64-year-old housewife, is admitted to the hospital with a diagnosis of hypertension. Questions 22 through 27 refer to this situation.

22 Mrs. Johnson is receiving methyldopa hydrochloride (Aldomet) intravenously for control of hypertension. Her blood pressure, before the infusion started, was 150/90. Fifteen minutes after the infusion is started her blood pressure rises to 180/100. The response to the drug would be described as a(n):
1. Synergistic response
2. Individual hypersusceptibility
3. Allergic response
4. Paradoxical response

23 To assess the effectiveness of Aldomet in lowering blood pressure levels, the nurse would take Mrs. Johnson's pulse and blood pressure:
1. Thirty minutes after giving the drug
2. Immediately after she gets out of bed
3. After she has been supine for 5 minutes
4. Prior to giving the drug

24 Mrs. Johnson's serum potassium level is low and she is placed on a cardiac monitor. She is to receive 40 mEq potassium chloride in 1000 ml of 5% dextrose in water IV. The nurse analyzes the monitor pattern to obtain a baseline for evaluating progress. The monitor pattern would show:
1. Shortening of the QRS complex
2. Elevation of the ST segment
3. Increased deflection of the Q wave
4. Lowering of the T wave

25 Mrs. Johnson's IV medication inadvertently runs in rapidly. The physician prescribes insulin added to a 10% dextrose in water solution. The rationale for the prescription is:
1. Glucose and insulin increase the metabolic rate and accelerate potassium excretion
2. Potassium moves into body cells with glucose and insulin
3. Increased potassium causes a temporary slowing of pancreatic production of insulin
4. Increased insulin accelerates excretion of glucose and potassium

26 Mrs. Johnson's condition has improved, and methyldopa (Aldomet) is being given orally. When explaining why orthostatic hypotension occurs, the nurse should base the response on knowledge that the drug causes vasodilation by:
1. Depleting acetylcholine
2. Decreasing adrenal release of epinephrine
3. Stimulating histamine release
4. Interrupting norepinephrine release

27 When discussing the plan for taking Aldomet at home, the nurse would tell Mrs. Johnson that orthostatic hypotension may be modified by:
1. Lying down for 30 minutes after taking the drug
2. Avoiding tasks that require high energy expenditures
3. Wearing support hose continuously
4. Sitting on the edge of the bed a short time before arising

28 The primary cause of essential hypertension is:
1. Generalized arteriosclerosis
2. Unresolved grief
3. Kidney failure
4. Unexpressed rage

29 Which mechanism mediates long-term (day-to-day, week-to-week) blood pressure regulation?
1. Fight or flight response
2. Adjustment of urinary output
3. Nervous system baroreceptors
4. Capillary fluid shifts

30 Patients receiving propranolol hydrochloride (Inderal) should be told they might:
1. Experience dizziness with strenuous activity
2. Have a flushing sensation for a few minutes after taking the drug
3. Notice acceleration of the heart rate after eating a heavy meal
4. Have pounding of the heart for a few minutes after taking the drug

31 Mr. Evere, a 69-year-old retired musician, was admitted to the intensive care unit with a diagnosis of Adams-Stokes syndrome. Symptoms most likely include:
1. Syncope and low ventricular rate
2. Flushing and slurred speech
3. Cephalalgia and blurred vision
4. Nausea and vertigo

32 The lethal arrhythmia that often requires immediate intervention by the nurse is:
1. Atrial fibrillation
2. Auricular flutter
3. Second-degree heart block
4. Ventricular fibrillation

33 Pulse pressure is the:
1. Difference between the apical and radial rates
2. Force exerted against an arterial wall
3. Degree of ventricular contraction in relation to output
4. Difference between systolic and diastolic readings

Situation: *Mr. Josh is admitted with a diagnosis of possible tuberculosis or pneumonia. Several diagnostic tests are performed. Questions 34 through 40 refer to this situation.*

34 As a general rule, which of the following tests is most valuable in the selection of an antibiotic?
1. Susceptibility test
2. Tissue culture test
3. Serologic test
4. Sensitivity test of organism

35 Acid-fast rods found in sputum are presumed to be:
1. Influenza virus
2. *Bordetella pertussis*
3. Diphtheria bacillus
4. *Mycobacterium tuberculosis*

36 As a result of pulmonary tuberculosis, Mr. Josh has a decreased surface area for gaseous exchange in his lungs. Oxygen and carbon dioxide are exchanged in the lungs by:

1. Active transport
2. Diffusion
3. Filtration
4. Osmosis

37 Mr. Josh says the physician told him his tidal volume is slightly diminished and asks the nurse what this means. The nurse explains that tidal air is the amount of air:
1. Exhaled normally after a normal inspiration
2. Exhaled forcibly after a normal expiration
3. Forcibly inspired over and above a normal inspiration
4. Trapped in the alveoli that cannot be exhaled

38 Mr. Josh has been receiving streptomycin sulfate daily for 1 week. He is being discharged and the physician plans to have him come to the clinic for administration of the drug twice a week. The spaced dosage is planned to:
1. Increase compliance with the therapy plan
2. Lessen risk of adverse effects of the drug on neural tissue
3. Minimize disruption of the rest hours required for recovery
4. Lessen tissue trauma from injections while resistance is low

39 Vitamin B_6 is given with isoniazid (INH) because it:
1. Improves the nutritional status of the patient
2. Enhances tuberculostatic effect of isoniazid
3. Provides the vitamin when isoniazid is interfering with natural vitamin synthesis
4. Accelerates destruction of remaining organisms after inhibition of their reproduction by isoniazid

40 After Mr. Josh has been receiving streptomycin sulfate for 2 weeks, he states that he is "walking like a drunken seaman." The nurse withholds the drug and promptly reports the problem to the physician because the signs may be a result of drug effect on the:
1. Cerebellar tissue
2. Peripheral motor end-plates
3. Vestibular branch of the eighth cranial nerve
4. Internal capsule and pyramidal tracts

Situation: *Mr. Arlo has come to the emergency room with shortness of breath, which occurred suddenly while he was getting dressed. He also has a history of emphysema. The physician diagnoses a spontaneous pneumothorax. Questions 41 to 48 refer to this situation.*

41 The probable cause of a spontaneous pneumothorax is:
1. Rupture of a subpleural bleb
2. Pleural friction rub
3. Tracheoesophageal fistula
4. Puncture wound of the chest wall

42 Besides dyspnea, which of the following symptoms is generally associated with a spontaneous pneumothorax?
1. Increased chest motion
2. Unilateral chest pain
3. Hematemesis
4. Mediastinal shift toward the involved side

43 Mr. Arlo questions the nurse as to what has happened to his lung. The nurse bases the explanation on the understanding that:
1. The heart and great vessels shift to the affected side
2. There is a greater negative pressure within the chest cavity
3. Inspired air will move from the lung into the pleural space
4. The other lung will collapse if not treated immediately

44 If Mr. Arlo has suffered a complete pneumothorax, there is danger of a mediastinal shift. If such a shift occurs, it may lead to:
1. Increased volume of the unaffected lung
2. Infection of the subpleural lining
3. Rupture of the pericardium or aorta
4. Decreased filling of the right heart

45 Mr. Arlo becomes extremely drowsy; his pulse and respirations increase. The nurse should suspect:
1. Elevated Po_2
2. Respiratory alkalosis
3. Hypercapnia
4. Hypokalemia

46 In addition to calling the physician, the nurse should:
1. Place the patient on his unaffected side
2. Administer 60% O_2 via Ventimask
3. Prepare for IV administration of electrolytes
4. Give 2 L O_2 per minute via nasal cannula

47 The physician inserts a chest tube in the right side and attaches it to a 2-bottle closed drainage system. In caring for Mr. Arlo, the nurse should:
1. Administer morphine sulfate, since the patient will be agitated
2. Apply a thoracic binder to prevent tension on the tube
3. Clamp the tubing to prevent a rapid decline in pressure
4. Observe for fluid fluctuations in the underwater glass tube

48 Complete lung expansion before the removal of chest tubes is evaluated by:
1. Absence of additional drainage
2. A decrease in adventitious sounds
3. Return of normal tidal volume
4. Comparison of chest radiographs

49 The poisonous nature of carbon monoxide (CO) results from:
1. Its preferential combination with hemoglobin
2. Its tendency to block CO_2 transport
3. Is inhibitory effect on vasodilation
4. The bubbles it tends to form in blood plasma

50 With an oxygen debt, muscle shows:
1. High levels of calcium
2. Low levels of lactic acid
3. High levels of glycogen
4. Low levels of ATP

51 If breathing is deliberately stopped in a person:
1. The individual will soon die of suffocation
2. Rising oxygen concentrations will stimulate the breathing center
3. Accumulated CO_2 will force resumption of breathing
4. Increased N_2 concentration will have a toxic effect

52 Patients with fractured mandibles usually have them immobilized with wires. The life-threatening problem that can develop postoperatively is:
1. Vomiting
2. Infection
3. Osteomyelitis
4. Bronchospasm

53 A patient of yours has a temperature of 99.8° F. This is the same as a temperature of:
1. 37.7° C
2. 38.2° C
3. 37.0° C
4. 36.5° C

54 A patient with pyrexia will be expected to have:
1. Dyspnea
2. Elevated blood pressure
3. Increased pulse rate
4. Precordial pain

55 The chief complaint in a patient with Vincent's angina is:
1. Chest pain
2. Shortness of breath
3. Bleeding and ulcerations in mouth
4. Shoulder discomfort

56 After undergoing surgery for removal of impacted molars, the patient should be instructed to notify the physician if there is:
1. Pain and swelling after 1 week
2. Tenderness in the mouth when chewing
3. Pain associate with swallowing
4. Foul odor to the breath

57 A patient who undergoes a submucosal resection should be observed carefully for:
1. Occipital headache
2. Periorbital crepitus
3. Spitting up or vomiting of blood
4. White areas of healing sublingually

Situation: Mr. Fink, a soft drink vendor, enters the hospital with diarrhea, anorexia, weight loss, and abdominal cramps. A tentative diagnosis of colitis has been made. He is scheduled for a sigmoidoscopy and barium enema. Questions 58 through 65 refer to this situation.

58 In eliciting a health history the nurse bases the interview on the knowledge that colitis is commonly associated with:
1. Chemical stress
2. Endocrine stress
3. Psychologic stress
4. Physiologic stress

59 Which of the following symptoms of fluid and electrolyte imbalance caused by Mr. Fink's symptoms should the nurse report immediately?
1. Extreme muscle weakness and tachycardia
2. Development of tetany with muscle spasms
3. Nausea, vomiting, and leg and stomach cramps
4. Skin rash, diarrhea, and diplopia

60 Specific nursing responsibility in preparing Mr. Fink for his diagnostic procedures includes:
1. Administering soapsuds enemas till clear
2. Giving castor oil the afternoon before
3. Withholding food and fluid for 8 hours
4. Ensuring his understanding of what is to happen

61 Prior to the barium enema, Mr. Fink is to receive an enema. How should he be positioned when receiving the enema?
1. Sims position
2. Knee-chest position
3. Mid-Fowler position
4. Back lying position

62 What is the maximum safe height at which the container of fluid can be held when administering an enema?
1. 30.5 cm (12 inches)
2. 37 cm (15 inches)
3. 46 cm (18 inches)
4. 66 cm (26 inches)

63 During administration of the enema Mr. Fink complains of intestinal cramps. The nurse should:
1. Give at a slower rate
2. Lower the height of the container
3. Stop until cramps are gone
4. Discontinue the procedure

64 The visualization of the GI tract after a barium enema is made possible by:
1. The high x-ray absorbing properties of barium
2. Barium physically coloring the intestinal wall
3. The high x-ray transmitting properties of barium
4. The chemical interaction between barium and the electrolytes

65 To decrease GI irritability, the nurse should teach Mr. Fink to minimize use of:
1. Triglycerides and amino acids
2. Milk products and cola drinks
3. Table salt and rice products
4. Sugar products and proteins

Situation: *Mr. Brown is admitted to the hospital with delirium tremens. His physician prescribes bed rest, and he is receiving paraldehyde, thiamine chloride, and nicotinic acid. Questions 66 through 70 refer to this situation.*

66 On Mr. Brown's admission, the nurse should assign him to a:
1. One-bed room next to the bathroom
2. Two-bed room at the quiet end of the unit
3. One-bed room next to the nurses' station
4. Two-bed room next to the nurses' station

67 The nurse understands that paraldehyde is given to combat which of Mr. Brown's problems?
1. Fluid and electrolyte
2. Detoxification from alcohol
3. Emotional
4. Motor and sensory

68 When Mr. Brown is able to eat, the diet ordered for him is:
1. High protein, low carbohydrate, low fat
2. Protein to tolerance, moderate fat, high calorie, high vitamin, soft
3. High carbohydrate, low saturated fat, 1800 calories
4. Low protein, high carbohydrate, high fat, soft

69 A high-calorie diet fortified with vitamins will prevent damage to which organ that detoxifies alcohol?
1. Kidneys
2. Liver
3. Pancreas
4. Adrenals

70 Mr. Brown requires thiamine chloride and nicotinic acid because these vitamins are needed for the maintenance of:
1. Good circulation
2. The nervous system
3. Prothrombin formation
4. Elimination

Situation: *Mrs. Smith is admitted to the hospital with an acute attack of ulcerative colitis. She has been very worried about her 2 small children and calls her mother frequently for help. She recently pleaded with her mother to come and live with them. Mr. Smith objects to this, goes out alone quite often, and does not seem to take an interest in the children. Questions 71 through 77 refer to this situation.*

71 The nurse will understand the emotional aspects of these disorders more readily if the "stress" functions of the _____ are recognized.
1. Cerebral cortex and thyroid gland
2. Sympathetic nervous system and pancreas
3. Autonomic nervous system and adrenal glands
4. Central nervous system and hypothalamus

72 To give complete nursing care to Mrs. Smith, the nurse should:
1. Understand the patient's emotional conflict
2. Recognize his or her own feelings toward this patient
3. Talk with the patient's husband and mother
4. Develop rapport with the patient's physician

73 The nurse recognizes that the prognosis for Mrs. Smith will remain guarded until:
1. A surgical procedure is performed to remove the somatic factor
2. Her husband accepts her desire to have her mother move in with them
3. Her emotional conflicts are resolved
4. She reaches her 40s and endocrine activity is decreased

74 Which of the following symptoms should the nurse expect when assessing Mrs. Smith on admission?
1. Diarrhea, anorexia, weight loss, abdominal cramps, anemia
2. Anemia, hemoptysis, weight loss, abdominal cramps
3. Fever, anemia, nausea and vomiting, leukopenia, diarrhea
4. Leukocytosis, anorexia, weight loss

75 The physician orders daily stool examinations. Mrs. Smith is also scheduled for a sigmoidoscopy and barium enema. Stool examinations are ordered to determine:
1. Culture and sensitivity
2. Occult blood and organisms
3. Ova and parasites
4. Fat and undigested food

76 A serious complication of this disease is:
1. Hemorrhage
2. Perforation
3. Obstruction
4. Ileus

77 Mrs. Smith's initial hospital diet is residue free during the acute stage. Which food combination should the nurse indicate as the best choice for her?
1. Cream soup and crackers, omelet, mashed potatoes, roll, orange juice, coffee
2. Stewed chicken, baked potato with butter, strained peas, white bread, plain cake, milk
3. Baked fish, macaroni with cheese, strained carrots, fruit gelatin, milk
4. Lean roast beef, buttered white rice with egg slices, white bread with butter and jelly, tea with sugar

78 An adult intolerance to milk, found mostly in black populations, is caused by a genetic deficiency of the enzyme:
1. Sucrase
2. Lactase
3. Maltase
4. Amylase

79 Mrs. Aster is diagnosed as having a hiatus hernia. She tells you she is having difficulty sleeping at night. Appropriate intervention is:
1. Suggesting a large glass of milk before retiring
2. Eliminating carbohydrates from the diet
3. Sleeping on 2 or 3 pillows
4. Administering antacids such as sodium bicarbonate

Situation: Dr. Kinsey was found in a coma in his room at the large hospital where he had begun his residency. There was a strong odor of acetone on his breath. He is married and 28 years of age. His wife, Jane, states that he is a diabetic and recently switched to Orinase on his own instead of taking insulin as prescribed. Health records submitted did not reveal that Dr. Kinsey had diabetes mellitus. Emergency measures were instituted immediately. Questions 80 through 86 refer to this question.

80 Oral hypoglycemic agents may be used for diabetic patients with:
1. Ketosis or impending coma

2. Mature onset
3. Juvenile onset
4. Obesity

81 Dr. Kinsey has omitted pertinent information from his health record because:
1. Physicians with diabetes are not accepted for residency in many hospitals
2. He is unable to handle the psychologic stress related to alterations in body functioning
3. He needs assistance in developing a more favorable adaptation to this stress
4. Diabetics often have lapses of memory

82 Diabetic coma results from an excess accumulation in the blood of:
1. Nitrogen from protein catabolism, causing ammonia intoxication
2. Ketones from rapid fat breakdown, causing acidosis
3. Glucose from rapid carbohydrate metabolism, causing drowsiness
4. Sodium bicarbonate, causing alkalosis

83 The most common cause of diabetic ketoacidosis is:
1. Presence of infection
2. Increasing insulin dose
3. Inadequate food intake
4. Emotional stress

84 An independent nursing action which should be included in the plan of care for this patient is:
1. Regulating insulin dosage according to the amount of ketones found in the urine
2. Withholding glucose in any form until the ketoacidosis is corrected
3. Observing for signs of hypoglycemia
4. Giving fruit juices, broth, and milk as soon as the patient is able to take fluids orally

85 The nurse suspected hypokalemia when she observed which of the following symptoms?
1. Edema, bounding pulse, confusion
2. Apathy, weakness, abdominal distention
3. Sunken eyeballs, Kussmaul breathing, thirst
4. Spasms, diarrhea, irregular pulse rate

86 Important to both Dr. Kinsey and his wife, Jane, is an understanding that his diet for management of his diabetes:
1. Is based on nutritional requirements that are the same for all patients
2. Can be planned around a wide variety of commonly used foods
3. Should be rigidly controlled to avoid similar emergencies
4. Must not include combination dishes and processed foods, since they have too many variable seasonings

87 A basic concept of rehabilitation is defined by which of the following statements?
1. Rehabilitation is a specialty area with unique methods for meeting the patient's needs
2. Rehabilitation is not necessary for most patients be-

cause they will return to their usual activities following hospitalization

3. Rehabilitation needs, immediate or potential, are exhibited by all patients with a health problem

4. Rehabilitation needs are best met by the patient's family and community resources

88 Carbohydrates provide one of our main fuel sources for energy. Which of the following carbohydrate foods provides the quickest source of energy?
1. A slice of bread
2. A glass of orange juice
3. A glass of milk
4. Chocolate candy bar

89 An untreated diabetic may lapse into a coma because of acidosis. This acidosis is directly caused by an increased concentration in the blood of:
1. Glucose
2. Lactic acid
3. Glutamic acid
4. Alpha-keto acids

90 How should a fractional urine specimen be removed from a retention catheter?
1. Cleanse the drainage valve and remove from the collection bag
2. Disconnect and drain into a clean catheter
3. Wipe the catheter with alcohol and drain into a sterile test tube
4. Use a sterile syringe to remove from a clamped, cleansed catheter

91 Which of the following secretes an antidiuretic substance important for maintaining fluid balance?
1. Anterior pituitary
2. Adrenal cortex
3. Adrenal medulla
4. Posterior pituitary

92 As the amount of antidiuretic hormone in blood increases:
1. Glomerular filtration tends to decrease
2. Tubular reabsorption of potassium and water increases
3. Tubular reabsorption of sodium and water increases
4. Urine concentration tends to decrease

93 The posterior pituitary gland secretes antidiuretic hormone (ADH), which influences normal kidney function by stimulating the:
1. Glomerulus to control the quantity of fluid passing through it
2. Glomerulus to withhold the proteins from the urine
3. Nephron tubules to reabsorb water
4. Nephron tubules to reabsorb glucose

94 Two body systems that interact with the bicarbonate buffer system to preserve the normal body fluid pH of 7.4 are the:
1. Respiratory and urinary systems
2. Muscular and endocrine systems
3. Skeletal and nervous systems
4. Circulatory and urinary systems

Situation: Mrs. Thompson, age 39, was admitted to the hospital with a diagnosis of Addison's disease. She exhibited the following signs and symptoms: muscular weakness, anorexia, emaciation, GI distress, generalized dark pigmentation, hypotension, hypoglycemia, low sodium and high potassium levels, and a loss of libido. Questions 95 through 102 refer to this situation.

95 The hypotension can be explained by the fact that Addison's disease involves a disturbance in the production of:
1. Glucocorticoids
2. Androgens
3. Mineralocorticoids
4. Estrogens

96 The nurse should observe Mrs. Thompson closely for signs of infectious complications because there is a disturbance of function in the:
1. Proinflammatory effect
2. Antiinflammatory effect
3. Metabolic effect
4. Electrolytic effect

97 The emaciation, muscular weakness, and fatigue are due to disturbance of function in:
1. Protein anabolic effect
2. Electrolytic effect
3. Diurnal effect
4. Masculinizing effect

98 An important aspect of nursing care specific for Mrs. Thompson is:
1. Encouraging exercise
2. Providing a variety of diversional activities
3. Permitting as much activity as the patient desires
4. Protecting from exertion

99 Therapy for Mrs. Thompson is aimed chiefly at:
1. Restoring electrolyte balance
2. Improving carbohydrate metabolism
3. Increasing lymphoid tissue
4. Increasing eosinophils

100 Mrs. Thompson's treatment included a high-protein high-calorie diet with extra salt. As a means of encouraging her to eat, the nurse explained the reasons for this diet therapy as follows:
1. Extra salt is needed to replace the amount being lost due to lack of sufficient aldosterone to conserve sodium
2. Increased vitamins are needed to supply energy to help her regain lost weight
3. Increased protein is needed to heal the adrenal tissue and thus cure the disease
4. Increased amounts of potassium are needed to replace renal losses

101 Prior to discharge the physician prescribes hydrocortisone, 10 mg t.i.d., and fludrocortisone, 0.1 mg q.d. The nurse expects hydrocortisone to:
1. Prevent hypoglycemia and permit Mrs. Thompson to respond to stress
2. Increase amounts of angiotensin II to raise Mrs. Thompson's blood pressure

3. Control excessive loss of potassium salts
4. Decrease cardiac arrhythmias and dyspnea

102 The nurse should teach Mrs. Thompson to consult her physician immediately if she experiences which of these symptoms related to fludrocortisone therapy?
1. Fatigue, particularly in the afternoon
2. Increased frequency of urination
3. Rapid weight gain and dependent edema
4. Unpredictable changes in mood

Situation: *Mrs. Louis is admitted to the hospital with the diagnosis of Cushing's syndrome: Questions 103 through 108 refer to this situation.*

103 The nurse understands that the cause of Cushing's syndrome is most commonly:
1. Deprivation of adrenocortical hormones
2. Insufficient ACTH production
3. Hyperplasia of the adrenal cortex
4. Pituitary hypoplasia

104 Glucocorticoids and mineralocorticoids are secreted by the:
1. Pancreas
2. Hypophysis cerebri
3. Adrenal glands
4. Gonads

105 Which symptoms would the nurse expect when assessing Mrs. Louis?
1. "Buffalo hump" and hypertension
2. Dehydration and menorrhagia
3. Pitting edema and frequent colds
4. Migraine headache and dysmenorrhea

106 A bilateral adrenalectomy is schedules. Prior to surgery, steroids are administered to Mrs. Louis. The nurse understands the reason for this is to:
1. Compensate for sudden lack of these hormones following surgery
2. Increase the inflammatory action to promote scar formation
3. Foster accumulation of glycogen in the liver
4. Facilitate urinary excretion of salt and water following surgery

107 Which of the following drugs should the nurse be prepared to administer to Mrs. Louis on the day of surgery and in the immediate postoperative period?
1. Regular insulin
2. ACTH
3. Hydrocortisone succinate (Solu-Cortef)
4. Pituitary extract (Pituitrin)

108 An adrenalectomy is performed. Postoperatively, until regulated by steroid therapy, Mrs. Louis may show symptoms of:
1. Hyperglycemia
2. Sodium retention
3. Potassium excretion
4. Hypotension

109 Rapid adjustments made by the body during an emergency are associated with the increased activity of which gland?
1. Pituitary
2. Thyroid
3. Adrenal
4. Pancreas

Situation: *Mrs. Dreck is admitted with a history of abdominal pain, chills, nausea, and a purulent vaginal discharge. She is diagnosed as having pelvic inflammatory disease. Questions 110 through 114 refer to this situation.*

110 The nurse should assist Mrs. Dreck to the:
1. Sims position
2. Fowler position
3. Lithotomy position
4. Supine position with knees flexed

111 Mrs. Dreck menstruates regularly every 30 days. Her last menses started on January 1. When will she most probably ovulate next?
1. January 5 or 6
2. January 15
3. January 17
4. January 28

112 The incubation period for syphilis is about:
1. 72 hours
2. 1 week
3. 2 months
4. 2 to 6 weeks

113 The most sensitive and reliable treponemal antibody test for syphylis is the:
1. Wasserman test
2. VDRL test
3. Kahn test
4. FTA-ABS test

114 At which stage is syphilis not considered contagious?
1. Primary
2. Tertiary
3. Secondary
4. Incubation

115 The term *condylomata acuminata* refers to:
1. Veneral warts
2. Cancer of epididymis
3. Herpes zoster
4. Scabies

116 A disease produced by a gram-negative diplococcus that generally invades the urogenital tract is:
1. Cholera
2. Syphilis
3. Gonorrhea
4. Chancroid

117 Acute salpingitis is most commonly the result of:
1. Abortion
2. Gonorrhea
3. Hydatidiform mole
4. Syphilis

118 A disease that can arise from normal microbial flora, especially after prolonged antibiotic therapy, is:
1. Moniliasis or candidiasis
2. Scarlet fever
3. Q fever
4. Herpes zoster

119 Gram-negative diplococci found in a vaginal smear are presumed to be:
1. Gonococci
2. Meningococci
3. Pneumococci
4. *Treponema pallidum*

120 Which of the following tests might the physician perform to determine the underlying cause of uterine pain?
1. Endometrial smear
2. Laparoscopy
3. Tubal insufflation
4. Estradiol level

Situation: *Mr. Saul, a 68-year-old retired civil service employee, is admitted to the hospital via the emergency service. He was found unconscious 30 minutes prior to admission. The physical examination reveals right hemiplegia. Tentative diagnosis is cerebral vascular accident. Questions 121 through 125 refer to this situation.*

121 In observing Mr. Saul the nurse should check for signs of increased intracranial pressure. Which one of the following combinations of symptoms is indicative of increased intracranial pressure?
1. Slow bounding pulse, rising blood pressure, elevated temperature, stupor
2. Rapid weak pulse, fall in blood pressure, low temperature, restlessness
3. Weak rapid pulse, normal blood pressure, intermittent fever, lethargy
4. Slow bounding pulse, fall in blood pressure, temperature below 36° C (97° F), stupor

122 Since Mr. Saul is unconscious, the nurse should expect him to be:
1. Unable to react to painful stimuli
2. Incontinent of urine and feces
3. Incapable of spontaneous motion
4. Incapable of hearing

123 Mr. Saul regains consciousness and has expressive aphasia. As a part of the long-range planning, the nurse would:
1. Help the family to accept the fact that Mr. Saul cannot participate in verbal communication
2. Wait for Mr. Saul to verbalize his needs regardless of how long it may take
3. Begin associating words with physical objects
4. Help Mr. Saul accept this disability as permanent

124 Urinary retention and overflow, a frequent problem of the stroke patient, is evidenced by:
1. Decrease in total amount of urine voided
2. Frequency from inability to empty bladder
3. Continual incontinence
4. Oliguria and edema

125 Which of the following hospital methods is the most useful for the nurse to employ in encouraging patients to void?
1. Having the patient listen to running water
2. Warming a bedpan
3. Placing the patient's hands in warm water
4. Providing privacy

Situation: *Ellen Smith, a 76-year-old woman, is admitted to the rehabilitation unit following a stroke. She is bedridden and aphasic. The morning after her admission the physician orders an indwelling catheter, since she has been incontinent during the night. Questions 126 through 132 refer to this situation.*

126 It is learned from the daughter that her mother had not been incontinent while at home, and she insisted that the nurse had failed to communicate with her mother. This is an example of:
1. Treatment without consent of the patient, which is an invasion of rights
2. A catheter inserted for the patient's benefit
3. Inability to obtain consent for treatment because the patient was aphasic
4. A treatment that does not need special consent

127 Mrs. Smith has left hemiplegia. The nurse contributes to her rehabilitation by:
1. Making a referral to the physical therapist
2. Not moving the affected arm and leg unless necessary
3. Beginning active exercises
4. Positioning Mrs. Smith to prevent deformity and decubiti

128 The nurse can best prevent footdrop in a patient for whom bed rest has been prescribed by the use of:
1. Boards
2. Blocks
3. Cradles
4. Sandbags

129 Mrs. Smith's emotional responses to her illness would probably be determined by:
1. Her premorbid personality
2. The location of her lesion
3. The care she is receiving
4. Her ability to understand her illness

130 Mrs. Smith's position should be changed:
1. Every hour
2. Every 2 hours
3. Every 4 hours
4. Every 6 hours

131 In aiding Mrs. Smith to develop independence, the nurse should:
1. Demonstrate ways she can regain independence in activities
2. Reinforce success in tasks accomplished
3. Establish long-range goals for the patient
4. Point out her errors in performance

Situation: Mr. Smith is a 60-year-old man who is admitted to the hospital with a diagnosis of idiopathic trigeminal neuralgia (tic douloureux). Questions 160 through 166 refer to this situation.

160 In planning the nursing care for Mr. Smith, the nurse would:
1. Emphasize the importance of mouth care
2. Be alert to prevent dehydration or starvation
3. Initiate exercises of the jaw and facial muscles
4. Apply iced compresses to the affected area

161 The nurse would expect Mr. Smith to exhibit:
1. Uncontrollable tremors of the eyelid
2. Excruciating facial and head pain
3. Unilateral muscle weakness
4. Multiple petechiae

162 Which of the following symptoms should the nurse also expect Mr. Smith to demonstrate?
1. Exhaustion and fatigue due to extreme pain
2. Excessive talkativeness due to apprehension
3. Hyperactivity due to medications received
4. Prolonged periods of sleep broken only by external stimuli

163 In planning care for Mr. Smith, the nurse must:
1. Avoid walking swiftly past the patient
2. Discontinue oral hygiene temporarily
3. Massage both sides of the face frequently
4. Keep the patient in the prone position

164 Mr. Smith tells the nurse he is taking all 4 of the medications listed. The nurse should be aware that the one used to treat trigeminal neuralgia is:
1. Carbamazepine (Tegretol)
2. Allopurinol (Zyloprim)
3. Morphine sulfate
4. Ascorbic acid

165 Surgery, with cutting of the nerve, is performed. Which of the following would be an unusual occurrence after surgery?
1. Development of herpes simplex
2. Recurrence of the pain, which will gradually decrease
3. Development of a crawling or tingling sensation in the area
4. Loss of muscle power in the area

166 In discharge planning for Mr. Smith, the nurse should counsel the patient to:
1. Perform facial exercises
2. Have regular dental checkups
3. Avoid stressful situations
4. Chew food on the affected side

167 Electric stimulation by the use of a peripheral nerve implant or dorsal column stimulator is used in intractable pain. The nurse should explain that after surgery:
1. The patient should not take tub baths
2. The device may interfere with the television remote control
3. Analgesics will no longer be necessary
4. The transmitter must be worn externally

168 A procedure done to relieve intractable pain in the upper torso is:

1. Chondrectomy
2. Cordotomy
3. Rhizotomy
4. Wolfgang's procedure

169 When the fluid in a bottle is allowed to flow into a person intravenously:
1. Chemical energy is converted to kinetic energy
2. Potential energy is converted to kinetic energy
3. Potential energy is converted to chemical energy
4. Kinetic energy is converted to potential energy

170 An important function of the albumin of the blood is:
1. Red blood cell formation
2. The activation of white blood cells
3. Blood clotting
4. The development of the colloid osmotic pressure

171 The capillary endothelium is a selectively permeable membrane. Which of the following molecules cannot easily pass through it?
1. O_2 and CO_2
2. Plasma proteins
3. Glucose, O_2, and CO_2
4. Ions, amino acids, and water

172. The reabsorption of water from glomerular filtrate (in the kidney tubules), the flow of water between the intracellular and interstitial compartments, and the exchange of fluid between plasma and interstitial fluid spaces are caused by what important physical process?
1. Dialysis
2. Active transport
3. Osmosis
4. Diffusion

Situation: Mr. McGee, a 31-year-old private in the Marines recently returned from Southeast Asia after a 13-month tour of duty, complains of chills along with a high fever. On the basis of the history and physical examination, the physician believes the most likely diagnosis is malaria. Questions 173 through 179 refer to this situation.

173 The most important diagnostic test in malaria is:
1. Smear of peripheral blood
2. Blood leukocyte count
3. Erythrocyte sedimentation rate
4. Splenic puncture

174 The nurse is reviewing Mr. McGee's physical examination and laboratory test. An important finding in malaria is:
1. Splenomegaly
2. Leukocytosis
3. Elevated sedimentation rate
4. Erythrocytosis

175 Mr. McGee asks the nurse how he could have prevented the disease. The nurse should explain that prophylaxis for the control of malaria includes:
1. Vaccination
2. Patient isolation
3. Prompt detection and effective treatment
4. Antibiotic therapy

176 Blackwater fever occurs in some cases of malaria. The nurse should observe Mr. McGee for:
1. Diarrhea
2. Coffee ground emesis
3. Low-grade fever
4. Dark red urine

177 A serious complication of acute malaria is:
1. Anemia and cachexia
2. Congested lungs
3. Changes in water and electrolyte balance
4. Impaired peristalsis

178 In caring for Mr. McGee, the nurse should know that:
1. Peritoneal dialysis is usually indicated
2. He should be awakened only for nourishment after a paroxysm
3. Attention should be focused on rest and nourishing food between paroxysms
4. Isolation is necessary to prevent cross infection

179 Because Mr. McGee has a chloroquine-resistant malaria, the physician orders 650 mg of quinine dihydrochloride to be given over an 8-hour period by IV drip in 1000 ml of normal saline. The IV equipment is calibrated at 20 drops per milliliter. To deliver the correct dosage, the solution must be set to flow at the rate of:
1. 10 drops/min
2. 21 drops/min
3. 34 drops/min
4. 42 drops/min

180 Whenever quinine is used, the nurse should be alert to symptoms of severe cinchonism, which are:
1. Tinnitus, decreased auditory acuity, nausea
2. Deafness, vertigo, and severe visual, GI, and central nervous system disturbances
3. Pruritus, urticaria, and difficulty in breathing
4. Leg cramps, fever, and swollen painful joints

181 After several days of IV therapy, the physician replaces the IV injection with quinine sulfate, 2 g per day in divided doses. The nurse should administer this medication after meals to:
1. Delay its absorption
2. Minimize gastric irritation
3. Decrease stimulation of appetite
4. Decrease its antiarrhythmic action

182 Which of the following statements is true concerning successful drug therapy against *Plasmodium falciparum* infections?
1. The infections can generally be eliminated
2. Transmission by the *Anopheles* mosquito can occur
3. The infections are controlled
4. Immunity will prevent reinfection

Situation: *Walter Sams, a 75-year-old man, enters the hospital with benign prostatic hypertrophy for further tests and a prostatectomy. Questions 183 through 187 refer to this situation.*

183 The nurse insists that a medication for sleep be taken at 9 P.M. even though the patient tells her he never went to sleep this early and would like the medication delayed. Later the patient awakens and is confused. He tries to get out of bed and in so doing falls, fracturing his hip. Legally:
1. Hospital policy requires that sleep medications be given at 9 P.M. and *respondeat superior* applies
2. Patient's rights have precedence over hospital policy or physician's orders
3. The time the medication was given has nothing to do with the confusion
4. When the physician orders a medication, it must be given at the scheduled time unless the nursing supervisor authorizes differently

184 The definitive diagnosis of benign prostatic hypertrophy is arrived at by:
1. Biopsy of prostatic tissue
2. Pap smear of prostatic fluid
3. Rectal examination
4. Serum phosphatase studies

185 Which of the following tests might be ordered to estimate the effect of Mr. Sams' illness on his kidneys?
1. PSP, urea clearance, urine concentration
2. Sulkowitch, catecholamines, urine dilution
3. Bence Jones protein, urine concentration, albumin
4. Microscopic porphyrins, urinalysis

186 While caring for Mr. Sams, the nurse is aware that benign prostatic hypertrophy (BPH):
1. Usually becomes malignant
2. Predisposes to hydronephrosis
3. Is a congenital abnormality
4. Causes an elevated acid phosphatase

187 Mr. Sams had a suprapubic prostatectomy with continuous bladder irrigations. When caring for a patient with a continuous bladder irrigation, the nurse should:
1. Measure urinary specific gravity
2. Record hourly outputs
3. Include irrigating solution on intake and output records
4. Exclude irrigating solution from any 24-hour urine tests ordered

188 Ammonia is excreted by the kidney to help maintain:
1. Low bacterial levels in the urine
2. Osmotic pressure of the blood
3. Acid-base balance of the body
4. Normal red blood cell production

189 What structure encircles the male urethra?
1. Bulbourethral gland
2. Epididymis
3. Prostate gland
4. Seminal vesicle

Situation: *Miss Jenner has chronic renal failure. Questions 190 through 194 refer to this situation.*

190 Miss Jenner is not responding to treatment. Dialysis may be performed to remove waste products from the blood. The main indication for dialysis is:

1. Increase in blood pressure
2. High and rising potassium levels
3. Ascites
4. Acidosis

191 The artificial kidney machine primarily makes use of the physical principle of:
1. Filtration
2. Osmosis
3. Diffusion
4. Dialysis

192 Miss Jenner, who is receiving hemodialysis for chronic renal failure, is especially prone to develop:
1. Peritonitis
2. Renal calculi
3. Bladder infection
4. Serum hepatitis

193 In caring for Miss Jenner, who has had an arteriovenous shunt inserted for hemodialysis, the nurse would:
1. Notify the physician if a bruit is heard in the cannula
2. Use strict aseptic technique when giving shunt care
3. Cover the entire cannula with an elastic bandage
4. Take the blood pressure every 4 hours from the arm that contains the shunt

194 A nurse working in a hemodialysis unit runs a high risk of developing:
1. Type A viral hepatitis
2. Infectious hepatitis
3. Type B viral hepatitis
4. Hemolytic hepatitis

Situation: Mr. Carson is hospitalized with severe right flank pain, general weakness, and fever. He has a history of recurrent urinary tract infection, and the formation of renal calculi is suspected. The physician orders a 200-mg calcium diet for 3 days to be monitored with urinary calcium tests. Questions 195 through 201 refer to this situation.

195 In caring for patients with renal calculi, the most important nursing action is to:
1. Record blood pressure
2. Strain all urine
3. Limit fluids at night
4. Administer analgesics every 3 hours

196 What background knowledge helps the nurse understand the reasons for this strict 200 mg calcium diet?
1. Excessive calcium intake has little influence on renal stone formation
2. The thyroid hormone controls the serum levels of calcium and phosphorus
3. If calcium excretion is lowered on the test diet, hyperparathyroidism can be identified as the cause of the calculi
4. If calcium excretion is still elevated on the test diet, dietary influences can be ruled out

197 Mr. Carson's calcium balance studies following his test diet are negative. His diet order is increased to 400 mg calcium—a general low-calcium diet level. Which of the following foods would be allowed on his diet?

1. Vanilla ice cream with chocolate syrup and nuts
2. Salmon loaf with cheese sauce
3. Chocolate pudding
4. Roast beef with baked potato

198 The name of the procedure for the removal of a bladder stone is:
1. Cystolithiasis
2. Cystolithectomy
3. Cystometry
4. Cryoextraction

199 Diet therapy for renal calculi of calcium phosphate composition would probably be:
1. High calcium and phosphorus, alkaline ash
2. High calcium and phosphorus, acid ash
3. Low purine
4. Low calcium and phosphorus, acid ash

200 Mr. Carson will be taking sulfisoxazole (Gantrisin) at home. The nurse instructs him to:
1. Measure and record urine output
2. Strain urine for crystals and stones
3. Maintain the exact time schedule for drug taking
4. Stop the drug if his urinary output increases

201 If Mr. Carson's renal stones had been of calcium oxalate composition, which of the following diets would the nurse have been expected to teach the patient?
1. Low in calcium and oxalate, acid ash
2. Low in calcium and oxalate, alkaline ash
3. Low in methionine, acid ash
4. Low in purines, alkaline ash

Situation: Mrs. Harvey has an acute episode of right-sided heart failure and is receiving furosemide (Lasix). Questions 202 through 208 refer to this situation.

202 The physician has prescribed aspirin for her arthritic pain. When Mrs. Harvey asks why she is not receiving the same aspirin dosage she usually takes, the nurse's response would be based on knowledge that:
1. Aspirin in large doses after an acute stress episode increases the bleeding potential
2. Use of furosemide and aspirin concomitantly increases formation of uric acid crystals in the nephron
3. Competition for renal excretion sites by the drugs causes increased serum levels of aspirin
4. Aspirin accelerates metabolism of furosemide and decreases the diuretic effect

203 The symptoms that Mrs. Harvey most likely displayed on admission are:
1. Dyspnea, edema, fatigue
2. Weakness, palpitations, nausea
3. Fatigue, vertigo, and headache
4. A feeling of distress when breathing

204 Mrs. Harvey has edema during the day and it disappears at night. The patient states it is not painful and is located in the lower extremities. The nurse should suspect:
1. Pulmonary edema
2. Right-sided heart failure

3. Myocardial infarction
4. Lung disease

205 Pitting edema in the lower extremities occurs with this problem because of the:
1. Increase in tissue colloid osmotic pressure
2. Increase in the tissue hydrostatic pressure at the arterial end of the capillary bed
3. Decrease in the plasma colloid osmotic pressure
4. Increase in the plasma hydrostatic pressure at the venous end of the capillary beds

206 The nurse can best assess the degree of edema in an extremity by:
1. Checking for pitting
2. Weighing the patient
3. Measuring the affected area
4. Observing intake and output

207 The nurse notes that Mrs. Harvey's abdomen is distended. The nurse should realize that the patient with congestive heart failure develops ascites because of:
1. Increased pressure within the circulatory system
2. Rapid diffusion of solutes and solvents into plasma
3. Rapid osmosis from tissue spaces to cells
4. Loss of cellular constituents in blood

208 Mrs. Harvey's condition worsens. The physician has ordered CVP readings q. 2 h. Which of the following is true of CVP?
1. A high reading may be indicative of dehydration
2. A normal reading is 60 to 120 mm of water
3. The zero point of the manometer is level with the midaxilla
4. The patient must be kept flat in bed while the catheter is in place

209 Which of the following is most likely to occur in a patient with unresolved edema?
1. Thrombus formation
2. Tissue ischemia
3. Proteinemia
4. Contractures

210 The mercurial diuretics alter active transport systems in the kidney tubules, resulting in increased excretion of sodium and, secondarily, water. The principle explaining the secondary water loss (diuresis) is:
1. Osmosis
2. Diffusion
3. Filtration
4. Active transport

211 Mrs. Johnson has a urinary tract infection and is receiving chlorothiazide (Diuril). The planned therapeutic effect of the drug is to:
1. Decrease the amount of fluid reabsorption in Henle's loop
2. Increase the excretion of sodium and chloride
3. Decrease the reabsorption of potassium
4. Increase the glomerular filtration rate

212 Shock is:
1. Failure of peripheral circulation
2. An irreversible phenomenon
3. Always caused by decreased blood volume
4. A fleeting reaction to tissue injury

213 Common symptoms of Buerger's disease are:
1. Burning pain precipitated by cold exposure, fatigue, blanching of skin
2. Easy fatigue of part, continuous claudication
3. General blanching of skin, intermittent claudication
4. Intermittent claudication, burning pain after exposure to cold

214 Patients with peripheral vascular disease are instructed to stop smoking because the nicotine:
1. Dilates the peripheral vessels, causing a reflex constriction of visceral vessels
2. Constricts the peripheral vessels and increases the force of flow
3. Constricts the collateral circulation, dilating the superficial vessels
4. Constricts the superficial vessels, dilating the deep vessels

215 In chronic occlusive arterial disease the precipitating cause for ulceration and gangrenous lesions often is:
1. Poor hygiene
2. Stimulants such as coffee, tea, or cola drinks
3. Emotional stress
4. Trauma from mechanical, chemical, or thermal sources

Situation: Mr. Wolfsmith, a 46-year-old executive, is admitted with chest pain and shortness of breath. A diagnosis of myocardial infarction is made. Questions 216 through 223 refer to this situation.

216 Mr. Wolfsmith is placed in the C.C.U., where the nurse will observe for one of the more common complications of myocardial infarction, which is:
1. Cardiac arrhythmia
2. Anaphylactic shock
3. Cardiac enlargement
4. Hypokalemia

217 To ascertain Mr. Wolfsmith's diagnosis, tests for which the nurse would prepare him include:
1. Paul-Bunnell, serum potassium
2. LDH, CPK, SGOT
3. Sedimentation rate, SGPT
4. Serum calcium, APPT

218 Mr. Wolfsmith is in the coronary unit on a cardiac monitor. The nurse observes ventricular irritability on the screen. The medication that might be administered for this would be:
1. Digoxin (Lanoxin)
2. Lidocaine
3. Furosemide (Lasix)
4. Levarterenol bitartrate (Levophed)

219 The nurse observes Mr. Wolfsmith's monitor and identifies asystole. This arrhythmia requires nursing attention because the heart is:

1. Beating very rapidly
2. Not beating
3. Beating irregularly
4. Beating slowly

220 A cardiac arrest code is called for Mr. Wolfsmith. During a cardiac arrest, the nurse and the arrest team must keep in mind the:
1. Time the patient is anoxic
2. Heart rate of the patient before arrest
3. Age of the patient
4. Emergency medications available

221 When it is discovered that Mr. Wolfsmith has no carotid pulse or respirations, the nurse:
1. Clears the airway
2. Gives 4 full lung inflations
3. Compresses the lower sternum 15 times
4. Checks for a radial pulse

222 There are 2 nurses performing CPR on Mr. Wolfsmith. During performance of cardiopulmonary resuscitation with 2 people, the rate of ventilation to cardiac compression is:
1. 1:5
2. 1:10
3. 2:15
4. 4:15

223 The nurse performing cardiac compression on Mr. Wolfsmith is aware that it is essential to exert a vertical downward pressure, which depresses the lower sternum at least:
1. 1.3 to 2 cm (½ to ¾ inch)
2. 2 to 2.5 cm (¾ to 1 inch)
3. 2.5 to 4 cm (1 to 1½ inches)
4. 4 to 5 cm (1½ to 2 inches)

---

224 Blood samples from the right atrium, right ventricle, and pulmonary artery are analyzed for their oxygen content during cardiac catheterization. Normally:
1. All contain about the same amount of oxygen
2. All contain less CO_2 than does pulmonary vein blood
3. Pulmonary artery blood contains more oxygen than the other samples
4. All contain more oxygen than does pulmonary vein blood

225 Many vitamins and minerals regulate the chemical changes of cell metabolism by acting in a coenzyme role. This means that the vitamin or mineral:
1. Is not a part of the enzyme controlling a particular reaction
2. May be a necessary catalyst present for the reaction to proceed
3. Forms a new compound by a series of complex changes
4. Prevents unnecessary reactions by neutralizing the controlling enzyme

226 Because fat is insoluble in water, it cannot travel freely in the blood. Therefore the main type of compound formed to serve as a vehicle of transport is:

1. Triglyceride
2. Plasma protein
3. Phospholipid
4. Lipoprotein

227 The food group lowest in natural sodium is:
1. Meat
2. Milk
3. Vegetables
4. Fruits

228 The terms *saturated and unsaturated,* when used in reference to fats, indicate degrees of:
1. Color
2. Taste
3. Hardness
4. Digestibility

229 When the transport fat compounds accumulate in abnormal levels in the blood, the diet may be modified as one effort to control them. The foods most affected by such diet therapy would be:
1. Vegetable oils
2. Fruits
3. Grains
4. Animal fats

230 The breakdown of triglyceride molecules can be expected to produce:
1. Urea nitrogen
2. Amino acids
3. Simple sugars
4. Fatty acids

231 Cholesterol is important in the human body for:
1. Bone formation
2. Blood clotting
3. Cellular membrane structure
4. Muscle contraction

232 Cholesterol is frequently discussed in relation to atherosclerosis. It is a substance that:
1. All persons would be better off without because it causes the disease process
2. Circulates in the blood, the level of which responds usually to dietary substitutions of unsaturated fats for saturated fats
3. Is found in many foods, both plant and animal sources
4. May be controlled entirely by eliminating food sources

Situation: *Mr. Psanka is admitted from the emergency room in acute respiratory distress resulting from an asthmatic attack. Questions 233 through 239 refer to this situation.*

233 In which position should the nurse place Mr. Psanka to facilitate maximum air exchange?
1. High Fowler
2. Semi-Fowler
3. Orthopneic
4. Supine with pillows

234 Inhalation of isoproterenol (Isuprel), 1:200 p.r.n., is prescribed for which of the following reasons?
1. To increase bronchial secretions
2. To decrease blood pressure
3. To produce sedation
4. To relax bronchial spasm

235 During therapy with isoproterenol Mr. Psanka complains of palpitation, chest pain, and a throbbing headache. In view of these symptoms, which of the following statements represents the most appropriate nursing action?
1. Reassure Mr. Psanka that these effects are temporary and will subside as he becomes accustomed to the drug
2. Withhold the drug until additional orders are obtained from the physician
3. Tell him not to worry; he is experiencing expected side effects from the medicine
4. Ask him to relax; then instruct him to breathe slowly and deeply for several minutes

236 Mr. Psanka's pulmonary function studies are abnormal. The nurse should realize that one of the most common complications of chronic asthma is:
1. Atelectasis
2. Emphysema
3. Pneumothorax
4. Pulmonary fibrosis

237 Emphysema causes a failure in oxygen supply because of:
1. Infectious obstructions
2. Respiratory muscle paralysis
3. Pleural effusion
4. Loss of aerating surface

238 When the alveoli lose their normal elasticity, the nurse teaches Mr. Psanka exercises that lead to effective use of the diaphragm because:
1. Mr. Psanka has an increase in the vital capacity of his lungs
2. The residual capacity of the lungs has been increased
3. Inspiration has been markedly prolonged and difficult
4. Abdominal breathing is an effective compensatory mechanism that is spontaneously initiated

239 Respiratory acidosis may occur as a result of a long-term problem in oxygen maintenance when:
1. The carbon dioxide is not excreted
2. Any localized tissue necrosis occurs as a result of poor oxygen supply to the area
3. Hyperventilation occurs, even if the cause is not physiologic
4. There is a loss of carbon dioxide from the body's buffer pool

240 Cutting the left phrenic nerve results in:
1. Relief of pain in the left side of the chest
2. Paralysis of the left side of the diaphragm
3. Collapse of the right lung
4. Paralysis of the diaphragm on the opposite side

241 Air rushes into the alveoli as a result of:
1. The rising pressure in the alveoli
2. The rising pressure in the pleura
3. The lowered pressure in the chest cavity
4. The relaxation of the diaphragm

242 A nurse will use an Ambu bag in the intensive care unit when:
1. The patient is in ventricular fibrillation
2. A surgical incision with copious drainage is present
3. Respiratory output must be monitored at intervals
4. There is respiratory arrest

243 In suctioning a tracheostomy the nurse must remember that it is important to:
1. Initiate suction as the catheter is being withdrawn slowly
2. Insert catheter until cough reflex is stimulated
3. Untie the neck tapes while cleansing the skin edge of the wound
4. Remove the inner cannula before inserting the suction catheter

244 A patient has an anaphylactic reaction within the first half hour after an IV infusion containing penicillin is started. Problems occurring during an anaphylactic reaction are the result of:
1. Decreased cardiac output and dilation of major blood vessels
2. Bronchial constriction and decreased peripheral resistance
3. Respiratory depression and cardiac standstill
4. Constriction of capillaries and decreased cardiac output

245 Occurrence of an anaphylactic reaction after receiving penicillin indicates that a patient has:
1. An acquired atopic sensitization
2. Passive immunity to the penicillin allergen
3. Antibodies to penicillin acquired after prior use of the drug
4. Developed potent bivalent antibodies when the IV administration was started

246 A patient has an urticarial response after taking ampicillin (Polycillin) orally for 3 days. Diphenhydramine hydrochloride (Benadryl) is administered to:
1. Destroy histamine in tissues and reverse the urticarial response
2. Inhibit release of vasoactive substances and dilate tissue capillaries
3. Metabolize histamine and inhibit release of substances causing intense itching
4. Complete with histamine for receptors and interfere with vasodilation

247 This patient may also be given penicillinase (Neutrapen) to:
1. Displace penicillin from receptor sites
2. Counteract the effects of penicillin in tissues
3. Destroy the penicillin allergen
4. Maintain therapy with a nonallergenic form of penicillin

248 The most important aspect of hand washing is:
1. Water
2. Soap
3. Friction
4. Time
249 Vitamin K is essential for normal blood clotting because it promotes:
1. Ionization of blood calcium
2. Platelet aggregation
3. Fibrinogen formation by liver
4. Prothrombin formation by liver
250 Prophylaxis for serum hepatitis includes:
1. Enteric precautions applied to infected individuals
2. Screening of blood donors
3. Case finding and treatment of infection
4. Patient isolation
251 In the patient with serum hepatitis the earliest indication of parenchymal damage to the liver usually is:
1. Elevation in transaminase
2. Rise in bilirubin
3. Alteration in proteins
4. Rise in alkaline phosphatase

Situation: Mrs. Carter, the mother of 2 children, has infectious hepatitis. Questions 252 through 254 refer to this situation.

252 Mrs. Carter's children are being given gamma globulin to provide passive immunity, which:
1. Stimulates production of short-lived antibodies
2. Stimulates the lymphatic system to produce large numbers of antibodies
3. Provides antibodies that neutralize the antigen
4. Accelerates antigen-antibody union at hepatic sites
253 The physician has prescribed phenobarbital sodium (Luminal) for Mrs. Carter. The nurse tells Mrs. Carter to contact the physician if she notices:
1. Decreased tolerance to common foods, constipation
2. Diarrhea, rash on the upper part of her body
3. Anal pruritus, orthostatic, hypotension
4. Loss of appetite, persistent lethargy
254 When caring for Mrs. Carter the nurse should take special precautions to:
1. Use caution when bringing food tray to patient
2. Wear mask and gown before entering the room
3. Use gloves when removing the patient's bedpan
4. Prevent droplet spread of infection

255 GI bleeding can be treated medically by infusing medication through an arterial line. The drug commonly used for this purpose is:
1. Phytonadione (Aquamephyton)
2. Neostigmine (Prostigmin)
3. Propantheline (Pro-Banthine)
4. Vasopressin (Pitressin)
256 A patient who may develop pernicious anemia is one who:
1. Has diabetes
2. Had a gastrectomy
3. Has hemorrhaged
4. Practices poor dietary habits
257 An antrectomy would most likely be done for a patient with a diagnosis of:
1. Trigeminal neuralgia
2. Otosclerosis
3. Gastric ulcers
4. Cataracts

Situation: Dr. Grove, a single, 25-year-old professor of mathematics at a major university, is hospitalized for bleeding gastric ulcers. A conservative regimen is being followed at present. At an early age it became apparent that Dr. Grove was a genius. His capabilities were encouraged to develop to their fullest potential by his mother. He graduated from high school summa cum laude at the age of 13 and at the age of 19 had received a Ph.D. degree in mathematics. Dr. Grove lives at home with his aging mother. Questions 258 through 262 refer to this situation.

258 Dr. Grove describes his pain as:
1. A dull ache radiating to the left side
2. An intermittent colicky flank pain
3. A generalized abdominal pain intensified by moving
4. A gnawing sensation relieved by food
259 Analysis of factors resulting in psychologic conflict for Dr. Grove reveals:
1. An unconscious need to be dependent
2. The drive to excel in whatever he does
3. Conversion of emotional tension due to chronic repressed hostility
4. Many feelings that are deep in the unconscious
260 Despite initiation of therapy, Dr. Grove continues to be apprehensive and restless. Nursing action should include:
1. Telling him everything will be all right
2. Administering antibiotics as ordered
3. Explaining the importance of rest
4. Administering sedatives as ordered
261 What is the basic goal underlying Dr. Grove's conservative regimen?
1. To increase roughage and bulk
2. To eliminate chemical, mechanical, and thermal irritation
3. To provide optimum amounts of all nutrients
4. To provide psychologic support by offering a wide variety of foods
262 If Dr. Grove has lost enough blood to develop a mild anemia, which of the following drugs may be used in treatment of this condition?
1. Dextran
2. Cari-Tab Softabs
3. Salts of iron
4. Vitamin B_{12}

263 Prolonged anemia or polycythemia may eventually place strain on a patient's heart. The concept underlying this strain is:
1. Pressure

2. Surface tension
3. Viscosity
4. Temperature

264 In caring for the patient with an ileostomy the nurse would:
   1. Expect the stoma to start draining on the third post-operative day
   2. Explain that the drainage can be controlled with daily irrigations
   3. Anticipate that emotional stress can increase intestinal peristalsis
   4. Encourage the patient to eat foods high in residue

265 If the ileum is removed surgically, the individual may suffer from anemia because:
   1. The hemopoietic factor is absorbed only in the terminal ileum
   2. Folic acid is absorbed only in the terminal ileum
   3. Iron absorption is dependent on simultaneous bile salt absorption in the terminal ileum
   4. The trace elements copper, cobalt, and nickel, required for hemoglobin synthesis, occur only in the ileum

266 Which of the following types of sports should a patient with an ileostomy avoid?
   1. Track events
   2. Swimming
   3. Skiing
   4. Football

267 How far into the rectum should a rectal catheter be inserted?
   1. 5 cm (2 inches)
   2. 10 cm (4 inches)
   3. 15 cm (6 inches)
   4. 20 cm (8 inches)

268 A rectal tube is sometimes inserted for the relief of distention. What is the minimal time it should remain in place to be effective?
   1. 15 minutes
   2. 30 minutes
   3. 45 minutes
   4. 60 minutes

Situation: Mrs. Graham has a diagnosis of possible bowel obstruction. She complains of nausea, is vomiting dark bile material, and has severe crampy, intermittent, abdominal pain. Her physician suspects the bowel obstruction is caused by an intussusception. Questions 269 through 275 refer to this situation.

269 An intussusception is:
   1. Kinking of the bowel onto itself
   2. Telescoping of a proximal loop of bowel into a distal loop
   3. A band of connective tissue compressing the bowel
   4. A protrusion of an organ or part of an organ through the wall that contains it

270 A flat plate radiograph of the abdomen is ordered. The nurse recognizes that the patient should receive:
   1. Nothing by mouth for 8 hours

2. A low soapsuds enema
3. No special preparation
4. A laxative the evening before the x-ray film is taken

271 Surgery is performed; Mrs. Graham is found to have a perforated appendix with localized peritonitis rather than an intussusception. In view of this finding, how would the nurse position Mrs. Graham postoperatively?
   1. Semi-Fowler
   2. Trendelenburg
   3. Sims
   4. Dorsal recumbent

272 Four days after surgery Mrs. Graham has not passed any flatus and there are no bowel sounds. Despite the fact that her abdomen has become more distended, she feels little discomfort. Paralytic ileus is suspected. In this condition there is an interference caused by:
   1. Impaired blood supply
   2. Impaired neural functioning
   3. Perforation of the bowel wall
   4. Obstruction of the bowel lumen

273 Mrs. Graham is convalescing from abdominal surgery when she develops thrombophlebitis. Which of the following signs would indicate this complication to the nurse?
   1. Severe pain on extension of an extremity
   2. Pitting edema of the lower extremities
   3. Intermittent claudication
   4. Warm, tender area on the leg

274 Mrs. Graham is receiving Dicumarol, a coumarin derivative. Which of the following tests would be most specific for calculating daily dosage of anticoagulant?
   1. Prothrombin time
   2. Clotting time
   3. Bleeding time
   4. Sedimentation rate

275 Which of the following drugs would you expect the physician to order if symptoms of Dicumarol overdose are observed?
   1. Iron-dextran (Imferon)
   2. Heparin
   3. Vitamin K
   4. Protamine sufate

Situation: Alice, a 45-year-old college student, is admitted to the hospital for diabetic acidosis. Questions 276 through 282 refer to this situation.

276 The cause of Alice's symptoms is a:
   1. Sudden increase in the concentration of cholesterol in the extracellular compartment
   2. Physiologic phenomenon following the ingestion of too much highly acidic food
   3. Rise in the pH of the blood to a point above 7.5
   4. Decrease in the pH of the blood to a point below 7.3

277 Several laboratory tests are done. Alice's symptoms lead the nurse to expect the blood test to reveal:
   1. Low sugar, decreased acidity, low CO_2 combining power

2. Elevated sugar, normal acidity, high CO_2 combining power
3. Elevated sugar, increased acidity, low CO_2 combining power
4. Low sugar, increased acidity, high CO_2 combining power

278 The type of insulin that will be used during the emergency treatment of the acidosis and until Alice is eating regularly is:
1. Isophane insulin suspension (NPH insulin)
2. Insulin injection (regular insulin)
3. Insulin zinc suspension (lente insulin)
4. Protamine zinc insulin suspension

279 After blood studies and observation of urinary volume, the physician orders potassium chloride, 20 mEq, to be added to the IV solution. The primary purpose for administering this drug to Alice is:
1. Replacement of potassium deficit
2. Treatment of hyperpnea
3. Prevention of flaccid paralysis
4. Treatment of cardiac arrhythmias

280 In the exchange system of dietary management, which of the following is *not* equivalent?
1. 1 scoop ice milk = 1 slice bread
2. 1 oz cheese = 1 cup milk
3. 1 egg = 1 oz meat
4. 1 slice bacon = 2 Tbsp cream

281 Alice and her family members should be taught the use of glucagon. The primary use of glucagon is to treat:
1. Diabetic acidosis
2. Insulin-induced hypoglycemia
3. Idiosyncratic reactions to insulin
4. Hyperinsulin secretion related to neoplasm

282 Alice's nursing plan includes that before discharge she will know how to give herself insulin, adjust the dosage, understand her diet, and test her urine. She progresses well and is discharged 10 days following admission. Legally:
1. The physician was responsible and the nurse should have cleared her care with him
2. The nurse was properly functioning as a health teacher
3. The visiting nurse should do health teaching in the home
4. A family member should have been taught also to administer the insulin

283 The main function of adipose tissue in fat metabolism is synthesizing and:
1. Using lipoproteins for fat transport
2. Storing triglycerides for energy reserves
3. Regulating cholesterol production
4. Releasing glucose for energy

284 A young man is brought to the hospital in a coma. It is discovered that he is diabetic. He is given an IV containing insulin, glucose, and potassium. The solution contains potassium because potassium ions in the extracellular fluid must be replenished since they:

1. Are carried with glucose to the kidneys and excreted in the urine in increased amounts
2. Enter the intracellular fluid because of the generalized anabolism induced by insulin and glucose
3. Are rapidly lost from the body by copious diaphoresis present during coma
4. Are quickly used up during the rapid series of catabolic reactions stimulated by insulin and glucose

285 When teaching a patient about an oral hypoglycemic medication, the nurse should emphasize the significance of:
1. Manifestations of toxicity
2. Untoward reactions
3. Taking it regularly and on time
4. Increasing dosage when necessary

286 Which of the following represents a normal pH for arterial blood?
1. 7.0
2. 7.30
3. 7.42
4. 7.50

Situation: Mr. Pierce, a patient who has acromegaly and diabetes mellitus, has had a hypophysectomy. Questions 287 through 291 refer to this situation.

287 An oversecretion of which hormone produces acromegaly?
1. Growth hormone
2. Thyroid hormone
3. Thyroid-stimulating hormone
4. Testosterone

288 Which of the following will *not* be true of Mr. Pierce after his hypophysectomy? He will:
1. Be sterile for the rest of his life
2. Have to take cortisone (or similar preparation) for the rest of his life
3. Have to take thyroxin (or similar preparation) for the rest of his life
4. Require larger doses of insulin than he did preoperatively

289 Increased blood concentration of cortisol (hydroxycortisone):
1. Decreases the anterior pituitary secretion of ACTH
2. Makes the body less able to resist stress successfully
3. Tends to accelerate wound healing
4. Tends to decrease liver gluconeogenesis

290 Following the hypophysectomy the nurse should observe Mr. Pierce for signs of:
1. Urinary retention
2. Bleeding at suture site
3. Increased intracranial pressure
4. Respiratory distress

291 The nurse knows that most of the hormones present in the body at any given time were secreted from the endocrine glands:
1. 24 hours ago
2. 4 to 6 hours ago

3. More than 72 hours ago
4. 8 to 12 hours ago

292 Mrs. Peters enters the hospital for exploratory abdominal surgery. She is 3 months pregnant and has been informed that there are many dangers involved. The nurse has her sign a consent form for an exploratory laparotomy. Cancer of the uterus is discovered and a hysterectomy is performed. On returning from surgery Mrs. Peters is informed that her uterus was removed. She sues the hospital, the surgeon, and the nurse. The decision in this case will be based on the fact that:
1. The patient received inadequate information to give consent
2. The surgeon has the legal right to do what was deemed necessary in surgery
3. General consent forms signed on admission are sufficient
4. Consent for exploratory surgery implies permission for removing organs if this is justified

293 Which one of the following operative procedures would result in surgical menopause?
1. Bilateral oophorectomy
2. Partial hysterectomy
3. Bilateral salpingectomy
4. Tubal ligation

294 Hot flashes are caused by:
1. Overstimulation of the adrenal medulla
2. Accumulation of acetylcholine
3. Cessation of pituitary gonadotropins
4. Hormonal stimulation of the sympathetic system

295 Menopause is the cessation of menstrual function. One of the reasons given is:
1. An increase in the secretion of progesterone from the follicles in the ovary
2. A decrease in the production of prostaglandins
3. The inability of the ovary to respond to gonadotropic hormones
4. A decrease in gonadotropin in the blood

296 Ovulation occurs when:
1. The blood levels of FSH and LH are high
2. The endometrial wall is sloughed off
3. Progesterone level is high
4. Oxytocin level is high

297 High concentration of estrogens in the blood:
1. Causes ovulation
2. Inhibits anterior pituitary secretions of FSH
3. Is one of the causes of osteoporosis
4. Stimulates lactation

Situation: Mr. Davis is a 55-year-old man who has suffered a cerebral vascular accident. He has right-sided paralysis and is dysphagic and dysphasic. His nursing care includes frequent monitoring of vital signs. Questions 298 through 304 refer to this situation.

298 Mr. Davis' temperature should be taken:
1. Orally

2. In the groin
3. Rectally
4. In the axilla

299 Mr. Davis is experiencing difficulty in:
1. Swallowing
2. Focusing
3. Writing
4. Understanding

300 Mr. Davis' dysphasia requires initial provision for:
1. Routine hygienic needs
2. Prevention of aspiration
3. Effective communication
4. Liquid formula diet

301 Blood pressure should not be taken on Mr. Davis' right arm because circulatory impairment may:
1. Precipitate the formation of a thrombus
2. Hinder restoration of function
3. Produce inaccurate readings
4. Cause excessive pressure on the brachial artery

302 Three days after admission Mr. Davis has a nasogastric tube inserted and is prescribed a liquid formula diet 6 times daily. For the first day the amount of liquid administered at one time should not exceed:
1. 150 ml
2. 250 ml
3. 350 ml
4. 450 ml

303 The formula temperature most compatible for administration is:
1. Chilled
2. Body
3. Room
4. 42° C (108° F)

304 The nurse should administer the tube feeding slowly to reduce the hazard of:
1. Indigestion
2. Regurgitation
3. Flatulence
4. Distention

305 The optic chiasm:
1. Receives nerve impulses from the optic tracts
2. Is the space posterior to the lens with the consistency of jelly
3. Is a crossing of some optic nerves in the cranial cavity
4. Is the cavity in which the eyeball is fixed

306 A feeling of pleasantness or unpleasantness, varying in degree from mild to intense, occurs when sensory impulses reach the:
1. Basal ganglia
2. Cerebral cortex
3. Hypothalamus
4. Thalamus

307 An arterial anastomosis present at the base of the brain is the:
1. Volar arch
2. Brachiocephalic sinus

3. Circle of Willis
4. Brachial plexus

308 Which part of the ear contains the receptors for hearing?
1. Cochlea
2. Middle ear
3. Tympanic cavity
4. Utricle

309 The ear bones that transmit vibrations to the oval window of the cochlea are found in the:
1. Outer ear
2. Inner ear
3. Middle ear
4. Eustachian tube

310 An injury or infection that would cause nerve deafness would most likely be to the:
1. Cochlear nerve
2. Vestibular nerve
3. Trigeminal nerve
4. Vagus nerve

311 The medulla has centers for:
1. Control of sexual development
2. Fat metabolism, temperature regulation, water balance
3. Voluntary movements, taste, skin sensations
4. Control of breathing, heartbeat, blood vessel diameter

312 The part of the brain that exerts reflex control of respiration is the:
1. Medulla and pons
2. Cerebral cortex
3. Hypothalamus
4. Cerebellum

313 A labyrinthectomy is frequently performed to treat Ménière's syndrome. The result of this procedure is:
1. Absence of pain
2. Permanent deafness
3. Anosmia
4. Reduction of tinnitus

314 Otosclerosis is the most common cause of conductive hearing loss. Which of the following statements is true?
1. The patient is usually unable to hear bass tones
2. Air conduction is more effective than bone conduction
3. Hearing aids usually restore hearing
4. Stapedectomy is the procedure of choice

Situation: Mr. Bloom, a 56-year-old baker, was admitted to the hospital 5 weeks ago with a fractured skull and concussion. Two weeks after admission he exhibited evidence of increasing intracranial pressure. Questions 315 through 320 refer to this situation.

315 Mr. Bloom has been receiving dexamethasone (Decadron) during the past 3 weeks for control of cerebral edema. The planned effect of the drug is to:
1. Increase fluid removal from the tissues
2. Reduce CSF secretion by the choroid plexus
3. Increase elasticity of the ventricle walls
4. Suppress production of antibodies

316 While Mr. Bloom is receiving dexamethasone (Decadron) the nurse is testing his urine for sugar and acetone every 4 hours because the drug:
1. Lowers the renal threshold for glucose
2. Mobilizes liver stores of glycogen
3. Accelerates protein breakdown and liberates excess glycogen
4. Has a glucose component, which raises the blood sugar level

317 Mr. Bloom has been taking Maalox while he is receiving dexamethasone. The antacid is prescribed because dexamethasone is a drug that:
1. Irritates the gastric mucosa
2. Stimulates gastric production of hydrochloric acid
3. Increases gastric acidity and slows emptying time
4. Increases pepsin-induced erosion of the gastric mucosa

318 Mr. Bloom has several loose bowel movements and the physician changes his antacid prescription to Amphojel. The change is made because:
1. Maalox and dexamethasone act synergistically to increase fluid content of the intestine
2. Amphojel increases the bulk of feces and slows peristalsis
3. Amphojel neutralizes larger amounts of the hydrochloric acid that causes diarrhea
4. Maalox contains a magnesium component that stimulates peristalsis

319 Mr. Bloom complains about the chalky taste of Amphojel. He states that he would rather take bicarbonate of soda as he does at home. The nurse tells him it is not advisable to take bicarbonate of soda regularly. This statement is based on knowledge that bicarbonate of soda:
1. Causes distention by producing carbon dioxide in the stomach
2. Is absorbed from the stomach, and the sodium component causes ankle edema
3. Is absorbed from the stomach and may cause alkalosis
4. Causes rebound hyperacidity after initial neutralization of hydrochloric acid

320 The physician states that he plans to reduce Mr. Bloom's dexamethasone dosage gradually and to continue him on a lower maintenance dosage during the next few weeks. The nurse explains to the patient that the reason for the gradual dosage reduction is to allow:
1. Production of adrenocorticotropic hormone (ACTH)
2. Return of cortisone production by the adrenal glands
3. Time to observe for return of increased intracranial pressure
4. Building of glycogen and protein stores in liver and muscle

321 Energy stored as ATP, ADP, and other high-energy compounds is formed chiefly by:
1. Oxidation of glucose
2. Hydrolysis of fats

3. Respiration
4. Peptidation

322 Neostigmine bromide (Prostigmin) is used for the diagnosis of myasthenia gravis because this drug will cause a temporary:
1. Increase in symptoms
2. Drying of the mouth and throat
3. Increase in blood pressure
4. Increase in muscle strength

Situation: Mrs. Pring, a 34-year-old mother of 5 children, has been diagnosed as having rheumatoid arthritis. Mrs. Pring is being admitted to the hospital because of a recent flare-up of symptoms. She has been taking aspirin and steroids for the past year. Questions 323 through 326 refer to this situation.

323 Daily blood work is ordered for Mrs. Pring during the first 3 days of her hospitalization. Which of the following symptoms may indicate a complication of the prolonged use of these medications?
1. Elevated sedimentation rate
2. Leukepenia
3. Elevated C-reactive protein
4. Hypochromic, normocytic anemia

324 While taking a nursing history from Mrs. Pring, the nurse promotes communication by:
1. Asking questions that can be answered by a simple ''yes'' or ''no''
2. Telling the patient there is no cause for alarm
3. Asking ''why'' and ''how'' questions
4. Using broad, open-ended statements

325 Mrs. Pring questions the nurse as to the source of her disease. The nurse is aware that this is a disease of:
1. Bones
2. Joints
3. Purine metabolism
4. Connective tissue

326 Gold salts may be used to treat rheumatoid arthritis. A serious side effect of this drug is:
1. Cardiac decompensation
2. Kidney damage
3. Persistent nausea
4. Pulmonary emboli

327 Allopurinol is used to treat gout. The objective of therapy is to:
1. Increase uric acid excretion
2. Decrease uric acid production
3. Prevent crystallization of uric acid
4. Decrease synovial swelling

328 One drug that may be prescribed and that has long been known to be of value in the prevention and treatment of acute attacks of gout is:
1. Hydrocortisone
2. Colchicine
3. Phenylbutazone (Butazolidin)
4. Probenecid (Benemid)

329 Systemic lupus erythematosus (SLE) is a collagen disease characterized by which of the following signs?
1. Butterfly rash
2. Inflammation of small arteries
3. Muscle mass degeneration
4. Firm skin fixed to tissue

330 Mrs. Laukhardt is diagnosed as having scleroderma. Although no cause has been determined for this disorder, it is thought to be a defect in:
1. Amino acid metabolism
2. Sebaceous gland formation
3. Autoimmunity
4. Ocular motility

331 Mrs. Laukhardt discusses her prognosis with the nurse. She states, ''I'm sure I'll live to a ripe old age. It's not too serious.'' In responding, the nurse should bear in mind that 50% of the patients with this disease:
1. Recover completely
2. Die within 6 months to 1 year
3. Succumb within 3 years
4. Have extended remissions

Situation: Mrs. Grey is a 45-year-old woman who has been admitted to the hospital with a diagnosis of open-angle chronic glaucoma. Questions 332 through 339 refer to this situation.

332 Which of the following symptoms is Mrs. Grey most likely to exhibit first?
1. A sudden, complete loss of vision
2. Impairment of peripheral vision
3. Sudden attacks of acute pain
4. Constant blurred vision

333 The nurse explains to Mrs. Grey that the chief aim of medical treatment in chronic glaucoma is:
1. Controlling intraocular pressure
2. Dilating the pupil to allow for an increase in the visual field
3. Allowing for healing process by resting the eye
4. Preventing secondary infections that may add to the visual problem

334 When the ciliary muscles contract:
1. They bring about convergence of both eyes
2. They close the eyelids
3. They focus the lens on distant objects
4. They focus the lens on near objects

335 Which of the following would not prove dangerous for Mrs. Grey?
1. Use of sedatives
2. Release of emotions by crying
3. Use of atropine in any form
4. Severe bouts of constipation

336 Mrs. Grey should be advised to:
1. Use eyewashes on a regular basis
2. Use laxatives daily
3. Keep an extra supply of eye medication on hand
4. Have prescriptions filled when necessary

337 Drugs instilled in the eye are said to be administered by which of the following methods?

1. Topical
2. Intraocular
3. Injection
4. Insufflation

338 A systemic drug that may be prescribed to produce diuresis and inhibit formation of aqueous humor is:
1. Acetazolamide (Diamox)
2. Bendroflumethiazide (Naturetin)
3. Chlorothiazide (Diuril)
4. Demecarium bromide (Humorsol)

339 Which one of the following drugs is likely to be prescribed to relieve symptoms if Mrs. Grey develops an inflammatory reaction in the eye?
1. Nitrofurazone (Furacin)
2. Sulfisoxazole (Gantrisin)
3. Neomycin
4. Cortisone

Situation: Miss Renee, 32 years old, is admitted to the emergency room with second-degree burns over 40% of her body and face, which she received when her nightgown caught fire. A urinary catheter is inserted. Questions 340 through 345 refer to this situation.

340 Because of the burns, her condition would be considered:
1. Good
2. Fair
3. Poor
4. Critical

341 Which of the following would not be a problem during the first few hours after the incident?
1. Edema of the larynx and trachea
2. Maintenance of blood volume
3. Rapid decrease in the leukocyte count
4. Pain

342 In the immediate shock period after Miss Renee's injury, nutritional care is centered on replacement therapy by IV fluids. Which of the following would not be anticipated?
1. Colloid (protein) through blood or plasma transfusions or by the use of plasma expanders such as dextran
2. Electrolytes, sodium and chloride, by use of a saline solution such as lactated Ringer's solution
3. Potassium added to replace losses
4. Water (dextrose solution) to cover additional insensible losses

343 It can be anticipated that the physician will wish to prevent tetanus from developing. If it is impossible to determine whether Miss Renee has been immunized against tetanus, which of the following preparations would produce passive immunization for several weeks with minimal danger of allergic reactions?
1. Tetanus antitoxin
2. Tetanus toxoid
3. Tetanus immune globulin
4. DPT vaccine

344 Sulfisoxazole (Gantrisin), which is often used to combat urinary tract infections, belongs to which of the following groups of drugs?
1. Antiseptics
2. Analgesics
3. Uricosurics
4. Sulfonamides

345 When the urinary catheter is removed, Miss Renee is unable to empty her bladder. Drugs used to relieve urinary retention include which of the following?
1. Bethanechol (Urecholine)
2. Pilocarpine hydrochloride
3. Carbachol injection
4. Neosporin

346 The best first-aid treatment for acid burns on the skin is to wash them with water and then apply a solution of:
1. Sodium hydroxide
2. Sodium chloride
3. Sodium bicarbonate
4. Sodium sulfate

347 A good first-aid treatment for an alkali (base) burn is to wash it with water and then flood it with:
1. A weak acid
2. A weak base
3. A solution of salt
4. Alcohol

348 The average adult human body has what percent of water?
1. 80
2. 60
3. 40
4. 20

349 The receptors for the regulation of body water through detection of osmotic pressure are located in the:
1. Hypothalamus
2. Neurohypophysis
3. Kidney tubules
4. Blood

350 Which play(s) the major role in maintaining fluid balance?
1. Heart
2. Kidneys
3. Liver
4. Lungs

351 The weight of extracellular body fluid is approximately 20% of the total body weight of an average individual. Which component of the extracellular fluid contributes the greatest portion to this amount?
1. Interstitial fluid
2. Plasma fluid
3. Fluid in body secretions
4. Fluid in dense tissue

352 The most important electrolyte of intracellular fluid is:
1. Calcium
2. Sodium
3. Potassium
4. Chloride

353 Which of the following body fluids makes up 40% to 50% of the total body weight?
1. Intracellular
2. Extracellular
3. Intravascular
4. Interstitial

354 Which of the following statements correctly compares blood plasma and interstitial fluid?
1. Both contain the same kinds of ions
2. Plasma contains slightly more of each kind of ion than does interstitial fluid
3. Plasma exerts lower osmotic pressure than does interstitial fluid
4. The main cation in plasma is sodium, whereas the main cation in interstitial fluid is potassium

355 Which statement is true?
1. Glomeruli are small arteries present in the kidneys
2. The volume of urine secreted is regulated mainly by mechanisms that control the glomerular filtration rate
3. An increase in the hydrostatic pressure in Bowman's capsule tends to increase the glomerular filtration rate
4. A decrease in blood protein concentration tends to increase the glomerular filtration rate

356 Which palliative method of urinary divergence is sometimes used for patients with advanced kidney disease?
1. Ileostomy
2. Nephrostomy
3. Cecostomy
4. Ureterostomy

357 The major disadvantage of an ileal conduit is that:
1. Stool continuously oozes from it
2. Absorption of nutrients is diminished
3. Peristalsis is greatly decreased
4. Urine drains from it continuously

Situation: Mrs. Virginia Wolfsmith is admitted to the hospital with a diagnosis of left hydronephrosis. She is scheduled for a left nephrectomy. Questions 358 through 362 refer to this situation.

358 The physician orders meperidine (Demerol), 50 mg, and atropine, gr $\frac{1}{150}$ IM, preoperatively for Mrs. Wolfsmith before the nephrectomy. Knowing that these 2 drugs are compatible and available in multidose vials, the nurse would *best* administer them by:
1. Drawing each up in a separate syringe
2. Drawing up saline to dilute both drugs
3. Drawing up the atropine and then the Demerol in the same syringe
4. Drawing up Demerol and then atropine in the same syringe

359 After the nephrectomy Mrs. Wolfsmith arrives in the recovery room with a plastic airway in place. In observing the patient for signs of hemorrhage, the nurse must be certain to:
1. Keep her nail beds in view at all times
2. Report any increase in blood pressure immediately
3. Observe her for hemoptysis when suctioning
4. Turn her to observe dressings

360 In the recovery room, while caring for Mrs. Wolfsmith who has received a general anesthesia, the nurse should notify the physician if:
1. The patient pushes out the airway
2. The respirations are regular but shallow
3. The systolic blood pressure drops from 130 to 100 mm Hg
4. The patient has snoring respirations

361 Which of the following nursing actions during the immediate postoperative period has the highest priority for Mrs. Wolfsmith?
1. Checking vital signs every 15 minutes
2. Maintaining a patent airway
3. Recording intake and output
4. Observing for hemorrhage

362 Which of the following is the *least* accurate method to estimate Mrs. Wolfsmith's drainage postoperatively?
1. Counting saturated 4 × 4-inch gauze pads
2. Measuring drainage that has seeped through the dressing
3. Wringing saturated 4 × 4 pads into a graduated container
4. Weighing saturated dressings

Situation: Miss Stewart was admitted to the hospital with complaints of hematuria, frequency, urgency, and pain on urination. She stated that she has had this problem for several days. Questions 363 through 365 refer to this situation.

363 The admitting diagnosis would most likely be:
1. Cystitis
2. Pyelitis
3. Nephrosis
4. Pyelonephritis

364 Miss Stewart is receiving methenamine mandelate (Mandelamine) and ammonium chloride. The primary reason for administering the 2 drugs concurrently is that ammonium chloride:
1. Improves methanamine mandelate effect on bacteria by acidifying the urine
2. Promotes healing of irritated bladder mucosa
3. Interacts with methenamine mandelate to decrease crystal and stone formation
4. Decreases bladder irritation by acidifying the urine

365 Miss Stewart has a higher risk of developing cystitis than does a man. This is due to:
1. Hormonal secretions
2. Length of the urethra
3. Juxtaposition of the bladder
4. Altered urinary pH

Situation: Mr. Everett has been admitted to the C.C.U. with a tentative diagnosis of bundle branch block. Questions 366 through 370 refer to this situation.

366 When observing the patient's cardiac monitor the nurse would expect:

1. Absence of P waves
2. Widening of QRS complex to 0.12 second or greater
3. Inverted T waves
4. Sagging ST segment

367 The physician has scheduled Mr. Everett for a pacemaker insertion. The pacing catheter will be inserted into a large vein such as the subclavian and advanced so that the electrode is positioned in the:
1. Superior vena cava
2. Left atrium
3. Right ventricle
4. SA node

368 The nurse realizes that a pacemaker is used in some patients to serve the function normally performed by the:
1. Accelerator nerves to the heart
2. AV node
3. Bundle of His
4. SA node

369 While the pacemaker catheter is being inserted, Mr. Everett's heart rate drops to 38. Which of the following drugs might the nurse expect the physician to order?
1. Digoxin (Lanoxin)
2. Lidocaine (Xylocaine)
3. Atropine
4. Procainamide (Pronestyl)

370 The physician has inserted a permanent demand pacemaker. In patient teaching, the nurse should:
1. Instruct the patient to sleep on 2 pillows
2. Inform the patient that the pacemaker will function continuously at a set rate
3. Instruct the patient to take his pulse daily and keep accurate records
4. Encourage the patient to reduce his former level of activity

---

371 Prompt treatment is most essential for a patient with:
1. Head injury
2. Ventricular fibrillation
3. Penetrating abdominal wound
4. Fractured femur

372 In charting notes describing a patient's heart rate, the nurse uses the term bradycardia. This describes:
1. A grossly irregular heartbeat
2. A heart rate of over 90 per minute
3. A heartbeat that has regular "skipped" beats
4. A heart rate of under 60 per minute

Situation: Mr. McNabb, a 65-year-old self-employed grocer, is admitted to the hospital with congestive heart failure and pulmonary edema. His treatment includes oxygen by mask, digoxin, chlorothiazide (Diuril), and a low-sodium diet. He is dyspneic, apprehensive, and restless. Questions 373 through 379 refer to this situation.

373 Mr. McNabb would be most comfortable with the oxygen set at:
1. 12 to 14 L
2. 5 to 7 L
3. 2 to 4 L
4. 16 to 18 L

374 Safety precautions are especially important in Mr. McNabb's room because oxygen:
1. Is flammable
2. Has unstable properties
3. Increases apprehension
4. Supports combustion

375 The nurse attempts to allay Mr. McNabb's anxiety, since restlessness:
1. Decreases the amount of oxygen available
2. Interferes with normal respiration
3. Increases the cardiac workload
4. Produces elevation in temperature

376 When instituting oxygen therapy, the nurse recognizes that the method of oxygen administration least likely to increase apprehension in the patient is:
1. Catheter
2. Cannula
3. Tent
4. Mask

377 After receiving a sedative, Mr. McNabb says to the nurse, "I guess you are too busy to stay with me." The best response in this circumstance is:
1. "I have to see other patients."
2. "The medication will help you rest soon."
3. "I have to go now but I will come back in 10 minutes."
4. "You will feel better; I will adjust your oxygen mask."

378 Before giving Mr. McNabb digoxin, the nurse should measure the:
1. Radial pulse in one arm
2. Apical heart rate
3. Radial pulse in both arms
4. Difference between apical and radial pulses

379 In addition to its cardiotonic action, the digitalis preparations also promote diuresis. As a result, Mr. McNabb can be seriously depleted of:
1. Calcium
2. Phosphates
3. Potassium
4. Sodium

---

380 Swan-Ganz catheters are inserted to give the medical team information on:
1. Stroke volume
2. Left-sided heart failure
3. Venous pressure
4. Cardiac output

381 Pulmonary edema is most likely to occur in an individual with:
1. Mitral stenosis
2. Calcification and incomplete closure of the tricuspid valve
3. Severe arteriosclerosis of the coronary arteries
4. Pulmonary valve stenosis

Situation: Mr. Singer, a patient with terminal cancer, is in the final stage of his illness. Questions 382 through 388 refer to this situation.

382 Mr. Singer is receiving prednisone and other chemotherapeutic agents and is placed in protective isolation. The administration of corticosteroids to control the symptoms of one disease can cause infections because of all the following *except:*
  1. Interference with the inflammatory response of the body
  2. Prevention of the production of leukocytes
  3. Promotion of the growth and spread of enteric viruses
  4. Stoppage of antibody production in lymphatic tissue
383 During Mr. Singer's chemotherapeutic course, he may develop soreness in the mouth and anus because:
  1. The side effects of the chemotherapeutic agents tend to concentrate in these body areas
  2. The entire GI tract is involved because of the direct irritating effects of chemotherapy
  3. These tissue are poorly nourished because the patient is anorectic
  4. These tissues normally divide rapidly and are damaged by the chemotherapeutic agent
384 In caring for Mr. Singer the nurse realizes that sink faucets in his room are considered contaminated because:
  1. They are not in sterile areas
  2. Water encourages bacterial growth
  3. They are opened with dirty hands
  4. Large numbers of people use them
385 On one occasion Mr. Singer says to the nurse, "If I could just be free of pain for a few days, I might be able to eat more and regain strength." In reference to the stages of dying, the patient indicates:
  1. Rationalization
  2. Frustration
  3. Bargaining
  4. Depression
386 When Mr. Singer reaches the point of acceptance in the stages of dying, it may be manifested in his behavior by:
  1. Euphoria
  2. Detachment
  3. Apathy
  4. Emotionalism
387 Mr. Singer drank 7½ oz of orange juice, 6 oz of tea, and 8 oz of eggnog. The calculated intake is:
  1. 515 ml
  2. 645 ml
  3. 625 ml
  4. 585 ml
388 The best nursing approach in dealing with Mr. Singer is to:
  1. Ignore his behavior
  2. Point out the reality of the situation
  3. Join him, since denial is his only defense
  4. Recognize and accept the behavior at this point

389 Characteristic behavior in the initial stage of a patient's coping with dying includes:
  1. Asking for additional medical consultations
  2. Ringing a call light as soon as the nurse has left the room
  3. Criticism of medical care
  4. Sleeping for long periods
390 The family is likely to require more understanding during which stage of the patient's dying?
  1. Denial
  2. Anger
  3. Depression
  4. Acceptance
391 The nurse can best help a patient in the stage of acceptance by:
  1. Allowing unrestricted visiting
  2. Being around and not necessarily speaking
  3. Explaining all that is being done
  4. Allowing the patient to cry
392 A form of folic acid is being administered intramuscularly during intra-arterial chemotherapy with methotrexate. The drug is being administered intramuscularly to:
  1. Provide levels of folic acid required by blood-forming organs
  2. Provide the metabolite required for destruction of cancer cells
  3. Provide folic acid, which acts synergistically with antineoplastic drugs to destroy cancer cells
  4. Increase production of phagocytic cells required to remove debris liberated by disintegrating cancer cells
393 Antibiotic therapy is administered along with extensive and prolonged chemotherapy primarily because chemotherapeutic agents destroy rapidly growing cells in the:
  1. Blood
  2. Lymph
  3. Liver
  4. Bone marrow

Situation: Mr. Lange, a 36-year-old delicatessen clerk, is admitted with a pulmonary embolism. Questions 394 through 398 refer to this situation.

394 Mr. Lange is receiving an anticoagulant for a pulmonary embolism. Which of the following drugs is contraindicated for patients receiving anticoagulants?
  1. Isoxsuprine (Vasodilan)
  2. Chloral hydrate
  3. Chlorpromazine (Thorazine)
  4. Aspirin
395 Which of the following actions would the nurse initiate with Mr. Lange as a measure to prevent further emboli?
  1. Encourage deep breathing and coughing
  2. Use of the knee gatch when positioning the patient
  3. Limit the fluid intake of the immobilized patient
  4. Encourage patient to move his legs while confined to bed

396 The nursing care plan should include observations of Mr. Lange for:
1. Headache
2. Epistaxis
3. Nausea
4. Chest pain

397 Mr. Lange begins to expectorate blood. The nurse describes this episode as:
1. Hematuria
2. Hematemesis
3. Hematoma
4. Hemoptysis

398 Mr. Lange becomes dyspneic. In which position should the nurse place him?
1. Trendelenburg
2. Sims
3. Orthopneic
4. Supine

---

399 In which of the following postoperative patients is there the least likelihood of developing a pulmonary embolism? The patient with a(n):
1. Prostatectomy
2. Hysterectomy
3. Saphenous vein ligation
4. Appendectomy

400 A bilirubin level above 2 mg/100 ml blood volume could be indicative of:
1. Hemolytic anemia
2. Low oxygen-carrying capacity of erythrocytes
3. Pernicious anemia
4. Decreased rate of red cell destruction

401 One of the main functions of bile is to:
1. Produce an acid condition
2. Provide vitamins
3. Emulsify fats
4. Split protein

Situation: Mrs. Smith, a 45-year-old, rather obese mother of 5 children, is admitted to the emergency room complaining of nausea, belching, gas, and right upper quadrant pain that was not relieved by taking Alka-Seltzer. She states that she has had attacks for the past several years, especially after eating fatty or fried foods. After a series of diagnostic tests, the patient is prepared for surgery. A cholecystectomy and choledochotomy are performed. Mrs. Smith is reluctant to cough or move. Questions 402 through 408 refer to this situation.

402 Mrs. Smith experiences discomfort after ingesting fatty foods because:
1. The liver was manufacturing inadequate bile
2. Fatty foods are hard to digest
3. Obstruction of the common bile duct prevented emptying of the bile into the intestine
4. She did not eliminate fatty foods from her diet

403 A patient with obstruction of the common bile duct may show a prolonged bleeding and clotting time because:

1. The extrinsic factor is not absorbed
2. Vitamin K is not absorbed
3. The ionized calcium level falls
4. Bilirubin accumulates in the plasma

404 Cholecystography is performed to:
1. Detect obstruction at the ampulla of Vater
2. Observe patency of the common bile duct
3. Determine the concentration ability of the gallbladder
4. Distinguish stone formation from other types of obstruction

405 Mrs. Smith had an interference in bile utilization caused by cholecystitis. The ejection of bile into the alimentary tract is controlled by which of the following hormones?
1. Cholecystokinin
2. Secretin
3. Gastrin
4. Enterocrinin

406 Mrs. Smith has a Penrose drain inserted. The nurse caring for her in the recovery room notices that the dressing has become soiled with a brownish red fluid. The nurse should:
1. Change the dressing
2. Reinforce the dressing
3. Apply an abdominal binder
4. Remove the tape and apply Montgomery straps

407 Postoperatively Mrs. Smith suddenly complains of numbness in the right leg and a "funny feeling" in the toes. The nurse should first:
1. Elevate the legs and tell her to stay in bed
2. Rub her legs to start circulation and place a warm blanket on her
3. Tell her she has been staying in bed too much and encourage ambulation
4. Tell her to remain in bed and notify the physician

408 When Mrs. Smith is able to eat solid food, which of the following special diets should be ordered?
1. High in protein and calories to promote wound healing
2. Low in fat to avoid painful contractions in the wound area
3. Low in protein and carbohydrate to avoid excess calories and help her lose weight
4. High in fat and carbohydrate to meet energy demands

Situation: Mrs. McCann, a 93-year-old widow, has been admitted to the hospital from a nursing home. She has been complaining of severe lower abdominal pain, anorexia, nausea, and vomiting for the past 24 hours. History and physical examination reveal a thin, elderly white woman in remarkably good physical and mental condition except for the present complaints. The most likely cause of Mrs. McCann's illness is thought to be sigmoid diverticulitis. After the appropriate diagnostic workup and preparation for surgery, an exploratory laparotomy is performed. Surgery confirms the admitting diagnosis but also reveals a large silent giant ulcer in the stomach, which requires a subtotal gastrectomy (Billroth I). Mrs. McCann does well after the surgery but on the fifth postoperative day develops severe abdominal pain with distended abdomen, a markedly elevated WBC, and temperature of

39.5° C (103° F) rectally. She is taken to the O.R. once again, where plication for a leak in the duodenostomy is performed. Questions 409 through 414 refer to this situation.

409 The primary reason for performing surgery in the first instance is most likely that:
1. Diverticulitis in some instances is difficult to differentiate from carcinoma except surgically
2. Of the symptoms exhibited by the patient on admission
3. The complication—perforation—had occurred with resultant abscess formation or generalized peritonitis
4. Surgery is usually indicated for patients with a diagnosis of diverticulitis

410 One of the major problems after this type of surgery is the prevention of pulmonary complications. The nurse can best achieve this by:
1. Encouraging deep breathing and coughing to counteract voluntary diaphragm splinting
2. Promoting frequent turning, moving, and deep breathing to mobilize bronchial secretions
3. Ambulating to increase respiratory exchange
4. Administering IPPB q. 4 h.

411 A gastrectomy following severe stomach ulceration may eventually be associated with pernicious anemia because:
1. Vitamin B_{12} is only absorbed in the stomach
2. The stomach parietal cells secrete the intrinsic factor
3. The hemopoietic factor is secreted in the stomach
4. Chief cells in the stomach secrete the extrinsic factor

412 In caring for a patient with a nasogastric tube attached to suction, the nurse should:
1. Irrigate the tube with physiologic saline
2. Allow the patient to have small chips of ice or sips of water unless nauseated
3. Use sterile technique in irrigating the tube
4. Withdraw the tube quickly when decompression is terminated

413 Because Mrs. McCann's skin is extremely dry, flaky, wrinkled, sagging, and sallow, an important nursing measure is to:
1. Avoid daily bathing but use emollients
2. Bathe her once or twice a week and use emollients
3. Bathe when necessary and use emollients
4. Use emollients for skin care

414 The wisest guideline for Mrs. McCann's diet would be:
1. No oral feedings for a prolonged period
2. Gradual resumption of small, easily digested feedings
3. At her age allow anything she wants at any time
4. Give nothing by mouth and depend on IV feedings indefinitely

Situation: Mr. Gray is admitted to the hospital with extensive carcinoma of the descending portion of the colon with metastasis to the lymph nodes. Questions 415 through 422 refer to this situation.

415 The operative procedure that would probably be performed is a(an):
1. Cecostomy
2. Ileostomy
3. Colectomy
4. Colostomy

416 The nurse administers neomycin sulfate to Mr. Gray preoperatively to:
1. Decrease the possibility of postoperative urinary tract infection
2. Increase the production of vitamin K
3. Destroy intestinal bacteria
4. Decrease the incidence of any secondary infection

417 The nurse protects the skin surrounding the colostomy opening by using:
1. Petroleum jelly
2. Alcohol
3. Aluminum paste
4. Mineral oil

418 After surgery Mr. Gray asks what effect the surgery will have on his sexual relationships. The nurse should tell him that:
1. Sexual relationships must be curtailed
2. He should tell his partner about his surgery prior to sexual activity
3. He will be able to resume normal sexual relationships
4. The surgery will temporarily decrease his sexual impulses

419 In teaching Mr. Gray to care for the colostomy, the nurse should advise him to irrigate it at the same time every day and to choose a time:
1. When he can be assured of uninterrupted bathroom use at home
2. That approximates his usual daily time for elimination
3. About halfway between the 2 largest meals of the day
4. About 1 hour before breakfast

420 If, during the colostomy irrigation, Mr. Gray complains of abdominal cramps, the nurse should:
1. Lower the container of fluid
2. Discontinue the irrigation
3. Clamp the catheter for a few minutes
4. Advance the catheter about 2.5 cm (1 inch)

421 When performing the colostomy irrigation, the nurse inserts the catheter into the stoma:
1. 5 cm (2 inches)
2. 10 cm (4 inches)
3. 15 cm (6 inches)
4. 20 cm (8 inches)

422 When teaching Mr. Gray to irrigate his colostomy, the nurse indicates that the distance of the container above the stoma should be no more than:
1. 45 cm (18 inches)
2. 15 cm (6 inches)
3. 25 cm (10 inches)
4. 30 cm (12 inches)

423 The 2 main sites for handling fat metabolism are the liver and adipose tissue. Of its several functions concerning fat, the main role of the liver is:

1. The production of phospholipids
2. Oxidizing fatty acids to produce energy
3. Converting fat to lipoproteins for rapid transport out into the body
4. Storing fat for energy reserves

424 A readily available form of energy, although limited in amount, is stored in the liver by conversion of glucose to:
1. Glycogen
2. Glycerol
3. Tissue fat
4. Amino acids

425 An important material produced in the liver and stored in the gallbladder is needed to prepare food fats for change to usable fuel forms. This material is:
1. Lipase
2. Amylase
3. Bile
4. Cholesterol

Situation: Mr. Weinberg is admitted to the hospital with cirrhosis of the liver and malnutrition. Questions 426 through 431 refer to this situation.

426 Mr. Weinberg begins to develop slurred speech, confusion, drowsiness, and tremors. With these symptoms his diet would be limited to:
1. 20 g protein, 2000 calories
2. 80 g protein, 1000 calories
3. 100 g protein, 2500 calories
4. 150 g protein, 1200 calories

427 Mr. Weinberg has a swollen appearance as a result of the edema and ascites. The ascites is caused by:
1. Portal hypertension
2. Kidney malfunction
3. Decreased production of potassium
4. Diminished plasma protein

428 The symptoms of portal hypertension are largely caused by:
1. Infection of the liver parenchyma
2. Fatty degeneration of Kupffer cells
3. Obstruction of the portal circulation
4. Obstruction of the cystic and hepatic ducts

429 What complication is most likely to occur when a patient has portal hypertension?
1. Perforation of the duodenum
2. Hemorrhage from esophageal varices
3. Liver abscess
4. Intestinal obstruction

430 Mr. Weinberg's long-standing poor nutrition, especially his deficiency of protein, has led to:
1. Fat accumulation in the liver tissue
2. Coagulation of blood in microcirculation
3. Tissue anabolism and positive nitrogen balance
4. Decreased bile in the blood

431 The nurse expects weight loss in a patient receiving IV administration of 5% dextrose in water due to:

1. Insufficient carbohydrate intake
2. Lack of protein supplementation
3. Insufficient intake of water-soluble vitamins
4. Increased concentration of electrolytes in cells

Situation: Mrs. Green, a known diabetic, has been admitted to the hospital in diabetic acidosis. Blood gases are determined immediately. Questions 432 through 438 refer to this situation.

432 In her state of uncompensated acidosis, which of the following might represent Mrs. Green's arterial blood pH?
1. 6.9
2. 7.2
3. 7.45
4. 7.48

433 Larger than normal amounts of acetoacetic acid have been entering Mrs. Green's blood as one of the indirect results of her insulin deficiency. Like lactic acid and other nonvolatile acids, acetoacetic acid is buffered in the blood chiefly by:
1. Carbon dioxide
2. Potassium salt of hemoglobin
3. Sodium bicarbonate
4. Sodium chloride

434 As a result of excessive acetoacetic acid:
1. Mrs. Green's blood pH remains unchanged
2. Mrs. Green's blood pH increases slightly
3. The carbonic acid content of Mrs. Green's blood remains unchanged
4. The sodium bicarbonate content of Mrs. Green's blood decreases and its carbonic acid content increases

435 The insulin given to Mrs. Green in this emergency would be:
1. Protamine zinc
2. Globulin
3. NPH
4. Regular

436 Initially, when the acidosis is controlled, NPH insulin, 40 units each morning, is prescribed for Mrs. Green. NPH insulin (100 U = 1 ml) is available. To give 40 units, using a regular syringe, the nurse should withdraw:
1. 6 minims
2. 12 minims
3. 20 minims
4. 40 minims

437 The nurse knows that glucagon is given with 50% dextrose in the treatment of hypoglycemia because it:
1. Provides more storage of glucose
2. Increases blood sugar levels
3. Stimulates release of insulin
4. Inhibits glycogenesis

438 When Mrs. Green is discharged, she is receiving isophane insulin suspension (NPH) daily and also is receiving insulin injection (regular insulin) when her urine test is positive. In instructing Mrs. Green the nurse should teach her to:

1. Mix the insulins in any required dosage in the same syringe
2. Give the insulins separately unless the ratio of dosage is greater than 1:1
3. Give the insulins in the same syringe when the ratio is 1:1
4. Administer the insulins in separate syringes using different sites for injection

---

439 Glucose is an important molecule to a cell because this molecule is primarily used for:
1. The building of cell membranes
2. The synthesis of proteins
3. Extraction of energy
4. Building the genetic material

440 The source of glucose for maintaining blood glucose at normal levels at all times is:
1. Ingested food
2. Intestinal hydrolysis
3. Liver glycogen
4. Gluconeogenesis

441 Early treatment of diabetic acidosis will include administration of:
1. Potassium
2. IV fluids
3. NPH insulin
4. Sodium polystyrene sulfonate (Kayexalate)

442 As the patient recovers from diabetic acidosis:
1. The precipitating cause of the coma must be investigated to prevent a recurrence
2. The cause of his condition should be reviewed with him so he understands how to avoid a recurrence
3. Teaching will be necessary to help him accept his disease
4. He will need assistance in obtaining a clear conception of the general character of diabetes

443 When glucagon is administered for reversal of the hypoglycemic state, it acts by:
1. Liberating glucose from hepatic stores of glycogen
2. Competing for insulin and blocking its action at tissue sites
3. Providing a glucose substitute for rapid replacement of deficits
4. Supplying glycogen to the brain and other vital organs

444 The fuel glucose is delivered to the cells by the blood for production of energy. The hormone controlling the use of glucose by the cell is:
1. Thyroxine
2. Growth hormone
3. Adrenal steroids
4. Insulin

445 If a routine urine specimen cannot be sent immediately to the laboratory, the nurse should:
1. Discard and collect a new specimen later
2. Store on "dirty" side of utility room
3. Refrigerate the specimen
4. Take no special action

446 Which of the following nursing actions is most needed when collecting a 24-hour urine specimen?
1. Weighing the patient before starting
2. Checking if any preservatives are needed
3. Placing collection jar in ice
4. Checking intake and output

Situation: Mrs. Butler had a radical mastectomy and will start chemotherapy while hospitalized. Questions 447 through 449 refer to this situation.

447 The nurse is aware that many of the chemotherapeutic agents cause:
1. Increased hemoglobin count and hematocrit
2. Bone marrow depression
3. Decreased sedimentation rate
4. Leukocytosis

448 Mrs. Butler's pathology report shows metastatic adenocarcinoma. She is to receive doxorubicin (Adriamycin), which modifies the growth of cancer cells by:
1. Preventing folic acid synthesis
2. Changing the osmotic gradient in the cell
3. Inhibiting RNA synthesis by binding DNA
4. Increasing the permeability of the cell wall

449 Because of problems occurring in 80% of the patients receiving Adriamycin, the nuse will observe Mrs. Butler for evidence of:
1. Nausea or vomiting, tachycardia
2. Hair loss, erythema of the oral mucosa
3. Decreased appetite, necrosis at the IV site
4. Low blood pressure, decreased vital capacity

---

450 Tumors of connective tissue are classified as:
1. Osteoblastomas
2. Collagenomas
3. Sarcomas
4. Carcinomas

451 Which of the following is the most frequently occurring brain tumor?
1. Pituitary adenoma
2. Neurofibroma
3. Glioma
4. Meningioma

452 Teratomas are tumors that originate in:
1. Muscle cells
2. The embryo
3. The bone marrow
4. Multiple sites

453 When counseling a patient after a vasectomy, the nurse should advise the patient that:
1. It requires at least 10 ejaculations to clear the tract of sperm
2. Recanalization of the vas deferens is impossible
3. Unprotected coitus is possible within a week to 10 days
4. Some impotency is to be expected for several weeks

Situation: *Mrs. O'Reilly, 62 years of age, has been admitted to the hospital after having had a cerebral vascular accident resulting in left hemiplegia. Questions 454 through 461 refer to this situation.*

454 The nurse identifies left hemiplegia by the following observations:
1. Paralysis of the left lower extremity
2. Paralysis of the left arm, left leg, and left side of the face
3. Paralysis of the left arm and left side of the face
4. Paralysis of the left arm, left leg, and right side of the face

455 When the nurse brings in the dinner tray, Mrs. O'Reilly is staring blankly at the wall and states that she feels like half a person. Specific nursing care of Mrs. O'Reilly should be directed at:
1. Including her in all decisions
2. Helping her explore her feelings
3. Distracting her from self-pity
4. Preventing contractures and decubiti

456 Mrs. O'Reilly has been incontinent of feces. When establishing a bowel training program, the nurse must remember that the most important factor is the:
1. Patient's previous habits in the area of diet and use of laxatives
2. Timing of elimination to take advantage of the gastro-colic reflex
3. Use of medication to induce elimination
4. Planning with the patient a definite time for attempted evacuations

457 Developing independence is a primary goal for Mrs. O'Reilly. The nurse plans to achieve this by:
1. Demonstrating ways she can regain independence
2. Establishing long-range goals for the patient
3. Reinforcing success in tasks accomplished
4. Pointing out her errors and helping her correct them

458 Mrs. O'Reilly's daughter threatens to sue when her mother develops a large decubitus ulcer after she insisted on lying on her back for long periods. She is very upset and blames the nurses. The decision in this suit would take into consideration the fact that:
1. The nurse should uphold the patient's right not to be moved
2. Decubitus ulcers frequently occur in immobilized patients
3. Patients should be turned at least every 2 hours
4. Nurses are not responsible to the patient's family

459 Which of the following drugs is likely to be used to treat Mrs. O'Reilly's decubitus ulcer?
1. Chymotrypsin
2. Hyaluronidase (Wydase)
3. Penicillinase
4. Dextranomer (Debrisan)

460 The nurse suspects Mrs. O'Reilly has become impacted when she states:
1. "I don't have much of an appetite."
2. "I have a lot of gas pains."

3. "I feel like I have to go and just can't."
4. "I haven't had a bowel movement for 2 days."

461 What assessment by the nurse is a further indication of the probable presence of a fecal impaction?
1. Tympanites
2. Decreased number of bowel movements
3. Fecal liquid seepage
4. Bright red blood in the stool

462 Which lobe of the cerebral cortex registers general sensations such as heat, cold, pain, and touch?
1. Frontal
2. Occipital
3. Parietal
4. Temporal

463 The relay center for sensory impulses is the:
1. Medulla oblongata
2. Hypothalamus
3. Cerebellum
4. Thalamus

464 The internal organs of humans, such as the bladder and the esophagus, are most directly under the control of the:
1. Peripheral nervous system
2. Central nervous system
3. Autonomic nervous system
4. Spinal cord

465 Stimulation of the vagus nerve results in:
1. Tachycardia
2. Dilation of the bronchioles
3. Slowing of the heart
4. Coronary artery vasodilation

Situation: *Mr. Ray, a 67-year-old retired plumber, falls and is unable to get up. His daughter calls an ambulance, and he is brought to the emergency room, where it is found that he has a fracture of the neck of the left femur. Mr. Ray is admitted to the orthopedic unit, put in Buck's extension, and prepared for surgery the next day. Questions 466 through 471 refer to this situation.*

466 On examination of Mr. Ray, the nurse would expect to find:
1. Shortening of the affected extremity with internal rotation
2. Shortening of the affected extremity with external rotation
3. Abduction with external rotation
4. Adduction with internal rotation

467 The nurse should know that, following a fracture of the neck of the femur, the desirable position for the limb is
1. External rotation with flexion of the knee and hip
2. External rotation with extension of the knee and hip
3. Internal rotation with extension of the knee
4. Internal rotation with flexion of the hip and knee

468 The nurse should explain to Mr. Ray that the chief reason for applying Buck's extension is to:
1. Help reduce the fracture and to relieve muscle spasm and pain

2. Keep him from turning and moving in bed
3. Prevent contractures from developing
4. Maintain the limb in a position of external rotation

469 Part of the nursing care of Mr. Ray is assessment of peripheral pulses. The important characteristics when assessing the peripheral pulses are:
1. Contractility and rate
2. Color of skin and type of spasms
3. Amplitude, symmetry, and rhythm
4. Local temperature and visible pulsations

470 When Mr. Ray is ready to walk with crutches after the hip pinning, he will probably be taught:
1. Four-point crutch walking
2. Two-point crutch walking
3. Swing-through gait
4. Three-point crutch walking

471 Which of the following principles should the nurse use in teaching Mr. Ray the 4-point gait once bone regrowth has occurred?
1. Most of weight should be supported by the axillae
2. Elbows should be maintained in rigid extension
3. The patient must be able to bear weight on both legs
4. The affected extremity should be kept about 15 cm (6 inches) off the ground

Situation: Mrs. Newt, a 35-year-old housewife and the mother of 5 young children, ages 6 months to 15 years, is involved in a serious auto accident on the highway when her car skids on the wet pavement, striking the concrete partition. She is taken to a hospital, where it is determined that she has multiple trauma, possible fractured skull, fractures of the fifth and sixth cervical and the tenth, eleventh, and twelfth thoracic vertebrae, as well as a ruptured spleen and hematuria. Questions 472 through 478 refer to this situation.

472 A splenectomy was necessary because:
1. The spleen is a highly vascular organ
2. Rupture of the spleen is frequently associated with diseases of the liver and blood
3. The spleen is the largest lymphoid organ in the body
4. An enlarged spleen causes such discomfort or disability as to justify its removal

473 Because of the nature of the particular surgery, in the immediate postoperative period the nurse should observe Mrs. Newt for:
1. Hemorrhage, abdominal distention
2. Peritonitis, pulmonary complications
3. Shock, infection
4. Intestinal obstruction, bleeding

474 When planning care for Mrs. Newt, the nurse should:
1. Observe patient for signs of brain injury
2. Place patient in Trendelenburg position if in shock
3. Check for hemorrhaging from oral cavity
4. Observe for decreased intracranial pressure and temperature

475 Following surgery the nurse should observe Mrs. Newt for the depletion of which of the following electrolytes?

1. Sodium
2. Calcium
3. Chloride
4. Potassium

476 The nurse can expect Mrs. Newt to complain of:
1. Excessively moist respirations
2. Pain on inspiration
3. Shortness of breath
4. Pain on expiration

477 Since Mrs. Newt has hematuria, the nurse should observe her for:
1. Diarrhea
2. Symptoms of peritonitis
3. Gross blood in the urine
4. Acetone in urine

478 Hematuria in this instance probably means that there has been injury to the:
1. Kidneys
2. Ureters
3. Bladder
4. Urethra

479 The protein of blood involved with immune responses is:
1. Hemoglobin
2. Albumin
3. Globulin
4. Thrombin

480 Fragments of cells in the bloodstream that break down on exposure to injured tissue and begin the chain reaction leading to a blood clot are known as:
1. Red blood cells
2. Platelets
3. Leukocytes
4. Erythrocytes

481 With respect to human blood cells, sodium chloride solution of 0.85% strength is:
1. Isotonic
2. Hypertonic
3. Hypotonic
4. Isomeric

482 Which stage of sleep is associated with psychologic rest?
1. Stage 1
2. REM sleep
3. Stage 2
4. Stage 4

483 The action of bulk to promote defecation is a consequence of the:
1. Irritating effect of fiber on the bowel wall
2. Tendency of smooth muscle to contract when stretched
3. Direct chemical stimulation of the colonic musculature
4. Action of the multiflora of the large intestine

484 The physical law explaining the greatly increased venous return accompanying mild vasoconstriction underlies the use of:
1. Adrenaline in treating shock

2. Rotating tourniquets in pulmonary edema
3. Sympathectomy in treating hypertension
4. Digoxin to increase cardiac output

Situation: Mr. Anthony has second- and third-degree burns and is to receive a skin graft over the third-degree burn of his arm. Questions 485 through 490 refer to this situation.

485 The graft is taken from his left buttock. This is referred to as a(n):
1. Homograft
2. Autograft
3. Heterograft
4. Allograft

486 A pigskin graft is often applied to burned areas. This is known as a(n):
1. Homograft
2. Allograft
3. Heterograft
4. Isograft

487 Which of the following laboratory tests will best reflect loss of fluid due to burns?
1. Blood pH
2. Sedimentation rate
3. Hematocrit
4. BUN

488 In a burned patient the relationship between body surface area and fluid loss is:
1. Directly proportionate
2. Inversely proportionate
3. Equal
4. Unrelated

489 Which of the following medications should a burned patient receive as soon after admission as possible?
1. Phytonadione (Aquamephyton)
2. Gamma globulin
3. Tetanux toxoid
4. Isoproterenol (Isuprel)

490 Mr. Anthony is to have mafenide (Sulfamylon) cream applied to his burned areas. A serious side effect of Sulfamylon therapy is:
1. Renal shutdown
2. Hemolysis of RBCs
3. Metabolic acidosis
4. Curling's ulcer

Situation: Mr. Neil has undergone a transurethral resection and returns to the unit with an indwelling urinary catheter. Questions 491 through 493 refer to this situation.

491 When irrigating the patient's catheter, the nurse would avoid which one of the following?
1. Using surgical aseptic technique
2. Allowing solution to flow in by gravity
3. Having irrigating solution at room temperature
4. Aspirating irrigating solution with a bulb syringe

492 The solution of choice for maintaining patency of an indwelling catheter is:
1. Isotonic saline
2. Hypotonic saline
3. Sterile water
4. Genitourinary irrigating solution

493 When irrigating Mr. Neil's catheter the nurse should:
1. Instill the fluid under pressure
2. Obtain and use sterile equipment
3. Aspirate to ensure return flow
4. Warm the solution to body temperature

Situation: Miss Fleming, a 35-year-old executive secretary, is hospitalized for treatment of hypertension. Her orders include bed rest with bathroom privileges, low-sodium diet, reserpine (Serpasil), and chlordiazepoxide (Librium). She has been active in both her business and social life, usually having a cocktail before dinner and smoking a pack of cigarettes daily. Miss Fleming expresses disgust for her regimen and dissatisfaction with the nursing care. Questions 494 through 500 refer to this situation.

494 Miss Fleming's behavior is probably a manifestation of her:
1. Denial of illness
2. Response to cerebral anoxia
3. Reaction to hypertensive medications
4. Fear of the health problem

495 The nurse should administer the Librium as ordered because it:
1. Promotes rest
2. Induces sleep
3. Produces hypotension
4. Reduces hostility

496 Miss Fleming has been receiving Librium, 10 mg q.i.d., for the past 5 days. The nurse should question giving the medication if the patient exhibits:
1. Muscle twitching
2. Blurred vision
3. Hypotension
4. Extreme drowsiness

497 Miss Fleming is receiving Serpasil because it is an effective:
1. Diuretic
2. Hypnotic
3. Antihypertensive
4. Tranquilizer

498 To avoid an error of parallax when taking a patient's blood pressure, the nurse should:
1. Use a narrow cuff
2. Stand close to the manometer
3. Elevate the patient's arm on a pillow
4. Read at eye level

499 Miss Fleming has been told she must stop smoking and eliminate her predinner cocktail. The nurse discovers a pack of cigarettes in Miss Fleming's bathrobe. The best course of action to take at this time is to:
1. Report the situation to the head nurse

2. Let the patient know you found them
3. Discard them and say nothing to her
4. Call the physician and request directions

500 When Miss Fleming is being overtly verbally hostile, the most appropriate nursing response is:
1. Reasonable exploration of situations
2. Complete withdrawal from her behavior
3. Silent acceptance of her behavior
4. Verbal defense of your position

Situation: Mrs. Campenella, an 80-year-old widow, is admitted with congestive heart failure and pulmonary edema. Questions 501 through 505 refer to this situation.

501 To help alleviate Mrs. Campenella's distress, the nurse should:
1. Elevate the lower extremities
2. Place the patient in orthopneic position
3. Encourage frequent coughing
4. Prepare for modified postural drainage

502 When a patient is admitted to the coronary care unit with a diagnosis of acute pulmonary edema, the nurse should be prepared for:
1. Postural drainage
2. Inhalation therapy
3. Rotating tourniquets
4. Wet phlebotomy

503 Mrs. Campenella is receiving furosemide (Lasix) and digoxin. Nursing care for her includes observation for symptoms of electrolyte depletion caused by:
1. Sodium restriction
2. Inadequate oral intake
3. Continuous dyspnea
4. Diuretic therapy

504 To help assess Mrs. Campenella's condition, a CVP catheter is inserted. In taking a central venous pressure reading the nurse should place the patient:
1. Horizontal
2. In a low Fowler position
3. Side lying, on affected side
4. Side lying, opposite to manometer

505 Since Mrs. Campenella will be staying with her daughter for the summer, the nurse suggests that her room be air conditioned. This is because:
1. The internal body temperature drops below 37° C (98.6° F)
2. The heart is relieved of the strain of pumping blood through many miles of blood vessels in the skin
3. The increased circulation in the skin causes excess body heat to radiate away
4. The increased circulation in the skin gives the heart the exercise it needs

Situation: Mr. Rogers, with a long history of emphysema, is now terminally ill with cancer of the esophagus. His plan of care includes a soft diet, modified postural drainage, and IPPB treatments

b.i.d. He is weak, dyspneic, emaciated, and apathetic. Questions 506 through 512 refer to this situation.

506 Nursing care plans for Mr. Rogers should give priority to:
1. Diet and nutrition
2. Hygiene and comfort
3. Body mechanics and posture
4. Intake and output

507 Mr. Rogers expresses aversion to his meals and eats only small amounts. The nurse should provide:
1. Only foods he likes in small portions
2. Supplementary vitamins to stimulate appetite
3. Nourishment between meals
4. Small portions more frequently

508 The term used to describe Mr. Roger's response to food most accurately is:
1. Anorexia
2. Anoxia
3. Apathy
4. Dysphagia

509 To obtain maximum benefits after postural drainage, Mr. Rogers should be:
1. Placed in a sitting position to provide drainage
2. Encouraged to cough deeply
3. Placed on an IPPB machine
4. Encouraged to rest for 30 minutes before coughing

510 Mr. Roger's pain and dyspnea are increasing in severity. The physician has ordered 100 mg meperidine q. 4 h. and oxygen p.r.n. In preparing Mr. Roger's medication, the nurse should know that meperidine is commonly available for dispensation as:
1. Darvon
2. Doriden
3. Demerol
4. Narcan

511 The nurse administers nasal oxygen at 2 L/minute. The nurse should observe Mr. Rogers closely for:
1. Hyperemia and increased respirations
2. Cyanosis and lethargy
3. Anxiety and tachycardia
4. Drowsiness and decreased respirations

512 Mr. Rogers has a 44-year-old wife, a 16-year-old daughter in high school, and a 20-year-old son in college. They visit him frequently. In view of Mr. Roger's extreme weakness and dyspnea, nursing care plans should include:
1. Limiting family visiting hours to the evening before sleep
2. Allowing self-activity whenever possible
3. Encouraging family to feed and assist him
4. Planning all necessary care at one time with long rests in between

Situation: Mr. Ergotano, 50 years old, recently came from Italy with his wife to visit with American relatives. While here, he is admitted to the hospital complaining of anorexia, loss of weight, abdominal distention, and passage of abnormal stools. The most likely diagnosis on the basis of history and physical examination is cancer of the stomach or malabsorption syndrome. Neither Mr. Ergotano nor his wife speaks any English. Their trip to America was sponsored by relatives. Questions 513 through 520 refer to this situation.

513 To determine the correct diagnosis, extensive diagnostic studies are performed. Tests in connection with cancer of the stomach include:
1. X-ray examination
2. CBC
3. Thorn test
4. Gastroscopy

514 Mr. Ergotano appears frightened and Mrs. Ergotano is near hysteria. Identifying their emotional state and being unable to communicate with only rudimentary sign language, the nurse should:
1. Give them a booklet with Italian translations of English medical terms
2. Call an Italian-speaking employee from another part of the hospital when necessary
3. Reduce communication to the bare essentials
4. Permit an American relative to stay with Mr. and Mrs. Erogotano at all times

515 An IV of 1000 ml 5% dextrose in water each shift is started on admission to correct fluid imbalance. The infusion set delivers 10 drops per milliliter. To regulate the rate of flow so that the solution would be infused over an 8-hour period, the nurse would select which of these rates of flow?
1. 160 drops per minute
2. 60 drops per minute
3. 20 drops per minute
4. 40 drops per minute

516 Later the physician changes the order to keep vein open. What is the longest possible period of time that 1 bottle of 1000 ml of 5% dextrose in water to keep a vein open can be infused without producing untoward effects?
1. 6 hours
2. 12 hours
3. 18 hours
4. 24 hours

517 Differential diagnosis establishes that Mr. Ergotano has nontropical sprue. Striking clinical improvement is noted after administration of:
1. A gluten-free diet
2. Folic acid
3. Corticotropin
4. Vitamin B$_{12}$

518 Because malabsorption syndrome seems to be present, a trial period on a sprue diet is ordered for Mr. Ergotano. He is not allowed to have:
1. Wheat, rye, or oats
2. Rice or corn
3. Milk or cheese
4. Fruit or fruit juices

519 A typical food combination served to Mr. Ergotano on this diet would be:
1. Creamed turkey on toast, rice, green peas, milk
2. Roast beef, baked potato, carrots, tea
3. Cheese omelet, noodles, green beans, coffee
4. Baked chicken, mashed potatoes with gravy, zucchini, Postum

520 Since Mr. Ergotano's nutritional status is poor, the nurse should:
1. Encourage meats at mealtime and high protein snacks
2. Keep the patient n.p.o., since he has diarrhea
3. Allow whatever foods he will eat from the diet
4. Institute IV therapy to improve hydration

---

521 What is the usual stimulant for the respiratory center?
1. Calcium ions
2. Carbon dioxide
3. Lactic acid
4. Oxygen

522 Oxygen dissociation from hemoglobin and therefore oxygen delivery to the tissues are accelerated by:
1. A decreasing oxygen pressure in the blood
2. A decreasing oxygen pressure and/or an increasing carbon dioxide pressure in the blood
3. An increasing oxygen pressure and/or a decreasing carbon dioxide pressure in the blood
4. An increasing carbon dioxide pressure in the blood

523 An anaerobic spore-forming rod that produces an exotoxin in canned food is:
1. *Salmonella typhosa*
2. *Clostridium botulinum*
3. *Clostridium tetani*
4. *Escherichia coli*

524 The most important method of preventing amebic dysentery is:
1. Proper pasteurization of milk
2. Killing biting gnats
3. Proper sewage disposal
4. Tick control

525 Ketone bodies appear in the blood and urine when fats are being oxidized in great amounts. This condition is associated with:
1. Starvation
2. Alcohol intoxication
3. Positive nitrogen balance
4. Bone healing

Situation: *Mrs. Evans, a 60-year-old homemaker, is admitted because of possible intestinal obstruction. A Cantor tube has been inserted and attached to suction. Questions 526 through 531 refer to this situation.*

526 A serious danger to which Mrs. Evans is exposed because of intestinal suction is excessive loss of:
1. Protein enzymes
2. Energy carbohydrates
3. Water and electrolytes
4. Vitamins and minerals

527 Critical assessment of Mrs. Evans includes observation for:
1. Dehydration
2. Excessive salivation
3. Edema
4. Belching

528 The solution of choice used to maintain patency of the Cantor tube is:
1. Hypertonic glucose
2. Isotonic saline
3. Hypotonic saline
4. Sterile water

529 Mrs. Evans is scheduled for a colostomy after diagnostic workup. Her anxiety is overt and realistic. The most effective way to help Mrs. Evans at this point is to:
1. Encourage her to express her feelings
2. Reassure her that many people cope with this problem
3. Explain the procedure and postoperative course
4. Administer a sedative and tell her to rest

530 The primary step toward long-range goals in Mrs. Evans' rehabilitation is her:
1. Mastery of techniques of colostomy care
2. Readiness to accept her altered body function
3. Knowledge of the necessary dietary modifications
4. Awareness of available community resources

531 Mrs. Evans has a transverse colostomy. When inserting the catheter, the nurse should:
1. Use an oil-base lubricant
2. Direct it toward patient's right side
3. Apply gentle but continuous force
4. Instruct the patient to bear down

532 Prolonged bed rest after surgery appears to promote hemostasis, particularly in the deep veins of the calves. The most likely pathologic result of such hemostasis may be thrombus formation and:
1. Cerebral embolism
2. Dry gangrene of a limb
3. Pulmonary embolism
4. Coronary occlusion

533 The absorption of fluids by gauze is explained by the principle of:
1. Diffusion
2. Osmosis
3. Capillarity
4. Dialysis

534 An attack of pancreatitis can be precipitated by heavy drinking because:
1. Alcohol promotes the formation of calculi in the cystic duct
2. The pancreas is stimulated to secrete more insulin than it can immediately produce
3. The alcohol alters the composition of enzymes so they are capable of damaging the pancreas
4. Alcohol increases enzyme secretion and pancreatic duct pressure and causes backflow of enzymes into the pancreas

535 Surgery may be needed to excise a pseudocyst of the pancreas. A pseudocyst of the pancreas:
1. Is filled with pancreatic enzymes
2. Contains necrotic tissue and blood
3. Is a pouch of undigested food particles
4. Is generally a malignant growth

536 A hormone that simulates the flow of pancreatic juice is:
1. Cholecystokinin
2. Enterocrinin
3. Enterogastrone
4. Pancreozymin

537 The major digestive changes in fat are accomplished in the small intestine by a lipase from the pancreas. This enzymatic activity:
1. Easily breaks down all the dietary fat to fatty acids and glycerol
2. Splits off all the fatty acids in only about 25% of the total dietary fat consumed
3. Synthesizes new triglycerides from the dietary fat consumed
4. Emulsifies the fat globules and reduces their surface tension

538 Secretin and pancreozymin are hormones secreted by the:
1. Duodenum
2. Pancreas
3. Adrenals
4. Liver

Situation: Mr. Smith, a 36-year-old father of 2 children, is admitted to the hospital after an episode of vomiting "coffee-ground" material. The tentative diagnosis is peptic ulcer. Questions 539 through 545 refer to this situation.

539 Most peptic ulcers occurring in the stomach are in the:
1. Pyloric portion
2. Body of the stomach
3. Cardiac portion
4. Esophageal junction

540 The physician orders propantheline (Pro-Banthine) for Mr. Smith. Pro-Banthine is an anticholinergic drug whose main action is to:
1. Neutralize gastric acidity
2. Increase gastric motility
3. Reduce the pH of gastric contents
4. Delay gastric emptying

541 Mr. Smith does not respond to conservative therapy, and a vagotomy and partial gastrectomy are scheduled. Mr. Smith is returned to the unit from the recovery room with IV solutions running and a nasogastric tube in place. Later that evening you note that there has been no nasogastric drainage for ½ hour. Physician's orders state: "Irrigate nasogastric tube p.r.n." Which of the following actions would you employ? Insert:
1. 30 ml of normal saline and withdraw slowly
2. 15 ml of distilled water and disconnect suction for 30 minutes
3. 20 ml of air and clamp off suction for 1 hour
4. 50 ml of saline and increase pressure of suction

542 A vagotomy:
1. Increases heart rate
2. Hastens gastric emptying
3. Eliminates pain sensation
4. Decreases secretions in the stomach

543 Intravenous orders for Mr. Smith state that he is to receive 1000 ml of fluid every 8 hours. If the equipment you are using delivers 15 drops/minute, you would regulate the flow at approximately:
1. 60 drops/min
2. 15 drops/min
3. 23 drops/min
4. 31 drops/min

544 When preparing an IV piggyback medication for Mr. Smith, the nurse is aware that it is essential to:
1. Rotate the bag after adding the medication
2. Use strict sterile technique
3. Use exactly 100 ml fluid to mix medication
4. Change needle prior to adding medication

545 During the convalescent period the nurse sets up a health teaching program designed specifically to meet Mr. Smith's needs. This plan would include:
1. A thorough explanation of the dumping syndrome and how to limit or prevent it
2. A warning to avoid all gas-forming foods
3. Encouragement to resume his previous eating habits as soon as possible
4. An explanation of the therapeutic effect of a high-roughage diet

Situation: Mrs. McNeer has been diagnosed as having Graves' disease. Radioactive iodine is prescribed to decrease the activity of the thyroid, but this therapy is unsuccessful. Questions 546 through 554 refer to this situation.

546 The nurse knows Mrs. McNeer is:
1. Not radioactive and can be handled as any other individual
2. Highly radioactive and should be isolated as much as possible
3. Mildly radioactive and should be treated with standard precautions
4. Not radioactive but may still transmit some dangerous radiations and must be treated with precautions

547 Mrs. McNeer would probably be placed on a:
1. High-calorie diet with supplementary feeding
2. High-roughage diet with supplementary nourishment
3. Regular diet with nourishment between meals
4. Soft, easily digested, nourishing diet

548 The physician decides to do a thyroidectomy. Which medication can the nurse expect the physician to prescribe pior to surgery to decrease the size and vascularity of the thyroid gland?
1. Propylthiouracil
2. Liothyronine sodium (Cytomel)
3. Lugol's iodine solution
4. Potassium permanganate

549 To evaluate possible laryngeal nerve injury following a thyroidectomy, the nurse should, on an hourly basis:
1. Swab the patient's throat to test gag reflex
2. Ask the patient to swallow
3. Ask the patient to speak
4. Have the patient hum a familiar tune

550 While taking Mrs. McNeer's blood pressure the nurse notices she is pale and has spasms of her hand. The nurse prepares for replacement of:
1. Potassium chloride
2. Magnesium
3. Calcium
4. Bicarbonate

551 The nurse suspects accidental removal of the parathyroids, which causes:
1. Tetany and death
2. Adrenocortical stimulation
3. Myxedema
4. Hypovolemic shock

552 Calcium is required because parathormone is the hormone that tends to:
1. Accelerate bone breakdown with release of calcium into the blood
2. Decrease blood calcium concentration and relieve tetany
3. Decrease blood phosphate concentration and increase calcium levels
4. Increase calcium absorption into bone and remove calcium from the blood

553 Overall calcium balance in the body is maintained between 2 sets of balances: (1) absorption-excretion, regulating the amount that will be absorbed; and (2) deposition-mobilization of bone tissue, regulating the amount for building of bone and withdrawing from bone. This dynamic homeostasis is controlled by which 2 interbalanced regulatory agents?
1. Vitamin A and thyroid hormone
2. Ascorbic acid and growth hormone
3. Phosphorus and ACTH
4. Vitamin D and parathyroid hormone

554 The hormone that tends to decrease calcium concentration in the blood is:
1. Aldosterone
2. Thyrocalcitonin
3. Parathyroid hormone
4. Thyroid hormone

555 Underproduction of thyroxin produces:
1. Myxedema
2. Acromegaly
3. Cushing's disease
4. Graves' disease

556 The rate of oxidation in all the body cells is regulated primarily by which gland?
1. Pituitary
2. Thyroid
3. Adrenal
4. Pancreas

Situation: Mrs. Garvin is admitted for treatment of cancer of the cervix. Questions 557 through 561 refer to this situation.

557 An early symptom of cancer of the cervix that should have brought Mrs. Garvin to the gynecologist is:
   1. Bloody spotting after intercourse
   2. Foul-smelling discharge
   3. Abdominal heaviness
   4. Pressure on the bladder

558 Mrs. Garvin is to have a radium implant. When caring for Mrs. Garvin, the nurse would:
   1. Spend as much time with the patient as possible
   2. Have the patient void q. 2 h.
   3. Use rubber gloves when giving the patient a bath
   4. Maintain the patient in isolation

559 Radium is stored in lead containers because:
   1. Chemical heat is produced when radium disintegrates
   2. The lead absorbs the harmful radiations
   3. Radium is a heavy substance
   4. Lead prevents disintegration of the radium

560 In caring for Mrs. Garvin after the radium implant, the nurse would:
   1. Collect and store urine for examination by nuclear medicine methods
   2. Wear a lead apron when giving care
   3. Restrict visitors to a 10-minute stay
   4. Avoid giving IM injections into the gluteal muscle

561 Before discharge the nurse would explain to Mrs. Garvin the importance of:
   1. Eating a diet high in fat
   2. Taking daily multivitamin supplements
   3. Returning for medical follow-up care
   4. Limiting daily fluid intake

562 During the ovulation phase of the menstrual cycle, ovulation is caused by secretion of:
   1. Follicle-stimulating hormone
   2. Luteinizing hormone
   3. Estrogen
   4. Progesterone

563 The large amount of progesterone secreted during the secretory phase of the menstrual cycle is responsible for:
   1. Sustaining the thick endometrium of the uterus
   2. The regulation of menstruation
   3. The onset of ovulation
   4. The incidence of capillary fragility

564 The hormones responsible for the proliferation phase of menstruation are:
   1. Luteinizing hormone and progesterone
   2. Follicle-stimulating hormone and estrogen
   3. Lactogenic hormone and progesterone
   4. Luteinizing hormone and estrogen

565 Eve is 15 years old and has complained of persistent dysmenorrhea. The nurse should encourage her to:
   1. Practice relaxation of abdominal muscles
   2. Have a gynecologic exam
   3. Maintain daily activities
   4. Eat a nutritious diet containing iron

566 When a young woman complains of especially severe abdominal cramps for a day or two each month at the time of menstruation, the nurse should suspect:
   1. Hypocalcemia
   2. Hyperglycemia
   3. Hypernatremia
   4. Hypokalemia

Situation: Mrs. Johns tells the nurse preparing her for surgery that she is ''terribly scared.'' Questions 567 through 569 refer to this situation.

567 The nurse knows that which one of the following statements does *not* accurately describe the autonomic nervous system?
   1. Both sympathetic and parasympathetic impulses continually play on most visceral effectors
   2. Sympathetic impulses tend to stimulate and parasympathetic impulses tend to inhibit the functioning of any visceral effector
   3. The autonomic nervous system does not function autonomously but is regulated by impulses from the hypothalamus and other parts of the brain
   4. Visceral effectors (i.e., cardiac muscle, smooth muscle, glandular epithelial tissue) receive impulses only via autonomic neurons

568 In caring for Mrs. Johns, the nurse observes which of the following indications of sympathetic control:
   1. Constriction of pupils
   2. Skin pallor
   3. Dry skin
   4. Pulse rate of 60

569 Which of the following indicate(s) parasympathetic dominance?
   1. Excess epinephrine secretion
   2. Excess hydrochloric acid secretion
   3. Constipation
   4. Goose pimples

570 Neural impulses travel in one direction because:
   1. Polarization occurs laterally
   2. Axons secrete acetylcholine
   3. Sodium pump does not work in reverse
   4. Cholinesterase acts along the entire axon

571 The terminals of axons supplying skeletal muscle:
   1. Release acetylcholine
   2. Release ATP
   3. Release cholinesterase
   4. Release epinephrine

Situation: Mrs. Smith is admitted with a diagnosis of partial occlusion of the left common carotid artery. She is an epileptic and has been taking phenytoin (Dilantin) for 10 years. Questions 572 through 576 refer to this situation.

572 In planning her care it is most important that the nurse:
   1. Place an airway, suction, and restraints at her bedside

2. Ask her to remove her dental bridge and eyeglasses
3. Obtain a history of seizure incidence
4. Observe her for evidence of increased restlessness and agitation

573 Mrs. Smith is scheduled for an arteriogram at 10 A.M. and is to have nothing by mouth before the test. Her phenytoin (Dilantin) is scheduled for administration at 9 A.M. The nurse should:
   1. Administer the drug with 30 ml of water at 9 A.M.
   2. Give the same dosage of the drug rectally
   3. Omit the 9 A.M. dose of the drug
   4. Ask the physician if the drug can be given IV

574 Mrs. Smith is scheduled to receive phenytoin (Dilantin), 100 mg, orally at 6 P.M. She is having difficulty swallowing capsules since the arteriogram. The nurse should:
   1. Open the capsule and sprinkle the powder in a cup of water
   2. Give her 4 ml of phenytoin suspension containing 125 mg/5 ml
   3. Obtain a change in the prescribed administration route to allow IM administration
   4. Insert a rectal suppository containing 100 mg phenytoin

575 The nursing history indicates that Mrs. Smith neglects her personal hygiene. The nurse plans health teaching and emphasizes meticulous oral hygiene because phenytoin (Dilantin):
   1. Causes hypertrophy of the gums
   2. Irritates the gingiva and destroys tooth enamel
   3. Increases alkalinity of the oral secretions
   4. Increases plaque and bacterial growth at the gum lines

576 Mrs. Smith will receive folic acid at home. The most likely reason for continuing the drug is:
   1. Folic acid will prevent neuropathy caused by phenytoin
   2. Folic acid improves absorption of iron from foods
   3. Folic acid content of common foods is inadequate to meet her needs
   4. Phenytoin inhibits folic acid absorption from foods

Situation: Mrs. Burt is unconscious when admitted to the hospital. Questions 577 through 583 refer to this situation.

577 Mrs. Burt's right eye stays open and its pupil appears dilated. Nonconduction by which cranial nerve would explain the fact that Mrs. Burt cannot close her right eye?
   1. Second
   2. Third
   3. Fourth
   4. Seventh

578 Nonconduction by which cranial nerve would explain Mrs. Burt's dilated right pupil?
   1. Second
   2. Third
   3. Fourth
   4. Seventh

579 Mrs. Burt's mouth is drawn over to the left, a fact suggesting nonconduction by which cranial nerve?
   1. Left facial
   2. Right facial
   3. Left abducent
   4. Right trigeminal

580 Tendon reflexes, for example, the knee-jerk on the right side of Mrs. Burt's body, are found to be exaggerated. Therefore which of the following structures must still be conducting impulses?
   1. Anterior horn neurons
   2. Basal ganglia
   3. Pyramidal tracts
   4. Upper motoneurons

581 When Mrs. Burt regains consciousness, she has a spastic paralysis of the right side of her body. Spasticity results from nonconduction by certain:
   1. Extrapyramidal pathways
   2. Lower motoneurons
   3. Spinothalamic tract fibers
   4. Pyramidal tract fibers

582 Mrs. Burt's physician performs a lumbar puncture. To do this procedure, he inserts a needle into the:
   1. Aqueduct of Sylvius
   2. Foramen ovale
   3. Subarachnoid space
   4. Pia mater

583 Which of the following conducts impulses initiated by stimulation of pain receptors?
   1. Lateral spinothalamic tracts
   2. Posterior white columns
   3. Reticulospinal tracts
   4. Ventral spinothalamic tracts

Situation: Mrs. Purcell is a 72-year-old woman with Parkinson's disease. Questions 584 through 588 refer to this situation.

584 This disease is caused by:
   1. Disintegration of the myelin sheath
   2. Degeneration of neurons of the basal ganglia
   3. Decreased acetylcholine levels at synapses
   4. Degeneration of the corpora quadrigemini

585 Which of the following would the nurse expect Mrs. Purcell to exhibit?
   1. Grand mal seizures
   2. Decreased intelligence
   3. A flattened affect
   4. Changes in pain tolerance

586 Levodopa is prescribed for Mrs. Purcell. The nurse should know that this drug:
   1. Is poorly absorbed if given with meals
   2. May cause a side effect of orthostatic hypotension
   3. Must be monitored by weekly laboratory tests
   4. Causes an initial euphoria followed by depression

587 Levodopa appears to be useful in treating Parkinson's disease because it can:
   1. Replace the dopamine in the brain cells

2. Cause regeneration of injured thalamic cells
3. Increase acetylcholine production
4. Improve myelination of neurons

588 Coordination of skeletal muscles and equilibrium are controlled by the:
   1. Medulla oblongata
   2. Hypothalamus
   3. Cerebellum
   4. Thalamus

---

589 Rehabilitating exercises carried out under water use:
   1. Water pressure
   2. Water vapor
   3. Water's buoyant force
   4. Water temperature

Situation: Mr. Brown is a 68-year-old retired widower who lives alone. He has a 10-year history of arthritis and has just been admitted to the hospital in an acute episode. Questions 590 through 594 refer to this situation.

590 In planning the nursing care for Mr. Brown, the nurse would take into consideration the fact that:
   1. If redness and swelling of a joint occur, they signify irreversible damage
   2. Bony ankylosis of the joint is irreversible and causes immobility
   3. Inflammation of the synovial membrane will rarely occur
   4. Complete immobility is desired during the acute phase of inflammation

591 A regimen of rest, exercise, and physical therapy will:
   1. Help prevent the crippling effects of the disease
   2. Prevent arthritic pain
   3. Provide for the return of joint motion after prolonged loss
   4. Halt the inflammatory process

592 The occurrence of a chronic illness that limits major activity is:
   1. Present to the same degree in every age group
   2. Greatest in children because of the prevalence of congenital defects
   3. Greatest in the older age group
   4. Greatest in the middle years of life

593 Mr. Brown reports that over the years the following diet suggestions have been given him for his arthritis. Which of the following recommendations for his daily diet should the nurse reinforce?
   1. Yogurt and blackstrap molasses
   2. Wheat germ and yeast
   3. A variety of meats, fruits, vegetables, milk, cereal grains
   4. Multiple vitamin supplements in large doses

594 The nurse understands the joints that would most likely be involved in a patient with osteoarthritis are the:
   1. Fingers and metacarpals
   2. Hips and knees

3. Ankles and metatarsals
4. Cervical spine and shoulders

---

595 Psoriasis is characterized by:
   1. Shiny, scaly lesions
   2. Pruritic lesions
   3. Multiple petechiae
   4. Erythematous macules

596 Treatment of psoriasis usually involves:
   1. Avoiding exposure to the sun
   2. Potassium permanganate baths
   3. Topical application of steroids
   4. Debridement of necrotic placques

597 When caring for a patient with scabies, the nurse should be aware that scabies is:
   1. Highly contagious
   2. Caused by a fungus
   3. Associated with other allergies
   4. A chronic problem

598 Which system does the disease pemphigus vulgaris affect?
   1. Gastrointestinal
   2. Reproductive
   3. Neuromuscular
   4. Integumentary

Situation: Following a car accident Harry Martin, a 26-year-old high school math teacher, is diagnosed as having quadriplegia. He is critically ill and needs specific services and equipment; therefore he is admitted to the hospital's intensive care unit. Questions 599 through 603 refer to this situation.

599 Harry is placed on a Stryker frame because it:
   1. Allows horizontal turning of the patient
   2. Promotes body functions
   3. Allows vertical turning of the patient
   4. Helps prevent deformities

600 Before releasing the pivot pins and turning the Stryker frame, the nurse should:
   1. Tell the patient to hold on to the bottom part of the frame
   2. Observe the patient for signs of hypotension
   3. Secure all bolts and straps to ensure patient safety
   4. Get another nurse, since this procedure requires 2 people

601 Two weeks after his accident Harry's physical condition has stabilized. He is overcoming his initial health crisis but still has special needs that could not be met on a general unit; therefore Harry is transferred to the intermediate care unit. Progressive patient care means:
   1. Providing specialized nursing care using an episodic approach
   2. Utilizing a variety of services and facilities to provide specialized care, depending on a patient's individual needs
   3. Transferring patients from an area of greater intensive care to an area of lesser intensive care

4. Providing total nursing care by using the latest techniques and technology

602 Three weeks after his injury Harry is placed on a tilt table for 1 hour while the head of the table is elevated to a 20-degree angle. Each day the angle is gradually increased. The tilt table is used to:
1. Facilitate turning
2. Prevent pressure sores
3. Promote hyperextension of the spine
4. Prevent loss of calcium from the bones

603 The majority of patients with quadriplegia are taught to use wheelchairs because:
1. They usually are not and never will be functional walkers
2. It assists them in overcoming orthostatic hypotension
3. Their lower extremities are paralyzed but they have the strength in the upper extremities for self-propulsion
4. It prepares them for bracing and crutch walking

Situation: Mr. Amond, age 84, is admitted to the hospital with the following signs and symptoms: severe dyspnea, marked generalized edema of lower extremities, penis, scrotum, back, and abdomen, confusion, irritability, and frequent complaint of low back pain. Three months earlier he had been hospitalized for acute urinary retention, at which time a transurethral prostatectomy (TURP) was done, followed by bilateral orchidectomy and radiation therapy when the pathology report revealed carcinoma of the prostate. Laboratory findings indicate markedly elevated chemistries. Corticosteroids are currently being administered. Questions 604 through 610 refer to this situation.

604 In cancer of the prostate it is possible to follow the course of the disease through the study of:
1. Serum acid phosphatase
2. Creatinine
3. Blood urea nitrogen
4. Nonprotein nitrogen

605 Bladder irritability may follow radiation therapy. A sign of this complication would probably be:
1. Polyuria
2. Dribbling
3. Hematuria
4. Dysuria

606 Mr. Amond requests the urinal at frequent intervals but either does not void or voids in very small amounts. This is most likely due to:
1. Renal failure
2. Edema
3. Retention
4. Suppression

607 A urinary retention catheter is inserted. If Mr. Amond complains of persistent discomfort in the bladder and urethra, the nurse most likely should do which of the following first?
1. Check the patency of the catheter
2. Notify the physician at once

3. Milk the tubing gently
4. Irrigate the catheter with prescribed solutions

608 The nurse can best prevent the contamination from retention catheters by:
1. Forcing fluids
2. Cleansing around the meatus periodically
3. Perineal cleansing
4. Irrigating the catheter

609 A Foley catheter operates by the principle of:
1. Inertia
2. Diffusion
3. Osmosis
4. Gravity

610 Mr. Amond experiences difficulty in voiding after the catheter is removed because of:
1. Interruption in normal voiding habits
2. Nervous tension
3. Remaining effects of anesthetics
4. Toxic symptoms from chemotherapy

---

611 Torsion of the testes requires immediate surgical correction because:
1. Irreversible damage occurs after a few hours
2. There is no other way to control the pain
3. Swelling is excessive and the testicle may rupture
4. The reduction in testicular blood flow leads to rapid death of sperm

Situation: Mr. Arnold is admitted to the C.C.U. with a diagnosis of acute pulmonary edema. The physician has ordered rotating tourniquets. Questions 612 through 618 refer to this situation.

612 When rotating tourniquets are used, the nurse should remember that:
1. The automatic tourniquets occlude arterial blood flow
2. The tourniquets are simultaneously applied to 4 limbs
3. The tourniquets are rotated every 15 minutes
4. The tourniquets are rotated 2 at a time

613 The rotating tourniquet technique is effective for:
1. Decreasing arterial flow of blood to the body
2. Restricting visceral flow in the internal body cavities
3. Decreasing venous flow of blood to the heart
4. Increasing the flow of blood through the capillaries

614 Mr. Arnold's respirations are rapid and he appears extremely anxious. The nurse should be aware that the medication most frequently used to relieve anxiety and apprehension in the patient with pulmonary edema is:
1. Hydroxyzine (Atarax)
2. Sodium phenobarbital
3. Chloral hydrate
4. Morphine sulfate

615 An example of a rapidly acting diuretic that can be administered intravenously to patients with acute pulmonary edema is:
1. Spironolactone
2. Ethacrynic acid
3. Chlorothiazide
4. Chlorthalidone

302 MOSBY'S COMPREHENSIVE REVIEW OF NURSING

616 Mr. Arnold is receiving aminophylline intravenously to relieve pulmonary edema. The nurse should observe him for:
1. Decreased pulse rate
2. Decreased urinary output
3. Hypotension
4. Visual disturbances

617 Mr. Arnold's condition worsens; he is intubated and placed on a mechanical ventilator. Central venous pressure must be monitored. In caring for Mr. Arnold, the nurse understands that:
1. The patient should not be taken off the ventilator for the central venous pressure readings
2. The fluid level in the manometer fluctuates with each respiration
3. Blood should not be easily aspirated from the central venous pressure line
4. The zero mark on the manometer should be at the level of the diaphragm

618 The physician orders an IV digitalis preparation. Which of the following preparations is only administered intravenously?
1. Digoxin
2. Gitalin
3. Deslanoside
4. Digitalis leaf

Situation: Mr. Rush is admitted to the coronary care unit with atrial fibrillation and a rapid ventricular response. The nurse prepares for cardioversion. Questions 619 through 625 refer to this situation.

619 Cardioversion is a procedure that is used to convert certain arrhythmias to normal rhythm. In addition to atrial fibrillation, which of the following arrhythmias is an indication for cardioversion?
1. Ventricular fibrillation
2. Premature ventricular contractions
3. Ventricular tachycardia
4. Ventricular standstill

620 When ventricular fibrillation occurs in a coronary care unit, the first person reaching the patient should:
1. Initiate cardiopulmonary resuscitation
2. Defibrillate the patient
3. Administer sodium bicarbonate intravenously
4. Administer oxygen

621 To overcome the potential danger of inducing ventricular fibrillation during cardioversion, the nurse should ensure that:
1. The energy level is set at its maximum level
2. The synchronizer switch is in the "on" position
3. The skin electrodes are applied after the T wave
4. The alarm system of the cardiac monitor is functioning simultaneously

622 The portion of the cardiac monitor that is related to the alarm system for extremes in the heart rate is called the:

1. Oscilloscope
2. Voltmeter
3. Pacemaker
4. Synchronizer

623 Cardioversion is only temporarily successful. Mr. Rush again develops atrial fibrillation. The physician has prescribed quinidine sulfate (Quinicardine) and digoxin (Lanoxin). The nurse should understand that the goal of the drug therapy plan is to:
1. Decrease atrial irritability and slow transmission of impulses through the AV node
2. Stimulate SA node control of conduction and shorten the refractory period of atrial tissue
3. Suppress irritability of atrial and ventricular myocardial tissue
4. Slow SA node firing rate and decrease irritability of the atrial myocardial tissue

624 When taking Mr. Rush's apical pulse the nurse should place the stethoscope:
1. Between the sixth and seventh ribs at the left midaxillary line
2. Between the third and fourth ribs and to the left of the sternum
3. In the fifth intercostal space along the left midclavicular line
4. Just to the left of the median point of the sternum

625 Mr. Rush is receiving digoxin (Lanoxin). Because he will continue taking the drug after discharge, the nurse should be primarily concerned with:
1. Taking his apical pulse before drug administration and teaching him how to count his pulse rate
2. Observing him for return of normal cardiac conduction patterns and for adverse effects of the drug
3. Observing him for changes in cardiac rhythm and planning activity at home based on his tolerance
4. Monitoring vital signs and encouraging gradual increase in activities of daily living

Situation: Mrs. Oliver is hospitalized with coronary heart disease. She is receiving IV fluids, her vital signs are checked q. 4 h., and bed rest and medications, including digitalis and a sedative, are prescribed. She does not seem to be acutely ill but her prognosis is guarded. Questions 626 through 632 refer to this situation.

626 The nurse who has been caring for Mrs. Oliver for several days notes cyanosis and a change in respiration. The nurse starts oxygen administration immediately. Which of the following statements is correct?
1. Oxygen had not been ordered and therefore should not be administered
2. The physician should have been called for an order before oxygen was begun
3. The symptoms were too vague for the nurse to diagnose a need for oxygen
4. The nurse's observations were sufficient to begin administration of oxygen

627 Mrs. Oliver asks what the coronary arteries have to do with her angina. In determining her answer, the nurse should take into consideration that the coronary arteries:
1. Carry reduced oxygen-content blood to the lungs
2. Carry blood from the aorta to the myocardium
3. Supply blood to the endocardium
4. Carry high-oxygen-content blood from the lungs toward the heart

628 After activity Mrs. Oliver states she has anginal pain. The nurse should realize that angina pectoris is a sign of:
1. Myocardial ischemia
2. Myocardial infarction
3. Coronary thrombosis
4. Mitral insufficiency

629 Mrs. Oliver's condition improves. Nitroglycerin is prescribed for anginal pain prn. When teaching Mrs. Oliver how to use nitroglycerin, the nurse tells her to place 1 tablet under her tongue when she has pain and to repeat the dose in 5 minutes if pain persists. The nurse should also tell her to:
1. Place 2 tablets under her tongue when intense pain occurs
2. Place 1 tablet under her tongue 3 minutes before activity and repeat the dose in 5 minutes if pain occurs
3. Swallow 1 tablet and place 1 tablet under her tongue when pain is intense
4. Place 1 tablet under her tongue when pain occurs and use an additional tablet after the attack to prevent recurrence

630 The nurse would tell Mrs. Oliver that she should suspect her nitroglycerin tablets to have lost their potency when:
1. Slight tingling is absent when the tablet is placed under her tongue
2. Onset of relief is delayed but the duration of relief is unchanged
3. Pain occurs even after taking the tablet prophylactically to prevent its onset
4. Pain is unrelieved but facial flushing is increased

631 In addition to a decreased apical rate, which one of the following symptoms would the nurse teach the patient to be alert for as an indication to withhold the digitalis?
1. Decreased urinary output
2. Singultus
3. Chest pain
4. Blurred vision

632 When discharged, Mrs. Oliver will continue to take a diuretic and digitalis. The nurse reviewing Mrs. Oliver's diet would be especially careful to look for adequate sources of potassium because:
1. Under conditions of hyperglycemia digitalis exerts toxic effects on the heart
2. Potassium is a necessary ion for normal body function
3. Under conditions of hypokalemia, digitalis exerts toxic effects on the heart
4. Potassium is a cofactor for several important enzymes

633 When cardiovascular disease is a concern, reduction of the saturated fat in an ulcer diet may be desired and substitutes made of polyunsaturated fat. In such a case which of the following foods should *not* be allowed?
1. Whole milk
2. Special soft margarine
3. Corn oil
4. Fish

634 If you were instructing a cardiac patient on a high-unsaturated fatty acid diet, which of the following foods should be increased in the diet?
1. Liver and other glandular organ meats
2. Enriched whole milk
3. Red meats, such as beef
4. Vegetable oils, such as corn oil

635 Thromboplastin is found in:
1. Plasma
2. Erythrocytes
3. Platelets
4. Bile

636 When blood clots, what soluble substance becomes an insoluble gel?
1. Fibrin
2. Fibrinogen
3. Prothrombin
4. Thrombin

637 An ion that acts as a catalyst in blood clotting is:
1. Fe^{+++}
2. Ca^{++}
3. F^-
4. Cl^-

638 A rocking bed promotes circulation and breathing through which of the following principles?
1. Centrifugal force
2. Inertia
3. Momentum
4. Gravity

639 The efficacy of the abdominal-thoracic thrust (Heimlich maneuver) to expel a foreign object in the larynx demonstrates the gas volume related to the individual's:
1. Vital capacity
2. Residual volume
3. Tidal volume
4. Inspiratory reserve volume

640 Mrs. Jesse is manifesting a diminished urine output after cardiac surgery. Her serum potassium level is elevated and the physician has prescribed polystyrene sodium sulfonate (Kayexalate) and sorbitol orally. This drug combination will:
1. Remove potassium ions from serum and provide carbohydrate for nutrition
2. Stimulate transfer of potassium ions and increase coupling with the resin
3. Allow exchange of sodium ions for potassium ions and increase intestinal water content
4. Increase solubility of polystyrene sodium sulfonate and facilitate its absorption

Situation: Mrs. Simone is admitted to the unit with a diagnosis of liver cirrhosis and hepatic coma. Questions 641 through 645 refer to this situation.

641 One classic sign of hepatic coma is:
1. Elevated cholesterol
2. Bile-colored stools
3. Flapping hand tremors
4. Depressed muscle reflexes

642 Which of the following skin characteristics might be exhibited by Mrs. Simone?
1. Uremic "frost"
2. Urticaria
3. Hemangioma
4. Icterus

643 The ascites seen in cirrhosis is in part due to:
1. Increased plasma colloid osmotic pressure due to excessive liver growth and metabolism
2. The escape of lymph into the abdominal cavity directly from the inflamed liver sinusoid
3. Compression of the portal veins with resultant increased backpressure in the portal venous system
4. The decreased levels of ADH and aldosterone due to increasing metabolic activity in the liver

644 Liver cirrhosis may promote varicose veins because of:
1. Toxic irritating products released into the blood from the diseased organs
2. Increased plasma hydrostatic pressure in veins of the extremities
3. Decreased plasma protein concentration resulting in pooling of blood in the venous system
4. Ballooning of the vein walls due to decreased venous pressure and incompetent valves

645 The physician's decision to order neomycin enemas for Mrs. Simone is based on the results of which of the following laboratory tests?
1. Culture and sensitivity
2. Serum glutamic-pyruvic transaminase
3. White blood count
4. Ammonia level

646 The portal vein can be identified as the one that:
1. Brings blood away from the liver
2. Brings venous blood from the intestinal wall to the liver
3. Enters the superior vena cava from the cranium
4. Is located superficially on the anteromedial surface of the thigh

647 A vitamin necssary for the synthesis of prothrombin by the liver is:
1. Vitamin K
2. Vitamin B$_{12}$
3. Vitamin D
4. Vitamin C

648 Jaundiced patients are susceptible to postoperative hemorrhage because their blood does not clot normally. Why?
1. Excess bile salts in blood inactivate prothrombinase and prevent formation of thrombin from prothrombin
2. Excess bile salts in blood inhibit liver synthesis of prothrombin
3. Excess bile salts in blood inhibit synthesis of vitamin K and prothrombin in the liver
4. Lack of bile in intestines causes inadequate vitamin K absorption, which causes inadequate prothrombin synthesis by liver

649 Miss McGill was admitted to the hospital for diagnostic tests, which included blood and stool. The blood samples were drawn by the laboratory technician. The patient was told that a stool specimen was necessary. However, she was not told a total specimen was necessary and she saved only a small amount. When it was noted that a whole specimen was not available, the test was cancelled. This necessitated an additional day in the hospital. The patient is very disturbed and insists on not paying for the additional day because of the error. In situations such as this:
1. The order for a total specimen should have been written by the physician
2. A full explanation of tests or treatments is the right of the patient, and the nurse was negligent
3. Tests do go wrong, and hospital personnel are not responsible unless there is gross negligence
4. The patient is responsible for the hospital bill and must pay

650 Which of the following statements are true about the sources of vitamin K?
1. Vitamin K is found in a wide variety of foods, so there is no danger of deficiency
2. Vitamin K can easily be absorbed without assistance, so all that is consumed is absorbed
3. Vitamin K is rarely found in dietary food sources, so a natural deficiency can easily occur
4. Almost all vitamin K sufficient for metabolic needs is produced by intestinal bacteria

Situation: Mrs. Eve, a 40-year-old housewife, is admitted to the hospital with a history of vomiting, tarry stools, ascites, and long-standing poor nutrition due to excessive alcohol intake. Her admitting diagnosis is bleeding esophageal varices. After emergency treatment the plan of therapy involves preparing Mrs. Eve for a portal-caval anastomosis. Questions 651 through 658 refer to this situation.

651 The pathophysiologic problem in cirrhosis of the liver causing esophageal varices is:
1. Dilated veins and varicosities
2. Portal hypertension
3. Ascites and edema
4. Loss of regeneration

652 Medical management that may be used to control the hemorrhage includes all *but:*
1. Aminocaproic acid (Amicar)
2. Balloon tamponade
3. Gastric suctioning
4. Iced lavage

653 Neomycin may be adminstered to prevent formation of:
1. Urea
2. Ammonia
3. Bile
4. Hemoglobin

654 If intubation is favored, the type of tube most likely to be used is:
1. Sengstaken-Blakemore
2. Miller-Abbott
3. Andersen
4. Levin

655 Characteristic signs that are a direct result of liver insufficiency may include:
1. Anuria
2. Fetor hepaticus
3. Globus hystericus
4. Blepharospasm

656 In an effort to prevent hepatic coma, it may become necessary to:
1. Eliminate protein from the diet
2. Eliminate carbohydrate from the diet
3. Give Fleet enemas
4. Prepare for emergency surgery

657 When Mrs. Eve is able to eat, the diet ordered for her is:
1. High-protein, low-carbohydrate, low-fat
2. Low-sodium, protein to tolerance, moderate-fat, high-calorie, high-vitamin, soft
3. High-carbohydrate, low–saturated fat, 1200 calories
4. Low-protein, low-carbohydrate, high-fat, soft

658 Mrs. Eve begins to develop slurred speech, confusion, drowsiness, and a flapping tremor. With these evidences of impending hepatic coma, her diet is changed to:
1. 20 g protein, 2000 calories
2. 70 g protein, 1200 calories
3. 80 g protein, 2500 calories
4. 100 g protein, 1500 calories

Situation: Mr. Greene, a 56-year-old married construction worker, has been in the hospital for 2 weeks with a diagnosis of cerebral thrombosis. His symptoms include aphasia, right-sided paresis, and loss of the gag reflex. Questions 659 through 664 refer to this situation.

659 Due to the location of the lesion, Mr. Greene has expressive aphasia. As part of the long-range planning, the nurse should:
1. Help the family to accept the fact that Mr. Greene cannot be verbally communicated with
2. Wait for Mr. Greene to verbalize his needs regardless of how long it may take
3. Begin associating words with physical objects
4. Help Mr. Greene accept this disability as permanent

660 Since Mr. Greene was comatose on admission, the nurse would expect him to:
1. Not be able to react to painful stimuli
2. Be incontinent

3. Be capable of purposeful motion
4. Have twitching or picking motions

661 Since one of the primary nursing objectives is maintenance of the airway, the nurse should place Mr. Greene in which of the following positions initially?
1. Sims
2. Prone
3. Semi-Fowler
4. Orthopneic or Fowler

662 Mr. Greene is still confined to bed rest, and, even though his physician has not ordered physical therapy for him, the nurse may institute:
1. Active exercises of all extremities
2. Passive range of motion exercises
3. Light weight-lifting exercises of the right side
4. Exercises that would actively capitalize on returning muscle function

663 Mr. Greene's wife insists on doing everything for him when she visits. After she leaves, Mr. Greene seems to be quite depressed. The nurse should assume that:
1. Mr. Greene feels guilty about being a burden to his wife
2. This depression is a natural outcome of his illness
3. Mr. Greene feels the loss of his independence
4. Mr. Greene is losing faith in the future

664 Mrs. Greene seems unable to accept the idea that her husband must be encouraged to do things for himself. The nurse may be able to work around these feelings by:
1. Telling Mrs. Greene to let her husband do things for himself
2. Letting Mrs. Greene know that the nursing staff has full responsibility for the patient's activities
3. Letting Mrs. Greene assume the responsibility as she sees fit
4. Asking Mrs. Greene for her assistance in planning the activites most helpful to the patient

Situation: Mr. Brown suffered severe head injuries in an automobile accident. Questions 665 through 672 refer to this situation.

665 Because Mr. Brown is still unconscious when placed on a stretcher to be moved from the emergency room to the intensive care unit, the nurse makes sure his arms do not hang down over the edge of the cart. By taking this precaution the nurse prevents injury to which plexus?
1. Basilic
2. Brachial
3. Celiac
4. Solar

666 Injury to which of the following parts of the brain is particularly likely to cause death?
1. Medulla
2. Midbrain
3. Pons
4. Thalamus

667 Mr. Brown's temperature, soon after admission to the hospital, registered 39° C (102.2° F), a fact suggesting injury of the:
1. Hypothalamus
2. Pallidum
3. Temporal lobe
4. Thalamus

668 After Mr. Brown recovers consciousness, he complains of hearing ringing noises, a fact suggesting injury of:
1. Cranial nerve VI (abducent)
2. Cranial nerve VIII (vestibulocochlear)
3. Frontal lobe
4. Occipital lobe

669 Mr. Brown has a grand mal seizure. The physician prescribes phenytoin (Dilantin) to control the seizures. The expected effect of this drug is to:
1. Alter the permeability of the cell membrane to potassium
2. Control nerve impulses originating in the motor cortex
3. Prevent depression of the central nervous system
4. Produce an antispasmodic action on the muscles

670 Mr. Brown's condition has stabilized and he is transferred out of the intensive care unit. The nurse should automatically place at the bedside:
1. A sphygmomanometer
2. Oxygen equipment
3. A padded tongue blade
4. A rubber or plastic airway

671 Mr. Brown questions the nurse regarding the scheduling of his medication. The nurse informs him that the medications:
1. Can usually be stopped after a year's absence of seizures
2. Need to be taken only in periods of emotional stress
3. Will probably have to be continued for life
4. Will prevent the occurrence of seizures

672 Mr. Brown had no paralysis after his accident, a fact suggesting no injury to the:
1. Basal ganglia
2. Parietal lobe
3. Precentral gyrus
4. Postcentral gyrus

Situation: Mrs. Crane, a 32-year-old woman who has intermittently been having painful, swollen knee and wrist joints during the past 3 months, is being admitted to the hospital for treatment of rheumatoid arthritis. Questions 673 through 676 refer to this situation.

673 One would expect the physician to order the following diet for Mrs. Crane:
1. High protein
2. Salt free
3. General diet, supplemented with vitamins and iron
4. Bland diet

674 Which of the following medications would the nurse expect to be prescribed to relieve the pain in Mrs. Crane's knees?
1. Codeine, 30 mg, every 4 hours
2. Aspirin, 0.6 g, every 4 hours
3. Codeine, 30 mg, every 4 hours p.r.n
4. Nembutal, 90 mg, every hour

675 To prevent deformity of the knee joint, the physician will:
1. Immobilize the joint in a cyclinder cast for a period of several weeks
2. Discourage use of the knee joint
3. Encourage motion of the joint within limits of pain
4. Put the patient on a bed rest regimen

676 Mrs. Crane asks the nurse why the physician may inject hydrocortisone into the knee joint. The nurse explains that the most important reason for doing this is to:
1. Prevent ankylosis of the joint
2. Reduce inflammation
3. Provide psychotherapy
4. Relieve pain

677 Which of the following terms does not refer to hypertrophic arthritis?
1. Degenerative
2. Nonankylosing
3. Heberden's nodes
4. Marie-Strümpell

678 The synovial fluid of the joints minimizes:
1. Velocity of movements
2. Friction in the joints
3. Efficiency
4. Work output

679 Mrs. Paul is hospitalized for an acute exacerbation of rheumatoid arthritis. In talking with the nurse, she states that she does not want cortisone even if it is prescribed by the physician. Later the nurse attempts to administer cortisone that has been ordered by the physician. When Mrs. Paul asks what the medication is, the nurse gives an evasive answer. The patient takes the medication and later finds that she has been given cortisone. She states that she intends to sue. The decision in this suit would take into consideration the fact that:
1. A physician's order takes precedence over a patient's preference
2. The patient has insufficient knowledge to make such a decision
3. The nurse is required to answer the patient truthfully
4. The nurse should have notified the physician

680 The type of membrane that lines the knee joint is called the:
1. Serous
2. Synovial
3. Mucous
4. Epithelial

681 If the nurse finds the supply of Darvocet-N100 depleted but the patient needs this medication urgently, the most appropriate action would be to:

1. Give two capsules of Darvon
2. Borrow a tablet of Darvocet-N100 from the supply belonging to another patient
3. Ask the pharmacist to refill the prescription immediately
4. Ask the patient if he can wait another hour until the next delivery from the pharmacy is scheduled

Situation: *Mr. Fritz, a 32-year-old car salesman, suffered a spinal cord injury in an auto accident, resulting in paraplegia. Questions 682 through 688 refer to this situation.*

682 Good nursing care of Mr. Fritz will provide that he be turned every 2 hours. This is necessary mainly to:
1. Keep the patient comfortable
2. Prevent pressure sores
3. Improve circulation in the lower extremities
4. Prevent flexion contractures of all the extremities
683 Which measure would *not* prevent contractures of the joints of Mr. Fritz's lower extremities?
1. Changing bed position every 2 hours
2. Maintaining proper bed positions
3. Passively moving the extremities through ROM several times daily
4. Providing the patient with active exercise instructions
684 Mr. Fritz questions the need for a tilt table. The nurse explains that the tilt table is used to help:
1. Prevent hypertension
2. Prevent pressure sores
3. Prevent loss of calcium from long bones
4. Encourage increased activity
685 Formation of urinary calculi is a complication that may be encountered by the paraplegic patient. A factor that contributes to this condition is:
1. High fluid intake
2. Increased intake of calcium
3. Inadequate kidney function
4. Increased loss of calcium from the skeletal system
686 Rehabilitation plans for Mr. Fritz:
1. Should be considered and planned for early in his care
2. Are not necessary, since he will return to his usual activities
3. Should be left up to the patient and his family
4. Are not necessary, since he will not be able to work again
687 Since Mr. Fritz has paraplegia, the nurse recognizes that one major early problem will be:
1. Use of mechanical aids for ambulation
2. Patient education
3. Quadriceps setting
4. Bladder control
688 The nurse may expect that Mr. Fritz will have some spasticity of the lower extremities. To prevent the development of contractures, careful consideration must be given to:
1. Proper positioning
2. Use of a tilt board

3. Active exercise
4. Deep massage

Situation: *Mr. Wilson has a herniated lumbar disc. Questions 689 through 693 refer to this situation.*

689 Mr. Wilson generally experiences a sudden increase in pain when he:
1. Sits on cold surfaces
2. Lies prone with knees flexed
3. Sneezes
4. Stands for extended periods
690 He is to undergo a myelogram before surgery. Which of the following will *not* be necessary when caring for Mr. Wilson postoperatively?
1. A thorough neurologic watch
2. Maintenance of a horizontal position
3. Encouragement of fluids to replace CSF
4. Application of cold compresses distal to the puncture
691 In caring for Mr. Wilson after the laminectomy, the nurse should be least concerned with which patient need?
1. Keeping the patient flat in bed
2. Turning the patient from side to side
3. Ambulating the patient with a back brace
4. Assessing for symmetry of movement
692 The main postoperative complication that the nurse should observe for following the laminectomy is:
1. Spasms of the bladder
2. Pain referred to the flanks
3. Compression of the cord
4. Cerebral edema
693 When caring for a patient with a cervical laminectomy, in contrast to caring for a patient with a lumbar laminectomy, the nurse:
1. Should provide range of motion exercise early during the postoperative period
2. Has the added responsibility of removing oral secretions
3. Should maintain the patient's head in a flexed position
4. Must keep the patient's head at a 45-degree angle from the spine

Situation: *Mrs. Elliot is a 52-year-old woman admitted to the hospital with the diagnosis of cancer of the cervix. She is scheduled for a hysterectomy and insertion of radium. She returns to the floor from the recovery room with a Foley catheter in place and vaginal packing. The packing is to be removed in 24 hours. Questions 694 through 697 refer to this situation.*

694 The nurse checking the perineum finds the packing protruding from the vagina. The immediate action to take is to report this situation to the physician at once because the:
1. Packing is radioactive
2. Purpose of the packing is to increase the distance between the insert and the rectum and/or bladder

3. Packing must be removed
4. Purpose of the packing is to prevent bleeding

695 In caring for Mrs. Elliot the nurse would do all of the following *except:*
   1. Plan the care to limit the time spent at or close to the bedside
   2. Limit Mrs. Elliot's activity so as not to dislodge the radium insert
   3. Check all bed linen carefully before discarding
   4. Spend as much time as possible in close contact with Mrs. Elliot to alleviate her anxiety

696 Which symptoms observed by the nurse following radium insertion are indicative of a radium reaction?
   1. Nausea and vomiting
   2. Pain and elevation of temperature
   3. Restlessness and irritability
   4. Vaginal discharge

697 Which of the following should the nurse avoid when assisting with radium removal?
   1. Handling the radium carefully with long forceps
   2. Cleaning radium carefully in ether or alcohol using long forceps
   3. Charting the date and hour of removal and the total time of treatment
   4. Handling the radium carefully wearing foil-lined rubber gloves

Situation: Mr. Piter has developed acute renal failure and uremia. Questions 698 through 703 refer to this situation.

698 Metabolic acidosis develops in renal failure as a result of:
   1. Depression of respiratory rate by metabolic wastes causing carbon dioxide retention
   2. Inability of renal tubules to secrete hydrogen ions and conserve bicarbonate
   3. Inability of renal tubules to reabsorb water to achieve dilution of the acid contents of the blood
   4. Impaired glomerular filtration causing retention of sodium and metabolic waste products

699 Of the following, which is most important in maintaining the fluid and electrolyte balance of the body?
   1. Urinary system
   2. Respiratory system
   3. Antidiuretic hormone (ADH)
   4. Aldosterone

700 Mr. Piter is to receive a modified Giordano-Giovannetti dietary regimen. This diet is based on which of the following principles?
   1. A high-protein intake ensures an adequate daily supply of all amino acids to compensate for losses
   2. Essential and nonessential amino acids are necessary in the diet to supply materials for tissue protein synthesis
   3. Urea nitrogen cannot be used to synthesize amino acids in the body, so all the nitrogen for amino acid synthesis must come from the dietary protein

4. If the diet is low in protein and supplies only essential amino acids, the body will use the excess urea nitrogen to synthesize the nonessential amino acids needed for tissue protein production

701 Mr. Piter complains of tingling of the fingers and toes and muscle twitching. This is caused by:
   1. Acidosis
   2. Potassium retention
   3. Calcium depletion
   4. Sodium chloride depletion

702 Mr. Piter becomes confused and irritable. The nurse realizes that this behavior may be caused by:
   1. An elevated BUN
   2. Hypernatremia
   3. Limited fluid intake
   4. Hyperkalemia

703 To gain access to a vein and an artery, an external shunt may be given to patients who require hemodialysis. The most serious problem with an external shunt is:
   1. Clot formation
   2. Septicemia
   3. Sclerosis of vessels
   4. Exsanguination

---

704 Women are more susceptible to urinary tract infections because of:
   1. Poor hygienic practices
   2. Length of the urethra
   3. Continuity of the mucous membrane
   4. Inadequate fluid intake

705 Which statement is false?
   1. When renal blood pressure falls below normal the kidneys release a substance called renin into the blood
   2. The substance renin from the kidneys changes a normal blood protein to a substance that tends to constrict blood vessels
   3. Glucose is reabsorbed into the blood only in the proximal tubules
   4. Urine always has an acid reaction

706 Severe albuminuria may cause edema because of the:
   1. Rise in plasma hydrostatic pressure
   2. Fall in plasma colloid osmotic pressure
   3. Fall in tissue hydrostatic pressure
   4. Rise in tissue colloid osmotic pressure

Situation: Mrs. Green underwent a cholecystectomy. Questions 707 through 711 refer to this situation.

707 When changing Mrs. Green's dressing, the nurse is careful not to introduce microorganisms into the surgical incision. This is an example of what kind of asepsis?
   1. Concurrent
   2. Medical
   3. Wound
   4. Surgical

708 Signs of obstructive jaundice include:
   1. Dark-colored urine, clay-colored stools, itchy skin

2. Straw-colored urine, putty-colored stools, yellow sclerae

3. Inadequate absorption of fat-soluble vitamin K

4. Light amber urine, dark brown stools, yellow skin

709 To promote healing of the large incision, Mrs. Green's physician would order daily doses of which of these vitamins?

1. Ascorbic acid
2. Mephyton
3. Vitamin B_{12} complex
4. Vitamin A

710 Mrs. Green is prone to upper respiratory tract complications because of:

1. Lowering of resistance due to bile in the blood
2. Invasion of the bloodstream by infection from the biliary tract
3. Proximity of the incision to the diaphragm
4. Length of time required for the surgery

711 Because vitamin A is fat soluble, it requires a helping agent for absorption. This agent is:

1. Lipase
2. Amylase
3. Hydrochloric acid
4. Bile

712 Advocating megadoses of vitamin A must be questioned because:

1. The vitamin cannot be stored, and the excess amount would saturate the general body tissues
2. The vitamin is highly toxic even in small amounts
3. The liver has a great storage capacity for the vitamin, even to toxic amounts
4. Although the body's requirement for the vitamin is very large, the cells can synthesize more as needed

713 Most of the work of changing raw fuel forms of carbohydrates to the refined usable fuel glucose is accomplished by enzymes located in the:

1. Mouth
2. Stomach mucosa
3. Small intestine
4. Large intestine

714 Calculate the intake-output of the following patient for an 8-hour period:

8 A.M.: IV with D5W running and 900 ml left in bottle
8:30 A.M.: 150 ml urine voided
9 A.M. to 3 P.M.: q. 3 h. intervals 200 ml gastric tube formula and 50 ml H_2O; no aspirate obtained until final feeding; 25 ml at this time
8 A.M. to 4 P.M.: vitamin solution, 10 ml q. 4 h.
1 P.M.: 220 ml voided
3:15 P.M.: 235 ml voided
4 P.M.: IV with 550 ml left in bottle

1. Intake, 930 ml; output, 650 ml
2. Intake, 1050 ml; output, 680 ml
3. Intake, 1080 ml; output, 595 ml
4. Intake, 1130 ml; output, 630 ml

715 Excessive loss of gastric juice caused by gastric lavage or pernicious vomiting can lead to:

1. Acidosis
2. Alkalosis
3. Loss of osmotic pressure of the blood
4. Loss of oxygen from the blood

716 The correct patient position for the insertion of a gavage tube is:

1. High Fowler
2. Mid-Fowler
3. Low Fowler
4. Supine

Situation: Mrs. Gorham, a 56-year-old woman, is admitted for repair of a cystocele and rectocele. She has 9 children: 3 are married, 2 are away at college, and 4 are still at home. The youngest child is 17 years old. Her husband is a Civil Service worker. Questions 717 through 720 refer to this situation.

717 In taking the health history, which of the following symptoms should the nurse expect Mrs. Gorham to experience?

1. Sporadic bleeding accompanied by abdominal pain
2. Stress incontinence, feeling of low abdominal pressure
3. Heavy leukorrhea, pruritus
4. Change in acidity level of the vagina, leukorrhea, spotting

718 Rectocele and cystocele are usually due to:

1. Relaxation of musculature of the pelvic floor
2. Injury during childbirth
3. Infection of the bladder
4. Trauma in repair of an episiotomy or laceration

719 Based on Mrs. Gorham's age and parity, the nurse expects the surgery done will most likely be:

1. Insertion of a pessary
2. Abdominal hysterectomy
3. Vaginal hysterectomy
4. Colporrhaphy

720 Mrs. Gorham returned from the operating room with a Foley catheter in place. The reason for the catheter was to prevent all the following *except:*

1. Retention with overflow
2. Bleeding following surgery
3. Pressure on the suture line
4. Loss of bladder tone

721 The main blood supply to the uterus is directly from the:

1. Uterine and ovarian arteries
2. Uterine and hypogastric arteries
3. Ovarian arteries and the aorta
4. Aorta and the hypogastric arteries

722 The following hormones are respnsible for the menstrual cycle:

1. Estrogen and progesterone
2. Gonadotropins
3. Gonadotropins and estrogen
4. Gonadotropins, estrogen, and progesterone

Situation: *Mrs. Thomas, 62 years of age, is admitted to the hospital complaining of nausea, vomiting, weight loss of 20 pounds in 2 months, and periods of constipation and diarrhea. A diagnosis of carcinoma of the colon is made. Questions 723 through 729 refer to this situation.*

723 A sigmoidoscopy is performed as a diagnostic measure. The nurse should place Mrs. Thomas in which position for this examination?
1. Prone
2. Lithotomy
3. Sims
4. Knee-chest

724 As part of the preparation of Mrs. Thomas for the sigmoidoscopy, the nurse should:
1. Withhold all fluids and foods for 24 hours before the examination
2. Explain to the patient that a chalklike substance will have to be swallowed
3. Administer an enema the morning of the examination
4. Provide a container for collection of a stool specimen

725 During the preoperative shaving preparation Mrs. Thomas starts to cry and says, "I'm sorry you have to do this messy thing for me." The choice response for a nurse at this time is:
1. "I don't mind it."
2. "Nurses get used to this."
3. "This is part of my job."
4. "You are upset."

726 For which of the following reasons is neomycin especially useful prior to colon surgery?
1. It is effective against many organisms
2. It acts systemically without delay
3. It will not affect the kidneys
4. It is poorly absorbed from the GI tract

727 The physician performs a colostomy. Postoperative nursing care should include:
1. Having the patient change her own dressing
2. Keeping the skin around the stoma clean and dry
3. Limiting fluid intake
4. Withholding all fluids for 72 hours

728 A person who has a permanent colostomy:
1. Needs special clothing
2. Has to limit activities
3. Will have to dilate the stoma periodically
4. Needs to be on a bland, low-residue diet

729 When at home, Mrs. Thomas' diet should be:
1. As close to normal as possible
2. Rich in protein
3. Low in fiber content
4. High in carbohydrate

Situation: *Mr. and Mrs. Lund, a retired couple who spent the winter in Florida, flew back to New York to see their newest grandson. On returning to their apartment after a family dinner, Mrs. Lund, age 72, tripped over a rug in the foyer. X-ray films at the hospital reveal a fracture of the acetabulum. Mrs. Lund's gen-*eral state of health appears good except for the necessity to take enemas periodically. Questions 730 through 735 refer to this situation.*

730 A fracture of the acetabulum most likely involves which of the following parts of the femur?
1. Head
2. Shaft
3. Neck
4. Trochanteric region

731 Mrs. Lund expresses concern about the treatment she will need. The nurse should be aware that the treatment of choice in this instance will probably be:
1. Insertion of a hip prosthesis with traction
2. Hip pinning or nailing
3. Application of a spica cast
4. Skeletal traction

732 To prevent pulmonary and circulatory complications, the nurse should make sure that Mrs. Lund is:
1. Turned from side to side every 5 hours
2. Ambulated as soon as the effects of anesthesia are gone
3. Turned on the unaffected side every 2 hours
4. Permitted to be up in a chair as soon as the effects of anesthesia are gone

733 Mrs. Lund has an Austin-Moore prosthesis inserted. After surgery the nurse should *not* routinely place Mrs. Lund:
1. On her affected side
2. On her unaffected side
3. In a low semi-Fowler position
4. In a supine position

734 Since Mrs. Lund is accustomed to taking enemas periodically to avoid constipation, the nurse should:
1. Arrange to have enemas ordered
2. Realize that enemas will be necessary because the normal conditioned reflex has been lost
3. Offer Mrs. Lund a large glass of prune juice in warm water each morning
4. Arrange to have laxatives ordered

735 Elderly patients have a high incidence of hip fractures because of:
1. Carelessness
2. Fragility of bone
3. Rheumatoid diseases
4. Sedentary existence

Situation: *Joan Yeats, 16 years of age, comes to the clinic because of severe burning on urination, persistent vaginal discharge, and irritation of the vulva. On examination, the vulva and vagina appear red and irritated and there is profuse greenish yellow discharge. A cervical culture and smear are taken. The smear reveals a gonorrheal infection. Questions 736 through 740 refer to this situation.*

736 The causative organism of gonorrhea is:
1. *Treponema pallidum*
2. Gonococcus

3. *Staphylococcus* organism
4. Döderlein's bacillus

737 The nurse understands that gonorrhea is highly infectious and:
1. Is easily cured
2. Can produce sterility
3. Occurs very rarely
4. Is limited to the external genitalia

738 In relation to the public health implications of this condition, the nurse would be most interested in:
1. The reasons for Joan's promiscuity
2. Interviewing Joan's parents to find out how she got this infection
3. Finding Joan's contacts
4. Instructing Joan in birth control measures

739 The drug of choice for the treatment of gonorrhea is:
1. Penicillin
2. Actinomycin
3. Chloramphenicol
4. Colistin

740 The nurse tells Joan that the drug therapy can be expected to:
1. Cure the infection
2. Prevent complications
3. Control its transmission
4. Reverse pathologic changes

Situation: Mrs. Bond, 35 years of age, has undergone a midthigh amputation following injury in an automobile accident. Questions 741 through 746 refer to this situation.

741 To promote early and efficient ambulation, the nurse would:
1. Place pillows under the stump
2. Encourage the patient to lie supine
3. Turn the patient to the prone position frequently
4. Keep backrest elevated

742 When Mrs. Bond is allowed to be up, the nurse should teach her to:
1. Keep her hip in extension and adduction
2. Keep her hip raised with stump elevated
3. Lift her shoulder and hip of affected side when taking a step
4. Walk with crutches until stump is completely healed

743 Before ambulation is started, which of the following activities will make walking with crutches easier?
1. Frequent use of the trapeze to strengthen the biceps muscles
2. Push-up exercises with sawed-off crutches to strengthen the triceps, finger flexors, wrist extensors, and elbow extensors
3. Doing isometric exercises of the hamstring muscles while sitting in a chair until circulatory status is stable
4. Keeping limb in extension and abduction to prevent contractures

744 Which crutch gait should the nurse teach to the patient with a single leg amputation and wearing a prosthesis?

1. Tripod crutch gait
2. Four-point gait
3. Three-point gait
4. Swing-through crutch gait

745 In preparing Mrs. Bond for ambulation with crutches, the nurse should *not* instruct her to:
1. Stand and maintain balance
2. Ambulate several hours a day for practice
3. Do active exercises for muscle strengthening
4. Sit down and stand up

746 Rehabilitation of Mrs. Bond should begin:
1. Before the surgery
2. During the convalescent phase
3. On discharge from the hospital
4. When she is ready for a prosthesis

Situation: Mrs. Uri is 45 years old. She has 3 children ages 12, 9, and 5 years. She is admitted to the hospital with complaints of severe metrorrhagia and menorrhagia of 1 year's duration. She was found to have a submucous myoma 6 months ago and has been carefully examined monthly. On the last examination, a week ago, the myoma was found to have grown appreciably, and she was told that a hysterectomy was necessary. Questions 747 through 750 refer to this situation.

747 The term *metrorrhagia* refers to:
1. Periods of severe bleeding in between menstrual periods
2. Severe bleeding during each menstrual period
3. Presence of occult blood in vaginal discharge
4. Spotting or staining at time of ovulation

748 Mrs. Uri expresses concern about having a hysterectomy done at her age because she has heard from friends that she will undergo severe symptoms of menopause after surgery. Based on the patient's knowledge, the most appropriate response for the nurse to make should be:
1. "This is something that does occur in older women on occasion, but you don't have to worry about it."
2. "It's too bad you did not discuss this with your doctor. I really can't give you any kind of information about this."
3. "You were misinformed. This never happens following this type of surgery. Your friend probably had a different diagnosis."
4. "Some women occasionally experience exaggerated symptoms of menopause. This is usually transitory, since the ovaries are mainly responsible for maintenance of the hormone balance."

749 Mrs. Uri wants to know if it would be wise for her to take hormones right away to prevent symptoms. The most appropriate response should be:
1. "It is best to wait; you may not have any symptoms at all."
2. "You have to wait until symptoms are severe; otherwise, hormones will have no effect."
3. "This is something you should discuss with your physician, since it is important for him to know how you feel and what your concerns are."

4. "Isn't it comforting to know that hormones are available if you should need them?"

750 Mrs. Uri, when being prepared for the night, starts to sob a little and says, "I told my husband today that after this operation I will only be half a woman. He reassured me, but I know that was just a front." The most appropriate response would be:
   1. "You feel this operation will have an effect on how your husband feels about you as his wife?"
   2. "You know of course that this is silly. I wish you would not worry about such irrelevant things. The main thing is that you have to get well quickly."
   3. "It must be frightening to know that your husband rejects you as a woman."
   4. "I think I'll call your physician. He might want to postpone the operation until you and your husband have adjusted better to the outcomes of a hysterectomy."

751 Which of the following indicates the need for oral contraceptives?
   1. A history of hypertension
   2. A diagnosis of cardiac insufficiency
   3. A history of repeated abortions
   4. An irregular menstrual cycle

752 Compact bone is stronger than cancellous bone because of its greater:
   1. Volume
   2. Size
   3. Weight
   4. Density

753 An overexercised muscle that has an insufficient oxygen supply may become sore from a buildup of:
   1. Butyric acid
   2. Lactic acid
   3. Acetoacetic acid
   4. Acetone

Situation: Mr. Styles is brought to the ophthalmologist's office by his wife. He has minimum vision in his left eye and tells the nurse, "I'm sure it's a cataract; my brother just had cataract surgery." Questions 754 through 757 refer to this situation.

754 A cataract is:
   1. A thin film over the cornea
   2. A crystallinization of the pupil
   3. An opacity of the lens
   4. An increase in the density of the conjunctiva

755 After a patient has cataract surgery, the nurse should:
   1. Encourage coughing and deep breathing
   2. Discourage the patient from vigorously brushing teeth and hair
   3. Keep the patient in the supine position with sand bags on each side of the head
   4. Encourage eye exercises to strengthen the ocular musculature

756 After examination the physician informs Mr. Styles that he has a detached retina. Retinal detachment is a:
   1. Separation between the photoreceptor and neural layers of the retina
   2. Separation between the sensory portion of the retina and the pigment layer
   3. Consequence of optic-retinal atrophy
   4. Separation of the choroid and optic chiasm

757 The goal of surgery for the treatment of a detached retina is to:
   1. Create a scar that aids in healing retinal holes
   2. Graft a healthy piece of retina in place
   3. Promote growth of new retinal cells
   4. Adhere the sclera to the choroid layer

758 The vision cycle in the eye requires vitamin A. Here the vitamin functions as:
   1. A necessary component of rhodopsin (visual purple), which controls light-dark adaptations
   2. A part of the rods and cones that controls color blindness
   3. The material in the cornea that prevents cataract formation
   4. An integral part of the retina's pigment—melanin

759 Vitamin A is a fat-soluble vitamin produced by humans and other animals from its precursor carotene-provitamin A. One of the main sources of this vitamin is:
   1. Skim milk
   2. Leafy greens
   3. Oranges
   4. Tomatoes

760 The preferred treatment for malignant melanoma of the eye is:
   1. Chemotherapy
   2. Radiation
   3. Cryosurgery
   4. Enucleation

Situation: Mrs. Prior, 35 years of age, had her third baby 6 months ago and is returning for a routine gynecologic examination. The doctor finds a small erosion of the cervix. He cauterizes the area and tells her to douche once daily with 3 tablespoons of vinegar to 2 quarts of water. Questions 761 through 765 refer to this situation.

761 Erosions of the cervix are common when:
   1. There has been a long labor
   2. The cervix stretches during delivery and there is an unhealed laceration
   3. The cervix is not dilated completely and delivery occurs
   4. The normal acidity of the vagina is altered

762 Douches are ordered for Mrs. Prior primarily to:
   1. Keep the vaginal canal clean and free of bacteria
   2. Promote healing by heat and elimination of sloughed tissue

3. Promote healing by altering the pH of the vagina
4. Make her comfortable

763 When receiving a douche, the best position for Mrs. Prior to assume would be the:
1. Knee-chest
2. Sims
3. Dorsal
4. Fowler

764 Mrs. Prior should be instructed to direct the douche nozzle:
1. Downward
2. Upward
3. Downward and backward
4. Backward and upward

765 Early treatment of cervical erosion is performed specifically to prevent:
1. Infections of the reproductive system
2. Cancer of the cervix
3. Metrorrhagia
4. Further erosions from occurring

766 When giving oral tetracycline to a patient, the nurse should:
1. Provide orange or other citrus fruit juice with the medication
2. Offer antacids 30 minutes after administration if GI side effects occur
3. Provide medication an hour before or after milk products have been ingested
4. Carefully monitor the total dosage to pregnant women and children

767 The primary reason for the ease of penetration of the needle through the tissue when administering an IM injection is:
1. The force used by the nurse when inserting the needle
2. The extremely high pressure developed at the tip of the needle due to its very small area
3. The softness of the tissue compared with the hardness of the needle
4. The long, slender shape of the needle

768 The end products of protein digestion—amino acids (the ''building blocks'')—are absorbed from the small intestine by:
1. Simple diffusion because of their small size
2. Active transport with aid of vitamin B_6 (pyridoxine)
3. Osmosis caused by their greater concentration in the intestinal lumen
4. Filtration according to the osmotic pressure direction

769 A complete protein, a food protein of high biologic value, is one that contains:
1. All 22 of the amino acids in sufficient quantity to meet human requirements
2. All 8 of the essential amino acids in correct proportion to meet human needs
3. The 8 essential amino acids in any proportion, since the body can always fill in the difference needed

4. Most of the 22 amino acids from which the body will make additional amounts of the 8 essential amino acids needed

770 Twenty-two amino acids are involved in total body metabolism building and rebuilding various tissues. Of these, 8 are essential amino acids. This means that:
1. The body cannot synthesize these 8 amino acids and thus they must be obtained in the diet
2. These 8 amino acids are essential in body processes and the remaining 14 are not
3. These 8 amino acids can be made by the body because they are essential to life
4. After synthesizing these 8 amino acids the body uses them in key processes essential for growth

771 Phospho-Soda is classified as which of the following types of cathartics?
1. Bulk forming
2. Saline
3. Emollient
4. Stimulant

772 Infection with Group A beta-hemolytic streptococci is associated with:
1. Rheumatoid arthritis
2. Infectious hepatitis
3. Spinal meningitis
4. Rheumatic fever

773 The common factor of puerperal sepsis, scarlet fever, otitis media, bacterial endocarditis, rheumatic fever, and glomerulonephritis is that all:
1. Can be easily controlled through childhood vaccination
2. Result from streptococcal infections that enter via the upper respiratory tract
3. Are noncontagious, self-limiting infections by spirilla
4. Are caused by parasitic bacteria that normally live outside the body

774 The darkening of tissue seen in the various forms of gangrene is due to the breakdown of hemoglobin with subsequent formation of:
1. Ferrous sulfide
2. Ferric chloride
3. Heme
4. Insoluble proteins

775 A solution containing 1 gram-equivalent weight of solute in 1 L of solution is called:
1. An isotonic solution
2. A normal solution
3. A molar solution
4. A saturated solution

776 Noble Manor, a 21-year-old patient, admits himself to the psychiatric unit for help in coping with the realities of life and activities of daily living. He develops severe pain in the right lower quadrant and is diagnosed as having acute appendicitis. In preparing Noble for an appendectomy, you will:
1. Ask him to sign his own preoperative consent after he is informed of the procedure and required care

2. Phone his next of kin to come in to sign his consent because he is on a psychiatric unit
3. Have 2 physicians, the surgeon and the psychiatrist, sign for the surgery, since it is an emergency procedure
4. Have 2 nurses witness the operative consent as the patient signs it

777 The best definition of a tort is:
1. Doing something that a reasonable person under ordinary circumstances would not do
2. The application of force to the person of another by a reasonable individual
3. An illegality committed by one person against the property or person of another
4. An illegality committed against the public and punishable by the law through the courts

778 Intentional torts are:
1. Malpractice and assault
2. False imprisonment and battery
3. Negligence and invasion of privacy
4. Malpractice and negligence

779 Nurses are protected from all legal action when they:
1. Report incidences of suspected child abuse to the appropriate authorities identified in legislation and policies
2. Administer CPR measures on an unconscious child pulled from a swimming pool
3. Offer first aid at the scene of an automobile-bus accident
4. Offer health teaching regarding family planning

780 Regulating the practice of nursing has as its primary purpose the protection of:
1. The public
2. Practicing nurses
3. Professional standards
4. The employing agency

Situation: Mrs. Franklin, age 33 years, is a known epileptic whose seizures are controlled by phenytoin. She is receiving IV heparin sodium and oral warfarin sodium (Coumadin) concurrently for a partial occlusion of the left common carotid artery. Questions 781 through 785 refer to this situation.

781 Mrs. Franklin expresses concern about why she needs both drugs. The nurse's explanation is based on knowledge that the plan:
1. Immediately provides maximum protection against clot formation
2. Allows clot dissolution and prevents new clot formation
3. Permits the administration of smaller doses of each drug
4. Provides anticoagulant intravenously until the oral drug reaches its peak effect

782 After Mrs. Franklin has received IV heparin sodium for 3 days, the drug is discontinued. The nurse continues to observe her closely during the early days of treatment with Coumadin because:

1. Coumadin action is greater in patients with epilepsy
2. Seizures increase the metabolic degradation rate of Coumadin
3. Coumadin affects the metabolism of phenytoin
4. Phenytoin increases the clotting potential

783 Mrs. Franklin is being discharged from the hospital at the end of the week. When discussing problems that relate to adverse effects of Coumadin, the nurse will tell her to consult with the physician if which one of the following problems occurs?
1. Increase in transient ischemic attacks
2. Excess menstrual flow
3. Swelling of ankles
4. Decreased ability to concentrate

784 Mrs. Franklin's prothrombin levels have been somewhat unstable when checked in the clinic laboratory. The nurse interviews her to identify factors contributing to the problem. The first question asked deals with her:
1. Intake of vitamin tablets or capsules
2. Use of sleeping medications
3. Use of analgesics
4. Compliance with the plan for taking Coumadin

785 Mrs. Franklin calls the clinic nurse after her weekly prothrombin test to find out if her oral anticoagulant dosage is to be changed. She mentions that her sleeping medication, secobarbital sodium (Seconal), is gone but she plans to get more when she comes for her appointment in 3 days. The nurse tells her to come for a refill today because:
1. Absence of sleep may precipitate seizures
2. Discontinuance of the drug may affect the prothrombin level
3. She may have withdrawal symptoms because she has been taking the drug for 3 weeks
4. Her seizure control is dependent on the combined action of phenytoin (Dilantin) and the barbiturate

786 A patient who complains of tinnitus is describing a symptom that is:
1. Functional
2. Prodromal
3. Objective
4. Subjective

787 Patients with general paresis are usually treated by:
1. Behavior modification
2. Major tranquilizers
3. Penicillin
4. Electroconvulsive therapy

788 Comprehension of which of the following principles is most beneficial in establishing routine patterns of defecation?
1. The gastrocolic reflex initiates peristalsis
2. Inactivity produces muscle atonia
3. Increased fluid promotes ease of evacuation
4. Increased potassium is needed for normal neuromuscular irritability

789 The nurse explains that during a pulmonary function test

the respiratory therapist will ask the patient to breathe normally in order to measure his:
1. Vital capacity
2. Tidal volume
3. Inspiratory reserve
4. Expiratory reserve

Situation: *Mrs. Row is seen at the gynecology clinic because of profuse vaginal discharge, pruritus, and burning. A smear for microscopic examination is taken and reveals the presence of Trichomonas vaginalis. Questions 790 through 792 refer to this situation.*

790 A trichomonal infection is caused by which organism?
1. Fungus
2. Yeast
3. Spirochete
4. Protozoon

791 Mrs. Row would be treated on medication and douches with:
1. Physiologic saline to decrease the pH of the vagina
2. Vinegar to decrease the pH of the vagina
3. Sodium bicarbonate to increase the pH of the vagina
4. Tap water to increase the pH of the vagina

792 Which oral drug is most likely to be prescribed for treatment of *Trichomonas vaginalis?*
1. Gentian violet
2. Penicillin
3. Metronidazole (Flagyl)
4. Nystatin

793 Spermatogenesis occurs:
1. During embryonic development
2. Immediately following birth
3. At the time of puberty
4. At any time following birth

794 The testes are suspended in the scrotum to:
1. Facilitate the passage of sperm through the urethra
2. Protect the sperm from the acidity of urine
3. Protect the sperm from high abdominal temperatures
4. Facilitate their maturation during embryonic development

Situation: *Mrs. Vale is 42 years old and the mother of 2 children, ages 3 and 7. She is admitted to the hospital because of spotting between menstrual periods. The bleeding increases during intercourse and when straining at defecation. Her admission diagnosis is possible cervical polyps, and she is scheduled for a dilation and curettage (D & C) and polypectomy. The nurse admitting her notes that she is pale, wringing her hands, and unable to sit still but not speaking unless asked a direct question. From these observations the nurse deduces that Mrs. Vale is very anxious. Questions 795 through 800 refer to this situation.*

795 To help Mrs. Vale express her anxieties, the best approach for the nurse to use would be to:
1. Tell Mrs. Vale that there is no need to worry; a polypectomy and a D and C are considered minor surgery

2. Say, "I can tell that something is troubling you. It might help to talk about it."
3. Tell Mrs. Vale that it is normal for her to be anxious; everybody is fearful, even though there is no reason to worry
4. Ask, "What are you really upset about, Mrs. Vale?"

796 Mrs. Vale finally tells the nurse that she believes she has cancer because the physician told her that he would have to remove the polyps and wait for laboratory reports. The best response of the nurse would be:
1. "No operation is done without specimens being sent to the laboratory; that's strictly routine."
2. "Of course you don't have cancer; polyps are always benign. The laboratory report is simple routine."
3. "Worrying today is not going to help you at all. It will only interfere with your rest, and you need to be relaxed for the surgery."
4. "It is very upsetting to have to wait for a laboratory report. It might help you to know that most of the time polyps are not cancerous."

797 The nurse knows that cervical polyps:
1. Are usually benign, but curettage of the uterus is always done to rule out malignancy
2. Are usually malignant, and curettage is always done
3. Do not cause bleeding until they are malignant
4. Are frequently the precursors of uterine cancer

798 Following surgery the laboratory reports reveal a stage O lesion. According to the International Federation of Gynecology and Obstetrics, stage O is indicative of:
1. Carcinoma in situ
2. Carcinoma strictly confined to cervix
3. Early stromal invasion
4. Parametrial involvement

799 The most common site for cancer cell growth in the cervix is at the:
1. Internal os and endocervical glands
2. External os and regional nodes
3. Columno squamous junction of the internal and external ossa
4. Junction of the cervix and lower uterine segment

800 After her discharge from the hospital, Mrs. Vale is asked to return in 1 month for an excisional conization of the cervix or a hysterectomy. This is done because:
1. Mrs. Vale is anxious about her condition and needs time to make her decision
2. Cervical cancer is slow growing so there is no need to hurry
3. In the preinvasive stage the prognosis is excellent if treatment is performed
4. This time is needed to rule out pregnancy

Medical-Surgical Nursing Answers and Rationales

1. (2) The hypothesis is the identification of the nursing problem after patient assessment. (c)*
   (1) Intervention follows formulation of the hypothesis and the plan of care.
   (3) Evaluation of data occurs prior to hypothesis formation.
   (4) Evaluation of care is the last phase of the nursing process; occurs after intervention.

2. (4) The primary nurse provides or oversees all aspects of care, including assessment, implementation, and evaluation of that care. (b)
   (1) Title given to a specially prepared nurse in one very specific clinical role.
   (2) The head nurse oversees all the staff and patients on a unit and coordinates care.
   (3) A clinician is an expert teacher or practitioner in the clinical area.

3. (2) Immunization programs prevent the occurrence of disease and are considered a primary intervention. (b)
   (1) This is a secondary intervention.
   (3) This is a tertiary intervention.
   (4) This is a tertiary intervention.

4. (4) Specimens can be analyzed for specific information, which is objective. (c)
   (1) Direct observations without precise measurements are subjective.
   (2) The history from a patient's family is subjective data.
   (3) The patient's verbal history of the illness is subjective data.

5. (4) When a plan does not adequately produce the desired outcome, the plan should be changed. (b)
   (1) Patient response is the determinant, not the nursing hypothesis.
   (2) Various methods may have the same outcome; effectiveness is most important.
   (3) Time is not relevant in the revision of a care plan.

6. (3) The nursing process is more than identifying a nursing problem. It is a step-by-step process that scientifically provides for patient-nursing needs. (b)
   (1) Incomplete; the nursing process goes beyond identification of a problem.

---

*Letters indicating the difficulty of the questions appear next to the answers. The letter *a* signifies that more than 75% of the students answering the question answered it correctly; *b* signifies that between 50% and 75% of the students answering the question answered it correctly; and *c* signifies that between 25% and 50% of the students answering the question were correct.

(2) Incomplete; goal establishment is one aspect of the nursing process.
(4) Incomplete; implementation of care is one aspect of the nursing process.

7. (3) The initial step in any process using problem solving is the collection of data. (a)
   (1) Nursing needs can be determined only after assessment.
   (2) Goals are set after nursing needs are established.
   (4) Evaluation is the last phase of the process.

8. (3) Feedback permits the patient to ask questions and express feelings and allows the nurse to verify patient understanding. (b)
   (1) Team conferences are subject to all members' evaluations of a patient's status.
   (2) Medical assessment does not necessarily include nurse-patient relationships.
   (4) Nurse-patient communication should be evaluated by the patient's verbal and behavioral responses.

9. (1) The first action should be to remove the victim from a source of further injury. (b)
   (2) This wound would be treated after patency of the airway is verified and the patient is moved from danger.
   (3) Breathing is the priority once further injury is avoided.
   (4) Preventing further injury and reestablishing breathing are the priorities.

10. (2) To avoid additional spinal cord damage, the victim must be moved only with great care. Moving a person whose spinal cord has been injured could cause irreversible paralysis. (b)
    (1) A back injury is suspected; therefore the patient should not be moved.
    (3) A back injury precludes changing the patient's position.
    (4) A flat board would be indicated; however, one rescuer could not move the patient alone.

11. (4) This position is useful in treating shock since it promotes gravity-induced venous return. Warmth and fluids are also supportive to the patient. (a)
    (1) These are not methods used in the treatment of shock.
    (2) This is not a method used in the treatment of shock; may also cause burns.
    (3) Promotes venous pooling, which compounds shock.

12. (3) People in panic could initiate the panic reaction in those who appear to be in control. (c)
    (1) Depressed people will be calm and not affect others.
    (2) Euphoric individuals would not adversely affect others.
    (4) Comatose individuals will not cause panic in others.

13. (2) This group would succumb quickly to severe blood loss if dressings as indicated were not applied. (c)
    (1) These patients could wait for treatment per the triage routine.

(3) These patients could wait for treatment per the triage routine.

(4) These patients could wait for treatment per the triage routine.

14. (2) *Clostridium welchii,* which causes muscular decay releasing gas, is the specific causative agent for gas gangrene. (a)

  (1) *Clostridium tetani* enters the body via puncture of the skin and affects the nervous system; no development of gas occurs in tissue.

  (3) *Clostridium botulinum* contaminates food which is ingested causing botulism.

  (4) Caused by *Bacillis anthracis,* not *Clostridium.*

15. (2) Tetanus antitoxin provides antibodies, which confer immediate passive immunity. (c)

  (1) Antitoxin does not stimulate production of antibodies.

  (3) This is an example of passive immunity.

  (4) Passive immunity, by definition, is not long lasting.

16. (1) In active immunity, plasma cells provide antibodies in response to a specific antigen. (c)

  (2) Eosinophils are involved in phagocytosis of antigen-antibody complexes.

  (3) Lymphocytes are white blood cells that become plasma cells.

  (4) Erythrocytes (red blood cells) carry oxygen in the bloodstream.

17. (3) Painless enlargement of the cervical lymph nodes is often the first sign of Hodgkin's disease, a malignant lymphoma of unknown etiology. (c)

  (1) Inguinal enlargement occurs later.

  (2) Axillary enlargement occurs after cervical.

  (4) Mediastinal involvement follows after the disease progresses.

18. (2) For reasons unknown, Hodgkin's disease occurs most frequently between 15 and 30 years of age. (b)

  (1) Less common in children.

  (3) Uncommon during middle years.

  (4) Uncommon in later years.

19. (2) Radiation exposure may lead to depression of the bone marrow, with subsequent insufficient WBCs to combat infection. (b)

  (1) Red cell production is decreased by radiation.

  (3) Bone structure is not affected by treatment; pathologic fractures may occur in response to disease.

  (4) There is no increase in the number of cells; therefore viscosity is not increased.

20. (1) Depression of the bone marrow interferes with hemopoiesis and results in anemia. (a)

  (2) Radiation causes increased susceptibility to infection as a result of the decreased number of white blood cells.

  (3) Pathologic fractures result from the disease, not the treatment.

  (4) There is a decrease in the number of cells and therefore a decrease in viscosity.

21. (3) Radiation in controlled doses is therapeutic. When uncontrolled or in excessive amounts, it is carcinogenic. (a)

  (1) Therapeutic doses are helpful in whatever areas are being treated.

  (2) Nutritional status of the cells does not influence radiation's effect.

  (4) Physical status does not affect the outcome of radiation therapy.

22. (4) A paradoxical response to a drug is directly opposite the desired therapeutic response. (c)

  (1) This response involves drug combinations that enhance each other.

  (2) A response to a drug that is more pronounced than the response observed in most of the population.

  (3) An allergic response induces an allergen-antibody reaction.

23. (2) Many antihypertensive agents lower peripheral vascular resistance and may cause orthostatic hypotension. Therefore blood pressure should be monitored in both a supine and an upright position. (c)

  (1) This is too short a time for determination of the drug's effect.

  (3) Change in position causes hypotension; when a position has been maintained for 5 minutes, the blood pressure has probably stabilized.

  (4) Assessment prior to administration will not yield information related to effectiveness.

24. (4) Hypokalemia causes a flattening of the T wave of the ECG because of its effect on muscle function. (c)

  (1) Hypokalemia widens the QRS complex.

  (2) Hypokalemia depresses the ST segment.

  (3) Hypokalemia does not deflect the Q wave.

25. (2) Potassium follows insulin into the cells of the body, thereby raising the cellular potassium and preventing fatal arrhythmias. (c)

  (1) Potassium is not excreted as a result of this therapy; it shifts into the intracellular compartment.

  (3) The potassium level has no effect on pancreatic insulin production.

  (4) Insulin does not cause excretion of these substances.

26. (4) Methyldopa decreases tissue concentrations of norepinephrine and interferes with its release in response to sympathetic stimulation. Therefore the vasoconstriction caused by norepinephrine is inhibited. (c)

  (1) Does not cause vasodilation.

  (2) Does not affect adrenal release of epinephrine.

  (3) Does not stimulate histamine release.

27. (4) Sitting on the edge of the bed before getting up is recommended because it gives the body a chance to adjust to the effects of gravity on circulation in the upright position. (b)

  (1) This would not prevent episodes of orthostatic hypotension.

  (2) Energetic tasks do not increase hypotension.

  (3) Support hose would not be worn continuously and would not prevent hypotension.

28. (4) Unexpressed rage or anger affects the sympathetic nervous system, precipitating the release of epinephrine and norepinephrine, constricting the blood vessels, and thus raising arterial blood pressure. (b)
    (1) May contribute; not the primary cause.
    (2) May contribute; not the primary cause.
    (3) Although the renin-angiotensin mechanism may contribute, kidney failure is not the primary cause of hypertension.

29. (2) If there is a decrease in urinary output with increased conservation of body fluid, the blood pressure will be increased and vice versa. (c)
    (1) This may cause a short-term increase but does not have a long-term effect.
    (3) These cause a rapid response; short-term effect.
    (4) These cause a rapid response; short-term effect.

30. (1) Because propranolol (Inderal) competes with catecholamines at the beta-adrenergic receptor sites, the normal increase in heart rate and contractility in response to exercise does not occur. This, combined with the drug's hypotensive effect, may lead to dizziness. (c)
    (2) Rapid systemic side effects do not occur with this drug.
    (3) The drug does not increase heart rate.
    (4) Rapid, systemic side effects do not occur.

31. (1) Adams-Stokes syndrome is a result of complete atrioventricular block. The ventricles take over the pacemaker function in the heart, but at a much slower rate than that of the SA node. As a result there is decreased cerebral circulation, causing syncope. (a)
    (2) These are symptoms of a cerebrovascular accident.
    (3) These symptoms are unrelated to Adams-Stokes.
    (4) These do not occur with the Adam-Stokes syndrome.

32. (4) Both ventricular fibrillation and ventricular standstill are death-producing arrhythmias because the heart is not functioning as a pump. Immediate action is required or death will occur as a result of anoxia to the brain and other vital organs. (a)
    (1) Not a lethal arrhythmia.
    (2) Similar to atrial fibrillation and not lethal.
    (3) May require intervention and insertion of a pacemaker but not lethal.

33. (4) Pulse pressure is obtained by subtracting the diastolic from the systolic readings after the blood pressure has been recorded. (a)
    (1) This is not pulse pressure; it is pulse deficit.
    (2) This is only a partial factor in determining pulse pressure; it is not the pulse pressure itself.
    (3) This is not pulse pressure.

34. (4) A culture and testing of the antibiotic sensitivity of secretions or drainage identify the causative organism (culture) and the antibiotics to which the organism is particularly sensitive or resistant. (a)
    (1) A test to determine whether a pathogen is virulent.

(2) A test for viral activity.
(3) A test for antibody content.

35. (4) This is the causative organism of tuberculosis and is acid fast. (a)
    (1) Not an acid-fast organism.
    (2) Not an acid-fast organism.
    (3) Not an acid-fast organism.

36. (2) The respiratory membrane, consisting of the alveolar and capillary walls, is extremely thin. This thinness facilitates exchange of respiratory gases without the need for additional energy. (a)
    (1) This mechanism is utilized when energy is required to move matter against the concentration gradient.
    (3) A process to prevent passage of certain-sized particles.
    (4) Diffusion of water through a selective membrane.

37. (1) Tidal air is defined as the amount of air exhaled normally after a normal inspiration. (b)
    (2) This is the expiratory reserve volume (ERV).
    (3) The volume of air that can be forcibly inspired over and above a normal inspiration is the inspiratory reserve volume (IRV).
    (4) This is the residual air volume.

38. (2) Because of potential damage to the eighth cranial (vestibulocochlear) nerve, the dosage is regulated according to the combination of drugs prescribed and the severity of the illness. (b)
    (1) Dosage spacing does not increase compliance with the regimen.
    (3) Although rest is important, this is not the rationale behind spacing doses.
    (4) Injection sites may be rotated to decrease tissue trauma.

39. (3) INH (isoniazid) often leads to pyridoxine (vitamin B_6) deficiency because it competes with the vitamin for the same enzyme. This is most often manifested by peripheral neuritis, which can be controlled by regular administration of vitamin B_6. (b)
    (1) A vitamin does not, in and of itself, improve nutritional status.
    (2) Pyridoxine does not enhance the effect of INH.
    (4) Pyridoxine does not destroy organisms.

40. (3) Streptomycin is ototoxic and may cause damage to the auditory and vestibular portions of the eighth cranial nerve. (c)
    (1) The drug does not adversely effect the cerebellum.
    (2) The motor end plates of the peripheral nervous system are not affected.
    (4) These cells and tracts of the nervous system are not affected.

41. (1) The etiology of a spontaneous pneumothorax is commonly the rupture of blebs on the lung surface. Blebs are similar to blisters. (b)
    (2) Pleural friction rub would result in pain on inspiration, not a pneumothorax.
    (3) A tracheoesophageal fistula would cause aspiration of food and saliva, resulting in respiratory distress.
    (4) The patient had no history of trauma.

42. (2) Sudden chest pain occurs on the affected side; may also involve the arm and shoulder. (b)
    (1) Decreased chest motion would occur because of failure to inflate the involved lung.
    (3) Bloody vomitus is unrelated to pneumothorax.
    (4) The shift is toward the unaffected side caused by pressure from the pneumothorax.

43. (3) As a person with a tear in the lung (e.g., a ruptured bleb) inhales, air moves through that opening into the pleural space. This creates a positive pressure and causes partial or complete collapse of the lung. (c)
    (1) Mediastinal shift occurs toward the unaffected side.
    (2) There is loss of intrathoracic negative pressure.
    (4) This is not an impending problem.

44. (4) Pressure within the pleural cavity causes a shift of the heart and great vessels to the unaffected side. This not only decreases the capacity of the unaffected lung but also impedes the filling of the right side of the heart and leads to a decreased cardiac output. (c)
    (1) The volume of the unaffected lung may decrease because of pressure from the shift.
    (2) Infection is not caused by a mediastinal shift.
    (3) This complication might occur in severe chest trauma, not in mediastinal shift.

45. (3) A pneumothorax results in decreased surface area for gaseous exchange. If the unaffected pleural regions cannot compensate, carbon dioxide builds up in the blood (hypercapnia). The patient becomes drowsy and may lose consciousness. The body attempts to compensate by increasing the respiratory and pulse rates and by the renal retention of bicarbonate. (c)
    (1) Carbon dioxide builds up in the blood, and the Po_2 is lowered because of the decreased surface area for gaseous exchange.
    (2) Acidosis occurs with elevated Pco_2.
    (4) Hypokalemia causes extreme muscle weakness, abdominal distension, and changes in the ECG pattern.

46. (4) Oxygen is supplied to prevent anoxia but cannot be given in higher concentrations because, in an individual with emphysema, a low Po_2 (not high Pco_2) is the only respiratory stimulus. (b)
    (1) This might increase the risk of mediastinal shift and interfere with expansion of the unaffected lung.
    (2) This concentration is too high for a patient with emphysema because it precipitates carbon dioxide narcosis.
    (3) This dependent action would require orders as to specific electrolytes.

47. (4) Fluctuations occur with normal inspiration and expiration until the lung is fully expanded. If these fluctuations do not occur, the chest tube may be clogged. The nurse should milk the chest tube q. 1 to 2 h. and avoid kinking the tube. (a)

    (1) The patient may not be agitated; morphine depresses respirations and is usually avoided; dependent function of the nurse.
    (2) The binder does not prevent tension on the tube; would be contraindicated, for it limits thoracic expansion.
    (3) The tube should be clamped only if ordered or if an air leak is suspected.

48. (4) Chest x-ray films or radiographs reveal the degree to which the lung fills the pleural cavity and also the presence of any mediastinal shift. (c)
    (1) The chest tubes may have minimal drainage; this is not an indicator.
    (2) These are not normal chest sounds and do not indicate the degree of lung expansion.
    (3) This would be an indicator of expansion of both lungs, and would not be specific to expansion of the affected side.

49. (1) Carbon monoxide (CO) binds with hemoglobin more avidly than does oxygen. The progressive results are dyspnea, asphyxia, and death. (b)
    (2) Carbon monoxide does not block carbon dioxide transport; it binds with hemoglobin.
    (3) Carbon monoxide inhibits oxygen transport, not vasodilation.
    (4) Carbon monoxide does not form bubbles in the blood plasma; bubbles in tissues are due to increased nitrogen, as in decompression sickness (bends).

50. (4) With an oxygen debt, a muscle would show primarily low levels of oxygen and low levels of ATP caused by the low levels of aerobic respiration and high levels of lactic acid formation. (c)
    (1) Low levels of calcium are present.
    (2) High levels of lactic acid are present.
    (3) Low levels of glycogen are present.

51. (3) Accumulated carbon dioxide (CO_2) will powerfully stimulate the breathing center of the brainstem, forcing resumption of respiration even if the person has fainted first. (b)
    (1) Increased carbon dioxide will stimulate breathing.
    (2) Rising carbon dioxide not oxygen will stimulate breathing.
    (4) Increased nitrogen will occur with changes in pressure, as in decompression sickness.

52. (1) Vomiting may result in aspiration of vomitus, since it cannot be expelled; this could cause pneumonia or asphyxia. (b)
    (2) This is not a life-threatening problem.
    (3) This is not a life-threatening problem.
    (4) This is not a life-threatening problem.

53. (1) $C° = \frac{5}{9} (F° - 32)$
    $= \frac{5}{9} (99.8 - 32)$
    $= \frac{5}{9} (67.8)$
    $= 37.7$ (b)
    (2) $38.2° C = 100.8° F$
    (3) $37.0° C = 98.6° F$
    (4) $36.5° C = 97.7° F$

54. (3) The pulse increases to meet increased tissue demands for oxygen in the febrile state. (a)
   (1) Fever may not cause difficulty breathing.
   (2) Blood pressure is not necessarily elevated in fever.
   (4) Pain is not related to fever.

55. (3) Vincent's angina (trenchmouth) is an infection of the mouth resulting in bleeding gums, pain on swallowing and talking, and fever. (c)
   (1) This symptom is related to angina pectoris, resulting from insufficient oxygenation of myocardial tissue, not Vincent's angina.
   (2) This symptom is related to angina pectoris, resulting from insufficient oxygenation of myocardial tissue, not Vincent's angina.
   (4) This symptom is related to angina pectoris, resulting from insufficient oxygenation of myocardial tissue, not Vincent's angina.

56. (1) Pain and swelling should subside prior to 1 week postoperative. Continued pain may indicate infection. (b)
   (2) Tenderness is expected during the postoperative period.
   (3) Painful swallowing may occur because of generalized trauma resulting from surgery and is to be expected.
   (4) The breath may have an odor because of dried blood in the oral cavity and is to be expected during the postoperative period.

57. (3) After a submucosal resection (SMR), hemorrhage from the nares is frequently detected by vomiting of blood that has been swallowed. (b)
   (1) Headaches in the back of the head would not be a complication of a submucosal resection.
   (2) The occurrence of crepitus would be caused by leakage of air into tissue spaces and is not usually a complication of SMR.
   (4) The tongue is not involved in this surgery.

58. (3) Personality and psychologic stresses cause pathologic changes that influence the development of ulcerative colitis. (b)
   (1) Although this may be another causative factor, psychologic stress is more commonly associated with this disease.
   (2) Although this may be another causative factor, psychologic stress is more commonly associated with this disease.
   (4) Although this may be another causative factor, psychologic stress is more commonly associated with this disease.

59. (1) Potassium, the major intracellular cation, functions with sodium and calcium to regulate neuromuscular activity and contraction of muscle fibers, particularly heart muscle. In hypokalemia these symptoms develop. (b)
   (2) These symptoms would indicate hypocalcemia, which does not generally occur in colitis.
   (3) Nausea and vomiting might occur with prolonged potassium deficit; however, not an early sign; leg and abdominal cramps occur with potassium excess, not deficit.
   (4) These symptoms are not indicative of an electrolyte imbalance.

60. (4) To promote understanding and allay anxiety, all diagnostic tests should be explained to the patient. (b)
   (1) Preparations for the test may vary depending on the patient's condition.
   (2) Preparations for the test may vary depending on the patient's condition.
   (3) Preparations for the test may vary depending on the patient's condition.

61. (1) To take advantage of the anatomic position of the sigmoid colon and the effect of gravity, the patient should be placed in a left Sim's position for the enema. (b)
   (2) This position does not facilitate the flow of fluid into the sigmoid colon by gravity.
   (3) This position does not facilitate the flow of fluid into the sigmoid colon by gravity.
   (4) This position does not facilitate the flow of fluid into the sigmoid colon by gravity.

62. (3) If the height of the enema fluid container above the anus is increased, the force and rate of flow also increase. If the container is raised excessively, damage to the mucosa may result and the procedure will be much more difficult for the patient to tolerate. (b)
   (1) The enema container can be held up to 30.5 cm above the anus and still be considered within safe limits.
   (2) The enema container can be held up to 37 cm above the anus and still be considered within safe limits.
   (4) This would be too high and could cause mucosal injury.

63. (3) Administration of additional fluid when a patient complains of abdominal cramps adds to discomfort because of additional pressure. By clamping the tubing a few minutes the nurse allows the cramps generally to subside and the enema can be continued. (b)
   (1) Slowing the rate decreases pressure but does not reduce it entirely.
   (2) This will reduce the solution flow, which will decrease pressure but not reduce it entirely.
   (4) Cramps are not a reason to discontinue the enema entirely; temporary clamping of the tubing usually relieves the cramps and the procedure can be continued.

64. (1) Since the soft tissues of the GI tract lack sufficient quantities of x ray–absorbing atoms (as are naturally present in the dense calcium salts of bone), an x ray–absorbing coating of barium is used for radiologic studies. (c)
   (2) Barium does not color the intestinal wall.
   (3) Barium absorbs x rays.
   (4) No interaction with electrolytes.

65. (2) Milk and the caffeine in cola are chemically irritating to the intestinal mucosa. They also promote secretion of gastric juice. (b)
    (1) These are absorbed slowly and are not irritating.
    (3) Salt helps retain water and rice produces bulk, both of which aid elimination.
    (4) Too general; except for those that contain lactose sugars, products containing sugar generally are not irritating to the mucosa; protein also is not irritating.

66. (3) Proximity to the nurses' station is vital. The patient must be observed frequently, since behavior is unpredictable. (a)
    (1) The patient may be unable to ambulate safely to the bathroom; this choice does not indicate proximity of the room to the nurses' station.
    (2) Sharing a room with another patient would be disturbing to the other patient; a room far from the nurses' station would prevent close observation.
    (4) Sharing a room with another patient would be disturbing to the other patient.

67. (4) Paraldehyde is a sedative that is ordered to reduce psychomotor stimuli. (b)
    (1) Fluid and electrolyte balance is unaffected by this drug.
    (2) Detoxification is a slow process and is not affected by sedation.
    (3) Emotional problems are masked, not resolved, through sedation.

68. (2) Protein helps correct severe malnutrition; moderate fat limits the need for bile; a high-calorie, high-vitamin diet prevents tissue breakdown. (b)
    (1) A diet high in protein, carbohydrates, and calories is needed to improve nutritional status.
    (3) This diet does not offer enough fat or calories.
    (4) A high-protein diet is essential in repairing tissues and restoring nutritional status.

69. (2) The liver detoxifies alcohol and is the organ most often damaged in chronic alcoholism. The high-calorie diet prevents tissue breakdown, which produces additional amino acids and nitrogen. (a)
    (1) These organs are not involved in detoxification of alcohol.
    (3) This organ is not involved in detoxification of alcohol.
    (4) These glands are not involved in detoxification of alcohol.

70. (2) Thiamine and nicotinic acid help convert glucose for energy and therefore nerve activity. (a)
    (1) These vitamins are not related to circulatory activity.
    (3) Vitamin K, not thiamine and niacin, is essential for the manufacture of prothrombin in the liver.
    (4) These vitamins do not affect elimination.

71. (3) The parasympathetic nervous system (a branch of the autonomic nervous system) causes increased GI motility and secretions. The adrenal cortex releases glucocorticoids, which also stimulate the GI tract, increasing the acidity of the secretions. (b)
    (1) They do not affect involuntary muscles of the colon.
    (2) While the adrenal cortex releases glucocorticoids, which stimulate the GI tract, increasing the acidity of secretions, the sympathetic nervous system decreases GI motility.
    (4) These do not affect involuntary muscles of the colon.

72. (2) The nurse must actively try to understand his or her own feelings and prejudices, since these will affect the ability to assess a patient's behavior objectively. (b)
    (1) Understanding a patient's emotional conflict can be accomplished only after dealing with one's own feelings.
    (3) Information from significant others is beneficial, but only after a nurse is able to deal with his or her own feeling.
    (4) The health team members should work together for the benefit of all patients.

73. (3) Ulcerative colitis is linked to psychoemotional stress and generally is exacerbated when conflicts exist. (c)
    (1) There is no physiologic change that can be made surgically to alter the disease; an ileostomy may be done to rest the small intestine.
    (2) This may be only one factor that is causing psychologic conflict.
    (4) Endocrine activity is not the only causative factor.

74. (1) Glucocorticoids and acetylcholine tend to increase peristalsis, causing cramping and diarrhea with subsequent weight loss. As ulceration occurs, loss of blood leads to anemia. (b)
    (2) Hemoptysis (coughing up blood from the respiratory tract) is not a related symptom.
    (3) Fever may not be a symptom and leukopenia (deficiency in number of leukocytes) does not occur.
    (4) Leukocytosis or increased leukocytes in the blood is not common in this disease.

75. (2) Occult blood in the stool could indicate active bleeding; the stool should also be examined for microorganisms to detect early infections that could easily become systemic by spread through the damaged intestinal mucosa. (b)
    (1) This situation does not warrant culturing.
    (3) No indication that parasites are present; situation does not warrant this examination.
    (4) Situation does not warrant these examinations.

76. (2) As a result of chronic irritation, the colon becomes thin and may perforate. (b)
    (1) Bleeding may vary from a small amount to hemorrhage; this is not the most serious complication.
    (3) Obstruction would not occur as the result of this disease.
    (4) Paralytic ileus may be a complication of surgical interventions involving the intestines or of perforation.

77. (4) This is a low-residue diet and is necessary in the acute phase of ulcerative colitis to prevent irritation of the colon. (c)
    (1) The juice in this diet contains cellulose, which is not absorbed and irritates the colon; cream soup contains lactose, which is irritating to the colon.
    (2) Milk contains lactose, which is irritating to the colon and contraindicated in colitis.
    (3) Milk contains lactose, which is irritating to the colon and contraindicated in colitis.
78. (2) Milk and milk products are not tolerated well because they contain lactose, a sugar that is converted to galactose by lactase. (c)
    (1) Sucrose is not a milk sugar.
    (3) Maltose is not a milk sugar.
    (4) This enzyme assists digestion of starch, which is not a milk sugar.
79. (3) Sleeping on pillows raises the upper torso and prevents reflux of the gastric contents through the hernia. (a)
    (1) Milk would be digested early in the night and symptoms might return.
    (2) This would have no effect on the mechanical problem of the stomach's entering the thoracic cavity.
    (4) The effect of antacids is not long lasting enough to promote a full night's sleep.
80. (2) Oral hypoglycemics may be helpful when some functioning of the beta cells exists, as in adult-onset diabetes. (a)
    (1) Rapid-acting regular insulin is needed to reverse ketoacidosis.
    (3) Juvenile-onset diabetics have no function of the beta cells.
    (4) Obesity as a symptom does not offer enough information to determine the status of beta-cell function.
81. (2) Many people are ashamed or have a distorted body image when they know they have a long-term disorder. (b)
    (1) Diabetes does not constitute a valid reasoning for not hiring an individual.
    (3) The stress is his feelings about diabetes not the diabetes itself.
    (4) Lapses in memory are not common in diabetes until advanced vascular changes occur in the brain.
82. (2) Ketones are given off when fat is broken down for energy. (a)
    (1) Diabetes does not interfere with removal of nitrogenous wastes.
    (3) Carbohydrate metabolism is hampered in the diabetic.
    (4) Sodium bicarbonate may be administered to correct the acid-base imbalance resulting from ketoacidosis; acidosis is due to excess acid not excess base bicarbonate.
83. (1) Infection increases the body's metabolic rate, and insulin is not available for increased demands. (b)

(2) Increased insulin dose will lead to insulin shock if diet is not increased as well.
(3) This would result in insulin shock.
(4) Although emotional stress will affect glucose levels, diabetic ketoacidosis will rarely result.
84. (3) During treatment for acidosis the patient may develop hypoglycemia; careful observation for this complication should be made by the nurse, even without an order. (b)
    (1) The regulation of insulin is dependent on the physician's orders for coverage.
    (2) Withholding all glucose may cause insulin shock; monitoring glucose is indicated to prevent this.
    (4) Whole milk and fruit juices contain large amounts of carbohydrates, which are contraindicated in this period immediately following ketoacidosis.
85. (2) Hypokalemia promotes mental confusion and apathy with poor muscle contractions and weakness; these effects are related to the diminished magnitude of the neuronal and muscle cell resting potentials. Abdominal distention results from flaccidity of the abdominal musculature. (b)
    (1) These are signs of sodium excess.
    (3) These are signs of diabetic ketoacidosis.
    (4) These are signs of hyperkalemia.
86. (2) Each patient should be given an individually devised diet selecting commonly used foods from the American Diabetic Association exchange diet; family members should be included in the diet teaching. (b)
    (1) Nutritional requirements are different for each individual depending on activity.
    (3) Rigid diets are difficult to comply with; substitutions should be offered.
    (4) Seasonings do not affect diabetics.
87. (3) All nursing intervention aims to assist an individual in maximizing capabilities and coping with modifications in life-style. (b)
    (1) Rehabilitation is a commonality in all areas of nursing practice.
    (2) Rehabilitation is necessary to help a patient return to a previous level of functioning after illness or surgery.
    (4) Too limiting; all resources, including the private physician, acute care facilities, etc., that can be beneficial to patient rehabilitation should be utilized.
88. (2) Orange juice has a higher proportion of simple sugars, which are readily available for conversion to energy. (c)
    (1) Bread contains carbohydrates, which require longer time to digest since they must be converted to simple sugars.
    (3) Milk contains fat and protein, which require longer digesting time, and lactose, which is a disaccharide.
    (4) Candy bars do not contain the high proportion of simple sugars found in orange juice; also contain fat, which takes longer to digest.

89. (4) The ketones produced excessively in diabetes are acetoacetic acid, beta-hydroxybutyric acid, and acetone. The major ketone, acetoacetic acid, is an alpha-ketoacid; lowers the blood pH (acidosis). (c)
   (1) Not an acid; does not change the pH.
   (2) Produced as a result of muscle contraction; not unique to diabetes.
   (3) This is a product of protein metabolism.

90. (4) The urinary catheter and drainage bag should always remain a closed sterile system; fractional urine should be drawn only from the catheter not the collection bag. (a)
   (1) This would not yield a fresh specimen indicating present sugar and acetone levels.
   (2) The system should remain closed so there will be fewer microorganisms entering the urinary system.
   (3) The system should remain closed so there will be a decreased possibility of urinary system infection.

91. (4) Antidiuretic hormone (ADH), from the posterior pituitary, promotes water uptake by the kidney tubules; the result is decreased urinary output—an antidiuretic effect. (c)
   (1) Does not produce ADH.
   (2) Does not produce ADH; the antidiuretic effect from the aldosterone that is secreted by the adrenal cortex is a secondary, osmotic effect of sodium reabsorption and not a direct antidiuretic effect (as is caused by ADH).
   (3) Does not produce ADH.

92. (3) Reabsorption of sodium and water in the tubules decreases urinary output and retains body fluids. (c)
   (1) Water reabsorption increases.
   (2) Potassium reabsorption is not increased.
   (4) Urine concentration increases as water is reabsorbed.

93. (3) Antidiuretic hormone aids the body in retaining fluid by causing the nephrons to reabsorb water. (b)
   (1) The glomeruli are not affected.
   (2) The glomeruli are not affected.
   (4) Reabsorption of glucose is not affected, only the reabsorption of water.

94. (1) The respiratory and urinary systems interact with the bicarbonate buffer system to preserve the normal body pH of 7.4 (7.35 to 7.45). Consider the following equation:

$$CO_2 + H_2O \rightleftarrows H_2CO_3 \rightleftarrows H^+ + HCO_3^-$$

Increased respiration blows off carbon dioxide and pulls the equation to the left; this decreases H^+ and the pH rises (less acidity). Decreased respiration results in carbon dioxide buildup, which pushes the equation to the right; this increases H^+ and the pH falls (more acidity). Similarly, the kidneys either conserve or excrete bicarbonate, which respectively shifts the equation to the left or to the right, thereby helping to adjust the pH. (a)
   (2) Interaction does not maintain pH.
   (3) Interaction does not maintain pH.
   (4) Although the circulatory system carries fluids and electrolytes to the kidneys, it does not interact with the urinary system to regulate plasma pH.

95. (3) Mineralocorticoids, such as aldosterone, cause the kidneys to retain sodium ions (Na^+). With Na^+, water is also retained, serving to elevate blood pressure. Absence of this hormone thus causes hypotension. (b)
   (1) The major effect of glucocorticoids, such as hydrocortisone, is on glucose, not on sodium and water metabolism; absence of this hormone would not cause significant hypotension.
   (2) Androgens are produced by the adrenal cortex; they have an effect similar to that of the male sex hormones: they do not affect blood pressure.
   (4) Estrogen is a female sex hormone produced by the ovaries, does not affect blood pressure.

96. (2) Because of a deficit of glucocorticoids, patients with Addison's disease have decreased ability to resist infection. (b)
   (1) Because of diminished glucocorticoid production, there is a decreased inflammatory effect.
   (3) Glucocorticoids are involved with metabolism; however, they do not affect susceptibility to infection.
   (4) In this disorder there is hyponatremia and hyperkalemia; however, these do not alter the defense against infection.

97. (1) Glucocorticoids help maintain blood sugar and liver and muscle glycogen content. A deficiency of glucocorticoids causes hypoglycemia, resulting in breakdown of protein and fats as energy sources. (c)
   (2) Emaciation results from diminished protein and fat stores and hypoglycemia, not from an alteration in electrolytes.
   (3) The diurnal rhythm of blood concentrations of cortisone, which start to rise around midnight and peak at 6 A.M., has no affect on emaciation.
   (4) Masculinization does not occur in this disease.

98. (4) Exertion, either physical or emotional, places additional stress on the adrenal glands, which may precipitate an addisonian crisis. (b)
   (1) Low levels of adrenocortical hormones will cause fatigue, and exercise may result in crisis due to increased metabolic demands.
   (2) Diversional activities are important to all patients not just those with Addison's disease.
   (3) Because of the limits imposed by the adrenal disease, the amount of exercise that the patient may desire may not be consistent with the amount she can tolerate.

99. (1) Lack of mineralocorticoids causes hyponatremia, hypovolemia, and hyperkalemia. Dietary modification, as well as administration of cortical hormones, is aimed at correcting these electrolyte imbalances. (a)

(2) Although glucocorticoids are involved in metabolic activities, including carbohydrate metabolism, the primary aim of therapy is to restore electrolyte imbalance. Lack of electrolyte balance is life threatening.

(3) Lymphoid tissue does not change in this disease.

(4) There is no disturbance in the eosinophil count.

100. (1) Lack of mineralocorticoids (aldosterone) leads to loss of sodium ions in the urine and subsequent hyponatremia. (a)

(2) Vitamins are not energy producing.

(3) This disease is caused by idiopathic atrophy of the adrenal cortex; tissue repair of the gland is not possible.

(4) Potassium intake is not encouraged since hyperkalemia is a problem because of insufficient mineralocorticoids.

101. (1) Hydrocortisone is a glucocorticoid that has antiinflammatory action and aids in metabolism of carbohydrate, fat, and protein, causing elevation of blood sugar. Thus it enables the body to adapt to stress. (b)

(2) Lack of angiotensin II is not the cause of hypotension in this disorder.

(3) Potassium salts are retained in Addison's disease.

(4) Cardiac arrhythmias are due to electrolyte imbalances, and dyspnea is due to cardiovascular hypotension; neither is affected by hydrocortisone.

102. (3) Fludrocortisone acetate (Florinef) has a strong effect on sodium retention by the kidneys, which leads to fluid retention (weight gain and edema). (a)

(1) Fatigue may occur in Addison's disease and is not related to cortisone therapy.

(2) Fluid retention, and hence decreased urination, may occur.

(4) Mood swings frequently occur with fludrocortisone therapy; not an indication of a problem.

103. (3) Hyperplasia of the adrenal cortex leads to increased secretion of cortical hormones, which causes signs of Cushing's syndrome. (c)

(1) Cushing's syndrome results from excessive cortical hormones.

(2) ACTH stimulates production of adrenal hormones. Inadequate ACTH would result in addisonian symptoms.

(4) This malfunction of the pituitary would result in Simmond's disease (panhypopituitarism), which has symptoms similar to Addison's disease.

104. (3) Glucocorticoids (e.g., cortisone) and mineralocorticoids (e.g., aldosterone) are secreted by the adrenals. (a)

(1) The pancreas secretes insulin and glucagon.

(2) The anterior hypophysis secretes STH, FSH, LH, LTH, TSH, and ACTH.

(4) The gonads secrete testosterone (primarily in males) and estrogen and progesterone (primarily in females).

105. (1) Cushing's syndrome results from excess adrenocortical activity. Signs include slow wound healing, buffalo hump, hirsutism, weight gain, hypertension, acne, moon face, thin arms and legs, and behavioral changes. (c)

(2) Menorrhagia (excessive menstrual bleeding) and dehydration do not occur; menses may cease or be scanty because of virilization; water balance is maintained by mineralocorticoid production.

(3) Pitting edema does not occur except when congestive heart failure is present and severe. There is no increase in frequency of colds since the ability to adapt to pathogens is not affected.

(4) Menses may become irregular or scanty, and headaches are not caused by this syndrome.

106. (1) Adrenal steroids help an individual adjust to stress. Unless received from external sources, there would be no hormone available to cope with surgical stresses after adrenalectomy. (c)

(2) The inflammatory effect of the adrenals would be obliterated after removal.

(3) Glucose (glycogen) stores will be utilized after surgery to adapt to surgery. Insulin is the hormone that facilitates conversion of glucose to glycogen.

(4) Steroids would result in fluid retention not loss.

107. (3) Hydrocortisone succinate (Solu-Cortef) is a glucocorticoid. A patient undergoing bilateral adrenalectomy must be given adrenocortical hormones so that adjustment to the sudden lack of these hormones which occurs with this surgery can take place. (c)

(1) Insulin is produced by the pancreas, and its function is not altered by this surgery.

(2) Since adrenal glands are removed, ACTH will have no target gland on which to act.

(4) Since the surgery is on the adrenals, not the pituitary gland, secretion of pituitary hormones will not be affected.

108. (4) Adrenal insufficiency results after an adrenalectomy, causing hypotension due to fluid and electrolyte alterations. (b)

(1) Hypoglycemia may be a problem stemming from the loss of glucocorticoids.

(2) Hyponatremia may occur because of the lack of mineralocorticoid production.

(3) Potassium ions (K^+) may be retained because of the lack of mineralcorticoids.

109. (3) The adrenal glands, stimulated by the sympathetic nervous system, secrete epinephrine during stressful situations. The ensuing alarm reaction involves rapid adjustment of the body to meet the emergency situation. (a)

(1) There may be modification in secretion of pituitary hormones, but it is not directly related to meeting emergency situations.

(2) There may be modification in secretion of thyroid hormones, but it is not directly related to meeting emergency situations.

(4) There may be modification in secretion of pancreatic hormones, but it is not directly related to meeting emergency situations.

110. (2) The Fowler position facilitates localization of the infection by pooling pelvic drainage. (b)
   (1) This position does not make use of gravity to promote drainage of exudate.
   (3) This position does not make use of gravity to promote pelvic drainage.
   (4) This position does not make use of gravity to promote pelvic drainage.

111. (3) The time between ovulation and the next menstruation is relatively constant, about 14 days; variations in the total cycle time are due to variations in the preovulatory phase. Within a 30-day cycle the first 15 days are preovulatory, ovulation occurs on day 16, and the next 14 days are postovulatory. Ovulation therefore occurs on January 17. (b)
   (1) This is within the first 15 days and is the preovulatory phase.
   (2) This is within the first 15 days and is the preovulatory phase.
   (4) This is within the last 14 days of the cycle and is postovulatory.

112. (4) Although the usual incubation period of syphilis is about 3 weeks, clinical symptoms may appear as early as 9 days or as long as 3 months after exposure. (b)
   (1) The normal incubation period is 21 days.
   (2) The normal incubation period is 21 days.
   (3) The normal incubation period is 21 days.

113. (4) The FTA-ABS test utilizes fluorescent treponemal antibody to confirm a diagnosis of syphilis. (c)
   (1) Although convenient for screening, a complement fixation test using nonspecific antigen may give false-positives (e.g., glandular fever, SLE) and false-negatives with late syphilis.
   (2) A nonspecific (nontreponemal) antibody test convenient for screening; may give false-positives (e.g., glandular fever, SLE) and false-negatives with late syphilis.
   (3) A nonspecific (nontrepnemal) antibody test convenient for screening; may give false-positives (e.g., glandular fever, SLE) and false-negatives with late syphilis.

114. (2) The tertiary stage is noncontagious; tertiary lesions contain only small numbers of treponemes; fatal cases involve the aorta, CNS, or eye. (c)
   (1) The primary stage lasts 8 to 12 weeks; the chancre is teeming with spirochetes, and the individual is contagious.
   (3) Duration of secondary stage variable (about 5 years); skin and mucosal lesions contain spirochetes, and the individual is highly contagious.
   (4) The incubation stage lasts 2 to 6 weeks; spirochetes proliferate at entry site, and the individual is contagious.

115. (1) Condylomata acuminata are variably sized cauliflower-like warts occurring principally on the genitals or the anogenital skin or mucosa of both females and males; they are generally associated with poor hygiene. (c)
   (2) Condylomata acuminata are warts occurring on the genitals or the anogenital skin or mucosa of both males and females; the epididymis is part of the male reproductive system and is an internal structure.
   (3) Herpes zoster is an acute vesicular skin infection caused by the varicella-zoster virus (VZV).
   (4) Scabies is an infestation of the skin by *Sarcoptes scabiei* (itch mite).

116. (3) The gonococcus *Neisseria gonorrhoeae* possesses fastidious growth requirements that are met by the columnar epithelium of the urethra, prostate, seminal vesicles, and epididymis in males and the urethra, endocervix, fallopian tubes, and Skene and Bartholin glands in females. (b)
   (1) The causative organism is *Vibrio cholerae*.
   (2) The causative organism is *Treponema pallidum*.
   (4) The causative organism is *Haemophilus ducreyi*.

117. (2) Gonorrhea frequently is an ascending infection and affects the fallopian tubes. (b)
   (1) Would not cause inflammation of the fallopian tubes.
   (3) Not an infection, an aberrant growth; would not cause inflammation of the fallopian tubes.
   (4) If untreated, may spread to the nervous system via the bloodstream; does not usually cause ascending infection of the fallopian tubes.

118. (1) The *Candida* genus consists of several species of fungi commonly found in the mouth, sputum, vagina, and stools of otherwise normal people. Candidiasis (*Candida* infection) arises in certain individuals when local resistance is decreased through prolonged antibiotic therapy or with certain diseases (e.g., diabetes) and debilitating conditions (e.g., drug addiction). (a)
   (2) *Streptococcus* organisms would be responsive to antibiotic therapy and are not considered part of the normal flora.
   (3) *Coxiella burnetii*, a rickettsia, is not part of the normal flora; spread by contact with infected animals, drinking contaminated milk, or the bite of a vector tick.
   (4) Herpes is not part of the normal flora.

119. (1) *Neisseria gonorrhoeae* is a gram-negative diplococcus commonly infecting the urogenital tract of both males and females. (b)
   (2) Associated with infections of the brain and spinal cord.
   (3) Associated with infections of the respiratory tract.
   (4) A spirochete that causes syphilis.

120. (2) Laparoscopy involves direct visualization of the uterus via fiberoptics. The procedure is carried out through a stab wound below the umbilicus. (a)

(1) This test would give information on tissue abnormalities.

(3) This procedure involves blowing air through the fallopian tubes to test for patency.

(4) This test yields data on hormone levels; usually done prior to delivery.

121. (1) Increased intracranial pressure places tension on the brainstem, causing signs such as increased systolic blood pressure, slow bounding pulse, elevated temperature, and changes in the respiratory pattern. (b)

(2) These combinations of symptoms are not found when vital brain centers are subjected to increased pressure.

(3) These combinations of symptoms are not found when vital brain centers are subjected to increased pressure.

(4) These combinations of symptoms are not found when vital brain centers are subjected to increased pressure.

122. (2) An unconscious individual loses voluntary control of the sphincters surrounding the urethra and anus. (b)

(1) Unconscious patients may react to various degrees of pain.

(3) Motion (although often purposeless) is possible in coma.

(4) This cannot be assumed; hearing is often the last sense to be lost.

123. (3) It is important to help the patient who has expressive aphasia regain maximum communicative abilities early during the hospital stay; this action provides reinforcement. (b)

(1) Some abilities do return, and therefore the family should not be discouraged.

(2) This approach may increase patient frustration and anxiety.

(4) Although expectations should be realistic, improvements are possible and should be encouraged.

124. (2) Atony permits the bladder to fill without being able to empty. As pressure builds within the bladder, the urge to void occurs and just enough urine is eliminated to relieve the pressure and the urge to void. The cycle is repeated as pressure again builds. Thus small amounts are voided without emptying the bladder. (c)

(1) Total amount of urine produced and voided would be unchanged.

(3) Continual incontinence would not occur if urine were retained.

(4) These might be signs of renal failure.

125. (4) A strange environment, as well as the anxiety associated with private body functions like elimination, interferes with the patient's ability to relax the urinary sphincter to void. (a)

(1) This method might be helpful in some situations; however, it does not take into account the common anxiety of voiding in a strange environment.

(2) This might be helpful in some situations; however, it does not take into account the common anxiety of voiding in a strange environment.

(3) This might be helpful in some situations; however, it does not take into account the common anxiety of voiding in a strange environment.

126. (4) This is considered a routine procedure to meet basic physiologic needs and is covered by a consent signed at the time of admission. (c)

(1) This treatment does not require special consent.

(2) The catheter is inserted to aid the health team in assessing the patient.

(3) This treatment does not require special consent.

127. (4) After a CVA the patient should be repositioned frequently, and passive ROM exercises should be instituted to prevent deformity. (b).

(1) The nurse is not directly assisting the patient.

(2) This would increase deformities and atrophy.

(3) Active exercises require a physician's order.

128. (1) Footboards provide a broad flat surface that helps to keep the foot in a position of dorsiflexion. (a)

(2) Blocks elevate the frame of the bed and have no effect on position of the feet.

(3) Cradles keep linen off of the patient's abdomen and legs but do nothing to position the feet.

(4) Sandbags help prevent lateral movement of an extremity or the head.

129. (1) Although the patient who has suffered a CVA is expected to be emotionally labile, the major factors determining the reaction to illness are past experiences and coping mechanisms. (a)

(2) The site of the CVA may influence behavior but would not affect the patient's emotional response to the disease.

(3) Although care is important, basic coping mechanisms and personality are already established.

(4) Emotional response is not dependent on one's ability to understand the underlying physiologic causes of disease.

130. (2) Change of position every 2 hours helps prevent the respiratory, urinary, and cutaneous complication of immobility. (a)

(1) Turning may raise intracranial pressure; doing it this frequently may be contraindicated in the early stages.

(3) Too protracted a period in one position increases the potential for respiratory, urinary, and neuromuscular impairment; prolonged physical pressure increases the possibility of skin breakdown.

(4) Too protracted a period in one position increases the potential for respiratory, urinary, and neuromuscular impairment; prolonged physical pressure increases the possibility of skin breakdown.

131. (2) To aid in motivation, the nurse should focus on the positive aspects of the patient's progress. (c)

(1) Having individuals actually perform is more beneficial than telling or showing them what to do.

(3) Short-term attainable goals provide positive reinforcement for the patient; goal setting should be done by the patient or shared with the nurse.

(4) This negative reinforcement may result in discouragement.

132. (1) As part of the rehabilitative process after a CVA, patients must be encouraged to participate in their own care to the extent to which they are able and to extend their abilities by establishing short-term goals. (b)

(2) Making the patient feel helpless discourages independence.

(3) A patient with a CVA may have dysphagia, and rapid entry may cause aspiration as well as indigestion.

(4) Meal time is an excellent opportunity to develop an effective nurse-patient relationship.

133. (3) The vessels branching from the circle of Willis provide excellent collateral circulation for the brain; partial blockage of one vessel is compensated by flow through other vessels. (b)

(1) This is not collateral circulation.

(2) This is not collateral circulation.

(4) These take blood away from the brain.

134. (2) After removal of an arterial obstruction by endarterectomy, adequate circulation may be monitored by observation of skin color, pulses, and skin temperature. (b)

(1) Bowel habits would not be altered after surgery.

(3) Turgor would be affected by changes in hydration.

(4) Appetite does not change as a result of vascular surgery.

135. (4) Polycythemia vera results in pathologically high concentrations of erythrocytes in the blood; increased viscosity increases the tendency toward thrombosis. (b)

(1) Hypertension is usually related to narrowing or sclerosing of arteries, not to increased number of blood cells.

(2) There is an increased number of RBCs in polycythemia; their immaturity is not related to the increased viscosity.

(3) The fragility of blood cells does not affect the viscosity of the blood.

136. (4) Vitamin C is an intercellular cement substance. (c)

(1) Function of vitamin A.

(2) Function of vitamin K.

(3) Function of vitamin D.

137. (3) According to the Nurse Practice Act, a nurse may independently test human responses to actual or potential health problems. (c)

(1) Providing supportive care is an independent, not dependent, function of the nurse.

(2) Active exercises must be ordered by the physician.

(4) Wound debridement is performed by the physician.

138. (1) Viscosity, a measure of a fluid's internal resistance to flow, is increased as the number of red cells suspended in plasma increases. (a)

(2) Number of cells does not affect the blood pH.

(3) RBCs do not affect immunity.

(4) The hematocrit would be higher.

139. (2) Some weight-bearing on the uninvolved leg helps maintain its muscle tone. (c)

(1) This is an unacceptable rationale for care.

(3) Speed is not important when ambulating.

(4) There is less danger of injury when the "good leg" is maintaining strength.

140. (1) Supports the fracture site; the involved leg must be maintained in alignment, avoiding adduction. (a)

(2) Comfort is not the most important reason for positioning.

(3) Adduction, not flexion contractures, are of most concern after surgery.

(4) Although friction is decreased when skin does not interface with skin, this is not the reason for separating the thighs and lower limbs.

141. (3) To prevent nerve damage in the axillary area, the palms should take all the weight. (a)

(1) Pressure in the axillary area causes nerve damage to the brachial plexus.

(2) Pressure in the axillary area causes nerve damage to the brachial plexus.

(4) Not explicit as to what extremities are being referred to; weight bearing on the affected lower extremity is initially contraindicated.

142. (3) After a fracture, if blood supply is cut off or impaired, necrosis of the bone may occur from lack of oxygen and nutrient perfusion. (c)

(1) *Aseptic* indicates that infection is not present.

(2) Immobilization does not cut off circulation to the bone; it may cause contractures.

(4) Early weight bearing at the fracture site might result in trauma to bone; circulation would not be impaired.

143. (3) This type of contracture frequently occurs when the patient lies in bed with knees bent and thighs not abducted. (b)

(1) Although foot-drop is a problem for all patients confined to bed rest, hyperextension of the knee is not possible.

(2) These two anatomic positions cannot occur at the same time.

(4) This does not describe a contracture.

144. (1) Intramedullary nails are used to maintain bone alignment and provide support along the femur's length. (c)

(2) Since these orthopedic problems do not affect the shaft of a long bone, a nailing device is not appropriate.

(3) Since these orthopedic problems do not affect the shaft of a long bone, a nailing device is not appropriate.

(4) Since these orthopedic problems do not affect the shaft of a long bone, a nailing device is not appropriate.

145. (1) Paralysis of the sympathetic vasomotor nerves after administration of spinal anesthesia results in dilation of blood vessels, which causes a subsequent drop in blood pressure. (c)
    (2) These receptors are sensitive to oxygen and carbon dioxide tension; not related to postural hypotension; not affected by spinal anesthesia.
    (3) The cardiac accelerator center neurons in the medulla regulate heart rate; not related to postural hypotension; not affected by spinal anesthesia.
    (4) Strength of cardiac contractions not affected by spinal anesthesia and postural hypotension.
146. (1) Turning the patient to the side promotes drainage of secretions and prevents aspiration, especially when the gag reflex is not intact. This position also brings the tongue forward, preventing it from occluding the airway in the relaxed state. (a)
    (2) This position is sometimes used in shock to increase venous return, not generally for a postoperative patient.
    (3) Increases the risk of aspiration; this position may flex the neck in an individual who is not alert, interfering with respirations.
    (4) The risk of aspiration is increased when this position is assumed by a semialert patient.
147. (3) Since pain is an all-encompassing and often demoralizing experience, the patient should be kept as pain free as possible. (b)
    (1) Motivation is difficult when a patient is in severe pain.
    (2) Concentration on learning something is difficult when a patient is in severe pain.
    (4) Pain can usually be managed medically; surgery is used to correct deformity and facilitate movement.
148. (1) A latex test can determine autoimmune rheumatoid factor in the blood. (a)
    (2) Lipase is an enzyme that catalyzes the breakdown of lipids; test used to diagnose pancreatic problems.
    (3) Bence Jones protein is a urine test helpful in diagnosing multiple myeloma.
    (4) Alkaline phosphatase is a blood test to determine phosphorus activity; generally used in diagnosing liver and biliary tract disorders and identifying periods of active bone growth or metastasis of cancer to bone.
149. (3) Heat causes muscles to relax, and therefore injury during exercise can be minimized. (c)
    (1) Active or passive exercises may be indicated depending on the patient's tolerance.
    (2) Avoiding exercise will increase the destructive effects of immobility.
    (4) Active or passive exercises may be indicated depending on the patient's tolerance.
150. (1) The nurse's positive attitude encourages and motivates the patient. (a)
    (2) This attitude on the part of the nurse may discourage the patient's ability to attain highest goals.
    (3) This attitude on the part of the nurse may discourage the patient's ability to attain highest goals.
    (4) Care plans should contain as many objectives as necessary.
151. (1) A long-range goal should be to involve the patient in many activities of daily living; such a program can help reestablish the patient in former life-style (b)
    (2) There is no indication that the patient is unemployed or unable to work.
    (3) There is no indication that the patient needs an assisting device; a walker is safer because it has four points and a wide base of support.
    (4) There is no indication that the patient is unable to care for herself or live with her family.
152. (2) Braces would restrict movement of the joint, causing increased deformity. (a)
    (1) This activity increases functional use of the affected part.
    (3) This activity increases functional use of the affected part.
    (4) This activity increases functional use of the affected part.
153. (1) Laminar air flow decreases the risk of bone infection, since potentially contaminated air continuously flows away from the sterile field, decreasing the concentration of airborne pathogens. (c)
    (2) The procedure is performed at one time.
    (3) The lithotomy position is used for gynecologic procedures; the side-lying position is generally used for hip surgery.
    (4) Surgery is generally considered when destruction of the femoral head and acetabulum is extensive.
154. (4) Warm compresses (at or slightly above body temperature) dilate blood vessels, increasing blood flow to the area and decreasing edema. (c)
    (1) This temperature is too cool to increase blood flow to the area.
    (2) This temperature is too cool to increase blood flow to the area.
    (3) This temperature is too cool to increase blood flow to the area.
155. (1) The temperature range for tepid applications is slightly below body temperature. (c)
    (2) This temperature is too cool to be considered tepid.
    (3) This temperature is too cool to be considered tepid.
    (4) This temperature is too cool to be considered tepid.
156. (4) Conduction is the conveyance of energy such as heat, cold, or sound by direct contact. (a)
    (1) Direct contact is not necessary to convey heat by radiation.
    (2) This is the transfer of heat by air circulation (e.g., by fans or open windows).
    (3) This refers to retention of heat not its transfer.
157. (4) Cold reduces the sensitivity of receptors for pain in the skin. In addition, local blood vessels constrict, limiting the amount of interstitial fluid and its related pressure and discomfort. (b)

(1) Local cold applications do not depress vital signs.

(2) Local blood vessels constrict.

(3) Local cold applications increase blood viscosity.

158. (4) The woman is unconscious. Although her husband can consent, he has no legal power to refuse a treatment for her unless he was previously given power of attorney; the court can make a decision for her. (b)

(1) This alternative does not have a legal basis, and the nurse could be held liable.

(2) This alternative does not have a legal basis, and the nurse could be held liable.

(3) This alternative does not have a legal basis, and the nurse could be held liable.

159. (2) Since their mental status prevents total awareness of reality, confused or delirious patients may protect themselves by assimilating small amounts of information at a time. (b)

(1) Confusion or delirium is not synonymous with brain destruction.

(3) A patient may be aware of surroundings; but perception may be inaccurate.

(4) Although this statement is true, teaching principles must be altered when dealing with a confused patient who can not handle the complex.

160. (2) The pain may prevent the patient from ingesting anything by mouth. (b)

(1) Mouth care is important for all patients.

(3) Exercises will have no effect.

(4) Hot or cold foods or compresses should be avoided because they may trigger a painful attack.

161. (2) Tic douloureux, also referred to as trigeminal neuralgia, is an inflammation of the fifth cranial (trigeminal) nerve, which innervates the midline of the face and head. (c)

(1) The oculomotor (or third, not the fifth) cranial nerve innervates the eyelid.

(3) Pain, not weakness, occurs in this disease.

(4) Petechiae are minute subcutaneous hemorhages; not present in this disorder.

162. (1) Severe constant pain, emotional stress, muscle tensing, and diminished nutritional intake can lead to exhaustion and fatigue. (c)

(2) The patient may be very quiet for fear of precipitating an attack.

(3) Pain medications do not normally cause hyperactivity.

(4) Because patients are apprehensive and feeling pain, prolonged periods of sleep usually do not occur.

163. (1) The nurse should avoid swiftly walking past the patient, since drafts or even slight air currents can initiate pain. (c)

(2) Oral hygiene is important in preventing infection.

(3) Massaging may trigger an attack and should be avoided.

(4) The patient may assume any position of comfort, but pressure on the face while in the prone position may trigger an attack.

164. (1) Carbamazepine (Tegretol) is a nonnarcotic analgesic, anticonvulsive drug used to control pain in trigeminal neuralgia and to abort future attacks. It sometimes eliminates the need for surgery. (c)

(2) Allopurinal is used in the treatment of gout.

(3) Morphine is a narcotic analgesic that will relieve severe pain but will not prevent its recurrence; prolonged frequent use is contraindicated because of possible addiction.

(4) Ascorbic acid is vitamin C. This vitamin is found in high concentrations in the adrenal gland and is utilized when the body is subject to stress as occurs with pain.

165. (2) Recurrence of pain would be unusual since the nerve is severed, resulting in permanent anesthesia. (a)

(1) Herpes simplex may develop because of injury to the gasserian ganglion, hyperthermia, or dehydration.

(3) These symptoms can result when the sensory root of the trigeminal nerve is sectioned.

(4) Severance of the nerve interferes with muscle innervation.

166. (2) Since neurectomy eliminates sensations, the patient must be counseled to get regular dental checkups to prevent local infection from becoming systemic. (c)

(1) Facial exercises are not indicated for patients with this disease.

(3) Stressful situations should have no effect on the condition after surgery.

(4) Food should be chewed on the unaffected side, since after surgery chewing would be difficult on the affected side.

167. (4) Electrodes are attached to sensory nerves or over the dorsal column; a transmitter is worn externally and, by electric stimulation, may be used to interfere with the transmission of painful stimuli as needed. (c)

(1) Patients may bathe when the transmitter is disconnected.

(2) The device should not interfere with a remote control apparatus.

(3) The patient may need analgesics in conjunction with the transmitter.

168. (3) A rhizotomy is the resection of posterior nerve roots to eliminate nerve impulses associated with severe pain from the thoracic area (as in lung cancer). (c)

(1) A chondrectomy is the surgical excision of a cartilage.

(2) A cordotomy is the surgical interruption of pain-conducting pathways in the spinal cord.

(4) This is a fictitious procedure.

169. (2) The fluid in a bottle hung over a person lying down possesses potential energy. When that fluid is allowed to run into the person intravenously, its potential energy is then converted to kinetic energy (energy of motion). (c)

(1) No chemical reaction occurs when fluid drips into a vein.

(3) No chemical reaction or formation of new substances occurs when fluid runs into a vein.

(4) Energy is not being stored in this action; rather stored energy is converted to energy of motion.

170. (4) Blood albumin, a protein, establishes the plasma colloid osmotic pressure because of its high molecular weight and size. (b)

(1) Red cell formation (erythropoiesis) occurs in red marrow and can be related to albumin only indirectly; albumin is the blood transport protein for thyroxin, which stimulates metabolism in all cells, including those in red bone marrow.

(2) Albumin does not activate WBCs; white blood cells are activated by antigens and substances released from damaged or diseased cells.

(3) Blood clotting involves blood protein fractions other than albumin; for example, prothrombin and fibrinogen are within the alpha and beta globulin fractions.

171. (2) Plasma proteins do not easily pass through the capillary endothelium; however, the slight leakage through the capillary endothelium is important and results in edema if not corrected (one of the lymphatic system's functions is to return "leaked" plasma proteins to the blood). (a)

(1) Oxygen and carbon dioxide pass through the capillary endothelium easily.

(3) Glucose, oxygen, and carbon dioxide pass through the capillary endothelium easily.

(4) Ions, amino acids, and water pass through the capillary endothelium easily.

172. (3) Osmosis is the diffusion of water through a selectively permeable membrane. Such membranes include cellular membranes and capillary walls. Osmosis occurs in the kidney tubules and in all capillary beds. (a)

(1) Dialysis is the diffusion of small molecules, other than water, down their concentration gradients through a selectively permeable membrane.

(2) Active transport is the movement of molecules against a concentration gradient and requires energy input; osmosis and diffusion are passive processes.

(4) Diffusion is the process by which particulate matter in a fluid moves from an area of greater concentration to an area of lesser concentration.

173. (1) Malaria is caused by the protozoan parasite *Plasmodium*. Plasmodia appear in the bloodstream during chills and fever. (b)

(2) White blood cells are not affected; this is not an infectious process but an infestation.

(3) Malaria is not an inflammation or infection but an infestation of parasites.

(4) Parasites in various stages are most easily identified in a smear of erythrocytes. The spleen enlarges because of destruction of the parasitized erythrocytes and accumulation of pigment.

174. (1) Parasites invade the erythrocytes, subsequently dividing and causing the cell to burst. The spleen enlarges from the sloughing of red blood cells. (c)

(2) WBCs (leukocytes) are not increased in number.

(3) Malaria is an infestation not an infection or inflammation.

(4) RBCs (erythrocytes) are not increased in number.

175. (3) Although it is not possible to prevent infection once an individual is bitten by an infected mosquito, early treatment with quinine sulfate, a selective parasiticide, can arrest disease and prevent recurrence. (b)

(1) No vaccine is available.

(2) Isolation is not required; contracted by bite of infected *Anopheles* mosquito.

(4) Antibiotic therapy is ineffective against this parasite.

176. (4) *Plasmodium falciparum* in persons who have been treated with quinine causes hemoglobinuria, intravascular hemolysis, and renal failure as a result of destruction of red blood cells. (c)

(1) This symptom is unrelated to the development of blackwater fever.

(2) This symptom is unrelated to the development of blackwater fever.

(3) This symptom is unrelated to the development of blackwater fever.

177. (3) Fluid and electrolyte disturbances occur because of fever, profuse diaphoresis, vomiting, and diarrhea. (c)

(1) This symptom is not associated with complications of malaria.

(2) This symptom is not associated with complications of malaria.

(4) This symptom is not associated with complications of malaria.

178. (3) Maintaining adequate nutritional and fluid balance is essential to life and must be accomplished during periods when intestinal motility is not too excessive so absorption can occur. (b)

(1) Peritoneal dialysis is not generally used in the treatment of malaria.

(2) The patient should be provided maximum rest and given nourishment upon awakening.

(4) Infection may occur only through direct serum contact or a bite from an infected *Anopheles* mosquito.

179. (4) $$\frac{1000 \text{ ml} \times 20 \text{ drops per ml}}{8 \text{ hr} \times 60 \text{ min}} =$$
$$\frac{20000}{480} = 42 \text{ drops/min}$$
(a)

(1) This rate would be too slow.

(2) This rate would be too slow.

(3) This rate would be too slow.

180. (2) Signs of cinchonism, such as tinnitus, headache, dizziness, and nausea, indicate that the maximum therapeutic level of quinine has been attained. (c)

(1) Tinnitus and auditory status are affected by maximum levels of quinine; however, nausea not a symptom.

(3) These are not signs of cinchonism.

(4) These are not signs of cinchonism.

181. (2) Quinine administered orally can cause gastric irritation, resulting in nausea and vomiting. By administering such a medication after meals the nurse minimizes its irritating effect. (c)

(1) Absorption of the drug is not significantly affected by pc administration.

(3) Appetite is not affected by this drug as long as gastric irritation is avoided.

(4) Quinidine sulfate or gluconate, also derived from cinchona bark, is given as an antiarrhythmic.

182. (1) Quinine sulfate is used in malaria when the plasmodia are resistant to the less toxic chloroquine. However, a new strain of *Plasmodium*, resistant to quinine, must be treated with a combination of quinine (quick acting), pyrimethamine, and sulfonamide (slow acting). (b)

(2) This would not occur if drug therapy is successful.

(3) The aim of therapy is to eliminate the asexual erythrocytic parasite, which is responsible for the symptoms, not to control them.

(4) Reinfection can occur with a different species or strain of *Plasmodium*.

183. (2) The patient still had the right to make decisions regarding hours of sleep and time of medication. The concept of invasion of rights or intrusion applies. (b)

(1) *Respondeat superior* (let the master respond) indicates that employers may be liable for torts committed by employees within their employment. In this case the patient has the right to make decisions about his care.

(3) Although this statement may be true, it has no bearing on the legality of the situation.

(4) Sleeping medications are to be given at the patient's bedtimes, not at the convenience of the nursing staff.

184. (1) A definitive diagnosis of the cellular changes associated with benign prostatic hypertrophy is made by biopsy with subsequent microscopic evaluation. (c)

(2) This test would not yield a definitive diagnosis because malignant cells might not be present in the fluid.

(3) Palpation of the prostate gland is not a definitive diagnosis; it only reveals size and configuration.

(4) This would give information as to the activity of phosphorus in the body; however, no definitive diagnosis could be made.

185. (1) The phenolsulfonphthalein test (PSP) and urea clearance test evaluate the kidneys' ability to excrete a particular substance from the blood. The urine concentration or specific gravity is an indicator of the kidney's ability to concentrate urine. (b)

(2) These tests are not generally ordered (as grouped) to determine kidney disease.

(3) These tests are not generally ordered (as grouped) to determine kidney disease.

(4) These tests are not generally ordered (as grouped) to determine kidney disease.

186. (2) Inability to empty the bladder, as a result of pressure exerted by the enlarging prostate on the urethra, causes a backup of urine into the ureters and finally the kidneys (hydronephrosis). (b)

(1) It is uncommon for BPH to become malignant.

(3) BPH develops over the patient's life span; it is not congenital.

(4) This level is elevated in prostatic carcinoma.

187. (3) The total amount of irrigation solution instilled into the bladder is eliminated with urine and therefore must be subtracted from the total output to determine the volume of urine excreted. (b)

(1) An accurate specific gravity cannot be obtained when irrigating solutions are being instilled into the bladder.

(2) Hourly outputs are indicated only if there is concern about renal failure or oliguria.

(4) Twenty-four hour urine tests would not be accurate if the patient was receiving continuous irrigations.

188. (3) The excreted ammonia combines with hydrogen ions (H^+) in the glomerular filtrate to form ammonium ions (NH_4^+), which are excreted from the body. This mechanism helps rid the body of excess H^+, maintaining acid-base balance. (b)

(1) Ammonia is formed by the decomposition of bacteria in the urine; ammonia excretion is not related to the process and does not control bacterial levels.

(2) Osmotic pressure is not affected by excretion of ammonia.

(4) Ammonia excretion does not affect hemopoiesis.

189. (3) The prostate gland is a tubuloalveolar gland shaped like a ring, with the urethra passing through its center. (a)

(1) Lies below the prostate.

(2) Lies along the top and sides of the testes.

(4) On the posterior surface of the bladder.

190. (2) Protein breakdown liberates cellular potassium ions (K^+), leading to hyperkalemia, which can cause cardiac arrhythmia and standstill. The failure of the kidneys to maintain a balance of K^+ is the main indication for dialysis. (b)

(1) Dialysis is not a treatment for hypertension; this is usually controlled by antihypertensive medication and diet.

(3) Ascites occurs in liver disease and is not an indication for dialysis.

(4) Dialysis is not the usual treatment for acidosis. This usually responds to administration of alkaline drugs.

191. (4) Hemodialysis exposes the blood to a solution that contains normal concentrations of nutrients and low

concentrations of waste products; the blood and dialyzing solution are separated by a selectively permeable membrane. The diffusion of small molecules (wastes) from the blood to the dialyzing solution is an example of dialysis. (c)

(1) Use of hydrostatic pressure to pass water and solute through a permeable membrane.

(2) Osmosis is the diffusion of water through a selectively permeable membrane.

(3) Movement of solute particles in the direction of a pressure gradient from an area of greater concentration to an area of lesser concentration.

192. (4) Serum hepatitis is transmitted by blood or blood products. The hemodialysis and routine transfusions needed for a patient in renal failure constitute a great risk of exposure. (b)

(1) Peritonitis is a danger in peritoneal dialysis.

(2) Renal calculi are not a complication of hemodialysis; they often occur in patients confined to prolonged bed rest because of demineralized bones.

(3) Dialysis does not involve the bladder and would not contribute to the development of a bladder infection.

193. (2) Insertion of an arteriovenous shunt represents a break in the first line of defense against infection, the skin. An infection of an arteriovenous shunt can be avoided by strict aseptic technique. (a)

(1) A bruit is normally auscultated by virtue of the increased arterial pressure in the area.

(3) An elastic bandage would interfere with examination of the site.

(4) To prevent damage to the shunt, blood pressure should not be measured in the affected arm.

194. (3) Homologous serum hepatitis is caused by the B virus and is transmitted by contact with the blood of carriers of the disease. (c)

(1) Infectious or type A hepatitis is spread by contaminated food or water.

(2) Infectious or type A hepatitis is spread by contaminated food or water.

(4) This is a fictitious disease.

195. (2) Urine is strained to determine whether any calculi or calcium gravel has been passed. (a)

(1) Blood pressure assessment is of no particular importance to the patient with kidney stones.

(3) Fluids should be encouraged to promote dilute urine and facilitate passage of the calculi.

(4) Administration of analgesics is a dependent function.

196. (4) Dietary intake of calcium, as well as parathormone excretion, will increase calcium blood levels. (c)

(1) Calcium intake through the diet may affect the blood calcium levels.

(2) Parathyroid hormone controls the serum calcium levels.

(3) This is not conclusive evidence that parathyroidism is the cause.

197. (4) Roast beef and a baked potato have only moderate amounts of calcium compared with the other choices. (b)

(1) Ice cream is made with milk and is high in calcium.

(2) Cheese is high in calcium.

(3) Pudding is made with milk and is high in calcium.

198. (2) Cystolithectomy refers to the removal of bladder stones. (c)

(1) Cystolithiasis denotes the presence of stones in the bladder.

(3) Cystometry is the process of measuring the bladder's pressure and capacity.

(4) Cryoextraction refers to the use of subfreezing temperatures in the removal; generally used in cataract extraction.

199. (4) Calcium and phosphorus are components of these stones and should therefore be avoided. Also an acid environment is not favorable to their development. (a)

(1) Diets high in calcium must be avoided.

(2) Diets high in calcium must be avoided.

(3) This diet is indicated for patients with gout.

200. (1) To prevent crystal formation, the patient should have sufficient intake to produce a liter of fluid per day while taking this drug. (b)

(2) Straining urine is not indicated when a patient is taking a urinary antibiotic.

(3) The drug need not be taken at a strict time daily.

(4) Urinary decrease is of concern, since it may indicate urinary failure. If fluids are forced, the patient's output should increase.

201. (1) Calcium oxalate renal stones can be prevented by adhering to a diet low in ash, calcium, and oxalate. (b)

(2) Alkaline ash restriction will have no effect on production of these renal stones.

(3) Methionine is an essential amino acid and must be included in the diet.

(4) Purines are catabolized to uric acid and must be avoided in gout.

202. (3) Because furosemide (Lasix) and aspirin compete for the same renal excretory sites, salicylate toxicity may occur even with lower dosages. (c)

(1) This response does not take into account the other drug that the patient is receiving.

(2) Although furosemide has a uricosemic effect similar to that of the thiazide diuretics, it is not potentiated by aspirin.

(4) Aspirin does not effect the metabolism of Lasix.

203. (1) Congestive heart failure is the failure of the heart to pump adequately to meet the needs of the body, resulting in a backward buildup of pressure in the venous system. Adaptations by the body include edema, ascites, hepatomegaly, tachycardia, dyspnea, and fatigue. (a)

(2) These symptoms might be indicative of coronary insufficiency or infarction.

(3) These symptoms are generally not related to a specific disorder.

(4) This vague complaint is not specific to CHF; it might be indicative of a variety of pulmonary conditions.

204. (2) Right-sided heart failure causes increased pressure in the systemic venous system, which leads to a fluid shift into the interstitial spaces. Because of gravity, the lower extremities are first affected in an ambulatory patient. (b)

(1) Pulmonary edema results in severe respiratory distress and peripheral edema.

(3) Myocardial infarction itself does not cause peripheral edema.

(4) Pulmonary disease would not result in varying degrees of edema.

205. (4) In right-sided heart failure blood backs up in the systemic capillary beds; the increase in plasma hydrostatic pressure shifts fluid from the intravascular compartment to the interstitial spaces, causing edema. (b)

(1) This would occur with crushing injuries or if proteins were pathologically shifting from the intravascular compartment to the interstitial spaces.

(2) Increased fluid pressures within the tissue would result in fluid shifts into the intravascular compartment.

(3) Although a decrease in colloid osmotic pressure can cause edema, it is due to lack of protein intake not increased hydrostatic pressure associated with right-sided heart failure.

206. (3) Measuring an area is an objective assessment and is not subject to individual interpretations. (b)

(1) Assessing for pitting is a subjective technique.

(2) Although monitoring the intake and output helps in assessing fluid balance, it does not determine the degree of edema in a specific extremity.

(4) Although assessing fluid balance by weighing a patient is important, it does not determine the degree of edema in a specific extremity.

207. (1) Failure of the right ventricle causes an increase in pressure in the systemic circulation. To equalize this pressure, fluid moves into the tissues, causing edema, and into the abdominal cavity, causing ascites. (c)

(2) The opposite results when there is an increase in hydrostatic pressure.

(3) Ascites is the accumulation of fluid in an extracellular space not intracellular.

(4) There is no loss of cellular constituents of blood in right-sided heart failure.

208. (3) The CVP is a measure of the pressure within the right atrium. For an accurate reading the zero point must be level with the right atrium. This is at approximately the midaxillary line. (a)

(1) A high reading is indicative of circulatory overload.

(2) A normal CVP reading ranges from approximately 2 to 8 mm Hg.

(4) The patient must be supine when the reading is taken.

209. (2) Oxygen perfusion is impaired during prolonged edema, leading to tissue ischemia. (b)

(1) This is not a complication resulting from long-term edema.

(3) This is not a complication resulting from long-term edema.

(4) This is not a complication resulting from long-term edema.

210. (1) The presence of excess solute (Na^+) in the nephric tubules effectively decreases the water concentration of the glomerular filtrate and urine; water passively diffuses (osmosis) from the kidney tubule cells into the urine to equalize the water concentration. (b)

(2) Diffusion is not specific to fluid; osmosis is.

(3) Filtration refers to solutes; none are being passed.

(4) Active transport requires energy; water is passively diffused from the tubule cells to the urine.

211. (2) Chlorothiazide (Diuril) affects electrolyte absorption in the nephron, causing an increased excretion of sodium and chloride. (b)

(1) Loop diuretics (e.g., furosemide, ethacrynic acid) inhibit the reabsorption of sodium and chloride at the ascending loop of Henle.

(3) Most diuretics cause loss of potassium; however, potassium-sparing diuretics, such as spironolactone, decrease this loss.

(4) Osmotic diuretics affect the glomerular filtration rate.

212. (1) Shock may have different etiologies (e.g., hypovolemic, cardiogenic, septic, anaphylactic) but always involves a drop in blood pressure and failure of the peripheral circulation because of sympathetic nervous system involvement. (b)

(2) Shock can be reversed by the administration of fluids, plasma expanders, and vasoconstrictors.

(3) Hypovolemia is only one cause; shock may also be septic, cardiogenic, or anaphylactic; always involves a drop in blood pressure.

(4) It may be a reaction to tissue injury but has many different etiologies (e.g., hypovolemia, sepsis, anaphylaxis).

213. (4) Buerger's disease (thromboangiitis obliterans) is characterized by vascular inflammation, usually in the lower extremities, leading to thrombus formation. As a result of impaired circulation, there is burning pain and intermittent claudication. (a)

(1) These symptoms are not related to thromboangiitis obliterans.

(2) These symptoms are not related to thromboangiitis obliterans.

(3) These symptoms are not related to thromboangiitis obliterans.

214. (2) Constriction of the peripheral blood vessels and the resulting increase in blood pressure impair circulation and limit the amount of oxygen being delivered to body cells, particularly in the extremities. (a)
    (1) Nicotine constricts rather than dilates peripheral vessels.
    (3) Nicotine constricts rather than dilates peripheral vessels.
    (4) Nicotine constricts all peripheral vessels, not just superficial ones; its primary action is to cause spasm; will not dilate deep vessels.

215. (4) Injured tissue cannot heal properly because of cellular deprivation of oxygen and nutrients; ulceration and gangrene may result; diminished sensation decreases awareness of injury. (b)
    (1) Poor hygiene is only one stress that may cause tissue trauma; not an inclusive answer.
    (2) Caffeine stimulates the cerebral cortex; does not contribute to ulceration or deprivation of oxygen.
    (3) Emotional stress does not cause tissue injury; however, because of vasoconstriction, it may prolong healing.

216. (1) Myocardial infarction (MI) may cause increased irritability of tissue or interruption of normal transmission of impulses. Arrhythmias occur in about 90% of patients after MI. (b)
    (2) Anaphylactic shock is due to an allergic reaction, not to MI.
    (3) Cardiac enlargement is a slow process and is not a complication that can be observed.
    (4) Hypokalemia may result when patients are taking cardiac glycosides and diuretics; a complication associated with therapy, not pathologic entity related to MI itself.

217. (2) LDH, CPK, and SGOT are enzymes released into the blood from cardiac muscle cells when the myocardium is damaged. (a)
    (1) The Paul-Bunnell test identifies heterophilic antibodies in infectious mononucleosis; would not be specific for myocardial infarction.
    (3) The sedimentation rate identifies the presence of inflammation or infection; not specific; SGPT identifies tissue destruction; more specific for liver injury.
    (4) APPT refers to the ability of blood to clot, not to the presence of myocardial infarction.

218. (2) Lidocaine hydrochloride (Xylocaine) decreases the irritability of the ventricles and is used in the treatment of ectopic beats originated by a ventricular focus. (b)
    (1) Digoxin slows and strengthens ventricular contractions; it will not rapidly correct ectopic beats.
    (3) Furosemide (Lasix), a diuretic, does not affect ectopic foci. (b)
    (4) Levarterenol bitartrate (Levophed) is a sympathomimetic and is indicated in cases of cardiogenic shock.

219. (2) Asystole refers to the absence of atrial and ventricular contractions, which can cause death within minutes. (b)
    (1) This would be tachycardia if the heart rate was 100 to 150 beats per minute.
    (3) The heartbeat has ceased in asystole.
    (4) This might be bradycardia (less than 60 beats per minute) or heart block (a partial or complete interruption in transmission of impulses from the sinoatrial node to the ventricles).

220. (1) Irreversible brain damage will occur if a patient is anoxic for more than 4 minutes. (a)
    (2) Prior heart rate is of minimal importance. Rhythm is more significant.
    (3) The age of the patient does not affect the code.
    (4) Although a variety of emergency medications must be available, their administration is ordered by the physician.

221. (1) Resuscitative efforts are futile unless an airway is patent so that oxygen expired by the resuscitator can reach the alveoli. (a)
    (2) Prior to pulmonary resuscitation, the airway must be clear.
    (3) This would not be done until the airway was clear and 4 breaths had been given.
    (4) The nurse has already checked the carotid pulse; this action would waste valuable time.

222. (1) When 2 people implement CPR, one inflates the lungs and the other performs cardiac compression. A ratio of 1 breath per 5 compressions, with a rate of 60 compressions per minute, is considered most effective. (a)
    (2) This is an incorrect ratio for CPR with 2 people.
    (3) This is the ratio for CPR with 1 administrator.
    (4) This is an incorrect ratio for CPR with either 1 or 2 people.

223. (4) The sternum must be depressed at least 3.7 to 5 cm (1½ to 2 inches) to compress the heart adequately between the sternum and vertebrae and simulate cardiac pumping action. (c)
    (1) This distance is ineffectual.
    (2) This distance is ineffectual.
    (3) This distance is ineffectual.

224. (1) Blood samples from the right atrium, right ventricle, and pulmonary artery would all be about the same with regard to oxygen concentration. Such blood contains slightly less oxygen than does systemic arterial blood. (b)
    (2) Contain slightly more carbon dioxide than does blood in the pulmonary vein, which has had some of its CO_2 expelled into the alveoli.
    (3) Contains the same amount as do samples from the right atrium and right ventricle.
    (4) Contain less oxygen than does the pulmonary vein, which will carry oxygenated blood to the circulation.

225. (2) A coenzyme is a nonprotein substance that, in the presence of a suitable enzyme, serves as a catalyst in chemical changes. (a)
    (1) A coenzyme is a nonprotein that combines with an apoenzyme to form a complete enzyme.
    (3) A series of complex changes is not involved in formation of the enzyme controlling a particular reaction.
    (4) The coenzyme does not neutralize the enzyme.

226. (4) Lipoproteins are simple proteins combined with lipid to facilitate circulation of fat in the blood. (b)
    (1) A triglyceride is insoluble in water.
    (2) Plasma proteins do not contain fat.
    (3) A phospholipid is insoluble in water.

227. (4) Fruits contain less natural sodium than do other foods. (b)
    (1) Meat is higher in natural sodium than is fruit.
    (2) Milk is higher in natural sodium than is fruit.
    (3) Vegetables are higher in natural sodium than is fruit.

228. (3) Saturated fats found in animal tissue are more dense than unsaturated fats, which are found in vegetable oils. (c)
    (1) This characteristic of food has no bearing on fat content.
    (2) This characteristic of food has no bearing on fat content.
    (4) The denseness of fat has nothing to do with digestibility.

229. (4) Animal fats are high in dense saturated fats. (a)
    (1) Vegetable oils contain unsaturated fats.
    (2) Fruits do not contain saturated fats.
    (3) Grains do not contain saturated fats.

230. (4) Since triglycerides are made up of fatty acids bonded (esterified) to glycerol, their breakdown releases fatty acids as well as glycerol. (a)
    (1) Triglycerides do not contain urea nitrogen.
    (2) Triglycerides do not contain amino acids.
    (3) Triglycerides do not contain simple sugars.

231. (3) Cholesterol is an absolutely essential structural and functional component of most cellular membranes. That it is associated with atherosclerotic plaques does not detract from its essential functions in membrane structure and steroid hormone metabolism. (b)
    (1) Not essential for bone formation; calcium, phosphorus, and calciferol are.
    (2) Not necessary for blood clotting; calcium and vitamin K are.
    (4) Not involved in muscle contraction; potassium, sodium, and calcium are.

232. (2) Cholesterol is a sterol found in tissue; is attributed in part to diets high in saturated fats. (a)
    (1) Cholesterol is needed for the synthesis of bile salts, adrenocortical and steroid sex hormones, and provitamin D.
    (3) Only animal foods furnish dietary cholesterol.
    (4) Cholesterol is also produced by the body.

233. (3) The orthopneic position is a sitting position that permits maximum lung expansion for gaseous exchange, since the abdominal organs do not provide pressure against the diaphragm and gravity facilitates the descent of the diaphragm. (b)
    (1) This position does not maximize lung expansion to the same degree as the orthopneic position.
    (2) This position does not maximize lung expansion to the same degree as the orthopneic position.
    (4) Does not permit the diaphragm to descend by gravity, and pressure of the abdominal organs against the diaphragm limits its movement.

234. (4) Isoproterenol stimulates the beta receptors of the sympathetic nervous system, causing bronchodilation and increased rate and strength of cardiac contractions. (b)
    (1) Expectorants mobilize respiratory secretions.
    (2) Antihypertensives and diuretics help decrease blood pressure.
    (3) Barbiturates and hypnotics produce sedation.

235. (2) Isoproterenol is a sympathomimetic catecholamine that causes increased heart contraction (positive inotropic effect) and increased heart rate (positive chronotropic effect). If toxic levels are reached, side effects occur and the drug should be withheld until the physician is notified. (c)
    (1) False reassurance; this is not a true statement, and the drug will have to be withheld until the physician is notified.
    (3) False reassurance; this is not a true statement, and the drug will have to be withheld until the physician is notified.
    (4) Breathing exercises are helpful in allaying a patient's anxiety; however, the drug may be producing side effects and should be withheld.

236. (2) As a result of the narrowed airways, exhalation is difficult, leaving air trapped in the lung. Distention of alveolar walls to accommodate this volume leads to emphysema. (b)
    (1) Atelectasis is the collapse of lung tissue.
    (3) Pneumothorax is the term that describes the collapse of a lung.
    (4) Pulmonary fibrosis is a condition in which fibrous connective tissue spreads over normal lung tissue.

237. (4) Destruction of the alveolar walls leads to diminished surface area for gaseous exchange and an increased CO_2 level in the blood. (b)
    (1) Infectious obstructions occur in conditions in which microorganisms invade lung tissue; emphysema is not an infectious disease.
    (2) Muscle paralysis may occur in diseases affecting the neurologic system; emphysema does not affect the neurologic system; therefore it is not a neurologic disease.
    (3) Pleural effusion occurs when there is seepage of fluid into the thoracic cavity; this does not occur with emphysema.

238. (2) Loss of elasticity causes difficult exhalation, with subsequent air trapping. Patients who have emphysema are taught to use accessory abdominal muscles and to breathe out through pursed lips to help keep the air passages open until exhalation is complete. (b)
   (1) There will be decreased vital capacity.
   (3) Expiration is difficult because of air trapping and poor elasticity.
   (4) Diaphragmatic breathing is a learned mechanism that is beneficial.
239. (1) Retention of carbon dioxide after exhausting the available bicarbonate ions as buffers will cause a lower pH (respiratory acidosis). (b)
   (2) Tissue necrosis is due to localized tissue anoxia and will not cause the systemic response of respiratory acidosis; this is due to excessive carbonic acid resulting from a respiratory insufficiency.
   (3) Hyperventilation will cause respiratory alkalosis.
   (4) The loss of carbon dioxide reduces the body's level of carbonic acid, causing respiratory alkalosis.
240. (2) The phrenic nerves conduct motor impulses to the diaphragm; cutting one phrenic nerve will paralyze the portion of the diaphragm innervated by that nerve. (c)
   (1) Phrenic nerves are motor not sensory nerves.
   (3) Phrenic nerves take motor impulses to the diaphragm not the lungs.
   (4) Paralysis of the diaphragm will result on the same side.
241. (3) Thoracic pressure is reduced because thoracic volume is increased as the diaphragm descends. (c)
   (1) Rising pressure in the alveoli and the intrapleural space or relaxation of the diaphragm expels air from the alveoli.
   (2) Rising pressure in the alveoli and the intrapleural space or relaxation of the diaphragm expels air from the alveoli.
   (4) Contraction of the diaphragm causes inspiration.
242. (4) An Ambu Bag is a piece of equipment that can be compressed at regular intervals by hand for temporary ventilation of the patient in respiratory arrest. (a)
   (1) Ventricular fibrillation requires immediate defibrillation.
   (2) Wound drainage bags, not an Ambu Bag, may be used for gross incisional drainage.
   (3) The Ambu Bag is used to ventilate a patient, not to measure respiratory output.
243. (1) During suctioning of a patient, negative pressure (suction) should not be applied until the catheter is ready to be drawn out because, in addition to the removal of secretions, oxygen is being depleted. (b)
   (2) A cough reflex may be absent or diminished in some patients; the catheter should be inserted approximately 12 cm (4 to 5 inches) or just past the end of the tracheostomy tube.

(3) Skin care is not involved in suctioning; may be part of tracheostomy care; tapes are untied only when being changed.
   (4) The inner cannula is not removed during suctioning; it may be removed during tracheostomy care.
244. (2) Hypersensitivity to a foreign substance can cause an anaphylactic reaction. Histamine is released, causing bronchial constriction, increased capillary permeability, and dilation of arterioles. This decreased peripheral resistance is associated with hypotension and inadequate circulation to major organs. (c)
   (1) Dilation of arterioles occurs.
   (3) These are the problems that result from bronchial constriction and vascular collapse.
   (4) Arterioles dilate, capillary permeability increases, and eventually vascular collapse occurs.
245. (3) Hypersensitivity results from the production of antibodies in response to exposure to certain foreign substances (allergens). Prior exposure is necessary for the development of these antibodies. (c)
   (1) Not a sensitivity reaction to penicillin; hayfever and asthma are atopic conditions caused by atopens.
   (2) It would be an active immunity.
   (4) Antibodies have been developed in a prior exposure to the allergen, in this case penicillin.
246. (4) Diphenhydramine hydrochloride (Benadryl), like other antihistamines, competes with histamine at receptor sites. This alleviates the effects of histamine, which include increased dilation and permeability of capillaries (the cause of urticaria). (c)
   (1) Benadryl does not destroy histamine; it competes with histamine at receptor sites.
   (2) Benadryl does not have these actions; histamine dilates capillaries.
   (3) Benadryl does not metabolize histamines.
247. (3) Penicillinase alters the structure of the penicillin molecule so it loses its antibiotic and allergenic capabilities. (c)
   (1) Not the action of penicillinase; penicillin's molecular structure is altered by this drug.
   (2) Penicillinase does not counteract tissue effects; it inactivates circulating penicillin.
   (4) Drug is used only to inactivate circulating penicillin.
248. (3) Soap and water reduce surface tension, facilitating the removal of microorganisms by friction. (b)
   (1) Although these aspects of handwashing are important, without friction they would have little or no value.
   (2) Although these aspects of handwashing are important, without friction they would have little or no value.
   (4) Although these aspects of handwashing are important, without friction they would have little or no value.
249. (4) Vitamin K, synthesized by the bacterial flora of the intestine, promotes the liver's synthesis of prothrombin, an important blood clotting factor. (c)

(1) Vitamin K does not affect calcium ionization.

(2) Vitamin K does not promote platelet aggregation.

(3) Vitamin K does not promote fibrinogen formation.

250. (2) Prevention of serum hepatitis from blood transfusions can be accomplished through screening donors. (b)

(1) Enteric precautions are indicated for individuals with infectious hepatitis.

(3) This is not a preventive measure.

(4) Isolation is not indicated for individuals with serum hepatitis.

251. (1) This is an enzyme that is released early in the course of liver damage. (c)

(2) This is not an early sign of liver damage.

(3) This is not an early sign of liver damage.

(4) This is not an early sign of liver damage.

252. (3) Gamma globulin, an immune globulin, contains most of the antibodies circulating in the blood. When injected into an individual, it prevents a specific antigen from entering a host cell. (b)

(1) Does not stimulate antibody production.

(2) Does not stimulate antibody production.

(4) Does not affect antigen-antibody function.

253. (4) Phenobarbital depresses the CNS, particularly the motor cortex, producing side effects such as lethargy, loss of appetite, depression, and vertigo. (b)

(1) These are not side effects of phenobarbital.

(2) These are not side effects of phenobarbital.

(3) These are not side effects of phenobarbital.

254. (3) The virus is present in the stool of patients with infectious hepatitis, so special handling is required. The virus may also be present in the urine and in the nasotracheal secretions of such patients. (b)

(1) Bringing food to a patient requires no precautions; however, disposable utensils should be used because the patient's nasotracheal secretions contain the virus.

(2) Infectious hepatitis is not usually transmitted via the air.

(4) Infectious hepatitis is not usually transmitted via the air.

255. (4) Pitressin is a vasoconstrictor that is used with great success in controlling GI bleeding. (c)

(1) Aquamephyton is vitamin K; it promotes formation of prothrombin in the liver; although this action would be helpful, it would take too long to be of value in an emergency situation.

(2) Neostigmine inhibits cholinesterase, permitting acetylcholine to function; used primarily for myasthenia gravis.

(3) Pro-Banthine is a gastrointestinal anticholineric; it decreases motility but has no effect on bleeding.

256. (2) Removal of the fundus of the stomach destroys the parietal cells that secrete intrinsic factor (needed to complex with vitamin B_{12} as a preliminary to its absorption in the ileum). (c)

(1) Diabetes has no effect on intrinsic factor.

(3) Hemorrhaging may cause anemia; however, pernicious anemia occurs when intrinsic factor is not produced.

(4) Dietary intake has no effect on the production of intrinsic factor.

257. (3) The antrum is responsible for gastrin production, which stimulates hydrochloric acid (HCl) secretion; its removal reduces HCl secretion and thus reduces irritation of the gastric mucosa. (c)

(1) A resection of the fifth cranial nerve would be done in trigeminal neuralgia.

(2) A stapedectomy, mobilization of the stapes, or a prosthetic implant would be used with otosclerosis.

(4) Removal by means of a laser beam, cryotechnique, or surgery is used when cataracts occur.

258. (4) The act of eating allows the hydrochloric acid in the stomach to work on and be neutralized by food rather than irritate the gastric mucosa. (b)

(1) These symptoms are not specific to gastric ulcers.

(2) This may indicate renal colic.

(3) Generalized symptoms not specific to gastric ulcers.

259. (1) Peptic ulcers may occur in an individual in whom there is a conflict between a strong drive for independence and an unconscious need to be dependent. (c)

(2) These psychologic states are not involved in the etiology of peptic ulcer.

(3) These psychologic states are not involved in the etiology of peptic ulcer.

(4) Does not include many feelings; involves the unconscious need to be dependent.

260. (4) The patient should be encouraged to rest mind and body; sedatives may be indicated to achieve this goal. (b)

(1) False reassurance is psychologically damaging.

(2) Antibiotics will have no direct effect on the patient's anxiety.

(3) Knowledge itself does not always reduce anxiety.

261. (2) Irritation of the mucosa may cause increased bleeding or perforation and therefore should be avoided. (b)

(1) Bulk and roughage may irritate the mucosa and should be decreased.

(3) All patients' diets should be nutritionally balanced; this is not specific to Dr. Grove's problem.

(4) Psychologic support is not the primary goal; efforts should be made to include foods that are psychologically beneficial, but not at the expense of foods that are nonirritating to the mucosa.

262. (3) Iron is needed in the formation of hemoglobin. (b)

(1) Dextran is a plasma volume expander; does not affect erythrocytes.

(2) Cari-Tab Softabs are vitamin supplements intended to promote the development of a carries-free dentition.

(4) Vitamin B_{12} is a fat-soluble vitamin that must be supplemented when an individual has pernicious anemia.

263. (3) The heart may be strained by prolonged anemia because the blood's decreased viscosity eases its return to the heart from the peripheral vessels. In accordance with Starling's law, the greater volume of blood returning to the heart will stretch it and result in greater cardiac output. The increased blood viscosity occurring in polycythemia forces the heart to strain to maintain adequate peripheral blood flow; the heart must exert greater force to propel the more viscous blood through the circulatory system. (a)
    (1) Pressure is not involved; the terms anemia and polycythemia both refer to the number of cells present in a given volume (viscosity).
    (2) Surface tension is not involved; the terms anemia and polycythemia both refer to the number of cells in a given volume (viscosity).
    (4) Temperature is not involved; the terms anemia and polycythemia both refer to the number of cells present in a given volume (viscosity).

264. (3) Emotional stress of any kind can stimulate peristalsis and thereby increase the volume of drainage. (b)
    (1) The stoma will start to drain within the first 24 hours after surgery.
    (2) Ileostomy drainage is liquefied and continuous, so irrigations are not indicated.
    (4) The patient should be encouraged to eat a diet as normal as possible.

265. (1) Vitamin B_{12} (extrinsic factor) combines with intrinsic factor, a substance secreted by the parietal cells of the gastric mucosa; forming hemopoietic factor. Hemopoietic factor is only absorbed in the ileum, from which it travels to bone marrow and stimulates erythropoiesis. (c)
    (2) Folic acid is not absorbed in the terminal ileum.
    (3) Iron absorption does not occur in the ileum.
    (4) Trace elements are not absorbed in the ileum.

266. (4) Trauma to the abdominal wall and to the stoma should be avoided, so contact sports are contraindicated. (a)
    (1) Trauma to the abdominal wall is a minimal risk in this sport.
    (2) Trauma to the abdominal wall is a minimal risk in this sport.
    (3) Trauma to the abdominal wall is a minimal risk in this sport.

267. (2) A rectal catheter should be inserted approximately 10 cm (4 inches) since this will be far enough to pass the rectal sphincter. (b)
    (1) Five-centimeter (2-inch) insertion will not allow the tube to pass the sphincter.
    (3) Deep insertion may cause damage to the intestinal mucosa.
    (4) Deep insertion may cause damage to the intestinal mucosa.

268. (2) A rectal tube promotes maximum benefits in 30 minutes. This allows adequate time for gas to escape. (b)

(1) Fifteen minutes is not adequate time to permit removal of flatus.
(3) After 30 minutes there would be minimal release of flatus.
(4) After 30 minutes there would be minimal release of flatus.

269. (2) Intussusception is the telescoping or prolapse of a segment of the bowel within the lumen of an immediately connecting part. (a)
    (1) Volvulus is a twisting of the bowel onto itself.
    (3) Adhesions are bands of scar tissue that can compress the bowel.
    (4) Herniation is the term that describes protrusion of an organ through the wall that contains it.

270. (3) A flat plate film of the abdomen visualizes abdominal organs as they are. (b)
    (1) The patient may eat and drink as tolerated.
    (2) No bowel preparation is indicated.
    (4) Now bowel preparation is indicated.

271. (1) The semi-Fowler position aids in drainage and prevents spread of infection throughout the abdominal cavity. (b)
    (2) The Trendelenburg position would contribute to the spread of infection and throughout the abdominal cavity.
    (3) The Sims position is generally used for administration of enemas, or rectal examination; would not be helpful in draining the area.
    (4) The dorsal recumbent position would not allow for lower body drainage.

272. (2) Paralytic ileus occurs when neurologic impulses are diminished, as from anesthesia, infection, or surgery. (a)
    (1) Interference in blood supply would result in necrosis of the bowel.
    (3) Perforation of the bowel would result in pain and peritonitis.
    (4) Obstruction of the bowel lumen would initially cause increased peristalsis and bowel sounds.

273. (4) Thrombophlebitis is inflammation of a vein that occurs with the formation of a clot. Signs include pain (especially on dorsiflexion of the foot), redness, warmth, tenderness, and edema. (a)
    (1) Pain occurs on flexion of the foot (Homan's sign).
    (2) Pitting edema does not occur in thrombophlebitis.
    (3) Intermittent claudication (pain and limping when walking) may occur with peripheral vascular disease.

274. (1) Coumarin derivatives are ordered day by day, based on the prothrombin time of the patient. This test gives a good index of the individual's clotting ability. (b)
    (2) Clotting time is the time required for blood to form a clot; not used for dosage calculation.
    (3) Bleeding time is the time required for blood to cease flowing from a small wound; not used for coumarin dosage calculation.

(4) Sedimentation rate is a test used to determine the presence of inflammation or infection; not indicative of clotting ability.

275. (3) Dicumarol depresses prothrombin activity and inhibits the formation of several of the clotting factors by the liver. Its antagonist is vitamin K, which is involved in prothrombin formation. (c)
  (1) Imferon is an iron supplement, not an antidote for coumarin.
  (2) Heparin is an anticoagulant.
  (4) Protamine sulfate is the antidote for heparin overdose.

276. (4) In the absence of insulin, which facilitates the transport of glucose into the cell, the body breaks down proteins and fats to supply energy ketones, a byproduct of fat metabolism. These accumulate, causing metabolic acidosis (pH < 7.35). (b)
  (1) Cholesterol level has no effect on the development of acidosis.
  (2) The pH of food ingested has no effect on the development of acidosis.
  (3) This would indicate a state of alkalosis.

277. (3) In the absence of insulin, glucose cannot enter the cell or be converted to glycogen; so it remains in the blood. Breakdown of fats as an energy source causes an accumulation of ketones, which results in acidosis. The lungs, in an attempt to compensate for lowered pH, will blow off CO_2 (Kussmaul respirations). (c)
  (1) Hyperglycemia and increased acidity would be present.
  (2) High acidity and a low CO_2 combining power would be present.
  (4) Hyperglycemia and a low CO_2 combining power would be present.

278. (2) Regular insulin is rapid acting and is used to meet a patient's current insulin needs, as in diabetic coma or in coverage for fractional urine test results. (b)
  (1) These are both intermediate acting insulins, which have an onset of 4 to 8 hours; in diabetic acidosis the individual needs rapid-acting insulin.
  (3) These are both intermediate-acting insulins, which have an onset of 4 to 8 hours; in diabetic acidosis the individual needs rapid-acting insulin.
  (4) PZI is a long-acting insulin, with an onset of 4 to 8 hours and a peak of 14 to 20 hours.

279. (1) Once treatment with insulin for diabetic ketoacidosis is begun, potassium ions reenter the cell, causing hypokalemia; therefore potassium, along with the replacement fluids, is generally supplied. (b)
  (2) Treatment with potassium would not correct this.
  (3) Flaccid paralysis would not occur in diabetic ketoacidosis; potassium replaces that which has reentered the cell after insulin therapy.
  (4) Knowing the relationship of insulin and potassium, the nurse should recognize that treatment with KCl is prophylactic, aborting any development of arrhythmias.

280. (1) Ice milk is a dairy product, whereas bread is not. (b)
  (2) This exchange is from the same food group and supplies approximately equal amounts of nutrients.
  (3) This exchange is from the same food group and supplies approximately equal amounts of nutrients.
  (4) This exchange is from the same food group and supplies approximately equal amounts of nutrients.

281. (2) Glucagon is an insulin antagonist produced by the alpha cells in the islets of Langerhans. It causes the breakdown of glycogen and protein to glucose. (b)
  (1) Acidosis occurs when there is a high sugar level; therefore glucagon is not indicated.
  (3) Glucagon is not indicated in idiosyncratic reactions to insulin.
  (4) Glucagon would be ineffective in the pathologic condition indicated.

282. (2) The Nurse Practice Act states that the nurse will do health teaching and administer nursing care supportive to life and well-being. (a)
  (1) Health teaching is an independent function of the nurse.
  (3) The teaching was essential prior to discharge.
  (4) The patient is responsible for her own care.

283. (2) A triglyceride comprises 3 fatty acids and a glycerol molecule. When energy is required, the fatty acids are mobilized from adipose tissue for fuel. (b)
  (1) This is not the function of adipose tissue in fat metabolism.
  (3) This is not a function of adipose tissue; cholesterol produced in liver.
  (4) This is not the function of adipose tissue; its main function is storage.

284. (2) Insulin stimulates cellular uptake of glucose and also stimulates the membrane-bound pump for sodium and potassium ions (Na^+ and K^+), leading to influx of K^+ into insulin's target cells. The resulting hypokalemia is offset by parenteral administration of K^+. (c)
  (1) Hypokalemia may occur because the K^+ move back into the cells as dehydration is reversed.
  (3) Hypokalemia may be caused by the movement of K^+ back into the cells as dehydration is reversed.
  (4) Anabolic reactions are stimulated by insulin and glucose administration; K^+ are drawn into the intercellular compartment, necessitating a replenishment of extracellular potassium.

285. (3) Since oral hyperglycemics stimulate the islets of Langerhans to produce insulin, a regular interval between doses should be maintained. (a)
  (1) Manifestations of toxicity should be taught but not emphasized because occurrence of toxicity is low and the nurse may needlessly cause anxiety.
  (2) Untoward reactions should be taught but not emphasized because occurrence of untoward reactions is low and the nurse may needlessly cause anxiety.
  (4) The dosage should be regulated by the physician.

286. (3) Blood has a narrow pH range of 7.35 to 7.45. Venous blood (pH 7.35) is more acidic and closer to 7.35 than is arterial blood, which is normally closer to a pH of 7.45. (a)
  (1) This is very acidic and needs immediate treatment.
  (2) This is slightly acidic for both arterial and venous blood.
  (4) This is alkaline and needs treatment.

287. (1) Somatotropin promotes growth by accelerating amino acid transport into cells. Oversecretion after full growth and epiphyseal closure results in acromegaly, with enlargement of bones and overlying soft tissue in the feet, hands, lower jaw, and cheeks. Growth hormone also increases blood glucose levels. (b)
  (2) This causes hyperthyroidism; not produced by hypophysis.
  (3) Would increase stimulation of the thyroid gland.
  (4) Oversecretion would affect secondary sexual characteristics.

288. (4) The hypophysis cerebri (pituitary) does not directly regulate insulin release. This is controlled by blood glucose levels. Since somatotropin release will stop after the hypophysectomy, any elevation of blood glucose caused by somatotropin will also stop. (a)
  (1) This effect may be expected after a hypophysectomy since follicle-stimulating hormone and follicle-stimulating hormone releasing factor will no longer be present to stimulate spermatogenesis.
  (2) ACTH, which stimulates glucocorticoid secretion by the adrenal glands, is absent and cortisone will have to be administered.
  (3) Thyroid-stimulating hormone will not be present, extrinsic thyroxin will have to be taken.

289. (1) ACTH is released in response to decreased blood levels of cortisol. The ACTH then stimulates release of more adrenocortical hormone. (c)
  (2) Cortisol assists the body in adapting to stress.
  (3) Cortisol has antiinflammatory properties, which delay wound healing.
  (4) As a glucocorticoid it increases gluconeogenesis in the liver.

290. (3) Because of the location of the pituitary gland, there is swelling in the brain after the gland's removal. This edema may result in increased intracranial pressure. (c)
  (1) This may follow any surgery and is not a specific occurrence following cranial surgery.
  (2) This may follow any surgery and is not a specific occurrence following cranial surgery.
  (4) Although this may be the result of pressure on the medulla caused by increased intracranial pressure, it is not an initial sign of ICP.

291. (2) Endocrine gland secretions (hormones) are inactivated by the liver and other tissues fairly rapidly; continuous hormonal secretion by the endocrine glands is regulated by immediate feedback controls, and the body's metabolism is always close to being suitable to the body's immediate needs. (b)
  (1) This time interval does not represent secretory patterns of the endocrine glands.
  (3) This time interval does not represent secretory patterns of the endocrine glands.
  (4) This time interval does not represent secretory patterns of the endocrine glands.

292. (1) Uninformed consent constitutes an artificial consent. Sufficient information was not given. (b)
  (2) The surgeon may do what is necessary if an informed consent is obtained for all eventualities.
  (3) This is not sufficient to cover invasive procedures or surgery.
  (4) Informed consent covers only that which is covered by the consent.

293. (1) The ovaries are responsible for producing the female sex hormones estrogen and progesterone. A bilateral oophorectomy causes an abrupt cessation in the production of most of these hormones (the adrenal cortex produces small quantities of female sex hormones) and results in surgical menopause. (b)
  (2) Hysterectomy is the removal of the uterus, and ovarian function is unaffected.
  (3) Salpingectomy is the removal of the fallopian tubes, and ovarian function is unaffected.
  (4) Tubal ligation is the surgical severing of the fallopian tubes to produce sterility, and ovarian function is unaffected.

294. (4) Depletion of ovarian hormones causes vasomotor instability. Periodic systemic vasodilation is then triggered by the sympathetic nervous system, causing the feeling of warmth. (c)
  (1) Hot flashes may be associated with understimulation of the adrenals.
  (2) Acetylcholine does not cause hot flashes; it is the chemical mediator of cholinergic nerve impulses.
  (3) Gonadotropins do not cause hot flashes; they stimulate the function of the testes and ovaries.

295. (3) The lack of utilization of gonadotropin by the ovaries causes an elevation of gonadotropin in the blood. Ovarian function is diminished; there is little or no follicular activity. (c)
  (1) There would be a decrease in secretion of progesterone.
  (2) There would be an increase in prostaglandins.
  (4) There would be an increase in gonadotropin in the blood, for it is not used by the ovaries.

296. (1) Ovulation occurs when the blood levels of both follicle-stimulating hormone and luteinizing hormone (FSH and LH) are relatively high, but it is the surge of LH secretion in midcycle that is responsible for ovulation. (a)
  (2) When the endometrial wall is built up.
  (3) When the progesterone level is low.
  (4) Not related; this stimulates ejection of milk into the mammary ducts.

297. (2) High levels of plasma estrogen inhibit pituitary secretion of FSH; this effect appears to be mediated by the hypothalamus and its releasing factors. (c)
(1) LH (luteinizing hormone) causes ovulation.
(3) Low concentrations of estrogen may precipitate demineralization of bone.
(4) Lactogenic hormone (prolactin) stimulates lactation.

298. (3) Rectal temperature is the most accurate. (a)
(1) Oral temperature is contraindicated since dysphagia may cause excessive salivation.
(2) Groin temperature is less accurate since it is affected by room temperature.
(4) Axillary temperature is less accurate since it is affected by room temperature.

299. (1) Dysphagia is difficulty in swallowing. (a)
(2) Focusing with the eyes is unrelated to dysphagia and dysphasia (difficulty speaking).
(3) Writing is unrelated to dysphagia and dysphasia.
(4) Understanding information is unrelated to dysphagia and dysphasia.

300. (3) Dysphasic patients have difficulty communicating verbally, and alternate means may be indicated. (b)
(1) An important aspect of care but not related to dysphasia.
(2) An important aspect of care but not related to dysphasia.
(4) An important aspect of care but not related to dysphasia.

301. (3) The paralyzed side has decreased muscle tone, which affects blood pressure readings. (b)
(1) Taking blood pressure does not precipitate the formation of thrombi.
(2) Return of function to the affected extremity is not affected by taking blood pressure; if it occurs, it is due to resolution of inflammation or resorption of blood in the area of the infarct.
(4) There is no difference when pressure is exerted on the brachial artery in either arm.

302. (2) To prevent distention and/or aspiration, the maximum amount of fluid administered at the first tube feeding is 250 ml. (c)
(1) More fluid than this can be administered safely.
(3) This amount of fluid would be excessive for initial tube feedings.
(4) This amount of fluid would be excessive for any tube feeding.

303. (2) Although tube feedings are often administered at room temperature, formula at body temperature is tolerated best. (b)
(1) Chilled feedings may cause gastric distress.
(3) Room temperature feedings are tolerable, but those at body temperature are better received.
(4) Hot feedings may cause gastric distress.

304. (2) Since the cardiac sphincter of the stomach is slightly opened because of the nasogastric tube, rapid feeding could result in regurgitation. (b)
(1) Indigestion is not hazardous to the patient.

(3) Speed of feeding does not cause flatulence; administration of air may.
(4) Distension can be diminished by avoiding the instillation of air with the feeding.

305. (3) The optic chiasm is the point of crossover of some optic nerve fibers in the cranial cavity at the base of the brain. The optic tracts conduct nerve impulses from the optic chiasm to other brain regions. (b)
(1) Optic tracts conduct nerve impulses from the optic chiasm.
(2) This is the vitreous body.
(4) The orbit is the cavity in which the eyeball is fixed.

306. (4) The thalamus associates sensory impulses with feelings of pleasantness and unpleasantness; therefore it is partly responsible for emotions. The cortical limbic system is also involved in expression of emotions. (c)
(1) Located in the cerebrum; controls all conscious functions.
(2) Outer layer of the cerebrum; controls mental functions.
(3) Controls body temperature and serves as a neural pathway.

307. (3) The arteries communicating (anastomosing) at the base of the brain are referred to as the circle of Willis. (b)
(1) Anastomosis of blood vessels located in the palm of the hand.
(2) A single large branch of the aorta.
(4) Nerve communication network in the region of the neck and axilla.

308. (1) Dendrites of the cochlear nerve terminate on the hair cells of the organ of Corti in the cochlea. (a)
(2) Contains bones (malleus, incus, stapes).
(3) Part of the middle ear that contains the auditory ossicles; area between the tympanic membrane and the bony labyrinth.
(4) A membranous sac that communicates with the semicircular canals of the ear.

309. (3) The ear bones that transmit and amplify air pressure waves from the tympanic membrane to the oval window of the cochlea are located in the inner ear. The tympanic membrane separates the outer from the middle ear. (b)
(1) Consists of the pinna and outer ear canal.
(2) The organ of Corti, chochlea, and semicircular canals are found in the inner ear.
(4) Connects the middle ear and nasopharynx; helps maintain the balance of air pressure.

310. (1) Since the organ of hearing is the organ of Corti, located in the cochlea, nerve deafness would most likely accompany damage to the cochlear nerve. (b)
(2) The vestibular nerve would affect balance.
(3) The trigeminal nerve would affect chewing movements.
(4) The vagus nerve would affect voice production.

311. (4) The medulla, part of the brainstem just above the foramen magnum, is concerned with vital functions. (b)
  (1) Sexual development controlled by the hypothalamus and the pituitary at puberty.
  (2) Temperature and water balance are controlled by the hypothalamus.
  (3) Voluntary movements are mediated through the somatomotor area of the frontal cerebral lobe. The opercular-insular area of the parietal cerebral lobe is concerned with taste sensations. (a)

312. (1) One of the centers for reflex control of respiration is in the medulla. Another important reflex respiratory center is in the pons. The other brain regions—cerebral cortex, hypothalamus, and cerebellum—may influence respiration but not so directly as the centers in the medulla and pons. (a)
  (2) Center of control for all conscious functions.
  (3) Control and integration of higher autonomic functions; influences respiration but not so directly as the centers in the medulla and pons.
  (4) Center for coordination and equilibrium.

313. (2) The labyrinth is the inner ear and consists of the vestibule, cochlea, semicircular canals, utricle, saccule, cochlear duct, and membranous semicircular canals. A labyrinthectomy is performed to alleviate the symptom of vertigo but results in deafness, since the organ of Corti and cochlear nerve are located in the inner ear. (b)
  (1) There is no pain associated with Ménière's syndrome.
  (3) Anosmia is loss of the sense of smell and would not be affected by surgery to the ear.
  (4) Ménière's syndrome does not produce tinnitus.

314. (4) In otosclerosis there is an overgrowth of bone in the middle ear, fusing the 3 ossicles. Removal of the stapes eliminates this obstruction. (b)
  (1) All tones are diminished or lost in otosclerosis, not just the base tones.
  (2) Bone conduction is better than air conduction in otosclerosis.
  (3) Since the ossicles can no longer vibrate and conduction is impaired, hearing aids are of little value.

315. (1) Decadron is a corticosteroid that acts on the cell membrane to prevent the normal inflammatory responses as well as stabilize the blood-brain barrier. (c)
  (2) This is not an effect of corticosteroid therapy.
  (3) This is not an effect of corticosteroid therapy.
  (4) This is not an effect of corticosteroid therapy.

316. (2) Dexamethasone (Decadron) increases glucogenesis, which may cause hyperglycemia. (c)
  (1) The renal threshold for glucose is not affected by Decadron.
  (3) Protein breakdown is not accelerated by Decadron.
  (4) Decadron does not contain a glucose component.

317. (2) Decadron increases the production of hydrochloric acid, which may cause GI ulcers. Patients should also be instructed to take Decadron with meals. (c)
  (1) Decadron is not irritating to the mucosa.
  (3) Stomach emptying time may be increased by Decadron.
  (4) Decadron does not affect the pepsin-induced erosion of the mucosa.

318. (4) To help prevent ulcer formation in the gastric mucosa, peristalsis and gastric motility should not be increased. (c)
  (1) This statement regarding Maalox and dexamethasone is not true.
  (2) This statement regarding Amphojel is not true.
  (3) This statement regarding Amphojel is not true.

319. (3) Prolonged use of sodium bicarbonate may cause systemic alkalosis as well as retention of sodium and water. (a)
  (1) This statement is inaccurate in describing the effects of sodium bicarbonate.
  (2) This statement is inaccurate in describing the effects of sodium bicarbonate.
  (4) This statement is inaccurate in describing the effects of sodium bicarbonate.

320. (2) Any hormone normally produced by the body must be withdrawn slowly to allow the appropriate organ to adjust and resume production. (b)
  (1) Production of ACTH is not affected.
  (3) Although important, this is not the reason for gradual withdrawal of the drug.
  (4) Although important, this is not the reason for gradual withdrawal of the drug.

321. (1) The aerobic oxidation of glucose occurring in the mitochondrion produces 38 moles of ATP for every mole of glucose oxidized. (b)
  (2) Digestion not hydrolysis of fats.
  (3) This activity involves gaseous exchange.
  (4) This is the formation of peptide bonds.

322. (4) Prostigmin, an anticholinesterase drug, causes temporary relief of symptoms of myasthenia gravis in patients who have the disease and is therefore an effective diagnostic aid. (b)
  (1) There is a decrease in symptoms.
  (2) Excessive salivation may occur.
  (3) Hypotension may occur.

323. (2) Prolonged use of steroids may cause leukopenia as a result of bone marrow depression. (c)
  (1) Sedimentation rate is elevated when infection is present; not associated with the medications.
  (3) CRP (C-reactive protein) is present in acute inflammatory diseases and necrosis; not associated with the medications.
  (4) This is the term given anemias that are characterized by decreased concentration of hemoglobin in erythrocytes; not a sequela of the use of aspirin or steroids.

324. (4) Open-ended questions provide a millieu in which people can verbalize their problems rather than be placed in a situation of forced response. (a)
  (1) Direct questions do not open or promote communication.
  (2) False reassurance is detrimental to the nurse-patient relationship and does not promote communication.
  (3) This can be threatening to the patient, who may not have the answer to these questions.
325. (4) Rheumatoid arthritis is a chronic systemic disease with inflammatory and degenerative changes in the body's connective tissue. (c)
  (1) Bones are not the focus of this disease.
  (2) It is connective tissue in the area of the joints that is affected.
  (3) Purine metabolism is affected in gout.
326. (2) Gold salts, bound to plasma proteins, are distributed irregularly throughout the body; but the highest concentration occurs in the kidneys. The slow excretion of gold salts cannot keep up with their intake; they accumulate in the kidneys, causing damage. (b)
  (1) This is not a side effect associated with gold salts, such as Myochrysine.
  (3) This is not a side effect associated with gold salts, such as Myochrysine.
  (4) This is not a side effect associated with gold salts, such as Myochrysine.
327. (2) Allopurinol interferes with the final steps in uric acid formation by inhibiting the production of xanthinoxidase. (a)
  (1) This drug acts to prevent the formation of uric acid.
  (3) This drug acts to prevent the formation of uric acid.
  (4) Allopurinol has no effect on swelling of the synovial membranes.
328. (2) Colchicine decreases the formation of lactic acid, which may promote the deposition of uric acid in the joints. It also decreases the inflammatory response. (b)
  (1) Hydrocortisone is an antiinflammatory; not used to treat gout.
  (3) Butazolidin (phenylbutazone) is a nonsteroid analgesic; used for pain management in arthritis.
  (4) Benemid (probenecid) acts to inhibit the reabsorption of urate in the kidneys and, therefore, decreases uric acid in the blood; not useful in the treatment of acute gout but rather of chronic gout.
329. (1) The connective tissue degeneration of SLE leads to involvement of the basal cell layer, producing a butterfly rash over the bridge of the nose and in the malar region. (b)
  (2) This occurs in polyarteritis nodosa, a collagen disease affecting the arteries and nervous system.
  (3) This occurs in muscular dystrophy, which is characterized by muscle wasting and weakness.
  (4) This occurs in scleroderma and may advance until the patient has the appearance of a living mummy.
330. (3) Scleroderma is an immunologic disorder characterized by inflammatory, fibrotic, and degenerative changes. (c)
  (1) This is not involved in the development of scleroderma.
  (2) This is not involved in the development of scleroderma.
  (4) This is not involved in the development of scleroderma.
331. (3) Not only the skin but also the major organs are affected, including the heart, lungs, liver, kidneys, and intestine. Death usually occurs from cardiac arrest, renal failure, or cachexia. (c)
  (1) The disease is fatal, with no known cure. Treatment with corticosteroids may prove helpful.
  (2) Depending on the patient's condition, death does not come rapidly since the disease spreads slowly to major organs.
  (4) The disease is fatal, with no known cure. Treatment with corticosteroids may prove helpful.
332. (2) Open angle glaucoma has an insidious onset, with increased intraocular pressure causing pressure on the retina and blood vessels in the eye. Peripheral vision is decreased as the visual field progressively diminishes. (b)
  (1) Occlusions of the central retinal artery would cause a sudden loss of vision.
  (3) Pain occurs in acute angle closure, not open angle, glaucoma.
  (4) This may be accompanied by untreated acute angle closure glaucoma.
333. (1) In glaucoma the intraocular pressure is elevated and must be returned to normal. (b)
  (2) Dilation of the pupils may cause a further increase in pressure by obstructing the canal of Schlemm; increased pressure reduces the visual field and leads to blindness.
  (3) Resting has no effect on this condition, for it will not decrease the pressure.
  (4) Increased intraocular pressure can lead to blindness; reducing pressure is the priority.
334. (4) The contraction permits the lens to return ot its normal bulge, decreasing focal length and allowing focus on near objects. (c)
  (1) The rectus and oblique muscles of the eye are involved in convergence.
  (2) The ciliary muscles are intrinsic (within the eyeball); the third cranial nerve (oculomotor), an extrinsic nerve, controls movements of the eyelid.
  (3) In this case the ciliary muscles would relax.
335. (1) Sedatives have no effect on the intraocular pressure. (b)
  (2) Would raise the intraocular pressure.
  (3) Would raise the intraocular pressure.
  (4) Would raise the intraocular pressure.
336. (3) Since continued use of eyedrops is indicated, an extra supply should always be available. (b)

(1) Eye washes (collyria) have no effect on the disease.

(2) Laxatives should not be taken on a routine basis.

(4) Since treatment must be maintained for life, extra medication should be available so the supply does not run out.

337. (1) Eye medications are applied directly to the eye. (a)

(2) Intraocular drugs are given for severe infections by an ophthalmologist.

(3) This route is not used for ocular medications.

(4) This route is not used for ocular medications.

338. (1) Acetazolamide (Diamox) is a carbonic anhydrase inhibitor that decreases the inflow of aqueous humor and controls intraocular pressure. (c)

(2) This diuretic has no effect on the eye.

(3) This diuretic has no effect on the eye.

(4) This strong miotic does not affect the production of aqueous humor.

339. (4) Cortisone, a steroid, stabilizes lysosomal membranes, inhibiting the release of proteolytic enzymes during inflammation. This antiinflammatory drug also maximizes vasoconstrictor effects. (b)

(1) An antibiotic, which would not decrease an inflammatory reaction.

(2) An antibiotic, which would not decrease an inflammatory reaction.

(3) An antibiotic, which would not decrease an inflammatory reaction.

340. (4) A second-degree burn over 30% of the body is considered critical. Shock, infection, electrolyte imbalance, and respiratory distress are life-threatening complications that can occur. (a)

(1) Burns involving less than 30% of the body surface of older children and adults under 50 years of age are generally less severe; the condition would be rated accordingly.

(2) Burns involving less than 30% of the body surface of older children and adults under 50 years of age are generally less severe; the condition would be rated accordingly.

(3) Burns involving less than 30% of the body surface of older children and adults under 50 years of age are generally less severe; the condition would be rated accordingly.

341. (3) The leukocyte count would not be affected in the first few hours. (b)

(1) Inhalation of hot air can cause tracheal edema.

(2) Replacement of fluids and electrolytes is essential in all burned patients.

(4) Pain is present in first-degree and second-degree burns, since the sensory nerves are not damaged.

342. (3) Potassium replacement is generally not indicated in the management of burns because hyperkalemia results from the liberation of potassium ions (K^+) from the injured cells. (c)

(1) This will be given with Ringer's and dextrose solutions in various combinations depending on the patient's needs.

(2) This will be given with colloidal and glucose solutions in various combinations depending on the patient needs.

(4) This will be given with colloidal Ringer's solution in various combinations depending on the patient's needs.

343. (3) Tetanus immune globulin provides antibodies against tetanus. This is used if the patient has never received tetanus toxoid or antitoxin, which confer active immunity (the body makes its own antibodies in response to the antigen). (c)

(1) Administration would produce active immunity.

(2) Administration would produce active immunity.

(4) DPT vaccine—diphtheria and tetanus toxoid combined with pertussis vaccine—produces active immunity.

344. (4) Sulfisoxazole (Gantrisin) is a short-acting sulfonamide. It has an antibacterial effect by acting as an antimetabolite and interfering with the microorganism's ability to manufacture folic acid. (a)

(1) Gantrisin is an antimicrobial not an antiseptic.

(2) Gantrisin is an antimicrobial; does not relieve pain.

(3) Gantrisin is an antimicrobial; does not inhibit the reabsorption of uric acid.

345. (1) Bethanechol chloride (Urecholine) improves the muscle tone of an atonic bladder, facilitating micturition. (c)

(2) Pilocarpine hydrochloride is a miotic, used in the treatment of glaucoma.

(3) Carbachol is a miotic, used in the treatment of glaucoma.

(4) Neosporin is a urinary tract antibiotic; does not aid in increasing bladder muscle tone.

346. (3) Application of a solution of sodium bicarbonate (a mild alkali) after a thorough flushing with water is the best way to treat acid-splashed skin, since the alkali will neutralize residual acid on the skin. (b)

(1) Although sodium hydroxide is also an alkali and would neutralize acid, it is too strong and can also cause burns.

(2) Sodium chloride is a neutral salt, which would serve no immediate first-aid benefit.

(4) Sodium sulfate is a neutral salt, which would serve no immediate first-aid benefit.

347. (1) This first-aid treatment will chemically neutralize residual alkali still on the skin. It will not reverse the chemical damage already done by the alkali (burns) but will minimize additional chemical change. (a)

(2) A weak base will not neutralize alkaline substance.

(3) This is a neutral substance; will not neutralize base.

(4) This is a neutral substance; will not neutralize base.

348. (2) The average adult human body is about 60% water. A newborn infant's body is about 80% water and reaches the 60% figure approximately 1 year after birth. (a)

(1) The percent for a newborn infant.

(3) The percent for the elderly may be as low as 40%.
(4) This represents complete dehydration of tissues.
349. (1) The osmoreceptors are located in the hypothalamus. Under conditions of dehydration they stimulate the neurohypophysis to release ADH into the blood. (b)
(2) This is the posterior lobe of the pituitary gland and is the source of antidiuretic hormone (ADH).
(3) The kidney tubules are the target organ for ADH; they reabsorb more water from the glomerular filtrate.
(4) Not a receptor for alterations in osmotic pressure.
350. (2) The kidneys regulate fluid balance by adjusting the amount of fluid reabsorbed from the glomerular filtrate. (b)
(1) Primarily a pump for the movement of blood.
(3) Does not play a major role in fluid balance.
(4) The role of the lungs is minimal.
351. (1) Interstitial fluid constitutes about 16% of body weight, which is 10 to 12 L in an adult male of 68 kg (150 lb). (b)
(2) 4% of body weight (2.8 L).
(3) This is derived from extracellular fluid and is calculated as part of the 20% of the total body weight.
(4) Part of the intracellular component.
352. (3) The concentration of potassium is greater inside the cell and is extremely important in establishing a membrane potential, a critical factor in the cell's ability to function. (b)
(1) Calcium is the most abundant electrolyte in the body; 99% is concentrated in the teeth and bones.
(2) Sodium is the most abundant cation of the extracellular compartment.
(4) Chloride is an extracellular anion.
353. (1) Approximately 25 of the 40 L of body fluid are in the cells. (c)
(2) Makes up 20%.
(3) Makes up 4%.
(4) Makes up 16%.
354. (1) Blood plasma and interstitial fluid are both part of the extracellular fluid and are of the same ionic composition. (b)
(2) Composition is the same.
(3) Osmotic pressure is the same.
(4) Ionic composition the same; the main cation of both would be sodium.
355. (4) Since the plasma colloid osmotic pressure (COP) opposes glomerular filtration, a decrease in blood proteins will increase the glomerular filtration rate (GFR). (b)
(1) Glomeruli are clusters of capillaries.
(2) Volume is determined by the amount of water reabsorbed in the tubules.
(3) Does not affect the glomerular filtration rate.
356. (2) A balloon tube is inserted into the renal pelvis to drain urine, necessitating an incision into the kidney (nephrostomy). (c)

(1) Ileostomy is the surgical implantation of the ileum into the abdominal wall; it is not related to urinary disease.
(3) Cecostomy is the surgical creation of a temporary opening into the cecum to relieve obstruction; not done for urinary problems.
(4) Ureterostomy is the surgical implantation of the ureter in the abdominal wall; would be performed if the bladder was involved.
357. (4) The ureters are implanted in a segment of the ileum, and urine drains continually because there is no sphincter. (b)
(1) No feces are present in an ileal conduit.
(2) Nutrients are not normally absorbed from urine as it passes from the kidneys.
(3) Ileal conduits are not neurologically innervated; therefore no peristalsis exists.
358. (4) When two compatible drugs are being mixed, if one is a narcotic it should be drawn up first. This prevents contaminating the bottle of narcotic with atropine. (c)
(1) Separate injections will cause undue discomfort to the patient and break the skin unnecessarily.
(2) These drugs are not available in powdered form; no need to dilute.
(3) The atropine may contaminate the Demerol vial, which is undesirable.
359. (4) Because of the anatomic position of the incision, drainage would flow by gravity and accumulate under the patient lying in the supine position. (b)
(1) Nail beds would indicate peripheral perfusion, not early hemorrhage.
(2) Blood pressure decreases in hemorrhage, and pulse increases.
(3) Respiratory hemorrhage is not common after kidney surgery.
360. (3) A drop in blood pressure, rapid pulse, cold clammy skin, and oliguria are all signs of shock, which, if not treated promptly, can lead to death. (a)
(1) An expected response; the patient will push out the airway as the effects of anesthesia subside.
(2) Shallow respirations are common because of the depressant effects of anesthesia.
(4) Snoring respirations are common because of the depressant effects of anesthesia.
361. (2) Maintenance of a patent airway is always the priority, since airway obstruction impedes breathing and may result in death. (c)
(1) This is important in the patient's postoperative care; however, oxygenation is the priority.
(3) This is important in the patient's postoperative care; however, oxygenation is the priority.
(4) This is important in the patient's postoperative care; however, oxygenation is the priority.
362. (3) Dressings retain an undetermined amount of drainage, which would lead to an inaccurate reading. (c)

(1) Counting of saturated pads allows for some degree of objectivity in the assessment, but it is not the most accurate.

(2) Measuring drainage that has seeped through is not as accurate as weighing; however, it does allow for more objective measurement.

(4) Weighing dressings is the most accurate method of estimating postoperative drainage. The nurse must subtract the dry weight of the dressings to determine fluid loss.

363. (1) Cystitis is an inflammation of the bladder that causes frequency, urgency, pain on micturition, and hematuria. (a)

(2) Pyelitis is an inflammation of the pelvis of the kidney, causing flank pain, chills, fever, and weakness.

(3) Nephrosis is a kidney condition in which there is proteinuria, hypoalbuminemia, and edema.

(4) Pyelonephritis is a diffuse pyogenic infection of the pelvis and parenchyma of the kidney that causes flank pain, chills, fever, and weakness.

364. (1) Ammonium chloride causes metabolic acidosis. As a result the kidneys secrete the excess hydrogen ions, increasing the acidity of the urine. An acid urine is essential for the antibacterial action of methenamine mandelate (Mandelamine). (c)

(2) Ammonium chloride is an acidifier and thus does not promote healing.

(3) There is no effect on uric crystal stone formation by combining these drugs.

(4) By acidifying the urine this drug enhances the antibacterial action of methenamine mandelate; it does not decrease bladder irritation.

365. (2) Since the female urethra is shorter than the male urethra, the bacteria can more easily invade the bladder. (a)

(1) Hormonal secretions have no effect on the development of bladder infections.

(3) The position of the bladder is the same in males and females.

(4) Urinary pH is within the same range in both males and females.

366. (2) Bundle branch block interferes with the conduction of impulses from the AV node to the ventricle supplied by the affected bundle. Conduction through the ventricles is delayed, as evidenced by a widened QRS complex. (c)

(1) P waves, produced when the SA node fires to begin a cycle, are present in bundle branch block.

(3) Changes in the T waves and/or ST segments usually occur as a result of cardiac damage.

(4) Changes in the T waves and/or ST segments usually occur as a result of cardiac damage.

367. (3) The pacemaker (PM) electrode is inserted via the venous system into the right ventricle, where PM-generated impulses can directly stimulate the ventricles. (c)

(1) The pacing catheter must directly stimulate the ventricles; this site is too far from the ventricles.

(2) The pacing catheter must directly stimulate the ventricles; the left atrium cannot transmit the impulse.

(4) Stimulation of the SA node would be inadequate because of inability of the left bundle branch to transmit the impulse to the Purkinje fibers of the left ventricle.

368. (4) The SA node is the heart's natural pacemaker. An electronic pacemaker is used in some persons to supply an impulse that stimulates the heart to more efficient action. (a)

(1) Sympathetic fibers to the heart; do not act as a pacemaker to initiate and regulate the heartbeat.

(2) Modified cardiac muscle, which receives impulses from the SA node and conducts them to the ventricular walls via the bundle of His and Purkinje fibers.

(3) Special cardiac muscle, which receives impulses from the AV node and conducts them to the ventricular walls.

369. (3) Atropine blocks vagal stimulation of the SA node, resulting in an increased heart rate. (c)

(1) Lanoxin (digoxin) slows the heart rate; hence would not be indicated in this situation.

(2) Lidocaine hydrochloride (Xylocaine) decreases myocardial sensitivity and would not increase heart rate.

(4) Procainamide hydrochloride (Pronestyl) is an antiarrhythmic drug; would not stimulate the heart rate.

370. (3) A demand pacemaker functions only when the heart rate falls below the set rate of the pacemaker. The patient can detect pacemaker malfunctions by monitoring the pulse rate and noting a drop below the set rate. (b)

(1) The patient need not alter previous sleeping habits.

(2) Demand pacemakers function only when the heart rate drops below a predetermined level.

(4) Normal activity may be resumed when healing has occurred.

371. (2) Ventricular fibrillation will cause irreversible brain damage and then death within minutes because the heart is not pumping blood. Defibrillation or CPR (until defibrillation is possible) must be initiated immediately. (a)

(1) Although this condition requires prompt treatment, a patient will live if treatment is withheld for several minutes.

(3) Although this condition requires prompt treatment, a patient will live if treatment is withheld for several minutes.

(4) Although this condition requires prompt treatment, a patient will live if treatment is withheld for several minutes.

372. (4) Bradycardia refers to a heart rate of less than 60 per minute. It may be a physiologic adaptation to long-term exercise, cardiac disease, or digitalis toxicity. (a)

(1) This condition is described as an arrhythmia; whereas bradycardia is also considered an arrhythmia, the rhythm is usually regular.
(2) Tachycardia is the term used for rapid heart rates.
(3) This is called a bigeminal rhythm.

373. (2) Five to seven liters provide enough oxygen without altering the patient's blood gases, which would cause increased respiratory distress. (b)
(1) Higher concentrations of oxygen may depress CO_2 and raise O_2 concentrations, interfering with the impetus to breathe.
(3) Is insufficient for an individual with congestive heart failure and pulmonary edema.
(4) Higher concentrations of oxygen may depress CO_2 and raise O_2 concentrations, interfering with the impetus to breathe.

374. (4) An open flame or spark from static electricity (e.g., leather-soled shoes, wool, silk, nylon and Dacron blankets, ungrounded electric appliances) can initiate an explosion and fire in the presence of higher than normal oxygen levels. (a)
(1) Oxygen is not flammable; however, it increases the rate of combustion.
(2) Oxygen is not unstable.
(3) Oxygen does not increase apprehension; by reducing dyspnea and shortness of breath, it usually reduces apprehension.

375. (3) Irritability and restlessness increase the metabolic rate (and the heart rate) and blood pressure. This complicates congestive heart failure. (a)
(1) Restlessness does not affect oxygen supply.
(2) Restlessness does not interfere with respiration; if anything, it increases respirations.
(4) Restlessness alone usually does not elevate the body temperature.

376. (2) Oxygen via nasal cannula is the most comfortable and least intrusive, since the cannula extends minimally into the nose. (a)
(1) This method is oppressive, and patients complain of feeling ''suffocated'' when it is used.
(3) This method is oppressive, and patients complain of feeling ''suffocated'' when it is used.
(4) This method is oppressive, and patients complain of feeling ''suffocated'' when it is used.

377. (3) The patient is made to feel that the nurse cares about him personally and will have time for his special emotional needs. Such an approach allays anxiety and reduces emotional stress, which is beneficial in cases of cardiovascular disease. (a)
(1) Indicates a lack of interest in the patient; interferes with developing an effective nurse-patient relationship.
(2) Does not respond to patient's need; cuts off communication.
(4) Does not respond to patient's need; cuts off communication.

378. (2) Since digoxin slows the heart, the apical pulse should be counted for 1 minute prior to administra-

tion. If the apical rate is below 60 (bradycardia), digoxin should be withheld since its administration could further depress the heart rate. If the heart rate is above 120, digoxin should be withheld because the patient may be in digitalis toxicity. (a)
(1) Not as accurate as apical pulse; the patient may also have an atrial arrhythmia, which would not be detected with the radial rate alone.
(3) Not as accurate as apical pulse; the patient may also have an atrial arrhythmia, which would not be detected with the radial rate alone.
(4) This is the pulse deficit; not an indicator of heart rate.

379. (3) Potassium is lost with the urine during diuresis. Hypokalemia, in turn, predisposes the patient to digitalis toxicity. (a)
(1) This electrolyte is not lost as a result of digitalis-induced diuresis.
(2) This electrolyte is not lost as a result of digitalis-induced diuresis.
(4) This electrolyte is not lost as a result of digitalis-induced diuresis.

380. (2) The Swan-Ganz catheter is placed in the pulmonary artery. Information regarding left ventricular function is obtained when the catheter balloon is inflated. (c)
(1) Information on stroke volume, the amount of blood ejected by the left ventricle with each contraction, will not be provided by a Swan-Ganz catheter.
(3) Central venous pressure is measured via a catheter that is inserted through the superior vena cava into the right atrium. It is attached to a water manometer.
(4) Circulation time is measured by injecting a tasteable substance into a vein and noting the time it takes to travel to the tongue.

381. (1) Mitral stenosis impairs blood flow from the left atrium to the left ventricle. This backs up blood into the pulmonary veins and lungs. The result may be pulmonary edema. (c)
(2) Tricuspid disease may cause jugular vein distention and hepatic congestion.
(3) Coronary arteriosclerosis may cause angina.
(4) Pulmonic stenosis tends to cause a bulging of the intraventricular septum.

382. (3) These agents are classified as antiinflammatory or immunosuppressive. Glucocorticoids interfere with the body's response to microorganisms but do not directly promote the spread of enteroviruses. (a)
(1) Interferes with the release of enzymes responsible for the inflammatory response.
(2) Immunosuppressant action causes bone marrow depression, which decreases the number of WBCs.
(4) Interferes with antibody production.

383. (4) Many chemotherapeutic agents function by interfering with DNA replication associated with normal cellular reproduction (mitosis). The normal rapid mitoses of the stratified squamous epithelium of the

mouth and anus result in their being powerfully affected by the drugs. (b)

(1) Chemotherapeutic agents affect the cells that are most rapidly proliferating, which include not only the cells of the GI epithelium but also those of the bone marrow and hair follicles.

(2) Effect not due to direct irritation; most agents are administered parenterally.

(3) State of nourishment would be applicable to all cells; although anorexia is common, this patient may not be anorexic.

384. (3) Unwashed hands are considered contaminated and are used to turn on sink faucets. The use of foot pedals or a paper towel barrier prevents recontamination of washed hands. (c)

(1) They are not considered contaminated for this reason; areas cannot be sterile.

(2) Although bacterial growth is facilitated in moist environments, this is not the reason why sinks are considered contaminated.

(4) It has nothing to do with the number of people; it is related to being touched by contaminated hands.

385. (3) Bargaining is one of the stages of dying in which the patient promises some type of desirable behavior in exchange for temporary postponement of death. (a)

(1) Rationalization is a defense mechanism in which attempts are made to justify or explain an action or feeling.

(2) Frustration is a subjective experience, a feeling of being thwarted, but not one of the stages of dying.

(4) Classified as the fourth stage, depression represents the grief experienced as the individual recognizes his fate.

386. (2) When an individual reaches the point of being able intellectually and psychologically to accept death, anxiety is reduced and he becomes detached from his environment. (c)

(1) Although resigned to death, the individual is not euphoric.

(3) Although detached, the client is still concerned and may use this time constructively.

(4) At the stage of acceptance, the client is no longer angry or depressed.

387. (2) Since 1 oz equals approximately 30 ml and the patient drank a total of 21.5 oz, 21.5 × 30 yields the answer in milliliters. (a)

(1) An incorrect calculation; too low.

(3) An incorrect calculation; too low.

(4) An incorrect calculation; too low.

388. (4) Denial, bargaining, and detachment are coping mechanisms often needed by the patient, especially when facing a devastating illness, and should be accepted by the nurse. (a)

(1) Ignoring the behavior does not convey a willingness to listen and denies the patient's feelings.

(2) Coping mechanisms are needed by the patient as psychologic protection and must not be taken from him until he is able to replace one for another.

(3) Reinforcement of denial will inhibit the individual's transition toward acceptance.

389. (1) Seeking other opinions to disprove the inevitable is a form of denial employed by individuals having illnesses with a poor prognosis. (b)

(2) Indiscriminant use of the call bell is often indicative of a fear of being alone, not denial, which is the first coping mechanism generally used.

(3) Criticism that is unjust is often characteristic of the stage of anger.

(4) Sleeping long periods is common during the depression experience as one moves toward acceptance.

390. (4) In the stage of acceptance the patient frequently detaches himself from the environment and may become indifferent to family members. In addition, the family may take longer to accept the death than does the patient. (c)

(1) Denial is often exhibited by both patient and family at the same time.

(2) Although the family may not understand the anger, dealing with the resultant behavior may serve as a diversion.

(3) During this stage the family is often able to offer emotional support, and sometimes false reassurances, thus fulfilling one of their needs.

391. (2) The nurse's presence communicates concern and provides an opportunity for the patient to initiate communication if needed. Silence is an effective interpersonal technique that permits the patient to direct the content and extent of his verbalizations without the nurse's imposing on his privacy. (b)

(1) During acceptance the patient may not wish to have visitors, preferring time for personal reflection.

(3) Detached from his environment, the client may find that the details of various hospital procedures lose significance.

(4) Crying, which is so much a part of depression, usually ceases when the individual reaches acceptance.

392. (1) Methotrexate is a folic acid antagonist that can cause depression of bone marrow. This serious toxic effect is sometimes prevented by administration of folic acid. Some physicians advocate its administration after a course of methotrexate therapy so as not to interfere with methotrexate activity. (c)

(2) Folic acid is a metabolite and does not destroy cancer cells.

(3) Folic acid is a metabolite and does not destroy cancer cells.

(4) Methotrexate does not increase the production of phagocytes.

393. (4) Prolonged chemotherapy may slow the production of leukocytes in bone marrow and lymph nodes, thus suppressing the activity of the immune system.

Antibiotics may be required to help counter infections that the body can no longer handle easily. (b)

(1) Although leukocytes are circulating in both blood and lymph, these cells are more mature and thus more resistant to the effects of chemotherapy.

(2) Although leukocytes are circulating in both blood and lymph, these cells are more mature and thus more resistant to the effects of chemotherapy.

(3) The liver does not produce leukocytes.

394. (4) Aspirin can cause a lowered prothrombin blood level, increasing the risk of undesired bleeding that may occur with administration of anticoagulants. (a)

(1) Isoxsuprine hydrochloride is a vasodilator; it does not affect bleeding times.

(2) Chloral hydrate is a hypnotic; it does not affect bleeding times.

(3) Chlorpromazine is an antipsychotic it does not affect bleeding times.

395. (4) The patient who is immobilized must do exercises such as dorsiflexion of the feet to prevent venous stasis and thrombus formation. (a)

(1) Improves pulmonary function rather than prevents venous stasis.

(2) Actually promotes venous stasis by compressing the popliteal space.

(3) Limiting fluid intake may lead to hemoconcentration and subsequent thrombus formation.

396. (2) The high vascularity of the nose, combined with its susceptibility to trauma (e.g., sneezing, nose blowing), makes it a frequent region for hemorrhage. (a)

(1) This symptom is usually not associated with anticoagulant therapy.

(3) This symptom is usually not associated with anticoagulant therapy.

(4) This symptom is usually not associated with anticoagulant therapy.

397. (4) Hemoptysis is expectoration of blood-stained sputum derived from the lungs, bronchi, or trachea. (a)

(1) Refers to blood in the urine.

(2) Refers to vomiting of blood.

(3) Refers to a local accumulation of blood in the tissues.

398. (3) Orthopneic position refers to sitting up and leaning slightly forward. This drops the diaphragm, allowing the lungs more room for expansion. (a)

(1) The Trendelenburg position forces the diaphragm up, interfering with lung expansion.

(2) Horizontal positions do not allow the gravitational effect on the diaphragm and thus do not maximize air exchange.

(4) Horizontal positions do not allow the gravitational effect on the diaphragm and thus do not maximize air exchange.

399. (4) An appendectomy is a relatively simple operation; the patient is generally out of bed the same day. With an ambulatory patient there is less risk of ve-

nous stasis, a condition that predisposes the individual to thrombus formation and emboli. (a)

(1) May or may not be out of bed the same day depending on the surgical approach; mobility may be hampered by a Foley catheter.

(2) Although generally ambulated the first day postoperatively, the patient often is hampered by pain.

(3) Vein ligation is performed for varicose veins; the diseased vein is removed, placing an additional burden on the deep venous system and possibly increasing the risk of thrombi.

400. (1) Since an elevated plasma bilirubin level could indicate an increased rate of red cell destruction (bilirubin is a product of free hemoglobin metabolism), the individual may have a hemolytic anemia (e.g., sickle cell anemia, glucose 6-phosphate dehydrogenase deficiency). (b)

(2) Oxygen-carrying ability reflected by hemoglobin.

(3) Does not involve the destruction of red blood cells with subsequent liberation of bilirubin.

(4) The decreased destruction of red cells does not liberate bile pigment.

401. (3) The salts in bile act as detergents to break large fat droplets into smaller ones (emulsification), providing a larger surface area for the enzymatic action of fat-splitting enzymes (lipases). (a)

(1) Does not have an acid pH.

(2) No vitamins are present in bile; it emulsifies fat and thus assists in absorption of fat soluble vitamins.

(4) Does not act on proteins.

402. (3) When bile does not mix with foods in the intestine, emulsification of fats cannot occur and fat digestion is retarded. Stomach motility is also reduced, since increased stomach peristalsis is dependent on fat digestion in the small intestine. (b)

(1) The production of bile is unaffected.

(2) Once emulsified by bile, fatty foods are broken down by digestive enzymes.

(4) Although people with cholecystitis may refrain from eating fatty foods, the basic pathologic disorder remains unaltered.

403. (2) Vitamin K, a fat-soluble vitamin, is not absorbed from the GI tract in the absence of bile. Bile enters the duodenum via the common bile duct. (a)

(1) Extrinsic factor (cyanocobalamin) is a water-soluble vitamin; bile is not necessary for its absorption.

(3) Calcium is related to rhythmic muscle contraction not coagulation.

(4) Bilirubin is formed by the breakdown of hemoglobin and RBCs and is not related to coagulation.

404. (3) Cholecystography is an x-ray examination of the gallbladder after ingestion or IV injection of a radiopaque drug that is concentrated by the normally functioning gallbladder. (b)

(1) The ampulla of Vater is not visualized.

(2) The common bile duct is examined during choledochography.

(4) In the presence of biliary obstruction, the dye is poorly absorbed by the gallbladder so visualization is generally poor.

405. (1) Cholecystokinin is a widely distributed hormone whose functions include stimulation of gallbladder contraction and the release of pancreatic enzymes. It also functions as a neurotransmitter in the CNS. (b)
    (2) Promotes the production of bile by the liver and the secretion of pancreatic juice.
    (3) Stimulates the secretion of gastric juice.
    (4) Stimulates the secretion of intestinal juice (succus entericus).

406. (2) A drain is inserted to remove fluid, which could cause pressure on the operative site and delay healing. The nurse should anticipate drainage and reinforce the surgical dressings as needed. (a)
    (1) Changing a dressing unnecessarily increases the risk of infection as well as possible dislodgement of the drain.
    (3) An abdominal binder may be ordered prior to ambulation but would interfere with assessment of the dressing at this time.
    (4) Montgomery straps are utilized when frequent dressing changes are anticipated; not appropriate at this time.

407. (4) Localized sensory changes may indicate nerve damage, impaired circulation, or thrombophlebitis. Activity should be limited, and the physician notified. (a)
    (1) Symptoms may be indicative of a serious problem, and the physician must be notified.
    (2) Rubbing or massaging the legs is contraindicated because of possible dislodging of a thrombus if present.
    (3) Bed rest is indicated to prevent the possibility of further damage or creation of an embolus.

408. (1) Protein and calories are necessary for tissue building. (a)
    (2) The obstruction has been corrected; dietary fat intake is dependent on the individual's tolerance.
    (3) Protein and calories are necessary for tissue repair.
    (4) A high-fat diet is contraindicated since fat requires bile to be absorbed; spasms in the biliary system may result in pain.

409. (1) Carcinoma can be ruled out only by tissue biopsy, which is obtained during surgery. (c)
    (2) Symptoms could have been treated medically.
    (3) The complication was the reason for the second surgical intervention.
    (4) Diverticulitis can in most cases be treated by diet, rest, and antibiotic therapy.

410. (2) To promote drainage of different lung regions, patients should turn every 2 hours. Deep breathing inflates the alveoli and promotes fluid drainage. (b)
    (1) Coughing is a major cause of incisional pain, and

its desirability in the absence of accumulated secretions is questioned.
    (3) During physical efforts, individuals with abdominal incisions often revert to shallow breathing.
    (4) Administration of IPPB is a dependent function of the nurse.

411. (2) Pernicious anemia is due to a lack of vitamin B_{12}. Intrinsic factor, produced by the parietal cells of the gastric mucosa, is necessary for B_{12} absorption. (b)
    (1) B_{12} is absorbed in the ileum.
    (3) Intrinsic factor is secreted by the stomach; the hemopoietic factor is the combination of B_{12} and intrinsic factor.
    (4) Chief cells secrete the enzymes of the gastric juice.

412. (1) To ensure continued suction, the patency of the tube should be maintained. Physiologic saline is used to prevent fluid and electrolyte disturbances during irrigation. (a)
    (2) Ice chips and water represent fluid intake, which must be approved by the physician; being hypotonic in nature, such intake may lower the serum electrolytes.
    (3) The stomach is not considered a sterile body cavity, so medical asepsis is indicated.
    (4) Care must be taken to avoid traumatizing the mucosa.

413. (3) Overbathing and use of soap can cause increased dryness and skin breakdown. Emollients help relieve dryness. (b)
    (1) The need for bathing must be evaluated on an individual basis.
    (2) The need for bathing must be evaluated on an individual basis.
    (4) Use of emollients without simultaneous consideration of the effects of soap and excessive bathing is generally ineffective.

414. (2) After a subtotal gastrectomy, small frequent feedings are best tolerated. (a)
    (1) As soon as edema subsides, the individual is generally given an ounce of fluid per hour and then diet is gradually progressed.
    (3) Recuperation from gastric surgery may take up to 3 months.
    (4) IV therapy is not sufficient to provide the nutrients needed for healing unless hyperalimentation is employed.

415. (4) The location of the tumor will usually indicate whether a colostomy, creation of an opening proximal to the tumor between the colon and the skin surface, is needed. (a)
    (1) A cecostomy is the creation of an opening between the cecum and the skin surface; usually a temporary procedure.
    (2) An ileostomy is the creation of an opening between the ileum and the skin surface; would not be done.
    (3) A colectomy is the surgical removal of a portion of

the colon, with creation of an anastomosis; generally used in less extensive carcinoma.

416. (3) Neomycin sulfate is poorly absorbed from the GI tract and is often used for sterilization of the intestines prior to bowel surgery. (a)
   (1) Being poorly absorbed from the GI tract, neomycin sulfate does not affect urinary tract infections.
   (2) Because intestinal bacteria are destroyed, there is a decreased production of vitamin K.
   (4) Oral administration of neomycin primarily affects intestinal bacteria only.

417. (3) Preparations such as aluminum paste can be used on the skin around the stoma to prevent excoriation from the ostomy drainage. (a)
   (1) Petroleum jelly would interfere with adherence of any ostomy appliance.
   (2) Alcohol tends to dry out the skin and mucous membranes, leading to irritation and breakdown.
   (4) Mineral oil is not an effective skin protectant and could interfere with adherence of any appliance.

418. (3) Surgery on the bowel has no direct anatomic or physiologic effect on sexual performance. However, psychologic factors could hamper this function, and the nurse should encourage verbalization. (b)
   (1) There is no reason why sexual relationships must be curtailed.
   (2) Although his partner should understand the nature of the surgery, the focus at this time should be on the patient.
   (4) Although it may take several months to resume satisfying sexual relationships, the surgery has no direct physiologic effect.

419. (1) Ample time in the bathroom must be ensured for the actual irrigation process and fecal returns, which may not be immediate. (c)
   (2) The availability of adequate time takes precedence over any specific timing that may be convenient.
   (3) The availability of adequate time takes precedence over any specific timing that may be convenient.
   (4) The availability of adequate time takes precedence over any specific timing that may be convenient.

420. (3) The rapid rate of enema administration or ostomy irrigation often causes cramping. Additional fluid leads to more discomfort. Cramping will generally subside if the enema tubing is clamped for a few minutes; the procedure can then be continued. (b)
   (1) Lowering the container will decrease the rate of flow, but fluid will continue to enter the colon if the container remains above the stoma.
   (2) Discontinuing the irrigation could lead to ineffective evacuation of the colon.
   (4) Indiscriminant advancing of the catheter can injure the mucosa and does not affect cramping.

421. (2) This is far enough to direct the flow of solution into the bowel. (c)
   (1) Inadequate; fluid may leak back around the catheter.

(3) Insertion of 6 inches may cause trauma to the mucosa.
(4) Insertion of 8 inches may cause trauma to the mucosa.

422. (1) A colostomy irrigation is much like a tap water enema. The solution must be held high enough to allow it to flow into the bowel but not so high that it flows rapidly, or it can cause cramping or mucosal injury. (b)
   (2) Does not represent maximum height of the solution; may not ensure flow of solution into the bowel.
   (3) Does not represent maximum height of the solution; may not ensure flow of solution into the bowel.
   (4) Does not represent maximum height of the solution; may not ensure flow of solution into the bowel.

423. (3) In the liver a simple protein combines with a lipid to form a lipoprotein. Lipoproteins circulate freely in the blood and can be utilized easily and quickly in various metabolic processes. (c)
   (1) The liver does not phosphorolyze fat.
   (2) The liver does not oxidize fat.
   (4) Fat is stored in adipose tissue.

424. (1) The liver stores carbohydrates as glycogen, which is polymer of glucose. (a)
   (2) Glycerol is a by-product of lipids and combines with 3 fatty acids to form triglyceride molecules.
   (3) Fat is not stored in the liver.
   (4) Not a ready form of energy; combination of amino acids from protein.

425. (3) Fatty acids are insoluble and must combine with bile to form water-soluble substances. (a)
   (1) Lipase is a pancreatic enzyme.
   (2) Amylase, which digests starch, is found in saliva and pancreatic juice.
   (4) A component of bile. It is produced in the liver and stored in the gallbladder, but it is not the component of bile that emulsifies fats.

426. (1) The symptoms indicate hepatic coma. Protein is reduced according to tolerance, and calories are increased to prevent tissue catabolism. (a)
   (2) This represents a high-protein diet, which is contraindicated in hepatic coma.
   (3) This represents a high-protein diet, which is contraindicated in hepatic coma.
   (4) This represents a high-protein diet, which is contraindicated in hepatic coma.

427. (4) The liver manufactures albumin, the major plasma protein. A deficit of this protein will lower the osmotic pressure in the intravascular space, leading to a fluid shift. (c)
   (1) The enlarged liver compresses the portal system, causing increased rather than decreased pressure.
   (2) The kidneys are not the primary source of the pathologic condition. It is the liver's inability to manufacture albumin that maintains the colloid oncotic pressure.

(3) Potassium is not produced by the body, nor is its major function the maintence of fluid balance.

428. (3) With obstruction of the portal vein there is an increase in pressure in the abdominal veins, which empty into the portal system. These veins develop collaterals to circumvent the obstruction. The collaterals are usually in the paraumbilical, hemorrhoidal, and esophageal areas. (a)
   (1) Although viral hepatitis may predispose to the development of cirrhosis, which in turn causes portal hypertension, most often it does not.
   (2) Kupffer cells are part of the reticuloendothelial system, which helps prevent infection and does not primarily affect venous pressure.
   (4) Obstruction of these ducts blocks the flow of bile, causing obstructive jaundice.

429. (2) The elevated pressure within the portal circulatory system causes elevated pressure in areas of portal systemic collateral circulation (most important, in the distal esophagus and proximal stomach). Hemorrhage is a possible complication. (a)
   (1) Perforation of the duodenum is usually caused by peptic ulcers; not a direct result of portal hypertension or cirrhosis.
   (3) Liver abcesses may occur as a complication of intestinal infections; not related to portal hypertension.
   (4) Not related to portal hypertension; may be caused by manipulation of the bowel during surgery, peritonitis, neurologic disorders, or organic obstruction.

430. (1) Since lipoproteins, a combination of a fat and a simple protein, have not been formed because of poor protein intake, fat accumulation occurs in the liver. (c)
   (2) Individuals with cirrhosis of the liver tend to have bleeding tendencies (rather than clotting) because of the decreased synthesis of prothrombin.
   (3) Deficiency of protein results in the breakdown of tissue (catabolism) and a negative nitrogen balance.
   (4) Elevations of bile in the blood occur as a result of obstruction of hepatic ducts by the enlarged liver.

431. (2) IV fluids do not provide proteins required for tissue growth, repair, and maintenance. Therefore tissue breakdown occurs to provide the essential amino acids. (b)
   (1) Although each liter provides approximately 200 calories, additional liters can be infused to meet minimal energy requirements and prevent weight loss.
   (3) Weight loss is caused by insufficient intake of nutrients, which provide calories; vitamins do not provide calories.
   (4) An infusion of 5% dextrose in water may decrease the electrolyte concentration because of a fluid shift.

432. (2) The pH of blood is maintained within the narrow range of 7.35 to 7.45. When there is an increase in hydrogen ions (H^+), acidosis results and is reflected in the lower pH. (a)

(1) This is too acidic.
(3) This is within the normal range for pH.
(4) This is slightly alkaline.

433. (3) Sodium bicarbonate is a base and one of the major buffers in the body. (b)
   (1) Carbon dioxide is carried in aqueous solution as carbonic acid (H_2CO_3); an acid does not buffer another acid.
   (2) Potassium is not a buffer; only a base can buffer an acid.
   (4) Sodium chloride is not a buffer; it is a salt.

434. (4) The sodium bicarbonate–carbonic acid buffer system helps maintain the pH of the body fluids. In metabolic acidosis there is a decrease in bicarbonate due to retention of metabolic acids. Since there is a decrease in bicarbonate, the carbonic acid will increase to maintain the balance between these 2 buffers. (c)
   (1) The pH will become more acidic.
   (2) The pH will decrease, indicating an increased acid content.
   (3) The carbonic acid content increases as sodium bicarbonate decreases.

435. (4) Regular insulin is rapid acting and should be used when immediate action is desired. (b)
   (1) Long-acting insulin; not indicated in an emergency.
   (2) Not a form of insulin; a simple protein.
   (3) Intermediate-acting insulin; not indicated in an emergency.

436. (1) There are 100 units of insulin in 1 ml (or in 15 minims); 6 minims must be administered to provide the patient with 40 units of insulin. (b)

$$\frac{40\ U}{100\ U} = \frac{x\ \text{minims}}{15\ \text{minims}}$$
$$100x = 600$$
$$x = 6\ \text{minims}$$

   (2) This reflects a miscalculation and would be an overdose.
   (3) This reflects a miscalculation and would be an overdose.
   (4) This reflects a miscalculation and would be an overdose.

437. (2) Glucagon, an insulin antagonist produced by the alpha cells in the islets of Langerhans, leads to the conversion of glycogen to glucose in the liver. (b)
   (1) Does not stimulate the storage of glucose but rather its release by conversion of glycogen to glucose.
   (3) It is an insulin antagonist.
   (4) Stimulates glycogenolysis, the conversion of glycogen to glucose.

438. (1) Different types of insulin are compatible and are administered in the same syringe. However, the regular insulin is generally drawn up first because it is fast acting; and the possibility that a slower-acting insulin will enter the multidose vial is eliminated. (c)
   (2) Ratio does not affect compatibility.
   (3) Ratio does not affect compatibility.

(4) Unnecessary injections increase the risk of infection as well as cause additional discomfort.

439. (3) Glucose catabolism is the main pathway for cellular energy production. (b)
   (1) Glucose is not used directly for this process; ATP is the energy source.
   (2) Glucose is not used directly for this process; ATP is the energy source.
   (4) Glucose is not used directly for this process; ATP is the energy source.

440. (3) Ingested glucose not used immediately for energy needs is stored in the liver as glycogen and broken down when the blood glucose level falls (glycogenolysis). (a)
   (1) Not all foods provide glucose; ingested glucose may meet immediate needs but must be converted to glycogen for storage; glycogen is converted to glucose as needed.
   (2) This is digestion.
   (4) Formation of glucose from protein or fat.

441. (2) IV fluids are given to combat dehydration in acidosis and to keep an IV line open for administration of medications. When the electrolyte levels have been evaluated, potassium may be added if needed. (b)
   (1) In acidosis potassium ions (K^+) initially shift from intracellular to extracellular fluids, which results in hyperkalemia; as acidosis is corrected, hypokalemia may occur and then potassium may be administered.
   (3) This is an intermediate-acting insulin; rapid-acting insulin such as regular insulin is indicated in an emergency.
   (4) Not indicated; abnormally high serum potassium levels will revert once dehydration is corrected.

442. (2) To increase compliance with treatment, all patients should have an adequate understanding of their disease. (b)
   (1) The precipitating cause must be investigated immediately rather than be postponed until recovery.
   (3) Teaching does not ensure acceptance.
   (4) Individual knowledge varies; must be assessed before a teaching plan is established.

443. (1) Glucagon, produced by the alpha cells in the islets of Langerhans, is an insulin antagonist. It mobilizes glycogen storage in the liver, leading to an increased blood glucose level. (c)
   (2) Glucagon does not compete with insulin; it promotes the conversion of glycogen to glucose.
   (3) Glucagon is not a glucose substitute.
   (4) Stimulates an increase in blood glucose not glycogen.

444. (4) Insulin functions by facilitating the transport of glucose through the cell membrane and by increasing the deposits of glycogen in muscle. Both cellular glucose and muscle glycogen can be utilized for energy. (a)
   (1) Stimulates rate of oxygen consumption and thus the rate at which carbohydrates are burned; not the main controlling hormone.
   (2) Accelerates protein anabolism and stimulates growth.
   (3) Stimulates glyconeogenesis.

445. (3) Refrigeration retards the growth of bacteria and may preserve the specimen for several hours. (b)
   (1) Represents an unnecessary waste of time, effort, and money.
   (2) Growth of bacteria will alter the pH and the glucose and protein levels in the urine; must be refrigerated to retard growth.
   (4) Growth of bacteria will alter the pH and the glucose and protein levels in the urine; must be refrigerated to retard growth.

446. (2) The method of preservation can affect the test results. Depending on the purpose of the 24-hour study, the urine may be iced, kept with preservatives, or stored in a routine collection bag. (b)
   (1) Not necessary unless specifically ordered.
   (3) Although some specimens are preserved with this method, others require chemical preservative.
   (4) Not necessary unless specifically ordered.

447. (2) Most chemotherapeutic agents interfere with mitosis. The bone marrow consists of rapidly dividing cells, and therefore its activity is depressed. (a)
   (1) If bleeding occurs, the hemoglobin and hematocrit may be decreased because of the decreased number of thrombocytes.
   (3) The ESR generally increases in the presence of tissue inflammation or necrosis.
   (4) Because of bone marrow depression, leukopenia rather than leukocytosis can occur.

448. (3) Doxorubicin hydrochloride (Adriamycin) is a chemotherapeutic agent classified as an antibiotic. It achieves its therapeutic effect by inhibiting the synthesis of RNA. This effect blocks protein synthesis and cell division. (c)
   (1) Not a physiologic action of Adriamycin.
   (2) Not a physiologic action of Adriamycin.
   (4) Not a physiologic action of Adriamycin.

449. (1) Doxorubicin hydrochloride (Adriamycin), an antitumor antibiotic, causes nausea, diarrhea, and cardiac toxicity because it interferes with cell division. (c)
   (2) Hair loss occurs but is temporary and does not represent a life-threatening complication.
   (3) Anorexia may occur but is not a life-threatening complication; local necrosis not common.
   (4) Blood pressure and vital capacity are not directly affected but may be compromised secondarily to cardiomyopathy or arrhythmias.

450. (3) A sarcoma is defined as a malignant tumor whose cells resemble those of the supportive (connective) tissues of the body. (c)
   (1) Osteoblastomas are benign tumors of the bone.
   (2) Although collagen is the substance used to form the connective tissue, the term collagenoma is incorrect.

(4) Carcinoma refers to a malignant neoplasm of epithelial tissue.

451. (3) Gliomas account for about 45% of all brain tumors. (c)
(1) An adenoma is a tumor involving glandular tissue; may occur in the pituitary.
(2) Neurofibroma is a tumor of nerve tissue but is more common in the peripheral nervous system.
(4) Meningioma, which occurs in the meninges of the brain, accounts for about 20% of all brain tumors.

452. (2) A teratoma is defined as a neoplasm originating in the embryo composed of bizarre and chaotically arranged tissues that are embryologically and histologically foreign to the region in which the tumor occurs. (c)
(1) Malignant tumors originating in the muscle cells are myosarcomas.
(3) Neoplasms of the bone marrow are referred to as myelomas.
(4) Tumors generally originate in a primary site but if malignant may metastasize to involve multiple sites; not specific to teratomas.

453. (1) Some spermatozoa will remain viable in the vas deferens for a variable time after vasectomy. (c)
(2) Although it is considered a permanent form of sterilization, there has been some success reversing the procedure.
(3) Precautions must be taken to prevent fertilization until absence of sperm in the semen has been verified.
(4) The procedure does not affect sexual functioning.

454. (4) Cerebral damage on one side of the cortex causes alterations on the opposite side, since three fourths of the fibers originating in the cortex decussate (cross over) in the medulla before extending down the spinal cord. When there is cranial nerve damage, the same side of the body is affected, since the cranial nerves do not decussate but leave the cranial cavity by way of the small foramina in the skull. (c)
(1) Hemiplegia refers to paralysis of one side of the body; affects both extremities.
(2) Facial muscles on the same side as the cerebral lesion are paralyzed because they are innervated by the cranial nerves, which originate above the points where the spinal nerves decussate.
(3) Hemiplegia refers to paralysis of one side of the body; affects both extremities.

455. (2) Because of the profound effect of paralysis on body image, the nurse should provide the patient with an environment that permits exploration of feelings without judgment, punishment, or rejection. (a)
(1) An important part of nursing care; but not specific to the situation described.
(3) Attempts to distract the patient may be interpreted as denial of the patient's feelings and will not resolve the underlying conflict.
(4) An important part of nursing care; but not specific to the situation described.

456. (4) Bowel training is a program for the development of a conditioned reflex that controls regular emptying of the bowel. The key to success in a conditioning program is adherence to a strict time for evacuation based on the patient's individual schedule. (c)
(1) Although this should be considered, the cerebrovascular accident affects the responses of the patient by altering mobility, peristalsis, and sphincter control despite adherence to previous habits.
(2) The passage of food into the stomach does stimulate peristalsis but is only one factor that should be considered when planning a specific time for evacuation.
(3) The indiscriminate use of laxatives can result in dependency.

457. (3) Success is a basic motivation for learning. People receive satisfaction when a goal is reached. The more frequent the success, the greater is their satisfaction, which in turn motivates them to continue striving toward realistic goals. (b)
(1) An important part of teaching; but will not necessarily motivate the patient to attempt them.
(2) Progress toward long-range goals is often not readily apparent and may tend to discourage a patient.
(4) Constructive criticism is an important aspect in patient teaching; but if not tempered with praise, is discouraging.

458. (3) Reasonably prudent behavior in dealing with an immobile patient is to change the patient's position at least every 2 hours to relieve pressure on tissues and promote circulation. The nurse is negligent in not doing this. (b)
(1) When a capable patient refuses necessary health care despite explanation, his rights must be respected but he must also sign a document absolving health professionals of liability.
(2) Although decubitus ulcers may occur, nursing care must include preventive measures.
(4) The family is included in the health team.

459. (4) The absorbent action of Debrisan (dextranomer) helps clean decubitus ulcers and promotes healing. (c)
(1) Although the action has not been established, this drug is used to resolve inflammation resulting from accidental or surgical trauma.
(2) Used to promote diffusion of fluids in tissue during hypodermoclysis.
(3) Enzyme capable of inactivating penicillin.

460. (3) Because of the presence of feces in the colon, a patient with a fecal impaction has the urge but is unable to defecate. (a)
(1) Anorexia may occur with an impaction but may also be due to other conditions.
(2) Flatulence may occur as a result of immobility or obstruction; patients with impactions may be able to pass flatus along with liquid stool around the fecal mass.

(4) The frequency of bowel movements varies for individuals; it may be normal for this individual not to have a BM for several days.

461. (3) When the bowel is impacted with hardened feces, there is often seepage of liquid feces around the obstruction and thus uncontrolled diarrhea. (a)
   (1) The bowel may become distended if completely obstructed, but this is a late symptom if it occurs at all.
   (2) There is often frequent liquid bowel movements in the presence of an impaction.
   (4) This is indicative of lower GI bleeding.

462. (3) Sensory impulses from temperature, touch, and pain travel via the spinothalamic pathway to the thalamus and then to the postcentral gyrus of the parietal lobe, the somatosensory area. (a)
   (1) Area of abstract thinking and muscular movements.
   (2) Area where nerve impulses are translated into sight.
   (4) Area where nerve impulses are translated into sound.

463. (4) The thalamus receives sensory impulses from the spinothalamic tract and relays them to the cerebral cortex. (c)
   (1) Conducts impulses between the cord and brain.
   (2) Relays between the cortex and autonomic centers.
   (3) Involved in motor activity and coordination.

464. (3) The autonomic nervous system functions to regulate visceral effectors and maintain internal equilibrium. (b)
   (1) Conveys information from peripheral receptors to the central nervous system and information from the CNS to muscles and glands.
   (2) Concerned with overall control; consists of the brain and spinal cord.
   (4) Transmits impulses from the periphery to the brain and from the brain to the periphery; also integrates reflexes.

465. (3) Vagal stimulation slows the heart. The vagus is the principal nerve of the parasympathetic portion of the autonomic nervous system, and its axon terminals release acetylcholine. The response of the viscera to acetylcholine varies, but in general the organism is in a relaxed state. (c)
   (1) Function of the sympathetic nervous system (accelerator nerve); release of norepinephrine.
   (2) Stimulation of the sympathetic nervous system dilates bronchioles in the lungs; the vagus constricts them.
   (4) No parasympathomimetic fibers to the coronary blood vessels; sympathetic impulses dilate these vessels.

466. (2) As a result of the muscles' contracting and pulling on the 2 portions of bone, there is a characteristic shortening of the femur with external rotation of the extremity. (c)

(1) The extremity externally rotates as the muscles contract.
(3) Lateral motion of the leg does not occur.
(4) Lateral motion of the leg does not occur; the leg externally rotates.

467. (3) A fracture in the neck of the femur will cause shortening of the femur and external rotation. To correct this malalignment, the patient's leg should be extended and maintained in slight internal rotation. (c)
   (1) To reduce the fracture, it is necessary to maintain the leg in extension, counteracting the contraction of the quadriceps, which may cause overriding of bone fragments. External rotation of the thigh as a result of muscle contraction tends to misalign the bone fragments; therefore slight internal rotation or normal alignment is preferred.
   (2) External rotation of the thigh as a result of muscle contraction tends to misalign the bone fragments; therefore slight internal rotation or normal alignment is preferred.
   (4) To reduce the fracture, it is necessary to maintain the leg in extension, counteracting the contraction of the quadriceps, which may cause overriding of bone fragments.

468. (1) Buck's traction is frequently used in the treatment of a fractured hip to align the bones (reduction of fracture). If such traction were not employed, the muscles would go into spasm, shifting the bone fragments and causing pain. (b)
   (2) Although the affected extremity must be properly aligned, turning and moving the patient is still necessary.
   (3) Buck's traction is usually a temporary measure prior to surgery; contractures result from a shortening of the muscles by prolonged immobility.
   (4) External rotation is contraindicated and prevented by the use of sandbags or trochanter rolls.

469. (3) Assessment of any peripheral pulse should include the characteristics of the pulse (e.g., amplitude, rhythm, rate). Symmetry, the correspondence of homologous parts on opposite sides of the body, provides a way of assessing data that should be identical. (b)
   (1) Contractility is not a characteristic of pulse but of the vessel.
   (2) Color of skin and type of spasm are not pulse characteristics.
   (4) Local temperature is not a characteristic of pulse.

470. (4) The 3-point gait, which requires considerable arm strength, is used when a limb cannot bear weight. The affected leg and crutches are advanced together, and the strong leg swings through. (c)
   (1) Require weight bearing on both feet.
   (2) Require weight bearing on both feet.
   (3) Used for individuals who cannot move their lower extremities; does not simulate normal ambulation.

471. (3) In the 4-point gait the patient brings the left crutch forward first, followed by the right foot; then the right crutch is brought forward, followed by the left foot. Thus both legs must be able to bear some weight. (c)
    (1) Pressure on the axillae may damage nerves in the area.
    (2) Although the arms are extended to allow the hands to bear weight, the elbows are not maintained in this position.
    (4) Both extremities must be able to bear weight.

472. (1) Because of its great blood supply and general fragility, the spleen, when ruptured, must be removed to prevent possible hemorrhage. (b)
    (2) Although rupturing of the spleen may be a sequela of certain diseases (e.g., mononucleosis) the situation described involves trauma, which is a more common cause.
    (3) Does not explain the reason for removal.
    (4) Splenomegaly may not be associated with discomfort; functions of purification, antibody production, and erythrocyte storage are important but not essential.

473. (1) Because the spleen has such vascularity, hemorrhage may occur and result in abdominal distention. (c)
    (2) The incidence is not higher after splenectomy than after other abdominal surgery.
    (3) Although an elevated temperature is common, it is usually not the result of infection; the incidence of infection is not higher after splenectomy, except in children.
    (4) The incidence of obstruction is not higher than for other abdominal surgery.

474. (1) Head injuries can cause trauma to the brain; and the patient should be observed for signs of increased intracranial pressure (e.g., headache, dizziness, visual disturbances). (b)
    (2) The Trendelenburg position should be avoided because it will increase intracranial pressure.
    (3) Not indicated in this situation.
    (4) The intracranial pressure may increase after trauma because of bleeding and edema.

475. (4) Release of the adrenocortical steroids (cortisol) by the stress of surgery causes renal retention of Na^+ and excretion of K^+. Potassium can also be depleted by nasogastric suction. (b)
    (1) Although sodium may be depleted by nasogastric suction, retention by the kidneys generally balances this loss.
    (2) Not depleted by surgery or urinary excretion.
    (3) Not depleted by surgery or urinary excretion.

476. (2) On inspiration, excursion of the fractured ribs is limited. The ribs press against the pleura, causing pain. (b)
    (1) This is not to be expected; accumulation of secretions can be avoided by coughing and deep breathing.

(3) Since limited activity decreases oxygen consumption, shortness of breath is not a common complaint.
(4) Pain does not occur on expiration, for the lungs deflate and decrease pressure on the fractured ribs.

477. (3) Changes in the amount of blood in the urine may indicate progressive increases in kidney damage. (b)
    (1) This is unrelated to hematuria.
    (2) This is unrelated to hematuria.
    (4) This is unrelated to hematuria; associated with breakdown of adipose tissue.

478. (1) Hematuria occurs when there is kidney damage with leakage of erythrocytes through the glomerular filtration membrane. (b)
    (2) Although lesions of the ureters may be responsible for hematuria, blunt trauma to the kidneys is more common because of their proximity to the rib cage.
    (3) Although injury to the bladder is possible, blunt trauma to the kidneys is more common because of their proximity to the rib cage.
    (4) Although injury to the urethra is possible, blunt trauma to the kidneys is more common because of their proximity to the rib cage.

479. (3) The gamma globulin fraction in the plasma is the fraction that includes the antibodies. (a)
    (1) Hemoglobin carries oxygen.
    (2) Albumin helps regulate fluid shifts by maintaining the plasma oncotic pressure.
    (4) Thrombin is involved in clotting.

480. (2) Platelets (thrombocytes) adhere to the intima of damaged vessels within seconds after injury, releasing substances that promote hemostasis. (b)
    (1) Red blood cells play no role in clotting; they carry oxygen to all body cells.
    (3) Play no role in clotting; they protect the body against microorganisms.
    (4) Erythrocytes are red blood cells; they carry oxygen and play no role in coagulation.

481. (1) Isotonic solutions are those which cause no change in the cellular volume or pressure, since their concentration is equivalent to that of body fluid. (a)
    (2) Contains more than 0.85 g of sodium chloride in each 100 ml.
    (3) Contains less than 0.85 g of sodium chloride in each 100 ml.
    (4) Relates to 2 compounds that possess the same molecular formula but that differ in their properties or in the position of atoms in the molecules; isomers.

482. (2) REM (rapid eye movement) sleep is necessary for psychologic coping. The nurse should be aware that some medications affect this sleep stage and thereby alter emotional health. (b)
    (1) The individual is just drifting off to sleep; alpha brain waves are present.
    (3) The individual is in a light sleep and can be readily wakened; delta waves are interspersed with alpha waves.

(4) The individual is in a deep sleep and is difficult to arouse; delta brain waves predominate; stages 1 and 4 are associated with physiologic rest.

483. (2) Fiber absorbs water, swells, and consequently stretches the bowel wall, promoting peristalsis, mass movements, and defecation. Smooth muscle tends to contract when stretched because of the reflex activity of stretch receptors. (c)
    (1) Does not irritate the bowel wall.
    (3) There is no chemical stimulation.
    (4) Bacterial action is not involved in the process by which bulk stimulates defecation.

484. (1) Adrenalin is used to treat shock because the induced arterial constriction reduces blood pooling (vessels cannot hold as much blood) and increases venous return and cardiac output. (c)
    (2) Tourniquets constrict veins of the extremities, reduce venous return.
    (3) A sympathectomy interferes with autonomic vasoconstriction; reduces venous return.
    (4) Digoxin slows and strengthens the heartbeat; does not cause vasoconstriction.

485. (2) An autograft is one taken from an uninjured area of the same person's body. (b)
    (1) A homograft is skin taken from the same species.
    (3) A heterograft or xenograft is skin taken from a different species.
    (4) An allograft is skin taken from the same species.

486. (3) A heterograft or xenograft involves the grafting of tissues from a different species. (b)
    (1) A homograft is skin taken from the same species.
    (2) An allograft is skin taken from the same species.
    (4) This type of graft does not exist.

487. (3) An increased hematocrit level indicates hemoconcentration secondary to fluid loss. (b)
    (1) The pH levels reflect acid-base balance.
    (2) The sedimentation rate is not used as an indicator of fluid loss; indicates the presence of an inflammatory process.
    (4) May be used to indicate dehydration from burns, but interpretation can be complicated by other conditions accompanying burns that also cause elevation of the BUN.

488. (1) As the amount of tissue involved increases, there is greater extravasation of fluid into the tissues. Thus the relationship of fluid loss to body surface is directly proportional. Several formulas (e.g., the Evans, the Baxter, the Brooke Army Hospital) are used to estimate fluid loss based on percent of body surface burned. (b)
    (2) Incorrect; relationship is proportional.
    (3) Incorrect; relationship is proportional.
    (4) Incorrect; relationship is proportional.

489. (3) *Clostridium tetani* can develop in wounds in which there is dead tissue. (b)
    (1) Indicated for hypoprothrombinemia caused by deficiency of vitamin K; not related to burns.
    (2) Although provides passive immunity against certain infectious agents, not specifically indicated in the treatment of burns.
    (4) Adrenergic drug used in the treatment of bronchospasm and heart block.

490. (3) Mafenide (Sulfamylon) interferes with the kidneys' role in hydrogen ion excretion, resulting in metabolic acidosis. (c)
    (1) Not indicated as an adverse effect of this drug.
    (2) Not indicated as an adverse effect of this drug.
    (4) Not indicated as an adverse effect of this drug.

491. (4) Negative pressure such as suction should never be exerted on the bladder, since this might injure the sensitive tissue. The solution should be allowed to drain by force of gravity alone. (b)
    (1) Since the bladder is a sterile body cavity, surgical asepsis is required.
    (2) The solution is introduced by compressing the bulb of the irrigating syringe or by gravity; to prevent trauma, excessive pressure is avoided.
    (3) The solution is normally used at room temperature.

492. (1) Although other solutions may be ordered, irrigations of the bladder usually employ normal saline (0.9% NaCl), which is a solution of approximately the tonicity of normal body fluids. (b)
    (2) This is a hypotonic solution, which may be absorbed by body tissues.
    (3) This is a hypotonic solution, which may be absorbed by body tissues.
    (4) Genitourinary irrigants usually contain an antimicrobial agent such as neosporin; indiscriminant use of such agents leads to the emergence of resistant strains of microorganisms.

493. (2) The bladder is a sterile body cavity. Any time a solution or catheter is introduced into the urinary meatus, strict surgical asepsis is required. (b)
    (1) Excessive pressure can traumatize the lining of the urinary tract.
    (3) The negative pressure exerted during aspiration may cause trauma.
    (4) The solution is generally administered at room temperature.

494. (4) Patients adapting to illness frequently feel afraid and helpless and strike out at health team members as a way of maintaining control or denying their fear. (b)
    (1) There is no evidence that the patient denies the existence of her health problem.
    (2) Although disorders such as cerebral vascular accidents and atherosclerosis, which are associated with hypertension, may lead to cerebral anoxia, there is insufficient evidence to support this conclusion in this situation.
    (3) Although reserpine may cause agitation or depression, the behaviors described are more likely attributable to the patient's psychologic adjustment to the situation.

495. (1) Chlordiazepoxide (Librium) is an anxiolytic. It promotes muscle relaxation, reducing anxiety and facilitating rest. (b)

(2) This is a side effect of Librium due to its effect on the brainstem reticular formation, which controls the overall degree of central nervous system activity.

(3) This is a side effect of Librium due to its effect on the brainstem reticular formation, which controls the overall degree of central nervous system activity.

(4) The antianxiety effect of Librium may indirectly reduce hostility, but this is not the goal.

496. (4) Drowsiness is a side effect of Librium and indicates excessive depression of the central nervous system. (b)

(1) Although tremors are listed as a possible adverse reaction, hyporeactivity is more common.

(2) Not commonly attributed to chlordiazepoxide.

(3) This drug may cause hypotension.

497. (3) Reserpine is an antihypertensive because it reduces norepinephrine levels in the peripheral nerve endings. (a)

(1) Reserpine is an antihypertensive not a diuretic; diuretics produce fluid excretion.

(2) Reserpine is an antihypertensive not a hypnotic; hypnotics promote sleep.

(4) Reserpine is an antihypertensive not a tranquilizer; tranquilizers reduce muscle tension and anxiety.

498. (4) An improper reading of the level of mercury will be obtained if the reader is not perpendicular to the column. An error of parallax results when an object is displaced by an observer's altered position. (a)

(1) Too narrow a cuff can result in erroneously high readings; not an error of parallax.

(2) Standing close to the manometer is not explicit; there may or may not be a resultant error of parallax depending upon whether the examiner is perpendicular to the column of mercury.

(3) Elevating the arm above the level of the heart will result in an erroneously low reading; not an error of parallax.

499. (3) At this time the patient is using this behavior as a defense. Quiet acceptance can be an effective interpersonal technique, since it is nonjudgmental. (c)

(1) During periods of overt hostility, perceptions are altered, making it difficult to evaluate the situation rationally.

(2) Withdrawal signifies nonacceptance and rejection.

(4) The nurse may be the target of a broad array of emotions; by focusing on only behaviors that affect the nurse, the full scope of the patient's feelings are not considered.

500. (2) An honest nurse-patient relationship should be maintained so that trust can develop. (a)

(1) Although other health team members may need to be informed eventually, the initial action should concern only the nurse-patient relationship.

(3) Does nothing to establish communication about feelings or motivation behind behavior.

(4) Although other health team members may need to be informed eventually, the initial action should concern only the nurse-patient relationship.

501. (2) The orthopneic position allows maximum lung expansion because gravity reduces the pressure of the abdominal viscera on the diaphragm and lungs. (b)

(1) Elevation of the extremities should be avoided because it increases venous returns, placing an increased workload on the heart.

(3) Excessive coughing and mucus production is characteristic of pulmonary edema and does not need to be encouraged.

(4) Positioning for postural drainage does not relieve acute dyspnea; furthermore, it increases venous return to the heart.

502. (3) Application of rotating tourniquets keeps blood in the extremities, decreasing venous return, which reduces pulmonary artery pressure and relieves congestion. (b)

(1) Extreme dyspnea and congestion necessitate a high-Fowler position.

(2) At times oxygen must be delivered under pressure to overcome the pressure of the edema fluid, but this is less common and is generally the responsibility of the inhalation or respiratory therapist.

(4) A wet phlebotomy is used only occasionally to reduce venous return to the heart; a dry phlebotomy (rotating tourniquets) is usually effective.

503. (4) Diuretic therapy generally involves use of drugs that directly or indirectly increase urinary sodium excretion. Increased urinary excretion of sodium also promotes potassium loss. (a)

(1) Sodium restriction does not necessarily accompany administration of furosemide (Lasix).

(2) Unless otherwise ordered, oral intake is unaffected.

(3) Dyspnea does not directly result in a depletion of electrolytes.

504. (1) CVP is to be recorded when the patient is horizontal and the zero point of the manometer is at the midaxillary line (level of the right atrium). (a)

(2) Alters the relationship of the midaxillary line and right atrium; inaccurate readings will be obtained.

(3) Alters the relationship of the midaxillary line and right atrium; inaccurate readings will be obtained.

(4) Alters the relationship of the midaxillary line and right atrium; inaccurate readings will be obtained.

505. (2) With air conditioning, blood vessels in the skin remain partially constricted, preventing extensive blood flow through the skin. Such extensive skin blood flow would ordinarily occur in hot weather to promote radiation of heat from the body; however, the heart must then work to pump the blood through many extra miles of blood vessels in the skin. (a)

(1) Body temperature is maintained.

(3) There is decreased circulation to the skin, which makes it beneficial to the person with cardiopulmonary problems.

(4) There is decreased circulation to the skin, which makes it beneficial to the person with cardiopulmonary problems.

506. (2) Since Mr. Roger's condition is described as terminal, nursing priority should be directed toward providing comfort. (b)
    (1) Although these are important aspects of nursing care, provision of comfort retains priority in the care of a dying patient.
    (3) Although these are important aspects of nursing care, provision of comfort retains priority in the care of a dying patient.
    (4) Although these are important aspects of nursing care, provision of comfort retains priority in the care of a dying patient.

507. (4) Small meals are not as psychologically overwhelming and do not upset the stomach as easily. They are therefore better tolerated. (a)
    (1) Does not ensure adequate nutrition; if the portion size is decreased, frequency must be increased.
    (2) Administration of vitamins is a dependent nursing function.
    (3) If no attempts are made to decrease portions at regular mealtimes, aversion will usually persist.

508. (1) Anorexia refers to loss of appetite. (a)
    (2) Anoxia refers to lack of oxygen.
    (3) Apathy refers to lack of concern.
    (4) Dysphagia refers to difficulty swallowing.

509. (2) IPPB treatments loosen bronchial secretions and dilate the air passages, but coughing is needed to raise the secretions for expectoration. (a)
    (1) A sitting position will allow secretions to remain in the lungs unless coughing is encouraged.
    (3) IPPB is sometimes administered before postural drainage to loosen secretions so they can be more easily mobilized.
    (4) Rest should be encouraged only after coughing to bring up secretions mobilized by postural drainage.

510. (3) Meperidine hydrochloride is the generic name for Demerol. (a)
    (1) Propoxyphene hydrochloride is the generic name for Darvon.
    (2) Glutethimide is the generic name for Doriden.
    (4) Naloxone is the generic name for Narcan.

511. (4) Patients with COPD (chronic obstructive pulmonary disease) respond only to the chemical stimulus of low oxygen levels. Administration of high concentrations of oxygen will eliminate the stimulus to breathe, leading to decreased respirations and lethargy. (c)
    (1) High concentrations of oxygen will eliminate the stimulus to breathe, so the respiratory rate would decrease.
    (2) Cyanosis is caused by excessive amounts of reduced oxyhemoglobin; since oxygen is being administered, cyanosis may be reduced.
    (3) Rising carbon dioxide levels cause lethargy rather than anxiety.

512. (3) Since family members are old enough to understand his needs, they should be encouraged to participate in his care. (c)
    (1) Deprives the patient of support system.
    (2) Self-care increases oxygen utilization, causing fatigue and dyspnea.
    (4) Overworking the patient causes undue fatigue and dyspnea; frequent rest periods should be incorporated into the plan.

513. (4) Gastroscopy permits visualization of the stomach and biopsy of the tissue. (a)
    (1) Soft tissue is not visualized by x rays unless radiopaque substance is utilized.
    (2) CBC may provide a general index of the extent of occult bleeding but is not diagnostic of cancer of the stomach.
    (3) Screening test of adrenocortical function based on eosinophil response to ACTH administration.

514. (4) An American relative can serve as interpreter and provide emotional support and security. (b)
    (1) Translation of medical terminology does not suffice in establishing communication for reducing the strangeness of the environment; nor does it provide emotional support.
    (2) Such sporadic communication is less than therapeutic because interpersonal relationships do not develop.
    (3) Ongoing communication is an essential element of the nursing process.

515. (3) $\dfrac{\text{Amount to be infused} \times \text{Drop factor}}{\text{Time of infusion in minutes}}$ (a)
    (1) Incorrect calculations; too rapid; would infuse in approximately 1 hour.
    (2) Incorrect calculation; too rapid; would take between 2 and 3 hours to infuse.
    (4) Incorrect calculation; too rapid; would infuse in approximately 4 hours.

516. (4) Approximately 42 ml of fluid per hour would be infused. This is adequate to keep the vein open without causing circulatory overload; after 24 hours there is increased risk of contamination of the solution and the container should be changed. (b)
    (1) Provides fluid not needed by the patient; increased risk of circulatory overload or heart failure.
    (2) Provides fluid not needed by the patient; increased risk of circulatory overload or heart failure.
    (3) Provides fluid not needed by the patient; increased risk of circulatory overload or heart failure.

517. (1) Gluten, a cereal protein, appears to be responsible for morphologic changes of the intestinal mucosa in individuals with nontropical sprue (celiac disease). (b)
    (2) Folic acid, along with antimicrobial agents, is used to treat tropical sprue; causes dramatic improvement.
    (3) The use of corticosteroids may be advantageous

with either form of sprue; however, does not produce the same effect as specific treatements already described.

(4) Vitamin B_{12} may be administered if macrocytic anemia or achlorhydria develops; however, does not correct the major pathosis.

518. (1) Gluten is found in rye, wheat, and oat products. (a)
(2) Gluten is not found in these foods; they do not have to be avoided.
(3) Gluten is not found in these foods; they do not have to be avoided.
(4) Gluten is not found in these foods; they do not have to be avoided.

519. (2) These foods are low in gluten. (c)
(1) Flours used in the production of bread are high in gluten.
(3) Flours used in the production of noodles are high in gluten.
(4) Postum is a cereal drink high in gluten.

520. (1) The diet should be high in protein and calories, low in fat, and gluten free for individuals with nontropical sprue. Protein is needed for tissue rebuilding. (b)
(2) Diarrhea is caused by malabsorption, which accounts for the poor nutritional status; once the diarrhea is corrected, it is essential to compensate for poor nutrition.
(3) May prefer foods high in gluten, which would potentiate malabsorption.
(4) IV therapy does not provide all the necessary nutrients.

521. (2) The respiratory center in the medulla responds primarily to increased carbon dioxide concentration in the blood. (a)
(1) Not a stimulant for respiration; involved in transmission of neural impulses.
(3) Not a stimulant; a by-product of muscular activity.
(4) Normally not the primary stimulus to breathing; functions as a primary stimulus in individuals who have chronic hypercapnia.

522. (2) The lower the P_{O_2} and the higher the P_{CO_2}, the more rapidly oxygen dissociates from the oxyhemoglobin molecule. (c)
(1) Must be associated with an increase in carbon dioxide pressure.
(3) Oxygen dissociations would be decreased in this situation.
(4) Must be associated with a decrease in oxygen pressure.

523. (2) This is the organism that causes botulism. (a)
(1) *Salmonella*, a gram-negative rod, is not anaerobic.
(3) An anaerobic organism that causes tetanus.
(4) A normal inhabitant of intestines; not anaerobic.

524. (3) *Entamoeba histolytica,* the organism that causes amebic dysentery, is transmitted through excreta. (a)
(1) Organism not passed via milk.

(2) Organism not transmitted by gnats.
(4) Not a tick-borne disease.

525. (1) In starvation there are inadequate carbohydrates available for immediate energy, and stored fats are used in excessive amounts. (a)
(2) There is no fat in alcohol; no fat oxidation occurs.
(3) Does not require use of great amounts of fat.
(4) Does not require use of great amounts of fat; calcium is deposited to form callus.

526. (3) Fluid and electrolytes are lost through intestinal decompression; on a daily basis about one fifth the total body water is secreted into and almost completed reabsorbed by the GI tract. (a)
(1) Since the patient is kept n.p.o., there would be no stimulus to cause enzymes to be secreted into the GI tract.
(2) Dextrose in IV supplies some carbohydrates as a source of energy; would not be drawn from storage by intestinal decompression.
(4) Since the patient is being kept n.p.o., vitamins and minerals are not entering the GI tract and therefore are not lost.

527. (1) Dehydration is a danger because of fluid loss in GI suction. (b)
(2) Based on data provided, these symptoms are not likely to occur.
(3) Based on data provided, these symptoms are not likely to occur.
(4) Based on data provided, these symptoms are not likely to occur.

528. (2) Isotonic saline most closely resembles normal body fluids; will not cause an imbalance by pulling extra fluids and electrolytes out of the circulation. (a)
(1) Hypertonic solutions would draw fluids out of the circulation into the GI tract; glucose provides a medium for bacterial growth.
(3) Hypotonic solutions would allow absorption of fluid into the circulation, resulting in dilution of electrolytes and possible circulatory overload.
(4) Hypotonic solutions would allow absorption of fluid into the circulation, resulting in dilution of electrolytes and possible circulatory overload.

529. (1) Open communication lines are always important in relieving anxiety and reducing stress, which might interfere with postoperative recovery. (b)
(2) Reassurances do not allow for open communication, invalidating the emotions experienced by the patient.
(3) Learning does not occur when anxiety levels are too high.
(4) Does not acknowledge the patient's feelings and therefore does not deal with the source of her anxiety.

530. (2) The patient must be ready to accept changes in body image and function; this acceptance will facilitate mastery of the techniques of colostomy care, special diets, and optimistic utilization of community resources. (b)

(1) Specific knowledge can be imparted only when an individual is ready to learn; requires acceptance of a new body image.

(3) Specific knowledge can be imparted only when an individual is ready to learn; requires acceptance of a new body image.

(4) Specific knowledge can be imparted only when an individual is ready to learn; requires acceptance of a new body image.

531. (2) A transverse colostomy is an opening created in the transverse colon. The rectal tube should be pointed to the proximal intestine to evacuate the bowels. (b)

(1) A water-soluble lubricant is generally used to facilitate insertion.

(3) Continual force may traumatize the mucosa; lack of nerve endings diminishes sensation.

(4) There are no sphincters so bearing down is unnecessary.

532. (3) The pulmonary capillary beds are the first small vessels (capillary beds) that the embolus encounters once it is released from the calf veins. (b)

(1) Unlikely to occur because the embolus would enter the pulmonary system first.

(2) Gangrene occurs when the arterial rather than the venous circulation is compromised.

(4) Unlikely to occur; the embolus would enter the pulmonary system first.

533. (3) The absorption of fluids by gauze is due to the adhesion of water to the gauze threads. The surface tension of water causes contraction of the fiber, pulling fluid up the threads. (c)

(1) This is movement of molecules from high to low concentration.

(2) This refers to diffusion of water through a semipermeable membrane.

(4) Separation of substances in solution utilizing their differing rates of diffusion through a membrane.

534. (4) Alcohol stimulates pancreatic enzyme secretion and an increase in pressure in the pancreatic duct. The backflow of enzymes into the pancreatic interstitial spaces results in partial digestion and inflammation of the pancreatic tissue. (b)

(1) Although blockage of the bile duct with calculi may precipitate pancreatitis, this is not associated with alcohol.

(2) Alcohol does not deplete insulin stores; the demand for insulin is unrelated to pancreatitis.

(3) Although the volume of secretions increases, the composition remains unchanged.

535. (2) A pseudocyst of the pancreas is an abnormally dilated space that contains blood, necrotic tissue, and enzymes and is surrounded by connective tissue. (c)

(1) Incorrect definition of a pseudocyst.

(3) Incorrect definition of a pseudocyst.

(4) Incorrect definition of a pseudocyst.

536. (4) That is the unique function of pancreozymin, which is secreted by the duodenal mucosa. It particularly affects the production of amylase. (a)

(1) Cholecystokinin stimulates the flow of bile from the gallbladder.

(2) Enterocrinin increases intestinal juice secretion.

(3) Enterogastrone causes a lessening of gastric secretion and motility.

537. (2) Lipase is a pancreatic enzyme that aids in the digestion of fat. (c)

(1) Does not break down all dietary fat.

(3) Does not synthesize triglycerides.

(4) This is the function of bile.

538. (1) The duodenum secretes several digestion-related hormones, including secretin, which elicits sodium bicarbonate secretion from the pancreas, and pancreozymin, which elicits enzyme secretion from the pancreas. It also brings about gallbladder contraction and secretion of bile; in this function it is known as cholecystokinin. (b)

(2) The pancreas produces the hormone insulin.

(3) The adrenals produce glucocorticoids, mineralocorticoids, epinephrine, etc.

(4) The liver produces bile, which aids in the digestion of fat, but does not produce any hormones.

539. (1) Almost all peptic ulcers in the stomach develop along the lesser curvature of the antral (pyloric) region. About 85% of all peptic ulcers occur within the first 2 cm of the duodenum. These regions are most exposed to acid conditions. (b)

(2) Less exposed to gastric secretions.

(3) Less exposed to gastric secretions.

(4) Less exposed to gastric secretions; however, erosion may occur after repeated episodes of gastric reflux.

540. (4) Propantheline bromide (Pro-Banthine) reduces the motility of the GI tract and thereby facilitates healing. (c)

(1) It does not affect the pH of gastric secretions.

(2) It decreases motility.

(3) It does not affect the pH of gastric secretions.

541. (1) Physiologic normal saline is used in gastric irrigation to prevent electrolyte imbalance. Because of the fresh gastric sutures, slow and gentle irrigation should be performed. Most surgeons, however, prefer gastric instillations. (a)

(2) The purpose of irrigation is to maintain the patency of the tube for gastric decompression; with disconnection from suction a buildup of secretions and air can occur or the tube can be become blocked by viscous drainage.

(3) The purpose of irrigation is to maintain the patency of the tube for gastric decompression; with disconnection from suction a buildup of secretions and air can occur or the tube can become blocked by viscous drainage.

(4) Increasing the pressure may cause damage to the suture line.

542. (4) The vagus nerve stimulates the stomach to secrete hydrochloric acid. When it is severed, this neural

pathway is interrrupted and there will be a decrease in stomach secretions. (b)

(1) The portion of the vagus nerve that was severed innervated the stomach, not the heart; therefore the heart rate would not be affected.

(2) The vagus nerve controls hydrochloric acid secretion not gastric emptying; this is determined by the nature of foods being digested.

(3) The vagus nerve is not a sensory nerve.

543. (4) To calculate the rate of fluid infusion:

$$\frac{\text{Amount of fluid to be infused} \times \text{Drop factor}}{\text{Amount of time (minutes)}}$$

$$\frac{1000 \times 15}{8 \times 60} = \frac{15000}{480} = 31.25 \text{ drops/min} \quad \text{(b)}$$

(1) Incorrect calculation, resulting in excessive administration of fluid.

(2) Incorrect calculation, resulting in inadequate administration of fluid.

(3) Incorrect calculation, resulting in inadequate administration of fluid.

544. (2) Since IV solutions enter the body's internal environment, all solutions and medications utilizing this route must be sterile to prevent the introduction of microbes. (b)

(1) The medication can be mixed with the IV solution in many ways; sterility takes priority.

(3) The amount and type of solution depend on the medication; sterility takes priority.

(4) The needle does not have to be changed if sterility is maintained.

545. (1) Symptoms of dumping syndrome occur to some degree in about 50% of all individuals who have undergone gastrectomy or vagotomy. They include weakness, faintness, heart palpitations, and diaphoresis. It is therefore important to explain to Mr. Smith that such symptoms can be minimized by resting after meals in the semi-Fowler position and eating small meals, omitting concentrated and highly refined carbohydrates. (b)

(2) Gas-forming foods affect the intestines, not the stomach.

(3) Eating habits must be modified to prevent rapid emptying of the stomach.

(4) Modification of roughage is part of the management of intestinal rather than gastric disorders.

546. (3) An individual treated for a thyroid problem by intake of radioactive iodine (^{131}I) becomes mildly radioactive, particularly in the region of the thyroid gland, which preferentially absorbs the iodine. Such patients should be treated with standard precautions. (b)

(1) Since radioactive iodine is internalized, the patient becomes the source of radioactivity.

(2) The amount of radioactive iodine utilized is not enough to cause high radioactivity.

(4) Since radioactive iodine is internalized, the patient becomes the source of radioactivity.

547. (1) Because of the individual's increased metabolic rate, a high-calorie diet is needed to meet the energy demands of the body and prevent weight loss. (b)

(2) GI motility is increased and does not require the additional stimulus of increased roughage.

(3) Nutritional needs are increased by increased metabolism; additional calories are needed.

(4) Modification of the consistency is unnecessary.

548. (3) Lugol's solution adds iodine to the body fluids, exerting negative feedback on the thyroid tissue and decreasing its metabolism and vascularity. (a)

(1) This drug interferes with production of thyroid hormone but causes increased vascularity and size of the thyroid.

(2) This is a synthetic thyroid hormone; its use is contraindicated because there is already an excessive production of thyroid hormone.

(4) This is a topical antiseptic.

549. (3) During surgery, if the laryngeal nerves are injured bilaterally, the vocal cords will tighten, interfering with speech. If one cord is affected, hoarseness develops. This can be evaluated simply by having the patient speak every hour. (b)

(1) This ability is not influenced by laryngeal nerve damage.

(2) This ability is not influenced by laryngeal nerve damage.

(4) This ability is not influenced by laryngeal nerve damage.

550. (3) These signs may indicate tetany from calcium depletion. If this occurs after a thyroidectomy, one might suspect inadvertent removal of the parathyroids. (c)

(1) Symptoms associated with hypokalemia include muscle weakness and malaise.

(2) Symptoms associated with hypomagnesemia include tremor, neuromuscular irritability, and confusion.

(4) Symptoms associated with metabolic acidosis include deep rapid breathing, weakness, and disorientation.

551. (1) Parathyroid removal eliminates the body's source of parathyroid hormone, which functions to increase blood calcium. Consequently, normal decreases in blood calcium cannot be balanced by additions to the blood from calcium reservoirs in bone, increased calcium reabsorption from the kidney tubules, or increased intestinal calcium absorption. Low body fluid calcium tetanizes muscles, including the diaphragm, resulting in dyspnea, asphyxia, and death. (a)

(2) The parathyroids do not regulate the adrenal glands.

(3) Loss of the thyroid gland would upset thyroid hormone balance and might cause myxedema.

(4) The parathyroids are not involved in regulating plasma volume; the pituitary and adrenal glands are.

552. (1) Parathyroid hormone increases osteoclastic activity, resulting in breakdown of bone substance and release of calcium into the blood. (b)
   (2) It increases blood calcium and thereby will prevent tetany.
   (3) Although blood calcium does increase, blood phosphate also increases.
   (4) The hormone calcitonin, released by the thyroid gland, increases calcium incorporation into the bones.

553. (4) Parathormone increases the blood concentration of calcium by accelerating calcium absorption from the intestine, bones, and kidneys. Vitamin D is essential for calcium to be absorbed from the intestine. (b)
   (1) Vitamin A and thyroid hormone do not interact to regulate calcium levels. Vitamin A is essential for the normal function of epithelial cells and visual purple; calcitonin, from the thyroid gland, lowers serum calcium.
   (2) Ascorbic acid (vitamin C) and growth hormone do not interact to regulate calcium levels. Vitamin C promotes collagen production and the formation of bone matrix; growth hormone, produced by the anterior pituitary, controls the rate of skeletal growth.
   (3) Phosphorus and ACTH do not interact to regulate calcium levels. Phosphorus is a component of bone; ACTH, produced by the anterior pituitary, stimulates the adrenal cortex to secrete the corticosteroid hormones.

554. (2) Calcitonin, a thyroid gland hormone, prevents the reabsorption of calcium by bone. It also inhibits the release of calcium from bone. The net result is lowered serum calcium levels. (a)
   (1) Aldosterone regulates fluid and electrolyte balance by promoting the retention of sodium and water and the excretion of potassium.
   (3) Parathyroid hormone promotes the intestinal absorption of calcium and mobilizes calcium for the bones to increase blood calcium levels.
   (4) Although calcitonin lowers serum calcium levels, the other thyroid hormones (thyroxine and triiodothyronine) control the body's metabolic rate.

555. (1) Myxedema is the severest form of hypothyroidism. Decreased thyroid gland activity causes a reduced production of its hormones. (b)
   (2) Results from excess growth hormone in adults once the epiphyses are closed.
   (3) Results from excess glucocorticoids.
   (4) Results from excess not a deficiency of thyroid hormones.

556. (2) The thyroid gland produces thyroxine (T_4) and triiodothyronine (T_3), which help regulate oxidation in all body cells. (a)
   (1) Involved in secondary regulation by its secretion of TSH, which stimulates thyroid production of thyroxine and triiodothyronine.
   (3) The primary regulator is the thyroid; the adrenals

exert an influence on metabolism of carbohydrates in times of stress.
   (4) Regulates glucose metabolism by secretion of insulin.

557. (1) Any abnormal sign of vaginal bleeding may be indicative of cervical cancer and must be checked by a physician. (c)
   (2) Discharge becomes foul smelling only after there is necrosis and infection.
   (3) There are few nerve endings, so pain is a late symptom.
   (4) If pressure occurs, it is not an early symptom because the cancer must be extensive to cause pressure.

558. (4) During radiation therapy with radium implants the patient is placed in isolation so exposure to radiation by family and staff will be decreased. (a)
   (1) Excess exposure to radiation is hazardous to personnel.
   (2) An indwelling catheter is left in place to prevent bladder distention.
   (3) Rubber gloves will not protect the nurse from radiation.

559. (2) Radium atoms are unstable and spontaneously disintegrate into other atomic species. This disintegration produces potentially harmful radiation, which is absorbed by lead. (a)
   (1) Heat is not produced during spontaneous disintegration; radiation is.
   (3) Radium is not a heavy substance but an unstable one.
   (4) Disintegration of radium occurs in the lead containers.

560. (3) Time, distance, and shielding are the important factors in determining the amount of radiation the individual receives. Restriction of each visitor to a 10-minute stay minimizes the risk of exposure. Many institutions will not allow visitors while an implant is in place. (c)
   (1) Urine is not radioactive, so no precautions are indicated.
   (2) Lead aprons are effective shields against x rays but not against rays emitted by internal sources of radiation.
   (4) Radium implants will not affect the location of IM injections.

561. (3) Prior to discharge it is important for the nurse to instruct the patient to follow through with medical care at specified intervals. (b)
   (1) Although increased calories may be required, high-fat diets are not encouraged because of associated cardiovascular risks.
   (2) If diet is adequate, multivitamins are unnecessary.
   (4) Fluids are not reduced unless other cardiac or renal pathosis is present.

562. (2) A sharp rise in luteinizing hormone production triggers the rupture of the follicle and ovulation. (c)

(1) FSH stimulates the development of the graafian follicle.

(3) Estrogen stimulates the thickening of the endometrium.

(4) Progesterone prepares the endometrium for the implantation of the fertilized ovum.

563. (1) The function of progesterone is to relax the uterus and maintain a succulent endometrium to foster implantation of the fertilized ovum. (c)

(2) Menstruation is controlled by regulating factors from the hypothalamus and pituitary (FSH-RH, FSH, LH-RH, LH); these hormones stimulate the production of ovarian follicles, ovulation, estrogen, and progesterone by the ovarian cells.

(3) Ovulation is stimulated by increases in the levels of luteinizing hormone (LH) and estrogen.

(4) Capillary fragility is often associated with deficiency of vitamin C (ascorbic acid); progesterone is not responsible.

564. (2) Estrogen is found in the follicular fluid of the ovaries and aids in the growth of the endometrium. (b)

(1) Luteinizing hormone promotes the development of ovarian follicles as well as stimulates ovulation and the production of estrogen and progesterone; progesterone prepares the endometrium for implantation and the breasts for lactation.

(3) These hormones prepare the breasts for milk secretion (lactation).

(4) Luteinizing hormone promotes the development of ovarian follicles as well as stimulates ovulation and the production of estrogen and progesterone by the ovarian cells.

565. (2) Persistent pain of any kind is usually a symptom, and the patient should seek medical attention. (b)

(1) Voluntary relaxation of the abdominal muscles does not cause cessation of uterine contractions.

(3) Although diversion is a method to alter pain perception, the presence of pain requires investigation of possible causes.

(4) Although a nutritious diet is beneficial, iron does not prevent the pain of dysmenorrhea.

566. (1) Mild hypocalcemia sometimes occurs during menstruation. An increase in dietary calcium just before and during menstruation may eliminate or relieve the occasional abdominal cramps resulting from this temporary disorder. (c)

(2) Hyperglycemia (elevated blood glucose levels) is evidenced by polyruia, polydipsia, polyphagia, weight loss, and urine that is positive for sugar and acetone.

(3) Hypernatremia (elevated sodium levels) is evidenced by agitatition, tissue turgor, and oliguria.

(4) Hypokalemia (lowered potassium levels) is evidenced by malaise and muscle weakness.

567. (2) Although sympathetic impulses usually control most visceral effectors in times of stress, parasympathetic fibers likewise stimulate increased gastric contractions and increased peristalsis. Sympathetic fibers also inhibit organs such as the bladder and cause relaxation of this organ. (c)

(1) This statement is accurate.

(3) This statement is accurate.

(4) This statement is accurate.

568. (2) The sympathetic nervous system constricts the smooth muscle of blood vessels in the skin when a person is under stress. (a)

(1) Not under sympathetic control; the parasympathetic system constricts the pupils.

(3) The sympathetic system stimulates rather than inhibits secretion by the sweat glands.

(4) The parasympathetic system (vagus nerve) slows the pulse, and the sympathetic increases it.

569. (2) Parasympathetic nerves increase peristalsis and secretion of gastric hydrochloric acid. (b)

(1) Epinephrine is sympathomimetic.

(3) The parasympathetic nervous system increases intestinal motility, which would result in diarrhea.

(4) Goosebumps, caused by contraction of the musculi arrectores pilorum, are under sympathetic control; vasoconstriction is also under sympathetic control.

570. (2) Only axon terminals secrete acetylcholine, so nerve impulse propagation occurs in one direction only: from axon terminal to dendrite or cell body of the next neuron, or from axon terminal to effector organ (muscle or gland). The action of cholinesterase (to inactivate acetylcholine) has physiologic meaning only at the synapse, where acetylcholine is active; its presence all along the axon would not affect the direction of the nerve impulse. (b)

(1) Does not affect direction; polarization refers to the resting potential of the neuron when one side of the membrane is negatively and the other side positively charged.

(3) Does not affect the direction of the impulse; refers to the active movement of sodium ions into the cell and back across the membrane to the opposite side.

(4) Cholinesterase acts only at the synapse, inactivating acetylcholine at the myoneural junction.

571. (1) Axon terminals release acetylcholine at the myoneural junctions. As acetylcholine contacts the sarcolemma, it stimulates the muscle fiber to contract. (a)

(2) ATP is not produced by axons; it is a nucleotide that gives off energy when it loses a phosphate radical.

(3) Cholinesterase is released by muscle cells.

(4) Epinephrine is produced by the adrenal medulla and released by axons of the autonomic nervous system.

572. (3) Phenytoin (Dilantin) is an anticonvulsant, most effective in controlling grand mal seizures. Data collection before planning nursing care for a patient with epilepsy should always include a history of seizure incidence (type and frequency). (c)

(1) Although protection is important, restraints during a seizure often cause injury as a result of violent muscle contractions.

(2) Although these would be removed during a seizure, the patient's normal routines should be respected.

(4) Increased restlessness may be evidence of the prodromal phase in some individuals, but symptoms vary so widely that the history of the patient should be obtained.

573. (4) To achieve the anticonvulsant effect, therapeutic blood levels of phenytoin must be maintained. If the patient is not able to take the prescribed oral preparation, the physician should be questioned about alternate routes of administration. (b)

(1) The patient is kept n.p.o.

(2) The route of administration cannot be altered without physician approval.

(3) Omission would result in lowered blood levels, possibly below the necessary therapeutic level to prevent a seizure.

574. (2) When an oral medication is available in a suspension form, the nurse should use it for patients with dysphagia. (c)

(1) Since a palatable suspension is available, it is a better alternative than opening the capsule.

(3) Intramuscular injections should be avoided because of related risks of tissue injury and infection.

(4) The route of administration cannot be altered without physician approval.

575. (1) Gingival hyperplasia is a frequently occurring adverse effect of long-term phenytoin (Dilantin) therapy. The incidence can be decreased by meticulous oral hygiene. (c)

(2) This is not a direct effect of Dilantin.

(3) Gingival hyperplasia is a frequently occurring adverse effect of long-term phenytoin therapy. The incidence can be decreased by meticulous oral hygiene.

(4) Gingival hyperplasia is a frequently occurring adverse effect of long-term phenytoin therapy. The incidence can be decreased by meticulous oral hygiene.

576. (4) Phenytoin inhibits folic acid absorption and potentiates the effects of folic acid antagonists. Folic acid therapy is often helpful in correcting certain anemias that can result from administration of phenytoin. (Note: dosage must be carefully adjusted because folic acid diminishes the effects of phenytoin.) (c)

(1) Neurologic side effects include an elevation of the excitability threshold of neurons; not prevented by folic acid.

(2) Although folic acid plays a role in the formation of heme in hemoglobin, its prescription in this case is related to Dilantin.

(3) The description of this situation does not provide data to arrive at this conclusion.

577. (4) Lesions affecting the seventh cranial (facial) nerve cause paralysis of the eyelids. (c)

(1) The optic nerve is concerned with vision; lesions result in visual field defects and loss of visual acuity.

(2) The oculomotor nerve is concerned with pupillary constriction and eye movements; lesions result in ptosis, strabismus, and diplopia.

(3) The trochlear nerve is concerned with eye movements; lesions result in diplopia, strabismus, and head tilt to the affected side.

578. (2) The third cranial (oculomotor) nerve contains autonomic fibers that innervate the smooth muscle responsible for constriction of the pupils. (c)

(1) The optic nerve is concerned with vision; lesions result in visual field defects and loss of visual acuity.

(3) The trochlear nerve is concerned with eye movements; lesions result in diplopia, strabismus, and head tilt to the affected side.

(4) The facial nerve is concerned with facial expressions; lesions result in loss of taste and paralysis of the facial muscles and the eyelids (lids remain open).

579. (1) The facial nerve (seventh cranial) has motor and sensory functions. The motor function is concerned with facial movement, including smiling and pursing the lips. Nonconduction of either right or left will cause dropping on that side. (c)

(2) Nonconduction of the facial nerve on the right side would cause that side of the face to droop.

(3) Nonconduction of the left abducent nerve would prevent abduction of the left eye.

(4) Nonconduction of the trigeminal nerve would cause problems in mastication.

580. (1) Anterior horn neurons are also known as lower motoneurons. Their cell bodies are located in the anterior gray columns and are part of the reflex arc. (c)

(2) Basal ganglia are islands of gray matter in each cerebral hemisphere; not part of the reflex arc.

(3) Pyramidal tracts are motor nerve pathways from the brain that pass down the spinal cord to motor cells in the anterior horn; not part of the reflex arc.

(4) Upper motoneurons are neurons in the cerebral cortex that conduct impulses to the spinal cord or the motor nuclei of the cerebral nerves.

581. (1) Extrapyramidal or motor pathways assist in maintaining muscle tonus; injury usually involves some spasticity. (c)

(2) These are also known as anterior horn neurons; disruption causes flaccid paralysis.

(3) These make up sensory tracts.

(4) Pyramidal tract disorders result in either spastic or flaccid paralysis; spasticity if upper motor neurons involved, flaccidity if lower.

582. (3) This is the space between the arachnoid and the pia mater. It is filled with cerebrospinal fluid. (b)

(1) The cerebral aqueduct, between the third and fourth ventricles, in the midbrain.

(2) An opening in the atrial septum in the fetal heart.

(4) The innermost of the three meninges covering the brain and spinal cord.

583. (1) Pain and temperature sensations enter the posterior horns of the spinal cord, cross to the contralateral side, and travel upward via the spinothalamic tracts to the thalamus. There they synapse with other sensory neurons for transmission to the cortex. (c)
   (2) The location of the fasciculus gracilis, which is involved with pressure sensation.
   (3) Descending motor tracts. The lateral tracts facilitate impulse transmission to the skeletal muscles; the medial tracts inhibit transmission to the skeletal muscles.
   (4) Ascending tracts. They conduct impulses of crude touch, pain, and temperature.

584. (2) Parkinson's disease involves destruction of the neurons of the substantia nigra, caudate nucleus, and globus pallidus of the basal ganglia. The cause of this destruction is unknown. (b)
   (1) This pathologic condition is associated with multiple sclerosis.
   (3) This condition is believed to be associated with myasthenia gravis.
   (4) This condition would result in auditory and visual problems; not associated with Parkinson's disease.

585. (3) Destruction of the neurons of the basal ganglia results in decreased muscle tone. The masklike appearance and monotonous speech patterns can be interpreted as flat. (b)
   (1) Not associated with Parkinson's disease.
   (2) Not associated with Parkinson's disease.
   (4) Not associated with Parkinson's disease.

586. (2) Levodopa is the metabolic precursor of dopamine. It reduces sympathetic outflow by limiting vasoconstriction, which may result in orthostatic hypotension. (b)
   (1) Should be administered with food to minimize gastric irritation.
   (3) Although periodic tests to evaluate hepatic, renal, and cardiovascular therapy are required for prolonged therapy, whether these tests should be done on a weekly basis has not been established.
   (4) May produce either symptom, but no established pattern of such responses exists.

587. (1) Levodopa is the precursor of dopamine. It is converted to dopamine in the brain cells, where it is stored until needed by axon terminals; functions as a neurotransmitter. (b)
   (2) Not an action of L-dopa; neurons do not regenerate.
   (3) Not an action of L-dopa.
   (4) Not an action of L-dopa; once myelin is destroyed, it does not usually regenerate.

588. (3) The cerebellum coordinates muscular activity and promotes balance. The other brain regions govern motor, sensory, and higher integrative functions. (a)
   (1) Controls the heartbeat, blood pressure, and reflexes such as vomiting and coughing.
   (2) Involved in temperature regulation; controls and integrates the autonomic nervous system; intermediary

between the nervous and endocrine systems; associated with feelings of rage and aggression.
   (4) Controls conscious recognition of pain, temperature, and crude touch and pressure.

589. (3) Rehabilitating exercises carried out underwater minimize strain on the partially atrophied and painful joints. The buoyant force of the water makes the limbs easier to move. (b)
   (1) Exercises are carried out near the surface of the water, where the water pressure would have no effect.
   (2) Vapors are produced above water as a result of evaporation; do not facilitate exercise.
   (4) Water temperature would not assist movement.

590. (2) Rheumatoid spondylitis (Marie-Strümpell disease) is a chronic, progressive polyarthritis. Ossification of cartilage, particularly of the spine, causes fixation of the involved joints. (a)
   (1) Redness and swelling are symptoms of local inflammation; do not indicate irreversible damage.
   (3) Inflammation and thickening of the synovial membrane are characteristic of arthritis.
   (4) Although rest is essential, complete immobility would result in a loss of joint motion.

591. (1) ROM exercises must be instituted to maintain mobility of joints. However, overuse may prevent resolution of the inflammation. (a)
   (2) Pain may persist but cannot be allowed to legitimize inactivity.
   (3) Severely damaged joints may require prosthetic replacement.
   (4) Activity will not prevent the inflammatory process; may aggravate it.

592. (3) As a result of the normal stresses on the body, the incidence of chronic illness increases in the elderly population. (a)
   (1) Younger individuals have greater physiologic reserves.
   (2) Younger individuals have greater physiologic reserves.
   (4) Younger individuals have greater physiologic reserves.

593. (3) A balanced diet, consisting of the basic 4 food groups, is essential in maintaining good nutrition. (b)
   (1) Limiting the diet to particular foods does not provide all essential nutrients.
   (2) Limiting the diet to particular foods does not provide all essential nutrients.
   (4) If nutritional intake is adequate, multivitamins are unnecessary.

594. (2) Osteoarthritis affects the hips and knees first because they are the weight-bearing joints and undergo the most stress. (b)
   (1) Although the distal interphalangeal joints are frequently affected, the remaining interphangeal joints and metacarpals are not.
   (3) Although these are weight-bearing joints, normal

motion is not as great as in the hips and knees; thus there is less degeneration.

(4) These are not weight-bearing joints.

595. (1) Psoriasis is characterized by dry scaly lesions that occur most frequently on the elbows, knees, scalp, and torso. (a)

(2) Pruritis, if present at all, is generally mild.

(3) Petechiae are not characteristic.

(4) Erythematous flat spots on the skin as in measles; no scales are present.

596. (3) Steroids are applied locally and usually covered with plastic (or Saran Wrap) at night to reverse the inflammatory process. (b)

(1) Solar rays are used in the treatment of psoriasis.

(2) Potassium permanganate is an antiseptic astringent used on infected, draining, or vesicular lesions.

(4) The plaques are not necrotic and therefore do not require debriding.

597. (1) Scabies is caused by the itch mite (Acarus scabiei), the female of which burrows under the skin to deposit eggs. It is intensely pruritic and is transmitted by direct contact or, in a limited way, by soiled sheets or undergarments. (b)

(2) It is caused by the itch mite, a parasite.

(3) It is an infectious disease and is unrelated to allergies.

(4) Scabies is an acute infection.

598. (4) Pemphigus is primarily a serious disease characterized by large vesicles called bullae. Although potentially fatal, it has been relatively controlled by steroid therapy. (b)

(1) Pemphigus is a disease of the skin.

(2) Pemphigus is a disease of the skin.

(3) Pemphigus is a disease of the skin.

599. (1) The Stryker frame provides for horizontal changes of position to prone or supine while maintaining proper body alignment. (a)

(2) Although the frame itself does not directly promote body functions or prevent deformities, it does enable the nurse to turn the patient, which helps prevent complications of immobility.

(3) Vertical turning is not possible with a Stryker frame.

(4) Vertical turning is not possible with a Stryker frame.

600. (3) The main nursing principles in turning a patient on the Stryker frame are the maintenance of alignment and safety. Securing all bolts and straps ensures that the patient is snug yet comfortably wedged between the frames. (b)

(1) Many patients who require special beds such as the Stryker frame or an electric circular bed are not able to use their arms.

(2) Since the patient is being turned horizontally, hypotension is not a major problem.

(4) The procedure does not require two nurses unless such a protocol is established by the institution.

601. (2) Progressive patient care is based on the precept that different levels of patient needs require different services and facilities. The care provided is specialized and individualized to meet the patient's needs in an appropriate, continuous, and dynamic pattern. (b)

(1) This explanation does not focus on the changing needs of the patient, which is inherent in progressive patient care.

(3) It is only part of answer; does not recognize specialized needs; change does not always mean less intensive care.

(4) Progressive care makes use of these; but they are only part of what is involved in progressive care, which adapts itself to specialized and changing needs of the individual.

602. (4) During prolonged inactivity bone reabsoption proceeds faster than bone formation, and lack of therapeutic weight bearing on bone results in disuse atrophy. A tilt table provides gradual progressive weight bearing, which counters these effects. (c)

(1) Lateral turning is possible and necessary if a patient is immobile and does not require the use of a tilt table.

(2) The tilt table is used for scheduled periods in physical therapy; the nursing care required to prevent decubiti must be consistently performed frequently throughout all shifts.

(3) The tilt table does not cause hyperextension of the spine; the spine remains in normal body alignment.

603. (1) Patients with quadriplegia do not have and never will have the muscle innervation, strength, or balance needed for ambulation. (b)

(2) Orthostatic hypotension can be prevented by any upright positioning and does not necessarily require a wheelchair.

(3) Quadriplegia refers to paralysis of all four extremities.

(4) Bracing and crutch walking require muscle strength and coordination that a quadriplegic individual does not have.

604. (1) The serum acid phosphatase is elevated when the cancer extends beyond the prostate, whereas the serum alkaline phosphatase is elevated in bony metastasis. (b)

(2) Elevated BUN levels may be caused by impaired renal function as a result of blockage by an enlarged prostate but do not indicate that metastasis has occurred.

(3) Elevated creatine levels may be caused by impaired renal function as a result of blockage by an enlarged prostate but do not indicate that metastasis has occurred.

(4) Nonprotein nitrogen refers to waste products from metabolism of protein and includes urea, creatinine, uric acid, and ammonia.

605. (4) Dysuria, nocturia, and urgency are all signs of an irritable bladder after radiation therapy. (b)
  (1) Not an indication of baldder irritability.
  (2) Not an indication of bladder irritability.
  (3) Not an indication of bladder irritability.

606. (3) An enlarged prostate constricts the urethra, interfering with urine flow and causing retention. When the bladder fills and approaches capacity, small amounts can be voided. (b)
  (1) The urge to void is caused by stimulation of the stretch receptors as the bladder fills with urine; in renal failure little or no urine is produced.
  (2) Edema does not cause the patient to void frequently in small amounts; patients with edema void infrequently.
  (4) The urge to void is caused by stimulation of the stretch receptors as the bladder fills with urine; in suppression little or no urine is produced.

607. (1) Catheter patency ensures drainage and prevents bladder distention and other complications. Therefore patency of a catheter should be established prior to notifying the physician. (a)
  (2) Assessment is necessary prior to consultation with the physician.
  (3) Milking a catheter is appropriate when viscous rather than clear drainage is present (e.g., with chest tubes).
  (4) Irrigation is a dependent function and is avoided if possible because of associated risk of infection.

608. (2) Cleansing the urinary meatus and adjacent skin removes accumulated bacteria, limiting the possible introduction of microbes into the urinary tract. (c)
  (1) Although forcing fluids helps prevent urinary stasis and subsequent infection, the most common source of infection is microorganisms from the perineal area.
  (3) Cranberry juice helps acidify the urine to discourage the growth of bacteria but does not eliminate the potential source of infection as cleansing would.
  (4) Irrigations require opening the closed drainage system and allowing the entry of microorganisms; increases the risk of infection.

609. (4) The Foley catheter is always positioned so the level of the bladder with catheter inserted is higher than the level of the drainage container; gravity causes urine flow. (a)
  (1) Refers to a property of matter.
  (2) Passage of molecules from high concentration to low concentration.
  (3) Diffusion of water across a semipermeable membrane; not responsible for the flow of urine through a catheter.

610. (1) An indwelling catheter dilates the urinary sphincters, keeps the bladder empty, and short-circuits the normal reflex mechanism based on bladder distention. When the catheter is removed, the body must adapt to functioning once again. (b)
  (2) Although retention may result from any interruption in normal voiding habits, this is the only condition that applies in such a situation.
  (3) Although retention may result from any interruption in normal voiding habits, this is the only condition that applies in such a situation.
  (4) Although retention may result from any interruption in normal voiding habits, this is the only condition that applies in such a situation.

611. (1) When the testes are twisted, a decrease in their blood supply occurs. This can result in gangrene. (c)
  (2) Pain can be alleviated through the use of medication.
  (3) Although edema occurs, the testes do not rupture.
  (4) Sperm are continually produced, so their destruction is not the concern.

612. (3) The tourniquets must be rotated in a clockwise direction at 15-minute intervals so venous outflow in any one extremity is not occluded more than 45 minutes at a time. (b)
  (1) Arterial blood flow cannot be totally occluded, or cell death will occur.
  (2) One extremity is left without a tourniquet every 15 minutes.
  (4) Since tourniquets are applied to 3 of the 4 extremities, only one tourniquet is rotated at a time.

613. (3) Application of rotating tourniquets keeps blood in the extremities, decreasing venous return to reduce pulmonary artery pressure and relieve pulmonary congestion. (b)
  (1) The aim is to maintain adequate arterial flow to prevent tissue hypoxia.
  (2) Visceral blood flow is not primarily affected.
  (4) Capillary blood flow is not primarily affected.

614. (4) The exact mode of action of morphine sulfate is unknown. However, it has a rapid onset, lowers blood pressure, and decreases pulmonary reflexes, producing sedation. (c)
  (1) Hydroxyzine hydrochloride is generally used to control anxiety associated with less acute situations and is available in oral form only.
  (2) Phenobarbital has a slower onset than morphine and does not affect respirations and blood pressure to the same extent as morphine.
  (3) Chloral hydrate is a hypnotic but is not appropriate for the acute situation described.

615. (2) Ethacrynic acid interferes with the concentrating and diluting mechanism of the descending and ascending limbs of the renal tubule and the concentrating process in the collecting duct. It inhibits the active transport of chloride ions back into the blood. A copious and dilute urine high in chloride and sodium ions is excreted. (c)
  (1) Potassium-sparing diuretic; less potent than thiazide diuretics.
  (3) Although used in the treatment of edema and hypertension, this drug is not as potent as ethacrynic acid.

(4) Although used in the treatment of edema and hypertension, this drug is not as potent as ethacrynic acid.

616. (3) Aminophylline, a theophylline derivative, promotes diuresis and relaxes smooth muscles, resulting in hypotension. (b)
   (1) Side effects include sinus tachycardia.
   (2) Urine output is increased.
   (4) Not a side effect of the drug.

617. (2) The fluid level in the manometer fluctuates with respiration because the changes in thoracic pressure affect the pressure in the right atrium. (b)
   (1) The positive pressure of a ventilator alters the central venous pressure readings, so the ventilator must be removed when CVP is taken.
   (3) Although the CVP line is not used routinely for blood samples, blood can be easily aspirated.
   (4) To approximate the level of the right atrium, the ''O'' level should be even with the midaxillary line.

618. (3) Deslanoside (Cedilanid-D) can be administered slowly by IV infusion. (c)
   (1) This can never be administered intravenously.
   (2) This can never be administered intravenously.
   (4) This can never be administered intravenously.

619. (3) Cardioversion involves administration of precordial shock, which is synchronized with the R wave to interrupt the heart rate. It is used for atrial fibrillation, paroxysmal atrial tachycardia (PAT), and ventricular tachycardia when pharmaceutical preparations fail. The heart is stopped by the electric stimulation, and it is hoped that the SA node will take over as pacemaker. (c)
   (1) Since there are no R waves, the shock would not be delivered.
   (2) Premature ventricular contractions suggest irritable myocardium and generally respond well to antiarrhythmic agents.
   (4) Since there are no R waves, the shock would not be delivered.

620. (2) Ventricular fibrillation is a death-producing arrhythmia and, once identified, must be terminated immediately by precordial shock (defibrillation). This is usually a standing physician's order in a cardiac care unit. (c)
   (1) CPR is instituted only when defibrillation fails to terminate the arrhythmia.
   (3) Bicarbonate is administered to correct acidosis; does not take priority over defibrillation.
   (4) Oxygen is administered to correct hypoxia; does not take priority over defibrillation.

621. (2) The precordial shock during cardioversion must not be delivered on the T wave, or ventricular fibrillation may ensue. By placing the synchronizer in the ''on'' position, the physician presets the machine so it will not deliver the shock on the T wave. (b)
   (1) The energy level may be set from 50 to 400 watt-seconds.

(3) This will not ensure that the shock is not delivered on the T wave.
   (4) This will not ensure that the shock is not delivered on the T wave.

622. (2) The height of the ventricular complexes must be sufficient to be picked up by the voltmeter, which will sound an alarm if the heart rate is outside the high and low parameters. (c)
   (1) The oscilloscope is the screen on which the electrical signals from the heart are displayed.
   (3) The pulse generator (pacemaker) may be either an internal or an external device but is generally not part of the monitor.
   (4) The synchronizer is used only during cardioversion to ensure that the electric shock is delivered during the QRS complex.

623. (1) Atrial fibrillation is the rapid discharge of impulses from a focus other than the SA node. Since not all these impulses are transmitted through the AV node, the ventricular response varies. Quinidine inhibits discharge of electric impulses from such ectopic foci, whereas digoxin delays the conduction of impulses from the AV node, slowing down the rate of ventricular response to impulses from the atria. (b)
   (2) Digoxin increases vagal activity to slow the heart rate, and quinidine inhibits ion exchange across the cellular membrane; thus excitability of the atrial and ventricular myocardium is decreased, intraventricular and AV nodal conduction is slowed, and the refractory period is prolonged.
   (3) This is true of quinidine but doesn't explain the action of digoxin.
   (4) This is only partially true. Digoxin increases vagal activity to slow the heart rate, and quinidine inhibits ion exchange across the cellular membrane; thus excitability of the atrial and ventricular myocardium is decreased, intraventricular and AV nodal conduction is slowed, and the refractory period is prolonged.

624. (3) The apex of the heart is between the fifth and sixth ribs at the midclavicular line. It is closest to the chest wall here, so auscultation is easier. (b)
   (1) Although it may be possible to auscultate the heart in this area, it is usually easier to do so over the apex.
   (2) Although it may be possible to auscultate the heart in this area, it is usually easier to do so over the apex.
   (4) Although it may be possible to auscultate the heart in this area, it is usually easier to do so over the apex.

625. (1) Adverse effects of digoxin include many types of arrhythmias. An apical pulse rate less than 60 or above 120 contraindicates administration of the drug. Since the patient will be taking the medication at home, he must be taught to take his own pulse

and to contact the physician if the rate falls outside the parameters mentioned. (b)

(2) Since the patient will be assuming responsibility for drug administration at home, teaching is more of a priority than the nurse's observations.

(3) Since the patient will be assuming responsibility for drug administration at home, teaching is more of a priority than the nurse's observations.

(4) Since the patient will be assuming responsibility for drug administration at home, teaching is more of a priority than the nurse's observations.

626. (4) The Nurse Practice Act states that nurses diagnose human responses to actual or potential health problems. The nurse used her knowledge. (b)

(1) Since the patient's symptoms reflected an immediate need for oxygen, postponement of treatment could result in further deterioration of her condition.

(2) Since the patient's symptoms reflected an immediate need for oxygen, postponement of treatment could result in further deterioration of her condition.

(3) Since the patient's symptoms reflected an immediate need for oxygen, postponement of treatment could result in further deterioration of her condition.

627. (2) The 2 coronary arteries are the first branches of the aorta and carry blood with a high oxygen content to the myocardium. (c)

(1) They carry blood with high oxygen content to the myocardium.

(3) Carry blood with high oxygen content to the myocardium, not the endocardium.

(4) This is function of the pulmonary veins.

628. (1) Angina pectoris is the pain referred to the chest wall and caused by hypoxia of the cardiac muscle. (b)

(2) There is no cell death in angina.

(3) A coronary thrombosis is an aggregation of platelets, clotting factors, and blood cellular elements that reduces the lumen of the artery; may progress to a complete obstruction, resulting in a myocardial infarction.

(4) Mitral insufficiency refers to an incompetent mitral valve; could be only indirectly related to angina.

629. (2) Anginal pain, which can be anticipated during certain activities, may be prevented by dilating the coronary arteries immediately before engaging in the activity. (b)

(1) One tablet is generally administered at a time; doubling the dosage may produce severe hypotension and headache.

(3) The sublingual form of nitroglycerin is absorbed directly through the mucous membranes and should not be swallowed

(4) When the pain is relieved, rest will generally prevent its recurrence by reducing oxygen consumption of myocardium.

630. (1) Nitroglycerin tablets are affected by light, heat, and moisture. A loss of potency can be detected by absence of a tingling sensation when the tablet is

placed under the tongue or by its ineffectiveness in relieving pain. A new supply should be obtained immediately. (c)

(2) Does not necessarily indicate a loss of potency.

(3) Does not necessarily indicate a loss of potency.

(4) Does not necessarily indicate a loss of potency.

631. (4) In addition to GI disturbances, visual disturbances such as blurred vision may be evidence of digitalis toxicity. Heart rates over 120 may also indicate toxicity. (b)

(1) This is not a symptom of digitalis toxicity.

(2) This is not a symptom of digitalis toxicity.

(3) This is not a symptom of digitalis toxicity.

632. (3) Toxic levels of digitalis overstimulate the vagus nerve, leading to depressed conduction through the AV node (AV block of any degree) as well as SA node depression (sinus bradycardia). In addition, ectopic pacemakers are accelerated, leading to multiple premature beats. Such pathologic effects are enhanced by low serum potassium levels from diuretics, vomiting, and nasogastric drainage as well as by chronic arterial hypoxemia and impared renal function. (b)

(1) Untrue statement.

(2) True but not specific to the situation described.

(4) Vitamins act as coenzymes.

633. (1) Whole milk is high in saturated fat. (a)

(2) High in unsaturated fat.

(3) High in unsaturated fat

(4) Low fat content.

634. (4) Vegetable oils, like most lipids from plants, are high in unsaturated fats. (b)

(1) Meats are high in saturated fats.

(2) Animal-derived products such as milk are high in saturated fats.

(3) Meats are high in saturated fats.

635. (3) Thromboplastin is a substance released by platelets that initiates the clotting process by converting prothrombin to thrombin. (b)

(1) Plasma does not produce thromboplastin.

(2) RBCs do not produce thromboplastin.

(4) Bile does not contain thromboplastin.

636. (2) Fibrinogen is a soluble plasma protein that becomes the insoluble clot, fibrin, during the clotting process. (c)

(1) Fibrin is the insoluble gel formed from fibrinogen by the action of thrombin.

(3) Prothrombin is the precursor of thrombin; becomes fibrinogin.

(4) Thrombin is needed to convert fibrinogen to fibrin; also needed in platelet aggregation.

637. (2) Calcium acts as a catalyst to convert prothrombin to thrombin. Thrombin accelerates the formation of insoluble fibrin from the soluble fibrinogen. (c)

(1) Iron is essential for the synthesis of hemoglobin, which is not involved in clotting.

(3) Fluorine is a gas of the halogen group and is not

involved in clotting; sodium fluoride helps harden tooth enamel.

(4) Chloride is an extracellular anion that helps regulate osmotic pressure and combines with hydrogen to form hydrochloric acid; not involved with clotting.

638. (4) In the process of rocking, the Trendelenburg position facilitates venous return from the lower extremities; reverse Trendelenburg decreases the pressure of the abdominal organs on the diaphragm, allowing maximum lung expansion. (c)

(1) Refers to a force directed outward from a central point, such as the force responsible for the planets' orbiting the sun.

(2) Refers to the tendency of a body at rest to remain at rest or if in motion to remain so.

(3) Refers to the force of a moving object; equal to mass times velocity.

639. (2) The residual volume is the amount of air remaining in the lungs after maximum exhalation. (b)

(1) The force exerted by the abdominal thrust surpasses that which the individual is voluntarily capable of exerting; normally under the individual's control.

(3) The force exerted by the abdominal thrust surpasses that which the individual is voluntarily capable of exerting; normally under the individual's control.

(4) The force exerted by the abdominal thrust surpasses that which the individual is voluntarily capable of exerting; normally under the individual's control.

640. (3) Sodium polystyrene sulfonate, a cation exchange resin used in the treatment of hyperkalemia, will release sodium ions in the intestines in exchange for potassium ions. Sorbitol has a hyperosmotic effect in the intestinal tract concomitantly maintaining the liquid content of the feces and counteracting the constipating effect of the resin. (b)

(1) Does not provide carbohydrates.

(2) Does not reflect a combined effect.

(4) Sorbitol counteracts the constipating effect of resin.

641. (3) In hepatic coma there is an accumulation of nitrogenous wastes, which affect the nervous system. In the second stage of this disease there are flapping tremors and generalized twitching. (b)

(1) Elevated cholesterol levels not necessarily present.

(2) Hepatic coma includes CNS disturbances; the stool is often clay colored as a result of biliary obstruction by a cirrhotic liver.

(4) As encephalopathy progesses to coma, all reflexes are absent.

642. (4) Bile deposits will impart a yellowish tinge (jaundice or icterus) to the skin, often first observed in the sclerae. (c)

(1) Uremic frost is characteristic of renal failure.

(2) Urticaria (or hives) is generally characteristic of an allergic response.

(3) Hemangioma is a benign lesion composed of blood vessels.

643. (3) In cirrhosis of the liver fibrous scarring within the

liver parenchyma, most often from alcohol toxicity, compresses the portal veins and causes a backup of blood and increased pressure within the portal system. Ascitic fluid (interstitial fluid) forms in excess and seeps into the abdominal cavity, mainly from the surface of the liver. (b)

(1) Plasma osmotic pressure is decreased because of decreased albumin production.

(2) Lymph does not escape from the liver sinusoids.

(4) Secretion of ADH and aldosterone increases as renal blood flow decreases.

644. (2) The increased plasma hydrostatic pressure in the extremities resulting from heart failure or liver cirrhosis, possibly combined with a genetic weakness in the vein walls, may lead to varicose veins. (c)

(1) Toxins are not responsible for varicose veins.

(3) Decreased plasma protein causes fluid to move out of the vascular compartment into the interstitial spaces.

(4) Distention of venous walls occurs as a result of increased rather than decreased pressure.

645. (4) Increased ammonia levels indicate the inability of the liver to detoxify protein by-products. Neomycin reduces the amount of ammonia-forming bacteria in the intestines. (c)

(1) Culture and sensitivity testing would identify the presence of a microorganism and which medication would be effective in its erradication; would not be indicated in cirrhosis.

(2) Serum glutamic-pyruvic transaminase (SGPT) is a test to assess for liver disease but has no relationship to the need for neomycin enemas.

(3) White blood cells may indicate the presence of infection; however, this would have no relationship to the need for neomycin enemas.

646. (2) The hepatic portal vein carries blood from the capillary beds of the viscera (small and large intestinal walls, stomach, spleen, pancreas, gallbladder) to the sinusoids of the liver. The hepatic veins drain the liver sinusoids into the inferior vena cava. (b)

(1) Takes blood to the liver; the hepatic veins drain the liver sinusoids into the inferior vena cava.

(3) Enters from the capillary beds of the viscera.

(4) Enters from the capillary beds of the viscera.

647. (1) Prothrombin, which is normally present in the plasma, is synthesized in the liver in the presence of vitamin K from the amino acid glutamine. Vitamin K initiates the vital process of coagulation. (b)

(2) Needed for hemoglobin synthesis.

(3) Involved in calcium absorption and metabolism.

(4) Plays a role in collagen formation.

648. (4) Vitamin K is a fat-soluble vitamin and needs bile salts for its absorption from the upper segment of the small intestine. It is a catalyst in the carboxylation of glutamine to prothrombin. (c)

(1) Bile salts do not affect prothrombinase (thromboplastin).

(2) Bile salts do not inhibit the synthesis of prothrombin.

(3) The liver does not synthesize vitamin K; intestines do.

649. (2) This is negligence. The patient should have been informed. Also the nurse was responsible for collecting the specimen. (b)

(1) The physician prescribes the diagnostic test, but the proper collection and handling of specimens are the nurse's responsibility.

(3) Staff are liable for negligent actions.

(4) The hospital should assume the added expense incurred as a result of the negligent actions of its employees.

650. (4) Vitamin K is synthesized by intestinal bacteria but is also found in liver, egg yolks, cheese, tomatoes, and green leafy vegetables. (b)

(1) Vitamin K is found in a small variety of foods.

(2) Vitamin K is not easily absorbed; it is fat soluble and requires bile salts for its absorption.

(3) It is found in enough foods that a natural deficiency usually does not occur.

651. (2) Cirrhosis of the liver results in the development of extensive scar tissue within the liver structure; such scar tissue contracts around hepatic blood vessels, impeding blood flow and raising the pressure in the hepatic portal system. The physiologic response to slowly developing portal circulatory obstruction is the growth of collateral vessels linking portal veins with esophageal veins; as destruction progresses, the collaterals become so large that they bulge into the esophageal lumen and are called esophageal varices. (b)

(1) The varicosities are the result of increased portal pressure.

(3) Ascites and edema are the result of the liver pathophysiologic process, not the cause; the fluid is present in the interstitial spaces and abdominal cavity as a result of portal hypertension and decreased plasma protein.

(4) The liver regenerates; but in the case of cirrhosis, scar tissue is formed.

652. (3) Gastric suctioning provides an estimate of the extent of bleeding but does not control it. (a)

(1) Aminocaproic acid inhibits the fibrinolysis that may accompany hepatic cirrhosis.

(2) Balloon tamponade (Sengstaken-Blakemore tube) may be used to apply pressure against the bleeding varices.

(4) Iced saline is instilled via a nasogastric tube to control hemorrhage; cold promotes blood vessel constriction.

653. (2) Neomycin destroys intestinal flora, which breaks down protein and in the process gives off ammonia. Ammonia at this time is poorly detoxified by the liver and can build up to toxic levels. (b)

(1) Urea is a by-product of protein metabolism; formed in the liver as it detoxifies ammonia. The production of urea is hampered by severe liver damage and is unaffected by neomycin.

(3) Bile levels may be elevated because of biliary obstruction by the enlarged liver but are unaffected by neomycin.

(4) Hemoglobin levels may be lowered as a result of cirrhosis and bleeding but are not increased by administration of neomycin.

654. (1) This tube has an esophageal balloon that on inflation exerts pressure, which retards hemorrhage. (b)

(2) This is used for intestinal decompression.

(3) This is used for intestinal decompression.

(4) This is used for gastric decompression or gavage.

655. (2) The patient's breath has a sweet odor because the liver is not metabolizing the amino acid methionine. (b)

(1) Anuria is characteristic of renal failure.

(3) Sensation of a lump in the throat associated with acute anxiety; unrelated to liver disease.

(4) Refers to spasm of the eyelid associated with anxiety or cranial nerve pathosis; unrelated to liver disease.

656. (1) Since protein breakdown gives off ammonia, which cannot be detoxified by the liver, protein should be eliminated from the diet. (b)

(2) Carbohydrates are unrelated to protein breakdown and rising ammonia levels; eliminating carbohydrates would have no effect.

(3) A Fleet enema would not affect ammonia levels, which are associated with hepatic coma; a neomycin enema would limit intestinal flora, which breaks down protein, giving off ammonia.

(4) No surgical intervention would affect ammonia levels associated with hepatic coma.

657. (2) Low sodium controls fluid retention, blood pressure, and consequently edema; low protein controls ammonia formation in proportion to the liver's ability to detoxify ammonia in forming urea; moderate fat and high calories and vitamins help repair a long-standing nutritional deficit. (b)

(1) High-protein diets are contraindicated because of the liver's inability to detoxify ammonia.

(3) Regeneration of tissue requires a high-calorie diet; 1200 calories is too low.

(4) Since protein is required for tissue regeneration, restriction is based on the liver's ability to detoxify ammonia; a high-fat diet is avoided because of the related cardiovascular risks and increased need for bile.

658. (1) Because of the liver's inability to detoxify ammonia to urea, protein intake should be further restricted when coma is inevitable. (b)

(2) Normal intake of protein is 55 to 60 gm; this high-protein diet will further increase blood ammonia levels.

(3) Normal intake of protein is 55 to 60 gm; this high-protein diet will further increase blood ammonia levels.

(4) Normal intake of protein is 55 to 60 gm; this high-protein diet will further increase blood ammonia levels.

659. (3) Patients with aphasia must be encouraged to speak so that communication ability is regained. (b)

(1) Despite difficulty speaking, individuals with expressive aphasia can understand what is said to them.

(2) To avoid frustration, needs should be anticipated.

(4) Speech can usually be improved through therapy.

660. (2) A patient who is comatose loses voluntary control of elimination. (a)

(1) Since there are different levels of coma, the individual may respond to intense stimuli such as pain.

(3) Since cerebral functioning is depressed, purposeful or voluntary movement is absent.

(4) Twitching motions may be evidence of abnormal cerebral electrical activity; such seizurelike activity is present in only comatose individuals.

661. (1) Absence of a gag reflex is common after a CVA. To prevent aspiration, the patient is positioned on the side to allow gravity to drain mucus in the nasopharyngeal area away from the trachea. (b)

(2) Chest expansion is hindered in the prone position.

(3) This position allows the tongue to occlude the airway and encourages the aspiration of secretions if the gag reflex is not intact.

(4) This position allows the tongue to occlude the airway and encourages the aspiration of secretions if the gag reflex is not intact.

662. (2) Passive ROM exercises prevent the development of deformities and yet do not require any energy expenditure by the patient who is confined to bed. Instituting ROM exercises is an independent nursing function. (b)

(1) Bed rest is prescribed to decrease oxygen demands; active exercises markedly increase oxygen consumption.

(3) Bed rest is prescribed to decrease oxygen demands; active exercises markedly increase oxygen consumption.

(4) Bed rest is prescribed to decrease oxygen demands; active exercises markedly increase oxygen consumption.

663. (3) Changes in self-image and family role can initiate a grieving process with a variety of emotional responses. (a)

(1) This cannot be assumed from the situation described unless the patient's feelings are elicited.

(2) The ability to cope successfully with an illness varies widely between individuals.

(4) This cannot be assumed from the situation described unless the patient's feelings are elicited.

664. (4) To foster communication and cooperation, family members should be involved in planning and implementing care. (a)

(1) This intervention does not focus on Mrs. Green's feelings or needs.

(2) This intervention does not focus on Mrs. Green's feelings or needs.

(3) The nurse remains responsible; Mrs. Green may promote dependency of her husband to satisfy her own needs.

665. (2) The brachial plexus is a maze of nerves extending from the axilla to the neck in the shoulder area; trauma to the arm may also injure this plexus. (a)

(1) The basilar plexus is a venous plexus over the basilar part of the occipital bone; unrelated to the arms.

(3) The celiac plexus (solar plexus) is where the splanchnic nerves terminate; unrelated to the arms.

(4) The solar plexus, also known as the celiac plexus, is where the splanchnic nerves terminate; unrelated to the arms.

666. (1) The medulla contains the vital respiratory, cardiac, and vasomotor centers. (a)

(2) The midbrain deals with sensory input from the eyes and ears.

(3) Conducts impulses; reflex centers for cranial nerves V, VI, VII, VIII (trigeminal, abducent, facial, vestibulocochlear).

(4) Sensory impulses to sensations.

667. (1) The hypothalamus connects with the autonomic area for vasoconstriction, vasodilation, and perspiration and with the somatic centers for shivering; therefore it is an important area for regulating body temperature. (a)

(2) The pallidum is part of the basal ganglia; also called the globus pallidus. Together with the putamen, it compresses the lenticular nucleus; concerned with muscle tone, which is required for specific body movements.

(3) The temporal lobe is concerned with auditory stimuli; may also be involved with the sense of smell.

(4) Receives all sensory stimuli, except taste, for transmission to the cerebral cortex; also involved with emotions and instinctive activities.

668. (2) The eighth cranial nerve has two (2) parts—the vestibular nerve and the cochlear nerve. Sensations of hearing are conducted by the cochlear nerve. (a)

(1) Cranial nerve VI (abducent) is concerned with abduction of the eye.

(3) The frontal lobe is concerned with thinking, skeletal muscle tone, and biorhythms.

(4) The occipital lobe is concerned with sight, particularly shape and color.

669. (2) The primary site of action is the motor cortex, where seizure activity is limited by maintaining the sodium ion gradient of the neurons. (b)

(1) This incorrectly describes the pharmacologic action of Dilantin.

(3) This incorrectly describes the pharmacologic action of Dilantin.

(4) This incorrectly describes the pharmacologic action of Dilantin.

670. (4) The respiratory tract can be obstructed during a seizure, and therefore a plastic airway should be available at all times for patients with convulsive disorders. (b)

(1) Taking a blood pressure reading will not protect the patient; maintaining a patent airway is a priority.

(2) Oxygen does not prevent seizures, nor would it be used during a seizure because the individual does not breathe; if an airway is maintained, room air is usually sufficient after a seizure.

(3) The use of a tongue blade is losing popularity because of the danger of airway occlusion when the blade is forced into place.

671. (3) Seizure disorders are usually associated with marked changes in the electrical activity of the cerebral cortex, requiring prolonged or lifelong therapy. (b)

(1) Absence of seizures would probably be due to medication effectiveness rather than to correction of the pathophysiologic condition.

(2) A therapeutic blood level must be maintained through consistent administration of drug.

(4) Seizures may occur despite drug therapy; the dosage may need to be adjusted.

672. (3) The precentral gyrus is the most posterior convolution of the frontal lobe and the primary motor area. Other gyri also contain motor neurons. (c)

(1) The basal ganglia are islands of gray matter within the cerebral hemispheres; one activity with which they are concerned is muscle tone, required for specific body movement.

(2) The parietal lobes translate nerve impulses into sensations such as taste, touch, and temperature.

(4) The postcentral gyrus is the primary sensory area of the cerebral cortex; unrelated to motor activity.

673. (3) There are no dietary restrictions, but iron and vitamins should be encouraged to normalize any underlying nutritional deficiencies. (b)

(1) A normal protein intake should fulfill nutritional needs.

(2) Sodium retention is not a major complication, so a salt-free diet is not indicated.

(4) Bland diets are usually prescribed for gastric disturbances.

674. (2) Because of its antiinflammatory effect, aspirin is useful in treating arthritis symptoms. (a)

(1) Narcotics should be avoided because they promote dependency and do not affect the inflammatory process.

(3) Narcotics should be avoided because they promote dependency and do not affect the inflammatory process.

(4) Pentobarbital sodium (Nembutal) is a hypnotic not

an analgesic; normal adult dosage is 100 to 200 mg p.o.h.s.

675. (3) Exercise of involved joints is important to maintain optimal mobility and prevent buildup of calcium deposits. (c)

(1) Immobilization causes loss of joint mobility and contractures.

(2) Immobilization causes loss of joint mobility and contractures.

(4) Immobilization causes loss of joint mobility and contractures.

676. (2) Steroids have an antiinflammatory effect, which can reduce arthritic pannus formation. (c)

(1) Ankylosis refers to fusion of joints. It is only indirectly influenced by steroids, which exert their major effect on the inflammatory process.

(3) Not a use for the drug; steroids can cause mood swings.

(4) The relief of pain is incorporated into the antiinflammatory actions of steroids.

677. (4) Marie-Strümpell disease is synonymous with rheumatoid spondylitis, which involves fixation of joints (usually vertebral). (c)

(1) As the cartilage of the joints degenerates, there are hypertrophic changes of the bone edges, which eventually replace the articular cartilage.

(2) Ankylosis occurs in rheumatoid arthritis, not in hypertrophic or degenerative arthritis.

(3) Heberden nodules are the bony or cartilaginous enlargements of the distal interphalangeal joints that are associated with degenerative arthritis.

678. (2) Synovial fluid minimizes friction at joints by providing lubrication for the moving parts. (b)

(1) Synovial fluid increases the speed of movements.

(3) Synovial fluid increases the efficiency of joint movements.

(4) Synovial fluid increases work output.

679. (3) The patient has a right to know what medication she is receiving (informed consent). This also constitutes an invasion of the patient's rights. (b)

(1) The patient has a right to refuse treatment and a right for an explanation of treatment prior to its administration; that patient's right takes precedence over the doctor's order.

(2) This cannot be determined from the situation described; the patient should have been questioned about her reasons for refusing the drug to determine her level of understanding.

(4) The physician should have been notified only after the nurse had interviewed the patient to determine the reasons for her decision; this would have been the time to impart the appropriate information.

680. (2) Synovial joints, like the knee, shoulder, or articulations between the middle ear bones, are lined with synovial membrane. (a)

(1) Serous membrane does not line joints but rather areas such as the thoracic and abdominal cavities.

(3) Mucous membrane lines passages that open to the exterior of the body such as the mouth and the genitourinary tract.

(4) Epithelium covers the internal and external organs of the body, including the skin.

681. (3) The nurse should obtain the drug from the pharmacy to meet the patient's need for relief of pain immediately. (a)

(1) Other medication cannot be substituted without the physician's approval.

(2) To prevent recurrence of a similar situation, another patient's supplies should not be depleted.

(4) Requiring the patient to wait imposes unnecessary discomfort and may intensify the pain.

682. (2) Decubiti easily develop when a particular position is maintained; the body weight, directed continuously in one region, restricts circulation and results in tissue necrosis. (a)

(1) Patients often state that they are comfortable and wish to remain in one position.

(3) Since turning is usually done laterally, the circulation to the lower extremities is not dramatically affected.

(4) Proper positioning with supportive devices and ROM are more effective measures to prevent contractures.

683. (4) The paraplegic patient is unable to exercise actively. (c)

(1) Changing a position involves moving the extremities. Contractures develop as a result of prolonged immobility.

(2) The use of pillows, splints, and other supportive devices helps maintain alignment and prevent the shortening of muscle fibers associated with contractures.

(3) Passive ROM helps maintain joint mobility and muscle tone.

684. (3) Calcium leaves the long bones during periods of prolonged bed rest. The tilt table places the patient in an upright position, which provides for weight bearing. (b)

(1) The tilt table is used to prevent orthostatic hypotension by gradually allowing an individual who has been immobilized to adjust to an upright position.

(2) Although the pressure on bony prominences is altered, the use of the tilt table is not frequent enough to prevent the development of decubiti.

(4) The patient is carefully strapped to the table so that mobility is actually impaired to ensure safety.

685. (4) Calcium that has left the bones as a response to prolonged inactivity enters the blood and may precipitate in the kidneys, forming calculi. (b)

(1) Increased fluid intake is helpful in avoiding this condition by preventing urinary stasis.

(2) Calcium intake is usually limited to prevent the increasing risk of calculi.

(3) Calculi may develop despite adequate kidney function; kidney function may be impaired by the presence of calculi and the high incidence of urinary tract infections associated with urinary stasis or repeated catheterizations.

686. (1) To promote optimism and facilitate smooth functioning, all rehabilitation should begin on admission to the hospital. (a)

(2) Since paralysis is permanent, alterations in normal life-style are required.

(3) The patient and family are often unaware of options available in the health care system; the nurse should be available to provide necessary information and support.

(4) Since the paralysis is permanent, rehabilitation plans should be made.

687. (4) Because of the location of the micturition reflex center (in the sacral region of the spinal cord), bladder function may be impaired with lower spinal cord injuries. (b)

(1) Since there is no voluntary control over the lower extremities mobility is usually accomplished through the use of a wheelchair rather than ambulation.

(2) Plans for education are usually postponed until the patient has had a chance to deal with his feelings; high anxiety interferes with learning.

(3) These exercises require motor control, which the patient does not have.

688. (1) Correct positioning prevents the patient from assumming incorrect positions, which could result in contracture formation. (a)

(2) The tilt board is used primarily to prevent orthostatic hypotension or bone demineralization.

(3) Since he is paralyzed, active exercises are not possible.

(4) Deep massage may dislodge thrombi that have formed as a result of venous stasis.

689. (3) Sneezing, as well as lifting and straining, causes an increase in the intraspinal pressure, resulting in pain. (c)

(1) Does not affect the intraspinal pressure.

(2) Maximizes the intervertebral spaces, relieving pressure and pain.

(4) Although pain may increase as a result of compression of the vertebrae, the increase is gradual not sudden.

690. (4) Compresses are not required after a spinal puncture. (c)

(1) Careful assessment is required to detect possible injury to the spinal cord.

(2) To prevent severe headache, which may accompany the procedure, the head of the bed is not elevated and fluids are encouraged.

(3) To prevent severe headache, which may accompany the procedure, the head of the bed is not elevated and fluids are encouraged.

691. (3) Ambulation may be postponed for several days. The use of back braces or body casts varies. (b)
    (1) The bed is generally kept flat; prevents strain on the operative site.
    (2) The patient is log rolled from side to side; will prevent complications of immobility while vertebral alignment is maintained.
    (4) To detect damage or compression of the spinal cord, assessment of motor and sensory status is necessary.

692. (3) A laminectomy that involves the removal of portions of one or more vertebrae is generally done in conjunction with removal of a herniated disc. Inflammation from the trauma of surgery could lead to compression of the spinal cord, with consequent motor or sensory dysfunction. (b)
    (1) Urinary retention rather than spasticity may occur if pressure on the cord occurs as a result of edema or bleeding.
    (2) Pain is usually experienced at the operative site and in the legs as a result of edema around the cord.
    (4) Cerebral edema does not occur.

693. (2) Sore throat and oral secretions are additional problems of the patient after cervical laminectomy. (c)
    (1) Limited range of motion occurs after both operations.
    (3) To prevent strain on the operative site, flexion of the head is avoided.
    (4) The head of the bed may be only slightly elevated after a cervical laminectomy.

694. (2) Radium, a radioactive isotope, is used to destroy or delay the growth of malignant cells. Special care is taken to maintain normal tissue and not allow it to come closer to the radioactive substance than is necessary. Distance, along with time and shielding, is a way of limiting exposure. (b)
    (1) This is not true.
    (3) This is the physician's decision; it may be reinserted.
    (4) Not the purpose of vaginal packing; there should be no active bleeding with radium implants although there may be cellular sloughing.

695. (4) While the patient is receiving therapy, alpha, beta, and gamma rays will be emitted. Therefore the nurse should employ the principles of time, distance, and shielding when providing care. Extent of exposure to the patient must be monitored and kept within safe limits depending on the type and amount of rays emitted. (a)
    (1) To prevent excessive exposure, the nurse should plan effectively to limit the total patient contact time.
    (2) Normal activity must be limited so the implant will not become dislodged.
    (3) To ensure that any radium has not been inadvertently dislodged, the linen must be carefully examined.

696. (2) Pain and elevated temperature may indicate toxic effects. Excessive sloughing of tissue can cause hemorrhage or infection. (b)
    (1) Expected side effects of internal radiotherapy.
    (3) Expected side effects of internal radiotherapy.
    (4) Expected side effects of internal radiotherapy.

697. (4) Foil-lined rubber gloves do not provide adequate shielding from the gamma rays emitted by radium. (b)
    (1) Radium should be handled with long-handled forceps since distance helps limit exposure.
    (2) Radium should be handled with long-handled forceps since distance helps limit exposure.
    (3) The amount and duration of exposure are important in assessing the effect on the patient.

698. (2) Bicarbonate buffering is limited, hydrogen ions accumulate, and acidosis results. (c)
    (1) The rate of respirations increases in metabolic acidosis to compensate for a low pH.
    (3) The fluid balance does not significantly alter the pH.
    (4) The retention of sodium ions is related to fluid retention and edema rather than to acidosis.

699. (1) The kidneys are ultimately responsible for maintaining fluid and electrolyte balance by excretion or retention based on the body's needs. (b)
    (2) The lungs eliminate water and carbon dioxide only if excess carbonic acid (H_2CO_3) is present; their role in fluid and electrolyte balance is less extensive than the kidneys'.
    (3) Antidiuretic hormone has a direct effect on the nephrons, resulting in water retention.
    (4) Aldosterone will cause the retention of sodium ions by the nephrons and subsequent fluid retention.

700. (4) The Giordano-Giovannetti diet includes very low protein (20 g) and controlled potassium (1500 mg) daily. (b)
    (1) The diet used in the management of renal failure is low in protein because the kidneys are unable to eliminate the wastes products from the body.
    (2) The body is able to synthesize the nonessential amino acids.
    (3) Urea is a waste product of protein metabolism; the body is able to synthesize the nonessential amino acids.

701. (3) In renal failure, as the glomerular filtration rate decreases, phosphorus is retained. As hyperphosphatemia occurs, calcium is excreted. Calcium depletion (hypocalcemia) causes tetany. (b)
    (1) The symptoms described are not characteristic of this condition.
    (2) The symptoms described are not characteristic of this condition.
    (4) The symptoms described are not characteristic of this condition.

702. (1) An elevated blood urea nitrogen, indicating uremia, is toxic to the central nervous system and causes

mental cloudiness, confusion, and loss of consciousness. (a)

(2) Hypernatremia is associated with firm tissue turgor, oliguria, and agitation.

(3) If decreased fluid intake results in dehydration, it can cause fatigue, dry skin and mucous membranes, and rapid pulse and respiratory rates.

(4) Hyperkalemia is associated with muscle weakness, irritability, nausea, and diarrhea.

703. (4) Since an external shunt provides circulatory access to a major artery and vein, special safety precautions must be taken to prevent disconnection of the cannulas. Disconnection can cause unimpeded excessive blood loss and death. Clamps should be carried at all times by the patient in case this emergency should arise. (c)

(1) Although a potential complication, this does not pose the same immediate threat to life as does exsanguination.

(2) Although a potential complication, this does not pose the same immediate threat to life as does exsanguination.

(3) Although a potential complication, this does not pose the same immediate threat to life as does exsanguination.

704. (2) The length of the urethra is shorter in females than in males; therefore microorganisms have a shorter distance to travel to reach the bladder. The proximity of the meatus to the anus in females also increases this incidence. (b)

(1) Hygienic practices can be poor in males or females; however, the anatomic length of the urethra in females predisposes them to infection.

(3) Mucous membranes are continuous in both males and females and would not make a difference.

(4) Fluid intake may be adequate in both males and females and would not account for the difference.

705. (4) The kidneys help control blood pH. Therefore the pH of the urine will vary with the needs of the blood and the number of hydrogen ions excreted by the kidney tubules. (c)

(1) When renal blood flow is insufficient because of ischemia or hypotension, renin is released.

(2) Renin secretion initiates conversion of the protein angiotensinogen to angiotensin, which causes vasoconstriction.

(3) Glucose is reabsorbed from the urine by active transport in the proximal tubules.

706. (2) Since the plasma colloidal osmotic pressure (COP) is the major force drawing fluid from the interstitial spaces back into the capillaries, a drop in COP due to albuminuria results in edema. (c)

(1) Hydrostatic pressure is influenced by the volume of fluid and the diameter of the blood vessel, not by the presence of protein such as albumin.

(3) Hydrostatic tissue pressure is unaffected by alteration of protein levels; colloidal pressure is.

(4) The osmotic pressure of tissues is not affected.

707. (4) Intact skin is the first line of defense against entry of microorganisms. A surgical incision is a portal of entry, so a technique that requires the absence of all microorganisms is essential. (c)

(1) Concurrent disinfection refers to measures initiated to control the spread of infection while an infection is present; concurrent asepsis is incorrect terminology.

(2) Medical asepsis utilizes clean technique to minimize the spread of microorganisms; when there is a break in the skin, such technique is insufficient.

(3) Wound asepsis is incorrect terminology.

708. (1) These symptoms result from failure of bile to enter the intestines, with subsequent backup into the biliary system and diffusion into the blood. The bilirubin is carried to all body regions, including the skin (itching) and kidneys (excretion of bile-colored urine). The absence of bilirubin in the intestine results in clay-colored stools. (c)

(2) If bile levels in the bloodstream are high, there would be bile in the urine, causing it to have a dark color.

(3) Signs refer to objective findings of an examiner; the signs of inadequate absorption of vitamin K include ecchymosis, hematuria, and other bleeding.

(4) The urine would be dark, reflecting increased serum bilirubin levels, and the stools would not be brown because the bile pigments would not be present in the GI tract.

709. (1) Vitamin C (ascorbic acid) plays a major role in wound healing. It is necessary for the maintenance and formation of strong collagen, the major protein of most connective tissues. (b)

(2) Phytonadione (e.g., Mephyton) is vitamin K, which plays a major role in blood coagulation.

(3) Vitamin B_{12} is needed for red blood cell synthesis and a healthy nervous system.

(4) Vitamin A is important for the healing process; however, vitamin C cements the ground substance of supportive tissue.

710. (3) The location of the incision results in pain on inspiration or coughing. The subsequent reluctance to cough and deep breathe facilitates respiratory complications from retained secretions. (b)

(1) Bile does not impair inflammatory or immune responses.

(2) A cholecystectomy is usually performed to treat cholelithiasis or cholecystitis; there is generally an inflammatory not an infectious process.

(4) The duration of surgery is not longer than for other abdominal surgery.

711. (4) Bile, a natural antioxidant, helps stabilize the vitamin and prevents destruction by oxygen. In addi-

tion, it serves as a transport vehicle for fat through the intestinal wall. (c)
(1) Digestive enzyme for lipids.
(2) Digestive enzyme for starch.
(3) Stomach acid.

712. (3) Vitamin A is a fat-soluble vitamin that accumulates in the body and is not significantly excreted even if extremely large amounts are ingested. After prolonged ingestion of extremely large doses, toxic effects can occur. (b)
(1) Vitamin A can be stored in the liver.
(2) Vitamin is toxic only after prolonged large dosages.
(4) Vitamin A cannot be synthesized by the body.

713. (3) Pancreatic amylase (which enters the small intestine at the sphincter of Oddi) and sucrase, lactase, and maltase (which are released by epithelial cells covering the villi in the small intestine) are responsible for carbohydrate digestion. (c)
(1) Because of the presence of ptyalin in saliva, some starch digestion occurs in the mouth.
(2) Limited carbohydrate digestion occurs in the stomach; pepsin begins the digestion of proteins.
(4) Digestion of carbohydrates is completed prior to their arrival in the large intestine, which is concerned primarily with fluid reabsorption.

714. (4)

Intake (ml)		Output (ml)	
IV fluid	350	Voiding	
NG tube feeding	600	8:30 A.M.	150
		1:00 P.M.	220
Water	150	3:15 P.M.	235
Vitamin	30	Aspirated stomach contents	25
	1130		630

(c)
(1) Represents a miscalculation; too little intake and too much output.
(2) A miscalculation; too little intake and too much output.
(3) A miscalculation; too little intake and output.

715. (2) Excessive loss of gastric juice results in excessive loss of hydrochloric acid (HCl) and can lead to alkalosis; the HCl is not available to neutralize the sodium bicarbonate ($NaHCO_3$) secreted into the duodenum by the pancreas. The intestinal tract absorbs the excess HCO_3^-, and alkalosis results. (a)
(1) Loss of HCl will move the pH to a basic level.
(3) Gastric juice does not regulate osmotic pressure in the blood; the volume of blood would be altered not by loss of gastric juice but by severe dehydration.
(4) Oxygen is not drawn from the blood by gastric lavage.

716. (1) The high Fowler position promotes optimal entry into the esophagus aided by gravity. (c)
(2) Positions do not take full advantage of the effect of gravity.
(3) Positions do not take full advantage of the effect of gravity.

(4) Positions do not take full advantage of the effect of gravity.

717. (2) As the uterus drops, the vaginal wall relaxes. When the bladder herniates into the vagina (cystocele) and the rectal wall herniates into the vagina (rectocele), the individual feels pressure or pain in the lower back and/or pelvis. When there is an increase in intraabdominal pressure in the presence of a cystocele, incontinence results. (b)
(1) Not indicative of cystocele and rectocele.
(3) Not indicative of cystocele and rectocele; common with infection.
(4) Not indicative of cystocele and rectocele.

718. (1) Relaxation of the pelvic musculature causes the uterus to drop, with a subsequent relaxation of the vaginal walls, most often as a result of childbirth. A rectocele is protrusion of the rectal wall into the vagina, whereas a cystocele is protrusion of the bladder into the vaginal wall. (b)
(2) Does not cause either a rectocele or a cystocele.
(3) Does not cause either a rectocele or a cystocele.
(4) Does not cause either a rectocele or a cystocele.

719. (4) Since Mrs. Gorham is past the childbearing age, plastic surgical repair designed to tighten both the anterior and the posterior vaginal wall will probably be performed. (b)
(1) A pessary is a device employed for a prolapsed uterus.
(2) A hysterectomy is performed only if there is uterine disease.
(3) A hysterectomy is performed only if there is uterine disease.

720. (4) Because the bladder is continually empty when an indwelling catheter is in place, it loses tone. This is an expected but undesirable effect. (a)
(1) The effects of anesthesia and the inflammatory process may impede voiding, leading to urinary retention; a Foley catheter empties the bladder continuously, preventing retention.
(2) The effects of anesthesia and the inflammatory process may impede voiding, leading to urinary retention; distention then places pressure on the suture line; an indwelling catheter prevents retention.
(3) Urinary retention causes bladder distention and discomfort; an indwelling catheter promotes continuous bladder drainage.

721. (1) A generous supply of blood is carried by the uterine arteries (branches of the internal iliac arteries). The vaginal and ovarian arteries also supply the uterus with blood by anastomosing with the uterine vessels. (b)
(2) The hypogastric or internal iliac arteries supply the pelvic wall and viscera.
(3) The aorta does not supply the uterus directly.
(4) The hypogastric arteries (internal iliac) supply the pelvic wall and gluteal area, and the external branches (called uterine arteries) supply the uterus

and genitalia; the aorta doesn't supply the uterus directly.

722. (4) The gonadotropins, follicle-stimulating hormone (FSH) and luteinizing hormone (LH), are concerned with ovarian changes that produce ovulation. Estrogen levels are high between the end of menses and ovulation because of secretion from the developing follicle. Progesterone levels are high between ovulation and the onset of menses because of secretion from the corpus luteum. The hormones work in concert to stimulate the menstrual cycle. (a)
   (1) Without FSH and LH there is no cycle.
   (2) The gonadotropins must work in concert with estrogen and progesterone for the cycle to be completed.
   (3) Progesterone is required for the menstrual cycle to be completed.

723. (4) This position maximally exposes the rectal area and facilitates entry of the sigmoidoscope. It is prefered. (b)
   (1) Although prone refers to a face-down position, the rectal area is not exposed.
   (2) The lithotomy position is appropriate for gynecologic examinations.
   (3) The Sims position does not expose the rectal area to the same extent as the knee-chest position does but can still be used for a sigmoidoscopy if the patient is unable to maintain the knee-chest position.

724. (3) To permit adequate visualization of the mucosa during the sigmoidoscopy, the bowel must be cleansed with a nonirritating enema before examination. (a)
   (1) Since only the lower bowel is being visualized, keeping the patient n.p.o. is unnecessary and debilitating; clear liquids and a laxative may be given the day before to limit fecal residue.
   (2) The patient does not drink such a substance in preparation for a sigmoidoscopy.
   (4) Stool should be eliminated from the colon by an enema before the examination.

725. (4) The nurse should pick up all clues to patient anxiety and allow for verbalization. This response recognizes the pateint's feelings. (a)
   (1) This response negates the patient's feelings and presents a negative connotation about the procedure.
   (2) This response negates the patient's feelings and presents a negative connotation about the procedure.
   (3) This response focuses on the task rather than on the patient's feelings.

726. (4) Because neomycin is poorly absorbed from the GI tract, most remains in the intestines and exerts its antibiotic effect on the intestinal mucosa. In preparation for GI surgery the level of microbial organisms will be reduced. (a)
   (1) Neomycin is mainly effective in suppression of intestinal flora.
   (2) Since it is poorly absorbed from the GI tract, the systemic effect is minimal.
   (3) Neomycin is nephrotoxic.

727. (2) If the area is not kept both clean and dry, drainage from the colostomy can quickly cause a breakdown of the skin around the stoma. This, in combination with a warm moist surface, also predisposes the individual to infection. (a)
   (1) The patient is often unwilling to accept the altered body image and must be given time to adjust before participating actively in dressing changes.
   (3) Although oral fluids are withheld until peristalsis returns, it is essential that parenteral fluids be administered to replace the losses incurred by surgery.
   (4) Although oral fluids are withheld until peristalsis returns, it is essential that parenteral fluids be administered to replace the losses incurred by surgery.

728. (3) The stoma of a colostomy must be dilated with a lubricated, gloved finger to prevent strictures and subsequent obstruction. (b)
   (1) Clothing need not be special but should be nonconstricting.
   (2) Once healing has occurred, activity is not limited.
   (4) Diet should be as close to normal for the individual as possible; gas-forming foods should be avoided.

729. (1) Although foods that produce gas are generally avoided, the diet of an individual with a colostomy should be as close to normal as possible for optimal physiologic and psychologic adaptation. (b)
   (2) A high-protein diet is important until healing occurs; but a balanced diet generally meets nutritional needs for protein.
   (3) There is no need to limit fiber; it provides bulk necessary for unconstipated stools.
   (4) Since absorption of nutrients is unaffected, there is no need to increase carbohydrate intake.

730. (1) The acetabulum is the socket in the pelvis with which the head of the femur articulates. (b)
   (2) Does not articulate with the acetabulum; long bone of the femur (longest and strongest bone in the body).
   (3) No articulation with the acetabulum; part of bone between the head and shaft; commonly fractured in the elderly.
   (4) The greater and lesser trochanters bulge at the proximal end of the femur shaft; serve as attachment points for some buttock and thigh muscles.

731. (2) Nails, pins, plates, and screws maintain bone alignment while bone replacement (healing) occurs. (a)
   (1) A prosthesis can be used if an intracapsular fracture cannot be reduced satisfactorily with the use of pins or nails; internal fixation is used instead of traction, which would require prolonged immobilization.
   (3) A hip spica cast requires prolonged immobilization and increases the risk of complications associated with immobility.
   (4) Skeletal traction requires prolonged immobilization and increases the risk of complications associated with immobility

732. (3) Turning and periodic deep breathing promote drainage of and circulation in the lung alveoli, which helps prevent circulatory and pulmonary complications. To prevent strain and possible misalignment or pressure at the fracture site, patients should not be turned onto the affected side. (b)
   (1) The patient must be turned at least every 2 hours to help prevent the complication of immobility; 5 hours is too long to keep a patient in one position.
   (2) The patient is generally not allowed out of bed until at least 1 day postoperative, and then weight bearing is not permitted on the affected extremity.
   (4) The patient is generally not allowed out of bed until 1 to 3 days postoperative.
733. (1) Pressure on the operative site may cause unnecessary pain and impair circulation necessary for healing. (c)
   (2) Supine or on the unaffected side is the position of choice; however, a wedge, thigh spreader, or pillows must be used to maintain abduction of the affected thigh; adduction can result in displacement of the prosthesis.
   (3) This is acceptable since there is no stress placed on the operative site.
   (4) This is acceptable since there is no stress placed on the operative side.
734. (3) Prune juice and warm water can be administered prophylactically by the nurse to promote defecation. Prune juice irritates the bowel mucosa, stimulating peristalsis. Increased fiber in the diet may also improve intestinal motility. (b)
   (1) Routine use of enemas should be avoided because they promote dependency and can result in electrolyte imbalance.
   (2) Routine use of enemas should be avoided because they promote dependency and can result in electrolyte imbalance.
   (4) Routine use of laxatives promotes dependency.
735. (2) Bones become more fragile with advancing age because of osteoporosis, often associated with lower circulating levels of estrogens or testosterone. (a)
   (1) Carelessness is a characteristic applicable to certain individuals rather than to a developmental level.
   (3) Rheumatoid diseases certainly can affect the skeletal system but do not increase the incidence of hip fractures.
   (4) Although prolonged immobility is associated with bone demineralization, hip fractures occur in elderly individuals who are active.
736. (2) Gonorrhea is caused by a gram-negative diplococcus, *Neisseria gonorrhoeae*. (a)
   (1) Spirochete of syphilis.
   (3) Staphylococci are constantly present on the skin and in the upper respiratory tract; commonly cause suppurating infection.
   (4) A lactobacillus found in the vagina; does not cause gonorrhea.

737. (2) In males the inflammatory process associated with the infection may lead to destruction of the epididymis. In females the gonorrheal infection causes destruction of the tubal mucosa and eventually tubo-ovarian abscesses. (a)
   (1) Gonorrhea is difficult to treat.
   (3) Gonorrhea is a common sexually transmitted disease.
   (4) *Neisseria gonorrhoeae* will invade internal structures, particularly the epididymis in males and the fallopian tubes in females.
738. (3) Gonorrhea is a highly contagious disease transmitted through sexual intercourse. The incubation period varies, but symptoms usually occur 2 to 10 days after contact. Early effective treatment prevents complications. (a)
   (1) Contracting venereal disease is not necessarily indicative of promiscuity.
   (2) The parents may be unaware that their daughter has gonorrhea; the nurse knows the etiology of the disease.
   (4) Most birth control measures do not protect against the transmission of venereal disease.
739. (1) Penicillin inhibits the synthesis of bacterial cell walls. It is effective against *Neisseria gonorrhoeae*, a gram-negative diplococcus. (b)
   (2) Actinomycin is an antineoplastic agent.
   (3) Chloramphenicol is a broad-spectrum antimicrobial agent; however, it can cause bone marrow depression, so its use is limited to severe infections that do not respond to less toxic drugs.
   (4) Colistin sulfate is effective against most gram-negative enteric pathogens such as *Escherichia coli*.
740. (1) Penicillin is specific for *Neisseria gonorrhoeae* and eradicates the microorganism. (a)
   (2) If the disease progresses before diagnosis is made, complications such as sterility, valve damage, or joint degeneration may occur.
   (3) The individual may still contract gonorrhea.
   (4) If tubal structures, valves, or joints degenerate, the pathologic changes will not be reversed by antibiotic therapy.
741. (3) Flexion contracture of the hip can be prevented by routinely placing the patient in a prone position to extend the hip. (b)
   (1) This can cause flexion of the hip, which will result in a hip contracture and affect balance.
   (2) Lying in the supine position does not allow for full extension of the hip.
   (4) This can cause flexion of the hip, which will result in a hip contracture and affect balance.
742. (1) This position offsets the development of hip deformities due to contractures. It also maintains the correct center of gravity when the patient is upright. (b)
   (2) Promotes flexion contracture of the hip.

(3) May alter the center of gravity and cause a loss of balance.

(4) A prosthesis may be applied early in the postoperative period but requires a rigid dressing (cast) to prevent edema; ambulation can be facilitated by the use of a walker, crutches, parallel bars, or cane.

743. (2) Preparing muscles that will do the work in crutch walking is imperative. (b)

(1) The biceps are not the major muscles required for crutch walking.

(3) Strengthening the hamstring muscles will not assist in the use of crutches.

(4) The condition of the limb will not have a great influence on the ability to use crutches.

744. (2) A 4-point gait provides for weight bearing on all 4 extremities and maximum support during ambulation. (b)

(1) A 3-point gait is used when one extremity cannot bear weight.

(3) A 3-point gait is used when one extremity cannot bear weight.

(4) A swing-through gait does not simulate ambulation; it is used when the individual can bear weight but lacks the muscular control needed for ambulation without an assisting device.

745. (2) Practicing ambulation without proper preparation of ambulation techniques and strengthening the involved muscle groups would not be helpful in the rehabilitation process and could exhaust the patient. (a)

(1) Prior to ambulation the individual must be able to maintain balance.

(3) The muscles used for crutch walking are different from those used in normal ambulation; therefore they must be strengthened by active exercises prior to ambulation.

(4) Since different muscle groups are utilized, the patient must be instructed even about what seems to be simple maneuvers; transfer from a sitting to a standing position must be accomplished before ambulation.

746. (1) Rehabilitation should begin on admission; this includes preoperative discussion of the nature of the operation and rehabilitation techniques. (b)

(2) Too late; valuable time to rehabilitate is not utilized.

(3) Too late; valuable time to rehabilitate is not utilized.

(4) Too late; valuable time to rehabilitate is not utilized.

747. (1) Bleeding between periods is abnormal. The occurrence of bleeding other than during the menstrual period is known as metrorrhagia. (b)

(2) Menorrhagia is the term used to describe excessive bleeding during menstruation.

(3) The amount varies from spotting to frank bleeding; it is not occult.

(4) Bleeding may not be limited to ovulation.

748. (4) A hysterectomy involves only removal of the uterus. The ovaries, which secrete estrogen and progester-

one, are not removed. Therefore menopause will not be precipitated but will occur naturally. (b)

(1) If the ovaries were being removed, older women might have less severe symptoms than younger women; however, in this instance there would be no symptoms.

(2) The nurse should serve as a resource person; the comment does not answer the question.

(3) Incorrect; fails to point out the difference between myth and reality.

749. (3) The prescribing of medications is the legal responsibility of the physician. In addition, the use of hormones is controversial and depends on the physician's beliefs and the patient's needs. (b)

(1) This is an evasive response; the patient is left without direction.

(2) Hormones may be used to prevent the development of severe symptoms.

(4) This is an evasive response; does not answer the patient's question.

750. (1) This response reflects and verbalizes the patient's feelings in a nonjudgmental way. (a)

(2) Demonstrates a lack of acceptance of the patient's feelings.

(3) The husband did not indicate this; the patient's perception is altered by her own feelings.

(4) Such feelings are common and need to be verbalized; surgery should not be postponed.

751. (4) Oral contraceptives contain hormones that help regulate the menstrual cycle. (b)

(1) Because of associated complications, the use of oral contraceptives is contraindicated in the presence of cardiovascular disease.

(2) Because of associated complications, the use of oral contraceptives is contraindicated in the presence of cardiovascular disease.

(3) All methods of birth control, including sterilization, should be discussed.

752. (4) The greater density of compact bone makes it stronger than cancellous bone. Compact bone forms from cancellous bone by the addition of concentric rings of bone substance to the marrow spaces of cancellous bone; the large marrow spaces are reduced to haversian canals. (a)

(1) Not related to strength.

(2) Overall size does not determine strength.

(3) Weight alone is not a factor.

753. (2) The ache in muscles that have been vigorously worked without adequate oxygen supply is caused in part by the buildup of lactic acid. During rest the lactic acid is oxidized completely to carbon dioxide and water, providing ATP for further muscular contraction. (a)

(1) Butyric acid is not a product of muscle contraction; it is a fatty acid occurring in feces, urine, and perspiration.

(3) Acetoacetic acid is not a product of muscle contraction; it is a ketone body resulting from incomplete oxidation of fatty acids. It is also produced by the metabolism of lipids and pyruviates.

(4) Acetone is not a product of muscle contraction; it is a ketone body and a by-product of acetoacetic acid metabolism.

754. (3) A cataract is a clouding of the crystalline lens or its capsule. (b)
(1) Not included in the pathophysiology related to cataracts.
(2) Not included in the pathophysiology related to cataracts.
(4) Not included in the pathophysiology related to cataracts.

755. (2) Activities such as rigorous brushing of hair and teeth cause increased intraocular pressure and may lead to hemorrhage in the anterior chamber. (b)
(1) Coughing and deep breathing can increase intraocular pressure.
(3) The patient is generally permitted out of bed as soon as the effects of anesthesia have worn off.
(4) Weakening of the eye musculature is not related to cataracts.

756. (2) Retinal detachment is a separation between the sensory retina and the retinal pigment epithelium. These layers are not attached by any special structures and can separate as a result of various pathologic processes. (c)
(1) The statement does not explain the disease process involved.
(3) The statement does not explain the disease process involved.
(4) The statement does not explain the disease process involved.

757. (1) Scar formation seals the hole and promotes attachment of the 2 retinal surfaces. (c)
(2) This is not the treatment used; is formation of a scar by the use of lasers or surgical "buckling."
(3) The retina is part of the nervous system; does not regenerate or grow new cells.
(4) The sclera is not involved; the retina adjoins and is nourished by the choroid.

758. (1) Vitamin A is used in the formation of retinene, a component of the light-sensitive rhodopsin molecule. (a)
(2) Vitamin A does not influence color vision, which is centered in the cones.
(3) The cornea is a transparent part of the anterior portion of the sclera; a cataract is an opacity of the normally transparent crystalline lens. Vitamin A does not prevent cataracts.
(4) Melanin is a pigment of the skin.

759. (2) Deep green and yellow vegetables contain large quantities of the pigments α-, β-, and γ-carotene; β-carotene is the major chemical precursor of vitamin A in human nutrition. (a)

(1) Levels of vitamin A are higher in whole milk than in skim milk.
(3) Oranges are considered a good source of both vitamin C and potassium.
(4) Tomatoes are a good source of vitamin C.

760. (4) Malignant melanoma of the eye is an intraocular tumor that metatasizes rapidly; therefore enucleation—removal of the eye—is the treatment of choice. (c)
(1) Only palliative at best.
(2) Only palliative at best.
(3) Only palliative at best.

761. (4) Changes in the pH of the vaginal tract cause cellular alteration and destruction. (c)
(1) The direct effects of labor and delivery will not cause cervical erosion; erosion involves continuous inflammation or ulceration.
(2) The direct effects of labor and delivery will not cause cervical erosion; erosion involves continuous inflammation or ulceration.
(3) The direct effects of labor and delivery will not cause cervical erosion; erosion involves continuous inflammation or ulceration.

762. (3) Douches with acidic solutions such as vinegar and water bring back the normal pH of the vaginal tract. (a)
(1) The use of vinegar will only indirectly affect bacterial growth because it acidifies the environment.
(2) Although this may be a secondary benefit, a vinegar and water solution would not be required.
(4) Comfort may be enhanced by correcting the pathologic disorder, but it is not the main goal of the treatment.

763. (3) Dorsal recumbency takes advantage of the anatomic position of the vaginal tract and prevents undue retention or too rapid return of the douche. (a)
(1) Promote retention of the douche.
(2) Promote retention of the douche.
(4) Promotes rapid return of the douche before the therapeutic effect is achieved.

764. (3) This is the anatomic direction of the vaginal tract in the back-lying position. (b)
(1) The vaginal tract may be injured when the douche nozzle is not directed with consideration of normal anatomy.
(2) The vaginal tract may be injured when the douche nozzle is not directed with consideration of normal anatomy.
(4) The vaginal tract may be injured when the douche nozzle is not directed with consideration of normal anatomy.

765. (2) Erosion of the cervix frequently occurs at the squamocolumnar junction, the most common site for carcinoma of the cervix. (a)
(1) Infection may occur in the cancerous area accompanied by profuse, malodorous discharge; treatment of the erosion is done to prevent the cancer, not the secondary infection.

(3) This may be present as erosion develops into carcinoma; however, spotting may be the earliest sign; will be eliminated when the cancer is treated; treatment of the erosion done to prevent cancer from developing.

(4) Even though a cervical erosion is treated, another may occur and repeat treatment may be necessary.

766. (3) Any product containing aluminum, magnesium, or calcium ions should not be taken in the hours before or after an oral dose, since it decreases absorption by as much as 25% to 50%. (c)

(1) Citrus juice has no influence on this drug.

(2) Antacids will interfere with absorption of this drug.

(4) Pregnant women and young children are not given tetracycline because it causes discoloration of developing teeth.

767. (2) Since pressure is force developed per unit of area over which the force is applied, as the area decreases the pressure increases. The tip of a needle or the point of a knife has an extremely small area, and consequently a very high pressure can be developed for a given force. (c)

(1) Although some energy is required to insert the needle, the amount is very little because the area at the tip of the needle is so small.

(3) Although a factor, texture relationship is not the primary reason for ease of insertion; the small point in relation to energy developed at the point of insertion is the prime factor.

(4) The length and shape of the needle have no relevance to ease of penetration; the small point in relation to energy developed at the point of insertion is the prime factor.

768. (2) Amino acids are absorbed into the blood in the intestinal capillaries with the aid of vitamin B_6 via the energy-dependent system active transport. (b)

(1) Proteins are fairly large molecules; do not passively diffuse.

(3) Osmosis refers to the movement of water across a semipermeable membrane; does not apply to proteins.

(4) Osmosis refers to the movement of water across a semipermeable membrane; does not apply to proteins.

769. (2) Complete proteins contain sufficient amounts of all essential amino acids and are of animal origin. (b)

(1) Not all 22 but rather the 8 essential and 2 semiessential (arginine and histidine) are needed during growth.

(3) Sufficient amounts of all 8 essential must be present plus 2 semiessential (arginine and histidine), which are essential only during periods of growth.

(4) The body cannot make the essential amino acids; they must be present in foods ingested.

770. (1) These amino acids are needed to maintain life and are not produced by the body. (a)

(2) All amino acids are needed for metabolism; however, arginine and histidine are necessary for growth, but not during adulthood.

(3) The essential amino acids cannot be made by the body.

(4) The body does not synthesize these amino acids; they must be ingested in the diet.

771. (2) Phospho-Soda is a saline cathartic, increasing the osmotic pressure within the intestines so that body fluids are drawn into the bowel, stimulating bowel stretching, peristalsis, and defecation. (c)

(1) Bulk-forming laxatives are cellulose derivatives that remain in the intestinal tract and absorb water; cause bulk, which stimulates peristalsis.

(3) Emollients have a detergent action, softening the stool by facilitating its absorption of water.

(4) Stimulants irritate the mucosa so that peristalsis is increased.

772. (4) Antibodies produced against group A beta-hemolytic streptococci sometimes interact with antigens in the heart's valves, causing damage and symptoms of rheumatic heart disease. (b)

(1) Rheumatoid arthritis is thought to be an autoimmune disease; is not caused by microorganisms.

(2) Hepatitis is caused by several types of viruses, not bacteria.

(3) The most common causes of meningitis include *Streptococcus pneumoniae, Neisseria meningitides,* and *Haemophilus influenzae.*

773. (2) Streptococci are present on the skin at all times. They cause many infections common in humans. (b)

(1) Vaccinations are not available for most of these conditions; there is a scarlet fever antitoxin, but antibiotics have replaced it.

(3) All are caused by streptococci.

(4) The causative organism normally lives on the skin.

774. (1) In gangrene the release of iron from hemoglobin as the erythrocytes disintegrate in necrotic tissue results in ferrous sulfide formation, causing darkening of the tissues. (c)

(2) Ferric chloride is used as a reagent; it is also used topically as an antiseptic and astringent; not related to gangrene.

(3) Heme constitutes the pigment portion of the hemoglobin molecule, which gives blood its red color; does not cause the darkening of tissue associated with gangrene.

(4) Proteins are not insoluble.

775. (3) A 1 molar (1 M) solution contains 1 gram-molecular weight of solute per liter of solution. Molarity is not as informative as normality because the latter is based on the actual chemical-combining properties of the substance involved. (c)

(1) Deals with the osmotic pressure of two liquids; isotonic solutions have equal osmotic pressure.

(2) A 1 normal (1 N) solution is defined as containing 1 gram-equivalent weight of solute per liter of solution. In human body fluids the milliequivalent

($\frac{1}{1000}$ of the gram-equivalent) is a more convenient term for expressing concentration, since the gram-equivalent is rather large.

(4) A solution holding all the solute it can at a given temperature and pressure.

776. (1) Unless Mr. Manor has been certified as incompetent, he retains the right of informed consent. (c)

(2) Since the description of the situation provides no evidence of incompetence, the patient should sign his own consent.

(3) Since the description of the situation provides no evidence of incompetence, the patient should sign his own consent.

(4) Since the description of the situation provides no evidence of incompetence, the patient should sign his own consent.

777. (3) An individual is held legally responsible for actions committed against another individual or his property. (c)

(1) This is the definition of negligence.

(2) This is related to battery, which involves physical harm.

(4) This is the definition of a crime.

778. (2) False imprisonment and battery are wrongs committed by one person against another in a willful intentional way without just cause and/or excuse. (c)

(1) Malpractice, which is professional negligence, is classified as an unintentional tort; assault, which is knowingly threatening another, is an intentional tort.

(3) Negligence, which is classified as an unintentional tort, involves exposure of another's person or property to unreasonable risk of injury by acts of commission or omission; invasion of privacy is an intentional tort.

(4) Malpractice and negligence are both unintentional torts.

779. (1) The reporting of possible child abuse is required by law, and the nurse can remain anonymous. (b)

(2) Although the Good Samaritan Act protects health professionals, the nurse would still be responsible for acting as any reasonably prudent nurse would in a similar situation.

(3) Although the Good Samaritan Act protects health professionals, the nurse would still be responsible for acting as any reasonable prudent nurse would in a similar situation.

(4) The nurse is functioning in a professional capacity and therefore can be held accountable.

780. (1) Each state or province is charged with the responsibility of protecting the health and welfare of its populace, which it does by regulating nursing practice. (b)

(2) Although the members of the profession can also benefit from a clear description of their role, this is not the primary purpose of the law.

(3) Professional standards are established by the profession to assure quality care for the public.

(4) The employing agency does assume responsibility for its employees and therefore benefits from maintenance of standards, but this is not the purpose of the law.

781. (4) Coumarin anticoagulants are administered orally and take 2 or 3 days to achieve the desired decrease in prothrombin level. Heparin, which must be administered parenterally, has immediate effects. (c)

(1) This does not account for the reason for the administration of both drugs because coumarin derivatives will not exert an immediate therapeutic effect.

(2) These drugs do not dissolve clots already present.

(3) Since each drug affects a different part of the coagulating mechanism, dosages must be adjusted separately.

782. (3) Warfarin sodium (Coumadin) has been shown to inhibit the metabolism of phenytoin (Dilantin), which results in an accumulation of this drug in the body. (b)

(1) This is true only if the patient is receiving phenytoin to control the epilepsy.

(2) They do not have a significant effect on the metabolism of Coumadin.

(4) By potentiating the anticoagulant, phenytoin decreases clotting potential.

783. (2) Coumarin derivatives cause an increase in the prothrombin time, leading to an increased risk of bleeding. Any abnormal or excessive bleeding must be reported, since it may indicate toxic levels of the drug. (b)

(1) TIAs are not caused by bleeding, which is the primary concern in patients receiving anticoagulants.

(3) Edema is not caused by bleeding.

(4) Would not be caused by Coumadin.

784. (4) Compliance with the prescribed regimen, which includes taking the drug and having prothrombin times performed by the laboratory, is necessary for safe and effective warfarin sodium (Coumadin) therapy. The dosage of Coumadin is adjusted according to the prothrombin time; and if the patient fails to take the drug as prescribed, the tests are not reliable in monitoring the response to therapy. (a)

(1) Although some medications can affect the absorption or metabolism of Coumadin and also should be investigated, this is less likely to be a cause of fluctuations in laboratory values.

(2) Although some medications can affect the absorption or metabolism of Coumadin and also should be investigated, this is less likely to be a cause of fluctuations in laboratory values.

(3) Although some medications can affect the absorption or metabolism of Coumadin and also should be investigated, this is less likely to be a cause of fluctuations in laboratory values.

785. (2) Secobarbital sodium (as well as other barbiturates) decreases the body's response to warfarin sodium (Coumadin). As a result there is less suppression of prothrombin. (c)
   (1) Insomnia may increase seizure incidence, but methods to promote sleep other than barbiturates should be considered.
   (3) Serious withdrawal symptoms are unlikely in this situation; however, indiscriminant use of the drug should be avoided.
   (4) Secobarbital is not used to control seizures although other barbiturates such as phenobarbital may be prescribed for this purpose.

786. (4) A subjective symptom such as ringing in the ears can be felt only by the patient. (b)
   (1) The term is not generally used to describe a symptom; a functional disease is one in which there is alteration in function without physiologic changes.
   (2) Prodromal refers to symptoms that are early indications of a developing disease; there is insufficient information to decide this from the situation described.
   (3) An objective symptom refers to signs that can be assessed through direct physical examination.

787. (3) Massive doses of penicillin may limit CNS damage if treatment is started before neural deterioration from syphilis occurs. (c)
   (1) Weakness is not a behavior and is therefore not suitably treated with behavior modification.
   (2) Tranquilizers will generally increase weakness.
   (4) Electroconvulsive therapy is used in the treatment of certain psychiatric disorders.

788. (1) Since stomach distention (after eating) results in contractions of the colon (gastrocolic reflex) promoting defecation, establishing some regularity of meals that include adequate bulk or fiber will help establish routine patterns of defecation. (b)
   (2) Although increased fluid intake and activity facilitate elimination, in general, they do not help establish a pattern.
   (3) Although increased fluid intake and activity facilitate elimination, in general, they do not help establish a pattern.
   (4) Increased potassium is not needed for normal elimination.

789. (2) The tidal volume is the amount of air inhaled and exhaled while breathing normally. (b)
   (1) Air that can be forcibly expired after deep inspiration.
   (3) The maximum amount of air that can be inspired from the tidal inspiratory level.
   (4) The maximum amount of air that can be expired for the tidal expiratory level.

790. (4) *Trichomonas vaginalis* is a protozoan that favors an alkaline environment. (c)
   (1) A fungus is a simple parasitic plant; does not cause trichomonal infections.

(2) A yeast is a unicellular, usually oval, nucleated fungus; does not cause trichomonal infections.
(3) A spirochete is a motile spiral-shaped bacterium; does not cause trichomonal infections.

791. (2) Since *Trichomonas vaginalis* favors an alkaline environment, vinegar, an acid, is utilized to decrease the pH of the vagina. (c)
   (1) Normal saline will not alter the pH.
   (3) An increase in pH would create an environment conducive to the growth of microorganisms.
   (4) An increase in pH would create an environment conducive to the growth of microorganisms.

792. (3) Metronidazole (Flagyl) is a potent amebicide. It is extremely effective in eradicating the protozoan *Trichomonas vaginalis*. (c)
   (1) Gentian violet is a local antiinfective that is applied topically and may cause discoloration of the skin; particularly effective against *Candida albicans*.
   (2) Penicillin is administered for its effect on bacterial, not protozoal, infections.
   (4) Nystatin is an antifungal used for infections caused by *Candida albicans*.

793. (3) Primitive sex cells, called spermatogonia, are present in newborn males. At puberty these cells mature and form spermatozoa (spermatogenesis). (b)
   (1) Only immature cells are found during this period.
   (2) Spermatogonia or primitive sex cells are found at this time.
   (4) Does not occur until puberty.

794. (3) Sperm cells are very fragile and can be destroyed by heat, resulting in sterility. (b)
   (1) Sperm are motile, achieving this by motion of their flagella; they move from the epididymis to the vas deferens to the ejaculatory ducts to the urethra.
   (2) Sperm do not move through the urine; are found in semen.
   (4) During this period the testes are not suspended.

795. (2) This recognizes that the patient is upset and by indirect questioning helps facilitate communication. (b)
   (1) An assumption is being made about the basis for the behavior; does not focus on the patient's feelings.
   (3) False reassurances block communication.
   (4) The patient has not verbally indicated that she is upset and may be unaware of or unable to verbalize the actual cause of her emotions.

796. (4) This recognizes the patient's feeling of anxiety as valid; informing her honestly of a fact may help decrease the anxiety. (b)
   (1) The polyps may be cancerous; this is false reassurance and may inhibit the expression of feelings.
   (2) The polyps may be cancerous; this is false reassurance and may inhibit the expression of feelings.
   (3) Does not focus on the patient; feelings exist and will not disappear on command.

797. (1) Polyps are usually benign but should undergo biopsy, since epidermoid cancer occasionally arises from cervical polyps. (a)

(2) Untrue; polyps are usually benign.

(3) Bleeding may occur whether they are malignant or not.

(4) Untrue; polyps are rarely the percursors of uterine cancer.

798. (1) When the cancerous cells are completely confined within the epithelium of the cervix without stromal invasion, it is stage 0 and called carcinoma in situ or preinvasive carcinoma. (c)

(2) Stage I; lymph node metastasis about 10%.

(3) Stage Ia; minimal stromal invasion.

(4) Stage IIb; involves area around the broad ligaments but not the pelvic wall; extension to the corpus of the uterus.

799. (3) The endocervical surface is frequently altered by metaplasia or covered by a variant of squamous epithelium. It is thus called the transitional zone. This area is often distorted by eversion and laceration, especially in pregnancy. Therefore it is a frequent site for carcinoma. Erosion in this area most frequently leads to squamous cell carcinoma, accounting for 95% of cervical cancer. (c)

(1) Adenocarcinoma, accounting for only 5% of cervical cancers, may be found in the endocervical glands.

(2) Extension to lymph nodes is a later stage.

(4) The cervix is the lower portion of the uterus; the juncture of the uterine body with the cervical canal is called the internal os; erosion most frequently occurs distal to this point, between the external and internal, closer to the external.

800. (3) Conization (conical excision of the lesion), cryosurgery, and hysterectomy can be used in the treatment of squamous cell carcinoma in situ. If treatment is initiated during the preinvasive stage, it is 100% curable. (b)

(1) Although the postponement of surgery gives Mrs. Vale time to cope, the decision should not be delayed; conization would be done if later pregnancy is desired. Hysterectomy would preclude that possibility.

(2) Although it may take 5 to 10 years for preinvasive carcinoma to progress to invasive carcinoma, the prognosis is excellent if therapy is initiated during the preinvasive stage. The decision should not be delayed.

(4) Conization does not predispose to abortion and can be done during pregnancy.

3

Pediatric Nursing

Pediatric nursing encompasses the care of well and ill children, stressing preventive as well as restorative interventions. This section is divided into the descriptive age groups of childhood, that is, infancy, toddlerhood, preschool years, school-age years, and adolescence. Principles of growth and development, age-specific acheivements, health maintenance objectives, and disease-related states are discussed for each age category. Such an organization attempts to present the nursing of children as one that incorporates their physical and psychologic needs toward optimum promotion of health.

BASIC CONCEPTS

A. Children are individuals, not little adults, who must be seen as part of a family
B. Family-centered care is the objective in the care of children to provide total health maintenance
C. Children are influenced by genetic factors, home and environment, and parental attitudes
D. Chronologic and developmental ages of children are the most important contributing factors influencing their care
E. Prevention of illness and maintenance of health are the main thrusts in health care of children
F. Play is a natural medium for expression, communication, and growth in children

THE FAMILY
Structure of the Family

A. The basic unit of a society
B. Composition varies although one member is usually recognized as head
C. Usually share common goals and beliefs
D. Roles change within the group and reflect both the individual's and the group's needs
E. Status of members determined by position in family in conjunction with views of society

Functions of the Family

A. Reproduction—group developed to reproduce and rear members of a society
B. Maintenance to provide
   1. Clothing, housing, food, and medical care
   2. Social, psychologic, and emotional support for family members

3. Protection, since immaturity of young children necessitates that care be given by adults
4. Status—child is a member of a family that is also a part of the larger community
C. Socialization
   1. Child is "humanized" by introduction to social situations and instruction in appropriate social behaviors
   2. Self-identity develops through relationships with other family members
   3. Child learns appropriate sex roles and responsibilities
D. Growth of individual members toward maturity and independence

HUMAN GROWTH AND DEVELOPMENT
Principles of Growth

A. Traditional definition of growth is limited to physical maturation
B. Integrated definition includes functional maturation
C. Growth is complex with all aspects closely related
D. Growth is measured both quantitatively and qualitatively over a period of time
E. Although the rate is not even, growth is a continuous and orderly process
   1. Infancy—most rapid period of growth
   2. Preschool to puberty—slow and uniform rate of growth
   3. Puberty—growth spurt
   4. After puberty—decline in growth rate till death
F. There are regular patterns in the direction of growth and development, such as the cephalocaudal law (from head to toe) and the proximodistal law (from center of body to periphery)
G. Different parts of the body grow at different rates
   1. Prenatally—head grows the fastest
   2. During the first year—elongation of trunk dominates
H. Both rate and pattern of growth can be modified, most obviously by nutrition
I. There are critical periods in growth and development, such as brain growth during uterine life and infancy
J. Although there are specified sequences for achieving growth and development, each individual proceeds at own rate
K. Development is closely related to the maturation of the nervous system; as some primitive reflexes disappear, they are replaced by a voluntary activity such as grasp

Characteristics of Growth

A. Circulatory system
   1. Heart rate decreases with increasing age
      a. Infancy—130 beats per minute
      b. One year—100 to 110
      c. Childhood—80 to 100
      d. Adolescence to adulthood—70 to 85 (after maturity, women have slightly higher pulse rate than men)
   2. Blood pressure increases with age
      a. Ranges from 40 to 70 mm Hg diastolic to 65 to 140 mm Hg systolic
      b. These levels increse about 2 to 3 mm Hg per year beginning at age 7 years
      c. Systolic pressure in adolescence—higher in males than in females
   3. Hemoglobin
      a. Highest at birth, 17 g per 100 ml of blood; then decreases to 11.5 to 12 g per 100 ml by 1 year
      b. Fetal hemoglobin (60% to 90% of total hemoglobin) gradually decreases during the first year to less than 5%
      c. Gradual increase in hemoglobin level to 14.5 g per 100 ml between 1 and 12 years of age
      d. Level higher in males than in females
B. Respiratory system
   1. Rate decreases with increase in age
      a. Infancy—30 to 40 per minute
      b. Childhood—20 to 24 per minute
      c. Adolescence and adulthood—16 to 20 per minute
   2. Vital capacity
      a. Gradual increase throughout childhood and adolescence, with a decrease in later life
      b. Capacity in males exceeds that in females
   3. Basal metabolism
      a. Highest rate is found in the newborn
      b. Rate declines with increase in age, higher in males than in females
C. Urinary system
   1. Premature and full-term newborns have some inability to concentrate urine
   2. Glomerular filtration rate greatly increased by 6 months of age
   3. Glomerular filtration rate decreases after 20 years of age
D. Digestive system
   1. Stomach size small at birth, rapidly increases during infancy and childhood
   2. Peristaltic activity decreases with advancing age
   3. Blood sugar levels gradually rise from 75 to 80

mg per 100 ml of blood in infancy to 95 to 100 mg during adolescence

4. Premature infants have lower blood sugar levels than do full-term infants
5. Enzymes are present at birth to digest proteins and a moderate amount of fat but only simple sugars (amylase is produced as starch is introduced)
6. Secretion of hydrochloric acid and salivary enzymes increases with age until adolescence; then decreases with advancing age

E. Nervous system
   1. Brain reaches 90% of total size by 2 years of age
   2. All brain cells are present by end of the first year, although their size and complexity will increase
   3. Maturation of the brainstem and spinal cord follows cephalocaudal and proximodistal laws

PLAY
Purposes

A. Educational
B. Recreational
C. Physical development
D. Social and emotional adjustment
   1. Learn moral values
   2. Develop the idea of sharing
E. Therapeutic

Types

A. Active, physical
   1. Push-and-pull toys
   2. Riding toys
   3. Sports and gym equipment
B. Manipulative, constructive, creative, or scientific
   1. Blocks
   2. Construction toys such as erector sets
   3. Drawing sets
   4. Microscope and chemistry sets
   5. Books
C. Imitative, imaginative, and dramatic
   1. Dolls
   2. Dress-up costumes
   3. Puppets
D. Competitive and social
   1. Games
   2. Role playing

Criteria for Judging the Suitability of Toys

A. Safety
B. Compatibility
   1. Child's age

   2. Level of development
   3. Experience
C. Usefulness
   1. Challenge to development of the child
   2. Enhancing social and personality development
   3. Increasing motor and sensory skills
   4. Developing creativity
   5. Expressing emotions
   6. Achieving mastery
   7. Implementating therapeutic procedures

Criteria for Judging the Nonsuitability of Toys

A. Beyond the child's level of growth and development
B. Unsafe
C. Overstimulating; frustrating
D. Limited uses and transient value (see also play for each age group)
E. Foster isolation from peer group

The Infant
GROWTH AND DEVELOPMENT
Developmental Timetable

A. One month
   1. Physical
     a. Weight—gains about 150 to 210 g (5 to 7 oz) weekly during the first 6 months of life
     b. Height—gains about 2.5 cm (1 inch) a month for the first 6 months of life
   2. Motor
     a. May lift the head temporarily, but generally the head must be supported
     b. Holds the head parallel with the body when placed prone
     c. Can turn the head from side to side when prone or supine
     d. Asymmetrical posture dominates, such as tonic neck reflex
     e. Primitive reflexes still present
   3. Sensory
     a. Follows a light to midline
     b. Eye movements coordinated most of the time
     c. Visual acuity 20/100 to 20/50
   4. Socialization and vocalization
     a. Smiles indiscriminately
     b. Utters small throaty sounds
B. Two to 3 months
   1. Physical—posterior fontanel closed
   2. Motor
     a. Holds the head erect for a short time and can raise chest supported on the forearms

    b. Can carry hand or an object to the mouth at will

    c. Reaches for attractive objects but misjudges distances

    d. Grasp, tonic neck, and Moro reflexes are fading

    e. Can sit when the back is supported; knees will be flexed and back rounded

    f. Step or dance reflex disappears

    g. Plays with fingers and hands

  3. Sensory

    a. Follows a light to the periphery

    b. Has binocular coordination (vertical and horizontal vision)

    c. Listens to sounds

  4. Socialization and vocalization

    a. Smiles in response to a person or object

    b. Laughs aloud and shows pleasure in making sounds

    c. Cries less

C. Four to 5 months

  1. Physical—drools because salivary glands are functioning but the child does not have sufficient coordination to swallow saliva

  2. Motor

    a. Balances the head well in a sitting position

    b. Sits with little support; holds the back straight when pulled to a sitting position

    c. Symmetrical body position predominates

    d. Can sustain a portion of own weight when held in a standing position

    e. Reaches for and grasps an object with the whole hand

    f. Can roll over from back to side

    g. Lifts the head and shoulders at a 90-degree angle when prone

    h. Primitive reflexes (e.g., grasp, tonic neck, and Moro) have disappeared

  3. Sensory

    a. Recognizes familiar objects and people

    b. Has coupled eye mvements; accommodation is developing

  4. Socialization and vocalization

    a. Coos and gurgles when talked to

    b. Definitely enjoys social interaction with people

    c. Vocalizes displeasure when an object is taken away

D. Six to 7 months

  1. Physical

    a. Weight—gains about 90 to 150 g (3 to 5 oz) weekly during second 6 months of life

    b. Height—gains about 1.25 cm (½ inch) a month

    c. Teething may begin with eruption of 2 lower central incisors, followed by upper incisors

  2. Motor

    a. Can turn over equally well from stomach or back

    b. Sits fairly well unsupported, especially if placed in a forward-leaning position

    c. Hitches or moves backward when in a sitting position

    d. Can transfer a toy from one hand to the other

    e. Can approach a toy and grasp it with one hand

    f. Plays with feet and puts them in mouth

    g. When lying down, lifts head as if trying to sit up

    h. Transfers everything from hand to mouth

  3. Sensory

    a. Has taste preferences

    b. Will spit out disliked food

  4. Socialization and vocalization

    a. Begins to differentiate between strange and familiar faces and shows "stranger anxiety"

    b. Makes polysyllabic vowel sounds

    c. Vocalizes "m-m-m-m" when crying

    d. Cries easily on slightest provocation but laughs just as quickly

E. Eight to 9 months

  1. Motor

    a. Sits steadily alone

    b. Has good hand-to-mouth coordination

    c. Developing pincer grasp, with preference for use of one hand over the other

    d. Crawls and then creeps (creeping is more advanced because the abdomen is supported off the floor)

    e. Can raise self to a sitting position but may require help to pull self to feet

  2. Sensory

    a. Depth perception is beginning to develop

    b. Displays interest in small objects

  3. Socialization and vocalization

    a. Shows anxiety with strangers by turning or pushing away and crying

    b. Definite social attachment is evident—stretches out arms to loved ones

    c. Is voluntarily separating self from mother by desire to act on own

    d. Reacts to adult anger—cries when scolded

    e. Has imitative and repetitive speech, using vowels and consonants such as "Dadda"

f. No true words as yet, but comprehends words such as "bye-bye"
F. Ten to 12 months
  1. Physical
    a. Has tripled birth weight
    b. Upper and lower lateral incisors usually have erupted, for total of 6 to 8 teeth
    c. Head and chest circumferences are equal
  2. Motor
    a. Stands alone for short times
    b. Walks with help—moves around by holding onto furniture
    c. Can sit down from a standing position without help
    d. Can eat from a spoon and a cup but needs help; prefers using fingers
    e. Can play pat-a-cake and peek-a-boo
    f. Can hold a crayon to make a mark on paper
    g. Helps in dressing, such as putting arm through sleeve
  3. Sensory
    a. Visual acuity 20/50 +
    b. Amblyopia may develop with lack of binocularity
    c. Discriminates simple geometric forms
  4. Socialization and vocalization
    a. Shows emotions such as jealousy, affection, anger
    b. Enjoys familiar surroundings and will explore away from mother
    c. Fearful in strange situation or with strangers; clings to mother
    d. May develop habit of "security" blanket
    e. Can say 2 words besides *Dadda* or *Mama*
    f. Understands simple verbal requests, such as "Give it to me."
    g. Knows own name

PLAY DURING INFANCY (SOLITARY PLAY)

A. Mostly used for physical development
B. Toys need to be simple because of short attention span
C. Safety is chief determinant in choosing toys (aspirating small objects is one cause of accidental death)
D. Visual and auditory stimulation is important
E. Suggested toys
  1. Rattles
  2. Soft stuffed toys
  3. Mobiles
  4. Push-pull toys
  5. Simple musical toys
  6. Strings of big beads and large snap toys

HEALTH PROMOTION DURING INFANCY
Developmental Milestones Associated with Feeding

A. At birth the full-term infant has sucking, rooting, and swallowing reflexes
B. Newborn feels hunger and indicates desire for food by crying
C. At 1 month the infant has strong extrusion reflex
D. By 5 to 6 months the infant can use fingers to eat zwieback or toast
E. By 6 to 7 months the infant is developmentally ready to chew solids
F. By 8 to 9 months the infant can hold a spoon and play with it during feeding
G. By 9 months the infant can hold own bottle
H. By 12 months the child usually can drink from a cup, although fluid may spill and bottle may be preferred at times

Infant Nutrition

A. Nutrition as it affects growth
  1. Birth weight usually doubled by 5 months of age and tripled by 1 year (small babies may gain more weight in a shorter period)
  2. Growth during the first year should be charted to observe for comparable gain in length, weight, and head circumference
  3. Generally, growth charts demonstrate the percentile of the child's growth rate (below the fifth and above the ninety-fifth percentile are considered abnormal)
  4. Percentiles of growth curves must be seen in relation to
    a. Deviation from a steady rate of growth
    b. Hereditary factors of parents (size and body shape)
    c. Comparison of height and weight
  5. Satisfactory rate of growth judged by
    a. Weight and length (overweight and underweight constitute malnutrition)
    b. Muscular development
    c. Tissue tone and turgor
    d. General appearance and activity level
    e. Amount of crying and needed sleep
    f. Presence or absence of illness
    g. Mental status and behavior in relation to norms for the age
B. Proper feeding essential to growth and development
  1. General good nutrition that promotes growth but prevents overweight
  2. Prevention of nutritional deficiencies
  3. Prevention of GI disturbances, such as vomiting or constipation

4. Establishment of good eating habits later in life
5. Consistency of foods should progress from liquid to semisoft to soft to solids as the dentition and jaw develop

Guidelines for Infant Feeding

A. Breast milk is the most desirable complete diet for the first 6 months but requires supplements of fluoride (regardless of the fluoride content of the local water supply), iron by 6 months, and vitamin D if the mother's supply is deficient or the infant is not exposed to frequent sunlight
B. Iron-fortified commercial formula is an acceptable alternative to breast-feeding; requires fluoride supplements in areas where the fluoride content of drinking water is below 0.3 ppm (Table 3-1)
C. Breast milk or commercial formula is recommended for the first year, but after this age the infant can be given homogenized vitamin D–fortified whole milk; the use of milk with reduced fat content (skimmed or low-fat) is not recommended because increased quantities of solids would be required to supply the caloric needs, leading to overfeeding, and the high solute load would place excessive demands on the immature kidneys; in addition, essential fatty acids are missing
D. Solids can be introduced by about 6 months; the first food is often commercially prepared iron-fortified infant cereals; rice is usually introduced first because of its low allergenic potential; infant cereals should be continued until 18 months of age
E. With the exception of infant cereals, the order of introducing other foods is variable; recommended sequence is weekly introduction of other foods such as fruits, followed by vegetables, and then meats; breast-fed infants require more high-protein foods than those fed formula
F. First solid foods are strained, puréed, or finely mashed

Table 3-1. Supplemental fluoride dosage schedule (mg/day*)

	Concentration of fluoride in drinking water (ppm)		
Age	<0.3	0.3 to 0.7	>0.7
2 weeks to 2 years	0.25	0	0
2 to 3 years	0.50	0.25	0
3 to 16 years	1.00	0.50	0

From Committee on Nutrition, American Academy of Pediatrics: Pediatrics 63:150, 1979. Copyright American Academy of Pediatrics 1979.
*2.2 mg sodium fluoride contains 1 mg fluoride.

G. Finger foods such as toast, zwieback, raw fruit, or crisp-cooked vegetables are introduced at 6 to 7 months
H. Chopped table food or commercially prepared junior foods can be started by 9 to 12 months
I. Fruit juices should be offered from a cup as early as possible to reduce the development of nursing bottle caries
J. Method
1. Feed when the baby is hungry, after a few sucks of breast milk or formula
2. Introduce 1 food at a time, usually at intervals of 4 to 7 days, to allow for identification of food allergies
3. Begin spoon feeding by pushing food to back of the tongue, because of the infant's natural tendency to thrust tongue forward
4. Use a small spoon with straight handle; begin with 1 or 2 teaspoons of food; gradually increase to a couple of tablespoons per feeding
5. As the amount of solid food increases, the quantity of milk needs to be decreased to approximately 888 ml (30 oz) daily to prevent overfeeding
6. Never introduce foods by mixing them with the formula in the bottle
K. Weaning
1. Giving up the bottle or breast for a cup is psychologically significant, since it requires the relinquishing of a major source of pleasure
2. Usually, readiness develops during second half of the first year because of
a. Pleasure from receiving food by a spoon
b. Increasing desire for more freedom
c. Acquiring more control over body and the environment
3. Weaning should be gradual, replacing only 1 bottle at a time with a cup and finally ending with the nighttime bottle
4. If breast-feeding must be terminated before 5 or 6 months of age, a bottle should be used to allow for the infant's continued sucking needs; after about 6 months wean directly to a cup
L. Diseases or conditions during infancy with possible diet modifications
1. Diarrhea—sterile feedings, decreased fat and carbohydrate
2. Constipation—increased fluids, added prune juice or strained fruit, change in type of carbohydrate
3. Celiac disease (malabsorption syndrome)—sometimes due to gluten sensitivity; diet should be low in gluten, which is found in wheat, rye,

and oat grains, so these grains are eliminated and rice and corn are substituted
4. Allergy—individual diet modification according to specific food sensitivity; e.g., if milk allergy exists, substitute forms of soybean or meat formula preparations are used
5. Lactose intolerance—found in non-Caucasian races; lactose-free diet used with Nutramigen as a milk substitute
6. See inborn errors of metabolism for other disorders.

Immunizations (see Tables 3-2 and 3-3)

A. Specific characteristics of immunizations
1. Diphtheria toxoid—about 80% effective; febrile reaction more commonly seen in older children, so the adult-type Td (tetanus and diphtheria toxoid) given
2. Tetanus toxoid—nearly 100% effective; induces prolonged immunity
3. Pertussis vaccine (vaccine of whole organism)—least effective of DTP; has the most side effects
   a. Started early since no passive immunity from mother exists, as with diphtheria and tetanus
   b. Not given after the child's seventh birthday because of more severe reactions
4. Td, after 6 years of age—given routinely every 10 years and at 5-year intervals in the event of a possibly contaminated wound

5. Measles vaccine (live attenuated vaccine)—generally not given before 15 months of age because of the presence of natural immunity from mother; if given before 15 months of age, a second dose should be administered
6. Rubella given to children mainly to prevent occurrence of the disease in women during the first trimester of pregnancy
   a. Not given if pregnancy is suspected in the mother because of potential infection of the fetus
   b. Pregnancy must be prevented until 3 months after immunization of the child to eliminate danger to the fetus
7. Smallpox no longer routinely recommended in nonendemic areas, since the occurrence of fatal and severe reactions to the vaccination outweighs the risk of contracting the disease

B. General contraindications for immunizations
1. Presence of maternal antibodies
2. Administration of blood transfusion or immune serum globulin within 6 weeks
3. High fever, serious illness
4. Diseases in which immunity is impaired
5. Immunosuppressive therapy
6. Generalized malignancy such as leukemia
7. Allergy to egg protein
8. Neurologic problems such as convulsions during administration of pertussis vaccine

Table 3-2. Recommended schedule for active immunization of normal infants and children

Recommended age	Vaccine(s)	Comments
2 mo	DTP,[1] OPV[2]	Can be initiated earlier in areas of high endemicity
4 mo	DTP, OPV	2 mo interval desired for OPV to avoid interference
6 mo	DTP (OPV)	OPV optional for areas where polio might be imported (e.g., some areas of southwest United States)
12 mo	Tuberculin test[3]	May be given simultaneously with MMR at 15 mo
15 mo	Measles, mumps, rubella (MMR)[4]	MMR preferred
18 mo	DTP, OPV	Consider as part of primary series—DTP essential
4 to 6 yr[5]	DTP, OPV	
14 to 16 yr	Td[6]	Repeat every 10 yr for lifetime

From American Academy of Pediatrics: Report of the Committee on Infectious Diseases, ed. 19, Evanston, Ill., 1982, The Academy.
[1]DTP—Diphtheria and tetanus toxoids with pertussis vaccine.
[2]OPV—Oral (attenuated) poliovirus vaccine (contains poliovirus types 1, 2, and 3).
[3]Tuberculin test—Mantoux (intradermal PPD) preferred. The frequency of tests depends on the local epidemiology. Annual or biennial testing is recommended unless local circumstances dictate less frequent or no testing.
[4]MMR—Live measles, mumps, and rubella viruses in a combined vaccine.
[5]Up to the seventh birthday.
[6]Td—Adult tetanus toxoid (full dose) and diphtheria toxoid (reduced dose) in combination.
For all products used, consult the manufacturer's brochure for instructions on storage, handling, and administration. Biologics prepared by different manufacturers may vary, and those of the same manufacturer change from time to time. The package insert should be followed for a specific product.

Table 3-3. Recommended immunization schedules for infants and children not initially immunized at usual recommended times in early infancy

Timing	Preferred schedule	Alternatives no. 1	no. 2	no. 3	Comments
First visit	DTP no. 1, OPV no. 1, Tuberculin test (PPD)	MMR, PPD	DTP no. 1, OPV no. 1, PPD	DTP no. 1, OPV no. 1, MMR, PPD	MMR should be given no younger than 15 mo old
1 mo after first visit	MMR	DTP no. 1, OPV no. 1	MMR, DTP no. 2	DTP no. 2	
2 mo after first visit	DTP no. 2, OPV no. 2	—	DTP no. 3, OPV no. 2	DTP no. 3, OPV no. 2	—
3 mo after first visit	DTP no. 3	DTP no. 2, OPV no. 2	—	—	In preferred schedule, DTP no. 3 can be given if OPV no. 3 is not to be given until 10 to 16 mo
4 mo after first visit	DTP no. 3 (OPV no. 3)	—	(OPV no. 3)	(OPV no. 3)	
5 mo after first visit	—	DTP no. 3 (OPV no. 3)	—	—	OPV no. 3 optional for areas for likely importation of polio (e.g., some southwestern states)
10 to 16 mo after last dose	DTP no. 4, OPV no. 3, or OPV no. 4	DTP no. 4, OPV no. 3, or OPV no. 4	DTP no. 4, OPV no. 3, or OPV no. 4	DTP no. 4, OPV no. 3, or OPV no. 4	—
Preschool	DTP no. 5, OPV no. 4, or OPV no. 5	DTP no. 5, OPV no. 4, or OPV no. 5	DTP no. 5, OPV no. 4, or OPV no. 5	DTP no. 5, OPV no. 4, or OPV no. 5	Preschool dose not necessary if DTP no. 4 or no. 5 given after fourth birthday
14 to 16 yr old	Td	Td	Td	Td	Repeat every 10 yr

From American Academy of Pediatrics: Report of the Committee on Infectious Diseases, ed. 19, Evanston, Ill., 1982, The Academy.

Alternative no. 1 can be used in infants more than 15 mo old if measles is occurring in the community.

Alternative no. 2 allows for more rapid DTP immunization.

Alternative no. 3 should be reserved for infants whose access to medical care is compromised by poor compliance.

DTP = Diphtheria and tetanus toxoids with pertussis vaccine.

OPV = Oral, attenuated poliovirus vaccine contains types 1, 2, and 3.

Tuberculin test = Mantoux (intradermal PPD) preferred. The frequency of tests depends on the local epidemiology. Annual or biennial testing is recommended unless local circumstances dictate less frequent or no testing.

MMR = Live measles, mumps, and rubella viruses in a combined vaccine.

Td = Adult tetanus toxoid (full dose) and diphtheria toxoid (reduced dose) in combination.

For all products used, consult the manufacturer's brochure for instructions on storage, handling, and administration. Biologics prepared by different manufacturers may vary, and those of the same manufacturer change from time to time. The package insert should be followed for a specific product.

Accident Prevention

A. Accidents are one of the leading causes of death during infancy
   1. Mechanical suffocation causes most accidental deaths in children under 1 year of age
   2. Aspiration of small objects and ingestion of poisonous substances occurs most often during second half of the first year and into early childhood
   3. Trauma from rolling off a bed or falling down stairs can occur at any time
B. Teaching is an essential aspect—parents should never
   1. Leave plastic bags in the crib
   2. Restrain the infant with items that may choke
   3. Leave the infant alone on a high surface or near stairs without a proper gate
   4. Give the infant objects with sharp edges or detachable parts that can be swallowed
   5. Take the infant in an automobile without a restraining device (e.g., an approved infant car restraint)
   6. Leave any poisons in a place that the crawling infant can explore
   7. Leave burning cigarettes, candles, or incense within the infant's reach
   8. Leave electric sockets uncovered or without plastic plugs
   9. Place the crib near a window where the infant can fall or pull on blind cords

Nursing Responsibilities for Parental Guidance During the Infant's First Year

A. Birth
   1. Understand each parent's adjustment to the newborn, especially the mother's postpartal emotional needs
   2. Teach care of the infant and assist the parents to understand that the infant expresses its needs through crying
   3. Encourage the parents to establish a flexible schedule to meet the needs of the child and themselves
B. First 6 months
   1. Help the parents understand the infant's need for stimulation in environment
   2. Support the parents' pleasure in seeing the child's growing friendliness and social response, especially smiling
C. Second 6 months
   1. Prepare the parents for the child's "stranger anxiety"
   2. Encourage the parents to let the child cling to mommy or daddy and to avoid long separation from either
   3. Guide the parents concerning discipline because of the infant's increasing mobility
   4. Teach accident prevention because of the child's motor skills and curiosity
   5. Encourage the parents to leave the child with a suitable mother substitute to allow some free time
   6. Prepare for the introduction of solid foods

ACUTE AND CHRONIC HEALTH PROBLEMS
Hospitalization During Infancy

A. Reactions to parental separation (greatest from 6 months to 2 years of age)
   1. Protest
      a. Prolonged loud crying, consoled by no one but the parent or usual care giver
      b. Continually asks to go home
      c. Rejection of the nurse or any other stranger
   2. Despair
      a. Alteration in sleep pattern
      b. Decreased appetite and weight loss
      c. Diminished interest in environment and play
      d. Relative immobility and listlessness
      e. No facial expression or smile
      f. Unresponsive to stimuli
   3. Detachment or denial
      a. Cheerful undiscriminating friendliness
      b. Lack of preference for parents
B. Prevention of separation anxiety
   1. Encourage the parent to stay with the child in hospital or to visit as frequently as possible
   2. Provide a consistent care giver
   3. Provide individual attention, physical touch, sensory stimulation, and affection
   4. Prepare the parent for the child's reaction to separation
   5. Involve the parent in the child's care as much as possible
   6. If the parent is unable to visit, establish phone contact
   7. Establish routine similar to the child's home routine
   8. Provide the child with favorite items from home, for example, a blanket, a toy, or a bottle pacifier
   9. Maintain the child's familiarity with home by talking about the parents, having the child listen to a tape recording of family members' voices, and showing photographs of family members

10. When family members leave, stay with the child for comfort and to reassure the parents
11. Associate the parents' visits with familiar events, such as ''Mommy is coming after lunch''
12. Encourage the parents to visit at frequent intervals for shorter times, rather than one long visit

C. General problems in care of the infant
  1. Small size
    a. Body warmth and temperature control
    b. Maintenance of fluids—prone to edema, dehydration, and electrolyte imbalance
      (1) Infants have a higher percentage of extracellular fluid than do adults, which can be quickly excreted
      (2) Infants' kidneys are unable to concentrate urine
  2. Immature organ systems
    a. Primary defense mechanisms just developing—loss of antibodies from fetal life increases the infant's susceptibility to infection
      (1) Antibody levels lowest at 6 weeks to 2 months of age; then infants begin to develop their own system
      (2) Problem subsides as infants grow older
    b. Blood vessels still developing; increased fragility causes hemorrhage
    c. Some essential enzymes (e.g., glucuronyl transferase, which is necessary for conjugation of bilirubin) still developing—more chance for jaundice and brain damage

Reactions of Parents to a Defective Child

A. Parents exhibit a variety of responses, such as grief and mourning, chronic grief, and excessive use of defense mechanisms
B. Stages of chronic grief
  1. Shock and disbelief—parents tend to
    a. Learn about the deformity but deny the facts
    b. Feel inadequate and guilty
    c. Feel insecure in their ability to care for the child
    d. ''Doctor shop'' in hope of finding solutions
  2. Awareness of the handicap—parents tend to
    a. Feel guilty, angry, and depressed
    b. Envy well children—closely related to bitterness and anger
    c. Search for clues or reasons why this happened to them
    d. Reject and feel ambivalent toward the child
  3. Restitution or recovery phase—parents tend to
    a. See the child's defect in proper perspective
    b. Function more effectively and realistically

    c. Socially and emotionally accept the child
    d. Reintegrate family life without centering it around the handicapped child
C. Implications for nursing
  1. Helping parents gain awareness of the child's defect
    a. Learning cannot take place until awareness of the problem exists
    b. Help the parents develop an awareness through their own realization of the problem rather than identifying problem for them
    c. Help the parents see the problem by drawing attention to certain manifestations of the problem, such as failure to walk or talk
  2. Help the parents understand the child's potential ability and assist them in setting realistic goals
    a. Help them feel a sense of adequacy in parenting by emphasizing good care, identifying small steps in learning process of child, and acquainting them with parents of children with similar problems
    b. Teach them how to work with their handicapped child in simple childhood tasks of walking, talking, toileting, feeding, and dressing
    c. Teach them how to stimulate the child's learning of new skills
  3. Encourage the parents to treat the child as normally as possible
    a. Encourage them to avoid overprotection and to use consistent, simple discipline
    b. Help them become aware of the effects of this child on siblings who may resent the excessive attention given to this child
  4. Provide the family with an outlet for own emotional tensions and needs
    a. Acquaint them with organizations, especially parent groups, who have children with similar problems
    b. Be a listener, not a preacher
    c. Assist siblings who may fear the possibility of giving birth to children with similar defects

Congenital Anomalies

A. Chromosomal aberrations
  1. Down's syndrome, or mongolism
    a. Chromosomal causes
      (1) Trisomy 21—associated with advanced parental age (about a 2% risk over the age of 40); can occur earlier
      (2) Translocation 15/21—translocated chro-

mosome transmitted most often by the mother who is a carrier; age not a factor

    (3) Mosaicism—mixture of normal cells and cells that are trisomic for 21

  b. Resulting defects

    (1) Hypotonia

    (2) Congenital heart defects, particularly atrioventricular defects

    (3) Mental retardation—IQ frequently within trainable range

  c. Nursing considerations

    (1) Emotional support of parents

    (2) Genetic counseling appropriate for type of defect

    (3) Assisting parents in setting realistic expectations and goals for the child

    (4) Preventing infection, especially respiratory

    (5) Activity consistent with defects

    (6) Physical supervision and habilitation

    (7) Careful testing of intellectual functioning for guidance

    (8) Same principles as in care of the child with mental retardation and birth of a defective child

2. Trisomy 18

  a. Several physical anomalies of the head, ears, mandible, hands, feet, heart, and kidneys

  b. Failure to thrive and short survival; if survive, severe mental retardation

  c. Nursing considerations

    (1) Genetic counseling

    (2) Because of short survival, preparation of the parents for loss of their child

3. Turner's syndrome (gonadal dysgenesis)

  a. Chromosome monosomy (XO karyotype) in females

  b. Congenital malformations such as short stature, webbed neck, infantile genitalia, and developmental failure of secondary sexual characteristics at puberty

  c. Usually normal intelligence; problems in directional sense and space-form recognition

  d. Nursing considerations

    (1) Genetic counseling of parents

    (2) Preparation of child for lack of pubertal changes and need for hormonal replacement

    (3) Counseling with emphasis on adoption rather than on the person's inability to conceive

4. Klinefelter's syndrome

  a. Sex-chromosomal abnormality of XXY in males

  b. Physical characteristics—tall, skinny, long legs and arms, small firm testes, gynecomastia, and poorly developed secondary sex characteristics at puberty

  c. Behavioral disorders and mental defects often present

  d. Nursing considerations

    (1) Counseling with emphasis on positive aspects such as adoption or donor insemination

    (2) May also be a larger psychopathologic problem with need for counseling

B. Malformations (structural anomalies present at birth)

  1. Facial malformations

    a. Failure of union of embryonic structure of face

      (1) Fusion of maxillary and premaxillary processes between 5 and 8 weeks of fetal life

      (2) Palatal structures fuse between 9 and 12 weeks

    b. Cause unknown; evidence of hereditary influence

      (1) Incidence in general population is 1 in 800 births

      (2) If one child is born with a cleft lip or palate but no history of the anomaly in family, the chance that it will occur in the next child is about 4%.

      (3) If a history of either anomaly exists in one parent, there is about a 4% chance that the first child will have the defect

  2. Cleft lip

    a. Bilateral or unilateral; if unilateral, more common on the left side

    b. More common in males

    c. Can be of several degrees; complete cleft usually continuous with cleft palate

    d. Treatment is surgical repair, usually done soon after birth because of psychologic difficulties of the parents associated with the visual effects of the defect and the child's inability to meet sucking needs

    e. Nursing difficulties and interventions

      (1) Main difficulty is feeding

        (a) The child cannot form a vacuum with his mouth to suck but may be able to breast-feed (sometimes the breast fills the cleft, making sucking easier)

      (b) Should be fed with a soft large-holed nipple or rubber-tipped syringe placed on the top and side of the tongue, toward back of the mouth

      (c) Should be bubbled frequently because of swallowed air

    (2) Problem of swallowed air (mouth breather)

      (a) Distended abdomen, pressure against the diaphragm

      (b) Mucous membranes of the orpharynx become dried and cracked, leading to infection

      (c) The parent should be taught to give water after each feeding to cleanse the infant's mouth

    (3) Problem of infection from irritation of the lip

      (a) Infant's hands may need restraining

      (b) May need a pacifier to increase sucking pleasure

  f. Postoperative nursing care

    (1) Maintain a patent airway

      (a) Problem because of edema of the nose, tongue, and lips combined with the child's habit of breathing through the mouth

      (b) Proper equipment such as laryngoscope, endotracheal tube, and suction at or near the bedside

    (2) Cleanse the suture line to prevent crust formation and eventual scarring

    (3) Prevent crying, because of pressure on suture line (encourage the parent to stay with the infant)

    (4) Place the child supine with arm or elbow restraints

      (a) Change position to the side or sitting up, to prevent hypostatic pneumonia

      (b) Remove restraints only when supervised

    (5) Feeding (same as before surgery)

    (6) Support the parents by accepting and treating the child as normal

 3. Cleft palate

  a. More common in girls

  b. May involve the soft or hard palate and may extend into the nose, forming an oronasal passageway

  c. Age for repair is usually after the child has grown but before speech is well developed

  d. Nursing problems and interventions (only the differences from cleft lip care will be discussed)

    (1) Feeding

      (a) Feed upright to prevent aspiration

      (b) In severe cases, gavage feeding may be necessary

      (c) Encourage early use of spoon and cup

    (2) Infection, especially aspiration pneumonia

    (3) Speech

      (a) Palate is needed to trap air in the mouth

      (b) Tonsils usually not removed because they provide an additional mechanism to trap air

      (c) The child will need a speech appliance to help prevent guttural sounds if repair is delayed beyond speech development

    (4) Dental development

      (a) Excessive dental caries

      (b) Malocclusion from displacement of the maxillary arch

      (c) Need for proper dental hygiene and regular dental supervision

    (5) Hearing problems caused by recurrent otitis media (eustachian tube connects the nasopharynx and middle ear and easily transports foreign material to the ear)

  e. Postoperative nursing care—same as for cleft lip except

    (1) In maintaining a patent airway, try to avoid use of suction that traumatizes the operative site

    (2) Place the child in a prone Trendelenburg position to prevent aspiration and promote postural drainage

    (3) Avoid trauma to suture line by instructing child not to rub tongue on roof of mouth

    (4) Feeding

      (a) Liquid diet; no milk, because of curd formation on suture line

      (b) Avoid the use of straw or spoon

    (5) Need for emotional support of the parents is greater, since recovery is longer and the prognosis uncertain

4. Tracheoesophageal anomalies

  a. Absence of the esophagus

b. Atresia of the esophagus without a tracheal fistula
c. Tracheoesophageal fistula
d. The most common type of anomaly is proximal esophageal atresia combined with distal tracheoesophageal fistula
e. Signs and symptoms
  (1) Excessive drooling
  (2) Excessive mucus in nasopharynx causing cyanosis, which is easily reversed by suctioning
  (3) Choking, sneezing, and coughing during feeding, with regurgitation of formula through the mouth and nose
  (4) Inability to pass a catheter into the stomach
f. Treatment—surgical correction
g. Postoperative nursing care
  (1) Frequent suctioning of the mouth and pharynx
  (2) Provision of high humidity to liquefy thick secretions
  (3) Stimulation of crying and change of position to prevent pneumonia
  (4) Proper care of chest tubes if used
  (5) Maintenance of nutrition by oral parenteral, or gastrostomy method
  (6) Use of a pacifier if oral feedings are contraindicated
  (7) Need for comfort and physical contact, because hospitalization is usually long

5. Intestinal obstruction
  a. Signs alerting the nurse to life-threatening obstruction
    (1) Abdominal distention
    (2) Absence of stools, especially meconium in the newborn
    (3) Vomiting of bile-stained material; may be projectile
    (4) Cyanosis and weak grunting respirations from abdominal distention, causing the diaphragm to compress the lungs
    (5) Paroxysmal pain
    (6) Weak thready pulse

6. Imperforate anus
  a. Most common intestinal anomaly
  b. Failure of the membrane separating the rectum from the anus to absorb during eighth week of fetal life
  c. Fistulas within the vagina, urinary tract, or scrotum are common
  d. Diagnosed by
    (1) Failure to pass meconium stool
    (2) Inability to insert a catheter or small finger into the rectum
    (3) Abdominal distention
  e. Treatment—immediate surgical correction unless a fistula is present
  f. Postoperative nursing care—dependent on the type of surgery performed
    (1) Keep operative sites clean and dry, especially after passage of stool
    (2) If perineal sutures are present, position the infant on side rather than abdomen to prevent pulling legs up under the chest
    (3) Care of colostomy—prevent excoriation of the skin by frequent cleansing and use of a diaper held on by a belly binder
    (4) Instruct the parent about colostomy care (include avoidance of tight diapers and clothes around the abdomen)

7. Pyloric stenosis
  a. Congenital hypertrophy of muscular tissue of the pyloric sphincter, usually asymptomatic until 2 to 4 weeks after birth
  b. Clinical signs
    (1) Vomiting, progressively projectile
    (2) Non-bile-stained vomitus
    (3) Constipation
    (4) Dehydration and weight loss
    (5) Distention of the epigastrium, visible peristalsis, and palpable olive-shaped mass in the right upper quadrant
  c. Treatment generally surgical—the Fredet-Ramstedt procedure: longitudinal splitting of the hypertrophied muscle
  d. Postoperative nursing care
    (1) Same as for any abdominal surgery
    (2) Teach parents the specific feeding method
      (a) Give small frequent feedings and feed slowly
      (b) Hold the baby in a high Fowler position during feeding and place on the right side after feeding with head of bed slightly elevated
      (c) Bubble frequently during feeding and avoid unnecessary handling afterward

8. Megacolon (Hirschsprung's disease)
  a. Absence of parasympathetic ganglion cells in a portion of the bowel, which causes enlargement of the bowel proximal to the defect
  b. Clinical signs may occur gradually

(1) Constipation, or passage of ribbon or pelletlike stool

(2) Intestinal obstruction

c. Treatment

    (1) Medical

        (a) Use of laxatives, enemas

        (b) Dietary management—decrease bulk and residue

    (2) Surgical

        (a) Removal of aganglionic portion of the bowel

        (b) Colostomy if necessary

d. Nursing considerations

    (1) Teach parents the correct procedure for enemas (point out danger of water intoxication)

    (2) Use only isotonic solutions

    (3) Prepare isotonic saline by using 1 tsp table salt to 500 ml (1 pint) of tapwater.

    (4) Use the following suggested amounts:

Age	Amount (ml)
Infant	150 to 250
Small child	250 to 350
Larger child	300 to 500
Adolescent	500 to 750

    (5) General postoperative care

9. Diaphragmatic hernia

a. Protrusion of abdominal viscera through an opening into the thoracic cavity

b. Symptoms alerting the nurse

    (1) Severe respiratory difficulty with cyanosis

    (2) Relatively large chest, especially on the affected side

    (3) Failure of affected side of the chest to expand during respiration, absence of breath sounds

    (4) Relatively small abdomen

c. Treatment—immediate surgical repair

d. Nursing care

    (1) Gastric suction is used to remove secretions and swallowed air from the stomach and intestine before and after surgery

    (2) Preoperatively, to allow full expansion of the unaffected side, position the infant on affected side with the head elevated

    (3) Postoperatively, to decrease chances of swallowing air, the infant may be fed by gavage

10. Congenital laryngeal stridor (laryngomalacia)

a. A crowing sound during inspiration caused by different factors, most often related flabbiness of the epiglottis

b. May correct itself as the infant grows, or may necessitate tracheostomy to sustain life

c. Nursing problems and interventions

    (1) Feeding

        (a) Infant must be fed slowly; stop frequently to allow breathing and then reoffer bottle or breast

        (b) Proper nipple hole size and position at the breast are important in regulating flow

        (c) Parent needs help to learn correct feeding method

    (2) Breathing

        (a) Parents should be encouraged to listen to sound of stridor to detect a change

        (b) Needs to be protected from respiratory tract infection, which increases breathing difficulty

11. Choanal atresia

a. Embryonic membrane obstructing the posterior nares at junction with the nasopharynx

b. Bilateral obstruction causes mouth breathing and dyspnea that is relieved by crying and aggravated by sucking

c. Nursing problems and interventions are the same as for laryngeal stridor

12. Congenital heart defects

a. Normal circulatory changes that occur at or shortly after birth

    (1) Pulmonary circulation rapidly increases

    (2) Increased pressure from left side of the heart results in closure of the foramen ovale, ductus arteriosus, and ductus venosus

b. General signs and symptoms of congenital heart defects in children

    (1) Dypsnea, especially on exertion

    (2) Feeding difficulty and failure to thrive, often first signs discovered by the mother

    (3) Stridor or choking spells

    (4) Heart rate over 200, respiratory rate about 60 in the infant

    (5) Recurrent respiratory tract infections

    (6) In the older child, poor physical development, delayed milestones, and decreased exercise tolerance

    (7) Cyanosis, squatting, and clubbing of fingers and toes

(8) Heart murmurs

(9) Excessive perspiration

c. Classification of cardiac lesions

  (1) Acyanotic—shunt from left to right side of heart

    (a) No abnormal communication between pulmonary and systemic circulation

    (b) If such a connection exists, pressure forces blood from the arterial to the venous side of the heart, where it is reoxygenated

  (2) Cyanotic—shunt from the right to left side of the heart

    (a) Abnormal connection between the pulmonary and systemic circulations

    (b) Venous or unoxygenated blood enters the systemic circulation

    (c) Polycythemia (increase in the number of red blood cells) occurs as the body tries to compensate for inadequate supply of oxygen

    (d) Squatting or knee-chest position is preferred because it decreases venous return by occluding the femoral veins, which have a very low oxygen content; consequently a smaller volume of this blood enters the right ventricle so that the blood shunted into the aorta has a higher oxygen content; it also increases systemic vascular resistance, which diverts right ventricular blood from the aorta into the pulmonary artery, increasing pulmonary blood flow; this increases the amount of oxygenated blood in the left side of the heart and eventually into systemic circulation

    (e) Compensation and the nature of the defect cause clubbing of fingers and toes, retarded growth, and increased viscosity of blood; can lead to congestive heart failure

d. Types of acyanotic defects

  (1) Ventricular septal defect (VSD)

    (a) Abnormal opening between the 2 ventricles

    (b) Severity of the defect depends on size of the opening

    (c) High pressure in the right ventricle causes hypertrophy, with development of pulmonary hypertension

    (d) Blowing-type murmur heard throughout systole

    (e) Treatment procedure—close the opening in the septum

  (2) Atrial septal defect (ASD)—3 types

    (a) Ostium secundum defect, in which the hole is in the center of the septum

    (b) Ostium primum defect, in which there is inadequate development of the endocardial cushions

    (c) Sinus venosus defect, in which the superior portion of the atrial septum fails to form near the junction of the atrial wall with the superior vena cava

    (d) Murmur heard high on the chest, with fixed splitting of the second heart sound

    (e) Treatment procedure—close the opening in the septum

  (3) Patent ductus arteriosus (PDA)

    (a) Failure of the fetal connection between the aorta and pulmonary artery to close

    (b) Blood shunted from the aorta back to the pulmonary artery; may progress to pulmonary hypertension and cardiomegaly

    (c) Machinery type murmur heard throughout the heartbeat in the left second or third interspace

    (d) Treatment procedure—close the opening between the aorta and the pulmonary artery; in critically ill newborns, pharmacologic closure may be attempted with a prostaglandin inhibitor (e.g., indomethacin)

  (4) Coarctation of the aorta

    (a) In utero, failure of aorta to develop completely; stricture usually occurs below level of the aortic arch

    (b) Increased systemic circulation above the stricture—bounding radial and carotid pulses, headache, dizziness, epistaxis

    (c) Decreased systemic circulation below the stricture—absent femoral pulses, cool lower extremities

    (d) Increased pressure in aorta above

the defect causes left ventricular hypertrophy
(e) Murmur may or may not be heard
(f) Treatment procedure—resection of the defect and anastomosis of the ends of the aorta
(5) Aortic stenosis
(a) Narrowing of the aortic valve
(b) Causes increased work load on the left ventricle, and the lowered pressure in the aorta reduces coronary artery flow
(c) Treatment procedures—divide the stenotic valves of the aorta
(6) Pulmonary stenosis
(a) Narrowing of the pulmonary valve
(b) Causes decreased blood flow to the lungs and increased pressure to the right ventricle
(c) Treatment procedures—valvotomy
e. Types of cyanotic defects
(1) Tetralogy of Fallot—4 associated defects
(a) Pulmonary valve stenosis
(b) Ventricular septal defect, usually high on the septum
(c) Overriding aorta, receiving blood from both ventricles, or an aorta arising from the right ventricle
(d) Right ventricular hypertrophy
(e) Palliative treatment procedures
[1] Waterston-Cooley procedure: aorta to pulmonary artery anastomosis
[2] Blalock-Taussig procedure: subclavian artery to pulmonary artery anastomosis
(f) Complete repair—closure of the ventricular septal defect and resection of the infundibular stenosis, possibly with a pericardial patch to enlarge the right ventricular outflow tract.
(2) Transposition of the great vessels
(a) Aorta arises from the right ventricle, and pulmonary artery arises from the left ventricle
(b) Incompatible with life unless there is a communication between the 2 sides of the heart, such as an atrial septal defect, ventricular septal defect, or patent ductus arteriosus
(c) Palliative treatment procedures

[1] Blalock-Hanlen operation: surgical creation of an atrial septal defect
[2] Rashkind procedure: enlargement of an existing atrial septal defect by pulling a balloon through the defect (balloon septotomy) during a cardiac catheterization
[3] Pulmonary artery banding if a ventricular septal defect is present to decrease blood flow to the lungs and increase shunting of oxygenated blood intraventricularly to the aorta
[4] Creation of a systemic-pulmonary shunt if pulmonic stenosis is present
[5] Pharmacologic dilation of a patent ductus arteriosus with use of prostaglandins (e.g., Prostin VR)
(d) Complete repair
[1] Mustard's or Senning's procedure: removing the entire atrial septum and creating a new atrial septum from existing pericardium or a prosthesis that tunnels or baffles blood for more effective oxygenation, with creation of 2 new functionally correct atrial chambers
[2] Jatene operation: switching the great vessels to their correct anatomic placement with reimplantation of the coronary arteries
(3) Tricuspid atresia
(a) Absence of the tricuspid valve
(b) Incompatible with life unless there is a communication between the 2 sides of the heart, such as atrial septal defect, ventricular septal defect, or patent ductus arteriosus
(c) Palliative treatment procedures—same as for tetralogy of Fallot
(d) Complete repair—Fontan procedure: conversion of the right atrium into an outlet for the pulmonary artery, which involves placing a tubular conduit with a valve between the two and closing the atrial septal defect; physiologically corrects tri-

cuspid atresia by preventing any mixing of systemic blood in the left atrium and shunting the entire venous blood to the lungs for oxygenation

(4) Truncus arteriosus

  (a) Single great vessel arising from the base of the heart, serving as a pulmonary artery and aorta

  (b) Systolic murmur is heard, and a single semilunar valve produces a loud second heart sound that is not split

  (c) Palliative treatment—banding the pulmonary arteries as they arise from the truncus to decrease blood flow to lungs

  (d) Complete repair—Rastelli's operation: excising pulmonary arteries from aorta and attaching them to the right ventricle by means of a prosthetic valve conduit; septal defects also repaired

f. Treatment—besides surgical intervention, digitalization can be used to increase the efficiency of heart action

(1) Positive inotropic effect is achieved by increasing the permeability of muscle membranes to the calcium and sodium ions required for contraction of muscle fibrils

  (a) Forceful contraction during systole improves peripheral tissue perfusion

  (b) Chamber emptying allows additional venous blood to enter the cardiac chambers during diastole

(2) Negative chronotropic effect is achieved through an action mediated by the vagus nerve that slows firing of the SA node and impulse transmission through the AV node (negative dromotropic action)

(3) Drug preparations have the same qualitative effect on heart action but differ in potency, rate of absorption, amount absorbed, onset of action, and speed of elimination

  (a) Digitalis—longer onset, peak action, and half-life

  (b) Digoxin (Lanoxin)—rapid onset and peak action and short half-life; drug of choice in children, especially because the risk of toxicity is lessened by the shorter half-life

(4) Digitalization

  (a) Provides an initial loading dose for acute effect on the enlarged heart

  (b) After desired effect is achieved, the dosage is lowered to maintenance level, replacing the drug metabolized and excreted each day

(5) Adverse effects

  (a) Most frequent—nausea, vomiting, headache, drowsiness, insomnia, vertigo, confusion; all attributable to drug action at CNS sites; oral forms also cause nausea and vomiting by irritation of the gastric mucosa

  (b) Bradycardia attributable to drug-induced slowing of SA node firing

  (c) Arrhythmias are first evidence of toxicity in one third of patients; premature nodal or ventricular impulses; varying degrees of heart block caused by drug action that slows transmission of impulses through the AV node

  (d) Xanthopsia (yellow vision) caused by drug effect on the visual cones

  (e) Gynecomastia (mammary enlargement) in males resulting from the estrogen-like steroid portion of digitalis glycosides

(6) Considerations during therapy

  (a) Premature contractions elevate the audible apical rate and mask the pacemaker conduction rate; apical pulse is taken before administration and drug is withheld when pulse rate drops to 110 to 90 in infants and below 70 in older children

  (b) Immaturity of hepatic and renal systems in premature and newborn infants or depressed hepatic or renal function in children may result in cumulation

  (c) Since potassium ions are required for interaction of digitalis glycosides with sodium-potassium dependent membranes, the lowering of serum levels of potassium ions may foster digitalis toxicity

  (d) Since calcium ions act synergistically with digitalis on myocardial membranes, an elevation of serum calcium ion levels may increase sensitivity of cardiac muscle to digitalis action

(7) Drug interactions

  (a) Phenobarbital, phenytoin, and phenylbutazone, by induction of hepatic microsomal enzymes, accelerate metabolism of digitalis glycosides; serum levels are lower when the drugs are used concomitantly

  (b) Diuretics that cause hypokalemia may contribute to the incidence of serious arrhythmias when administered concurrently with digitalis glycosides; supplemental potassium may be used for replacement of losses, or potassium-sparing diuretics may be prescribed to prevent potassium ion losses

g. Nursing responsibilities

  (1) Correctly calculate the dosage of digoxin; usually prescribed in micrograms (1000 μg = 1 mg)

  (2) Take the apical pulse prior to administering the drug

  (3) Observe for signs of digitalis toxicity

  (4) Teach the parents home administration of digoxin

  (5) Help the parents cope with symptoms of the disease

    (a) During dyspneic/cyanotic spell, place the child in a side-lying knee-chest position, with the head and chest elevated

    (b) Keep the child warm; encourage rest and sleep

    (c) Decrease the child's anxiety by remaining calm

    (d) Feed the child slowly; allow frequent burping

    (e) Administer small, frequent meals

    (f) Introduce solids and spoon feeding early

    (g) Encourage the anorexic child to eat

    (h) Encourage parents to include others in the child's care to prevent their own exhaustion

  (6) Foster growth-promoting family relationships

    (a) Encourage family members to discuss their feelings about each other and the child's defect

    (b) Maintain expectations from all siblings as equal as possible

    (c) Provide consistent discipline, especially from infancy, to prevent behavioral problems

    (d) Encourage acceptable pursuits for the child

    (e) Discuss school entry with the teacher and school nurse

    (f) Guide parents to the eventual hazards of fostering overdependency

    (g) Help the parents feel adequate in their maternal-paternal roles by emphasizing growth and developmental progress of the child

    (h) Help the parents foster the child's development by stimulating the child to age-appropriate goals consistent with his activity tolerance

    (i) Provide social experiences for the child

h. Preoperative preparation

  (1) Main assessment factor in preparation of the child is the developmental and chronologic age

    (a) Explanation of the heart differs according to age of the child

    (b) Children 4 to 6 years of age know that the heart is in the chest, describe it as valentine shaped, and characterize its function by the sound of "tick tock"

    (c) Children 7 to 10 years of age do not see the heart as valentine shaped, know it has veins, have an idea of its function (e.g., "It makes you live"), but do not understand the concept of pumping

    (d) Children over 10 years of age have a concept of veins, valves, circulation, and why death occurs when the heart stops

  (2) Based on the principle that fear of the unknown increases anxiety

  (3) The same nurse should participate in preoperative and postoperative preparation as a source of support for the child and parents

  (4) Nurse must know what equipment is usual after open or closed heart surgery

  (5) Let the child play with equipment such as stethoscope, blood pressure ma-

chine, oxygen mask, suction, and syringes

(6) For the young child, especially the preschooler, use dolls and puppets to describe procedures

(7) Preparation for cardiac catheterization prior to surgery is essential as well

(8) For the young child, talk about the size of the bandage; for the older child, discuss the actual incision

(9) Familiarize the child with the postoperative environment such as recovery room and intensive care unit, stressing the strange noises there (e.g., the monitors)

(10) Have the child practice coughing, using blow bottles, and breathing on the IPPB machine

(11) Explain to the child why coughing and moving are necessary even though they may be uncomfortable

(12) Explain to the child what tubes may be used and what they will look like

(13) For more specific discussion of the aforementioned, see specific age groups under pediatric nursing

i. Preoperative assessment areas necessary for planning postoperative care

(1) Keep a sleep record so care can be organized around the child's usual rest pattern

(2) Constipation and straining after surgery must be avoided—this can be accomplished by

    (a) Knowing the child's elimination pattern

    (b) Knowing words the child uses

    (c) Having the child practice using a bedpan

(3) Record the level of activity and list favorite toys or games that require gradually increased exertion.

(4) Determine the child's fluid preferences for postoperative maintenance

(5) When recording vital signs, always indicate the child's activity at the time of measurement

(6) Observe the child's verbal and nonverbal responses to pain

(7) Specifics of postoperative care are similar to those for any major surgery

j. Adjustment of the child and family to correction of cardiac defect

(1) Improved physical status is often difficult for the child who has become accustomed to the sick role and its secondary gains

(2) Improved physical status of the child is also difficult for the parents, since it reduces child's dependency

(3) The child may have difficulty learning to relate to peers and siblings on a competitive basis

(4) The child can no longer use the disability as a crutch for educational and social shortcomings

(5) Parental expectations must be adjusted to accommodate the child's new physical vigor and search for independence

13. Spina bifida

a. Malformation of the spine in which the posterior portion of the laminae of the vertebrae fails to close; most common site is the lumbosacral area

(1) Spine bifida occulta—defect only of the vertebrae; spinal cord and meninges are intact

(2) Meningocele—meninges protrude through the vertebral defect

(3) Meningomyelocele—meninges and spinal cord protrude through the defect; most serious type

b. Associated defects include weakness or paralysis below the defect, bowel and bladder dysfunction, clubfeet, dislocated hip, and hydrocephalus

c. Arnold-Chiari syndrome—defect of the occipitocervical region with swelling and displacement of medulla into the spinal cord

d. Nursing problems and intervention (meningomyelocele)

(1) Infection because breakdown of the sac leaves the spinal cord open to the environment

    (a) Area must be kept clean, especially from urine and feces

    (b) Diaper is not used, but sterile gauze with antibiotic solution may be placed over the sac

(2) Associated orthopedic defects

    (a) Maintain function through proper position, which also decreases pressure on the sac

    (b) Clubfeet and dislocated hip—prone position, hips slightly flexed and abducted, feet hanging free of mattress, and a slight Trendelenburg slope to reduce spinal fluid pressure

(3) Feeding because of restriction in position; the child is usually fed prone; nurse should establish eye contact and encourage parents to visit and feed the child

(4) Elimination, especially infants with a neurogenic bladder

    (a) Credé method or slight pressure against the abdomen for complete emptying of the bladder

    (b) While the infant is prone, the nurse can apply pressure to the abdomen above symphysis pubis with sides of the fingers and counterpressure with thumbs against the buttocks

e. Postoperative nursing care

(1) Surgical repair of the sac may be done soon after birth to prevent infection and maintain neurologic function

(2) Care is same as for cardiac surgery, with emphasis on development of the child's abilities

(3) Head size should be measured to determine whether hydrocephalus is occurring

14. Hydrocephalus

a. Abnormal accumulation of cerebrospinal fluid within the ventricular system

(1) Noncommunicating—obstruction within the ventricles such as congenital malformation, neoplasm, or hematoma

(2) Communicating—inadequate absorption of CSF resulting from infection or trauma

b. Clinical signs

(1) Increasing head size in the infant because of open sutures and bulging fontanels

(2) Prominent scalp veins and taut shiny skin

(3) "Sunset" eyes (sclera visible above iris), bulging eyes, and papilledema of retina

(4) Head lag, especially important after 4 to 6 months

(5) Increased intracranial pressure—projectile vomiting not associated with feeding, irritability, anorexia, high shrill cry, convulsions

(6) Damage to the brain because increased pressure decreases blood flow to the cells, causing necrosis

c. Treatment

(1) Removal of the obstruction

(2) Mechanical shunting of fluid to another area of the body

    (a) Ventriculoatrial shunt—catheter from a lateral ventricle to the internal jugular vein to the right atrium of the heart

    (b) Ventriculoperitoneal shunt—catheter passed subcutaneously to the peritoneal cavity

d. General nursing problems and intervention

(1) Breakdown of scalp; infection and damage to the spinal cord

    (a) Proper positioning—place the infant in a Fowler position to facilitate draining of fluid; postoperative positioning should be flat with no pressure on the shunted side

    (b) When holding the child, support the neck and head

    (c) Observe shunt site (abdominal site in peritoneal procedure) for infection

(2) Increasing intracranial pressure

    (a) Careful observation, minimal use of sedatives or analgesics, which can mask signs

    (b) Frequent checking of the valve for patency

    (c) Pumping the valve per physician's orders to ensure proper functioning

(3) Nutrition

    (a) Frequent vomiting, irritability, lethargy, and anorexia decrease the intake of nutrients

    (b) All care should be done before feeding to prevent vomiting; infant should be held if possible

    (c) Observe for signs of dehydration

(4) Irritation of the eyes if eyelids incompletely cover corneas

e. Specific postoperative nursing care—similar to that for cardiac surgery except

(1) The child is usually kept in bed after surgery, with minimal handling to prevent damage to shunt

(2) Parents need much support

    (a) Continued shunt revisions are usually necessary as growth occurs

    (b) Usually very concerned about retardation

(3) Observe for brain damage by recording milestones during infancy

(4) Parental teaching must include
    (a) Pumping of the shunt
    (b) Signs of increasing intracranial pressure
    (c) Evidence of dehydration

15. Exstrophy of the bladder
   a. Entire lower urinary tract, from bladder to external urethral meatus, is outside the abdominal cavity
   b. May be accompanied by defects such as epispadias, undescended testes, or short penis in boys and a cleft clitoris or absent vagina in girls
   c. Treatment
    (1) Plastic surgery
    (2) Ileal conduit (also called ureteroileal cutaneous ureterostomy)—a small section of the ileum or colon is resected, and the remaining bowel is reanastomosed; one end of the resected bowel is sutured closed and the other end is attached to a small opening in the lower abdomen, forming a stoma; the distal ends of the ureters are severed from the bladder and attached to the ileum, which acts like a bladder, although there is no voluntary control in the regulation of voiding; the child wears an ileostomy appliance over the stoma, which collects the continuously flowing urine; in a young child diapers serve the same purpose as the collecting appliance
    (3) Cutaneous ureterostomy—the ureters are attached directly to the abdominal wall, usually at a site proximal to the level of the kidneys; 2 collecting appliances are worn over the bilateral openings
   d. Nursing problems and intervention
    (1) Parental teaching is vital, but objectives can be achieved only after the parents have accepted both the disorder and the long-term sequelae
    (2) Infection and the care of the skin
      (a) Scrupulous cleansing of the area, application of sterile petrolatum gauze, and care of the skin around the bladder
      (b) To avoid pressure over the area, clothing should be light
      (c) Frequent change of clothing because of odor
      (d) Care of the appliance that collects urine

16. Displacement of the urethral opening
   a. Hypospadias
    (1) In boys the urethra opens on the lower surface of the penis from just behind the glans to the perineum
    (2) In girls the urethra opens into the vagina
   b. Epispadias
    (1) Occurs only in boys
    (2) Urethra opens on dorsal surface of the penis; often associated with exstrophy of the bladder
   c. Nursing considerations
    (1) Repair is usually of concern to parents, who need an explicit explanation of the child's future functioning
    (2) Repair may be in several stages; the boy needs preparation for surgery and help in coping with adjustment to voiding in a sitting position
    (3) Defect can be a sign of ambiguous genitalia
    (4) Procreation may be interfered with in severe cases

17. Orthopedic deformities
   a. Clubfoot
    (1) Foot has been twisted out of position in utero
    (2) Most common type—talipes equinovarus: foot is fixed in plantar flexion (downward) and deviated medially (inward)
    (3) Treatment is most successful when started early, since delay causes muscles and bones of legs to develop abnormally, with shortening of tendons
    (4) Treatment and nursing measures in infancy
      (a) Denis Browne splint (a crossbar with shoes attached)
        [1] Encourage activity since success of the appliance depends on alternate kicking and extension of the baby's legs
        [2] Watch for circulatory impairment caused by swelling around ankles
        [3] Pick the child up frequently to prevent respiratory and other problems from immobility
      (b) Gentle repeated manipulation of the foot or forcible correction under anesthesia and application of a wedge cast

[1] Observe toes for signs of circulatory impairment; make sure toes are visible at the end of the cast

[2] Watch for signs of weakness and wear of the cast, especially if the child is allowed to walk on it

[3] For other areas of cast care, see treatment of a dislocated hip

[4] Main nursing objective is teaching parents all the aforementioned, stressing the need for follow-up care, which may be prolonged

(5) Follow-up care of the patient

  (a) Extended medical supervision is required, since there is a tendency for this deformity to recur (considered cured when the child is able to wear normal shoes and walk properly)

  (b) Care emphasizes muscle reeducation (by manipulation) and proper walking

  (c) Heels and soles of braces or shoes prescribed following correction must be kept in repair

  (d) Corrective shoes may have sole and heel lifts on lateral border to maintain proper position

b. Dislocated hip

(1) Head of the femur does not lie deep enough within the acetabulum and slips out on movement (may be caused by lack of embryonic development of the joint)

(2) Main clinical signs

  (a) Limitation in abduction of leg on the affected side

  (b) Asymmetry of gluteal, popliteal, and thigh folds

  (c) Audible click when abducting and externally rotating the hip on the affected side—Ortolani's sign

  (d) Apparent shortening of the femur—Galeazzi's sign

  (e) Waddling gait and lordosis when the child begins to walk

(3) Treatment—directed toward enlarging and deepening the acetabulum by placing the head of the femur within the acetabulum and applying constant pressure

  (a) Proper positioning—legs slightly flexed and abducted

    [1] Frejka pillow—a pillow splint that maintains abduction of the legs

    [2] Use of pillow or rolled diapers between the legs

    [3] Bryant's traction

    [4] Spica cast—from the waist to below the knees

  (b) Surgical intervention such as open reduction with casting

(4) Specific nursing problems and intervention when a spica cast is applied

  (a) Respiratory problems—hypostatic pneumonia

    [1] Need to change position from back to stomach frequently

    [2] Teach parents postural drainage and exerises such as blowing bubbles to increase lung expansion

    [3] Encourage parents to seek immediate medical care if the child develops congestion or cough

  (b) Infection and excoriation of skin

    [1] Observe for circulation of toes, pedal pulses, and blanching

    [2] Do not let the child put small toys or food inside cast

    [3] Gauze strips may be used inside cast as a scratcher

    [4] Alert parents to signs of infection, such as odor

    [5] Protect cast edges with adhesive tape or waterproof material, especially around perineum

    [6] Use diapers and plastic lining to minimize soiling of cast by feces and urine

  (c) Constipation from immobility

    [1] Parents should observe for straining on defecation and constipation

    [2] Increase fluids and roughage to prevent constipation

  (d) Nutrition

    [1] Provide small, frequent meals because of inflexibility of cast around waist

    [2] Adjust calorie intake, since less energy expenditure can lead to obesity

(e) Transportation and positioning

    [1] Use wagon or stroller with back flat

    [2] Protect child from falling when positioned

    [3] Child must not be picked up by the bar between the legs of the cast (use 2 people to provide adequate body support if necessary)

(f) Emotional needs

    [1] Since the child cannot be picked up and cuddled, touch should be used as much as possible

    [2] Stimulate and provide for play activities appropriate to age

(g) Parents need help and support

    [1] Directions should be written

    [2] Home visits should be routine, with telephone counseling available

    [3] Treatment may be prolonged, so follow-up care must be stressed

    [4] Prepare parents for the possible use of an abduction brace after the cast is removed

c. Developmental anomalies of the extremities

  (1) Polydactyly—extra digits

  (2) Syndactyly—partial or complete fusion of 2 or more digits

  (3) Amelia—absence of a limb

  (4) Treatment—if possible, early correction and preparation for use of a prosthesis

  (5) Nursing considerations

    (a) Recognize own reaction to the deformity

    (b) Accept the parents' reactions of guilt, anger, and hopelessness

    (c) Assist the parents in setting realistic goals for the child

    (d) Prepare the parents to answer the child's questions about the deformity and what it will mean in the future

C. Inborn errors of metabolism

  1. Phenylketonuria (PKU)

    a. Lack of the enzyme phenylalanine hydroxylase, which changes phenylalanine (essential amino acid) into tyrosine

    b. Transmitted by autosomal recessive gene

    c. Clinical symptoms

      (1) Mental retardation from damage to the nervous system by buildup of phenylalanine

        (a) Often noticed by 4 months of age

        (b) IQ is usually below 50 and most frequently under 20

      (2) Strong musty odor in urine from phenylacetic acid

      (3) Absence of tyrosine reduces the production of melanin and results in blond hair and blue eyes

      (4) Fair skin is susceptible to eczema

    d. Treatment

      (1) Prevention—test for PKU at birth

        (a) Guthrie blood test—effective in newborns; testing is recommended after 4 days of milk-based feeding; if testing is done during initial 24 hours, it should be repeated by the third week of life

        (b) Ferric chloride urine test—effective only when infant is over 2 weeks of age, when brain damage may have occurred

      (2) Dietary—low-phenylalanine: use Lofenalac as a milk substitute and restrict foods to those low in this amino acid (usually continued until the child is 6 to 8 years of age)

    e. Nursing considerations

      (1) Parents need help in understanding the disease and the role of diet

      (2) Genetic counseling

  2. Galactosemia

    a. Missing enzyme that converts galactose to glucose

    b. Transmitted by autosomal recessive gene

    c. Treatment—dietary, reduction of lactose: use a meat-base formula or Nutramigen as a milk substitute and restrict foods to those low in lactose (usually continued until the child is 7 to 8 years of age) followed by a relaxed modification throughout life

    d. Nursing considerations similar to those for phenylketonuria

Noncongenital Conditions

A. Surgical problems

  1. Intussusception

    a. Telescoping of 1 portion of the intestine into another; occurs most frequently at the ileocecal valve

    b. Clinical signs

(1) Healthy, well-nourished infant who wakes up with severe paroxysmal abdominal pain, evidenced by kicking and drawing legs up to the abdomen

(2) One or 2 normal stools, then bloody mucous stool ("currant jelly" stool)

(3) Palpation of a sausage-shaped mass

(4) Other signs of intestinal obstruction usually present

  c. Treatment

(1) Medical—reduction by hydrostatic pressure (barium enema)

(2) Surgical reduction; sometimes with intestinal resection

  d. Nursing considerations

(1) Same as those for any abdominal surgery

(2) Since the problem usually occurs when the child is 6 to 8 months of age, separation anxiety is acute and provision must be made for parent's frequent visits

B. Medical problems

1. Failure to thrive (FTT)—The term used to describe infants and children whose weight and sometimes height fall below the fifth percentile for their age; there are two distinct categories of FTT:

  a. Organic—result of a physical cause, such as congenital heart defects, neurologic lesions, microcephaly, chronic urinary tract infection, gastroesophageal reflux, renal insufficiency, malabsorption syndrome, endocrine dysfunction, or cystic fibrosis

  b. Nonorganic—caused by psychosocial factors, problem being between the child and the primary caregiver, usually the mother; in this situation the lack of physical growth is secondary to the lack of emotional and sensory stimulation (other terms include maternal deprivation, environmental deprivation, and deprivation dwarfism)

(1) Characteristics of nonorganic FTT children

(a) Growth failure—below the fifth percentile in height and weight

(b) Developmental retardation—social, motor, adaptive, language

(c) Apathy

(d) Poor hygiene

(e) Withdrawing behavior

(f) Feeding or eating disorders, such as vomiting, anorexia, voracious appetite, pica, rumination

(g) No fear of strangers (at the age when stranger anxiety is normal)

(h) Avoidance of eye-to-eye contact

(i) Wide-eyed gaze and continual scan of the environment ("radar gaze")

(j) Stiff and unyielding or flaccid and unresponsive

(k) Minimal smiling

(2) Characteristics of the parent providing care

(a) Difficulty perceiving and assessing the infant's needs

(b) Frustrated and angered at the infant's dissatisfied response

(c) Frequently under stress and in crisis, with emotional, social, and financial problems

(d) Often with marital disturbances (e.g., absent spouse or one who gives little emotional support)

(e) Tending to lead lonely, solitary lives with few outside interests or friends

(f) Experienced poor parenting as a child

  c. Nursing considerations

(1) The child needs a consistent care giver, who can begin to satisfy routine needs

(2) Provide optimum nutrients

(a) Make feeding a priority goal

(b) Keep an accurate record of intake to ensure ingestion of calculated daily calories

(c) Weigh daily and record to ascertain weight gain

(3) Introduce a positive feeding environment

(a) Assign one nurse for feeding

(b) Maintain a calm, even temperament; be persistent

(c) Provide a quiet, unstimulating environment

(d) Hold the young child for feeding

(e) Maintain eye-to-eye contact with the child

(f) Talk to the child by giving appropriate directions and praise for eating

(g) Follow the child's rhythm of feeding

(h) Establish a structured routine and follow it consistently

(4) Increase stimulation, appropriate to the child's present developmental level

(5) Provide the parent an opportunity to talk

(6) When necessary, relieve the parent of childrearing responsibilities until able and ready emotionally to support the child

(7) Demonstrate proper infant care by example, not lecturing (allow the parent to proceed at own pace)

(8) Supply the parent with emotional support without fostering dependency

(9) Promote the parent's self-respect and confidence by praising achievements with child

2. Sudden infant death syndrome—SIDS (crib death)

a. A definite syndrome with cause unknown

b. No. 1 cause of death in infants between 2 weeks and 1 year of age; incidence of 1 in every 350 live births

c. Peak age of occurrence—healthy infant 3 to 4 months of age

d. Higher incidence in:
(1) Premature infants
(2) Multiple births
(3) Newborns with low Apgar scores
(4) Infants with central nervous system disturbances

e. Feeding habits not significant; breast-feeding does not prevent SIDS

f. Five times greater incidence in siblings of SIDS children

g. Nursing considerations to assist parents
(1) Know signs of SIDS to distinguish it from child neglect or abuse; do or say nothing that instills guilt in the parents
(2) Reassure the parents that they could not have prevented the death or predicted its occurrence
(3) An autopsy should be done on every child to confirm diagnosis
(4) Visit the parents at home to discuss the cause of death and help them with their guilt and grief
(5) Refer the parents to a National Sudden Infant Death Syndrome Parent Group

3. Diarrhea
a. Symptom of a variety of conditions such as viral or bacterial infection or allergy
b. Metabolic acidosis from loss of water and electrolytes, which decreases available bicarbonate

c. Clinical manifestations
(1) Dehydration is severe when weight loss is greater than 10%
(2) Poor skin turgor and dry mucous membranes
(3) Depressed fontanels and sunken eyeballs
(4) Decreased urine output, increased specific gravity, and increased hematocrit
(5) Irritability, stupor, convulsions from loss of intracellular water and decreased plasma volume

d. Treatment and nursing considerations
(1) In severe diarrhea, medical treatment is necessary to correct fluid and electrolyte imbalance
(2) Isolate the infant until stool culture results are reported
(3) Identify the causative agent and institute proper therapy (antibiotics are used if a bacterial agent is present)
(4) Explain to the parents why antibiotics and an increase in food are ineffective in treating viral diarrhea
(5) Parents should be taught progressive increase in diet—alterations in diet may control mild diarrhea
(a) Clear fluids to decrease inflammation of the mucosa
(b) If tolerated, half-strength skim milk
(c) Regular diet of bland foods

4. Vomiting
a. Symptom of many conditions, such as poor feeding technique, chalasia (abnormal relaxation of the cardiac sphincter), or infections
b. Results in metabolic alkalosis from loss of hydrogen ion
c. Clinical signs
(1) Dehydration
(2) Tetany and convulsions in severe alkalosis, resulting from hypokalemia and hypocalcemia
d. Nursing considerations
(1) Care directed toward correction of the underlying problem
(2) Chalasia
(a) Thicken the consistency of foods given
(b) Feed in an upright position
(c) Maintain the upright position 20 to 30 minutes after feeding

5. Colic
   a. Paroxysmal intestinal cramps from accumulation of excessive gas
   b. May be caused by cow's milk sensitivity, but often no cause is found
   c. Treatment—directed toward correction of the underlying cause when identified
   d. Nursing considerations
      (1) Watch the parent feed the infant before attempting to counsel
      (2) Teach the parent to bubble the infant frequently and to position on its abdomen after feeding
      (3) Encourage the mother to take time away from the infant
6. Constipation
   a. Usually a result of diet, although may have a psychologic component
   b. Treatment should be dietary—enemas should be avoided
   c. If mineral oil is used, it should not be given with foods, since it decreases the absorption of nutrients
7. Respiratory tract infections
   a. Frequent cause of morbidity
   b. Acute infection may be bacterial or viral (refer to microbiology in medical-surgical chapter)
      (1) Acute nasopharyngitis (common cold)
      (2) Pneumonia
      (3) Bronchitis
      (4) Tonsillitis
      (5) Epiglottitis
      (6) Croup
      (7) Acute laryngotracheobronchitis
   c. General nursing care for respiratory conditions
      (1) Increase fluid intake
         (a) Prevents dehydration from fever and perspiration
         (b) Loosens thickened secretions
      (2) Increase humidity and coolness
         (a) Liquefies secretions
         (b) Decreases the febrile state and inflammation of the mucous membrane
         (c) Causes vasoconstriction and bronchiolar dilation
      (3) Promote nasal and pulmonary drainage
         (a) Clean the nares with a bulb syringe
         (b) Suction the oronasal pharynx
         (c) Postural drainage, clapping, and vibrating
      (4) Provide rest by decreasing stimulation

      (5) Increase oxygen
      (6) Tracheotomy if necessary (see medical-surgical nursing for general nursing care of tracheotomy)
8. Otitis media
   a. Acute infection of the middle ear; causative organism usually *Haemophilus influenzae, Staphylococcus* organism, or *Streptococcus* organism
   b. Symptoms of acute otitis
      (1) Pain—infant frets and rubs his ear or rolls his head from side to side
      (2) Drum bulging, red, may rupture; no light reflex
   c. Serous—accumulation of uninfected serous or mucoid matter in the middle ear; cause unknown
   d. Symptoms of serous otitis
      (1) No pain or fever, but "fullness' in the ear
      (2) Drum appears gray, bulging
      (3) May be loss of hearing from scarring of the drum
   e. Nursing considerations
      (1) Proper instillation of eardrops
         (a) If the child is under 3 years of age, pull the auricle down and back
         (b) Older child, pull the auricle up and back
      (2) Check for complications such as chronic hearing loss, mastoiditis, or possible meningitis
9. Meningitis
   a. Causative agent may be viral or bacterial, such as *Haemophilus influenzae, Neisseria meningitidis* or *Diplococcus pneumoniae*
   b. Clinical manifestations (more severe in bacterial)
      (1) Opisthotonos—rigidity and hyperextension of the neck
      (2) Headache
      (3) Irritability and high-pitched cry
      (4) Signs of increased intracranial pressure
      (5) Fever, nausea, and vomiting
   c. Nursing considerations
      (1) Provide for rest
      (2) Decrease stimuli from the environment (control light and noise)
      (3) Position on the side with head gently supported in extension
      (4) Institute respiratory isolation for bacterial meningitis
      (5) Decrease fluids because of meningeal edema

(a) Carefully record intake and output

(b) Monitor IV fluid

(6) Provide emotional support for the parents, since the child usually becomes ill very suddenly

(7) Administer antibiotic therapy as prescribed

10. Eczema
    a. Atopic manifestation of a specific allergen that may have an emotional component
    b. Most common during first 2 years of life
    c. Clinical manifestations
       (1) Erythema and edema from dilation of capillaries
       (2) Papules, vesicles, and crusts
       (3) Itching that may precipitate infection from scratching
       (4) Periods of remission and exacerbation
       (5) Seen mostly on cheeks, scalp, neck, and flexor surfaces of arms and legs
    d. Nursing considerations
       (1) Support the parents because this long-term problem is often discouraging, since the infant is difficult to comfort
       (2) Restrain hands to keep the infant from scratching when unsupervised, but provide supervised unrestrained play periods
       (3) Pick up frequently since the infant is irritable, fretful, and anorectic
       (4) Avoid using wool clothing or blankets
       (5) Provide the parent a list of foods permitted and omitted on an elimination or restricted diet
       (6) Instruct the parent how to apply topical ointments prescribed

11. Febrile convulsions
    a. Caused by elevation of temperature
    b. Usually occur in children between 6 months and 3 years of age
    c. Nursing considerations
       (1) Reduce fever with antipyretic drugs and sponge baths
       (2) General seizure precautions
          (a) Protect the child from injury; do not restrain; pad crib rails
          (b) Prevent the tongue from blocking the airway and protect it from injury
          (c) Record the time of seizure, duration, and body parts involved
          (d) Suction the nasopharynx and administer oxygen after the seizure as required
          (e) Observe the degree of consciousness and behavior after the seizure
          (f) Provide rest after the seizure
    d. For further discussion of convulsive disorders, see medical-surgical nursing

The Toddler

GROWTH AND DEVELOPMENT
Developmental Timetable

A. Fifteen months
   1. Motor
      a. Walks well alone by 14 months, with a wide-based gait
      b. Creeps upstairs
      c. Builds tower of 2 blocks
      d. Drinks from a cup and can use a spoon
      e. Enjoys throwing objects and picking them up
   2. Vocalization and socialization
      a. Can use 10 to 15 single words
      b. Has learned "No," which may be said while doing a requested demand
      c. Indicates when diaper is wet

B. Eighteen months
   1. Physical
      a. Growth has decreased and appetite lessened—"physiologic anorexia"
      b. Anterior fontanel is usually closed
      c. Abdomen protrudes, larger than chest circumference
   2. Motor
      a. Walks sideways and backward, runs well
      b. Climbs stairs or up on furniture
      c. Scribbles vigorously, attempting a straight line
      d. Drinks well from a cup, still spills with a spoon
      e. May begin to control bowel movements
   3. Vocalization and socialization
      a. Uses phrases composed of adjectives and nouns
      b. Has new awareness of strangers
      c. Begins to have temper tantrums
      d. Very ritualistic, has favorite toy or blanket, thumb-sucking may be at peak

C. Two years
   1. Physical
      a. Weight—about 11 to 12 kg (26 to 28 pounds)
      b. Height—about 80 to 82 cm (32 to 33 inches)
      c. Teeth—16 temporary
   2. Motor
      a. Gross motor skills quite well refined

  b. Can walk up and down stairs, both feet on one step at a time, holding onto rail

  c. Builds tower of 5 cubes or will make cubes into a train

  d. Control of spoon well developed

  e. Toilet trained during the daytime

 3. Sensory

  a. Accommodation well developed

  b. Visual acuity 20/40

 4. Vocalization and socialization

  a. Vocabulary of about 300 words

  b. Uses short 2-to-3-word phrases, also pronouns

  c. Obeys simple commands

  d. Still very ritualistic, especially at bedtime

  e. Can help undress self and pull on simple clothes

  f. Shows signs of increasing autonomy and individuality

  g. Does not share possessions, everything "mine"

D. Thirty months

 1. Physical

  a. Full set of 20 temporary teeth

  b. Decreased need for naps

 2. Motor

  a. Walks on tiptoe

  b. Stands on 1 foot

  c. Builds tower of 8 blocks

  d. Copies horizontal or vertical line

 3. Vocalization and socialization

  a. Beginning to see self as a separate individual from reflected appraisal of significant others

  b. Still sees other children as "objects"

  c. Increasingly independent, ritualistic, and negativistic

Major Learning Events

A. Toilet training—most important task of the toddler

 1. Physical maturation must be reached before training is possible

  a. Sphincter control adequate when the child can walk

  b. Able to retain urine for at least 2 hours

  c. Usual age for bowel training—24 to 30 months

  d. Daytime bowel and bladder control—during second year

  e. Night control—by 3 to 4 years of age

 2. Psychologic readiness

  a. Aware of the act of elimination

  b. Able to inform the parent of the need to urinate or defecate

  c. Desire to please the parent

 3. Process of training

  a. Usually begin with bowel, then bladder

  b. Accidents and regressions frequently occur

 4. Parental response

  a. Choose a specific word for the act

  b. Have a specific time and place

  c. Do not punish for accidents

B. Need for independence without overprotection; the parents should

 1. Be consistent—set realistic limits

 2. Reinforce desired behavior

 3. Be constructive, geared to teach self-control

 4. Punish immediately after a wrongdoing

 5. Punish appropriately

PLAY (PARALLEL PLAY)

A. The child plays alongside other children but not with them

B. Mostly free and spontaneous, no rules or regulations

C. Attention span is still very short, and change of toys occurs at frequent intervals

D. Safety is important; there is danger of

 1. Breaking a toy through exploration and ingesting small pieces

 2. Ingesting lead from lead-based paint on toys

 3. Being burned by potentially flammable toys

E. Imitation and make-believe play begins by end of the second year

F. Suggested toys

 1. Play furniture, dishes, cooking utensils, dress-up clothes

 2. Telephone

 3. Puzzles with a few large pieces

 4. Pedal-propelled toys, such as tricycle

 5. Straddle toys and rocking horse

 6. Clay, sandbox toys, crayons, finger paints

 7. Pounding toys, blocks

HEALTH PROMOTION DURING CHILDHOOD
Childhood Nutrition

A. Nutritional objectives

 1. Provide adequate nutrient intake to meet continuing growth and development needs

 2. Provide a basis for support of psychosocial development in relation to food patterns, eating behavior and attitudes

 3. Provide sufficient calories for increasing physical activities and energy needs

B. Diet—calorie and nutrient requirements increase with age

 1. Increased variety in types and textures of foods

 2. Increased involvement in the feeding process,

stimulation of curiosity about food environment, language learning
3. Consideration for the child's appetite, choices, motor skills

C. Possible nutritional problem areas
1. Anemia—increase foods containing iron (e.g., enriched cereals, meat, egg, green vegetables)
2. Obesity or underweight—increase or decrease calories; maintain core foods
3. Low intake of calcium, iron, vitamins A and C—usually caused by dietary fads
4. Often omitting breakfast before school
5. Influence of commercialism on selection of foods and emphasis on fast foods, "empty-calorie" snacks, and high-carbohydrate convenience foods

Accident Prevention

A. Leading cause of death in children over 1 year of age
B. Children under 5 years of age account for over half of all accidental deaths during childhood
C. More than half of accidental child deaths are related to automobiles and fire
D. Accidents can be viewed in terms of the child's growth and development, especially curiosity about the environment
1. Motor vehicle
a. Walking or running, especially after objects thrown into the street
b. Poor perception of speed, lack of experience to foresee danger
c. Child often unseen because of small size; can be run over by a car backing out of the driveway, or when playing in leaves or snow
d. Failure to restrain in a car (sitting in a person's lap, improper use of seat belts rather than appropriate car restraint)
2. Burns
a. Investigating—pulls a pot off the stove, plays with matches, inserts an object into wall socket
b. Climbing—reaches the stove, oven, ironing board and iron, cigarettes on the table
3. Poisons
a. Learning new tastes and textures, puts everything into mouth
b. Developing fine motor skills—able to open bottles, cabinets, jars
c. Climbing to previously unreachable shelves and cabinets
4. Drowning
a. Child and parents do not recognize the danger of water

b. Child is unaware of inability to breathe under water
5. Aspirating small objects and putting foreign bodies in ear or nose
a. Puts everything in mouth
b. Very interested in body and newly found openings
6. Fractures
a. Climbing, running, and jumping
b. Still developing sense of balance

E. Prevention, through parent education and child protection, is the goal

ACUTE AND CHRONIC HEALTH PROBLEMS
Hospitalization

A. Specific response of the toddler is separation anxiety (see hospitalization during infancy)
B. Toddler experiences basic fear of loss of love, fear of unknown, fear of punishment
C. Immobilization and isolation represent additional crises to the toddler
D. Nursing considerations in preparing parents and the child for hospitalization
1. Primary consideration is maintaining the parent-child relationship by preventing separation
2. Through assessment, establish routines and rituals that the child is accustomed to in the areas of
a. Toilet training
b. Feeding
c. Bathing
d. Sleep patterns
e. Recreational activities
3. Prepare the parent for regression of the child to previous modes of behavior and loss of newly learned skills
4. Hospitalization is usually not a time for teaching the child new skills
5. Allow the child's release of tension, especially aggression, through play (banging a drum, knocking blocks over, scribbling on paper)
6. Only minimal advance preparation of the child for hsopitalization is possible, since cognitive ability to grasp verbal explanation is limited

Burns

See medical-surgical nursing
A. Principles of treatment
1. Stop the burning process
a. Remove from source of danger
b. Remove smoldering clothes
c. For superficial burns, immerse the affected area in cool water
2. Administer prompt first aid

    a. Maintain a patent airway
    b. For first-degree burns, cleanse the area, apply sterile dressing soaked in sterile saline if possible
    c. Do not apply creams, butter, or any household remedies
    d. For severe burns (more than 10% of body) oral fluids are not given
  3. Transport the patient to a proper care facility
    a. Children are hospitalized with burns of 5% to 12% of body surface or more
    b. Large body surface in proportion to weight results in greater potential for fluid loss
    c. Shock—primary cause of death in first 24 to 48 hours
    d. Infection—primary cause of death after initial period
B. Nursing problems and interventions
  1. Fluid and electrolyte loss
    a. Greatest in first 24 to 48 hours because of tissue damage
    b. Immediate replacement of both fluids and electrolytes is essential
    c. Accurate measurement of both intake and output is critical (daily weights, diaper count, and weight)
    d. Determination of hematocrit, hemoglobin, and chemistries should be done daily to provide a guide for replacement
  2. Isolation
    a. The child has feelings of guilt and punishment
    b. Children under 5 years of age rarely understand the reason for isolation
    c. Furthers separation between parents and the child
    d. Encourage the child to express feelings
    e. Allow the child to play with gown, mask, and gloves so that they are less strange
  3. Touch deprivation
    a. Touch, a child's main means of comfort and security, is now painful
    b. Pleasurable touch must be reestablished (apply lotion to unaffected areas and let the child apply it to a doll)
    c. Prepare the child for baths and whirlpool treatments, which can be frightening and painful
  4. Nutrition
    a. High in protein, vitamins, and calories
    b. The child is frequently anorectic because of discomfort, isolation, emotional depression
    c. Provide the child food preferences when feasible; do not force eating or use it as a weapon; encourage parent participation
    d. Alter the diet as needs change, especially when high-calorie foods are no longer needed and can cause obesity
  5. Contractures
    a. Make moving a game; use play that utilizes the affected part, such as throwing a ball for arm movement
    b. Provide for proper body alignment; place the child so attention is focused on an object that will keep the body in specific position
    c. Do passive exercises during bath or whirlpool
  6. Body image
    a. For the younger child, more of a concern to parents (whose reactions are communicated to the child)
    b. For the older child, especially the adolescent, body damage is of great concern
    c. Emphasize what can be done to improve looks (plastic surgery, wigs, appropriate clothing, makeup)
  7. Pain
    a. Assessed by observing behavior of the young child rather than verbal complaints
    b. Distinguish pain from fear of dark, being left alone, or being in strange surroundings
    c. Administer analgesics prior to procedures; often narcotics may be required
C. Main nursing consideration—prevention
  1. Parent education especially in regard to the child's growth and development and specific dangers at each age level
  2. Child education regarding fire safety
    a. Tell the child to leave the house as soon as smoke is smelled or flames are seen, without stopping to retrieve a pet or toy
    b. Involve all members of the family in fire drills
    c. Demonstrate rolling rather than running if clothes are on fire
  3. Fire and burn prevention in the house
    a. Intelligent use of heaters, barbecue, and fireplace
    b. Children should be supervised at all times
    c. Maintain integrity of the electrical system
    d. Escape route must be maintained

Poisoning

A. Principles of treatment
  1. Terminate the exposure
    a. Empty the mouth of pills, plant parts, or other material

b. If the eyes and/or skin were involved, thoroughly flush them with tap water

c. If gasoline was spilled, remove contaminated clothing

d. If an inhalation poisoning, bring the victim into fresh air

2. Identify that a poisoning has occurred

   a. Call the local poison control center, emergency facility, or physician for immediate advice regarding treatment

   b. Save all evidence of poison (container, vomitus, urine, etc.)

3. Remove the poison

   a. Dilute with water

   b. Induce vomiting except as contraindicated:

     (1) If the person is comatose, in severe shock, or convulsing or has lost the gag reflex; any of these conditions can increase the risk of aspiration

     (2) If the poison is a low-viscosity hydrocarbon; once aspirated, it can cause a severe chemical pneumonitis

     (3) If the poison is a strong corrosive (acid or alkali); emesis of the corrosive redamages the mucosa of the esophagus and pharynx

   c. Administer ipecac syrup (15 ml with 1 to 2 glasses of water) if vomiting has not occurred; repeat once in 20 minutes

   d. Administer activated charcoal only *after* inducing vomiting

   e. Prepare appropriate equipment for potential medical use, such as gastric lavage

4. Prevent aspiration of vomitus

   a. Keep the child's head lower than the chest; place the head between the legs or position on the side

5. Observe for latent symptoms and complications of poisoning

   a. Treat as appropriate; e.g., institute seizure precautions, keep warm and position correctly in case of shock, reduce temperature if hyperpyrexic

6. Support the child and parent

   a. Keep calm and quiet

   b. Do not admonish or accuse the child or parent of wrongdoing

7. Prevent occurrence and/or recurrence

   a. Assess possible contributing factors in the occurrence of an accident, such as discipline, parent-child relationship, developmental ability, environmental factors, and behavior problems

   b. Institute anticipatory guidance for possible future accidents based on the child's age and maturational level

   c. Refer to a visiting nurse agency for evaluation of the home environment and the need for safety measures

   d. Provide assistance with environmental manipulation when necessary

B. Salicylate poisoning

1. One of the most common drugs taken by children

2. Toxic dose—4.4 gr per kilogram of body weight or 8 adult aspirins (32 baby aspirin) for a 9 kg child

3. Clinical signs of mild salicylate toxicity

   a. Ringing in the ears

   b. Dizziness

   c. Disturbances of hearing and vision

   d. Sweating

   e. Nausea

   f. Vomiting

   g. Diarrhea

   h. Delirium

4. Clinical signs of salicylate poisoning

   a. Hyperventilation—confusion, coma

   b. Metabolic acidosis—anorexia, sweating, increased temperature

   c. Bleeding, especially if chronic ingestion

5. Treatment

   a. Induce vomiting, gastric lavage, activated charcoal, saline cathartics

   b. IV fluids

   c. Vitamin K if bleeding

   d. Peritoneal dialysis in severe cases

6. Nursing considerations

   a. Identify the salicylate overdose

   b. Assist with removal of the drug and other therapies

     (1) Administer ipecac syrup

     (2) Assist with gastric lavage if appropriate

     (3) Administer activated charcoal after ipecac syrup

     (4) Administer a saline cathartic

     (5) Assist with peritoneal dialysis, hemodialysis, or exchange transfusion if necessary

     (6) Administer intravenous fluids as prescribed

     (7) Assess blood gases and serum electrolyte concentration frequently

     (8) Administer sodium bicarbonate, electrolytes, and vitamin K as indicated

     (9) Measure intake and output

    (10) Check urine specific gravity
    (11) Administer tepid sponge bath
    (12) Place on a cooling blanket
    (13) Observe vital signs frequently
    (14) Obtain serial blood and urine specimens
    (15) Assess the level of unconsciousness and other neurologic signs
    (16) Administer anticonvulsants
    (17) Implement seizure precautions
    (18) Insert a nasogastric tube to detect any gastric bleeding
    (19) Assess stools for occult blood (guaiac test)
  c. Support the child and parents
    (1) Explain procedures and tests according to developmental level of the child
    (2) Allow for expression of feelings
    (3) Provide comfort measures
    (4) Encourage parents to visit
    (5) Allow expression of feelings regarding circumstances related to the poisoning
    (6) Provide reassurance as appropriate
    (7) Keep informed of the child's progress
  d. Prevent salicylate poisoning
    (1) Educate the parents regarding safe storage of the family supply of aspirin
    (2) Teach parents to take aspirin or other drugs out of the sight of children
    (3) Teach children the hazards of ingesting nonfood items without supervision
    (4) Caution the family against leaving aspirin within reach of children
    (5) Caution against keeping large amounts of the drug on hand, especially children's varieties
    (6) Discourage transferring aspirin to containers without safety caps
    (7) Discuss problems of discipline and children's noncompliance
    (8) Instruct the parents regarding correct administration of aspirin for therapeutic purposes and to discontinue drug if evidence of mild toxicity

C. Acetaminophen poisoning
  1. Clinical signs of overdose
    a. Profuse sweating
    b. Nausea and vomiting
    c. Skin eruptions
    d. Weakness
    e. Cyanosis
    f. Slow, weak pulse
    g. Depressed respirations
    h. Decreased urine output
    i. Hypothermia
    j. Circulatory collapse
    k. Coma
  2. Treatment
    a. Induce vomiting with ipecac syrup, lavage
    b. Administer IV fluid
    c. Administer an antidote (acetylcysteine)
  3. Nursing considerations—goals are essentially the same as those discussed under salicylate poisoning
    a. Monitor the electrocardiograph
    b. Measure intake and output
    c. Measure and record the vital signs frequently
    d. Obtain blood for hepatic and renal function tests
    e. Support the child and family
    f. Prevent overdose

D. Petroleum distillates (hydrocarbons)
  1. Clinical signs of toxicity
    a. Gagging, choking, and coughing
    b. Nausea
    c. Vomiting
    d. Alterations in sensorium, such as lethargy
    e. Weakness
    f. Respiratory symptoms of pulmonary involvement
     (1) Tachypnea
     (2) Cyanosis
     (3) Substernal retractions
     (4) Grunting
  2. Vomiting is not induced—aspiration is a particular danger because of the risk of a chemical pneumonia
  3. Nursing considerations
    a. Identify ingestion of distillates
    b. Prevent further irritation
     (1) Avoid causing emesis
     (2) Implement gastric lavage or emesis *only* as indicated
    c. Support the child and family
    d. Prevent ingestion
     (1) Teach parents the proper storage of petroleum distillate products (kerosene, turpentine, gasoline, lighter fluid, furniture polish, metal polish, benzene, naphtha, some insecticides, cleaning fluid)

E. Corrosive chemicals
  1. Clinical signs of toxicity
    a. Severe burning pain in the mouth, throat, and stomach
    b. White, swollen mucous membranes, edema of the lips, tongue, and pharynx (respiratory obstruction)

c. Violent vomiting; hemoptysis, hematemesis
d. Signs of shock
e. Anxiety and agitation
2. Never induce vomiting, since regurgitation of the substance will cause further damage to the mucous membranes
3. Nursing considerations
   a. Identify ingestion
   b. Maintain a patent airway
      (1) Examine the pharynx for burns
      (2) Observe for respiratory difficulty
      (3) Provide an airway if necessary; have emergency equipment available
      (4) Administer steroids if prescribed
   c. Prevent further irritation
      (1) Avoid causing emesis
      (2) Dilute with water if advised
      (3) Give nothing by mouth except as ordered and tolerated
   d. Provide comfort and support to the child and family
      (1) Administer analgesics as needed
      (2) Remain with the child
      (3) Keep parents informed of the child's progress
   e. Prevent ingestion
      (1) Teach the parents proper storage of corrosive products (oven and drain cleaners, electric dishwasher granules, strong detergents)
F. Lead poisoning
   1. Most common between 18 months and 3 years of age, usually from eating lead chips from peeling paint or sucking on objects painted with lead-based paint
   2. Characteristics of the child and parents
      a. About 50% of mothers had habit of pica (eating nonfood substances)
      b. High level of oral activity in the child (e.g., use of pacifier, thumb-sucking)
      c. Oral gratification used as method of relieving anxiety in the child
      d. Maternal dependency, despair, passivity
         (1) Mother is absent from home
         (2) Mother present but unable to supervise the child
   3. Clinical manifestations (chronic ingestion)
      a. Loss of weight, anorexia
      b. Abdominal pain, vomiting
      c. Constipation
      d. Anemia, pallor, listlessness, fatigue
      e. Lead line on teeth; density of long bones

f. Behavior changes (impulsiveness, irritability, hyperactivity, or lethargy)
g. Headache, insomnia, joint pains
h. Brain damage, convulsions, death
i. Increased blood lead level
   (1) Normal—below 40 μg per 100 ml of blood
   (2) Borderline—below 60 μg per 100 ml of blood
   (3) Treatment begun—usually 60 μg or higher
   (4) Convulsions and irreversible brain damage—about 80 μg
4. Treatment
   a. Objective—reduce concentration of lead in the blood and soft tissue by promoting its excretion and deposition in bones
      (1) Calcium disodium edetate (Calcium Disodium Versenate)
         (a) Urine lead content monitored; peak excretion in 24 to 48 hours
         (b) Adverse effects—acute tubular necrosis, malaise, fatigue, numbness of extremities, GI disturbances, fever, pain in muscles and joints
      (2) Dimercaprol (BAL)
         (a) Generally used in conjunction with calcium disodium edetate
         (b) Adverse effects—local pain at the site of injection; may cause persistent fever in children receiving therapy; rise in blood pressure accompanied by tachycardia after injection
      (3) Use vitamin D, calcium, and phosphorus
   b. Prevention of further ingestion
5. Nursing considerations
   a. Prevention through education, proper housing, supervision of children
   b. Screening for these children by recognizing signs, especially behavior changes
   c. Careful planning for rotation of injection sites and preparation of the child
   d. Seizure precautions
   e. Discharge planning and follow-up care of the child
   f. Teach parents to prevent further ingestion

Fractures

See medical-surgical nursing
A. Greenstick fractures—incomplete break and bending of a long bone, occurring in young children because the bones are soft and not fully mineralized

B. Treatment of fractures—splint, traction, or cast
   1. Bryant's traction—for fractured femur
      a. Generally used for children under 2 years of age
      b. Legs are suspended vertically with buttocks slightly off bed and upper body maintaining countertraction
   2. Spica cast may be used for child of any age
C. Nursing considerations
   1. The child must be kept flat on back
   2. Restraining jacket may be necessary to prevent moving
   3. Provide activity to keep child occupied and entertained

Aspiration of Foreign Objects

A. Symptoms
   1. Substernal retractions
   2. Cough and inability to speak
   3. Increased pulse and respiratory rate
   4. Cyanosis
B. Treatment
   1. Immediate first aid if object is in the trachea
      a. Try to pull the object out if possible without forcing it further down
      b. Turn the small child upside down (head lower than chest) and deliver 4 quick sharp back blows with the heel of the hand; turn the infant over and deliver 4 quick chest thrusts using the technique for CPR
      c. Abdominal thrust (Heimlich maneuver)—grasp the victim from behind around the upper abdomen and squeeze, forcing the diaphragm up
   2. Medical removal by bronchoscopy
   3. Surgical relief by a tracheotomy below level of the object
C. Prevention
   1. Keep small objects such as balloons out of the child's reach
   2. Inspect large toys for removable objects
   3. Teach the child not to run or laugh with food or fluid in the mouth
   4. Avoid giving young children foods easily aspirated, such as nuts or hotdogs
   5. Teach the child to chew food well before swallowing

Battered Child Syndrome

A. Refers to both physical abuse and emotional neglect
B. Majority of abused children are under 4 years of age
C. About 70% to 80% of abuse is by parents
D. One theory—role reversal: a reversal of dependency role in which the parent turns to the child for nurturing and love
E. Characteristics of abusing parents
   1. Their own childrearing included abuse
   2. Have incorrect concept of what a small child is and can do
   3. Plagued by a deep sense of inferiority and lack of identity
   4. Tend to be young, immature, and dependent
   5. Frequently expect the child to provide them with nurturing and love
   6. Tend to be depressed, lonely people, yearning for love and understanding
   7. Have no outside resources for emotional support or relief from responsibility, especially in time of crisis; thus they take out their frustration on the child
F. How to identify child neglect or abuse
   1. The child has many unexplained injuries, scars, bruises
   2. Parents offer inconsistent stories explaining child's injuries when questioned
   3. Emotional response of parents is inconsistent with the degree of the child's injury
   4. Parents may resist or fail to be present for questioning
   5. The child exhibits physical signs of neglect—malnourished, dehydrated, unkempt
   6. The child cringes when physically approached
   7. The child responds in a manner that indicates avoiding punishment rather than gaining reward
G. Nursing considerations
   1. Main objective—protect the child from an abusing environment (nurse must be aware of child abuse laws)
   2. Be alert for clues that indicate child abuse
   3. Focus on helping parents with their own dependency needs
      a. Group therapy
      b. Home visiting
      c. Foster grandparents
   4. Help parents learn to control frustration through other outlets
   5. Educate parents about the child's normal needs and development, new modes of discipline, and realistic expectations
   6. Provide emotional support and therapy for the child since abused children frequently grow up to be abusing parents

Mental Retardation

A. Usually defined as low IQ (70 or below); about 3% of the population
B. American Association on Mental Deficiency defines subaverage IQ as 83 or 84 associated with impairment in adaptive behavior, which represents about 16% of population
C. Retardation can be further classified by the use of the following intelligence test scores (these numbers are approximate and should not be used in a fixed manner for diagnosis):
   1. Normal—90 to 110 IQ
   2. Slow—71 to 89 IQ
   3. Mildly retarded—50 to 70 IQ
      a. Educable—can achieve a mental age of 8 to 12 years
      b. Can learn to read, write, do arithmetic, achieve a vocational skill, and function in society
   4. Moderately retarded—36 to 49 IQ
      a. Trainable—can achieve a mental age of 3 to 7 years
      b. Can learn the activities of daily living, social skills; can be trained to work in a sheltered workshop
   5. Severely retarded—below 35 IQ
      a. Barely trainable—can achieve a mental age of 0 to 2 years
      b. Totally dependent on others and in need of custodial care
D. Causes
   1. Prenatal—heredity, PKU, Down's syndrome, severe malnutrition (relationship is under study), rubella
   2. Natal—kernicterus (high bilirubin level), intracranial hemorrhage, anoxia
   3. Postnatal—lead poisoning, meningitis, encephalitis, neoplasms, recurrent convulsions
E. Diagnosis
   1. Delayed milestones
      a. Infant fails to suck
      b. Head lag after 4 to 6 months of age
      c. Slow in learning self-help; slow to respond to new stimuli
      d. Slow or absent speech development
   2. Conditions that may lead to a false diagnosis of mental retardation
      a. Emotional disturbance, such as autism or maternal deprivation
      b. Sensory problems, such as deafness or blindness

   c. Cerebral dysfunctions, such as cerebral palsy, learning disorders, hyperkinesia, epilepsy
F. Characteristics of mentally retarded children
   1. Mental abilities are concrete—abstract ability is limited
   2. Lack power of self-appraisal
   3. Do not learn from errors
   4. Cannot carry out complex instructions
   5. Do not relate with peers—more secure with adults
   6. Comforted by physical touch
   7. Learn rote responses and socially acceptable behavior
   8. May repeat words (echolalia)
   9. Short attention span, but usually attracted to music
G. Nursing considerations
   1. Always deal with the child's developmental not chronologic age
      a. Educate the parent regarding developmental age
      b. When the child is nearing adolescence, sexual feelings accompany maturation and need to be explained according to the child's mental capacity
   2. Set realistic goals; teach by simple steps for habit formation rather than for understanding or transference of learning
      a. When teaching a skill, break the process down into simple steps that can be easily achieved
      b. Each step must be learned completely before teaching the child the next step
      c. Behavior modification is a very effective method of teaching these children
      d. Praise for accomplishment must be given to develop the child's self-esteem
   3. Discipline must remain simple, geared toward learning acceptable behavior rather than developing judgment
   4. Routines are the foundation of the child's lifestyle; hospitalization should be based on the child's normal schedule
   5. See parents' reaction to a defective child

Cerebral Palsy

A. Neuromuscular disability or difficulty in controlling voluntary muscles (caused by damage to some portion of the brain, with associated sensory, intellectual, emotional, or convulsive disorders)

B. Characteristics of cerebral palsy
  1. Affects young children, usually becoming evident before 3 years of age
  2. Nonprogressive, but persists throughout life
  3. Some motor dysfunction always present
  4. Mental deficiency may or may not be present
C. Major causes
  1. Anoxia of the brain caused by a variety of insults at or near the time of birth
  2. Infection of the central nervous system
D. Types—classified according to predominant clinical manifestation
  1. Spasticity (65%)—hyperactivity of muscle stretch reflex, which becomes worse with rapid passive motion
  2. Athetosis—slow, wormlike, involuntary purposeless movement
  3. Rigidity—persistent stiffness of the muscles on movement, which becomes less severe with rapid passive motion
  4. Ataxia—disturbance in the sense of balance
  5. Tremor—a rhythmic purposeless movement that becomes worse with excitement or intentional movement
  6. Flaccidity—decreased muscle tension
E. Clinical manifestations
  1. Difficulty in feeding, especially sucking and swallowing
  2. Asymmetry in motion or contour
  3. Delayed motor development and speech
  4. Excessive or feeble cry
  5. Any of the muscular abnormalities listed under types
F. Nursing problems and interventions
  1. Feeding
    a. Drooling results from difficulty in swallowing
    b. Use a spoon and blunt fork, with plate attached to the table, for easier self-feeding
    c. The child may require increased calories because of excessive energy expenditure, increased protein for muscle activity, and increased vitamins (especially B$_6$) for amino acid metabolism
  2. Relaxation
    a. Provide rest periods in an area with few stimuli
    b. Set limits and control activity level
  3. Safety
    a. Protect from accidents resulting from poor balance and lack of muscle control
    b. Provide helmet for protection against head injuries
    c. Always restrain in chair, bed, etc.
    d. Institute seizure precautions
  4. Play
    a. Keep safety as main objective
    b. Must not be overstimulating, should have educational value, appropriate to child's developmental level and ability
  5. Elimination
    a. Difficulty in toilet training because of poor muscle control
    b. May need special bowel and bladder training
  6. Speech
    a. Poor coordination of lips, tongue, cheeks, larynx, and poor control of diaphragm make formation of words difficult
    b. May need speech therapy
  7. Breathing
    a. Poor control of the intercostal muscles and diaphragm causes the child to be prone to respiratory tract infection
    b. Need to protect the child from exposure to infection as much as possible; be alert for symptoms of aspiration pneumonia
  8. Dental problems
    a. Problems in muscular control affect development and alignment of teeth
    b. Frequent dental caries occur; a great need for dental supervision and care
    c. The parent may have to be taught to brush the child's teeth because of muscular dysfunction
  9. Vision
    a. Common ocular problems such as strabismus and refractive errors may be related to poor muscular control
    b. Must look for such disorders to prevent further problems such as amblyopia
  10. Hearing problems may be present depending on the basic cause of the brain damage

Hearing Disorders

A. Types
  1. Conductive—loss from damage to middle ear
    a. Accounts for about 80% of reduced hearing
    b. Conductive loss of 30 dB or more may require a hearing aid
  2. Sensorineural—damage to inner ear structures of the auditory nerve
    a. Distortion in clarity of words
    b. Problem in discrimination of sounds
  3. Mixed conductive-sensorineural

4. Central auditory
    a. Not explained by other 3 causes
    b. The child hears but does not understand
B. Causes
    1. Maternal factors—rubella, syphilis
    2. Perinatal—anoxia, kernicterus, prematurity, excessive noise
    3. Postnatal—mumps, otitis media, head trauma, drugs such as streptomycin
C. Developmental and behavioral manifestations of hearing loss
    1. Lack of the Moro reflex in response to a sharp clap
    2. Failure to respond to loud noise
    3. Failure to locate a source of sound at 61 to 95 cm (2 to 3 feet) after 6 months of age
    4. Absence of babble by 7 months of age
    5. Inability to understand words or phrases by 12 months of age
    6. Use of gestures rather than verbalization to establish wants
    7. History of frequent respiratory tract infections and otitis media
D. Nursing considerations
    1. Detection—can and should be identified within the first year of life
    2. Specific guidelines for working with a deaf child
        a. Face the child to facilitate lipreading
        b. Do not walk back and forth while talking
        c. Have a good light on speaker's face
        d. Be level with the child's face and speak toward the good ear
        e. Always enunciate and articulate carefully
        f. Do not talk too loudly, especially if the loss is sensorineural
        g. Use facial expressions, since verbal intonations are not communicated
        h. Encourage active play to build self-confidence

Visual Disorders

A. Strabismus—imbalance of the extraocular muscles causing a physiologic incoordination of the eye
    1. A cause of blindness—amblyopia develops in the weak eye from disuse
    2. Must be corrected before 4 years of age to prevent blindness
    3. Treatment
        a. To force the weak eye to fixate—patch the good eye and exercise the weak eye
        b. Surgery to lengthen or shorten the extraocular muscles

B. Functional definition of blindness—visual loss of acuity to read print, must use braille, may have light perception
C. Causes other than strabismus
    1. Maternal—albinism, congenital cataracts, rubella, galactosemia
    2. Perinatal—retrolental fibroplasia
    3. Postnatal—trauma, diabetes, syphilis, tumor
D. Developmental and behavioral manifestations indicating a reduction in vision
    1. Retarded motor development
    2. Rocking for sensory stimulation
    3. Squinting, rubbing eyes
    4. Sitting close to television, holding book close to face
    5. Clumsiness, bumping into objects
E. Nursing considerations
    1. Early detection of loss
    2. Specific nursing intervention when working with a blind child
        a. Always talk so the child can hear clearly
        b. Use noise so the child can locate your position
        c. Help the child learn through other senses, especially touch through play activities
        d. Facilitate eating by
            (1) Arranging food on the plate at clock hours and teaching the child its location
            (2) Providing finger foods when possible
            (3) Providing a light spoon and deep bowl so the child can feel weight of food on spoon

Pinworms

Most common intestinal parasites
A. Children reinfect themselves by fingers to anus to mouth route
B. Can also be infected by breathing air-borne ova
C. Symptoms
    1. Severe pruritus of the anal area
    2. Vaginitis
    3. Irritability and insomnia
    4. Poor appetite and weight loss
    5. Eosinophilia
D. Diagnosis—cellophane tape test to isolate eggs from the anal area (must be done in morning before the first bowel movement)
E. Treatment—anthelmintics
    1. Hexylresorcinol (Caprokol, Crystoids)
        a. Paralyzes worms (hookworms, roundworms, pinworms, whipworms, threadworms, tapeworms, intestinal flukes), which are inactive when excreted

b. Adverse effects—burning sensation of skin, oral and anal mucous membrane
2. Methylrosaniline chloride—paralyzes pinworms, threadworms, and liver flukes
3. Piperazine citrate (Antepar Citrate, Multifuge, Ta-Verm, Vermidol)
    a. Paralyzes musculature of pinworms and roundworms by curare-like action
    b. Within 3 days pinworms are passed active and alive; roundworms paralyzed and alive
4. Pyrantel pamoate (Antiminth)
    a. Blocks neuromuscular transmission in roundworms, hookworms, pinworms
    b. Adverse effects—anorexia, nausea, vomiting, diarrhea, abdominal cramps, headache, dizziness, drowsiness, rash
5. Pyrvinium pamoate (Povan)
    a. Inhibits respiratory enzymes and anaerobic metabolism to inactivate pinworms, threadworms
    b. Adverse effects—nausea, vomiting, abdominal cramps; cyanine dye origin of the drug colors stool, emesis, and most materials bright red or orange
F. Nursing considerations
1. Prevent reinfestation
    a. The child should not be allowed to scratch anus; may need to wear mittens
    b. Fingernails should be kept short
    c. Should wear a tight diaper or underpants
    d. Wash anal area thoroughly at least once a day
    e. Change clothes daily; wash in hot water
    f. Air out bedroom, dust and vacuum house thoroughly
2. Teach parent administration of medication
    a. Overdose will not produce a quicker recovery
    b. Stools may turn bright red from medication

Anemia

A. Most prevalent nutritional disorder among children in the United States, caused by lack of adequate sources of dietary iron
1. Infant usually has iron reserve for 6 months
2. Premature infant lacks reserve
3. Children receiving only milk have no source of iron
B. Insidious onset, usually diagnosed because of an infection or chronic GI loss
C. Clinical manifestations
1. Pallor, weakness
2. Slow motor development
3. Poor muscle tone
4. Hemoglobin level below 11 g

D. Treatment
1. Food sources rich in iron
2. Iron replacement
    a. Oral iron sources
        (1) Drugs
            (a) Ferrocholinate (Chel-Iron, Ferrolip)
            (b) Ferrous fumarate (Ircon, Toleron)
            (c) Ferrous gluconate
            (d) Ferrous lactate (Ferro Drops)
            (e) Ferrous sulfate
        (2) Adverse effects—nausea, vomiting; fatalities in children who ingest enteric coated tablets, thinking they are candy
        (3) Drug interactions—ferrous sulfate binds tetracycline and decreases absorption; magnesium trisilicate decreases absorption of iron preparations
    b. Parenteral iron sources
        (1) Drugs
            (a) Iron-Dextran injection (Imferon)
            (b) Iron sorbitex (Jectofer)
        (2) Adverse effects—tissue staining (use Z tract for injection), fever, lymphadenopathy, nausea, vomiting, arthralgia, urticaria, severe peripheral vascular failure, anaphylaxis, secondary hematochromatosis
E. Nursing considerations
1. Prevention
    a. Teach pregnant women the importance of their iron intake
    b. Encourage feeding of iron-fortified infant cereal
    c. Introduce foods high in iron
2. Good nutrition and proper administration of supplemental iron
    a. Vitamin C aids absorption
    b. Hydrochloric acid aids absorption
    c. Oxalates, phosphate, and phytates decrease absorption
    d. Use a straw, since some liquid preparations stain teeth
    e. Discolors stools; may cause gastric irritation or constipation

Celiac Disease

A. Chronic intestinal malabsorption and inability to digest gluten, a protein found mostly in wheat and rye
B. Usually begins in infancy or toddler stage, but later in breast-fed infants
C. Clinical manifestations
1. Progressive malnutrition—secondary deficiencies: anemia, rickets

   a. Stunted growth
   b. Wasting of extremities
   c. Distended abdomen
  2. Steatorrhea—fatty, foul, frothy, bulky stools
  3. Celiac crisis—severe episode of dehydration and acidosis from diarrhea
D. Treatment—dietary
  1. Low in glutens; no wheat, rye, oats, or barley
  2. High in calories and protein
  3. Low fat
  4. Smooth, soft foods with low roughage and residue
  5. Small, frequent feedings; adequate fluids
  6. Vitamin supplements, all in water-miscible form
  7. Supplemental iron
E. Nursing considerations—parental education
  1. Protect the child from infection
  2. Strict adherence to dietary regimen
  3. Need for frequent follow-up supervision, home visits

Cystic Fibrosis of the Pancreas

A. Autosomal recessive disorder affecting the mucus-secreting glands
B. Pathology—defect is in overproduction of mucus or an absence of normal mucus-removing mechanism
  1. Pancreas—becomes fibrotic, with a decreased production of pancreatic enzymes
   a. Lipase—causes steatorrhea
   b. Trypsin—causes increased nitrogen in stool
   c. Amylase—inability to break down polysaccharides
  2. Intestines—increased mucus production prevents enzymes from reaching the duodenum, resulting in an inability to absorb fat
  3. Sweat glands—high electrolyte content of sodium and chloride (3 to 5 times higher than normal); chloride levels above 60 mEq/L are diagnostic
  4. Respiratory system—increased viscous mucus in the trachea, bronchi, and bronchioles resulting in
   a. Obstruction, interfering with expiration (emphysema)
   b. Infection
  5. Liver—possible cirrhosis from biliary obstruction, malnutrition, or infection
C. Clinical manifestations
  1. Based on above pathophysiology
  2. Similar to celiac disease
  3. Some early manifestations during infancy
   a. Meconium ileus at birth (about 15%)
   b. Failure to regain normal 10% weight loss at birth

   c. Presence of cough or wheezing during first 6 months of age
  4. Because of respiratory involvement, there may be clubbing of fingers, barrel-shaped chest, cyanosis, distended neck veins
  5. Cardiac enlargement, particularly right ventricular hypertrophy (cor pulmonale)
D. Nursing problems and interventions
  1. Prevention of respiratory tract infection
   a. Postural drainage, percussion, vibrating
   b. Aerosol therapy and additional oxygen as needed
   c. Use of expectorants and antibiotics
  2. Nutrition
   a. Replacement of pancreatic enzymes, given with cold food
   b. Replacement of fat-soluble vitamins in water-miscible form
   c. High-protein diet of easily digested food, normal fat, high calories
   d. Small frequent feedings
  3. Mobility and activity
   a. The child may have little tolerance for exertion
   b. Help the child regulate activity to own tolerance
   c. Provide frequent rest periods
  4. Body image
   a. Barrel-shaped chest, poor weight gain, thin extremities, bluish coloring, smell of stools, poor posture
   b. Encourage good hygiene and select clothes that compensate for protuberant abdomen and emaciated extremities
  5. Counseling
   a. Long-term problem causing financial and emotional stresses
   b. Illness can become a major controlling factor in the family
    (1) The child begins to recognize that wheezing brings attention and uses this knowledge
    (2) Parents can deal with such behavior by recognizing false attacks and using consistent discipline
   c. Encourage the family to join the Cystic Fibrosis Foundation

Sickle Cell Anemia

A. Autosomal recessive disorder affecting hemoglobin
B. Defective hemoglobin causes red blood cells to become sickle shaped and clump together under reduced oxygen tension

C. Clinical manifestations of a sickle cell crisis
   1. Severe pain in the abdomen, legs, and flank area
   2. Fever
   3. Anemia, pallor, weakness
   4. Vomiting, anorexia
   5. Convulsion, stiff neck, coma
   6. Jaundice
   7. Enlarged spleen, liver, heart
D. Nursing problems and interventions
   1. Prevention of crisis
     a. Avoid infection, dehydration, and other conditions causing strain on body, which precipitates a crisis; avoid the use of pneumococcal and meningococcal vaccines
     b. Avoid hypoxia
       (1) Avoid drugs that depress the respiratory center
       (2) Treat respiratory tract infections immediately
       (3) Administer additional oxygen with high humidity
     c. Avoid dehydration
       (1) May cause a rapid thrombus formation
       (2) Daily fluid intake should be calculated according to body weight (130 to 200 ml per kilogram [2 to 3 oz per pound])
       (3) During crisis, fluid needs to be increased, especially if the patient is febrile
   2. Care during crisis—provisions should be made for
     a. Adequate hydration (may need IV therapy)
     b. Proper positioning, careful handling
     c. Exercise as tolerated (immobility promotes thrombus formation and respiratory problems)
     d. Adequate ventilation
     e. Control of pain (avoid narcotics or barbiturates)
     f. Blood transfusions for severe anemia
   3. Genetic counseling
     a. Disorder mostly of blacks
     b. Parents need to know the risk of having other children with the trait or disease
     c. Screen young children for the disorder, since clinical manifestations usually do not appear before 6 months of age

β-Thalassemia (Cooley's Anemia)

A. Autosomal recessive disorder with varied expressivity
B. Basic defect seems to be a deficiency in the synthesis of β-chain polypeptides, which results in a decreased rate of production of the globin molecule

C. Clinical manifestations
   1. Severe anemia
   2. Unexplained fever
   3. Poor feeding
   4. Markedly enlarged spleen
   5. Enlarged abdomen, reflecting significant hepatomegaly
   6. Impaired physical growth
   7. Bone changes
     a. Enlarged head
     b. Prominent frontal and parietal bone bosses
     c. Prominent malar eminences
     d. Depressed bridge of the nose
     e. Oblique appearance of the eyes
     f. Enlarged maxilla with upward protrusion of the lip and upper central incisors
   8. Exercise intolerance
   9. Headache
   10. Listlessness
   11. Anorexia
D. Treatment
   1. Use of blood transfusions to maintain adequate hemoglobin levels
   2. Transfusions greatly increase the risk of hemosiderosis (excessive iron storage in various tissues of the body, especially the spleen, liver, lymph glands, heart, and pancreas) and hemochromatosis (excessive iron storage with resultant cellular damage)
   3. Iron-chelating agents such as deferoxamine (Desferal) are given to reduce iron storage
E. Nursing considerations
   1. Be alert for signs and symptoms in older infants or young children of Mediterranean descent (Italian, Greek, Syrian)
   2. Prevent infection
     a. Avoid contact with persons who have infections
     b. Administer prophylactic antibiotics
   3. Prevent complications
     a. Carry out careful observation during transfusion
     b. Administer chelating agents as ordered
     c. Administer folic acid
     d. Avoid activities that increase risk of fractures
     e. Observe for signs of cholecystitis in the adolescent
   4. Assist the child in coping with the disorder and its effects
     a. Explore the child's feelings about being different from other children
     b. Emphasize the child's abilities and focus on realistic endeavors

c. Encourage quiet activities, creative efforts, and ''thinking'' games
d. Emphasize good hygiene and grooming
e. Encourage interaction with peers
f. Help plan therapies and medical care so they do not interfere with the child's regular activities and social interaction
g. Assist the child with vocational planning
h. Introduce the child to other children who have adjusted well to this or a similar disorder
5. Support the parents
a. Explore feelings of guilt regarding the hereditary nature of the disease
b. Emphasize the need for the child to lead as normal a life as possible
c. Help the family deal with the potentially fatal nature of the disease
6. Prevent the occurrence of thalassemia
a. Refer for genetic counseling
b. Reinforce and clarify counseling information

The Preschool-Age Child
GROWTH AND DEVELOPMENT
Developmental Timetable

A. Three years
1. Motor
a. Walks backward
b. Rides a tricycle, using pedals
c. Walks upstairs, alternating feet
d. Begins to use scissors
e. Constructs a 3-block bridge
f. Can unbutton front or side button
g. Usually toilet trained at night
2. Sensory—visual acuity 20/30
3. Vocalization and socialization
a. Vocabulary of about 900 words; uses 8-to-9-word sentences
b. May have normal hesitation in speech pattern
c. Uses plurals
d. Begins to understand ideas of sharing and taking turns
4. Mental abilities
a. Little understanding of the past, present, or future or any aspect of time
b. Stage of magical thinking
B. Four years
1. Motor
a. Climbs and jumps well
b. Walks up and down stairs like an adult

c. Can button buttons and lace shoes
d. Throws ball overhand
2. Vocalization and socialization
a. Vocabulary of 1500 words or more
b. May have an imaginary companion
c. Tends to be selfish and impatient, but takes pride in accomplishments
d. Exaggerates, boasts, and tattles on others
3. Mental abilities
a. Reading readiness is present
b. Can repeat 4 numbers and is learning number concept
c. Knows which is the longer of 2 lines
d. Has poor space perception
C. Five years
1. Motor
a. Gross motor abilities well developed
b. Can balance on 1 foot for about 10 seconds
c. Can jump rope, skip, and roller skate
d. Can draw a picture of a person
e. Prints first name and other words as learned
f. Dresses and washes self
g. May be able to tie shoelaces
2. Sensory
a. Minimal potential for amblyopia to develop
b. Color recognition is well established
3. Vocalization and socialization
a. Vocabulary of about 2100 words
b. Talks constantly
c. Asks meaning of new words
d. Generally cooperative and sympathetic toward others
e. Basic personality structure is well established
4. Mental abilities (Piaget's phase of intuitive thought)
a. Beginning understanding of time in terms of days as part of a week
b. Can determine difference in weights
c. Has not mastered the concept that parts equal a whole regardless of their appearance

PLAY (COOPERATIVE PLAY)

A. Loosely organized group play where membership changes readily and rules are absent
B. Through play, the child deals with reality, learns control of feelings, and expresses emotions more through words than through actions
C. Play is still physically oriented but is also imitative and imaginary
D. There is increasing sharing and cooperation among preschool children, especially 5-year-olds
E. Suggested toys (same principles as discussed before)

1. Puppets
2. Addditional dress-up clothes, dolls, house, furniture, small trucks, animals, etc.
3. Painting sets, coloring books, paste, and cut-out sets
4. Illustrated books
5. Puzzles with large pieces and more shapes
6. Tricycle, swing, slide and other playground equipment

ACUTE AND CHRONIC HEALTH PROBLEMS
Hospitalization

A. Reaction of the child
   1. Fears about body image are now greater than fear of separation
   2. The fears include
      a. Intrusive experiences—needles, thermometer, otoscope
      b. Punishment and rejection
      c. Pain
      d. Castration and mutilation
B. Preparation
   1. Can prepare the child beforehand, since increased cognitive and verbal ability makes explanations possible
   2. General considerations for nursing intervention
      a. Should begin a few days before, but not too soon because of the poor concept of time
      b. Clarify cause and effect because of the child's phenomenalistic thinking (in the child's mind, proximity of 2 events relates them to each other)
      c. Explain routines of hospital admission but not all procedures at one time, since this would be overwhelming
      d. Play is an excellent medium for preparation (use dolls, puppets, make-believe equipment, dress-up doctor and nurse clothes)
      e. Provide time for play as an outlet for fear, anger, and hostility, as well as a temporary escape from reality
      f. Verbal explanation should be as simple as possible and always honest
      g. Add details about procedures, drugs, surgery, and the like as the child's cognitive level and personal experiences increase

Cancer

A. Second leading cause of death in children
B. Leukemia—principal type of cancer
   1. Peak incidence—3 to 4 years of age
   2. Malignant neoplasm of blood-forming organs
   3. In children, overproduction of immature leukocytes—blast-cell or stem-cell leukemia
      a. Lymphocytic—about 85% of cases; better prognosis than for myelogenous
      b. Myelogenous—about 10%; poorer prognosis
   4. Symptoms—caused by overproduction of immature nonfunctional cells
      a. Anemia—pallor, weakness, irritability
      b. Infection—fever
      c. Tendency toward bleeding—petechiae and bleeding into joints
      d. Pain in joints caused by seepage of serous fluid
      e. Tendency toward easy fracture of bones
      f. Enlargement of spleen, liver, lymph glands
      g. Abdominal pain and anorexia resulting in weight loss
      h. Necrosis and bleeding of gums and other mucous membranes
      i. Later symptoms—central nervous system involvement and frank hemorrhage
   5. Treatment objectives
      a. Induce remission by chemotherapy
         (1) Prednisone—steroid
         (2) Vincristine—plant alkaloid
         (3) Methotrexate—folic acid antagonist
         (4) 6-Mercaptopurine—purine antagonist
         (5) Cyclophosphamide—alkylating agent
         (6) Daunorubicin—cytotoxic antibiotic
      b. Prevent CNS involvement by use of irradiation and intrathecal methotrexate, because leukemic cells invade the brain but most antileukemic drugs do not pass the blood-brain barrier
      c. Transfusions to replace and provide blood factors such as platelets, white cells, and clotting factors
      d. See antineoplastic drugs in medical-surgical nursing
   6. Nursing considerations
      a. Prognosis—improving
         (1) Adjustment of parents may be difficult because of the potential long-term status of the illness
         (2) Must deal with the child's idea of death—discussion should be appropriate to level of understanding
            (a) Preschooler—concept that death is reversible; greatest fear is separation
            (b) Child 6 to 9 years of age—concept that death is personified; a person actually comes and removes the child

(c) Child over 9 years of age—adult concept of death as irreversible and inevitable

b. Treatment

(1) Be alert for and attempt to support the child experiencing side effects of drugs:

(a) Cytoxan—severe nausea and vomiting

(b) Vincristine—constipation, alopecia, neurotoxicity

(2) Prevent infection by means of protective isolation

(3) Handle the child carefully because of pain and hemorrhage; use narcotics for pain

(4) Provide gentle oral hygiene, soft, bland foods, and increased liquids

(5) Provide for frequent rest periods, quiet play

c. See behavioral sciences for further details on behavioral changes that result from physical illness

Nephrosis (Minimal Change Nephrotic Syndrome)

A. Pathology—abnormal, increased permeability of the glomerular basement membrane to plasma albumin

B. Cause unknown—theories include

1. Hypersensitivity

2. Antigen-antibody response (rationale for the use of glucocorticoids and other immunosuppressive drugs)

C. Peak incidence—2 to 5 years of age

D. Clinical manifestations

1. Generalized edema, especially genital, periorbital, and abdominal (ascites)

2. Proteinuria

3. Hypoproteinemia—poor general health, loss of appetite

4. Hyperlipemia

5. May also see symptoms usually associated with nephritis

a. Hematuria

b. Hypertension

E. Nursing problems and interventions

1. Infection—both disease state and drug therapy increase susceptibility

a. The child should be protected from others who are ill

b. Teach parents the signs of impending infection and encourage them to seek medical care

2. Malnutrition caused by loss of protein and poor appetite

a. Regular diet is usually allowed; added salt and salty foods discouraged

b. Protein is usually not adjusted; encourage the child to select foods from high-protein choices

c. Fluids may be restricted, but this generally causes more discomfort than benefit

3. Respiratory difficulty caused by ascites

a. Proper positioning—place in a Fowler position to decrease pressure against the diaphragm

b. Frequent change of position is vital because of dependent edema

4. Discomfort caused by edema, pressure areas

a. Positioning and skin care provide some relief

b. Support the genitalia if edematous

5. Change in body image caused by edema and steroids

a. Of greater concern as the child grows older

b. Emphasize clothes, hairdo, etc. that make the child attractive

c. Stress that "diets" will not help weight loss

6. Behavioral changes such as irritability and depression

a. Parents need to understand that mood swings are influenced by physical condition

b. Encourage the child to participate in own care

c. Encourage diversionary activities that provide satisfaction

Urinary Tract Infection

A. Very common in females because of anatomy of the lower urinary tract—urethra is short and meatus is close to the anus

B. Nursing considerations—teach prevention

1. Proper cleansing of genitalia (front to back)

2. Voiding when necessary as opposed to holding urine in bladder

3. Increased fluids, particularly those that acidify urine

4. Identification of asymptomatic infections

5. Use of showers instead of tub baths

Allergy

A. Altered tissue response to a substance that has been inhaled or ingested or that has contacted the skin

B. Most common types in children

1. Eczema

2. Allergic rhinitis

3. Asthma

C. General nursing considerations

1. Family history can be a significant factor
2. Comprehensive study of the child and environment essential
   a. Prepare the child for skin tests
   b. Study the environment in terms of emotional stresses as well as physical allergens
3. Teach the parents to eliminate allergenic substances and to administer drugs properly

D. Asthma
   1. Pathology
      a. Bronchiolar spasm
      b. Bronchiolar constriction
      c. Increased secretions
      d. Respiratory acidosis from buildup of carbon dioxide
   2. Clinical manifestations
      a. Wheezing, especially on expiration
      b. Labored breathing, cough, increased secretion
      c. Flaring nares, distended neck veins

E. Treatment for respiratory allergies
   1. Bronchodilators
      a. Theophyllines
         (1) Drugs
             (a) Aminophylline
             (b) Dyphylline (Dilor, Neothylline)
             (c) Oxtriphylline (Choledyl)
             (d) Theophylline (Aqualin, Elixophyllin)
         (2) Actions
             (a) Act directly on the bronchial smooth muscle to decrease spasm, relax smooth muscle of the vasculature
             (b) Direct stimulatory effect on the myocardium increases cardiac output, which improves blood flow to kidneys
             (c) Direct action on the renal tubules provides diuretic effect by increasing excretion of sodium and chloride ions
         (3) Adverse effects—oral forms cause gastric irritation
         (4) Considerations during therapy—cumulation of drug can occur unless dosage is regulated: parenteral drug must be administered slowly over a 4-to-5-minute period to avoid peripheral vasodilation (hypotension, facial flushing), cerebral vascular constriction (headache, dizziness), cardiac palpitation, and precordial pain
      b. Epinephrine hydrochloride—drug of choice in respiratory emergency, such as status asthmaticus
         (1) Actions
             (a) Effect is on the beta-adrenergic receptors in the bronchi; relaxes smooth muscle and increases respiratory volume
             (b) Inhalants cause vasoconstriction, which reduces congestion or edema
         (2) Adverse effects—cardiac palpitation; overuse of inhalants may cause "congestive rebound"
      c. Isoproterenol hydrochloride (Isuprel Hydrochloride, Proternol)
         (1) Action—similar to that of theophyllines
         (2) Adverse effects—action at cardiovascular beta receptors causes tachycardia, peripheral blood vessel dilation (hypotension)
      d. Metaproterenol (Alupent, Metaprel)
      e. Terbutaline (Bricanyl) has little effect on cardiac tissue
      f. Oral drugs that relax bronchi and decrease glandular and tissue fluid in the bronchi
         (1) Drugs
             (a) Methoxyphenamine hydrochloride (Orthoxine)
             (b) Phenylpropanolamine hydrochloride (Propadrine)
             (c) Pseudoephedrine hydrochloride (Sudafed)
         (2) Adverse effects—transient elevation in pulse and systolic blood pressure, dry oral tissues
      g. Cromolyn sodium (Aarane, Intal) acts primarily by preventing release of mediators of type I allergic reactions (histamine, slow-reacting substance of anaphylaxis) from sensitized mast cells; prophylactic use by inhaling capsule contents lessens bronchoconstriction
      h. Adverse effects common to bronchodilator group—anxiety, nervousness, tremors, nausea, vomiting, headache, dizziness
   2. Expectorants—increase the production of thinner, less viscid secretions that protect bronchial tissues
      a. Drugs
         (1) Calcium iodide
         (2) Glyceryl guaiacolate (Robitussin)
         (3) Iodinated glycerol (Organidin)
         (4) Potassium iodide (Enkide)
      b. Act to raise the osmolality of bronchial glandular secretions, causing fluids to move to dilute the secretions

c. Adverse effects—nausea, skin eruptions; long-term use of iodides may cause iodism (inflammation of respiratory tract tissues, skin eruptions, accumulation of fluid in nasal passages, lungs, eyelids)
  3. Corticosteroids
    a. Antiinflammatory effect diminishes the inflammatory component of asthma and reduces airway obstruction
    b. Used in status asthmaticus; however, less often for long-term control because of side effects
F. Nursing considerations
  1. Treatment—use of antispasmodic drugs and bronchodilators; parents must know how to give medication and why it must be given even if the child does not have an attack
  2. Good respiratory hygiene; teach parents postural drainage, need for increased fluids, and the use of a cool mist humidifier to provide high humidity in home
  3. Improved ventilating capacity
    a. Position in a high-Fowler, leaning slightly forward
    b. Teach breathing exercises and controlled breathing
  4. Proper environment
    a. Free of as many allergens as possible
    b. Avoid exertion, exposure to cold air, and people with infections
    c. Avoid as much as possible emotional factors that precipitate attacks

Mucocutaneous Lymph Node Syndrome (Kawasaki Disease)

A. Acute febrile illness of unknown etiology; The principal area of involvement is the cardiovascular system, with extensive perivasculitis of arterioles, venules, and capillaries, including the coronary arteries; panvasculitis and perivasculitis of the main coronary arteries may result in stenosis or obstruction with aneurysm formation, pericarditis, interstitial myocarditis and endocarditis, and phlebitis of the larger veins
B. Clinical manifestations
  1. Fever for 5 or more days
  2. Bilateral congestion of the ocular conjunctiva without exudation
  3. Changes of the mucous membranes of the oral cavity, such as erythema, dryness, and fissuring of the lips, oropharyngeal reddening, or "strawberry tongue"
  4. Changes in the extremities, such as peripheral edema, peripheral erythema, and desquamation of the palms and soles—particularly periungual peeling
  5. Polymorphous rash, primarily of the trunk
  6. Cervical lymphadenopathy
  7. Other signs, including diarrhea, photophobia, tympanitis, and arthralgia and arthritis, especially involving the larger joints such as elbows, wrists, knees, and ankles.
C. Treatment—primarily supportive and directed toward controlling fever, preventing dehydration, and minimizing possible cardiac complications
  1. Large doses of aspirin
  2. Corticosteriods
  3. Monitoring the cardiac status
D. Nursing considerations
  1. Administer aspirin to control fever; assess for early signs of toxicity
  2. Provide optimal nutrition
  3. Administer analgesics for joint pain if needed in addition to aspirin
  4. Monitor for any signs of heart disease, especially arrhythmias

Tonsillectomy and Adenoidectomy

Not done routinely, since lymphoid tissue helps prevent invasion of organisms
A. Indications for surgical removal
  1. Recurrent tonsillitis or otitis media
  2. Enlargement that interferes with breathing or swallowing
B. Contraindications for removal
  1. Occasional infections that clear up rapidly
  2. Cleft palate, hemophilia, or debilitating disease such as leukemia
C. Complications after surgery
  1. Hemorrhage—first 24 hours
    a. Frequent swallowing, bright red blood in the vomitus
    b. Restlessness
    c. Increased pulse rate, pallor
  2. Hemorrhage from sloughing of tissue—5 to 10 days postoperative
D. Nursing considerations
  1. Keep the child on the abdomen or side with head turned to the side
  2. After surgery the child should be given cool liquids, not red in color and not thick or mucus-producing
  3. Ask the child to talk; provide assurance that it is possible
  4. Ice collar to decrease edema
  5. Attempt to limit crying

The School-Age Child

GROWTH AND DEVELOPMENT
Developmental Timetable

A. Physical growth
   1. Permanent dentition, beginning with 6-year molars and central incisors at 7 or 8 years of age
   2. Growth has decreased, about 2.5 cm (1 inch) in height a year
   3. Tends to look lanky because bone development precedes muscular development
B. Motor
   1. Refinement of coordination, balance, and control is ocurring
   2. Motor development necessary for competitive activity becomes important
C. Sensory—visual acuity of 20/20
D. Mental abilities
   1. Readiness for learning, especially in perceptual organization—names months of year, knows right from left, can tell time, can follow several directions at once
   2. Acquires use of reason and understanding of rules
   3. Trial and error problem solving becomes more conceptual rather than action oriented
   4. Reasoning ability allows greater understanding and use of language
   5. Quantity conservation (Piaget)—knows that quantity remains the same even though appearance differs

PLAY
Play Activities Vary with Age

A. Number of play activities decreases while the amount of time spent in one particular activity increases
B. Likes games with rules because of increased mental abilities
C. Likes games of athletic competition because of increased motor ability
D. Should learn how to work as well as play, with a beginning appreciation for economics and finances
E. In beginning of school years, boys and girls play together but gradually separate into sex-oriented type of activities
F. Suggested play for 6-to-9-year-olds
   1. More housekeeping toys that work, doll accessories, paper doll sets, simple sewing machine, and needlework
   2. Simple work and number games (i.e., calling for increased skills)
   3. Physically active games such as hopscotch, jump rope, climbing trees
   4. Stamp collecting and the like building simple models
   5. Bicycle riding
G. Suggested play for 9-to-12-year-olds
   1. Handicrafts of all kinds
   2. Model kits, collections, hobbies
   3. Archery, dart games, chess, jigsaw puzzles
   4. Sculpturing materials such as pottery clay
   5. Science toys, magic sets

ACUTE AND CHRONIC HEALTH PROBLEMS
Diabetes Mellitus

A. Symptons—juvenile diabetes may be more severe and variable than diabetes in adults
   1. Onset—rapid, obvious
   2. Child usually thin, underweight; obesity does not appear to be a factor
   3. Increased thirst, fluid intake, appetite, and urinary output
   4. Hypoglycemia and ketoacidosis common
B. Differences between childhood and adult-onset diabetes
   1. Onset
      a. Rapid in children
      b. Insidious in adults
   2. Obesity
      a. Does not appear to be a factor in children
      b. Predisposing factor in adults
   3. Dietary treatment
      a. Rarely adequate for children
      b. Possible in one third of adults
   4. Oral hypoglycemics
      a. Contraindicated for children
      b. Helpful in one third of adults
   5. Insulin
      a. Almost universally necessary in children
      b. Necessary for only one third of adults
   6. Hypoglycemia and ketoacidosis
      a. Quite frequent in children
      b. More uncommon in adults
   7. Degenerative vascular changes
      a. Develop after adolescence in children
      b. May be present at the time of diagnosis in adults
C. Hypoglycemia—insulin shock
   1. Causes
      a. Overdose of insulin
      b. Decreased food intake
      c. Excessive physical exercise—increases muscle activity and movement of glucose into muscle cells

2. Signs
   a. Sweating, flushing, pallor
   b. Numbness, trembling, chilliness
   c. Unsteadiness, nervousness, irritability
   d. Hunger
   e. Hallucinations
   f. Late signs—convulsions, coma, death
3. Emergency treatment—immediate supply of readily available glucose

D. Hyperglycemia—ketoacidosis or diabetic coma
1. Causes
   a. Decreased insulin
   b. Emotional stress
   c. Fever
   d. Infection
   e. Increased food intake
2. Signs
   a. Weakness, drowsiness
   b. Lack of appetite, thirst
   c. Abdominal and/or generalized pain
   d. Acetone breath
   e. Late signs—Kussmaul breathing (deep, rapid respirations), cherry red lips, loss of consciousness, death
3. Treatment—hospitalizaion with administration of insulin

F. Peak incidence in the school-age group
1. Around 6 years of age
2. Around 12 years of age

G. Treatment
1. Control calorie, carbohydrate, fat, and protein intake
2. Insulin (see endocrine section in medical -surgical nursing)

H. Nursing problems and interventions—main objective is control of diabetes and education of child and family
1. Explain the differences between childhood and adult-onset diabetes to parents, who may think the child is faking because their own illness does not cause serious problems
2. Teach factors that affect insulin requirements and signs of insulin overdose and diabetic coma
   a. Give family a written list explaining symptoms
   b. Emphasize that sugar can be given if insulin shock is suspected but that insulin should *not be* increased if diabetic coma is developing
   c. Emphasize the need for close medical supervision
3. Infection—teach need for
   a. Good skin care, frequent baths
   b. Properly fitting shoes

c. Prompt treatment of any small cut
d. Protection from undue exposure to illness
4. Diet—should be well balanced, with fairly equal quantities of food eaten frequently and regularly, usually unrestricted within reason
5. Urine testing—child should learn how to do this to increase independence
6. Administration of insulin
   a. The child should be taught as early as motor and mental ability allows, usually by 7 or 9 years of age
   b. Explanations should be simple; diagrams for rotating sites should be used
   c. Periodic observation by an adult should be routine to discover faulty or careless technique

Hemophilia

A. Defects in clotting mechanism of blood—3 most common deficiencies
1. Factor VIII, classic hemophilia
2. Factor IX, Christmas disease
3. Factor XI

B. Hereditary influence—sex-linked recessive gene, classically occurring in males

C. Clinical manifestations
1. Prolonged bleeding from any wound
2. Bleeding into the joints (hemarthrosis), resulting in pain, deformity, and retarded growth
3. Anemia
4. Intracranial hemorrhage

D. Treatment
1. Control of bleeding
2. Prevention of bleeding with use of factor replacement
   a. Drugs that replace deficient coagulation factors
      (1) Antihemophilic factor (Hemofil)
         (a) Obtained from human sources
         (b) Provides concentrated factor VIII
      (2) Antihemophilic plasma
      (3) Factor IX complex (Konyne) contains factors II, VII, IX, X (concentrated)
   b. Adjunctive measures
      (1) Episilon-aminocaproic acid (Amicar) inhibits the enzyme that destroys formed fibrin and increases fibrinogen activity in clot formation
      (2) Fibrinogen (Parenogen) maintains plasma fibrinogen levels required for clotting materials
      (3) Thrombin supplies physiologic levels of

natural material at superficial bleeding sites to control bleeding

E. Nursing problems and interventions
  1. Bleeding
    a. Instruct the child and parents in the treatment of bleeding, especially of joints
      (1) Immobilization of the area
      (2) Compression of the area
      (3) Elevation of the body part
      (4) Application of cool compresses
    b. Appropriate activity that lessens the chance of trauma, which is often difficult since boys are so physically active
  2. Pain
    a. Avoid use of aspirin or phenylbutazone
    b. Control joint pain so the child uses extremity to prevent muscle atrophy
  3. Repeated hospitalizations—objective now is to strive for home care, with self-administration of coagulation factors such as cryoprecipitate
  4. Guilt of parents
    a. Provide counseling, since disease is genetic and parents need assistance
    b. Encourage parents to treat the child as normally as possible, avoiding overprotection or overpermissivesness

Rheumatic Fever

A. Collagen disease—characterized by damage to connective tissue and usually blood vessels
B. Cause unknown—frequently follows infection with group A beta hemolytic streptococci
C. One of chief causes of death in school-age children, peak incidence between 6 and 8 years of age, with familial incidence
D. Predisposing factors—crowded living conditions, general lack of hygiene, temperate climate, poor nutrition
E. Clinical manifestations
  1. Carditis—possible damage to the mitral valve
    a. Increased pulse rate, especially at night; poor pulse quality
    b. Low-grade fever in afternoon
    c. Anemia, pallor, weakness
    d. Anorexia, weight loss
    e. Increased respiratory rate
  2. Arthritis
    a. Enlarged joints, with migratory pain
    b. Joints red, hot, swollen, and tender; but deformity does not result
  3. Sydenham's chorea (St. Vitus' dance)
    a. Gradual onset
    b. Involuntary, purposeless movements

    c. Facial grimaces
    d. Restlessness and inability to maintain one position
    e. Emotional instability
  4. Subcutaneous nodules on extensor tendons of the hands, feet, elbows, scapulae, patellae, vertebrae
    a. Nonpainful
    b. Skin moves freely over the nodules
F. Laboratory findings
  1. Increased eyrthrocyte sedimentation rate
  2. Antistreptolysin-O titer
  3. Presence of C-reactive protein
  4. Aschoff bodies—in the heart, arteries, nodules
  5. Leukocytosis
G. Treatment—antibiotics to eradicate organism and prevent recurrence
  1. Penicillin preparations—drugs of choice
    a. Disrupt bacterial cell wall synthesis when new cells are forming by interfering with the synthesis and cross-linkage of mucopeptides in the final stage of cell wall synthesis
    b. Adverse effects—allergic reactions (highest incidence with parenteral administration)
      (1) Penicillinase (Neutrapen) used to inactivate circulating penicillin by its enzymatic action, which converts the drug to penicillic acid
      (2) Superinfection (e.g., *Candida* and *Pseudomonas* organisms in the vagina and the respiratory and intestinal tracts)
    c. Drug interactions—salicylates and sulfonamides compete with penicillin for nephron tubule transport sites for secretion from the blood; blocking may cause high blood levels of penicillin; probenecid (Benemid) is a sulfonamide used therapeutically with penicillin to slow tubular secretion and allow lower dosages of penicillin
  2. Erythromycins and similar drugs
    a. Compete for receptor sites on the ribosome unit to inhibit mRNA synthesis of protein required for reproduction
    b. Excretion route is in the bile through the intestine (90%), which allows their use with compromised renal function
    c. Adverse effects—GI disturbances (nausea, vomiting, pyrosis, diarrhea, abdominal pain, stomatitis, black tongue)
    d. Drug interactions—decrease tolerance to alcohol ingestion
  3. Sulfonamides—sulfadiazine

a. Actions
  (1) Substitution of a false metabolite for pa-raaminobenzoic acid, required in the bacterial synthesis of folic acid
  (2) Plasma protein-binding maintains tissue levels by liberating drug when tissue levels are low
  (3) Tenacious plasma protein binding may hold the drug until it reaches renal sites, producing high levels in tubule urine
  (4) Many forms require alkalinization of the urine and high fluid intake to maintain urine volume and decrease incidence of nephron crystals
  (5) Recycling of drug in the nephrons delays excretion and maintains blood levels of the drug
    (a) Tubule cells excrete the drug into tubular urine after removal from plasma protein-binding sites
    (b) Tubule cells also reabsorb the drug from tubular urine; drugs return to tissue and liver sites to be metabolized
    (c) Alkalinization of the urine slows recycling and increases excretion rate
b. Adverse effects—anorexia, nausea, vomiting (caused by gastric irritation and action at the vomiting center in the medulla), malaise, blood dyscrasias (leukopenia, thrombocytopenia, erythrocytopenia) and hypoprothrombinemia, allergic reactions (generalized skin eruptions, high fever, severe headache, stomatitis, conjunctivitis, rhinitis, destructive skin lesions, death can result), hepatotoxicity, kernicterus in fetus (replaces protein-bound bilirubin)
c. Drug interactions—enhances action of oral anticoagulants and methotrexate

H. Nursing problems and interventions
  1. Bed rest—to reduce workload of the heart in the presence of carditis
    a. Often difficult to maintain when the child is feeling better
    b. Encourage the child to do schoolwork and keep up with class
    c. Stimulate the development of quiet hobbies and collections
    d. Gradually increase activities when the pulse rate returns to normal
  2. Pain
    a. Handle painful joints carefully
    b. Maintain proper body alignment to prevent deformities
    c. Monitor need for pain medication and administer when necessary
  3. Nutrition
    a. Increase fluids
    b. Provide small, frequent, nutritious meals
  4. Emotional support
    a. Prevent invalidism by emphasizing abilities rather than limitations
    b. Maintain the child's status in home and school by keeping channels of communication open during illness
    c. Reassure the child that chorea is temporary
  5. Public health prevention
    a. Proper and prompt treatment of streptococcal infections with antibiotics
    b. School screening and health promotion programs
    c. Improvement of poor housing conditions
    d. Teach proper standards of hygiene

Juvenile Rheumatoid Arthritis

A. Collagen disease, cause unknown, may occur in response to stress
B. Clinical manifestations
  1. Joint enlargement
    a. Stiffness, pain, and limited motion, especially in morning on awakening
    b. Spindle-fingers—thick proximal joint with slender tip
  2. Low-grade fever
  3. Erythematous rash on the trunk and extremities
  4. Weight loss, fatigue, weakness
  5. Tachycardia
  6. Enlargement of the spleen, liver, and lymph nodes
C. Treatment
  1. Salicylates—used in large doses for antiinflammatory properties
    a. Drugs
      (1) Acetylsalicylic acid (aspirin)
      (2) Carbaspirin calcium (Calurin)
      (3) Choline salicylate (Arthropan)
      (4) Salicylamide (Amid-Sal, Liquiprin, Raspberin, Salamide, Salicim, Salrin)
      (5) Sodium salicylate
    b. Adverse effects—gastric irritation, salicylism with long-term use (visual disturbances, tinnitus, dizziness, mental confusion, diaphoresis, nausea, vomiting, intense thirst)
    c. Drug interactions
      (1) Salicylates have an intrinsic hypogly-

cemic effect and require a decrease in the dosage of oral hypoglycemics for diabetics (they displace sulfonylurea hypoglycemics from protein-binding sites, which causes a greater hypoglycemic effect)

(2) Salicylates decrease absorption of indomethacin from the intestinal tract and lower its effective circulating level

(3) Salicylates antagonize the effect of sulfinpyrazone and probenecid in reducing serum uric acid levels by inhibiting tubular excretion of uric acid

(4) Salicylates have a hypoprothrombinemic action and potentiate the effect of oral anticoagulants primarily by inhibiting platelet aggregation

2. Steroids
3. Physical therapy

D. Nursing problems and interventions
1. Joint deformity and pain
   a. Emphasize that aspirin must be taken regularly, even in periods of remission, to decrease inflammation and pain
   b. Promote proper body alignment and provide passive range of motion
   c. Encourage a warm bath in the morning to decrease stiffness and increase mobility
   d. Encourage exercises such as swimming
2. Acceptance of the disease by the family and child
   a. Encourage parents to accept the child's illness but to limit the use of the disease to foster dependency or control relationships
   b. Teach the family why aspirin is given in large dosages and why other medications are not used
3. Aspirin toxicity—demonstrated by tinnitus, vertigo, nausea, vomiting, sweating, and other signs of salicylate poisoning

Skin Infections

A. Pediculosis—lice
1. May infest the head, body, pubic area
2. Eggs (greenish, translucent oval bodies) attach to hair
3. Severe itching may lead to secondary infection
4. Treatment—special shampoo, use of a fine-toothed comb to remove nits, or eggs
5. Prevention
   a. Cleanliness
      (1) Teach proper hair care
      (2) Encourage frequent bathing and change of clothes
   b. Screening in schools to identify the source of infection

B. Scabies—produced by itch mite
1. Female burrows under the skin to lay eggs (usually in folds of skin)
2. Intensely pruritic—scratching can lead to secondary infection with the development of papules and vesicles
3. Treatment—all members of the family must be treated, since it is highly contagious
   a. Must wear clean clothes
   b. Must wash with sulfur or other special soap

C. Ringworm—fungus disease
1. Scalp (tinea capitis)
   a. Reddened, oval or round areas of alopecia
   b. Treated topically or orally with an antifungal drug such as griseofulvin
   c. Head should be covered to prevent spread of infection
2. Feet (athlete's foot, tinea pedis)
   a. Scaly fissures between toes, vesicles on sides of feet, pruritus
   b. Particularly common in summer; contracted in swimming areas and gymnasium locker rooms
   c. Prevention—do not walk barefooted, dry feet carefully, wear lightweight shoes to decrease heat, disinfect shoes and socks
   d. Treatment—griseofulvin, micronized (Fulvicin-U/F, Grifulvin V, Grisactin)
      (1) Acts as an analog of purine and is incorporated into new epithelial cells during synthesis of nucleic acids
      (2) Adverse effects—peripheral neuritis, vertigo, fever, dryness of mouth, arthralgia, mild transient urticaria, nausea, diarrhea, headache (may disappear as therapy continues), drowsiness, fatigue

D. Intertrigo—excoriation of any adjacent body surfaces caused by moisture and chafing (diaper rash)
1. Keep area clean and dry, rinse wastes from skin
2. Expose area to light and air
3. Apply bland ointment at night
4. Avoid strong alkalis such as bleach in clothes washing

E. Impetigo
1. Bacterial infection of skin by streptococci or staphylococci
2. Highly contagious; other areas of body frequently become infected
3. Treatment—antibiotics systemically and locally, isolate child, keep from scratching other areas of the body

Attention Deficit Disorder

A. Disturbance of central nervous system functioning in which specific motor, sensory, or intellectual impairment exists
B. Characteristics of children with an attention deficit disorder
   1. Difficulty with attention span
   2. May be hyperkinetic or underactive but are awkward and clumsy
   3. Impulsive acting out
   4. Problems with remembering, language, conceptualization, and perception
   5. Normal intellectual functioning
C. Nursing considerations—teach parent to
   1. Avoid overstimulation, provide frequent rest periods throughout day
   2. Structure situations to provide less frustration (play with only one other child rather than group)
   3. Provide firm and consistent discipline; ignore temper tantrums
   4. Learning is best done through play and use of concrete examples, such as 2 halves of an orange to teach fractions
   5. Provide exercises in perceptual-motor coordination and balance
   6. Structure learning experience to utilize the child's ability
   7. Provide opportunities so the child can experience success and satisfaction
   8. Administer drugs such as amphetamines to reduce hyperactivity

Reye's Syndrome

A. Acute encephalopathy with fatty degeneration of the liver
B. Cause unknown although there appears to be a relationship with antecedent viral infection and administration of aspirin
C. Clinical manifestations—prodromal symptoms include malaise, cough, rhinorrhea, or sore throat, followed by worsening cerebral signs as seen in the clinical stages:
   1. Stage I: Vomiting, lethargy, drowsiness
   2. Stage II: Disorientation, delirium, aggressiveness and combativeness, central neurologic hyperventilation (or sometimes shallow breathing), hyperactive reflexes, and stupor
   3. Stage III: Obtundence, coma, hyperventilation, cerebral decortication
   4. Stage IV: Deepening coma, decerebrate rigidity, loss of ocular reflexes, large fixed pupils, divergent eye movements

   5. Stage V: Seizures, loss of deep tendon reflexes, flaccidity, respiratory arrest
D. Treatment—determined by the clinical stage of the disease
   1. Stage I treatment is primarily supportive and directed toward restoring blood sugar levels, controlling cerebral edema, correcting acid-base imbalances, and eliminating factors known to increase intracranial pressure
   2. Stages II through V require invasive support, intracranial pressure monitoring and tracheal intubation with controlled ventilation; a radical approach is curarization and sedation.
E. Nursing considerations
   1. Continuously assess vital signs and neurologic status
   2. Assist with numerous invasive procedures
   3. Explain all therapies to the child (if alert) and parents
   4. Monitor intake and output and invasive equipment (intracranial line, central venous pressure)
   5. Support the family, who will be frightened by the sudden and critical nature of the illness.

Legg-Calvé-Perthes Disease (Coxa Plana)

A. Cause unknown; there is a disturbance of circulation to the femoral capital epiphysis producing an ischemic aseptic necrosis of the femoral head, epiphysis, and acetabulum
B. Clinical manifestations
   1. Persistent pain in the affected hip(s)
   2. Limitation of movement in the affected hip(s)
   3. Limp
C. Treatment—aim is to keep the head of the femur in the acetabulum and maintain a full range of motion with
   1. Non-weight-bearing devices such as an abduction brace, leg casts, or a leather harness sling that prevents weight bearing on the affected limb
   2. Use of abduction-ambulation braces or casts after a period of bed rest and traction
   3. Surgical reconstructive and containment procedures
D. Conservative therapy must be continued for 2 to 4 years, whereas surgical correction returns the child to normal activities in 3 to 4 months.
E. Nursing considerations
   1. Instruct the child and parents regarding what constitutes nonweight bearing (e.g., no standing or kneeling on the affected leg)
   2. Educate the child and parents regarding correct use of appliances
   3. Assist the child and family in selecting activities

according to the child's age, interests, and physical limitations
  a. Quiet games
  b. Hobbies such as collections, model building, crafts, indoor gardening
4. Encourage peer interaction
5. Involve the child in planning activities and therapy
6. Help the child determine alternatives to weight-bearing activity (e.g., scorekeeping, sideline ''coach'')
7. Help the child devise explanations for appliances and his inability to participate actively with peers

The Adolescent
GROWTH AND DEVELOPMENT
Developmental Timetable

A. Physical growth—includes the physical changes associated with puberty such as secondary sexual characteristics
B. Mental abilities
  1. Abstract thinking
    a. New level of social communication and understanding
      (1) Can comprehend satire and double meanings
      (2) Can say one thing and mean another
    b. Can conceptualize thought; more interested in exploring ideas than facts
    c. Can appreciate scientific thinking, problem solve, and theoretically explore alternatives
  2. Perception
    a. Can appreciate nonrepresentational art
    b. Can understand that the whole is more than the sum of its parts
  3. Learning
    a. Much longer span of attention
    b. Learns through inference, intuition, and surmise, rather than repetition and imitation
    c. Enjoys regressing in terms of language development by using jargon to suit changing moods
C. Social patterns
  1. Peer group identity
    a. One of the strongest motivating forces of behavior
    b. Extremely important to be part of the group and like everyone else in every way
    c. Clique formation; usually based on common

denominators such as race, social class, ethnic group, or special interests
  2. Interpersonal relationships
    a. Major goal is learning to form a close intimate relationship with the opposite sex
    b. Adolescents may develop crushes and worship many idols
    c. Time of sexual exploration and questioning of one's sexual role
  3. Independence
    a. By 15 or 16 years of age, adolescents feel they should be treated as adults
    b. Ambivalence—adolescent wants freedom but is not happy about corresponding responsibilities and frequently yearns for more carefree days of childhood
    c. Parental ambivalence and discipline problems are common as parents try to allow for increasing independence but continue to offer constructive guidance and enforce discipline

HEALTH PROMOTION
Adolescent Nutrition

A. Nutritional objectives
  1. Provide optimum nutritional support for demands of rapid growth and high energy expenditure
  2. Support development of good eating habits through variety of foods, regular pattern, good quality snacks (high in protein, low in refined carbohydrate, primarily sugar)
B. Nutrient needs increased in all respects, so adequate intakes of all nutrients should form basis of diet
C. Possible nutritional problems
  1. Low intakes of calcium, vitamin A and C, iron in girls
  2. Anemia—increase foods containing iron
  3. Obesity or underweight—decrease or increase calories as needed
  4. Skin problems—use well-balanced diet high in protein, vitamins, minerals
  5. Nutritional deficiencies related to
    a. Psychologic factors—food aversions, emotional problems
    b. Fear of overweight—crash diets, mainly in girls; cultural pressure
    c. Fad diets—caused by misinformation; need for sound counseling
    d. Poor choice of snack foods—usually high in sugar; use more fruit and protein forms
    e. Irregular eating pattern
  6. Additional stress of pregnancy—need high protein and calorie intake

D. Nutrition education may be made through association with teenagers' concerns about physical appearance, figure control, complexion, physical fitness, athletic ability

Accident Prevention

A. Appropriate education regarding sexual maturity, reproduction, and sexual behavior
B. Driver education
C. Education regarding use and abuse of drugs, especially alcohol
D. Education on health hazards associated with smoking

Problems of Adolescence

A. Accidents—still the no. 1 cause of death, with motor vehicle accidents causing the most fatalities
B. Suicide—one of chief causes of death among this age group
C. Drug abuse
D. Delinquency
E. Alcoholism
F. Pregnancy
G. Obesity
H. Acne
I. Anorexia nervosa
J. Many problems of adolescence similar to those of adults; see specific areas in psychiatric and medical-surgical nursing for further discussion

Scoliosis

A. Lateral curvature of the spine usually associated with a rotary deformity that eventually causes cosmetic and physiologic alterations in the spine, chest, and pelvis
B. Nonstructural scoliosis—curve is flexible and corrects by bending
C. Structural scoliosis—curve fails to straighten on side-bending; characterized by changes in the spine and its supporting structures
D. Cause in 70% of cases is "idiopathic"; probably transmitted as an autosomal dominant trait with incomplete penetrance
E. Clinical manifestations
  1. Prominence of one hip
  2. Deformity of the rib cage
  3. Prominence of one scapula.
  4. Difference in shoulder or scapular height.
  5. Curve in the vertebral spinous process alignment.
  6. Breasts appear unequal in size.
  7. Other clues
    a. Clothes do not fit right
    b. Skirt hems are uneven
F. Screening for scoliosis
  1. Have the child stand erect, clothed only in underpants (and bra if older girl) and observe from behind; note asymmetry of the shoulders and hips
  2. Have the child bend forward so the back is parallel with the floor; observe from the side, noting asymmetry or prominence of the rib
G. Diagnosis—confirmed by x-ray examination
H. Treatment—depending on severity of the curvature
  1. Curves of less than 30 degrees treated by exercises
  2. May also include the Milwaukee brace, an individually adapted steel and leather brace that extends from a chin cup and neck pads to the pelvis, where lumbar pads rest on the hips
    a. Worn 23 hours a day
    b. The child is gradually weaned from the brace over a 1-to-2 year period
    c. Brace then worn only at night until the spine is mature
  3. More severe curves usually require surgery—techniques consist of spinal realignment and straightening by way of external or internal fixation and instrumentation combined with bony fusion (arthrodesis) of the realigned spine
    a. Harrington rods
    b. Dwyer instrumentation
  4. Most severe scoliotic curvatures require traction devices and exercises for a time before spinal fusion to provide partial correction and more flexibility
I. Nursing considerations
  1. Check spine alignment as part of child assessment
  2. Reinforce and clarify explanations provided by the orthopedist
    a. Appliance
    b. Plan of care
    c. Activities allowed or restricted
    d. Child's and parents' responsibilities in therapy
  3. Examine skin surfaces in contact with the brace for signs of irritation; implement corrective action to treat or prevent skin breakdown
  4. Help in selection of the appropriate wearing apparel to wear over the brace and footwear to maintain proper balance
  5. Prepare for surgery if required

Bone Tumors

A. Osteogenic sarcoma
1. Most frequent bone tumor in children
2. Primary tumor site—diaphysis (shaft) of a long bone, especially the femur

B. Ewing's sarcoma
1. Most frequent sites—shaft of the long and trunk bones, especially the femur, tibia, fibula, humerus, ulna, vertebra, scapula, ribs, pelvic bones, and skull

C. Clinical manifestations
1. Localized pain in the affected site
2. Limp
3. Voluntary curtailment of activity
4. Inability to hold heavy objects
5. Weight loss
6. Frequent infection

D. Diagnosis
1. X-ray examination
2. Tomography (bone and lung)
3. Bone scan
4. Bone marrow aspiration
5. Surgical biopsy (Ewing's sarcoma)

E. Treatment
1. Osteogenic sarcoma—amputation of the affected bone followed by high-dose methotrexate or preoperative and postoperative use of chemotherapy with en bloc resection of the primary tumor followed by a prosthetic replacement
2. Ewing's sarcoma—intensive irradiation of the involved bone and chemotherapy

F. Nursing considerations
1. Prepare the child and family for probable amputation (osteogenic sarcoma)
   a. Employ straightforward honesty
   b. Avoid disguising the diagnosis with terms such as "infection"
   c. Emphasize lack of alternatives
   d. Answer questions regarding information presented by the surgeon and clarify any misconceptions
   e. Avoid overwhelming the child or parents with too much information
2. Prepare the child and family for radiotherapy (Ewing's sarcoma)
   a. Explain the procedure
   b. Remain with the child during the procedure
   c. Explain the undesirable side effects of radiotherapy
   d. Suggest and/or implement measures to reduce the physical effects of radiotherapy, such as selecting loose-fitting clothing over the irradiated areas to decrease additional irritation, protection of the area from sunlight and sudden changes in temperature (avoid ice packs, heating pads)
3. Prepare the child and family for chemotherapy
   a. Impress on the child the importance of therapy
   b. Explain the probable side effects of antimetabolites (e.g., nausea, hair loss)
4. Assist the child in adjusting to his disability
   a. Assist the child in becoming adept at using the appliances
   b. Help the child select clothing to camouflage the prosthesis
   c. Encourage good hygiene, grooming and sex-appropriate items to enhance appearance such as wig (for hair loss from antimetabolites), makeup, attractive, sex-appropriate clothing
   d. Allow the child time and opportunity to go through the grief process
   e. Allow for expression of feelings regarding the loss and the undesirable effects of chemotherapy
   f. Help the child cope with the side effects of chemotherapy and irradiation
   g. Encourage independence
5. Support the child and family
   a. Allow for expression of feelings
   b. Clarify misconceptions and provide technical information as needed
   c. Impress upon both child and family the need for continuing normal activities, interactions, and behaviors

Pediatric Nursing Review Questions

Situation: Mr. Crew, a nursing student, is doing therapeutic play with the children in the playroom of the well-baby clinic. To understand how to plan for children of various ages, he needs to have knowledge of their developmental norms. Questions 1 through 4 refer to this situation.

1 Mr. Crew observes that 2-year-old Mark:
1. Builds houses with blocks
2. Is very possessive of toys
3. Attempts to stay within the lines when coloring
4. Amuses himself with a picture book for 15 minutes

2 Mr Crew observes 4-year-old Colin having difficulty playing with the other children. He understands that it is normal for Colin to:
1. Exaggerate and boast to impress others
2. Have fierce temper tantrums and negativism
3. Engage in parallel or solitary play
4. Be almost totally dependent on parents

3 Fifteen-month-old Nadia is playing in the playpen. Mr. Crew observes her activities and realizes that her physical tasks are within the norms when she is able to:
1. Build a tower of 6 blocks
2. Stand in the playpen holding onto the sides
3. Throw all the toys out of the playpen
4. Walk across the playpen with ease

4 Mr. Crew would encourage two 6-year-old boys in the playroom to play with:
1. A board game
2. An erector set
3. Checkers
4. Clay

Situation: Mr. and Mrs B were emotionally upset when their baby girl Sue was born with a cleft palate and double cleft lip. Questions 5 through 9 refer to this situation.

5 How could the nurse give the most support to the parents?
1. Discourage them from talking about the baby
2. Encourage them to express their worries and fears
3. Tell them not to worry because the defect can be repaired
4. Show them postoperative photographs of babies who had similar defects

6 What is the most critical factor in the immediate care of Sue after repair of the lip?
1. Maintenance of a patent airway
2. Administration of drugs to reduce oral secretions
3. Administration of parenteral fluids
4. Prevention of vomiting

7 Additional nursing care for Sue after the surgical lip repair would include:
1. Placing the infant in a semisitting position
2. Keeping the infant from crying

3. Spoon-feeding for the first 2 days after surgery
4. Keeping the baby n.p.o.

8 At 2 years of age Sue returned for palate surgery. What is the most important factor in preparing her for this experience?
1. Her previous hospital visits
2. Gratification of all her wishes
3. Never leaving her with strangers
4. Assurance of affection and security

9 A toothbrush was not used on Sue immediately after palate surgery because:
1. The suture line might be injured
2. She was not accustomed to a brush at home
3. She had no teeth
4. It might be frightening to her

Situation: David, age 1 year, weighs 12.6 kg (28 pounds) but is pale and lethargic. His hemoglobin level is 5 g and he has an enlarged heart. When taking a nursing history from his mother, the nurse learns that he refuses food so she gives him a quart of milk per day from a bottle. Questions 10 through 16 refer to this situation.

10 The nurse suggests that his mother:
1. Put a large hole in the nipple and put baby food in with his milk
2. Take him to the metabolic clinic for a check-up
3. Immediately begin the weaning process
4. Give him finger foods such as raisins and chopped meat

11 David should have been started on solid foods by at least 5 or 6 months of age because:
1. His fetal reserve of iron was depleted
2. It would have taught him how to chew
3. His bone marrow activity had slacked off at this time
4. It would have helped control his weight

12 The most prevalent nutritional disorder among children in the United States is iron deficiency anemia. A major reason for this in young children is:
1. Overfeeding of milk
2. Lack of adequate iron reserves from the mother
3. Blood disorders
4. Introduction of solid foods too early for proper absorption

13 Anemia, a nutritional problem encountered in children and adults, involves several different nutrients. The nutrients include proteins, iron, vitamin B_{12}, and:
1. Carbohydrates
2. Thiamin
3. Calcium
4. Folic acid

14 Which of the following foods would you emphasize to David's mother as a source of iron to be included in his diet daily?
1. Orange juice
2. Lamb
3. Egg yolk
4. Milk

15 David's mother also states that he has 8 teeth and asks when she should take him to the dentist. For dental prophylaxis, the nurse encourages her to take him:
1. The next time another family member goes to the dentist
2. Before starting school
3. Between 2 and 3 years of age
4. When he begins to lose his deciduous teeth

16 Your background knowledge of the basic nutrients that act as partners in building red blood cells will form the basis for a teaching plan. These nutrient partners of iron are:
1. Calcium and vitamins
2. Carbohydrates and thiamine
3. Proteins and ascorbic acid
4. Vitamin D and riboflavin

Situation: Four-year-old Ann weighs 18 kg (40 pounds) and is in a private pediatric room on "hand and linen precaution." She was admitted for weight loss, anorexia, vaginitis, and insomnia. A diagnosis of pinworm infestation was made. Questions 17 through 21 refer to this situation.

17 The most effective time for the nurse to do a cellophane tape test for pinworms is:
1. At bedtime before bathing
2. Just following a bowel movement
3. Immediately after meals
4. Early morning before arising

18 Pinworms cause a number of symptoms besides anal itching. A rare sequela of pinworm infestation that the nurse would observe for is:
1. Pneumonitis
2. Stomatitis
3. Hepatitis
4. Appendicitis

19 Pyrvinium pamoate (Povan) is an effective single-dose drug to eliminate pinworms. How many milligrams will you give Ann if 5 mg per kilogram of body weight are ordered?
1. 90 mg
2. 18 mg
3. 40 mg
4. 200 mg

20 After administering pyrvinium pamoate (Povan) to Ann, it is important to alert the staff that a normal side effect of this drug is that it colors the stool or vomitus:
1. Dark brown
2. Light green
3. Bright red
4. Gentian blue

21 The nurse's decision to alert the staff is based on her knowledge that:
1. Irritation by pinworms in the rectum may cause ulceration and bleeding
2. The cyanine dye origin of the drug colors the stool
3. The stool contains hemoglobin-like metabolic products of disintegrating pinworms

4. The drug is irritating to the intestinal mucosa and may cause transient bleeding

Situation: Seven-year-old Johnny has been admitted for a tonsillectomy. Questions 22 through 24 refer to this situation.

22 An essential nursing action preoperatively is to:
1. Encourage parent to stay until Johnny goes to the operating room
2. Provide him with his favorite toy
3. Observe his ASO titer
4. Check for loose teeth and report to physician

23 The nurse suspects hemorrhage postoperatively when Johnny:
1. Snores noisily
2. Becomes pale
3. Complains of thirst
4. Swallows frequently

24 Johnny is complaining of pain in his throat. Which of the following medications for pain would be best for him at this time?
1. Aspirin, 300 mg
2. Tylenol, 300 mg
3. Phenobarbital, 15 mg
4. Demerol, 50 mg

Situation: Two-day-old Edward has a meningomyelocele. He is scheduled for surgery. Questions 25 through 27 refer to this situation.

25 Prior to the surgical correction, a primary nursing goal is to:
1. Observe for bowel and bladder dysfunction
2. Prevent infection
3. Prevent skin breakdown
4. Observe for increasing paralysis

26 After closure of Edward's meningomyelocele, it is essential that his nursing care include:
1. Decrease of environmental stimuli
2. Strict limitation of leg movement
3. Measurement of head circumference daily
4. Observation of serous drainage from the nares

27 To meet a major developmental need of Edward's the nurse should:
1. Provide a soft cuddly toy
2. Give him a pacifier
3. Warm his formula before feeding
4. Put a mobile over his crib

Situation: Eight-year-old John Kee is being discharged following treatment for sickle cell crisis. He is allowed to return to school and resume normal activities. Questions 28 through 32 refer to this situation.

28 The nurse explains to Mrs. Kee that a very important aspect of care for John at home should include:
1. At least 14 hours sleep per day
2. Rigorous exercise and play

3. Ingestion of large quantities of liquids

4. High-calorie diet

29 Infants with sickle cell anemia may not be diagnosed as having this disorder because of:

1. The presence of fetal hemoglobin during the first year of life

2. Compensation of increased hematocrit and hemoglobin if well fed

3. Absence of respiratory disorders

4. General good qealth and an excellent growth curve

30 The sickling process of the red blood cell occurs in conditions of:

1. Hemodilution

2. Hypoxia

3. Thrombocytopenia

4. Hypocalcemia

31 To prevent thrombus formation in capillaries, as well as other problems from stasis and clotting of blood in the sickling process, the main nursing intervention is:

1. Administration of oxygen

2. Increasing fluids by mouth and a humidifier

3. Complete bed rest

4. Use of heparin or other anticoagulants

32 Common nursing care that helps prevent both sickle cell crisis and celiac crisis is:

1. Limitation of activity

2. Protection from infection

3. High-iron, low-fat, high-protein diet

4. Careful observation of all vital signs

Situation: *Johnny Smith, 12 months of age, is brought to the pediatric health clinic for a regular physical assessment. Questions 33 through 36 refer to this situation.*

33 In reviewing his immunizations for the past 10 months the nurse would expect him to have been immunized against:

1. Measles, rubella, polio, tuberculosis, and pertussis

2. Polio, pertussis, tetanus, and diphtheria

3. Measles, mumps, rubella and tuberculosis

4. Pertussis, tetanus, polio, and measles

34 Mrs. Smith asks the nurse how the DTP injection works. The nurse, in formulating a response, recalls that in active immunity:

1. Blood antigens are aided by phagocytes in defending the body against pathogens

2. Protein antigens are formed in the blood to fight invading antibodies

3. Protein substances are formed by the body to destroy or neutralize antigens

4. Lipid agents are formed by the body against antigens

35 The measles immunization is usually routinely given after 15 months of age because of the:

1. Increased hazard of side effects in infants

2. Presence of maternal antibodies during the first year

3. Interference it causes with effectiveness of pertussis, diphtheria, and tetanus immunizations

4. Rare incidence of measles infection prior to 12 months of age

36 In terms of preventive teaching for a 1-year-old, the nurse would speak to Mrs. Smith about:

1. Adequate nutrition

2. Accidents

3. Sexual development

4. Toilet training

Situation: *Nancy Hand, a 5-year-old only child, is admitted to the hospital with rheumatic fever. She requires bed rest, a soft diet, liberal fluid intake, and ampicillin, 250 mg, p.o. q.i.d. She is restless and fretful and tells you that her legs hurt. Questions 37 through 44 refer to this situation.*

37 Nancy may be more comfortable if her:

1. Position is changed frequently

2. Bed is elevated at the head

3. Legs are supported on a pillow

4. Body alignment is maintained

38 The immediate priority in Nancy's nursing care is:

1. Nutrition

2. Rest

3. Exercise

4. Elimination

39 Nursing care likely to be most effective in alleviating Nancy's fretfulness is:

1. Giving her a jigsaw puzzle

2. Putting her in a room by herself

3. Letting her play with a doll

4. Reading a story to her

40 The best choice of between-meal nourishment for Nancy is:

1. Fresh fruit

2. Hard candy

3. Fruit gelatin

4. Creamed soup

41 The most serious complication that may threaten Nancy is:

1. Endocarditis

2. Pneumonitis

3. Tenosynovitis

4. Rheumatoid arthritis

42 When you bring Nancy her dinner tray she says, "I'm too sick to feed myself." You should tell her to:

1. Try to eat as much as she can

2. Be a big girl and not act like a baby

3. Let it go until she feels better

4. Wait 5 minutes and you will help her

43 Nancy's statement is most likely indicative of:

1. Immaturity

2. Lonesomeness

3. Regression

4. Temper tantrum

44 Nancy is apathetic about eating. Nursing care directed toward supporting her nutrition ought to include:

1. Providing diversional activity at mealtime

2. Eliminating all between-meal nourishment
3. Asking her parents to visit at mealtime
4. Giving her only the foods she likes best

Situation: Mrs. Bronson is informed that her infant daughter has phenylketonuria (PKU). Questions 45 through 49 refer to this situation.

45 Which of the following statements is true concerning PKU?
1. PKU is transmitted by an autosomal dominant gene
2. The infant is tested for PKU immediately after delivery
3. If untreated, mental retardation occurs
4. Treatment for PKU includes lifelong diet therapy

46 A test that was done on Baby Bronson in the nursery to detect PKU is:
1. Guthrie blood test
2. Ferric chloride urine test
3. Phenistix test
4. Clinitest serum phosphopyruvic acid

47 Primary treatment of an infant who has an inherited inborn error of metabolism consists mostly of:
1. Hormonal therapy
2. Dietary control
3. Enzyme replacement
4. Vitamin supplement

48 When teaching Mr. and Mrs. Bronson about their daughter's disorder, the nurse should state that:
1. Phenylalanine is not necessary for growth
2. Other amino acids can be increased to substitute for phenylalanine
3. A low-phenylalanine diet is required
4. Phenylalanine can be administered to correct the deficiency

49 In terms of dietary counseling, the parents need much help and support in adhering to specific regimens. A frequent question asked by parents is, "How long will my child have to be on this diet?" An appropriate response by the nurse is:
1. "Unfortunately, this is a life-long problem and dietary management must always be maintained."
2. "Usually, if the child does well for 1 year, she then can gradually begin eating regular foods."
3. "As of now, research shows that a child needs to be on this diet until she is about 6 to 8 years of age. Then she can gradually begin to eat other foods."
4. "No one knows, but why don't you discuss it with your doctor."

Situation: Mrs. Simmons brings 3-year-old Sam to the emergency room, indicating he has had a fever for several days, has held his neck rigid, and is now vomiting. While being examined he has a convulsion and is admitted to the pediatric unit. Questions 50 through 54 refer to this situation.

50 While instituting nursing measures to reduce Sam's fever, the nurse recognizes that an important consideration is to:
1. Monitor vital signs every 10 minutes
2. Force oral fluids
3. Measure output every hour
4. Limit exposure to prevent shivering

51 Febrile convulsions are common in children and:
1. Usually occur after the first year of life
2. The cause is usually readily identified
3. May occur in minor illnesses
4. Occur more frequently in females than males

52 The physician orders A.S.A., 150 mg, p.o., q. 4 h., p.r.n. for fever above 38° C (101° F). You have on hand A.S.A. labeled "1 tablet equals 1¼ gr." How many tablets should be administered?
1. ½ tablet
2. 1 tablet
3. 1½ tablets
4. 2 tablets

53 Sam is diagnosed as having meningococcal meningitis. The nurse observes Sam for the:
1. Identifying purpuric skin rash
2. Continual tremors of the extremities
3. Low-grade nature of the fever
4. Palatal paralysis and glossitis

54 The most serious complication of meningitis in young children is:
1. Hydrocephalus
2. Blindness
3. Peripheral circulatory collapse
4. Epilepsy

Situation: Three-month-old Matt Quincy is admitted to the hospital with bile-stained vomitus and abdominal distention. Questions 55 through 58 refer to this situation.

55 The nurse should also observe for:
1. Constant severe pain and absence of stools
2. Bounding pulse and hypotonicity
3. Paroxysmal pain and grunting respirations
4. High-pitched cry and weak thready pulse

56 Prior to surgery for the intestinal obstruction, Matt is kept n.p.o. and has a Levin tube in place. To calm Matt and also to meet his developmental needs best, the nurse should:
1. Allow him to suck on a pacifier
2. Hang a brightly colored mobile in his crib
3. Place him on his abdomen and permit him to crawl
4. Allow him to hold his favorite toy

57 Matt develops diarrhea postoperatively and is given IV fluids. The rate of flow must be observed often by the nurse to:
1. Avoid IV infiltration
2. Prevent increased output
3. Prevent cardiac embarrassment
4. Replace all fluids lost

58 When Mrs. Quincy returns to the surgical clinic for follow-up care, the nurse includes the following preventive suggestion in her teaching:
1. Remove all tiny objects from the floor
2. Keep crib rails up to the highest position
3. Cover electric outlets with safety plugs
4. Remove poisonous substance from low areas

Situation: Five-year-old Sam has been hospitalized with acute glomerulonephritis. Questions 59 through 62 refer to this situation.

59 The nurse observes Sam primarily for:
1. Polyuria, high fever
2. Dehydration, hematuria
3. Hypertension, circumocular edema
4. Oliguria, hypotension

60 When planning nursing care for Sam, the nurse realizes that he needs help in understanding his restrictions, one of which is:
1. Bed rest for at least 4 weeks
2. A bland diet high in protein
3. Daily doses of IM penicillin
4. Isolation from other children with infections

61 The average 5-year-old is incapable of:
1. Making decisions
2. Tying his shoelaces
3. Abstract thought
4. Hand-eye coordination

62 Sam loves to ride his bike, and his parents are very concerned about his activity when he returns home. You base your answer to them on the fact that after the urinary findings are nearly normal:
1. He must remain in bed for 2 weeks
2. Activity does not affect the course of the disease
3. He must not play active games
4. Activity must be limited for 1 month

Situation: Eight-year-old John has rheumatic fever. He has a low-grade fever in the afternoon, is anemic, and his shoulder, elbow, and knee joints are painful, hot, and enlarged. His therapy includes bed rest, and he is receiving large amounts of A.S.A. daily. Questions 63 through 65 refer to this situation.

63 During the acute phase, to help relieve the pain in John's joints, the nurse should maintain body alignment, support the joints with pillows, and:
1. Apply heat to the joints
2. Give passive range of motion exercises once a day only
3. Massage the extremities
4. Move him as little as possible

64 While John is in bed convalescing, he becomes very bored and irritable. The nurse plans activities that a school-age child would like and suggests he:

1. Play chess
2. Start a collection
3. Watch game shows on TV
4. Do arithmetic puzzles

65 John *must* remain in bed until his pulse rate and hemoglobin level are normal and the:
1. C-reactive protein is negative
2. Fever is decreased to 37.8° C (100° F)
3. Pain is totally gone from the joints
4. Rash has disappeared

Situation: Sue Green, a 2-year-old girl, is admitted to the pediatric unit with respiratory wheezing, dyspnea, and cyanosis. One of the tentative diagnoses is cystic fibrosis. Questions 66 through 72 refer to this situation.

66 Cystic fibrosis can predispose Sue to bronchitis mainly because:
1. Tenacious secretions obstruct the bronchioles and respiratory tract and provide a favorable medium for growth of bacteria
2. Increased salt content in saliva can irritate and necrose mucous membranes in nasopharynx
3. Neuromuscular irritability causes spasm and constriction of the bronchi
4. The associated heart defects of cystic fibrosis cause congestive heart failure and respiratory depression

67 The problem of cystic fibrosis is sometimes first noted by the nurse in the newborn nursery because of:
1. Increased heart rate
2. Abdominal distention
3. Excessive crying
4. Sternal retractions

68 Sue is small and underdeveloped for her age primarily because she:
1. Ingested little food for several months because of poor appetite
2. Was unable to absorb nutrients because of a lack of pancreatic enzymes
3. Secreted less than normal amounts of pituitary growth hormone
4. Developed muscular and bony atrophy from lack of motor activity

69 When caring for the child with cystic fibrosis the nurse should:
1. Promote postural drainage
2. Encourage active exercise
3. Prevent coughing
4. Provide small frequent feedings

70 The foul-smelling, frothy characteristic of the stool in cystic fibrosis results from the presence of large amounts of:
1. Sodium and chloride
2. Semidigested carbohydrates
3. Undigested fat
4. Lipase, trypsin, and amylase

71 Medications that will probably be used for Sue in her therapeutic regimen include:
1. A steroid and an antimetabolite
2. Antibiotics, a multivitamin preparation, and cough drops
3. Pancreatic enzymes and antibiotics
4. Aerosol mists, decongestants, and fat-soluble vitamins

72 In cystic fibrosis, frequent stools and tenacious mucus often produce:
1. Intussusception
2. Anal fissures
3. Meconium ileus
4. Rectal prolapse

Situation: Two-year-old Mike Cox is admitted to the hospital for the second surgical repair of his clubfoot. Mrs. Cox cannot stay overnight with her son, since visiting hours are restricted. On the morning after admission, Mike is standing in his crib crying. He refuses to be comforted and calls for his mother. Questions 73 through 76 refer to this situation.

73 The nurse approaches Mike to bathe him and he screams louder. This behavior is recognized as the stage of protest, and the nurse:
1. Picks him up and walks with him around the room
2. Sits by his crib and bathes him later when his anxiety decreases
3. Decides he really does not need a bath when he is this upset
4. Fills the basin with water and proceeds to bathe him

74 On the third postoperative day Mike begins to regress and lies quietly in his crib with his blanket. The nurse recognizes that Mike is in a stage of:
1. Denial
2. Mistrust
3. Rejection
4. Despair

75 During his second week of hospitalization, Mike smiles easily, goes to all the nurses happily, and no longer cries when his mother goes home. After leaving Mike's room, Mrs. Cox tells the nurse she is pleased that Mike is adjusting well. Before responding to Mrs. Cox, the nurse understands Mike's behavior and realizes that he:
1. Is repressing his feelings for his mother
2. Has established a routine and feels safe
3. Feels better physically so his behavior has improved
4. Has given up fighting and accepts the separation

76 The nurse explains the meaning of Mike's behavior to Mrs. Cox and tells her that after he goes home she should expect that:
1. Mike will miss the nurses and hospital routine
2. It will be easier for Mike to adjust to his home situation
3. Mike will continue his happy, normal behavior
4. It will take some time before the mother-child relationship is reestablished

Situation: Sara, 12 years old, was diagnosed at the orthopedic clinic as having idiopathic scoliosis. Proper exercising and avoidance of fatigue are essential components of Sara's care. Questions 77 through 79 refer to this situation.

77 Early in Sara's treatment the nurse can suggest which of the following sports as therapeutic?
1. Bowling
2. Swimming
3. Badminton
4. Golf

78 To assist her curvature correction, Sara is fitted with a Milwaukee brace. The nurse explains to Sara and her parents that the length of time the brace must be worn varies but it is usually worn until:
1. Cessation of bone growth at the time of physical maturity
2. The curvature of the spine is completely straightened
3. Pain on prolonged standing diminishes
4. The iliac crests are at equal levels

79 One of the earliest signs of sexual maturity in a young girl such as Sara is:
1. Interest in the opposite sex
2. Attention to grooming
3. An increase in the size of the external genitalia
4. The appearance of axillary and pubic hair

Situation: At 2 weeks of age Baby Williams begins to vomit after his feedings and is admitted to the hospital for observation with a tentative diagnosis of pyloric stenosis. Questions 80 through 84 refer to this situation.

80 The nurse was careful to note:
1. Signs of dehydration
2. Coughing and gagging after feeding
3. Quality of cry
4. Quality of stool

81 When vomiting is uncontrolled in an infant, the nurse should observe for signs of:
1. Tetany
2. Alkalosis
3. Acidosis
4. Hyperactivity

82 The maintenance of fluid and electrolyte balance is more critical in children than in adults because:
1. Renal function is immature in children
2. Cellular metabolism is less stable than in adults
3. The proportion of water in the body is less than in adults
4. The daily fluid requirement per unit of body weight is greater than in adults

83 What is the most critical factor confronting the nurse in the administration of IV fluids to a small, dehydrated infant?
1. Maintenance of the prescribed rate of flow
2. Maintenance of the fluid at body temperature
3. Calculation of the total necessary intake
4. Maintenance of sterility

84 Surgery is performed and Baby Williams' condition is stable. The nurse caring for him notices that his postoperative orders are similar to those for other infants having undergone such surgery and include:
1. Withholding of all feedings for the first 24 hours
2. Additional glucose feedings after the first 24 hours
3. Thickened formula 24 hours after surgery
4. Diluted formula feeding 24 hours after surgery

Situation: Karen Vale, a 5-year-old girl, is admitted to the hospital 1 week before surgery for tetralogy of Fallot. Questions 85 through 89 refer to this situation.

85 The defects associated with this heart anomaly include:
1. Right ventricular hypertrophy, atrial and ventricular defects, and mitral valve stenosis
2. Right ventricular hypertrophy, ventricular septal defect, stenosis of pulmonary artery, and overriding aorta
3. Origin of the aorta from the right ventricle and of the pulmonary artery from the left ventricle
4. Abnormal connection between the pulmonary artery and the aorta, right ventricular hypertrophy, and atrial septal defects

86 A common finding in most children with cardiac anomalies is:
1. Mental retardation
2. Cyanosis and clubbing of fingertips
3. A family history of cardiac anomalies
4. Delayed physical growth

87 Karen is to receive digoxin (Lanoxin) elixir, 0.010 mg, p.o. Based on developmental norms for a 5-year-old, the nurse would withhold the medication and notify the physician if the apical rate is below:
1. 60 beats per minute
2. 80 beats per minute
3. 90 beats per minute
4. 100 beats per minute

88 Karen's laboratory analysis indicates a high red blood cell count. This polycythemia can best be understood as a compensatory mechanism for:
1. Cardiomegaly
2. Low iron level
3. Low blood pressure
4. Tissue oxygen need

89 Karen undergoes heart surgery to repair the anomaly. Postoperatively it is essential that the nurse prevent which of the following?
1. Constipation
2. Unnecessary movement
3. Crying
4. Coughing

Situation: Johnny, a 10-year-old, is taken to the emergency room of the local hospital because he stepped on a nail. Questions 90 and 91 refer to this situation.

90 The puncture wound is cleansed, and a sterile dressing applied. While doing these tasks, the nurse asks the mother if Johnny has been immunized against tetanus. The reply is affirmative. Penicillin is administered, and the child sent home with instructions to return if there is any change in the wound area. A few days later, Johnny is admitted to the hospital with a diagnosis of tetanus. Legally:
1. The possibility of tetanus could not have been foreseen, since he had been immunized
2. The nurse's judgment was adequate in view of the patient's symptoms
3. Assessment by the nurse was incomplete and the treatment was inadequate
4. Hospital protocol should govern treatment in emergency room care

91 After Johnny's admission, one of the most important aspects of nursing care should be directed toward:
1. Maintaining body alignment
2. Encouraging high intake of fluid
3. Carefully monitoring urinary output
4. Decreasing external stimuli

Situation: Three-day-old Patty is diagnosed as having congenital hip dysplasia. Questions 92 through 94 refer to this situation.

92 An early sign able to be observed by the nurse in the newborn nursery is:
1. Limitation in adduction of the leg
2. Shortening of the leg on the unaffected side
3. Depressed dance reflex
4. Asymmetry of the gluteal folds

93 At 3 months of age Patty has a spica cast applied from below the axilla to below the knee. To prevent a serious complication that often occurs in infants in a spica cast, the nurse teaches Patty's parents to:
1. Seek immediate medical care if Patty develops a cough
2. Limit movement to prevent cast damage
3. Change Patty's diapers frequently
4. Feed Patty a low-calorie diet

94 When elevating Patty's head, the nurse is aware that it is important to:
1. Limit this position to 1 hour at a maximum
2. Raise the entire mattress and spring at the head of the bed
3. Use at least 2 pillows under her shoulders
4. Place folded diapers at the edge of the cast

Situation: Working on a cardiac care unit, the nurse will care for many children with a variety of congenital anomalies. Questions 95 through 98 refer to this situation.

95 Meg, 2 years old, has a cyanotic congenital heart disease. The nurse would expect to observe:
1. Edema in the extremities
2. An elevated hematocrit

3. Absence of pedal pulses

4. Orthopnea

96 Baby boy Vics has been found to have a patent ductus arteriosus, which is:

1. A narrowing of the pulmonary artery

2. An abnormal opening between the right and left ventricles

3. A connection between the pulmonary artery and the aorta

4. An enlarged aorta and pulmonary artery

97 The nurse is caring for a child with an acyanotic heart disease. A major *common* symptom of acyanotic heart disease is:

1. Polycythemia

2. Clubbing of fingers and toes

3. Severe retarded growth

4. The presence of an audible heart murmur

98 Alma has coarctation of the aorta. When taking her vital signs, the nurse can expect to observe:

1. Weak, thready radial pulses

2. Higher blood pressure in the upper extremities

3. Bounding femoral pulses

4. Notching of the clavicle

Situation: John, 17 years old, is admitted to the hospital because of minor injuries suffered in an automobile accident. During the examination the physician notices a rash on the skin and finds that John has suffered from a sore throat for several days. Based on the clinical examination the physician makes a tentative diagnosis of syphilis, pending a report on the serologic test. Questions 99 through 101 refer to this situation.

99 These symptoms are classified as which of the following stages of syphilis?

1. Primary

2. Latent

3. Infectious

4. Late

100 The report of the serologic test is reactive. In view of the clinical examination and history of exposure, the physician confirms the diagnosis of syphilis. The nursing care of the patient should include the following:

1. Thorough hand-washing after patient care

2. Isolation for 7 days

3. Autoclaving linens

4. Boiling dishes

101 John was exposed to syphilis through sexual contact with an infected person. It is important to locate the source of his infection and also persons whom he may have infected. Therefore all sexual contacts from how long ago should be located and examined?

1. Past 3 months

2. Past 6 months

3. Past 30 days

4. Past 3 weeks

Situation: Ten-year-old Jim Smith is admitted to the emergency room after a car accident. However, normal measures to stop his bleeding are unsuccessful, and, on further study, Jim is found to have a mild case of classic hemophilia. Mr. and Mrs. Smith are very concerned about this and wonder how it happened. Questions 102 through 104 refer to this situation.

102 The nurse should explain that:

1. Hemophilia is a sex-linked recessive disorder in which the mother is usually the carrier of the illness but is not affected by it

2. Hemophilia is a sex-linked dominant disorder in which the woman carries the trait

3. Hemophilia follows regular laws of mendelian inherited disorders such as sickle cell anemia

4. This disorder can be carried by either male or female but occurs in the sex opposite that of the carrier

103 Jim's parents are very worried about their other children, 2 girls and another boy, and want to know what the chances are concerning their having the disorder or being a carrier. An appropriate answer to this question would be that:

1. All the girls will be normal and the other son a carrier

2. Each son has a 50% chance of being a victim and each daughter a 50% chance of being a carrier

3. All the girls will be carriers and one half the boys will be victims

4. Each son has a 50% chance of being either a victim or carrier, and the girls will all be carriers

104 The most common site of internal bleeding in hemophiliacs is:

1. Cerebrum

2. Ends of the long bones

3. Intestines

4. Joints

Situation: Cara has rheumatic fever. Drug therapy includes the administration of sodium salicylate, 10 gr, 4 times daily. Questions 105 through 107 refer to this situation.

105 During the salicylate therapy the nurse should observe Cara for which of the following groups of symptoms?

1. Nausea, dizziness, edema, headache

2. Gastric distress, nausea, vomiting, tinnitus

3. Constipation, deafness, nausea, headache

4. Diarrhea, gastric distress, edema of the face

106 Sodium salicylate is classified as an:

1. Antibiotic and antipyretic

2. Analgesic and antipyretic

3. Analgesic and sedative

4. Antipyretic and hypnotic

107 In working with parents in the preventive aspects of rheumatic fever, the nurse would stress:

1. Prevention of exposure to childhood diseases

2. Early treatment of upper respiratory tract infections

3. Isolating the child with rheumatic fever from siblings

4. Early immunization

Situation: *Nellie, a newborn, is admitted to the pediatric unit with the diagnosis of choanal atresia. Questions 108 through 110 refer to this situation.*

108 Choanal atresia is an anomaly located in the:
1. Nasopharynx
2. Intestinal tract
3. Pharynx and larynx
4. Anal area

109 While feeding Nellie, the nurse notices that she:
1. Lacks a swallow reflex
2. Chokes on her feeding
3. Does not appear to be hungry
4. Takes only about half of her feeding

110 When reviewing the data recorded on Nellie's chart, what information might indicate to the nurse that the baby requires special attention?
1. Birth weight of 3500 g
2. 20 ml of milky-colored fluid was aspirated from her stomach
3. The infant has a positive Babinski reflex
4. The Apgar score at birth was 3

Situation: *Three-year-old Roger is admitted to the pediatric unit with a diagnosis of nephrosis. Questions 111 through 114 refer to this situation.*

111 The most important nursing intervention for Roger is:
1. Encouraging fluids
2. Regulating his diet
3. Maintaining bed rest
4. Preventing infection

112 As Roger gets older and has repeated attacks of nephrosis, it is most important for the nurse to help him develop:
1. Fine muscle coordination
2. Acceptance of possible sterility
3. A positive body image
4. The ability to test his own urine

113 During his nap, Roger wets the bed. The best approach by the nurse would be to:
1. Change his clothes and make no issue of it
2. Explain that big boys should try to call the nurse
3. Tell him to help you remake the bed
4. Change his bed, putting a rubber sheet on it

114 When providing nursing care to a preschool-age child, the nurse should remember that his greatest fear is of:
1. Isolation
2. Intrusive procedures
3. Death
4. Pain

Situation: *Mary is hospitalized with a severe asthma attack. Questions 115 through 118 refer to this situation.*

115 The acid-base imbalance complicating this condition is:
1. Respiratory alkalosis caused by the accelerated respirations and loss of carbon dioxide

2. Respiratory acidosis caused by the impaired respirations and increased formation of carbonic acid
3. Metabolic acidosis caused by excessive production of acid metabolites
4. Metabolic acidosis caused by the kidney's inability to help compensate for the increased carbonic acid formed

116 Mary is in a Croupette and is given prednisone, 15 mg, p.o. b.i.d. The nurse should:
1. Check her eosinophil count daily
2. Prevent exposure to infection
3. Keep Mary n.p.o.
4. Have her rest as much as possible

117 Mary has IV therapy of 5% dextrose in ½ normal saline started. Aminophylline is to run in via piggyback for 20 minutes every 8 hours. Before administering the drug, the nurse should:
1. Check her temperature
2. Monitor blood pressure
3. Administer oxygen
4. Take her pulse

118 When Mary's parents take her home, they should be taught to increase her fluid intake and to have her:
1. Avoid exertion and exposure to cold
2. Stay in the house for at least 2 weeks
3. Increase her calorie intake
4. Avoid foods high in fat

Situation: *Two-month-old Paul Carr is brought to the clinic, and a diagnosis of colic is made. Mrs. Carr appears exhausted. Questions 119 through 122 refer to this situation.*

119 The nurse realizes that Mrs. Carr needs help coping with Paul and suggests that she:
1. Provide Paul with warm sweetened tea when he begins to cry
2. Arrange for some time away from Paul each day to rest
3. Sit comfortably in a quiet darkened room to hold Paul when he cries
4. Give Paul a warm bath to calm him down

120 The behavior of an infant with colic is usually suggestive of:
1. Inadequate peristalsis resulting in constipation
2. A protective mechanism designed to rid the GI tract of foreign proteins
3. Paroxysmal abdominal pain due to excessive gas
4. An allergic response to certain proteins in milk

121 Paul returns with his mother for his 6-month check-up. When teaching Mrs. Carr how to prevent accidents when caring for her 6-month-old, the nurse should emphasize that this age child can usually:
1. Sit up
2. Stand while holding onto furniture
3. Roll over
4. Crawl lengthy distances

122 When Mrs. Carr returns with Paul for his 9-month check-up, she expresses concern about his development. The baby no longer has the same strong grasp that he had shortly after birth, nor does he have a similar response to startle that he had at an early age. The nurse should discuss with Mrs. Carr that:
1. Neurologic examination is desirable
2. Failure of these responses may be related to mental retardation
3. These responses are usually replaced by voluntary activity at 5 to 6 months of age
4. The infant needs additional sensory stimulation to aid in the return of these responses

Situation: Loren, age 14, is admitted to the hospital and is scheduled to undergo orthopedic surgery the following day. Questions 123 through 126 refer to this situation.

123 At the conclusion of visiting hours, Loren's mother hands the nurse a bottle of capsules and says, "These are for Loren's allergy. Will you be sure she takes one about 9 o'clock?" The nurse might best respond with which of the following statements?
1. "One capsule at 9 P.M.? Of course, I will give it to her.
2. "Did you ask the doctor if she should have this to-night?"
3. "I am certain the doctor knows about Loren's allergy."
4. "We will ask Loren's doctor to write an order so we can give this medication to her."

124 In relation to obtaining an informed consent, the nurse should remember that the adolescent:
1. Does not have the legal capacity to give consent
2. Is not able to make an acceptable or intelligent choice
3. Is able to give voluntary consent when parents are not available
4. Will most likely be unable to choose between alternatives when asked to consent

125 Postoperatively, Loren complains of pain and is given 15 mg of codeine sulfate as ordered q 3 to 4 h prn. Two hours after she is given this medication she complains of severe pain. The nurse should:
1. Administer another dose of codeine within 30 minutes, since it is a relatively safe drug
2. Tell Loren she cannot have any additional medication for 1 more hour
3. Report that Loren has an apparent idiosyncrasy to codeine
4. Request that the physician evaluate Loren's need for additional medication

126 About 8 hours later, Loren complains of itching. A drug that can be ordered to relieve this symptom is:
1. Chlorpheniramine (Chlor-Trimeton)
2. Nitrofurazone (Furacin)
3. Salicylanilide (Salinidol)
4. Hyaluronidase (Alidase)

Situation: Two-year-old Sue McMichael, fractures her femur and is placed in Bryant's traction. Questions 127 through 130 refer to this situation.

127 While caring for Sue, the nurse should know that Bryant's traction:
1. Helps by allowing the child to turn side to side
2. Is skin traction to the affected leg
3. Is skin traction and elevates the hips slightly from the bed
4. Is attached to a pin placed in the affected femur

128 Sue becomes constipated and the physician orders an isotonic enema. The nurse is aware that the maximum amount of fluid to be given a small child without a physician's specific order is:
1. 100 to 150 ml
2. 150 to 250 ml
3. 250 to 350 ml
4. 350 to 500 ml

129 One evening Sue screams and cries frequently, particularly after her mother's visit. Her loud crying disturbs others on the unit, and the nurse finds it impossible to quiet her. She is in a 4-bed room, adjacent to which is a storeroom large enough to hold a crib. When her crying is particularly loud and prolonged, the nurse puts her crib in the storeroom and closes the door. She is left there until her crying ceases, a matter of 30 or 45 minutes. Legally:
1. The other children had to be considered, so Sue needed to be removed
2. Sue needed to have limits set to control her crying
3. Sue had a right to remain in the room with the other children
4. Keeping the child by herself for more than 30 minutes was too long

130 Several days later, Mrs. McMichael asks the nurse what to do when Sue has her temper tantrums. The nurse suggests that Mrs. McMichael allow Sue another way of expressing her anger, such as the use of:
1. A ball and bat
2. A pounding board
3. Clay or Play-Doh
4. A punching bag

Situation: Karina, 7 years old, is to have an exploratory laparotomy and possible appendectomy. Questions 131 through 134 refer to this situation.

131 The physician orders atropine, gr 1/300, IM preoperatively. The vial reads "atropine 0.4 mg/ml." How much should the nurse administer?
1. 0.5 ml
2. 1 ml
3. 0.25 ml
4. 0.75 ml

132 Postoperatively, to help relieve Karina's anxiety, the nurse should:

1. Tell her a story about a girl with similar surgery
2. Allow her time to talk about her feelings
3. Provide her with bandage, tape, scissors, and a doll
4. Ask her mother to room with her for a few days

133 Karina begins thumb-sucking after her surgery. Although this was not Karina's behavior preoperatively, the nurse should:
1. Report this behavior to the physician
2. Distract her by playing checkers
3. Accept the thumb-sucking
4. Tell her thumb-sucking causes buck teeth

134 Karina develops a urinary tract infection. The physician orders a sulfonamide preparation. A major nursing responsibility when administering this drug is to:
1. Weigh the child daily
2. Administer the drug at the prescribed times
3. Give milk with the medication
4. Monitor the temperature frequently

Situation: Mr. Gioni, the father of 3 young children, is diagnosed as having tuberculosis. Questions 135 through 137 refer to this situation.

135 Members of the family who have a positive reaction to the tuberculin test are candidates for treatment with:
1. Old tuberculin
2. BCG vaccine
3. INH and PAS
4. Purified protein derivative of tuberculin

136 If a person has been exposed to tuberculosis but shows no signs or symptoms except a positive tuberculin test, prophylactic drug therapy is usually continued after the last exposure for a period of:
1. 3 weeks
2. 6 months
3. 1 year
4. 5 years

137 Children in the family who have been exposed to but show no evidence of tuberculosis:
1. Can be considered to be immune
2. Should be treated with INH and PAS
3. Are usually given massive doses of penicillin
4. Are given x-ray examinations every 6 months and observed for evidence of tuberculosis

Situation: The nurse in the outpatient pediatric clinic is talking to a group of parents whose children have been diagnosed as having attention deficit disorder. Questions 138 and 139 refer to this situation.

138 One of the major behavioral characteristics of children with attention deficit disorders is their:
1. Inability to use abstract thought
2. Overreaction to stimuli
3. Continued use of rituals
4. Retarded speech development

139 In helping the parents to cope with their children's behavior, the nurse suggests that one of their best approaches would be to:
1. Write a list of expectations to avoid confusion
2. Be consistent and firm about established rules
3. Avoid asking specific questions
4. Allow the child to set up his own routines

140 Play during infancy is:
1. Initiated by the child
2. A way of teaching how to share
3. More important than in later years
4. Mostly used for physical development

141 The primary task to be accomplished between 12 and 15 months of age is to learn to:
1. Use a spoon
2. Give up the bottle
3. Walk
4. Say simple words

142 Preschool children role play. This is an important part of socialization, since it:
1. Encourages expression
2. Helps children think about careers
3. Teaches children about stereotypes
4. Provides guidelines for adult behavior

143 Learning processes associated with a particular stage of development often are referred to as "developmental task." What is characteristic about these tasks?
1. There is no uniform time for learning a task
2. Tasks are learned at the same age in children
3. Tasks occur with predictable rhythm
4. Most development tasks are learned by school age

144 Parents can predispose their children to problems with nutrition by using food in early childhood as a means of:
1. Socializing
2. Reward and punishment
3. Aculturization
4. Teaching dicipline

145 The major influence on eating habits of the *early* school-age child is the:
1. Example of parents at mealtime
2. Food preferences of the peer group
3. Availability of food selections
4. Smell and appearance of food

146 Selection of drugs of choice for the treatment of pneumonia depends primarily on:
1. Selectivity of the organism
2. Tolerance of the patient
3. Preference of the physician
4. Sensitivity of the organism

147 Mrs. Legere and her son Johnny are seen at the clinic. They both have severe upper respiratory tract infections, and the physician plans to prescribe tetracycline (Achromycin). The nurse reminds him that Johnny is 6 years old and that Mrs. Legere is in her eighteenth week of

pregnancy. The data are important because the drug may cause:
1. Persistent vomiting when given to small children and pregnant women
2. Tooth enamel defects in children under 8 years of age and in the maturing fetus
3. Lower red blood cell production at times in their development when anemia is a common problem
4. Changes in the bone structure of young children and pregnant women

148 A viral infection characterized by red blotchy rash and Koplik's spots in the mouth is:
1. Rubeola
2. Rubella
3. Chickpox
4. Mumps

149 Under certain circumstances the virus that causes chickenpox can also cause:
1. Athlete's foot
2. Infectious hepatitis
3. Herpes zoster
4. German measles

150 Using live virus vaccines against measles is contraindicated in children receiving corticosteroids or antineoplastic or irradiation therapy because these children may:
1. Have had the disease or have been immunized previously
2. Be unlikely to need this protection during their shortened life span
3. Be allergic to rabbit serum, which is used as a base for these vaccines
4. Be susceptible to infection because of their depressed immune response

151 An injection consisting of bacterial cells that have been modified is:
1. A vaccine
2. An antitoxin
3. A toxoid
4. A toxin

152 A child comes to the hospital after exposure to diphtheria and is given antitoxin. This is what type of immunity?
1. Active natural immunity
2. Active artificial immunity
3. Passive natural immunity
4. Passive artifical immunity

153 Immunity by antibody formation during the course of a disease is:
1. Active natural immunity
2. Active artificial immunity
3. Passive natural immunity
4. Passive artificial immunity

154 A viral disease that begins with respiratory inflammation and skin rash and may result in grave complications is:
1. Rubeola
2. Rubella
3. Yellow fever
4. Chickenpox

155 Mary has received her primary immunizations, so her mother asks the nurse which ones she should receive prior to starting kindergarten. The nurse suggests the following booster doses:
1. DTP, TOPV
2. Measles, DTP
3. TOPV, rubella
4. DTP, tuberculin test

156 Occasionally infants are born without an immune system. They can live normally with no apparent problems during their first months after birth because:
1. Limited antibodies are produced by the fetal thymus during the eighth and ninth months of gestation
2. Antibodies are passively received from the mother through the placenta and milk
3. Limited antibodies are produced by the infant's colonic bacteria
4. Exposure to pathogens during this time can be limited

157 James, a 2-year-old child, is admitted to the hospital with a diagnosis of pneumonia. He is given antibiotics, forced fluids, and oxygen. James' temperature continued to rise until it reached 39.4° C (103° F). The nurse calls the physician at the mother's request, but the physician sees no cause for alarm or change in treatment, even though James has a history of convulsions during previous periods of high fever. Although the nurse is concerned, she takes no further action. Later James has a convulsion that results in neurologic impairment of the left arm and leg. Legally:
1. The nurse's actions did not derive from observations, patient's history, or scientific fact
2. The physician's decision takes precedence over the nurse's concern
3. High temperatures are common in children, and this situation presented little cause for undue concern
4. The physician is totally responsible for the patient's health history and treatment regimen

158 Four-year-old Bobby has a seizure disorder and has been taking phenytoin (Dilantin) for 3 years. An important nursing measure for Bobby would be to:
1. Offer the urinal frequently
2. Administer scrupulous oral hygiene
3. Check for pupillary reaction
4. Observe for flushing of the face

159 When teaching parents at the school about communicable diseases, the nurse reminds them that these diseases are serious, and the encephalitis can be a complication of:
1. Chickenpox
2. Pertussis
3. Poliomyelitis
4. Scarlet fever

160 A viral disease caused by one of the smallest human viruses that infect the motor cells of the anterior horn of the spinal cord is:
1. Rubeola
2. Rubella
3. Poliomyelitis
4. Chickenpox

161 A *Streptococcus* infection characterized by swollen joints, fever, and the possibility of endocarditis and death is:
1. Whooping cough
2. Measles
3. Tetanus
4. Rheumatic fever

162 A skin infection that can be a sequela of rheumatic fever or glomerulonephritis is:
1. Herpes simplex
2. Scabies
3. Intertrigo
4. Impetigo

163 A small toddler is admitted to the hospital because of sudden hoarseness and an insistence on continuous and somewhat unintelligible speech. In talking with the mother, the nurse will be particularly concerned about:
1. Acute respiratory tract infection
2. Undetected laryngeal abnormality
3. Respiratory tract obstruction due to a foreign body
4. Retropharyngeal abscess

164 An infection caused by the yeast *Candida albicans* often occurring in infants and debilitated individuals is:
1. Typhoid fever
2. Thrush
3. Malta fever
4. Dysentery

165 A mother talks to the nurse about her sick infant and she is disturbed because she did not realize the baby was ill. Which of the following is a major indication of illness in an infant?
1. Longer periods of sleep
2. Grunting and rapid respirations
3. Profuse perspiration
4. Desire for increased fluids during the feedings

166 Among the last signs of heart failure in the infant and child is:
1. Rapid respiratory rate in the supine position
2. Orthopnea
3. Tachypnea
4. Peripheral edema

167 A newborn of a few hours appears to be less cyanotic when he cries. The nurse should observe for:
1. Twitching of the body resulting from neural damage
2. Unequality of chest expansion associated with atelectasis
3. Alterations in heart rate associated with an atrioventricular septal defect
4. Sternal retractions of respiratory distress syndrome

168 A mother brings her week-old newborn to the clinic because he continually regurgitates. Chalasia is suspected. The nurse instructs the mother to:
1. Keep the infant prone following feedings
2. Not permit the infant to cry for prolonged periods
3. Keep the infant in a semisitting position, particularly after feedings
4. Administer a minimum of 8 oz of formula at each feeding

169 The best legal definition of assault is:
1. The application of force to another person without lawful justification
2. Threats to do bodily harm to the person of another person
3. A legal wrong committed by one person against the property of another
4. A legal wrong committed against the public and punishable by law through the state and courts

170 In legal terminology, the term battery means:
1. Doing something that a reasonable person with the same education or preparation would not do
2. A legal wrong committed by one person against the property of another
3. The application of force to the person of another person without lawful justification
4. Maligning the character of an individual while threatening to do bodily harm

171 Dietary treatment of PKU consists of a:
1. Low-phenylalanine diet
2. Phenylalanine-free diet
3. Dietary supplement for phenylalanine
4. Protein-free diet

172 Alan, age 3 months, has been diagnosed as having cretinism. If care is not instituted until after early infancy, he will probably:
1. Have myxedema
2. Be somewhat mentally retarded
3. Have abnormal deep tendon reflexes
4. Have thyrotoxicosis

173 Three-month-old Lisa is diagnosed as having cretinism. She is to receive thyroxine sodium, 0.35 mg, q.d. p.o. The medication is available in elixir form, 0.25 mg/ml. How many minims would the nurse give?
1. 16 minims
2. 21 minims
3. 18 minims
4. 20 minims

174 Three-year-old Karen Allen may have celiac disease. One symptom common in children with celiac disease is stools that are:
1. Large, frothy, dark green
2. Small, pale, mucoid
3. Large, pale, foul smelling
4. Moderate, green, foul smelling

175 Mrs. Joyce asks the nurse how to tell the difference between measles (rubeola) and German measles (rubella). The nurse tells Mrs. Joyce that with rubeola the child has:
1. A high fever and Koplik's spots
2. Symptoms similar to a cold, followed by a rash
3. Nausea, vomiting and abdominal cramps
4. A rash on the trunk with pruritus

176 The physician orders a tap water enema for 6-month-old Bart. The nurse considers that giving Bart an enema could:
1. Cause a fluid and electrolyte imbalance

2. Increase his fear of intrusive procedures
3. Result in shock from a sudden drop in temperature
4. Result in loss of necessary nutrients

177 Chickenpox can sometimes be fatal to children who are receiving which of the following medications?
1. Antibiotics
2. Steroids
3. Anticonvulsants
4. Insulin

178 The nurse explains to the parent group that the most important complication of mumps in postpubertal males is:
1. Decrease in libido
2. Hypopituitarism
3. Sterility
4. A decrease in androgens

179 Paula, a 3-year-old with eczema of the face and arms, has not heeded her nurse's warnings to "stop scratching—or else!" The nurse finds Paula scratching so intensely that her arms are bleeding. With great flurry, the nurse ties Paul's arms to the crib sides saying, "I'm going to teach you one way or another." In this situation, the nurse:
1. Had to protect Paula's skin and acted as any reasonably prudent nurse would do
2. Tried to explain to Paula and rightly expected her to understand and cooperate
3. Has used actions that can be interpreted as assault and battery
4. Has merely done her job with considerable accountability

180 Nancy, age 8, is receiving tetracycline (Achromycin). Her fever is down and secretions have lessened; but she is eating poorly, is withdrawn, lethargic, and irritable, and sobs readily. The nurse should promptly discuss the problem with the physician because:
1. She needs a higher food intake to fight the infection
2. Anemia is a frequent occurrence after infection and treatment with antibiotics
3. Concurrent bladder infection may be present as an extension of her gram-negative infection
4. Generalized physical symptoms and behavior problems may procede drug-induced liver damage

181 Fourteen-year-old Evelyn is severely hurt while on a skateboard and develops muscle contractures in all her limbs. She refuses to move, so the nurse should encourage her by:
1. Explaining that some pain is inevitable
2. Allowing friends to vist every day
3. Permitting her to make decisions regarding her care
4. Setting strict limits to increase her security

182 Nine-year-old Harold has a fractured femur and a full leg cast has just been applied. Which of the following observations made by the nurse should be reported to the physician immediately?
1. Pedal pulse of 90
2. Cast still damp and warm after 4 hours

3. Inability to move the toes
4. Increased urinary output

183 Two-year-old Jimmy swallowed kerosene from a soda bottle stored in the garage. Immediate treatment for ingestion of petroleum distillates is to have the child swallow:
1. Milk of magnesia
2. Strong tea
3. Weak salt solution
4. Mineral oil

184 A toddler has swallowed a liquid drain cleaner containing lye. The immediate intervention is to administer:
1. Syrup of ipecac
2. Two ounces of milk
3. Dilute vinegar solution
4. Sodium bicarbonate and water

185 Susan is found by her mother playing with an open bottle of diuretic tablets. The physician tells Susan's mother to give syrup of ipecac to Susan. The effect of the drug will be enhanced by:
1. Resting until vomiting occurs
2. Drinking 2 to 3 glasses of water
3. Actively playing until vomiting occurs
4. Stimulating the gag reflex

186 The primary reason for using prednisone in the treatment of acute leukemia in children is that it is able to:
1. Suppress mitosis in lymphocytes
2. Reduce irradiation edema
3. Decrease inflammation
4. Increase appetite and sense of well-being

187 A combination of drugs, which includes vincristine (Oncovin) and prednisone, is prescribed for a child with leukemia. The toxic symptom(s) that the nurse should expect are:
1. Neurologic
2. Irreversible alopecia
3. Anemia and fever
4. Gastrointestinal

188 Which of the following responses is unusual in infants subjected to prolonged hospitalization?
1. Lack or slowness of weight gain
2. Looking at ceiling lights rather than at persons caring for them
3. Limited emotional response to stimuli
4. Excessive crying and clinging when approached

189 A characteristic of infants and young children who have experienced maternal deprivation is:
1. Extreme activity
2. Proneness to illness
3. Responsiveness to stimuli
4. Tendency toward overeating

190 Naomi, 9 years old, is about to have surgery. The physician orders meperidine (Demerol), 20 mg, IM preoperatively. The container reads "50 mg/ml." How many minims would the nurse administer?
1. 4 minims
2. 6 minims

3. 8 minims
4. 10 minims

191 An infant scheduled for surgery is diagnosed as having a diaphragmatic hernia. A measure that a nurse would expect to be employed at this time includes:
1. Positive pressure oxygen by mask
2. Positive pressure oxygen by intratracheal tube
3. Increased oxygen concentration by any method
4. Humidity of 40%

192 It is expected that, after some surgical intervention for atelectasis, lung expansion will recur within:
1. An hour
2. 48 to 72 hours
3. 4 hours
4. 12 to 48 hours

193 Dina, 18 months old, is to receive 5% dextrose and Ringer's lactate, 1000 ml IV, in 24 hours. The drop factor of the minidropper is 60 drops/ml. The nurse should regulate the IV to run at:
1. 34 drops per minute
2. 38 drops per minute
3. 42 drops per minute
4. 21 drops per minute

194 When picked up by either the mother or the nurse, an 8-month-old infant screams. The scream seems to be that of pain. At his clinic visit the nurse will note and talk particularly to the mother about:
1. The infant's food and specific vitamins given to him, including vitamins C and D
2. Accidents and injuries and the importance of their prevention
3. Any other behavior of the infant that may have been noticed by the mother
4. Limiting the play time and activities that this infant has with other children in the family

195 Eleven-year-old Harry has gained weight. His mother is concerned that Harry, who loves sports, may become obese. The nurse:
1. Urges a decreased caloric intake
2. Explains this is normal for a preadolescent
3. Advises an increase in activity
4. Discusses the relationship of genetics and weight gain

196 Hepatitis occurs in sporadic cases and isolated outbreaks. Exposure to virus B homologous serum hepatitis (SH) may be expected to occur in hospitals because of which of the following?
1. Increased use of blood and blood products
2. Careless handling of excreta
3. Asymptomatic carriers
4. Increasing use of ventilating systems

197 Elouise, 8 months old, has a gastrostomy tube and is given 240 ml of tube feeding q. 4 h. One of the primary nursing responsibilities at the time of the feeding is to:
1. Elevate the tube 30 cm (12 inches) above the mattress
2. Give 10 ml of normal saline before and after feeding
3. Position on the right side after feeding
4. Open the tube 1 hour before feeding

198 Prior to administering a gastrostomy tube feeding to an infant, the nurse should:
1. Slowly instill 5 ml of water
2. Aspirate the tube
3. Provide the baby with a pacifier
4. Place in a semi-Fowler position

199 Sal has been admitted to the hospital for surgery to correct his congenital megacolon. Enemas are ordered preoperatively to cleanse the bowel. The nurse should use:
1. Soapsuds
2. Hypertonic phosphate
3. Isotonic saline
4. Tap water

200 If monocular strabismus is not corrected early enough:
1. Vision in both eyes will be diminished
2. Peripheral vision will disappear
3. Dyslexia will develop
4. Amblyopia develops in the weak eye

Pediatric Nursing Answers and Rationales

1. (2) Common developmental norms of the toddler, who is struggling for independence, are inability to share easily, egotism, egocentrism, and possessiveness. (b)
   (1) This task is too advanced for toddlers and more accurate for preschoolers.
   (3) This is true of 4-year-olds.
   (4) One characteristic of toddlers is their short attention spans; 15 minutes is too much to expect.

2. (1) Four-year-olds boast, exaggerate, and are impatient, noisy, and selfish. (c)
   (2) The tendency toward tantrums and negativism should have waned by the age of 4
   (3) Four-year-olds engage in more advanced cooperative play.
   (4) This is highly unusual for 4-year-olds as they are striving toward more initiative and less dependence.

3. (4) The child 9 to 12 months of age can stand alone with support. By 15 months his strength and balance improve, and he can stand and walk alone. (b)
   (1) This is not usually true until the child is 2 years old.
   (2) A 10-month-old is capable of this task.
   (3) Infants are very capable of this.

4. (2) Six-year-olds are aware of their hands as tools and enjoy building simple structures. (b)
   (1) This is more useful for an older, school age child, with a longer attention span and a better ability to follow instructions.
   (3) This is more useful for an older, school age child, with a longer attention span and a better ability to follow instructions.
   (4) This is more appropriate for preschoolers.

5. (2) Helps and encourages parents to put their fears and feelings into words. Once these sentiments are expressed, they can at least be examined and dealt with. (b)
   (1) This would not assist the parents in coping with the problem. Neither would it demonstrate the supportive and emphatic roles of the nurse.
   (3) This response lacks insight. Parents will worry about their infant anyway.
   (4) This may or may not be helpful.

6. (1) These children frequently have difficulty in handling secretions as well as breathing after surgery. Nursing measures such as using the partial side-lying position or gently aspirating secretions from the mouth or nasopharynx may be necessary to prevent aspiration and respiratory complications. (a)
   (2) This is not necessary.
   (3) Fluids are usually administered carefully by mouth.
   (4) Although this is important, maintaining a patent airway is essential.

7. (2) Crying should be prevented, since it places tension on the suture line. Frequently an appliance called a Logan bow is taped to the cheeks to relax the operative site, which helps prevent trauma. (b)
   (1) May also be positioned on the side and on the back with surveillance.
   (3) The feeding method of choice is by a rubber-tipped syringe or medicine dropper.
   (4) This is not necessary or desirable.

8. (4) The 2-year-old is still attached to and dependent on the parents. Fear of separation is a great stress. (b)
   (1) Most likely these will not be remembered accurately.
   (2) This is neither possible nor desirable.
   (3) This is not possible in a health care setting.

9. (1) A priority during the immediate postoperative period is protecting the operative site. (a)
   (2) Two-year-olds can brush their teeth.
   (3) Normal 2-year-olds have about 16 teeth; although tooth development may not be normal in these children, they usually have them.
   (4) A toothbrush should be a familiar sight to a 2-year-old and, therefore, not frightening.

10. (4) David is anemic. A diet of milk only is not sufficient to meet iron needs. Raisins and meat are high in iron, and finger foods are appropriate for toddlers. (b)
    (1) This is not appropriate for a 1-year-old, nor is it necessary or desirable.
    (2) Although medical care and monitoring will be required, the metabolic clinic is not the appropriate referral.
    (3) Weaning from the bottle is not the issue; supplementary iron intake is.

11. (1) Fetal iron reserves are depleted by the fourth to fifth month in the full-term infant and considerably earlier in the premature infant. When exogenous sources of iron are not supplied after depletion of fetal iron stores, iron-deficiency anemia results. (a)
    (2) Although this is true, it is not an important reason for starting solid foods earlier with this child.
    (3) The problem is not with bone marrow production of cells but with the production of hemoglobin.
    (4) Weight control by itself is not the major reason for starting solid foods; the overingestion of milk often seen in anemia frequently causes the infant to be overweight.

12. (1) Milk is a very poor source of iron. If fed in large amounts to the exclusion of solid foods after 4 to 6 months of age, iron-deficiency anemia results. (b)
    (2) Maternal iron stores are usually adequate for the infant's first 4 to 5 months.
    (3) This is not a major cause of anemia.
    (4) Lack of absorption and early introduction of solid foods are not commonly found as problems producing anemia in infants.

13. (4) Folic acid acts as a necessary coenzyme in the for-

mation of heme, the iron-containing protein in hemoglobin. (c)

(1) The production of red blood cells does not involve carbohydrates.

(2) This is a coenzyme in carbohydrate metabolism.

(3) Calcium is not involved in the production of red blood cells.

14. (3) Egg yolk is a rich source of iron and is easily digested by infants. (a)

(1) This does not contain iron.

(2) This contains iron in smaller amounts and is not so easily digestible as egg yolks.

(4) Milk is a poor source of iron.

15. (3) The child should be taken to the dentist between 2 and 3 years of age, when all the deciduous teeth (20) have erupted. (a)

(1) This is too soon.

(2) This is too late.

(4) This is too late.

16. (3) Proteins are essential for the synthesis of the blood proteins, albumin, fibrinogen, and hemoglobin. Ascorbic acid influences the removal of iron from ferritin (making more iron available for production of heme) and influences the conversion of folic acid to folinic acid. (b)

(1) These are not involved in building red blood cells.

(2) These are not involved in building red blood cells.

(4) These are not involved in building red blood cells.

17. (4) The adult pinworm lives in the rectum or colon and emerges onto the perirectal skin during hours of sleep, depositing her eggs during this time. (b)

(1) Pinworms attach to the bowel wall and do not emerge from the rectum at this time.

(2) Pinworms attach to the bowel wall and do not emerge from the rectum at this time.

(3) Pinworms attach to the bowel wall and do not emerge from the rectum at this time.

18. (4) The worm attaches itself to the bowel wall in the cecum and appendix and can damage the mucosa, causing appendicitis. (c)

(1) The pinworm does not migrate to the respiratory system.

(2) Although pinworms (and their ova) are ingested by mouth, they do not attach there; inflammation of the mouth is not a complication of pinworm.

(3) The pinworm does not migrate to the liver.

19. (1) Forty pounds = 18 kg. Therefore 5 mg per kilogram × 18 kg = 90 mg. (b)

(2) This is an inadequate dose.

(3) This is an inadequate dose.

(4) This is an overdose.

20. (3) Pyrvinium pamoate (Povan), a cyanine dye, is a deep red, relatively insoluble crystalline powder that stains the stool, vomitus, and most materials. (b)

(1) Incorrect answer; does not cause a brown color.

(2) Incorrect answer; does not cause a green color.

(4) Incorrect answer; does not cause a blue color.

21. (2) Pyrvinium pamoate (Povan), a cyanine dye, is a deep red relatively insoluble crystalline powder that stains the stool, vomitus, and most materials. In this instance, red-stained excreta would not be significant. (b)

(1) These complications do not occur with pinworms.

(3) This does not occur.

(4) Intestinal bleeding does not occur as a result of Povan administration.

22. (4) School-age children lose their primary teeth, which could be aspirated during surgery. The anesthesiologist must take special precautions to maintain patient safety. (a)

(1) This is important but not essential and not always possible.

(2) This is a comforting gesture but is not essential.

(3) There is no reason to obtain an ASO titer on Johnny.

23. (4) The seeping of blood from the operative site increases secretions, which the child adapts to by swallowing frequently. (b)

(1) Snoring can be expected in a child who is postoperative from a tonsillectomy.

(2) This may be a later sign of hemorrhage. Frequent swallowing would be an initial sign.

(3) The child has been n.p.o. for an extended time and is not able to ingest fluids easily because of his sore throat; as a result he will probably be thirsty.

24. (2) Acetaminophen relieves pain and does not cause bleeding tendencies, as does aspirin. The correct dose for this age is 300 mg. (c)

(1) Aspirin increases the clotting time and should be avoided.

(3) Phenobarbitol will not relieve the pain; it will only sedate the patient.

(4) Demerol may be given, although a narcotic is not usually necessary for children after tonsillectomy; however, 50 mg would be the normal dose for an adult.

25. (2) A meningomyelocele sac is thinly covered and can be partially open, allowing a portal of entry for organisms directly to the central nervous system. The sac should be protected. (b)

(1) A meningomyelocele will influence the patient's ability to control these functions, but control is not developed until the toddler and preschool years.

(3) Although this is always an important nursing measure, care of the sac is even more important.

(4) Although observation of paralysis is an important nursing measure, care of the meningomyelocele sac is of primary importance.

26. (3) The surgical closure of the sac eliminates the route by which the spinal fluid drains. Skull bones are soft and will expand as fluid increases, causing hydrocephalus. (b)

(1) There is no reason to decrease environmental stimuli for infants with hydrocephalus unless they also have seizures.

458 MOSBY'S COMPREHENSIVE REVIEW OF NURSING

(2) Most infants with meningomyelocele are partially or completely paralyzed in the lower extremities; careful range of motion exercises are one of the important parts of nursing care for these infants.

(4) This is not expected since damage to the meninges of the brain is not a factor in the surgical treatment of meningomyelocele.

27. (2) Sucking meets oral needs, which are primary during infancy. (c)

(1) Two-day-old infants are not yet developmentally capable of enjoying a soft, cuddly toy.

(3) This is not a developmental need.

(4) An infant of a few days is probably too young to focus well on a mobile; in addition, he will be placed in a prone or side-lying position postoperatively and thus would not be able to focus on the mobile.

28. (3) Fluids prevent dehydration. Under conditions of decreased oxygen, dehydration promotes the sickling of erythrocytes. (c)

(1) This is not necessary.

(2) Rigorous exercise will cause sickling.

(4) This is not necessary or helpful in sickle cell anemia.

29. (1) High levels of fetal hemoglobin prevent sickling of red blood cells. The newborn has from 44% to 89% fetal hemoglobin, but this rapidly decreases during the first year. (c)

(2) These will not affect the diagnosis of sickle cell anemia.

(3) Respiratory difficulties are not associated with sickle cell anemia except as a consequence of hypoxia during a crisis.

(4) The diagnosis of sickle cell anemia is made on the basis of hematologic tests; general health and growth are not affected initially.

30. (2) Under conditions of decreased oxygen the relatively insoluble hemoglobin S changes its molecular structure to form long slender crystals and eventually the crescent, or sickled, shape. (b)

(1) Hemodilution helps prevent sickling and is accomplished by encouraging fluids.

(3) The platelets are not involved in sickle cell anemia.

(4) This will not influence the sickling process.

31. (2) Sickling is related to the concentration of hemoglobin within the cell. Since hypertonicity of the blood plasma increases the intracellular concentration of hemoglobin, dehydration promotes sickling. (c)

(1) This will not prevent thrombus formation.

(3) Usually the child can dictate his activity level; although bed rest may be necessary during a crisis, complete bed rest is rarely necessary.

(4) Anticoagulants do not help prevent the trombus formation in sickle cell anemia.

32. (2) Both cause poor resistance. With sickling it is due to low oxygen levels, and with celiac disease it is due to malnourishment and immunologic defects. (b)

(1) Activity does not need to be limited in celiac disease; strenuous activity should be limited in sickle cell anemia.

(3) This specific diet is not particularly helpful for either sickle cell anemia or celiac disease.

(4) Vital signs will not be abnormal except during a crisis in either condition.

33. (2) The recommended immunization schedule for infants is administration of the combined diphtheria, pertussis, and tetanus vaccine and the trivalent oral polio virus at ages 2, 4, and 6 months. (b)

(1) Measles and rubella vaccines are not usually given until 15 months of age; tuberculosis vaccine is not given routinely to children.

(3) Measles, mumps, and rubella vaccines are not given until 15 months; tuberculosis vaccine is not routinely administered to children.

(4) Measles vaccine is not usually administered until the child is 15 months old.

34. (3) The body's immune system constructs proteins called antibodies that possess a specificity toward another protein called the antigen. The antibody may neutralize or damage the antigen and thus render it harmless. (c)

(1) Antigens are harmful to the body.

(2) Antibodies are produced to fight antigens.

(4) Antibodies are protein substances.

35. (2) Maternal antibodies to measles infection persist in the infant until approximately 15 months of age. (b)

(1) Side effects are no more common for infants than for toddlers.

(3) This has not been found to be true.

(4) This is true, but it is due to the presence of maternal antibodies.

36. (2) Because of the infant's increasing mobility, high level of oral activity, and relative lack of fear or appreciation for danger, accidents are the primary cause of death in children above 1 year of age. (c)

(1) This is best discussed with the mother prenatally or soon after delivery.

(3) This is too early for discussions of psychosexual development.

(4) This is too early for discussions about toilet training.

37. (3) Supporting and slightly flexing the knee with a pillow will relieve tension (and pain) in the joint; elevation of the leg will promote venous return, reducing joint swelling and pain. (b)

(1) Frequent position change will be painful.

(2) This will not help promote venous return in the legs or assist in relieving her leg pains.

(4) Body alignment alone will not help reduce the pain in her legs.

38. (2) Rest reduces the strain on the heart and minimizes metabolic needs during the acute, febrile stage of the disease. (a)

(1) This is not a priority, and the child will be anorexic during the febrile phase.

(3) The child with rheumatic fever is confined to bed rest and needs to reduce activity to prevent heart damage.

(4) Elimination is not usually a problem except as a result of immobility.

39. (4) Nonstrenuous, diversional activities involving interpersonal relationships with another person provide better support and resting conditions than does more active play. (a)

(1) A jigsaw puzzle is too complicated for a 5-year-old and does not provide her the human contact she needs.

(2) This will probably increase her fretfulness and does not provide the human contact she needs.

(3) Although a doll is appropriate for a 5-year-old, it does not provide the human contact she needs.

40. (3) A bland high-protein, high-carbohydrate diet provides adequate nutrition in the face of infection and fever. (a)

(1) This does not provide the protein needed for the healing process.

(2) These are empty calories.

(4) This is too heavy for a between-meal snack and contains fats, which are not helpful in the healing process.

41. (1) The attack by autoantibodies on the heart valves can cause immediate impairment of heart function and lifelong valvular insufficiency. (b)

(2) This is not a common complication; if it does occur, it is not serious and is easily treated.

(3) Although this may occur, it is not the most serious complication.

(4) This does not occur as a result of rheumatic fever.

42. (4) A few minutes will be enough time for Nancy to begin to feed herself. The nurse should provide both physical and emotional support, since the child's request for help indicates the need for dependence during a period of stress. (a)

(1) This does not provide the child the help she may need.

(2) A nurse should never make a statement like this; it can cause stress, feelings of guilt, and embarrassment to a sick child.

(3) It may be a while until the child feels better; in the meantime, she needs adequate nourishment to provide for healing.

43. (3) Regression is the retreat to a past level of behavior as a way of minimizing stress or controlling anxiety. Increased dependence, such as being fed by another person, is a form of regression (a)

(1) Her statement does not reflect immaturity.

(2) Although lonesomeness may be a factor, it is not the key one in her response.

(4) Her statement can hardly be construed as a temper tantrum.

44. (3) Dinner is frequently a family activity. Having her parents visit during mealtime may provide her with additional emotional, social, and physical support, resulting in an improved nutritional intake. (a)

(1) This will further inhibit her nutritional intake.

(2) This may not influence her overall intake.

(4) If given full rein, 5-year-olds will not select the most nutritional foods.

45. (3) In PKU the absence of the hepatic enzyme phenylalanine hydroxylase prevents normal metabolism (hydroxylation to tyrosine) of the amino acid phenylalanine. The increased fluid levels of phenylalanine in the body and the alternate metabolic byproducts (phenylketones) are associated with severe mental retardation (exact mechanism not known). (b)

(1) PKU is transmitted by an autosomal recessive gene.

(2) Testing for PKU cannot be done until after several days of milk ingestion.

(4) Children are usually treated until they are 8 years old, when most of the growth and development of the brain are complete.

46. (1) The Guthrie blood test reliably detects abnormal phenylalanine levels as early as 4 days of age, provided the infant has been fed a milk diet. (a)

(2) This is not used since it takes too long for the phenylpyruvic acid to appear in the urine. By this time (10 to 14 days), brain damage may have occurred.

(3) This is used for screening large groups of infants but cannot be used until after 6 weeks of age.

(4) This is an inappropriate test for PKU.

47. (2) The deficient product can be supplied. However, in most cases, limiting the intake of the substance the body cannot metabolize reduces toxic buildup. (b)

(1) Hormones are not involved in inborn errors of metabolism.

(3) This is not possible, for the genetic enzyme is intracellular.

(4) This will not help.

48. (3) It is hoped that reducing dietary phenylalanine will prevent brain damage. Diets are planned to attempt to maintain the serum phenylalanine level between 5 and 10 mg/100 ml. (c)

(1) Phenylalanine is essential for normal growth and development of the brain.

(2) There are no substitutes; phenylalanine is one of the essential amino acids.

(4) It is not possible to do this.

49. (3) Maintaining low phenylalanine levels is recommended until brain growth is almost completed, usually by 6 to 8 years of age. (b)

(1) Dietary management is necessary until the child is 8 years old.

(2) Dietary management is necessary until the child is 8 years old.

(4) This is untrue and is not helpful to the parents.

50. (4) Shivering increases the metabolic rate, which intensifies the body's need for oxygen and raises the body temperature. (c)

(1) Monitoring vital signs is not as important as taking affirmative action to prevent increases in fever.

(2) Forcing fluids is contraindicated because the child is vomiting.

(3) Although monitoring output will provide information about the patient's level of hydration, it is more important to take affirmative action toward preventing increases in fever.

51. (3) Febrile convulsions are not necessarily associated with major neurologic problems but often accompany high fever. Such convulsions may be partially accounted for by the overall brain immaturity in children. (b)

(1) Febrile convulsions are more common in the infant and young toddler.

(2) The cause of febrile convulsions is still uncertain.

(4) Boys are affected about twice as often as girls.

52. (4) First convert the grains to milligrams:

$$\frac{1 \text{ gr}}{60 \text{ mg}} \times \frac{1.25 \text{ gr}}{x \text{ mg}}$$

$$x = 75.00 \text{ mg}$$

Then perform the computation for the correct dosage:

$$\frac{150 \text{ mg}}{75 \text{ mg}} \times \frac{x \text{ tablets}}{1 \text{ tablet}}$$

$$75x = 150$$

$$x = 2 \text{ tablets} \qquad \text{(b)}$$

(1) This is an insufficient dose.

(2) This is an insufficient dose.

(3) This is an insufficient dose.

53. (1) Meningococcal meningitis is identified by its epidemic nature and purpuric skin rash. It is treated with sulfadiazine. (c)

(2) This is not characteristic of meningococcal meningitis.

(3) The fever of meningitis is usually high.

(4) This is not characteristic of meningococcal meningitis.

54. (3) Peripheral circulatory collapse (the Waterhouse-Friderichsen syndrome) is a serious complication of meningococcal meningitis due to bilateral adrenal hemorrhage. The resultant acute adrenocortical insufficiency causes profound shock, petechiae and ecchymotic lesions, vomiting, prostration, and hypotension. (b)

(1) Although this may occur, it is rare and not as serious as peripheral circulatory collapse.

(2) Although this may occur, it is not as serious a complication as peripheral circulatory collapse.

(4) Although this may occur, it is controllable and not as serious as peripheral circulatory collapse.

55. (3) Pain is paroxysmal due to peristaltic action. Abdominal distention pushes up the diaphragm, causing respiratory distress characterized by grunting respirations. (c)

(1) The pain of intestinal obstruction is paroxysmal.

(2) These symptoms do not usually accompany intestinal obstruction.

(4) These symptoms are not characteristic of intestinal obstruction.

56. (1) Sucking is a primary need of infancy. It decreases anxiety and does not interfere with gastric decompression. (b)

(2) This will probably not help to calm him.

(3) This will probably increase his pain from abdominal distension.

(4) This would be more helpful if Matt were a toddler.

57. (3) If the circulation is overloaded with too much fluid or the rate is too rapid, the stress on the heart becomes too great and cardiac embarrassment may occur. (b)

(1) This is important, but an infiltrated IV is not a serious complication.

(2) This is not a primary consideration in intestinal obstruction.

(4) Although fluid replacement is important, prevention of cardiac problems from fluid overload is critical.

58. (2) By 4 months of age infants are able to turn over and can easily fall from an inadequately guarded height. (a)

(1) Although Matt is capable of putting small things in his mouth, he is not yet able to crawl and would probably not be placed on the floor.

(3) At 4 months of age infants are not yet able to explore the environment to the point that electric outlets pose a problem.

(4) Matt is still too small and has not yet developed motor capabilities to get into containers of poison.

59. (3) The decreased filtration of plasma in the glomeruli results in an excess accumulation of water and sodium, producing edema that is first evident around the eyes. Hypertension is thought to be due to the hypervolemia, although its exact cause is unclear. (b)

(1) Neither of these is a sign of acute glomerulonephritis.

(2) Although hematuria is found, dehydration is not a sign of acute glomerulonephritis.

(4) Oliguria is not found with acute glomerulonephritis. The patient is usually hypertensive.

60. (4) During the acute stage, anorexia and the loss of protein lower the child's resistance to infection. (b)

(1) Bed rest is necessary only during the most acute stage; 4 weeks is too long.

(2) A bland diet is not necessary, and high protein should be avoided.

(3) Antibiotics are not necessary for all children with acute glomerulonephritis, only those with persistent streptococcal infections.

61. (3) Piaget stresses that age 7 is the turning point in mental development. New forms of organization appear at this age that mark the beginning of logic, symbolism, and abstract thought. (a)

(1) A toddler is capable of making simple decisions.

(2) A 5-year-old is capable of tying his shoes.

(4) An infant is capable of hand-eye coordination.

62. (2) When urinary test findings are normal, such as no evidence of hematuria or proteinuria, the child is allowed to resume his pre-illness activities. (b)

(1) Bed rest is unnecessary at this stage.

(3) This restriction is unnecessary.

(4) This restriction is unnecessary.

63. (4) During the acute phase, body movement causes pain and should therefore be avoided. Immobility in rheumatic fever does not lead to joint deformity, since the acute phase is not prolonged. (c)

(1) Applying heat to the joints of this child will aggravate the pain.

(2) This will aggravate the pain.

(3) This will exaggerate the pain.

64. (2) The child with rheumatic fever needs to be kept happy to decrease his oxygen needs. The school-age child has an interest in hobbies or collections of various kinds as a means of gathering information and knowledge about the world in which he lives. (b)

(1) This is too advanced for a normal 8-year-old.

(3) These would probably not interest an 8-year-old.

(4) This would not interest an 8-year-old.

65. (1) C-reactive protein, which indicates the presence of an inflammatory reaction, is never present in normal blood and disappears as the child's condition improves. (c)

(2) This is not a reason to confine the child to bed rest.

(3) Joint pains may persist for 2 weeks. Bed rest is indicated only for the most acute stage.

(4) This is not a reason to confine the child to bed rest.

66. (1) Cystic fibrosis is characterized by overproduction of viscid mucus by exocrine glands in the lungs. The mucus traps bacteria and foreign debris but adheres to the lining and cannot be expelled by the cilia, thus obstructing the airway and favoring growth of organisms and infection. (a)

(2) Although there is an increased sodium and chloride in the saliva, it does not irritate or necrose mucous membranes.

(3) Neuromuscular irritability of the bronchi does not occur in cystic fibrosis.

(4) Cardiac defects are not associated with cystic fibrosis.

67. (2) The first usual indication of cystic fibrosis is meconium ileus. The small intestine is blocked with a thick, tenacious mucilaginous meconium, usually near the ileocecal valve. This causes intestinal obstruction with abdominal distention, vomiting, and fluid and electrolyte imbalance. (b)

(1) This is not an early sign of cystic fibrosis.

(3) This does not have special significance in cystic fibrosis.

(4) This is not an early sign of cystic fibrosis.

68. (2) Production of tenacious mucus in the pancreatic ducts prevents the flow of digestive enzymes into the intestines. Thus fats, proteins, and (to a lesser extent) carbohydrates cannot be digested and absorbed. (b)

(1) Anorexia is not a usual problem found with cystic fibrosis.

(3) Cystic fibrosis does not influence the secretion of growth hormone.

(4) These are not problems associated with cystic fibrosis.

69. (1) In cystic fibrosis the mucous glands secrete thick mucoid secretions that accumulate, reducing ciliary action and mucus flow. Expectoration is greatly hindered. Postural drainage promotes the removal of mucopurulent secretions by means of gravity. (b)

(2) The nurse should encourage activities appropriate for the child's physical capacity; this will include helping him conserve energy during acute phases of his illness.

(3) Coughing should be encouraged.

(4) This is not necessary with cystic fibrosis.

70. (3) Because of a lack of the pancreatic enzyme lipase, fats remain unabsorbed and are excreted in excessive amounts in the stool. (a)

(1) This does not cause the foul smell of stools.

(2) This does not cause the foul smell of stools.

(4) These are the pancreatic enzymes, whose passage into the intestine is prevented by blocked pancreatic ducts.

71. (3) Pancreatic enzymes are given as replacement because of the lack of their production by the pancreas. Antibiotics are prescribed to prevent and control respiratory tract infection. (a)

(1) These are not indicated in the treatment of cystic fibrosis.

(2) These may be used but are not specific for cystic fibrosis.

(4) Mists and expectorants may be used; fat-soluble vitamins must be given in water-miscible preparations.

72. (4) Rectal prolapse is the most common GI complication and is due to wasting of perirectal supporting tissues, secondary to malnutrition. (c)

(1) Intussusception is not associated with cystic fibrosis.

(2) Anal fissures may or may not occur with cystic fibrosis.

(3) Meconium ileus is associated with cystic fibrosis in newborns and prevents the passage of stools.

73. (2) The nurse recognizes the child's protest over his mother's absence and tries to comfort him by staying near him until he feels more relaxed. The bathing can be postponed until he has had time to test out his environment and is less anxious. (b)

(1) This may frighten him more.

(3) This is probably true, although the nurse has not attempted to reduce anxiety.

(4) This action does not attempt to relieve the child's anxiety and will probably cause it to increase.

74. (4) The second stage of separation anxiety is despair, in which the child is depressed, lonely, and disinterested in his surroundings. (b)
    (1) The third stage of separation, denial or detachment, is a more advanced stage than that demonstrated in the situation.
    (2) The nurse must recognize that the child is suffering from separation anxiety, which does not include a stage of mistrust.
    (3) The nurse must recognize that the child is suffering from separation anxiety, which does not include a stage of rejection.
75. (1) Detachment is the result of trying to escape the emotional pain of desiring the mother by repressing feelings for her. (c)
    (2) This interpretation is not appropriate to the situation cited.
    (3) This response lacks insight.
    (4) This conclusion cannot be drawn from the situation cited.
76. (4) When the child has progressed to detachment as a method of coping with the separation, reunion of child and mother necessitates a period of reconciliation before the child is again willing to experience his emotional feelings because of his memory of the pain during their separation. (a)
    (1) Mike will not miss the nurses or the hospital routine.
    (2) Because he has suffered extreme separation anxiety, Mike will have some difficulty readjusting to his home.
    (3) Mike will probably demonstrate difficulty in his readjustment to his family.
77. (2) The hyperextension required in swimming aids in strengthening back muscles and increases deeper respirations, both of which are necessary prior to surgery and/or wearing a brace or cast. (a)
    (1) This will not be especially therapeutic for Sara.
    (3) This will not be especially therapeutic for Sara.
    (4) This will not be especially therapeutic for Sara.
78. (1) Continuing growth causes changes in muscle and bone structure and position. Adolescent girls have a rapid growth spurt. The brace is worn for 6 months after physical maturity, which is proved by x-ray examination to show cessation of bone growth. (b)
    (2) The Milwaukee brace is used to halt the progression of the curvature.
    (3) Pain is not usually a symptom with scoliosis.
    (4) This is not an appropriate criteron for removal of the Milwaukee brace.
79. (4) The hypothalamic-pituitary-gonadal-adrenal mechanism is responsible for the physiologic and structural changes that occur at puberty. In girls the adrenal glands secrete androgens that are responsible for the appearance of axillary and pubic hair, generally between 11 and 14 years of age. Menarche usually occurs 2 years after initial pubescent changes. (b)

(1) This is not a reliable indicator of sexual maturity.
(2) This is not an indicator of sexual maturity.
(3) This is not an appropriate indicator of sexual maturity in females or males.
80. (1) Hypertrophy of the pyloric sphincter, at the distal end of the stomach, causes partial and then complete obstruction. Nonprojectile vomiting progresses to projectile vomiting, which rapidly leads to dehydration. (c)
    (2) This can be expected with a tracheoesophageal fistula but not with pyloric stenosis.
    (3) The infant's cry is not affected by pyloric stenosis; there does not appear to be pain associated with this condition, except for the pain of hunger.
    (4) The quality of the stool is not usually affected by pyloric stenosis.
81. (2) In excessive vomiting there is an increased loss of hydrogen ions (hydrochloric acid), which leads to a lowered serum pH (metabolic alkalosis) and an excess of base bicarbonate. (b)
    (1) Although some calcium is lost through vomiting, it is highly unusual that the infant would develop tetany.
    (3) This is caused by a retention of hydrogen ions and a loss of base bicarbonates. In vomiting, base bicarbonates are retained and hydrogen ions are lost.
    (4) Hyperactivity is not associated with pyloric stenosis.
82. (4) The newborn's proportion of total body water is 20% greater than the adult's. It rapidly diminishes in the neonatal period and continues to decline steadily until about 2 years of age, when it almost equals that of the adult. In addition, infants have very little fluid volume reserve. (c)
    (1) Renal function is immature during infancy only.
    (2) Cellular metabolism in children is not less stable than in adults.
    (3) The proportion of total body water in children (up to 2 years) is 20% greater than in adults.
83. (1) An infant's intravascular compartment is fairly limited and cannot accommodate large volumes of fluid administered in a short time. Equipment such as minidroppers, volume control chambers, and infusion pumps should be used, since they help control or limit the volume of fluid to be infused. (b)
    (2) IV fluids can be administered at room temperature.
    (3) This is the physician's role.
    (4) This is important for everyone receiving IV fluids.
84. (4) Initial feedings of glucose in water or electrolyte solutions are given 4 to 6 hours after surgery. When clear fluids are retained, usually within 24 hours, diluted formula feedings are begun. (c)
    (1) This is not necessary.
    (2) This is not necessary.
    (3) The formula should be diluted 24 hours after surgery in a gradual attempt to return the infant to a full feeding schedule.
85. (2) Tetralogy of Fallot classically consists of 4 defects.

Three of them are anatomic—ventricular septal defect, pulmonic stenosis, and overriding aorta. The fourth defect, right ventricular hypertrophy, is secondary to increased resistance to blood flow in that ventricle. (b)
(1) Although right ventricular hypertrophy is correct, the other anomalies are not.
(3) These are the characteristics of transposition of the great vessels.
(4) Although the right ventricular hypertrophy is correct, the other anomalies are not.

86. (4) Oxygen is necessary for growth of cells. Decreased oxygen in the developing child causes a slow growth rate. (b)
(1) Mental retardation is not a common finding in children with congenital heart disease.
(2) Cyanosis and clubbing are not characteristic of most children with cardiac anomalies, only of those with the more serious forms.
(3) Cardiac anomalies are more often a result of prenatal, rather than genetic, factors.

87. (2) The purpose of digoxin (lanoxin) is to slow and strengthen the apical rate. The normal apical rate for a child of 5 years is 90 to 110 beats per minute. If the apical rate is already slow (10 to 20 beats below normal), administration of the drug could lower the apical rate to an unsafe level. (a)
(1) This rate is well below that which necessitates withholding Lanoxin for children; it is the correct rate for withholding Lanoxin in adults.
(3) This is within the normal range of the heart rate of 5-year-olds and does not necessitate withholding Lanoxin.
(4) This is within the normal range of the heart rate of 5-year-olds and does not necessitate withholding Lanoxin.

88. (4) Decreased tissue oxygenation stimulates erythropoiesis, resulting in excessive production of red blood cells. (a)
(1) This would not be a direct cause of polycythemia.
(2) This may or may not affect the production of red blood cells.
(3) This would not be a direct cause of polycythemia.

89. (1) Forceful evacuation results in the child's taking a deep breath, holding it, and straining (Valsalva maneuver). This increased intrathoracic pressure puts excessive strain on the heart sutures. (b)
(2) Activity is gradually increased postoperatively.
(3) Crying is not a problem after cardiac surgery; it may, in fact, help prevent respiratory complications.
(4) Coughing and deep breathing are essential for the prevention of postoperative respiratory complications.

90. (3) The nurse's data collection was not adequate because no questions were asked concerning the recency of the previous tetanus inoculation. The nurse failed to support the life and well-being of a patient. (c)

(1) It was essential to determine the recency of the immunization; for a "tetanus prone" wound, like a puncture from a rusty nail, some form of tetanus immunization is usually given.
(2) The nurse's assessment was not thorough in regard to determining the recency of immunization.
(4) This is usually a clinical decision.

91. (4) The slightest stimulation sets off a wave of very severe and very painful muscle spasms involving the whole body. Nerve impulses cross the myoneural junction and stimulate muscle contraction due to the presence of exotoxins produced by *Clostridium tetani*. (c)
(1) Body alignment is not an important consideration in tetanus.
(2) Oral intake of fluids may not be possible because of excessive secretions and laryngospasm.
(3) Monitoring output is not a major nursing concern with tetanus.

92. (4) Gluteal folds should be symmetric, as should all planes and folds of the body. Any abnormality of the hips will cause asymmetry and/or a shorter leg on the affected side. (a)
(1) In congenital hip dysplasia there is usually a limited abduction of the leg at the hip.
(2) The affected side is shorter.
(3) The dance reflex is not affected.

93. (1) Hypostatic pneumonia can develop from decreased activity. Also the cast prevents full chest expansion. (a)
(2) Cast damage, although problematic, is not a serious complication.
(3) Soiling of the cast with excreta, although problematic, is not a serious complication.
(4) This is not necessary or desirable.

94. (2) Pillows under the head or shoulders of a child in a spica cast will thrust the chest forward against the cast, causing discomfort and respiratory distress. Therefore, when elevation of the head is desired, the entire mattress and spring should be raised at the head of the bed. (b)
(1) There is no reason to place a time limit on this position.
(3) This will thrust the chest forward against the cast, causing discomfort and respiratory distress.
(4) This will not help in any way.

95. (2) Polycythemia, reflected in an elevated hematocrit level, is a direct attempt of the body to compensate for the decrease in oxygenation to all body cells due to the mixture of oxygenated and unoxygenated circulating blood. (c)
(1) Edema is not a common finding in cyanotic heart disease.
(3) This is characteristic of coarctation of the aorta, an acyanotic heart disease.
(4) This is not characteristic of cyanotic heart disease in children.

96. (3) In the fetus, oxygenated blood is shunted directly into the systemic circulation via the ductus arteriosus, a connection between the pulmonry artery and the aorta. Normally after birth the increased oxygen tension causes a functional closure of the ductus arteriosus. Occasionally, particularly in premature infants, this vessel remains open and is known as patent ductus arteriosus. (c)
    (1) This is known as pulmonic stenosis.
    (2) Patent ductus arteriosus does not involve ventricular septal defects.
    (4) This is not the problem in patent ductus arteriosus.

97. (4) In acyanotic heart disease there is a narrowing of the vessels and/or pinpoint holes in the septum of the heart that cause a murmuring sound as the blood is pumped through. (c)
    (1) This is not a common clinical finding in acyanotic heart disease.
    (2) Clubbing is a common finding in cyanotic heart disease.
    (3) This is not a common finding in acyanotic heart disease, for tissue perfusion is usually adequate.

98. (2) Coarctation of the aorta is a narrowing, usually in the thoracic segment, causing decreased blood flow below the constriction and increased blood volume above it. (c)
    (1) In coarctation of the aorta, radial pulses would be full and bounding.
    (3) In coarctation of the aorta, femoral pulses would be weak or absent and blood pressure in the lower extremities would be decreased.
    (4) This has nothing to do with coarctation of the aorta.

99. (3) Secondary syphilis, occurring 1 to 3 months after healing of the primary lesion and lasting for several weeks to as long as a year, is the stage at which the individual is most infectious. (b)
    (1) Primary syphillis is the stage of initial infection; it preceeds secondary syphillis.
    (2) This is the third stage of the disease.
    (4) This is the fourth or final stage.

100. (1) Syphilis is caused by a spirochete, *Treponema pallidum*. The organism is readily destroyed by mild disinfectants such as soap and water. (b)
    (2) Isolation is not necessary since the disease is transferred through direct contact with lesions, usually through intercourse.
    (3) The causative organism is transferred through direct contact with lesions.
    (4) The causative organism is transferred through direct contact with lesions.

101. (2) John's symptoms indicate that he is in the secondary stage, which begins from 6 weeks to 6 months after primary contact. Therefore a 6-month history is needed to ensure that all possible contacts and original contacts are located. (c)
    (1) Any time less than 6 months may miss contacts who could become infected.

(3) Any time less than 6 months may miss contacts who could become infected.
    (4) Any time less than 6 months may miss contacts who could become infected.

102. (1) Hemophilia is carried on the X chromosome but is recessive. Therefore the female is the carrier (a normal X_O and an affected X_H). If the male receives the affected X_H ($X_H Y_O$), the disease is manifest. (a)
    (2) Hemophilia is a sex-linked recessive disorder.
    (3) Hemophilia is carried by the female. Regular laws of mendelian inheritance are not sex-specific.
    (4) Only females carry the trait; only males have the disease.

103. (2) The mating of a carrier female ($X_O X_H$) and an unaffected male ($X_O Y_O$) results in the following possible offspring: a carrier female ($X_O X_H$), a normal female ($X_O X_O$), a normal male ($X_O Y_O$), or an affected male ($X_H Y_O$). (b)
    (1) For each child there is a 50% chance of being normal.
    (3) For each child there is a 50% chance of being affected.
    (4) Males cannot carry the trait; females have a 50% chance of being affected.

104. (4) Bleeding is greatly influenced by activity. Therefore hemorrhage into weight-bearing joints, especially the knees, is the most common site. (b)
    (1) This area is fairly well protected by the skull and less likely to be injured.
    (2) Bleeding from bones themselves is not common without other associated trauma.
    (3) This area is usually protected from the trauma of direct force in known hemophiliacs.

105. (2) Salicylates in large doses cause irritation of the gastric mucosa (gastric distress, nausea, vomiting) and also affect the CNS (tinnitus, dizziness, disturbances in hearing and vision). (a)
    (1) Although nausea and dizziness and severe headache may be associated with salicylate ingestion, edema is not.
    (3) Constipation is not a common problem associated with salicylates.
    (4) Edema is not a problem associated with salicylates.

106. (2) Salicylates act as analgesics by protecting peripheral pain receptors from bradykinin, a component in the inflammatory process. Salicylates act as antipyretics by affecting the heat-regulating center in the hypothalamus and increasing the elimination of heat through peripheral blood vessel dilation and evaporation of increased perspiration. (a)
    (1) Salicylates have no capacity to destroy or control a microorganism's effect.
    (3) Salicylates have no capacity to act as a sedative and calm individuals.
    (4) Salicylates have no capacity to act as a hypnotic and induce sleep.

107. (2) Rheumatic fever is almost always preceded by a

group A *Streptococcus* infection, which is most often associated with upper respiratory tract infections. Therefore upper respiratory tract infections should be treated early to prevent the development of rheumatic fever. (b)

(1) Childhood diseases are not caused by the organism associated with rheumatic fever.

(3) Rheumatic fever is believed to be an autoimmune disease resulting from nontreated streptococcal infections and is not itself communicable.

(4) Immunizations are not available to prevent this.

108. (1) Choanal atresia is a lack of an opening between one or both of the nasal passages and the nasopharynx. (c)

(2) Atresias associated with the GI tract include esophageal and intestinal atresia involving the ileum, jejunum, or colon.

(3) An atresia involving the pharynx and larynx is not commonly seen.

(4) Rectal atresia involves the rectum's ending in a pouch and the normal anal canal's opening into the other (nonconnected) end of the rectum.

109. (2) Since there is little or no opening between the nasal passages and the nasopharynx, the infant can breathe only through the mouth. When feeding, the infant cannot breathe without aspirating some of the fluid; this causes choking. (b)

(1) The swallowing reflex is normal.

(3) Since it is difficult if not impossible to eat, she will be very hungry.

(4) If choanal atresia is unilateral, there may be no symptoms and she will eat normally; if bilateral, sucking will be almost impossible.

110. (4) An Apgar score of 3 indicates neonatal distress and should signal the nurse that the infant requires close supervision and support. (b)

(1) Average birth weight is ubout 3200 gm.

(2) Infants often swallow in utero.

(3) A positive Babinski is normal through the age of 2 years.

111. (4) Infection is a constant threat because of poor general state of nutrition, tendency toward skin breakdown in edematous areas, corticosteroid therapy, and lowered immunoglobulin levels. (c)

(1) Fluid monitoring is important in determining whether restriction is indicated.

(2) Rather than regulating diet, the nurse should encourage intake of proteins and foods with high nutritional value.

(3) Bed rest may be used for severe stages, but generally ambulation is encouraged.

112. (3) Children with nephrosis have a characteristic pale, overweight appearance from the malnutrition and edema. They may become very sensitive about these changes as they grow older. (b)

(1) Engaging in usual childhood activities between attacks should promote normal development of fine muscle coordination.

(2) Sterility is not associated with nephrosis.

(4) Although this may be indicated, body image problems pose a much greater threat.

113. (1) Bed-wetting accidents are not uncommon in this age group, especially during hospitalization when regression may occur. Therefore the best approach is to ignore the event. (b)

(2) This may tend to make Roger feel guilty for his action.

(3) He may interpret this as punishment. Punishment for regressive behavior is inappropriate.

(4) Since skin breakdown is a concern, rubber sheets are contraindicated; they would hold moisture close to the skin.

114. (2) Fear of mutilation and intrusive procedures is most common at this age because of fantasies and active imagination. These children also connect illness with being bad and view intrusion as punishment. (c)

(1) Fear of insolation from peers is a problem for school-age children and adolescents.

(3) Death is seen as reversible and not final.

(4) A child this age usually has little previous contact with pain and therefore little experience upon which to base fear.

115. (2) The restricted ventilation accompanying an asthmatic attack limits the body's ability to blow off carbon dioxide. As carbon dioxide accumulates in the body fluids, it reacts with water to produce carbonic acid (H_2CO_3); the result is respiratory acidosis. (b)

(1) Asthma is a respiratory problem causing carbon dioxide retention. Respiratory alkalosis is caused by exhaling large amounts of carbon dioxide.

(3) The problem basic to asthma is respiratory, not metabolic.

(4) Asthma is a respiratory problem, not a metabolic one; metabolic acidosis can be produced by a gain of nonvolatile acids or a loss of base bicarbonate.

116. (2) Prednisone causes atrophy of the thymus, decreases the number of lymphocytes, plasma cells, and eosinophils in the blood, and decreases the formation of antibodies. Therefore it reduces the individual's resistance to certain infectious processes and viral diseases. Also, prednisone is an antiinflammatory drug that masks infection. (b)

(1) Eosinophil counts are often consistently elevated in children with asthma.

(3) Mary will need adequate hydration to assist with loosening and removing mucus from the lungs.

(4) Mary will limit her own activity based upon her respiratory status.

117. (2) Aminophylline relaxes the smooth muscle of the vasculature, causing peripheral vasodilation that can lead to hypotension. (b)

(1) Temperature changes will not be related to aminophylline administration.

(3) Oxygen therapy is not associated with drug administration.

(4) Epinephrine, also used in the treatment of asthma, may cause tachycardia.

118. (1) Cold can precipitate bronchospasm, and increased exercise depletes oxygen. (b)

(2) Asthma is a chronic condition. Return to usual activities after the acute stage is essential for normal growth and development.

(3) Although increased calories may be needed to support the child during a coexisting bacterial infection in the acute stage, by discharge a return to usual habits is indicated.

(4) Treatment of asthma does not involve a high-fat diet.

119. (2) Peak crying times are early evening and night, which exhaust the mother. She needs time away from the baby to rest and should be encouraged to hire a sitter or make some arrangements for time alone. (a)

(1) Many treatments, including this one, may not be effective; children do outgrow colic, so parents need support to help them manage until that time.

(3) Treatment is usually based on relieving abdominal cramping by stimulating peristalsis; quiet environments may help prevent, not treat, the problem.

(4) Providing warmth through a hot water bottle or heating pad over the abdomen may be helpful for some children but not for others.

120. (3) The traditional efforts to explain and treat colic center around control of gas in the intestinal tract that is causing the paroxysmal pain. (a)

(1) Colic is thought to be due to excessive fermentation and gas production.

(2) The exact cause of colic is not known.

(4) Excessive intake of carbohydrates may cause flatus, but diet changes rarely prevent colic attacks.

121. (3) Muscular coordination and perception are developed enough at 6 months so the infant can roll over. If unaware of this ability of the infant, the nurse could leave the child unattended for a moment to reach for something and the child could roll off the crib. (b)

(1) Sitting up unsupported is accomplished by most children at 7 to 8 months.

(2) Standing by holding on to furniture is accomplished by most children between 8 and 10 months.

(4) Crawling takes place at about 9 months of age.

122. (3) Touching the palms of the hands causes flexion of the fingers (grasp reflex); this usually lessens after 3 months of age. An unexpected loud noise causes abduction of the extremities and then flexion of the elbows (startle reflex); this usually disappears by 4 months of age. Persistence of primitive reflexes usually is indicative of a cerebral insult. (b)

(1) These changes are consistent with normal growth and development.

(2) The data do not support making this comment and would cause needless concern.

(4) Sensory stimulation at this age is directed toward experiences to add new motor, language, and social skills.

123. (4) By law, a nurse cannot administer medications without a prescription from a physician. This is a dependent function of the nurse. (a)

(1) The nurse cannot distribute medication without a physician's order.

(2) The nurse must get a doctor's order for the medication and cannot accept the parent's information alone.

(3) The nurse should not assume that the physician is aware of the problem.

124. (1) An individual is legally unable to sign a consent until age 18 years. The only exception is the emancipated minor, a minor who is self-sufficient or married. (a)

(2) Although the adolescent is capable of intelligent choices, it is the legality, not the acceptability or intelligence of the choice, that is at issue.

(3) Parents or guardians are legally responsible under all circumstances unless the adolescent is an emancipated minor.

(4) Adolescents have the capacity to choose between alternatives, but not the legal right in this situation.

125. (4) The nurse made the assessment that the medication was ineffective in relieving Loren's pain for the duration ordered. This information should be communicated to the physician for evaluation. (a)

(1) The doctor's order is for administration only every 3 to 4 hours. Legally it can be given only within these guidelines.

(2) The nurse should not ignore the patient's need for pain relief.

(3) There are no data to support this. The amount of medication was probably inadequate for her pain tolerance level.

126. (1) Chlorpheniramine (Chlor-Trimeton) is an antihistaminic that prevents histamine from reaching its site of action by competing for the receptors. (b)

(2) Nitrofurazone is a bactericidal agent used especially with burns.

(3) This is a salicylate-like agent.

(4) Hyaluronidase is a mucolytic enzyme that promotes diffusion and absorption of injected fluids, exudates, and transudates.

127. (3) The principle of Bryant's traction is bilateral 90 degree hip flexion. It is skin traction applied to the legs to decrease the fracture, maintain alignment, and immobilize both legs. (a)

(1) Bryant's traction requires the supine position.

(2) Bryant's traction is always applied bilaterally.

(4) Skeletal traction is applied to a pin in the affected extremity.

128. (3) No more than 300 ml of solution should be administered to an infant or child unless specifically or-

dered, since fluid and electrolyte balance in an infant or child is easily disturbed. (c)

(1) This quantity may be ordered for a small infant.

(2) This quantity may be ordered for an older or larger infant.

(4) This quantity is too large for small children.

129. (3) A patient cannot legally be locked in a room (isolated) unless there is a threat of danger involved either to the patient or to other patients. (b)

(1) Crying, although irritating, will not harm the other children.

(2) Sue is probably reacting to separation from her mother, which is common at this age.

(4) Legal limits rarely include time parameters.

130. (2) A pounding board is a safe toy for toddlers, since it is fairly large, easy to manipulate, and sturdy. A pounding board provides a way for anger to be sublimated. (b)

(1) Sue's motor and hand-eye coordination is too immature for using this.

(3) This is not as safe since toddlers may eat clay or Play-Doh.

(4) This would be appropriate for an older child with more mature motor coordination to compensate for a moving object.

131. (1) Using the formula, convert grains to milligrams (gr 1/300 = 0.2 mg); then use the formula:

$$\frac{0.2 \text{ mg}}{0.4 \text{ mg}} \times \frac{x}{1 \text{ ml}}$$

$$0.4x = 0.2$$
$$x = 0.5 \text{ ml (This will contain the desired dose of 0.2 mg atropine.)} \quad (c)$$

(2) This amount is too much according to calculations.

(3) This amount is too little according to calculations.

(4) This amount is too much according to calculations.

132. (3) Since young children have difficulty verbalizing their fears or anxiety, play is a therapeutic way for these feelings to be expressed. The school-age child also likes to role play. (b)

(1) Young school-age children are still somewhat egocentric and therefore interested in their own experiences and sensations.

(2) A child this age is unable to express feelings entirely through words.

(4) This may be helpful for a toddler or preschooler.

133. (3) Regression is normal in times of stress. It is a transient need that should be accepted, since it helps reduce anxiety. (a)

(1) This behavior is unrelated to medical progress.

(2) Distraction works only as long as it is employed.

(4) Cause (thumb sucking) and future effect (buckteeth) will not be meaningful to a 7-year-old.

134. (2) To maintain the desired blood level, the drug must be given in the exact amount at the times directed. If the blood level of the drug falls, the organisms

have an opportunity to build up resistance to the drug. (b)

(1) Weighing a patient is important with drugs that affect fluid balance such as Lasix.

(3) Giving medication with milk or meals is important with drugs such as Mandelamine that cause GI distress.

(4) Monitoring temperature would be important with antipyretic drugs.

135. (3) Isoniazid (INH) is the most potent tuberculostatic drug available at this time. It is given in conjunction with paraaminosalicylic acid (PAS), since PAS potentiates the action of INH as well as limits bacterial resistance to the drug. (b)

(1) Old tuberculin is one type of skin test used to detect tuberculosis.

(2) Bacille Calmette Guérin (BCG) vaccine is the only successful vaccine for tuberculosis to date, but greater protection is afforded by daily prophylactic administration of INH.

(4) Purified protein derivative (PPD) is a widely used skin test for detecting tuberculosis.

136. (3) Tubercle bacilli multiply in caseous lesions, which have a poor vascular supply. These areas receive lower levels of the drugs, and as a result therapy must be prolonged. (b)

(1) This length of therapy is insufficient to erradicate the bacilli.

(2) Because lower levels of drug reach caseous lesions, longer treatment periods are needed.

(4) Treatment for infected persons is usually 2 years.

137. (2) Family members who have been exposed are at high risk and should receive prophylactic therapy with INH and PAS. (b)

(1) Symptoms generally do not contribute significantly to a diagnosis of tuberculosis.

(3) Tubercle bacilli are not responsive to penicillin treatment.

(4) Prophylactic treatment is given to children with a high probability of exposure to tuberculosis.

138. (2) One practically universal characteristic of minimally brain damaged children is distractibility. They are highly reactive to any extraneous stimuli such as noise and movement and are unable to inhibit their responses to such stimuli. (c)

(1) Learning disabilities associated with minimal brain dysfunction are manifested in a variety of ways; loss of abstract thought is not a universal characteristic.

(3) Perseveration, the use of repetition in language or movement, is seen in some children.

(4) Delayed development of language skills is seen in varying degree and may include dyslexia (reading difficulty), dysgrammatism (speaking difficulty), and dysgraphia (writing difficulty) and/or delayed talking.

139. (2) Because of short attention span and distractibility, the specific limit setting consistently employed is

crucial toward providing an environment that promotes concentration, prevents confusion, and minimizes conflicts for the child. (a)

(1) Some children have difficulty reading.

(3) Questions are appropriate as long as alternatives are
limited.

(4) Parents need to manipulate the child's environment
so it is simplified, controlled, and predictable.

140. (4) Play during infancy (solitary) promotes physical development. For example, mobiles strengthen eye
movement, large beads promote fine finger movement, and soft toys encourage tactile sense. (a)

(1) Play during infancy is usually initiated by the parent.

(2) Children do not begin to share until the preschool
years.

(3) Play is important throughout childhood.

141. (3) Walking is the primary developmental task of this
age group. The other choices are not applicable to
this age group. (b)

(1) A child learns to use a spoon around 2 years of age.

(2) The ability to drink from a cup is not developed
until 18 months.

(4) Learning to walk takes precedence over learning to
talk; speaking is not a primary task at this age.

142. (1) Role playing encourages expression of feelings
through behavior, since children's ability to verbalize feelings is limited. (b)

(2) The preschooler is too young to think about careers.

(3) This may occur, but it is not a purpose of role playing.

(4) Although preschoolers may try to imitate adults,
providing guidelines for adult behavior is premature.

143. (1) Although there is a time range, there is no specific
time for a development task. (b)

(2) Children differ in the ages at which they learn tasks.

(3) Tasks are more often learned in spurts than at a uniform rhythm.

(4) The entire life cycle requires the learning of developmental tasks.

144. (2) If food is used early as praise or punishment, the
older child or adult will either undereat or overeat
at times of stress to decrease anxiety. (b)

(1) Eating is a social as well as a nutritional process.

(3) This does not usually cause nutritional problems.

(4) This is important for teaching good eating habits in
later life and, therefore preventing certain nutritional
problems.

145. (1) The early school–age child has become a cooperative member of the family and will mimic parents'
attitudes and food habits readily. (b)

(2) The peer group does not become highly influential
until later school age and during adolescence.

(3) This does not have a major influence on later eating
habits.

(4) This certainly has some influence, though not major, on later eating habits.

146. (4) When the causative organism is isolated, it is tested
for antimicrobial susceptibility (sensitivity) to various antimicrobial agents. When an organism is sensitive to a medication, the medication is capable of
destroying the organism. (b)

(1) Inappropriate answer.

(2) Although this is considered, the selection of drugs
is based primarily on the ability of the drug to destroy the specific organism.

(3) Although the physician's preference is considered,
the selection of drugs is based primarily on the ability of the drug to destroy the specific organism.

147. (2) The tetracyclines are not recommended during periods of tooth development (children under 8 years of
age or in pregnant women during the later half of
pregnancy) because they may permanently discolor
teeth yellow, gray, or brown. (b)

(1) This is not an expected complication of tetracycline.

(3) Anemia is not a common condition for 6-year-olds;
thrombocytopenia is a very rare complication.

(4) Tetracycline does not interfere with bone structure
of school-age children or pregnant women.

148. (1) Rubeola, or measles, is generally a viral-induced
childhood disease, diagnosed on or about the second
day by the presence of Koplik's spots on the oral
mucosa. (a)

(2) Rubella is manifested by a rash but not by Koplik's
spots.

(3) Chickenpox is manifested by a maculopapular rash;
no Koplik spots are present.

(4) Neither a rash nor Koplik's spots occur with
mumps.

149. (3) Invasion of the posterior (dorsal) root ganglia by the
same virus that causes chickenpox can result in
herpes zoster, or shingles. This may be due to reactivation of a previous chickenpox virus that has lain
dormant in the body or by fresh contact with an individual who has chickenpox. (a)

(1) Athlete's foot is caused by a fungus.

(2) Infectious hepatitis is caused by a virus, but not the
herpesvirus.

(4) German measles is caused by a virus, but not the
herpesvirus.

150. (4) Corticosteroids (e.g., cortisol) cause involution of
lymphatic tissue and resultant depression of the immune response. Antineoplastic drugs or high-energy
radiation preferentially destroys tissues with high
mitotic rates, including lymphatic tissue and bone
marrow, where antibody production and other immune responses take place. (a)

(1) Inappropriate answer; no more true for these than
for other children.

(2) This is not a reason to withhold immunizations.

(3) The measles vaccine does not contain rabbit serum.

151. (1) The injected bacteria in the vaccine have been so modified that they do not cause active infection but still elicit an immune response. (b)
(2) This is an antibody capable of neutralizing a specific toxin.
(3) This is a modified toxin, whose poisonous properties are destroyed but that is still capable of producing antibodies.
(4) This is a poisonous substance released from bacterial cells.

152. (4) In passive artificial immunity an antibody made in another organism is injected into the infected or presumed infected person to provide immediate immunity to the invading organism. (b)
(1) This type of immunity takes too much time to develop; this patient needs immediate protection.
(2) This type of immunity takes too much time to develop; this patient needs immediate protection.
(3) This type of immunity is probably not applicable in this case, for passive natural immunity is acquired from the mother and is effective only during the first few months of the child's life.

153. (1) In active, natural immunity the infected person's immune system responds to the invading organism by producing antibodies specific for the invader. (c)
(2) Active artificial immunity is acquired by the injection of antigens, after which the individual develops antibodies.
(3) Passive natural immunity is acquired by the fetus from the mother.
(4) Passive artificial immunity is acquired through injection of antibodies.

154. (1) Rubeola, or measles, produces coldlike respiratory symptoms and, after 3 or 4 days, a dark red macular or maculopapular skin rash. Complications include convulsions in young children and secondary infection with hemolytic streptococci, pneumococci, or staphylococci. Such infection can result in otitis media and pneumonia, which are especially dangerous in children under 2 years of age. (c)
(2) This is the most benign communicable disease of childhood; complications are rare.
(3) Yellow fever does not have respiratory complications.
(4) Chickenpox does not usually include respiratory inflammation, although pneumonia may occur as a complication.

155. (2) Adequate immunizations for normal preschool children include DTP and TOPV at 4 to 6 years. (c)
(1) Measles vaccine is normally given between 12 and 15 months of age.
(3) Rubella vaccine is normally given between 12 and 15 months of age.
(4) The tuberculin test is not an immunization.

156. (2) Antibodies received in utero through the placenta and in the newborn through the mother's milk provide the baby with immunity against most bac-

terial, viral, and fungal infections during the first several weeks after birth. Then, as the titer of maternal antibodies drops and is not replaced by the child's own antibodies, prolonged and repeated infection occurs. (a)
(1) This probably does not occur in children born without an immune system.
(3) Bacteria do not produce antibodies.
(4) This is not enough to prevent infection in these children.

157. (1) Since part of a nurse's responsibility is to foresee potential harm and prevent risks, it is imperative that the nurse not only take a health history and perform a physical assessment on each patient but also ensure the safety of the patient. (c)
(2) This is not true and cannot be accepted as a rationale for inaction.
(3) High temperatures are common in children but are nonetheless a valid cause for concern.
(4) The nurse and physician share interdependent roles in the assessment and care of patients.

158. (2) A common side effect of long-term phenytoin (Dilantin) therapy is hyperplasia of the gingiva. (c)
(1) Dilantin does not affect urinary output.
(3) Dilantin does not influence pupillary response.
(4) Dilantin does not cause flushing.

159. (1) Chickenpox, mumps, and rubeola are all caused by a virus and may be followed by encephalitis. (c)
(2) Pertussis is caused by a bacterium and does not result in encephalitis.
(3) Although polio is caused by a virus, it does not result in encephalitis.
(4) Scarlet fever is caused by a bacterium and does not result in encephalitis.

160. (3) Viral multiplication damages the anterior horn cells of the spinal cord with a typical irregular and asymmetric pattern. The cervical and lumbar regions contain more anterior horn cells, and therefore the extremities are more frequently affected than the trunk. (b)
(1) The virus for rubeola does not affect the motor cells of the anterior horn of the spinal cord.
(2) The virus for rubella does not affect the motor cells of the anterior horn of the spinal cord.
(4) The virus for chickenpox does not affect the motor cells of the anterior horn of the spinal cord.

161. (4) Rheumatic fever is an inflammatory disease involving the joints, heart, central nervous system, and subcutaneous tissue. It is believed to be an autoimmune process that causes connective tissue damage. (b)
(1) Whooping cough is not caused by a streptococcus and does not include the symptoms listed.
(2) Measles is caused by a virus and does not include the symptoms listed.
(3) Tetanus is not caused by a streptococcus and does not include the symptoms listed.

162. (4) Impetigo is a bacterial infection of the skin caused by streptococci or staphylococci. Group A hemolytic streptococci cause rheumatic fever and glomerulonephritis. (b)
     (1) This is a viral condition; not associated with rheumatic fever or glomerulonephritis.
     (2) This infectious condition of the skin is a result of infestation by mites; not associated with rheumatic fever or glomerulonephritis.
     (3) Intertrigo is a superficial dermatitis in the folds of the skin; not associated with rheumatic fever or glomerulonephritis.

163. (3) Respiratory tract obstructions usually occur in the larynx, trachea, or major bronchi (usually right). Hoarseness may indicate vocal cord injury. Unintelligible speech may indicate an interference in the flow of air out of the respiratory tract and/or obstruction or injury to the larynx. (b)
     (1) Acute respiratory infection usually has a gradual onset.
     (2) In view of the sudden onset of clinical signs and the age of the child, this is unlikely.
     (4) A retropharyngeal abscess would not produce the clinical signs listed.

164. (2) Thrush, also called moniliasis, usually affects the mucous membranes of the oral cavity, causing painful white patches. Individuals with immunologic deficiencies or those receiving prolonged antibiotic therapy are particularly susceptible to this organism. (b)
     (1) This is not caused by yeast, nor does it occur often in infants.
     (3) This is not caused by yeast and is not common in the U.S. or in infants.
     (4) This is usually caused by an ameba or a bacterium; is not common in infants.

165. (2) Grunting and rapid respirations are abnormal behaviors in the infant. Grunting is a compensatory mechanism whereby the infant attempts to keep air in the alveoli to increase arterial oxygenation; increased respirations increase the amount of oxygen and carbon dioxide exchange. (b)
     (1) This is not necessarily a sign of illness.
     (3) Sweating in infants is usually scanty because of immature functioning of the exocrine glands; profuse sweating is rarely seen in the sick infant.
     (4) This is not necessarily indicative of illness.

166. (4) In heart failure there is a decrease in the blood flow to the kidneys, causing sodium and water reabsorption and resulting in peripheral edema. The peripheral edema indicates severe cardiac decompensation. (b)
     (1) This may be an early attempt by the body to compensate for decreased cardiac output.
     (2) This may be an early attempt by the body to compensate for decreased cardiac output.
     (3) This may be an early attempt by the body to compensate for decreased cardiac output.

167. (2) Crying increases the amount of air being brought into the lungs. The flow of air coming into the lungs creates an increase in positive pressure, which helps expand the alveoli and improve gaseous exchange, thereby decreasing cyanosis. In atelectasis some of the alveoli do not expand, which is evidenced by a lack of chest expansion on the affected side. (c)
     (1) Decreasing cyanosis with crying is not indicative of neurologic damage.
     (3) The heart rate will not provide information about atrioventricular septal defects.
     (4) The signs of respiratory distress syndrome are much more severe than transient cyanosis.

168. (3) Chalasia is an incompetent cardiac sphincter, which allows a reflux of gastric contents into the esophagus and eventual regurgitation. Placing the infant in an upright position keeps the gastric contents in the stomach by gravity as well as limits the pressure against the cardiac sphincter. (b)
     (1) This will promote regurgitation.
     (2) This will probably have little effect on chalasia.
     (4) This will promote vomiting since it is too much formula for a week-old infant.

169. (2) Assault is a threat or an attempt to do violence to another. (c)
     (1) This is not the appropriate legal definition of assault.
     (3) Assault implies harm to persons rather than property.
     (4) This definition is too broad to describe assault.

170. (3) Battery means touching in an offensive manner or the actual injuring of another person. (b)
     (1) This definition is too broad to describe battery.
     (2) Battery refers to harm against persons instead of property.
     (4) Battery refers to actual bodily harm rather than threats of physical or psychologic harm.

171. (1) Because phenylalanine is an essential amino acid, it must be provided in quantities sufficient for promoting growth while maintaining safe blood levels. (c)
     (2) Phenylalanine is an essential amino acid and cannot be totally removed from the diet.
     (3) In PKU phenylalanine accumulates in the blood, causing irreversable CNS damage; additional phenylalanine must be avoided.
     (4) All proteins do not contain phenylalanine.

172. (2) Congenital cretinism is the result of insufficient secretion by the thyroid gland due to an embryonic defect. The decreased thyroid hormone has been affecting the infant since before birth during cerebral development, so it is likely that mental development will be retarded. Treatment prior to 3 months will limit damage. (b)
     (1) Myxedema is an alternate term for cretinism.
     (3) Treatment corrects abnormal responses.
     (4) This is a term for hyperthyroidism.

173. (2) $\dfrac{0.35 \text{ mg}}{0.25 \text{ mg}} \times \dfrac{x \text{ minims}}{15 \text{ minims}} = 21 \text{ minims}$ (b)

(15 or 16 minims = 1 ml)

(1) This is too low.
(3) This is too low.
(4) This is too low.

174. (3) This is due to the fact that celiac patients have a gluten-induced enteropathy and are unable to absorb fats from the intestinal tract. (b)
(1) Although stools are large and frothy, they lack color because of incomplete absorption.
(2) Stools are large and fatty or frothy, not mucoid.
(4) Stools are foul smelling, in large quantities, and without color because of incomplete absorption.

175. (1) Rubeola signs and symptoms include a high fever, photophobia, Koplik's spots (white patches on mucous membranes of the oral cavity), and a rash. Rubella usually does not cause a high fever, runs a 3-to-6-day course, and never causes Koplik's spots. (c)
(2) Some symptoms may be similar to those of a severe cold, but are associated with high fever.
(3) These symptoms are not associated with rubeola.
(4) The rash spreads over most of the body.

176. (1) Infants are almost 85% water in composition. An elevated temperature causes increased absorption of fluid via the bowel and may upset the balance of fluid. It could also interfere with potassiumion balance, the electrolyte that can be lost via the large intestine. (a)
(2) Preschoolers fear intrusive procedures.
(3) The temperature of the water should be regulated so this does not occur.
(4) The enema would remove only waste products from the bowel.

177. (2) Steroids have an antiinflammatory effect. It is believed that resistance to certain viral diseases, including chickenpox, is greatly decreased when the child is taking steroids regularly. (b)
(1) Since chickenpox is viral, antibiotics would have no effect.
(3) There is no known correlation between chickenpox and these drugs.
(4) There is no known correlation between chickenpox and insulin.

178. (3) Mumps can cause orchitis (inflammation of the testes) in males and oophoritis (inflammation of the ovaries) in females. Although rare, both can render the postpubescent child sterile. (b)
(1) This symptom is not associated with mumps.
(2) This symptom is not associated with mumps.
(4) This symptom is not associated with mumps.

179. (3) Assault is a threat or an attempt to do violence to another, and battery means touching an individual in an offensive manner or the actual injuring of another person. (a)

(1) Although the behavior (scratching) needs to be decreased, this can be done through mittens so as not to immobilize this age of child.
(2) A 3-year-old does not have the capacity to understand cause (scratching) and effect (bleeding).
(4) The nurse's behavior demonstrates anger and has not taken into account the growth and developmental needs of this age.

180. (4) Tetracycline is potentially hepatotoxic, especially in anyone with liver dysfunction, since it is metabolized in the liver. Signs of hepatotoxicity are lethargy, anorexia, behavioral changes, jaundice, and fatty necrosis. (c)
(1) The decreasing fever and secretions indicate that the infectious process is under control.
(2) Anemia may cause fatigue but is unassociated with withdrawal and irritability.
(3) Common symptoms of bladder infection include burning upon urination, frequency or hesitancy, abdominal pain, and low-grade fever.

181. (3) Decision making fosters and supports independence, a developmental need of the adolescent. It also increases a sense of self-worth and control. (b)
(1) Although this may be true, it is not motivating.
(2) This does not ensure movement but social interaction.
(4) Limit setting meets the security needs of young children.

182. (3) A plaster cast is not flexible and can inhibit circulation. Cold toes, loss of sensation in toes, pain, and inability to move toes should be reported to the physician immediately. (b)
(1) The normal pulse for a 9-year-old ranges from 70 to 110.
(2) It takes 24 to 48 hours for a plaster cast to dry.
(4) This may be related to increased fluid intake.

183. (4) Mineral oil coats the mucosal lining of the stomach and retards absorption of the poison. (c)
(1) Soap, baking soda, and milk of magnesia are all chemical antidotes that neutralize ingested acids.
(2) Strong tea only dilutes the substance to be absorbed and wastes precious treatment time.
(3) A weak salt solution provides no effective immediate treatment.

184. (3) Lye, a basic solution, is neutralized by administration of a weak acid such as vinegar. (c)
(1) This induces vomiting and would cause further burning of tissue when the lye was vomited back through the esophagus.
(2) Milk is useful to soothe irritated mucous membrane but will not inactivate the poison.
(4) Bicarbonate is used to neutralize acids.

185. (2) Ipecac exerts its effect through direct stimulation of the vomiting control center and local irritation of the gastric mucosa, which is enhanced through dilution of the drug in large quantities of fluid. (c)
(1) Resting has no effect on drug efficiency.

(3) The child should be kept calm and quiet.

(4) Ipecac works by stimulating the vomiting control center and local gastric irritation.

186. (3) Prednisone is a synthetic glucocorticoid that has an active antiinflammatory effect by stabilizing lysosomal membranes and thus inhibiting proteolytic enzyme release. (b)

(1) Prednisone has an antiinflammatory effect, which inhibits proteolytic enzyme release.

(2) Prednisone's antiinflammatory effects include inhibiting phagocytosis and preventing or suppressing other clinical evidence of inflammation.

(4) Increased appetite and aggravation of preexisting psychiatric conditions are adverse reactions of prednisone.

187. (1) Vincristine is highly neurotoxic, causing paresthesias, muscle weakness, ptosis, diplopia, paralytic ileus, vocal cord paralysis, and loss of deep tendon reflexes. (c)

(2) Alopecia is reversible with cessation of the drug.

(3) Hematologic effects are rare with vincristine.

(4) The most severe problems associated with vincristine are neurologic and neuromuscular.

188. (4) Excessive crying and clinging are the usual responses of an infant who expects to be comforted, not one who has been separated from a parent because of illness. (a)

(1) Prolonged hospitalization and separation from parenting can cause delayed growth or even death in infants.

(2) Inattentiveness to focus may be learned from failure to gain reponses from humans in previous experiences.

(3) Withdrawing active attention is the infant's way to "turn off" and may be learned from multiple failure in interactions with stimuli.

189. (2) Infants who have experienced maternal deprivation usually exhibit failure to thrive (i.e., weight below third percentile, developmental retardation, clinical signs of deprivation, and malnutrition). These physical and emotional factors predispose the infant to a variety of illness. (b)

(1) Infants who have experienced maternal deprivation are usually quiet and nonresponsive.

(3) Responsiveness to stimuli is limited or nonexistant.

(4) Weight below the third percentile is characteristic.

190. (2)

$$\frac{20 \text{ mg}}{50 \text{ mg}} \times \frac{x}{15 \text{ minims}}$$

$$50x = 300$$
$$x = 6 \text{ minims}$$
(15 or 16 minims = 1 ml) (a)

(1) This calculation is too low.

(3) This calculation is too high.

(4) This calculation is too high.

191. (1) This defect interferes with the normal diaphragmatic respirations of the newborn. Respirations are further affected by stomach and intestinal distension, a mediastinal shift, atelectasis, and the presence of abdominal organs in the thoracic cavity. Oxygen should be administered via positive pressure by a nonintrusive means such as mask or hood. (c)

(2) An intratracheal tube would be used when there is a concern of upper respiratory or other interference with oxygen reaching the lungs adequately.

(3) The least intrusive method which adequately delivers oxygen should be used.

(4) The defect interferes with normal respirations so oxygen is needed.

192. (4) Following a thoracotomy, negative intrathoracic pressure is reestablished and the alveoli reexpand within 12 to 48 hours. (b)

(1) This time is inadequate for reexpansion to occur.

(2) In some instances, reexpansion will occur sooner than 48 hours.

(3) This time is inadequate for expecting reexpansion.

193. (3)

$$\frac{\text{Total milliliters to be infused} \times \text{Drop factor}}{\text{Total time to be infused in minutes}}$$

$$\frac{1000 \times 60}{1440} \times \frac{60000}{1440} = 41.6 \text{ drops/minute}$$ (a)

(1) Calculations show this is too low to deliver 1000 ml in 24 hours.

(2) Calculations show this is too low to deliver 1000 ml in 24 hours.

(4) Calculations show this is too low to deliver 1000 ml in 24 hours.

194. (3) When the nurse takes a health history, any areas of concern should be explored fully before a nursing diagnosis is made. (a)

(1) Data are inadequate to focus immediately on nutrition.

(2) The nurse needs to gather more data to be able to determine the basis for the problem.

(4) More data are needed before recommendations can be made.

195. (2) Normally there may be a weight gain caused by the influence of hormones prior to the growth spurt. Also, 10-to-12-year olds eat an adult-size meal without the increased metabolic needs of adolescence. (b)

(1) This weight gain is normal and adequate calorie intake is needed for the growth spurt occuring in adolescents.

(3) Before advising increased activity, the nurse would need to assess Harry's present activity level.

(4) Family eating patterns have more effect on weight than do genetics.

196. (1) Hepatitis virus B is in the blood during the late incubation and acute stages of the disease. It may also persist in the carrier state for years. It is transmitted

when the blood of an infected individual comes in contact with the blood or mucous membranes of another individual. Posttransfusion hepatitis has been reduced now that the surface antigen of hepatitis B (HBsAg) can be identified in the blood of carriers of type B virus. (a)

(2) Hepatitis A is principally transferred through oral-fecal routes.

(3) Although the virus may persist in carriers, the principal mode of transmission is parenteral.

(4) Oral and venereal transmission is a less frequent mode of transmission.

197. (3) Positioning on the right side after feeding facilitates digestion because the pyloric sphincter is on this side and gravity aids in emptying the stomach. (c)

(1) The usual height for elevation of the gastrostomy tube when feeding an infant is 6 to 8 inches.

(2) It is standard procedure to flush the tube after the feeding to ensure that all the formula gets into the stomach.

(4) Feeding may proceed immediately after opening the tube.

198. (3) A pacifier should be given during the feeding to help the infant associate sucking with feeding and the sense of fullness. (b)

(1) Instilling water after the feeding clears the tube.

(2) Although aspiration may be used to ascertain residual stomach content before feeding, it is not necessary when feedings are well tolerated.

(4) Upright positioning is essential to prevent regurgitation or reflux and subsequent aspiration.

199. (3) Isotonic saline is compatible with body fluids. It is neither hypertonic nor hypotonic so it does not cause a change in osmotic pressure and upset the balance of intracellular and extracellular fluid and electrolytes. (b)

(1) Soap suds enemas are water with added soap products and therefore usually hypotonic; this can cause fluid shifts and overloads.

(2) This solution would cause excess fluid loss and therefore be dangerous.

(4) This hypotonic solution might cause fluid and electrolyte imbalances.

200. (4) Amblyopia is reduced visual acuity that may occur when an eye weakened by strabismus is not forced to function. (c)

(1) Only vision in the affected eye will be diminished.

(2) Depth and spatial perceptions are impaired when vision in one eye is severly impaired.

(3) The lack of binocularity could result in impaired depth and spatial perceptions, not dyslexia.

4

Maternity Nursing

This section, maternity nursing, covers reproductive problems and emphasizes the pubertal changes of adolescence; the normal processes of conception, embryologic development, pregnancy, labor, delivery, and postpartum developments; and family planning. In addition, the newborn and the mother are discussed in relation to prematurity, birth injuries, and complications of labor and delivery. Current topics such as abortion, infant narcotic addiction, venereal disease, and sterility are included.

Childbirth is a family experience. Humanity's basic needs for survival are centered in the family because without continuous love, physical contact, food, and stimulation of the senses, the infant would never survive. As each new member becomes a part of the family unit, interactions with the environment and other human beings become a part of early physical and emotional development. What is learned is determined by the kinds of stimulation received from the interactions occurring within the family. It is through this reciprocal give-and-take between the newborn and the family that each person becomes an individual, unique self.

Although childbearing patterns differ the world over, there are constants. In order of priority, they are: immediate physical contact between the infant and the parents; ability of the parents to give the infant love, food, and protection from the environment; the biologic need in men and women to reproduce; and the maturation and growth process that occurs in males and females in their changing roles as parents.

The unique and changing responsibilities in the life cycle event of parenthood can be a real crisis. The changes occurring in society, whether social, economic, technical, or political, directly affect the patterns of childbearing and childrearing. Parenthood today is given serious thought, since it concerns both the family and society with the emphasis on quality rather than quantity.

PUBERTY

A period during which the organs of reproduction mature and are prepared for their reproductive function

A. Physical and physiologic changes
1. In males
   a. Occur between 10 and 14 years of age; less dramatic than in female
   b. Heralded by deepening of voice and growth of body hair on the face, axillae, and genitalia
   c. Second year after onset—increased activity of sweat glands, spermatogenesis occurs with periodic erections and emissions of mature sperm
   d. Dramatic body growth spurt
   e. Ejaculation is beginning of fertility and end of puberty
2. In females
   a. Occur between 9 and 13 years of age
   b. Sudden enlargement of the breasts, growth of body hair on the axillae und genitalia; changes in size and vascularity of internal reproductive organs
   c. Heralded by first menstrual flow, called *menarche;* unlike the male's first ejaculation, many first menstrual cycles are anovulatory (infertile)
   d. Dramatic body growth more evident than in male
B. Psychologic changes
1. Age differences in maturation
2. Heterosexual interests—girls earlier than boys, girls interested in older boys

3. Emancipation struggles with parents—independence versus dependence
4. Need for belonging to a peer group
C. Menstrual cycle
1. Rhythmic reproductive cycle in females extending from the onset of a period of uterine bleeding to the onset of the next period of bleeding; mean cycle length is 28 days; normal range is 20 to 45 days per cycle
2. During each cycle several (about 20) follicles commence maturation, but usually only one reaches full maturity and ruptures its contained ovum (and some surrounding granulosa cells) into the abdominal cavity
3. The rhythmic menstrual cycles begin at puberty and cease at menopause
4. Menstrual cycle divided into 3 stages based on endometrial histologic makeup and may be correlated with concentration fluctuations in hypothalamic, hypophyseal, and ovarian hormones (which cause the endometrial and other reproductive tract histologic changes)
   a. First stage—menstruation or menses—lasts 4 to 6 days; characterized by endometrial hemorrhage with the discharge exiting through the vagina; estrogen and progesterone blood levels are relatively low; the FSH level is elevated and, combined with a steady low level of LH secretion, initiates ovarian estrogen secretion, leading to the second stage
   b. Second stage—follicular or proliferative—lasts 8 to 10 days culminating in ovulation; endometrium repairs and proliferates in preparation for possible implantation, and a single ovarian follicle approaches full maturation as the concentration of estradiol (the principal estrogenic hormone) in the blood rises; estradiol exerts a negative feedback on FSH secretion and a positive feedback on LH secretion (the latter hormone induces ovulation); estradiol's feedback effects are exerted on the hypothalamic secretion of FSH-RH and LH-RH (which control the hypophyseal secretion of FSH and LH)
   c. Third stage—luteal or secretory—final stage is 9 to 13 days and begins after ovulation; LH promotes formation of a temporary endocrine gland, the corpus luteum, from the ruptured follicle: granulosa and theca interna cells of follicle enlarge, divide into and occupy the cavity (antrum) of the follicle, and secrete progesterone and estrogen; progesterone stimulates the already proliferated endometrium to become glandular with a high glycogen-secreting potential (uterus now prepared for implantation); if fertilization does not occur, the corpus luteum functions for 7 to 8 days after ovulation and then involutes, becoming nonfunctional (corpus albicans) 10 to 12 days after ovulation; progesterone and estrogen blood levels drop, the negative feedback effect of estradiol on FSH is released, and the first stage begins again

MATERNITY CYCLE
Antepartal Period

A. Maturation, fertilization, and implantation
1. Maturation of ovum and sperm by mitosis and meiosis; reduction in chromosome number from 46 to 23
2. Fertilization occurs when ovum and sperm unite in distal portion of fallopian tube
3. Rapid division by cleavage without increase in cell size in 6 days (morula stage)
4. Implantation within 6 to 9 days generally in upper fundal portion of the uterus; in this blastocyst stage cells are arranged into 3 layers; ectoderm, mesoderm, endoderm
5. Trophoblastic stage—projection of villi into maternal tissue, later to become placenta, vehicle for exchange of nutrients and wastes
B. Growth and development of the baby (cephalocaudal)
1. 14 days—heart begins to beat; brain, early spinal cord, and muscle segments present
2. 26 days–tiny buds for arms appear
3. 28 days–tiny buds for legs appear
4. 30 days—embryo ¼ to ½ inch (0.6 to 1.2 cm) in length, definite form, beginning of umbilical cord is visible
5. 31 days—arm buds develop into hands, arms, and shoulders
6. 33 days—finger outlines present
7. 46 to 48 days—cartilage in upper arms replaced by first bone cells, amniotic fluid surrounds the fetus (amniotic fluid is a protective cushion, equalizes pressures, and facilitates the baby's movements for adequate growth and development)
8. 3 months (12 weeks)—fetus moves body parts, swallows, practices inhaling and exhaling, weighs 28 g (1 oz)
9. 4 to 5 months (16 to 20 weeks)—fetal movements felt by mother (known as quickening), weighs 170 g (6 oz), is 20 to 25 cm (8 to 10 inches) in length

10. 5 to 6 months (20 to 24 weeks)—hair growth on head, eyelashes and brow, skeleton hardens, eyelids closed, weighs 0.45 kg (1 lb), is 30.5 cm (12 inches) in length, fetal heart audible with fetoscope
11. 6 to 7 months (24 to 28 weeks)—eyelids open, amniotic fluid increases to 1 quart with a daily exchange of 6 gallons, weighs 0.5 kg (1¼ lb)
12. 7 to 8 months (28 to 32 weeks)—many fat deposits, weighs 0.45 to 0.7 kg (1 to 1½ lb)
13. 8 to 9 months (32 to 36 weeks)—stores protein for extrauterine life, gains 1.81 kg (4 lb)
C. Fetal circulation—differs from adult because of following accessory structures
   1. Placenta
      a. Organ of dual origin (maternal and embryonic portions) serving interchange of food and wastes between mother and embryo (or fetus) during pregnancy
      b. Villous portion of the chorion (chorion frondosum) and the portion of the uterine endometrium (called the decidua during pregnancy) directly underlying the implanted embryo (decidua basalis) constitute the placenta: chorionic villi project into placental sinuses (in decidua basalis) filled with maternal blood
      c. Placenta functions as the fetal digestive tract and also as fetal lungs, kidneys, and as a major endocrine gland (producing estrogens, progesterone, ACTH, growth hormone, and gonadotropic hormones HCG and HPL) (see endocrine system)
   2. Umbilical cord
      a. Inserted close to the central portion of the placenta and attached to fetus
      b. Has 1 vein (which transports nourishment) and 2 arteries (which transport wastes) between the mother and baby
      c. Wharton's jelly, a protective covering, surrounds the entire cord
   3. Foramen ovale is an opening between the right and left atria during fetal life, bypassing fetal lungs
   4. Ductus arteriosus is a connection between pulmonary trunk and aorta, also bypassing fetal lungs
   5. Ductus venosus is a connection between umbilical vein and ascending vena cava, bypassing fetal liver
   6. As a result of previously mentioned structures all blood in fetal heart is mixed blood; less than maximal O_2 saturation
   7. Only oxygenated blood in the fetus is at the immediate entrance of the umbilical vessel on entering the liver
D. Physical and physiologic changes in the mother during pregnancy; pregnancy is a normal physiologic process that affects all body systems and results in both objective and subjective changes; it is a stressful time requiring many adaptations
   1. Endocrine and reproductive systems
      a. Fatigue is a result of increased hormonal levels causing sodium and water retention and relaxation of smooth muscles
      b. Amenorrhea occurs, since the corpus luteum persists and ovulation is inhibited by the high levels of circulating estrogen and progesterone
      c. Breast changes such as fullness, tingling, soreness, darkening of the areolae and nipples occur along with an increase in hormonal levels
      d. Leukorrhea is increased as hormonal levels rise, and the increased acidity is a protection from bacterial invasion
      e. Changes in the uterus are circulatory, hormonal, and related to fetal growth
         (1) Softening of the cervix—Goodell's sign
         (2) Softening of the lower uterine segment—Hegar's sign
         (3) Purplish hue to the vaginal mucosa—Chadwick's sign
         (4) Changes in position of the uterus—first trimester uterus is in pelvic cavity, second and third trimester uterus is in abdominal cavity before lightening occurs
   2. Digestive system
      a. Reduction in hydrochloric acid interferes with gastric motility, causing nausea and vomiting
      b. Constipation is secondary to hypoperistalsis, lack of fluids, poor dietary habits, pressure of the enlarged uterus on internal organs, and effects of progesterone on muscle
   3. Excretory system
      a. Proximity of the uterus and bladder in early and late pregnancy causes urinary frequency
      b. Bladder tone is reduced by effects of hormones on smooth muscle
      c. Bladder capacity increases gradually to 1500 ml
      d. Increased urinary output results in lowered specific gravity
      e. Increased excretion of sugar caused by lowered renal threshold

f. Presence of gonadotropic hormones in the urine (used as basis for pregnancy tests)

4. Circulatory system
   a. Physiologic anemia occurs as a result of increased blood volume with no proportional increase in red blood cells
   b. Cardiac output increases 25% to 50% during pregnancy, peaking at 7 or 8 months
   c. Heart rate increases 10 beats per minute in the latter half of pregnancy—approximately 14,000 extra beats in 24 hours
   d. Edema of extremities common in the last 6 weeks of pregnancy because of stasis of blood
   e. Leg cramps are believed to result from an imbalance of the calcium/phosphorus ratio in the body and from pressure of the gravid uterus on nerves supplying lower extremities

5. Respiratory system
   a. At 36 to 38 weeks, pressure of the enlarged uterus on diaphragm and lungs may cause dyspnea that subsides when lightening occurs
   b. Oxygen consumption is increased by about 15% between the sixteenth and fortieth weeks, although there may be only a slight increase in vital capacity during pregnancy

6. Integumentary system
   a. Excretion of wastes through the skin causes diaphoresis
   b. Skin changes—darkening of the areolae, darkening patches on the face (chloasma), linea alba becomes nigra on the abdomen, striae on the abdomen and legs caused by skin stretching as pregnancy advances, erythematous changes on the palms and face in some women

7. Skeletal system—a softening of all ligaments and joints especially pubic symphysis and sacroiliac joint) caused by increased hormonal action of estrogens and relaxin

8. Nervous system—no specific changes unless related to nonpregnant state or stress of pregnancy

E. Course, signs, and diagnosis of pregnancy
   1. Estimated date of delivery—Naegele's rule—count back 3 months from the first day of the last normal menstrual period and add 7 days (9 calendar months, 270 days, or 10 lunar months, 290 days)
   2. Estimated gestational age—noninvasive techniques
      a. Fundal height
      b. Serum estriols
      c. Ultrasonography—term pregnancy can be diagnosed if biparietal diameter is greater than 9.8 cm
      d. Radiography (rarely done)—presence of distal femoral ossification centers indicate fetal age of 36 weeks; if proximal tibial centers are present, fetal age is 40 weeks
   3. Estimated gestational age—direct invasive techniques

      Amniocentesis—lecithin/sphyngomyelin ratio greater than 2 indicates adequate lung maturity for extrauterine life; if optical density of bilirubinoid pigments is 450 mm <0.01, gestational age is greater than 38 weeks; elevated creatinine levels also indicate fetal maturity
   4. Positive signs of pregnancy are auscultation of fetal heart tones (fetoscope or Doppler ultrasound), palpation of fetal parts, roentgenogram of fetal skeleton, and ultrasound scanning of fetus
   5. Diagnostic pregnancy tests—urine of pregnant women used to detect chorionic gonadotropin
      a. Animal tests—Friedman's, Aschheim-Zondek
      b. Chemical—Pregnosticon, Gravindex, or radioimmunoassay for chorionic gonadotropin

Prenatal Period

A. Medical supervision during pregnancy
   1. History, including medical, surgical, gynecologic and obstetric data; family history of hereditary and transmittable diseases such as diabetes, tuberculosis, heart disease
   2. Physical examination of the skin, thyroid, teeth, lungs, heart, and breasts, abdominal palpation, auscultation, height of fundus, vaginal examination, and pelvic evaluation (prior to last 4 weeks of pregnancy)
   3. Smears taken for monilial and trichomonal infections, Papanicolaou test done for cancer
   4. Blood pressure; weight; and urinalysis for acetone, albumin, and sugar done at intervals
   5. Blood specimens taken for typing, cross matching, Rh factor, serologic test for syphilis, and rubella titer; in addition, for black women, a sickle cell test should be done

B. Nutritional needs during pregnancy
   1. Consideration of preconceptional nutritional status; age and parity of mother, biologic interactions between mother, fetus, and placenta; and individual needs such as in times of stress

2. Weight gain should be evaluated with regard to the quality of gain (Is weight gain caused by edema or fat deposition?)
3. Severe caloric restriction during pregnancy is contraindicated, since it is a potential hazard to the mother and fetus
4. Weight reduction should never be started as a regimen during pregnancy
5. Restriction of sodium and administration of diuretics are potentially dangerous to the mother and fetus during pregnancy
6. Nausea and vomiting—limited fluids with meals, small frequent feedings, restricted fats, high carbohydrate
7. Constipation—increased fluids and residue or fiber; appropriate activity level
8. Consideration of the demands of pregnancy related to growth and development of the fetus during the various trimesters; provide adequate nutrition to meet increased maternal and fetal nutrient demands
    a. Increased calories to meet increased basal metabolic needs and spare protein for growth, to promote weight gain to support pregnancy (averages 11.4 kg, or 25 lb, but is individual according to need), and for lactation
    b. Increased protein to provide for growth demands
    c. Increased vitamins, especially folic acid supplement to prevent anemia
    d. Increased minerals with supplement of iron to prevent anemia
    e. Iodized salt to provide needed sodium and iodine
9. Lactating mother needs additional caloric requirements
10. Dietary assessment should be an integral part of prenatal care for every pregnant woman
11. Changes in dietary regimen should consider cultural, economic, and psychologic implications of food habits
12. Food guide may be based on basic 4 groups with
    a. Increased protein foods—1 qt milk, 2 eggs, 2 servings of meat, added cheese
    b. Additional servings from each of the remaining food groups—grains, vegetables, fruits
    c. Additional calories, protein, and fluids during lactation
C. Nursing goals to prepare parents for childbirth
    1. Assist the parents in understanding the anatomy and physiology of pregnancy, labor, and delivery
    2. Help the parents discuss and explore feelings related to childbearing and childrearing in attempting to alleviate fears
    3. Prepare the mother for the physical work of labor through the use of muscle and breathing exercises for the various phases of labor
    4. Identify parents' situational support systems
    5. Prepare the father for a coaching and supporting role during pregnancy, labor, and delivery
    6. Introduce families to health facilities available for continued health care of the family
    7. Discuss various childbirth preparation techniques such as Lamaze, Reade, and Bradley

Intrapartal Period

A. Labor—physiologic and mechanical process in which the baby, placenta, and fetal membranes are propelled through the pelvis and expelled from the birth canal
B. Anatomy of the bony pelvis
    1. Parts—ischium, ilium, sacrum, coccyx
    2. Joints—sacroiliacs, sacrococcygeal, symphysis pubis (all soften during pregnancy)
    3. Divisions—false pelvis supports the enlarged uterus in the abdominal cavity; true pelvis is the bony inner pelvis through which the baby must pass
    4. Diameters—at inlet: true conjugate (anteroposterior diameter), transverse (widest diameter at inlet), right and left oblique diameters; at outlet: conjugate diagonal (anteroposterior is widest diameter), transverse (one ischial tuberosity to the other)
    5. Classification of pelvis—gynecoid (normal female pelvis), android (male pelvis), anthropoid, and platypelloid
    6. Normal female pelvis has an ample pubic arch, curved sacrum, curved side walls, blunt ischial spines, and a movable coccyx
C. Attitude—relationship of fetal parts to each other
D. Presentation—baby's body part that engages in the true pelvis
    1. Cephalic (head)—vertex, brow, or face
    2. Breech—frank, complete, single, or double footling
    3. Shoulder—must be turned for delivery
E. Position—relationship of presenting parts to 4 quadrants of the mother's pelvis (the letters L and R are used for left or right; A and P for anterior or posterior; O for occiput; M for mentum or face; S for sacrum)

1. Vertex—occiput, L.O.A., L.O.P., R.O.A., R.O.P.
2. Face—chin (mentum), L.M.A., L.M.P., R.M.A., R.M.P.
3. Breech—sacrum, L.S.A., L.S.P., R.S.A., R.S.P.

F. Station—relationship of presenting part to the false and true pelves
   1. Floating—presenting part movable above the true pelvic inlet
   2. Engaged—suboccipitobregmatic diameter fixed into the pelvic inlet
   3. Station O—presenting part at level of the ischial spines—levels below spines +1, +2, +3; levels above spines −1, −2, −3

G. Signs and symptoms prior to true labor
   1. Lightening—baby drops down into the true pelvis
   2. Mother experiences Braxton Hicks contractions—painless tryout contractions in preparation for true labor
   3. Increased vaginal secretions
   4. Softening of cervix

H. Signs and symptoms of true labor
   1. Uterine contractions that increase in frequency, strength, and duration
   2. Bloody show—pressure of the presenting part on the cervix causes effacement and dilation of the cervix
   3. Rupture of the membranes

I. Mechanisms of labor—rotation of vertex presentation through the true pelvis
   1. Engagement, descent with flexion—at onset of labor, head descends and chin flexes on the chest
   2. Internal rotation—as labor contractions and uterine forces move the baby downward, the head internally rotates to pass through the ischial spines
   3. Extension—occiput emerges under the symphysis pubis and the head is delivered by extension
   4. External rotation—to allow for rotation of the shoulders to an anteroposterior position
   5. Lateral flexion—allows for delivery of the shoulders and body

J. Stages of labor
   1. First stage—from the onset of true labor to complete effacement and dilation of the cervix
   2. Second stage—from complete effacement and dilation of the cervix to birth of the baby
   3. Third stage—from birth of the baby through expulsion of the placenta
   4. Fourth stage—first hour following delivery

K. Changes in mother during labor
   1. First stage
      a. Latent phase—irregular contractions, cervix dilated 0 to 2 cm, mother excited and happy that labor has started, some apprehension
      b. Active phase—moderate to strong contractions 5 to 8 minutes apart, cervix dilates from 2 to 6 cm, bloody show, membranes may rupture, breathing techniques help in relaxing, medication may be necessary for discomfort, supportive measures by the husband or nurse (e.g., encouragement, praise, reassurance, keeping the mother informed of progress, providing rest between contractions, presence of a supporting person) help
      c. Transition phase—strong contractions 1 to 2 minutes apart (often last 60 to 90 seconds each with little or no rest in between), bloody show, mother becomes irritable, restless, agitated, highly emotional, belches, has leg tremors, perspires, pale white ring around mouth (circumoral pallor), flushed face, sudden nausea, and vomiting; generally lasts less than an hour
   2. Second stage—beginning with full dilation of the cervix and ending with birth of the baby, perineum bulges, pushing with contractions, grunting sounds, behavior changes from great irritability to great involvement and work, sleep and relaxation occur between contractions, leg cramps are common

L. Nursing care during labor and delivery
   1. Emotional support by the husband, nurse, or significant others
   2. Maintenance of asepsis
   3. Timing frequency, duration, and strength of contractions
   4. Auscultation or monitoring of fetal heart sounds as to rate, regularity, variability, accelerations, and early and late decelerations
   5. Positioning the mother on her left side to avoid supine hypotension to increase uterine perfusion
   6. Frequent observation of the perineum for show, rupture of membranes, and presenting part
   7. Check vital signs at frequent intervals
   8. Emergency equipment available for safe care of the mother and baby such as oxygen, blood, drugs
   9. Assessment of basic needs such as body fluids, bladder and bowel function
   10. Assist the mother with breathing techniques throughout labor

M. Induction and control of uterine contractions by pharmacologic agents
1. Oxytocin (Pitocin, Syntocinon, Uteracon)
    a. Used to induce labor by stimulation of characteristic rhythmic contraction and relaxation of the uterine muscles
    b. Administered IM after delivery of the anterior shoulder or IV after delivery of the baby to provide uterine contractions that complete expulsion of uterine contents and decrease bleeding from endometrial sites
2. Sparteine sulfate (Spartocin, Tocosamine)
    a. Used to stimulate uterine muscle contraction when inertia occurs during labor
    b. Adverse effects—lengthens the refractory period of cardiac muscle and may cause bradycardia
N. Danger signs and symptoms during labor
1. Tonic, strong, continuous contractions with sharp abdominal pain and, on palpation, abdomen taut and boardlike
2. Variations in rate, regularity, and tone of fetal heart sounds
3. Meconium-stained or excessive amount of amniotic fluid
4. Elevation or drop in blood pressure
5. Increase in pulse or temperature
6. Sudden excessive fetal movements
7. Bleeding, protrusion of umbilical cord or placenta
O. Nursing care immediately after delivery
1. Mother
    a. Palpate the fundus frequently for firmness and height in relation to umbilicus
    b. Keep the airway open if inhalation anesthesia has been given
    c. Monitor blood pressure and pulse; report fluctuations
    d. Check the perineum for vaginal and suture line bleeding
    e. Administer an oxytocic drug as ordered
    f. Administer a lactogenic inhibitor as ordered if bottle feeding preferred
    g. Administer RhoGAM as ordered if the mother is Rh negative and the baby is Rh positive and has a negative Coombs
2. Baby
    a. Clear the airway of mucus
    b. Observe frequently
    c. Use Apgar scoring to determine respiratory effort
    d. Maintain body heat
    e. Assess the newborn for visible anomalies
    f. Instill silver nitrate or other medication into each eye to prevent ophthalmia neonatorum
    g. Identify the mother and baby prior to leaving delivery room by use of prints and application of bands
    h. Leboyer technique—newborn immersed in a warm water bath in room with lights dimmed; mother, father, and newborn spend extra time together

Postpartal Period

Puerperium—6-week period following delivery in which the reproductive organs undergo physical and physiologic changes, a process called *involution;* because of the many physiologic and psychologic stresses of the postpartum period, there is a current trend to increase this period to 3 months following delivery and call it the fourth trimester of pregnancy
A. Systemic changes during the puerperium
1. Reproductive system
    a. Uterus—intermittent contractions bring about involution, after-contractions may cause discomfort necessitating analgesics
    b. Lochia—vaginal flow following delivery, changes from rubra to serosa in 1 week, then becomes alba (uterine lining regenerates with new epithelum in 2 or 3 days)
    c. Vagina practically returns to its prepregnant state through a healing of soft tissue und cicatrization
    d. Abdominal wall soft and flabby but eventually regains tone
    e. Breasts
        (1) As placenta is delivered, there is activation of luteinizing hormone in the anterior pituitary—secretion of prolactin also stimulates milk production
        (2) Posterior pituitary secretes pitocin, an oxytocic that initiates the letdown reflex with milk ejection as the baby suckles
        (3) Breast engorgement occurs on the second or third day because of vasodilation prior to lactation
2. Digestive system
    a. Added proteins and calories to replenish those lost with the process of involution
    b. Lactating mother needs added calories and fluids
    c. Roughage and exercise relieve constipation and distention
3. Circulatory system
    a. Blood volume usually back to normal by the third week after delivery

b. Blood fibrinogen levels increase during the first week

c. Increase in leukocytes, especially if labor was lengthy

d. Drop in hemoglobin and red blood count on the fourth postpartal day

4. Excretory system

   a. Increased urinary output, second to fifth postpartal day

   b. Bladder tone altered during pregnancy—retention with overflow may occur

   c. Activation of lactogenic hormone may result in lactose in the urine

   d. Excretion of nitrogen as involution occurs

5. Integumentary system—profuse diaphoresis as wastes are being excreted

B. Nursing care during the puerperium—nurse should

1. Use aseptic techniques in giving perineal care

2. Inspect the breasts for tissue and nipple breakdown, palpate to rule out growths (teach breast self-examination for continued health), support breasts with well-fitted brassiere

3. Teach the importance of handwashing in caring for self and baby (important for personnel to avoid cross contamination)

4. Observe vital signs—a temperature of 38° C (100.4° F) or above for 2 consecutive days (excluding first 24 hours after delivery) considered sign of beginning puerperal infection—bradycardia is a normal phenomenon following delivery

5. Palpate the fundus for firmness and descent below the umbilical level (involution normally follows a 1-finger breadth descent daily, by the fifth or sixth day fundus cannot be felt)—a fundus that is boggy indicates poor contractile power of uterus and results in bleeding

6. Administer oxytocic medication as ordered to promote involution

   a. Ergonovine maleate (Ergotrate)

   b. Methylergonovine maleate (Methergine)

   c. Maintain the uterus in a slightly contracted state that controls bleeding from intrauterine sites and maintains tone, rate and amplitude of rhythmic contractions required for involution of the uterus

7. Check lochia for color, amount, odor (foul odor indicates beginning infection); observe suture line for redness, ecchymosis, edema, or gapping

8. Promote bladder and bowel function

9. Encourage Kegal exercises to strengthen pubococcygeal muscles

10. Provide diet high in proteins and calories to restore body tissues

11. Ambulate early to prevent blood stasis

12. Observe for postpartal blues, which may be caused by a drop in hormonal levels on the fourth or fifth day

13. Meet the mother's needs to enable her to meet the baby's needs

14. Assist the mother with self-care and care of the baby as needed

15. Provide for group discussions on breast-feeding, infant care, etc.

C. Concepts basic to parent-infant relationships

1. Early and frequent parent-infant contact is essential for suvival (bonding)

2. Parenting abilities can be fostered and developed

3. Biologic changes that occur at puberty and during pregnancy influence the development of nurturance

4. Interaction between mother and child begins from the moment of conception and can be shared with the father

5. Love for the infant grows as the parents interacts and cares for the infant

6. As the parent gives to the infant and the infant receives, the parent in turn receives satisfaction from parenting tasks

7. Any disturbance in the give-and-take cycle sets up frustrations in both the parent and the infant

8. Parent behavior is learned and frequent parent-infant contact enhances the development of parenting abilities

THE NEWBORN
Family History

A. Chronic illness in the mother's or father's family

B. Previous medical-surgical illnesses of the mother and father

C. Age and present health status of the mother and father

D. History of previous pregnancies

E. Prenatal history

1. Medical supervision during pregnancy

2. Nutrition during pregnancy

3. Course of pregnancy—illnesses, medications taken or treatments required

4. Duration of gestation

5. Course and amount of sedation and anesthesia required

6. Type of delivery and significant events during the immediate period after delivery

7. Immediate response of newborn (Apgar score at 1 and 5 minutes following birth)

Parent-Child Relationships

A. Infant
1. Before the birth
   a. First 8 weeks is a period of rapid growth and development for fetus
   b. Any interference with maternal physiology may cause irreparable damage to fetus; no drugs should be taken during this period if possible
   c. Increased maternal hormonal action is necessary for continued implantation of fetus in the uterus
2. After the birth the baby has need for
   a. Contact with one person on a consistent basis
   b. Food, fondling, caressing, rocking, speaking, clothing, bathing, comfort, and protection from environment

B. Mothering and fathering are
1. Based on a biologic inborn desire to reproduce
2. Role concepts that begin with own childhood experiences
3. Primitive emotional relationships
4. Maturing processes
5. Conceptualizations of the physiologic and psychologic processes following infant's birth
6. Fostered by the parent-infant interaction that constantly reinforces gratification as needs are met and security develops
7. Abilities that are learned rather than innate

C. Parent-child relationships are affected by
1. Readiness for pregnancy
   a. Planned or unplanned
   b. Health status prior to pregnancy
   c. Financial status
   d. Determinants such as age, cultural backgrounds, number in the family unit
   e. Political forces
2. Nature of the pregnancy
   a. Health status during pregnancy
   b. Preparation for parenthood
   c. Support from family members and members of the health team
3. Character of the labor and delivery
   a. Length and pattern of labor
   b. Type and amount of analgesia received
   c. Support from family and health team
   d. Anesthesia during delivery
   e. Type of delivery
4. Period immediately after the birth
   a. Early parent-infant contact
      (1) Allow the mother to touch, fondle, and hold
      (2) Give the mother ample time to inspect and begin to identify with baby
      (3) Early give-and-take between parents and infant—rooming-in arrangement
      (4) Supportive nursing care in these beginning relationships
      (5) Identification of beginning disturbed relationships, with nursing intervention
   b. Significant phases
      (1) Taking-in phase—mother's needs have to be met before she can meet the baby's; behavior—talks about self rather than the baby, doesn't seem too interested in the baby, doesn't touch the infant, cries easily
      (2) Transition phase—characterized by the mother's starting to take hold, looking at and reaching for the baby, touching with fingertips, talking about the baby, etc.
      (3) Taking-hold phase—kisses, embraces, gives care to infant, eye contact, uses whole hand to make contact, calls the baby by name, etc.

Adaptation to Extrauterine Life

A. Immediate needs at the time of delivery
1. Aspiration of mucus to provide an open airway
2. Evaluation by use of Apgar score 1 and 5 minutes following birth (Table 4-1)
3. Maintenance of body temperature to prevent acidosis
4. Constant observation of physical condition
5. Eye care—prophylactic instillation of silver nitrate or other medication in each eye to prevent ophthalmia neonatorum

B. Appraisal of the newborn after delivery
1. Skin
   a. Body is normally pink with slight cyanosis of hands and feet for 24 hours (jaundice is abnormal during the first 24 to 48 hours of life)
   b. Check for abrasions, rashes, crackling, and elasticity, which indicates the status of tissue hydration; at times, milia (white pinpoint spots over the nose caused by retained sebaceous secretions), birthmarks, forceps marks, ecchymosis, or papules are present
2. Respirations are abdominal and irregular, with a rate of 30 to 50 per minute (retractions—depression of the sternum—are abnormal)
3. Head and sensory organs
   a. Head and chest circumference nearly equal to the crown-rump length; chest slightly smaller than head

Table 4-1. Apgar score chart*

Adaptation	0	1	2
Heart rate	Absent	Slow, below 100	Over 100
Respiratory effort	Absent	Weak cry	Strong cry
Muscle tone	Limp	Some flexion of extremities	Active motion
Reflex irritability	No response	Grimace	Cry
Color	Cyanotic, pale	Body pink, extremities cyanotic	Completely pink

*Scores: 7 to 10, good condition; 3 to 6, moderately depressed; 0 to 2, severely depressed.

   b. Symmetry of face—as the baby cries, sides of the face move equally

   c. Check the head for molding, abrasions, or skin breakdowns; observe for caput succedaneum—edema of soft tissue of the scalp; cephalhematoma—edema of the scalp caused by effusion of blood between the bone and periosteum; extend the head fully in all directions for adequacy in range of motion

   d. Observe the eyes for discharge or irritation; check the pupils for reaction to light, equality of eye movements (normally there is some ocular incoordination); check the sclerae for clarity, jaundice, or hemorrhage

   e. Nose—observe for patency of both nostrils

   f. Mouth—observe the gums and hard and soft palates for any openings—mucosa of the mouth normally clear (white patches that bleed on rubbing indicate thrush, a monilial infection)

   g. Ears—auricles open; vernix covers tympanic membrane, making otoscopic examination useless (ring bell close to ear—baby should stir); both eyes should be same level as ears; upper earlobes normally curved (flatness indicative of kidney anomaly)

4. Chest and abdomen

   a. Chest auscultation—only respiratory sounds should be audible (noisy crackling sounds abnormal); heart rate—regular 120 to 160 per minute (rubbing or unusual sounds abnormal)

   b. Abdomen

     (1) Listen to bowel sounds over the abdomen

     (2) Palpate the spleen with fingertips under the left costal margin—tip should be palpable

     (3) Palpate liver on the right side—normally 1 cm below the costal margin

     (4) Observe umbilical cord for redness, odor, or discharge

     (5) Palpate the femoral pulses gently at inner aspect of the groin—indicate intact circulation to extremities

5. Genitalia

   a. Boys

     (1) Palpate the scrotum for testes—at times undescended at birth, which is normal (must descend by puberty or sperm will be destroyed by high temperature within the abdominal cavity)

     (2) Enlargement of scrotum—indicates hydrocele (diagnosis affirmed by transparent appearance of the scrotum when a flashlight is held close to the scrotal sac)

     (3) Observe tip of the penis for the urinary meatus—epispadias, meatus on upper surface of the penis; hypospadias, meatus on lower surface

   b. Girls—observe the genitalia for labia and vaginal opening; edema of labia and bloody mucoid discharge normal, resulting from transfer of maternal hormones

6. Extremities

   a. Hands and arms—thumbs clenched in fist

     (1) Check for number and variation of fingers

     (2) Check the clavicle and scapulae while putting arm through normal range of motion; clicking or resistance indicates dislocation or fracture

     (3) Palpate for fractures; crepitation is indicative

   b. Feet and legs

     (1) Check toes, pattern and number

     (2) Adduct and abduct feet through range of motion; there should be no resistance or tightness

     (3) Flex both legs onto the lower abdomen; there should be no resistance or tightness

     (4) Place both feet on a flat surface and bend

the knees; knees should be at the same height (when unequal, known as Allis' sign, indicates hip dislocation)

7. Back—turn the baby on its abdomen, run a finger along the vertebral column; any separations or swellings indicative of spina bifida

8. Anus—patency confirmed with passage of meconium; inability to insert a rectal thermometer may be indicative of imperforate anus

9. Neuromuscular development—check reflexes
   a. Rooting—touch the baby's cheek; baby should root for finger
   b. Sucking—place an object close to the baby's mouth; baby should make an attempt to suck
   c. Grasp—place fingers in palm of the baby's hand and encircle palm with your hand; lift the infant off a firm surface, baby will grasp; infant's head will lag as baby is raised
   d. Babinski—run thumb up middle undersurface of infant's foot; toes will separate and flare-out
   e. Plantar—run thumb up the lateral undersurface of infant's foot; toes will curl downward
   f. Moro—making a loud, sharp noise close to the baby; will result in the baby's bringing both arms and legs close to the body as if in an embrace (disappears by 4 months of age)
   g. Crawl—when the baby is on a firm surface and turned on its abdomen, crawling movements will follow
   h. Step or dance—while the infant is supported under both arms, stepping movements will occur when feet are placed on a firm surface

C. Changes in the newborn during the first week of life
   1. Circulatory
      a. Tying of cord at birth brings changes in fetal circulation—closure of the foramen ovale and ductus arteriosus and obliteration of the umbilical arteries produce an adultlike circulation within 1 hour after birth.
      b. Heart rate regular; 120 to 180, but variable depending on the infant's activity; soft heart murmur common for first month of life
      c. Clotting mechanism poor because of low prothrombin concentration
      d. Liver immature (although large)—cannot destroy excessive red cells in the newborn, resulting in physiologic jaundice by third day
      e. Hemoglobin level high—14 to 20 g/100 ml of blood
      f. White blood count high—6000 to 22,000

   2. Respiratory—respirations diaphragmatic, irregular, abdominal; 30 to 50 per minute, quiet with periods of apnea
   3. Excretory
      a. Kidneys immature—newborn should void during first 24 hours (2 weeks of age voids 20 times daily), albumin and urates (brick red staining on diaper) common during first week because of dehydration
      b. Stools—first stool, black-green and tenacious, called *meconium;* by third day, becomes mixed with light yellow, called *transitional*
   4. Integumentary
      a. Lanugo—fine downy hair growth over the entire body
      b. Milia—small, whitish, pinpoint spots over the nose caused by retained sebaceous secretions
      c. Monogolian spots—blue-black discolorations on back, buttocks, and sacral region that disappear by first year
   5. Digestive
      a. Has stores of nutrients from intrauterine existence; therefore needs very little nourishment first few days
      b. Roots and sucks when anything is brought to mouth
      c. Digests simple carbohydrates, fats, and proteins readily
      d. Cardiac sphincter of stomach not well developed, therefore regurgitates if stomach is overfull
      e. Needs to be bubbled frequently to get rid of air bubbles in stomach
   6. Endocrine
      a. Metabolic—all newborns normally lose 10% of their body weight by first week of life
      b. Hormonal—enlargement of breasts in boys and girls is normal as a result of hormones transmitted to baby by mother
   7. Neural
      a. Central nervous system and brain not well developed—infant needs constant supply of oxygen
      b. Breathing, sucking, and crying are early neural activities necessary for the infant's survival

D. Needs of newborn
   1. Air for survival
      a. Suctioning of mucus as needed to maintain an open airway

b. Positioning—side lying to facilitate drainage of mucus

c. Observing any signs of air hunger (e.g., cyanosis, flaring of the nostrils, noisy respirations, sternal retractions) would warrant aspiration and administration of oxygen by inhalation

2. Warmth, comfort, and protection from the environment

   a. Keep in a heated crib until body temperature is stabilized to prevent chilling; baby is unable to shiver and must break down brown fat to produce energy for warmth; premature or skinny infants can be compromised by chilling because they have a paucity of brown fat available for breakdown

   b. Clothing should be loose, soft

   c. Crib should be firm and provide protection

   d. Skin should be kept clean and dry to maintain integrity

3. Human contact—body contact with another human is paramount for the newborn's survival; ministrations in giving care should be carried out with purpose and awareness of the importance of these early beginning relationships (talking, rocking, singing are an essential part of body contact with a newborn)

4. Food

   a. Initial weight loss of 10% of birth weight is normal and usually regained by tenth day of life

   b. Infant feeding usually delayed immediately after birth because of

      (1) General weakness and danger of aspiration

      (2) Reduced calorie requirement because of inactivity and low heat production of infant

   c. Newborn needs to ingest simple proteins, carbohydrates, fats, vitamins, and minerals for continued cell growth

   d. Fluid (130 to 200 ml per kilogram or 2 to 3 oz fluid per pound of body weight)

   e. Calories (110 to 130 calories per kilogram or 50 to 60 calories per pound of body weight)

   f. Protein (2.2 to 2.0 g per kilogram of body weight from birth to 6 months of age; 1.8 g per kilogram of body weight from 6 to 12 months of age)

5. Sleep—since sleep lowers body metabolism, it helps restore energy and assimilate nutriments for growth

Breast-Feeding

A. Advantages

1. Psychologic value of closeness and satisfaction in beginning mother-child relationship

2. Optimum nutritional value for infant

3. Economical and readily accessible

4. Greater immunity to infection

5. Infant is less likely to be allergic to mother's milk

6. Develops facial muscles, jaw, and nasal passages of infant, since stronger sucking is necessary

7. Assists in involution of uterus

8. Reduces chances of infection because of maternal antibodies present in colostrum and milk

B. Prerequisites

1. Psychologic readiness of mother is a major factor in successful breast-feeding

2. Adequate diet must be available prenatally and postnatally to ensure high quality milk

3. Suitable rest, exercise, and freedom from tension for mother will provide increased satisfaction for both her and the infant

4. Infant's sucking at the breast stimulates the maternal posterior pituitary to produce pitocin whose properties in the blood system constrict the lactiferous sinuses to move the milk down through the nipple ducts—known as the letdown reflex; a poor sucking reflex of the child will inhibit the letdown of milk; sucking also stimulates prolactin secretion

5. Absence of emotional stress in the mother, since anxiety inhibits the letdown reflex

C. Length of nursing period

1. Self-demand schedule is desirable

2. Length of feeding time is usually 20 minutes with greatest quantity of milk consumed in first 5 to 10 minutes

D. Feeding techniques

1. Mother and infant in comfortable position, such as semireclining or in rocking chair

2. Initiate feeding by stimulating rooting reflex (stroking cheek toward breast, being careful not to stroke other cheek, since this will confuse infant)

3. Burp or bubble baby during and after feeding to allow for escape of air by

   a. Placing baby over shoulder

   b. Sitting baby on lap, flexed forward

   c. Rubbing or patting back (avoid jarring baby)

4. Breast milk intake similar to formula intake

a. 130 to 200 ml of milk per kilogram (2 to 3 oz of milk per pound) of body weight

b. From ⅙ to ⅐ of baby's weight per day

5. After lactation has been established, occasional bottle-feeding can be substituted

6. Length of time for continuing breast-feeding is variable (may be discontinued when teeth erupt, since this can be uncomfortable for mother)

E. Care of breasts

1. Cleanse with plain water once daily (soap or alcohol can cause irritation and dryness)

2. Support breasts day and night with properly fitting brassiere

3. Nursing pads should be placed inside bra cup to absorb any milk leaking between feedings

4. Plastic bra liners should be avoided because they increase heat and perspiration and decrease air circulation necessary for drying of the nipple area

F. Contraindications

1. In mother
   a. Active tuberculosis
   b. Acute contagious disease
   c. Chronic disease such as cancer, advanced nephritis, cardiac disease
   d. Extensive surgery
   e. Narcotic addiction

2. In infant—cleft lip or palate or any other condition that interferes or prevents grasp of the nipple is the only real containdication

Bottle-Feeding

A. Advantages

1. Provides an alternative to breast-feeding

2. Less restrictive than breast-feeding; may meet needs of working mothers

3. Allows a more accurate assessment of intake

4. May be indicated in the presence of a congenital anomaly such as cleft palate

5. May be necessary for infants who require special formulas due to allergies or inborn errors of metabolism

B. Factors affecting success

1. Pasteuration of milk

2. Tuberculin testing of cows

3. Sanitation in milk handling

4. Adequate refrigeration and storage

5. Preparation under clean conditions and sterilization to prevent contamination

6. Formula designed to match nutrient ratio of breast milk composition: water dilution to reduce protein and mineral concentration; added carbohydrate to increase energy value

C. Types of formulas

1. Fresh whole or skimmed milk

2. Evaporated milk

3. Dried milks (whole or skimmed)

4. Commercial formulas

D. Preparation for bottle-feeding

1. Calculation of formula to yield 110 to 130 calories and 130 to 200 ml of fluid per kilogram of body weight

2. Proper preparation of formula by terminal heat method and feeding utensils (full 25 minutes of boiling)

3. Proper refrigeration of formula

4. Warming of formula before feeding by immersing bottle into warm water until approximately equal to body temperature (keep level of water in warmer below cap)

E. Feeding techniques

1. Always hold infant during feeding to provide warm body contact (bottle propping may contribute to aspiration of formula)

2. Hold bottle so nipple is always filled with milk to prevent excessive air ingestion

3. Adjust size of nipple hole to needs of baby (a premature infant needs a larger hole that requires less sucking)

4. After feeding and burping infant, place child on abdomen or side to aid digestion and prevent aspiration

5. Feeding should be offered on demand to meet the infant's needs

F. Comparison of breast milk and cow's milk

	Human milk	Cow's milk (whole)
Water	88%	88%
Protein	1.0% to 1.5%	3.5% to 4.0%
Sugar (lactose)	6.5% to 7.5%	4.5% to 5.0%
Fat	3.5% to 4.0%	3.5% to 5.0%
Minerals	0.15% to 0.25%	0.7% to 0.75%
Calories (per fluid ounce)	20	20

Self-Regulation Schedule

A. Each infant born with different degree of maturity and rhythm of needs

B. Superior to rigid schedule, but should be modified to meet needs of infant and parents

C. Usually fed every 4 hours, with a nighttime feeding for first month, although schedule and amount are highly variable

D. Feeding behavior and degree of satisfaction reflect psychologic development of child

E. Close mother-infant relationship in feeding process meets basic need of trust (Erikson's stage of trust)

DEVIATIONS FROM THE NORMAL MATERNITY CYCLE IN THE MOTHER
Pregnancy-Induced Hypertension (Toxemias of Pregnancy)

Characterized by a triad of symptoms: edema, elevation of blood pressure, and proteinuria
A. Classification (American Committee on Maternal Welfare)
1. Acute toxemia of pregnancy—onset after twenty-fourth week
   a. Preeclampsia—mild, severe
   b. Eclampsia—convulsions and/or coma associated with hypertension, proteinuria, and edema
2. Chronic hypertensive vascular disease with pregnancy
   a. Without superimposed acute toxemia (no exacerbation of hypertension or development of proteinuria occurs)
      (1) Hypertension known to have antedated pregnancy
      (2) Hypertension discovered in pregnancy (before the twenty-fourth week and with postpartal persistence)
   b. With superimposed acute toxemia
3. Unclassified toxemia (data insufficient to differentiate the diagnosis)
B. Guidelines for prevention of toxemia
1. Sound nutrition counseling during pregnancy and lactation—vitamins and minerals should complement a nutritious, protein-rich diet
2. An additional 30 to 60 mg of supplemental iron daily in the second and third trimester (continue for 2 to 3 months postpartally in breast-feeding mother)
3. Caloric intake should be increased 10% during pregnancy; severe calorie restriction is harmful during pregnancy
4. Restriction of sodium is harmful during pregnancy and can result in electrolyte imbalance and the elimination of essential nutritional components and may contribute to reduced circulatory volume
5. Diuretics are contraindicated during pregnancy, since they cause hypovolemia and deplete essential nutrients for mother and fetus
C. Treatment and nursing care in preeclampsia
1. High-protein diet
2. Ambulatory care—frequent visits to obstetrician
3. Instructions to report headaches, dizziness, blurring of vision, and scotoma
4. Sedatives to ensure rest and sleep
5. Blood chemistry—rise in hematocrit, uric acid, blood urea nitrogen, and decrease in CO_2 combining power indicate worsening of toxemia
6. Qualitative urinalysis—increase in albumin output and/or decrease in urinary output indicates worsening of toxemia
7. Administration of albumin concentrate increases renal flow by correcting the hypovolemia
8. Conserve energy to decrease metabolic rate
9. Assess anxieties and concerns
10. Monitor to protect mother and fetus (includes respiratory rate, pulse, fetal heart rate, weight, intake and output, blood pressure)
D. Treatment and nursing care for eclampsia
1. Hospitalization and complete bed rest
2. Check vital signs, fetal heart, irritability, restlessness, signs of labor
3. When the patient is receiving magnesium sulfate therapy, check frequently for depression of patellar reflexes and respirations (these side effects can be treated with the administration of calcium gluconate to the mother and levallorphan [Lorfan] to the newborn if respiratory depression occurs); magnesium sulfate also causes dizziness, diaphoresis, and vomiting
4. Emergency equipment for possible convulsion, equipment to maintain an open airway, suction and oxygen, sedatives such as morphine sulfate and sodium luminal, tracheotomy set readily available on unit
5. Once symptoms are under control, labor may be induced or emergency cesarean section performed
6. Insertion of a Foley catheter ensures accurate measurement of urinary output
7. Limitation of visitors and reduction of environmental stimuli
8. Daily blood chemistry testing

Bleeding During the Maternity Cycle

Bleeding is an abnormal sign indicating a possible interruption of pregnancy
A. First trimester bleeding
1. Abortion
   a. Interruption of pregnancy in which there is complete expulsion or partial expulsion (incomplete) of the products of conception
   b. May be sudden, spontaneous, or induced by some external mechanical force
   c. Treatment consists of bed rest, immediate blood count, blood typing, Rh incompatibilty, and cross matching with availability of blood

　　d. Vital signs and observing for signs of labor will indicate course of abortion and treatment

　　e. Complete abortion—24 to 48 hours observation for bleeding is imperative

　　f. Incomplete abortion—dilation and curettage performed to empty the uterus of retained products of conception; same observation as with complete abortion

　2. Ectopic pregnancy

　　a. Pregnancy in which implantation occurs outside the uterus (most frequent site is middle portion of fallopain tube, other sites are abdomen, ovaries, or cervix)

　　b. Early signs and symptoms are usually concealed

　　c. Pattern in tubal pregnancy is usually one in which spotting may occur after 1 or 2 missed menstrual periods, sharp lower right or left abdominal pain radiating to shoulder develops, concealed bleeding from site of rupture leads to sudden shock

　　d. Treatment is immediate blood replacement and surgical removal of ruptured fallopian tube

　3. Hydatidiform mole

　　a. An abnormal pregnancy in which there is a benign growth of the chorion

　　b. Spontaneous expulsion usually occurs between the sixteenth and eighteenth weeks of pregnancy

　　c. Toxemia symptoms are common

　　d. Diagnosis—suspected when uterus is excessively large for period of gestation and fetal parts are not palpable

　　e. Treatment—if spontaneous evacuation does not occur, evacuation by delicate curettage or hysterotomy is performed

　　f. Dangers include uterine perforation, hemorrhage, and infection

　　g. Continued follow-up of serum gonadotropin levels is imperative for 1 year to rule out metastasis from chorionic carcinoma (increased gonadotropin levels warrant immediate hysterectomy)

　　h. Preventing a new pregnancy is essential for 1 year

B. Third trimester bleeding

　1. Placenta previa

　　a. Implantation of the embryo in the lower uterine segment

　　b. Three types: marginal (placental edge is close to internal os), partial (placenta partially covers internal os), and central (placenta completely covers internal os)

　　c. Painless bleeding in the latter part of pregnancy is only symptom

　　d. Treatment is to control bleeding—cesarean section is/maybe performed

　2. Abruptio placentae

　　a. Premature separation of a normally implanted placenta

　　b. Symptoms—with partially detached placenta there is external vaginal bleeding; with totally detached placenta, there is concealed bleeding, excruciating abdominal pain, and a broadlike abdominal wall

　　c. Common in individuals with toxemia, essential hypertension, and an abnormally short umbilical cord

　　d. Treatment

　　　(1) Replacement of blood loss

　　　(2) With fetal distress—emergency cesarean section

　　　(3) Without fetal distress and in the presence of some cervical effacement and dilation—induction of labor may be attempted

C. Postpartal hemorrhage

　1. Bleeding in excess of 500 ml within the first 24 hours following delivery

　2. Frequent causes are uterine atony, vaginal and cervical lacerations, and retained placental fragments (bleeding occurring after 24 hours is usually caused by retained placental fragments)

　3. Treatment for atony—massage fundal portion of uterus, administer oxytocics, and, with severe blood loss, blood replacement

　4. Bleeding caused by retained placental fragments necessitates manual removal

　5. Vaginal and cervical lacerations require surgical repair

D. Nursing care of mother with bleeding during maternity cycle—the nurse should

　1. Institute measures to alleviate fear and anxiety

　2. Check vital signs frequently

　3. Observe for signs of labor and imminent delivery

　4. Monitor fetal heart if pregnancy is beyond twentieth week

　5. Explain the need for and maintain parenteral therapy

　6. Maintain asepsis to prevent infection

7. Consider and provide for patient's spiritual needs

Dystocia (Abnormal Labor)

A. Difficult labor—may be mechanical (contracted pelvis, obstruction in pelvis, malpresentation or position of the fetus) or functional (caused by faulty uterine contractions)
 1. Treatment for mechanical dystocia is cesarean section
 2. Treatment for functional dystocia is oxytocics to stimulate labor or cesarean section—deciding factors are length of labor, condition of mother and fetus, amount of cervical effacement and dilation, presentation, position, and station of presenting part
 3. Nursing care of mother in prolonged labor—the nurse should
  a. Observe for signs of maternal exhaustion such as elevation of body temperature, fruity odor to breath, diminished urinary output with positive acetone reaction
  b. Observe for signs of fetal distress
  c. Have oxygen, suction, and resuscitation equipment readily available
  d. Constantly monitor contractions, fetal heart, and vital signs when patient is receiving oxytocic stimulation
B. Precipitate labor—a rapid labor and delivery of less than 2-hour duration
 1. Hazards to mother are perineal laceration and postpartum hemorrhage
 2. Hazards to baby are anoxia and intracranial hemorrhage
 3. At times, a safe anesthesia may help slow down labor process
C. Labor induction—initiation of labor contractions by medical (oxytocic drugs) or mechanical means (artificial rupture of membranes)
 1. Elective induction may be done for medical or obstetric reasons: medical—diabetes, pyelonephritis; obstetric—toxemia, Rh incompatibility, polyhydramnios, abruptio placentae, premature rupture of membranes at term without onset of labor
 2. Medical methods of induction
  a. Sparteine sulfate (Tocosamine)—75 to 150 mg IM (series given every ½ hour, every hour, or every 2 hours)
  b. Oxytocin (Pitocin)—5 units in 1000 ml of 5% glucose in Ringer's lactate IV at 5 to 10 drops per minute or buccal Pitocin, 200 unit tablets, given in an hourly series

c. Prostaglandins given orally, intravenously, or vaginally
  d. Breast pumping can be used but is the least effective method
 3. Nursing care of mother undergoing induction of labor—the nurse should
  a. Prepare mother with explanation of treatment
  b. Vigilantly time contractions and monitor vital signs and fetal heart
  c. Constantly monitor IV flow rate
  d. Remain with patient at all times during induction
  e. Provide for blood typing, Rh compatibility, cross matching, and availability of blood
  f. Have oxygen, suction, and resuscitation equipment readily available
  g. Prepare for emergency cesarean section if necessary
D. Abdominal delivery (cesarean section)—delivery of baby via abdominal incision
 1. Indicated in cephalopelvic disproportion, dystocia, placenta previa and abruptio placentae, postmaturity, growths within the birth canal, diabetes, toxemia, Rh incompatibility, malpresentation, fetal distress
 2. Nursing care following cesarean section—the nurse should
  a. Encourage early ambulation to prevent blood stasis
  b. Check vital signs and fundus
  c. Observe abdominal dressing for drainage
  d. Encourage eating of solids to promote peristalsis (prevents distention)
  e. Record intake and output
  f. Give analgesics as ordered
E. Breech delivery—position of the baby in which the buttocks alone or the buttocks and feet descend through the birth canal first
Nursing care
 1. Monitor the fetal heart in upper quadrants
 2. Watch for prolapsed cord; if it occurs:
  a. Place the patient in a knee-chest or Trendelenburg position to keep presenting part away from the cord.
  b. Cover the cord with moist, sterile dressing to keep it from drying
 3. Observation of frank meconium causes no concern—results from contraction of the uterus on lower colon of the fetus
 4. Add Piper forceps to the delivery table if vaginal delivery is done

Childbirth Injuries

A. Episiotomy—incision into the perineum to facilitate delivery and prevent lacerations and overstretching of the pelvic floor
  1. Routine procedure—closed surgically
  2. Nursing care
     a. Keep area clean and dry
     b. Analgesics as ordered for comfort
     c. Heat and local spray medications
     d. Perineal exercise
B. Lacerations are tears of the perineum or vulva resulting from a difficult or precipitate delivery—characterized as first, second, third, or fourth degree depending on the amount of involvement
  1. Treatment—surgical repair
  2. Nursing care—same as above; however, healing is slower following repair of a laceration
C. Relaxations of the vaginal outlet—an overstretching of the perineal supporting tissues resulting from childbirth
  1. Cystocele—a herniation of anterior vaginal wall with the descent and protrusion of the bladder
  2. Rectocele—a herniation of the pararectal fascia into the vagina
     a. Signs and symptoms—backache, feeling of heaviness and bearing down in the lower abdomen, urinary stress incontinence, and constipation
     b. Treatment—Kegel's exercises for stress incontinence (after childbearing period is completed, vaginoplasty is done)
     c. Nursing care with vaginoplasty consists of keeping perineal area clean and dry with insertion of Foley catheter or suprapubic catheter, warm sitz baths once healing has begun, analgesics for discomfort, antibiotics to prevent infection, high-protein diet to promote tissue repair; ambulation may be delayed to promote healing but leg motion and deep breathing are essential
D. Uterine prolapse—condition in which the uterus is found in a position lower than normal resulting from stretching and tearing of tissues during childbirth
  1. Signs and symptoms—bearing-down sensation and a feeling of a dropping of the pelvic organs, leukorrhea with marked congestion of cervix or lacerations of exposed vaginal walls, frequency with retention, and eventually cystitis
  2. Treatment—dependent on age, desire for more children, and severity of symptoms; pessaries may be used as temporary measure; surgical intervention is usually a vaginal hysterectomy

E. Displacement of uterus—results from lesions of the pelvic organs or stretching and relaxation of the ligaments supporting the uterus (may be congenital or result from the trauma of childbirth)
  1. Signs and symptoms—backache, excessive bleeding during menstruation, sense of pressure or fullness
  2. Treatment—insertion of a pessary to relieve symptoms; severe symptoms warrant surgical intervention
F. Rupture of the uterus—usually occurs after the fetus reaches a viable size
  1. Causes—perforation during attempted abortion, rupture of a previous uterine scar, spontaneous rupture of an intact uterus with abdominal overdistention, labor induction
  2. Treatment—relieve symptoms of shock from hemorrhage and surgical intervention (the extent of surgical intervention depends on degree of rupture)

Medical Diseases During Pregnancy

A. Heart disease—90% of rheumatic origin, 10% congenital lesions or syphilis
  1. Normal hemodynamics of pregnancy that adversely affect the pregnant woman with heart disease
     a. Growing fetus needs increase in oxygen supply
     b. Accelerated heart rate of mother in latter half of pregnancy puts extra workload on her heart
     c. Steady increase in mother's blood volume during the 36 weeks of pregnancy
     d. Rise in cardiac output from the tenth week through the twenty-eighth week of pregnancy
     e. The increase in oxygen consumption with contractions during labor makes length of labor a significant factor
     f. The sudden tachycardia during delivery or the sudden bradycardia and the normal increase in cardiac output following delivery may cause cardiac arrest
  2. Review the functional and therapeutic classification of heart disease in a medical-surgical nursing text
  3. Management of mother with heart disease during pregnancy
     a. Extra rest and protection from infection
     b. Medical supervision by cardiologist
     c. Obstetric supervision by obstetrician
     d. Low-sodium, high-protein diet

e. Immediate reporting of fatigue, dyspnea, hemoptysis, or edema
f. Hospitalization for any cardiac embarrassment
g. Minimal analgesia and anesthesia during labor and delivery
h. Forceps should be used to limit pushing efforts of the mother, since pushing increases cardiac workload
i. Scopolamine is contraindicated, since it is a vasodilator that will affect hemodynamics
j. Oxytocics are administered cautiously if needed in IV solutions
k. Observation of vital signs during labor, delivery, and immediately following delivery
l. Prophylactic antibiotics are administered to prevent infection
m. Digitalis and diuretic therapy are instituted to prevent heart failure and pulmonary edema
n. Longer hospital stay to provide continued health supervision
4. Nursing care of the mother with heart disease
   a. Prenatal—health teaching, rest and diet counseling, referral to community agencies for family care, avoidance of stress, preparation for the stress of labor and delivery, teaching importance of preventing infection
   b. Intrapartal—early admission prior to start of labor, vital signs, observation for signs of heart failure and pulmonary edema, maintenance of the Fowler position, availability of oxygen, added support during labor, delivery in bed if necessary
   c. Postpartal—observation for respiratory distress, since there is an increase in cardiac output with tachycardia, monitoring of vital signs, rest and sedation to decrease heart action, referral to various agencies for family aid on discharge
B. Diabetes mellitus
   1. Normal physiology of pregnancy that affects the pregnant woman with diabetes
      a. Vomiting during pregnancy, especially in first trimester, decreases carbohydrate intake with resulting acidosis
      b. Increased activity of anterior pituitary decreases the tolerance for sugar
      c. Elevated basal metabolic rate and decrease in carbon dioxide combining power increase tendency toward acidosis
      d. Normal lowered renal threshold for glucose can result in glucosuria that might confuse diabetic picture
      e. Muscular activity during labor depletes glycogen; therefore carbohydrate intake must be increased
      f. During puerperium, hypoglycemia is common as involution and lactation occur
   2. Hazards of diabetes during pregnancy
      a. Often there is a history of repeated stillbirths and fetal deaths
      b. Babies are excessively large, weighing over 4000 g
      c. Neonatal deaths occur as a result of hypoxia, hypoglycemia, congenital anomalies, and premature labor
      d. Toxemia and hydramnios are common
   3. Nursing care of the mother with diabetes
      a. Early medical and prenatal supervision
      b. Prevention of acidosis
      c. Effective dietary regimen
      d. Awareness of signs and symptoms of acidosis and hypoglycemia
      e. Teaching hygiene and avoidance of stress
      f. Referral to a public health nurse for continuity in care
      g. Identification card on person
   4. Nursing care of the baby of a diabetic mother
      a. Keep the infant warm because of poor temperature control mechanisms
      b. Observe respiration (stomach aspiration imperative at time of delivery, since hydramnios inflates stomach, which pushes up and interferes with diaphragm)
      c. Observe for signs of hypoglycemia such as lethargy, poor sucking reflex, cyanosis, or muscular twitching
      d. Provide glucose water feeding to prevent acidosis (with poor sucking reflex, glucose should be given parenterally)
C. Acute and chronic pyelonephritis
   1. Acute pyelonephritis is a diffuse inflammatory process of interstitial connective tissue of kidney (nephron involved when infection is extreme)
   2. Most common organism is *Escherichia coli;* occasionally *Staphylococcus* and *Streptococcus* organisms
   3. Signs and symptoms are chills, fever, severe backache, tenderness over kidney region, rise in nonprotein nitrogen, decrease in phenolsulfonphthalein excretion and dye excretion on pyelography
   4. Nursing care of mother with pyelonephritis

    a. Adequate diet and rest

    b. Force fluids

    c. Sulfonamides and antibiotics

    d. Intake and output monitoring

    e. Sims' position to relieve pressure on uterus

    f. Teaching importance of health supervision and follow-up care after delivery

    g. Family planning avoids risk of early recurrence of pregnancy

D. Assessment techniques for high-risk pregnancy

  1. AFP—(alpha fetoprotein) blood test—elevated levels may identify the pregnant woman carrying a baby with neural tube defects (spina bifida and anencephaly); may also indicate twins; if the AFP is elevated for two samples, it is followed by ultrasonography and amniocentesis for further confirmation

  2. Ultrasonography—high-frequency sound wave testing; discerns placental location and gestational age by measurement of biparietal diameters

     Nursing care—the patient is encouraged to drink and refrain from voiding before the test to improve visualization

  3. Serum estriol levels—confirms healthy fetal-placental functioning

    a. Results—falling levels at term may be indicative of impending fetal stress; two or more tests necessary to make diagnosis

    b. Nursing care—encourage the mother to return for testing

  4. Nonstress test—to observe for accelerations of fetal heart rate in response to fetal movement

    a. Classification of results

      (1) Reactive—2 or more accelerations of FHR of 15 beats/minute lasting 15 seconds throughout any fetal movement; no intervention necessary

      (2) Nonreactive—no FHR acceleration or accelerations less than 15 seconds; further monitoring necessary with use of the oxytocin challenge test

      (3) Unsatisfactory—recording uninterpretable; test should be repeated in 24 hours

    b. Nursing care—observation of the fetal monitor; explanation of test to decrease the mother's anxiety

  5. Oxytocin challenge test (OCT)—to demonstrate whether a healthy fetus can withstand a decreased oxygen supply during the stress of a contraction produced by exogenous oxytocin (Pitocin); if late decelerations appear, the fetus may be compromised due to uteroplacental insufficiency

    a. Classification of results

      (1) Negative—no late decelerations with a minimum of 3 contractions in 10 minutes; indicates that the fetus has good chance of surviving labor

      (2) Positive—persistent and late decelerations occurring with more than half the contractions; indicates the need for considering premature intervention

      (3) Suspicious—late decelerations occurring in less than half of uterine contractions; test should be repeated in 24 hours.

    b. Nursing care—conscientious monitoring of the mother after the test to observe for possible initiation of labor

  6. Fetal scalp pH sampling—may be done during labor when fetal heart patterns begin to indicate distress; capillary blood samples are taken from the fetal scalp in utero

    a. Results—if acidosis present, immediate delivery of infant is indicated

    b. Nursing care—cleanse the vaginal area to avoid contamination when the test is done

DEVIATIONS FROM THE NORMAL MATERNITY CYCLE IN THE NEWBORN
Neonatal Respiratory Distress

A. Asphyxia neonatorum occurs when respirations are not well established within 60 seconds after birth as a result of anoxia, cerebral damage, or narcosis

  1. Prevention—early prenatal care, prenatal education, early management of deviations from the normal pregnancy, adequate medical management during labor and delivery

  2. Signs and symptoms—asphyxia livida: persistent generalized cyanosis, good muscle tone; asphyxia pallida: marked pallor, poor muscle tone

  3. Treatment—after initial resuscitation keep baby under very close observation for first 24 hours, keep equipment for intubation and oxygen administration readily available

B. Atelectasis—incomplete expansion of the lung or a partial or total collapse of the lung following initial expansion; common in prematurity, oversedation, damage to the respiratory center, or results from inhalation of mucus or amniotic fluid

  1. Signs and symptoms—cyanosis, rapid irregular respirations, flaring of the nostrils, intercostal or suprasternal retraction, grunting on expiration

  2. Treatment—maintain an open airway, administer oxygen with high humidity, stimulate respira-

tions by frequently changing baby's position, administer antibiotics as ordered to prevent infection

C. Hyaline membrane disease—condition in which a deficiency in surface-active (detergent-like) lipoproteins results in inadequate lung inflation and ventilation; common following cesarean section and in low birth weight infants
   1. Symptoms—cyanosis, dyspnea, and sternal retraction
   2. Treatment—keep the airway patent; keep the infant in an Isolette with oxygen and high humidity; administer antibiotics as ordered

Birth Injuries

A. Caput succedaneum—edema with extravasation of serum into scalp tissues caused by molding during the birth process; no treatment is necessary since it subsides in a few days

B. Cephalhematoma—edema of the scalp with effusion of blood between the bone and periosteum; reabsorption usually occurs in a few days

C. Intracranial hemorrhage—bleeding into cerebellum, pons, and medulla oblongata caused by a tearing of the tentorium cerebelli; occurs following prolonged labor, difficult forceps delivery, precipitate delivery, version or breech extraction
   1. Symptoms—abnormal respirations; cyanosis; sharp, shrill, or weak cry; flaccidity or spasticity; restlessness; wakefulness; convulsions; poor sucking reflex
   2. Treatment—keep in Isolette with oxygen, humidity, and minimal handling; place in a high Fowler position, administer vitamins C and K to control and prevent further hemorrhage; with impaired sucking reflex, gavage feeding is necessary; support of parents is vital because of guarded prognosis

D. Facial paralysis—asymmetry of face caused by damage to facial nerves from a difficult forceps delivery; temporary paralysis disappears in a few days

E. Erb-Duchenne paralysis (brachial palsy)—caused by a difficult forceps or breech extraction delivery; treatment depends on severity of paralysis; massage and exercise prevent contractures; when severe, splints and casts are applied

F. Dislocations and fractures are diagnosed by crepitation, immobility, and variations in range of motion; treatment depends on the site of fracture; therefore swaddling, positioning, splints, slings, or casts may be used; referral to a public health agency ensures continuity of care; if necessary, refer to community agencies

Infections

A. Thrush—mouth infection caused by *Candida albicans;* it may be transmitted as the baby passes through the mother's vaginal canal, by unclean feeding utensils, or improper handwashing techniques by staff or mother
   1. Symptoms are white patches on tongue, palate, and inner cheek surfaces that bleed on examination, and difficulty with sucking
   2. Treatment—oral administration of nystatin (Mycostatin), application of 1% gentian violet, isolation of baby and equipment to prevent cross contamination

B. Impetigo—infectious skin eruption characterized by vesicles or pustules caused by *Staphylococcus* or *Streptococcus* organisms; treatment consists of isolating infant, pHisoHex baths daily, breaking pustules with alcohol wipe, local application of gentian violet, neomycin, or bacitracin, and administration of antibiotics

C. Ophthalmia neonatorum—eye infection caused by the *Neisseria gonorrhoeae* transmitted from the genital tract during delivery or by infected hands of personnel; prophylactic eye care is administered to all infants at birth; treatment for the eye infection consists of prompt antibiotic therapy to prevent eye damage; isolation of the infant, sterilization of all equipment, and strict handwashing are imperative

D. *Staphylococcus* infection—prevented by reduction of transient personnel in nurseries, adequate crib spacing, and medical asepsis

E. Epidemic diarrhea—caused by *Escherichia coli* organism in stool; characterized by forceful, watery, yellow-green stool; dry skin; rapid weight loss and acidosis; treatment, oral antibiotics, replacement of fluids parenterally, isolation to prevent cross contamination

F. Syphilis—spirochetal infection characterized by maculopapular lesions of the palms of the hands and soles of the feet, restlessness, rhinitis, hoarse cry, enlargement of the spleen and palpable lymph nodes, enlarged ends of long bones on x-ray examination; penicillin is a specific treatment for syphilis with a 1-to-2-year follow-up
   1. Prenatal syphilis transmitted to fetus by the mother
   2. Incidence of fetal infection varies with stage of the disease in the mother at the time of pregnancy
   3. Fetus seldom infected prior to fourth month of pregnancy; Langhan's cells in chorion are protective barrier

4. Pregnant women treated immediately with penicillin (prior to the fourth month of pregnancy, fetus not infected; after fourth month, the longer the infection goes untreated the greater the damage to the fetus)
G. TORCH—acronym for the following infections:
T—Toxoplasmosis *(Toxoplasma gondii)*—can be acquired by eating raw or undercooked meat or contacting cat litter; organism crosses the placenta; severity of infection related to gestational age; can cause hydrocephalus, intracranial calcifications, or chorioretinitis in the infant
O—Others (syphilis [*Treponema pallidum*], gonorrhea [*Neisseria gonorrhoeae*]); see syphilis (F)
R—Rubella (rubella virus): greatest risk to the fetus when maternal infection occurs in first 12 weeks of gestation; baby may be born with encephalitis, ocular abnormalities, cardiac maldevelopment, and other defects; these infants may have active viral infection and should be isolated until pharyngeal mucus and urine are free of virus; for mothers who have not had rubella or who are serologically negative rubella vaccine should be given in the immediate postdelivery period
C—Cytomegalic inclusion disease (cytomegalovirus)—pregnant woman usually asymptomatic; this sexually transmitted infection may cause hemolytic anemia, hydrocephalus, microcephalus, intrauterine growth retardation, or neonatal death
H—Herpes genitalis (herpesvirus)—contracted by the mother during sexual relations; characterized by periods of exacerbations and remissions; first attack most severe; during active stage the infant must be delivered by cesarean section; if delivered vaginally, neonatal infection can be disseminated and result in death; surviving infants suffer central nervous system involvement

Congenital Abnormalities

Defects present at birth are structural or metabolic (birth injuries are not included); may be genetically determined or a result of environmental interference during intrauterine life (see pediatrics for congenital abnormalities)

Hemolytic Disease

Hemolytic disease, an ABO or Rh incompatibility with destruction of red cells and resulting anemia; caused by a transfer of incompatible blood from the fetal to the maternal circulation, with antibody formation in the mother; the antibodies are then transferred through the placental barrier to the fetus, with a resulting agglutination and destruction of red cells
A. Symptoms—jaundice within the first 24 hours of birth, anemia, enlargement of the liver und spleen, lethargy, poor feeding pattern, vomiting, tremors and convulsions indicative of kernicterus (signs of kernicterus are absence of Moro reflex, severe lethargy, apnea, high-pitched cry, and assuming an opisthotonos position)
B. Treatment—during pregnancy amniotic fluid determinations are done by chemical and spectrophotometric analysis; elevated readings warrant either intrauterine transfusion or induction of labor depending on the weeks of gestation; following delivery exchange transfusion is done on the infant to decrease the antibody level and increase red blood cells and hemoglobin levels
C. Prevention—RhoGAM, a preparation of Rh_o (D antigen) immune globulin is now given intramuscularly to the mother 72 hours after delivery or after abortion to prevent erythroblastosis fetalis in future pregnancies; mother must be negative for Rh antibodies to receive RhoGAM

Drug Dependence

A. Definition—infant born with physiologic dependence on drugs as a result of maternal drug use and/or abuse
B. Source—many preparations including
1. Alcohol
2. Morphine derivatives
3. Synthetic opiates
4. Methadone
C. Perinatal mortality—6 to 8 times higher than in normal control group
D. Withdrawal symptoms—appear soon after birth, depending on the length of maternal addiction, amount of drug taken, and time taken prior to birth
1. Jittery
2. Hyperactive
3. Shrill and persistent cry
4. Frequent yawning and sneezing
5. Tendon reflexes increased
6. Moro reflex decreased
7. If untreated, may develop fever, vomiting, diarrhea, dehydration, apnea, convulsions; death may result
E. Treatment—sedation and weaning from drugs
F. Nursing interventions
1. Careful monitoring of infant
2. Administering supportive care to prevent injury

3. Promoting mother-infant attachment
4. Assessing for long-term intervention

G. Fetal alcohol syndrome—may produce congenital defects and retardation

Low–Birth Weight Infant

A. Prevention
   1. Education of teenagers (prior to planning a family) in nutrition and general hygiene
   2. Education of teenagers to the hazards of drug use and smoking
   3. Adequate and early prenatal health supervision
   4. Provisions for adequate housing and financial aid to persons of lower socioeconomic means
   5. Adequate community agencies to facilitate available services to persons in need
   6. Higher prematurity rates and low birth weight babies are frequently associated with malnutrition and underweight in the mother

B. Definitions
   1. Classification of newborn infants is now made on the basis of gestational age as well as birth weight
   2. An infant born at term (37 weeks or over) is called full size; an infant born before term (36 weeks or less) is called premature or preterm
   3. A low birth weight infant is one who weighs 2500 g (5½ pounds) or less
   4. Full-term infant may be of low birth weight; premature infant need not be

C. Management of the mother in premature labor (before the thirty-seventh week of pregnancy)
   1. Preanesthetic medications should be minimal to prevent depression of the fetus (barbiturates and opiates are especially contraindicated, since they depress respirations, depleting oxygen to the fetus)
   2. Regional anesthesias are safer than general anesthesias
   3. Added support to the mother, since she is concerned with the baby's welfare
   4. Adequate preparation for the infant at birth; a heated Isolette and equipment for aspiration and resuscitation should be available
   5. The pediatrician should be present at the time of delivery to care for the infant

D. Management of the low birth weight infant immediately after delivery
   1. Aspiration of mucus to maintain an open airway is vital
   2. Absence of respirations necessitates direct laryngoscopy, tracheal aspiration, intubation, and mouth-to-tube insufflation
   3. Maintenance of body temperature is difficult because of heat loss by skin evaporation; heated Isolette is needed
   4. Aspiration of stomach contents at birth facilitates respirations and is often indicated for the low birth weight infant
   5. Infant should be moved to the nursery in the heated unit with oxygen and resuscitation equipment available

E. Differences in premature and full-size newborns
   1. Premature infant has less subcutaneous fat, therefore the skin is wrinkled, blood vessels and bony structures are visible, lanugo present on face, eyebrows are absent, and ears are poorly supported by cartilage
   2. Circumference of the head of the premature infant is quite large in comparison with the chest; the fontanels are small and bones are soft
   3. Skin color changes when premature infant is moved; upper half of the body pale and lower half red, known as harlequin color change
   4. Premature infant's posture is one of complete relaxation with marked flexion and abduction of the thighs; random movements are common with slightest stimulus
   5. Heat regulation poorly developed in the premature infant because of poor development of central nervous system; heat loss caused by large skin surface area; poorly developed respiratory center with diminished oxygen consumption causing asphyxia; weak heart action, therefore slower circulation and poor oxygenation; insufficient heat production caused by inadequate metabolism
   6. Respirations are not efficient in the premature infant because of muscular weakness of the lung and rib cage; retraction at xiphoid is evidence of air hunger; infant should be stimulated if apnea occurs
   7. Greater tendency toward capillary fragility and intracranial hemorrhage in the premature infant; red and white blood cell counts are low with resulting anemia during first few months of life
   8. Nutrition is difficult to maintain in the premature infant because of weak sucking and swallowing reflexes, small capacity of stomach, low gastric acidity, and slow emptying time of the stomach; the usual caloric intake of 110 to 130 calories per kilogram (50 to 60 calories per pound) of body weight may need to be increased to 200 to 220 calories per kilogram (100 calories per pound) for adequate growth and development

F. Nursing care of low birth weight and premature infants
 1. Observe for changes in respirations, color, and vital signs
 2. Check efficacy of Isolette—heat, humidity, and oxygen concentration
 3. Maintain aseptic technique to prevent infection
 4. Adhere to the techniques of gavage feeding for safety of infant
 5. Determine blood gases frequently to prevent acidosis
 6. Institute phototherapy should hyperbilirubinemia occur
 7. Support parents by letting them verbalize and ask questions to relieve anxiety
 8. Arrange follow-up before and after discharge by a visiting nurse
 9. Provide flexible and liberal visting hours for parents as soon as possible
 10. Allow parents to do as much as possible for the infant after appropriate teaching

INFERTILITY AND STERILITY
Definitions

A. Sterility—presence of an absolute factor that makes a person unable to produce offspring
B. Infertility—inability on the part of a couple to reproduce after consistent attempts for a 1-year period

Male Infertility and Sterility

A. Coital difficulties—chordee (painful downward curving erection) or marked obesity
B. Spermatozoal abnormalities—small ejaculatory volume, low sperm count, increased viscosity, reduced mobility of spermatozoa and/or more than 30% abnormal sperm forms
C. Testicular abnormalities—agenesis or degenesis of testes, cryptorchidism, poor maturation of the spermatozoa, physical injury due to trauma, irradiation, or increased temperature for prolonged periods
D. Abnormalities of the penis or urethra—hypospadias or urethral stricture
E. Prostate and seminal vesicle abnormalities—chronic prostatitis or seminal vesiculitis
F. Abnormalities of the epididymis and vas deferens—inflammation or closure
G. Severe nutritional deficiencies
H. Emotional factors

Female Infertility and Sterility

A. Endocrine disorders—pituitary, thyroid, or adrenal
B. Vaginal disorders—absence or stenosis of vagina, imperforate hymen, vaginitis
C. Cervical abnormalities—cervicitis obstruction by cervical polyps or tumors
D. Uterine abnormalities—hypoplasia, uterine neoplasms
E. Tubal disorders—obstruction (generally result of infection), perisalpingeal adhesions
F. Ovarian abnormalities—congenital abnormalities such as ovarian dysgenesis or agenesis, infections, tumors
G. Emotional problems—severe psychoneurosis or psychosis may cause anovulatory cycles
H. Coital factors—feminine hygiene preparations (including douches) that decrease vaginal pH may inactivate or destroy spermatozoa
I. Chronic disease states
J. Immunologic reactions to sperm
K. Nutritional factors such as a seriously faulty diet

Diagnostic Measures

A. Male—history, physical examination, semen analysis
B. Female—history, physical examination, CBC, sedimentation rate, serologic tests, urinalysis, serum protein-bound iodine, x-ray films of the chest, basal metabolic rate determination, Sims or Huhner tests, endometrial biopsy, tubal insufflation, hysterosalpingography, culdoscopy

Treatment

Depends on causative factor

Nursing Care

A. Apply principles of human relations and psychology
B. Listen to and discuss couple's particular problems, giving necessary support
C. Explain diagnostic procedure to alleviate anxiety and fear
D. Refer to visting nurse service for continuity in care

Drugs that Affect Gonadal Function and Fertility

A. Androgens are used to replace deficient hormones in males after puberty and before the climacteric to improve development of secondary sex characteristics or as single-incident therapy controlling lactogenic activity in the nonnursing mother
 1. Drugs
  a. Fluoxymesterone (Halotestin, Ora-Testryl, Ultandren)
  b. Methyltestosterone (Metandren, Neo-Hombreol-M, Oreton-M)
  c. Testosterone (Androlan, Andronaq, Hormale Aqueous, Malogen, Neo-Hombreol-F, Oreton, Sterotate)

d. Testosterone cypionate (Depo-Testosterone, Durandro, Malogen CYP, T-Ionate-P.A.)

e. Testosterone enanthate (Delatestryl, Malogen LA, Repo-Test, Testate, Testostroval-P.A.)

f. Testosterone propionate (Hormale Oil, Neo-Hombreol, Oreton Propionate, Testonate)

2. Adverse effects—adolescent males may have premature epiphyseal closure (decreased skeletal development, height stops increasing)

B. Estrogens primarily used to replace deficient hormones to control hormonal balance in menopausal or postmenopausal women or to maintain menses and fertility in females during reproductive years

1. Drugs

a. Chlorotrianisene (Tace)

b. Conjugated estrogens (Conestron, Conjutab, Equgen, Menotabs, Premarin, Theogen)

c. Dienestrol (DV, Synestrol)

d. Esterified estrogens (Amnestrogen, Estrifol, Evex, Femogen, Glyestrin, Menest, SK-Estrogens, Trocosone, Zeste)

e. Estradiol (Aquadiol, Progynon)

f. Estrone (Estrusol, Menformon [A], Theelin, Wynestron)

g. Ethinyl estradiol (Estinyl, Feminone, Lynoral, Palonyl)

h. Hexestrol

i. Methallenestril (Vallestril)

j. Promethestrol dipropionate (Meprane Dipropionate)

2. Adverse effects—anorexia, nausea, vomiting, tissue fluid accumulation

C. Conception enhancers

1. Menotropins (Pergonal) stimulate growth and maturation of ovarian follicles in women with deficient ovum production by creating an effect on ovarian follicles comparable to that of natural FSH and LH

2. Chorionic gonadotropin (A.P.L., Almetropin, Antuitrin-S, Chorex, Chorigon, Follutein, Glucotropin-Forte, Khorion, Libigen, Luton, Pregnyl, Riogon, Stemultrolin)

a. Administered concurrently to support LH effect on ovulation when follicle maturation has occurred

b. Adverse effects—20% of patients have multiple births

3. Clomiphene citrate (Clomid)

a. Used during the fifth to the tenth day of the menstrual cycle to stimulate release of FSH and LH in anovulatory women

b. Adverse effects—multiple births, visual changes, dizziness, light-headedness

FAMILY PLANNING
Goals

A. Maintain optimum emotional and physical health of the family

B. Involve both partners in planning family size

C. Inform the couple of available methods of birth control and give them the freedom of choice

Contraceptive Methods

A. Oral contraceptives—combined progestins and estrogens that suppress ovulation when taken as prescribed

1. Fixed combination program—provides the estrogen component of the combination tablet to suppress secretion of FSH; the progestins inhibit midcycle release of LH from the pituitary when tablets are taken from the fifth to the twenty-fifth day and a placebo tablet is taken the remaining 7 days

a. Ethinyl estradiol-ethynodiol diacetate (Demulen)

b. Ethinyl estradiol-norethindrone acetate (Norlestrin)

c. Ethinyl estradiol-norgestrel (Ovral)

d. Mestranol-ethynodiol diacetate (Ovulen)

e. Mestranol-norethindrone (Norinyl, Ortho-Novum)

f. Mestranol-norethynodrel (Enovid)

2. Adverse effects—thrombophlebitis; during the first 4 months can include headache, nausea, vomiting, breast fullness, depression, fatigue, brownish facial pigmentation, fluid retention, intermenstrual spotting, increased susceptibility to vaginal infection

B. Intrauterine devices (IUD)—mechanical devices inserted into isthmus of uterus; prevent pregnancy by increasing tubal motility so that ovum gets to uterus before lining is optimum for implantation; not as effective as oral contraceptives, since pregnancy may occur with device in place

C. Diaphragms—mechanical devices that fit over cervix and prevent sperm from entering cervical os

D. Condoms—rubber sheaths that cover penis and prevent semen from entering cervical os

E. Creams, jellies, foam tablets, and vaginal suppositories—spermicidal (generally low pH) preparations inserted into vaginal canal by applicator immediately prior to coitus (used in conjunction with the diaphragm and condom for added protection)

F. Coitus interruptus—withdrawal of the penis during sexual intercourse prior to ejaculation; least effective method

G. Rhythm—the plotting of the basal body temperature to determine fertile period, with abstinence from coitus during that time

Sterilization

A. Male—accomplished by surgical severance and suturing of the vas deferens, preventing ejaculation of sperm (vasectomy); after vasectomy, sperm are still produced; however, after 3 azoospermic specimens, sterility is achieved
B. Female—accomplished by abdominal laparotomy, laparoscopy, or culdoscopy; the fallopian tubes are severed and tied so there is no way the mature ovum can be impregnated by a mature sperm

Nursing Implications

A. Method of contraception—should be acceptable to the couple, since acceptability increases effectiveness
B. Ideal contraceptive—completely safe, free of side effects, reversible, easily obtainable, and inexpensive
C. Periodic physical examination of all women using oral or mechanical devices should include pelvic examination and Pap smear
D. Discussion groups—help couples expand their knowledge related to the anatomy and physiology of the reproductive systems
E. Assess couples individually and together prior to sterilization, since consideration of the physiologic and psychologic reactions to such procedures is vital

ABORTION
Methods of Induced Abortion

A. Vacuum aspiration—done under local paracervical, epidural, or general anesthesia in the first 12 weeks of pregnancy; the cervix is dilated and the products of conception are suctioned by a small hollow tube; the uterus is then curettaged to remove all fetal tissue
B. Dilation and curettage—performed during the first 12 to 14 weeks of pregnancy under local paracervical or general anesthesia; the cervix is dilated and uterus is curettaged
C. Saline injection—labor is induced when a pregnancy is 14 to 24 weeks in duration by injecting a sterile saline solution into the uterus by amniocentesis; labor usually begins within 20 to 36 hours after instillation of saline; produces a macerated fetus
D. Hysterotomy—performed after 16 weeks of pregnancy by surgically removing the fetus and placenta abdominally

E. Estrogen in high dosage after ovulation—disrupts the estrogen-progesterone balance that usually maintains the dense endometrial nutrient bed for fertilized ova
F. Dinoprost tromethamine (Prostin F_2 Alpha)
   1. Action—used during second trimester to trigger vasoconstrction and uterine concontractions that interfere with endocrine function of placenta
   2. Adverse effects—nausea, vomiting, diarrhea, pain at extrauterine sites, allergic reactions (not administered to patients with history of asthma)

Nursing Considerations

A. Be aware of own feelings about abortion—essential if the nurse is to intervene therapeutically with women having abortions
B. Nurse needs to encourage the patient's expression of frustration, fear, and anger
C. Nurse needs to be objective and support the woman's decision about abortion
D. Complete history and physical examination, complete laboratory workup, pelvic examination and Pap test, and a pregnancy test are essential for safe care prior to induced abortion
E. Postabortion counseling in contraceptive methods should be available
F. If prone to Rh sensitization, RhoGAM is given when patient's blood is negative for antibodies

Prerequisites for Abortion Facility (Recommended by the College of Obstetricians and Gynecologists)

A. Verification of the diagnosis and duration of pregnancy
B. Preoperative instructions and counseling
C. Recorded preoperative history and physical examination
D. Laboratory procedures usually required for hospitalization, such as blood typing and Rh factor
E. Prevention of Rh sensitization
F. A receiving facility where client is prepared and may receive necessary preoperative medication and be observed prior to treatment
G. Recovery facility for care and observation following surgery, with a qualified anesthetist in attendance
H. Postoperative instructions and follow-up including family planning
I. Adequate permanent records

GRIEF RESPONSES IN PREGNANCY
Causative Factors

A. Spontaneous abortion
B. Elective abortion

C. Ectopic pregnancy

D. Antenatal fetal death

E. Removal of a hydatidiform mole

F. Stillborn

G. Neonatal death

Emotional Responses

A. Guilt

B. Loss of self-esteem

C. Denial

D. Anger

Nursing Intervention

A. Assist the parents in ventilating their feelings of guilt and/or self-shame

B. Assist the parents in verbalizing their feelings about the dead fetus or infant

C. Support the parents if they want to see and/or hold the dead infant

D. Assess their support system and refer for assistance as required

MENOPAUSE

A period in a woman's life when there is gradual cessation of ovarian function and menstrual cycles

Physiologic Changes

A. Ovaries lose their ability to respond to gonadotropic hormones

B. Dramatic decrease in levels of circulating estrogens and progesterone, since the ovary has run out of follicles

C. Increased gonadotropin level in the blood, since production is no longer inhibited (negative feedback) by the ovaries; false-positive pregnancy test may occur

Symptoms

A. Somatic—atrophic changes in reproductive organs resulting in dyspareunia, weight gain, facial hair growth, cardiac palpitations, hot flashes, profuse diaphoresis, constipation, pruritus, faintness

B. Psychic—headache, irritability, anxiety over loss of reproductive function, sexual feelings, and feelings of womanliness

Treatment

A. Support system to deal with stress

B. For dyspareunia—vaginal estrogen creams

C. Tranquilizers and phenobarbital if necessary

D. Hormonal therapy only if absolutely necessary and when no history of malignancy is present

Nursing Care

A. Prepare the woman for the changes that may occur with menopause

B. Let the woman ventilate her feelings

C. Refer for medical supervision

AGENCIES PROVIDING PARENT-CHILD HEALTH SERVICES
Government

A. World Health Organization—founded in 1948 by United Nations; 100 or more countries exchange knowledge and collaborate on elevating level of health throughout the world

B. Children's Bureau—founded in 1972 under the Department of Health, Education and Welfare (now Health and Human Services); its purpose is to improve services for maintenance of health in mothers and children through research, care, and teaching

C. Department of Family and Children's Services (HHS)—federal monies for food, shelter, and medical services for dependent children

D. Women's Bureau—under the Department of Labor, provides supervision of places of employment for pregnant women

E. National Institutes of Health—monies provided for research on child health and human development

Private Organizations

A. La Leche League—international, organized in 1956 by mothers interested in fostering breast-feeding

B. International Childbirth Education Association—federation of groups and individuals interested in fostering family-centered maternity and infant care, and to create an interest in education for childbirth

C. American Society for Psychoprophylaxis in Obstetrics (A.S.P.O.)—responsible for teaching the Lamaze method in preparation for childbirth

Maternity Nursing Review Questions

1 The outermost membrane that helps form the placenta is the:
1. Amnion
2. Yolk sac
3. Chorion
4. Allantois

2 Progesterone is secreted in relatively large quantities by which of the following structures?
1. Corpus luteum
2. Adrenal cortex
3. Endometrium
4. Pituitary gland

3 The developing cells are called a fetus from the:
1. End of the second week to the onset of labor
2. Implantation of the fertilized ovum
3. Time the fetal heart is heard
4. Eighth week to the time of birth

4 The ischial spines are designated as an important landmark in labor and delivery because the distance between the spines is:
1. A measurement of the floor of the pelvis
2. A measurement of the inlet of the birth canal
3. The widest measurement of the pelvis
4. The narrowest diameter of the pelvis

5 Which of the following is *not* characteristic of prodromal labor?
1. Intensification of uterine contractions with walking
2. Failure of presenting part to descend
3. Lack of cervical effacement or dilation
4. Cessation of uterine contractions with walking

6 During pregnancy the volume of tidal air increases because there is:
1. Increased expansion of the lower ribs
2. A relative increase in the height of the rib cage
3. Upward displacement of the diaphragm
4. An increase in total blood volume

Situation: Mrs. Greene, a 22-year-old primigravida, is attending prenatal clinic. She has missed 2 menstrual periods. She relates that the first day of her last menstrual period was July 22. Questions 7 through 12 refer to this situation.

7 Mrs. Greene's estimated date of confinement would be:
1. May 5
2. April 29
3. April 15
4. May 14

8 As Mrs. Greene is being prepared for the pelvic examination, she complains of feeling very tired and sick to her stomach, especially in the morning. The best response for the nurse to make is:
1. "This is common during the early part of pregnancy. There is no need to worry."

2. "This is a common occurrence during the early part of pregnancy because of all the changes going on in your body."
3. "These are common occurrences during pregnancy with all the body changes; can you tell me how you feel in the morning?"
4. "Perhaps you might ask the doctor when he arrives."

9 Mrs. Greene works as a secretary in a large office. Her job has implications for her plan of care during pregnancy. The nurse would most likely recommend that Mrs. Greene:
1. Ask for a break in the morning and afternoon so she can elevate her legs
2. Inform her employer that she cannot work beyond the second trimester
3. Ask for a break in the morning and afternoon for added nourishment
4. Try to walk about every few hours of her work day

10 The physician performs a pelvic examination and discovers that Mrs. Greene has a normal female pelvis, with the sacrum:
1. Well hollowed, coccyx movable, spines not prominent, pubic arch wide
2. Flat, coccyx movable, spines prominent, pubic arch wide
3. Deeply hollowed, coccyx immovable, pubic arch narrow, spines not prominent
4. Flat, coccyx movable, spines prominent, pubic arch narrow

11 Mrs. Greene is concerned because she has read that nutrition during pregnancy is important for proper growth and development of the baby. She wants to know something about the foods she should eat. The nurse should:
1. Give her a list of foods so she can better plan her meals
2. Assess what she eats by taking a diet history
3. Emphasize the importance of limiting salt and highly seasoned foods
4. Instruct her to continue eating a normal diet

12 Mrs. Greene states, "I'm worried about gaining too much weight because I've heard it's bad for me." The nurse should respond:
1. "Yes, weight gain causes complications during pregnancy."
2. "Don't worry about gaining weight. We are more concerned if you don't gain enough weight to ensure proper growth of your baby."
3. "The pattern of your weight gain will be of more importance than the total amount."
4. "If you gain over 15 pounds, you'll have to follow a low-calorie diet."

13 The uterus rises out of the pelvis and becomes an abdominal organ at about the:
1. Eighth week of pregnancy
2. Eighteenth week of pregnancy
3. Tenth week of pregnancy
4. Twelfth week of pregnancy

Situation: Mrs. Bey is pregnant and requests an abortion. Questions 14 through 17 refer to this situation.

14 During the salinization method of elective abortion, the nurse should be alert for side effects such as:
1. Oliguria
2. Thirst
3. Bradycardia
4. Edema

15 After the salinization procedure the patient should be told that labor will probably begin within:
1. Two hours after the procedure
2. Several minutes following the procedure
3. Eight hours after the procedure
4. Twenty-four to 72 hours after the procedure

16 When Mrs. Bey returns to the clinic, she asks about an intrauterine device for birth control. The nurse explains that the copper intrauterine device provides contraception by:
1. Blocking the cervical os
2. Increasing the mobility of the uterus
3. Setting up a nonspecific inflammatory cell reaction
4. Preventing the sperm from reaching the fallopian tube

17 The nurse should also explain that the most common problem encountered by patients using an IUD is:
1. Development of vaginal infections
2. Discomfort associated with coitus
3. Spontaneous expulsion of the device
4. Perforation of the uterus

18 Most spontaneous abortions are caused by:
1. Physical trauma
2. Germ plasma defects
3. Unresolved stress
4. Congenital defects

19 In the dilation and suction evacuation method of elective abortion, laminarias are used in the dilation stage of the procedure because:
1. They are stronger in action than instruments
2. Dilation occurs within 2 hours
3. Less anesthesia is necessary with this method
4. They are hygroscopic and expand

Situation: Mrs. Johnson is in her first trimester and comes to the prenatal clinic. She has a cold and appears to be farther into her pregnancy than the history indicates. Questions 20 through 25 refer to this situation.

20 Mrs. Johnson asks if it is all right to take aspirin. The best advice the nurse can give to a pregnant woman in her first trimester is to:
1. Avoid all drugs, including aspirin, and refrain from smoking and ingesting alcohol
2. Take only prescription drugs, especially in the second and third trimesters
3. Cut down on drugs, alcohol, and cigarettes
4. Avoid smoking and all drugs except aspirin when needed, and limit alcohol to no more than 1 oz daily

21 Mrs. Johnson delivers twins during the seventh month, and they are diagnosed as having hyaline membrane disease. The principle underlying the respiratory distress of these infants is:
1. Surface tension
2. Pascal's principle
3. Second law of thermodynamics
4. Archimedes' principle

22 When caring for Mrs. Johnson's twins, the nurse should:
1. Keep them prone to prevent aspiration
2. Keep them in a high-humidity environment
3. Reduce oxygen concentration to prevent eye damage
4. Reduce caloric intake to decrease metabolic rate

23 While considering nursing measures to foster parent-child relationships, the nurse should be aware that the most important factor at this time is the:
1. Duration and difficulty of labor
2. Anesthesia during labor
3. Health status during pregnancy
4. Physical condition of the twins

24 Mrs. Johnson might experience postpartal hemorrhage for all the following reasons. However, the most common one is:
1. Retained secundines
2. Lacerations of the cervix
3. Atony of the uterus
4. Secondary infections

25 Overstretching of perineal supporting tissues as a result of childbirth can bring about a rectocele. The most common symptom is:
1. Protrusion of the bladder into the vagina
2. Crampy abdominal pain
3. Urinary stress incontinence
4. Recurrent urinary tract infections

Situation: Mrs. Unger delivers a baby spontaneously. Questions 26 through 31 refer to this situation.

26 Immediate critical observation for Apgar scoring includes:
1. Respiratory rate
2. Heart rate
3. Presence of meconium
4. Evaluation of Moro reflex

27 Within 3 minutes after birth the normal heart rate of the infant may range between:
1. 100 and 180
2. 130 and 160
3. 120 and 140
4. 100 and 130

28 Within this same period the normal respiratory rate may be as high as:
1. 100
2. 80
3. 60
4. 50

29 The nurse may best obtain a Moro reflex by:
 1. Creating a loud noise suddenly
 2. Changing the infant's equilibrium
 3. Stimulating the infant's feet
 4. Grasping the infant's hand

30 The Moro reflex response is marked by:
 1. Extension of arms
 2. Extension of the legs and fanning of the toes
 3. Adduction of arms
 4. Abduction and then adduction of the arms

31 Asymmetric Moro reflexes are frequently associated with:
 1. Cerebral or cerebellar injuries
 2. Cranial nerve damage
 3. Brachial plexus, clavicle, or humerus injuries
 4. Down's syndrome

Situation: Mrs. Cohen, a 26-year-old primigravida, comes to the prenatal clinic during the first trimester. She states she weighed 47.6 kg (105 lb) before her pregnancy and currently weighs 49.4 kg (109 lb). Questions 32 through 36 refer to this situation.

32 Mrs. Cohen is concerned about regaining her figure after delivery and wishes to diet during pregnancy. The nurse should advise Mrs. Cohen that:
 1. Dieting is recommended to make delivery easier
 2. Indequate food intake during pregnancy can cause some congenital anomalies
 3. Dieting is recommended to lessen the incidence of stillbirth
 4. Inadequate food intake during pregnancy can cause toxemia

33 The nurse should provide dietary teaching for Mrs. Cohen because:
 1. Pregnant women must adhere to a specific pregnancy diet
 2. Different sources of essential nutrients are favorite foods in different cultural groups
 3. Most weight gain during pregnancy is fluid retention
 4. Dietary allowances should not increase during pregnancy

34 During the seventh month of pregnancy Mrs. Cohen exhibits dependent edema. The nurse explains the treatment for fluid retention during pregnancy, which is:
 1. Adequate fluid and a low-salt diet
 2. Adequate fluid and elevation of the lower extremities
 3. A low-salt diet and elevation of the lower extremities
 4. Judicious use of diuretics and elevation of the lower extremities

35 Mrs. Cohen develops painless vaginal bleeding during the last trimester. The nurse realizes that this may be caused by:
 1. Abruptio placentae
 2. Frequent intercourse
 3. Placenta previa
 4. Excessive alcohol ingestion

36 Although the causative factors are not clear, 40% to 50% of all patients with abruptio placentae also have:
 1. Polyhydramnios
 2. Hypertension
 3. Diabetes
 4. Cardiac arrhythmias

37 The inner membrane that provides a fluid medium for the embryo is the:
 1. Amnion
 2. Yolk sac
 3. Chorion
 4. Allantois

38 First fetal movements felt by the mother are known as:
 1. Ballottement
 2. Engagement
 3. Lightening
 4. Quickening

39 Growth is most rapid during which phase of prenatal development?
 1. Implantation
 2. First trimester
 3. Second trimester
 4. Third trimester

40 The chief function of progesterone is the:
 1. Establishment of secondary male sex characteristics
 2. Rupturing of follicles for ovulation to occur
 3. Development of female reproductive organs
 4. Preparation of the uterus to receive a fertilized ovum

Situation: Mrs. Elliot, 9 weeks pregnant, visits the obstetric clinic complaining of severe nausea and vomiting. Questions 41 through 47 refer to this situation.

41 Which of the following factors is unrelated to hyperemesis gravidarum?
 1. High levels of chorionic gonadotropin
 2. Decreased secretion of free hydrochloric acid
 3. Preestablished stress-involved GI disturbances
 4. Incidence of polyhydramnios

42 Mrs. Elliot asks the nurse if she can continue to have sexual relations. The nurse's response is based on the knowledge that coitus during pregnancy would be contraindicated only in the presence of:
 1. Leukorrhea
 2. Gestation of 30 weeks or more
 3. Premature rupture of membranes
 4. Increased fetal heart rate

43 On her expected date of delivery Mrs. Elliot has a bloody show but contractions have not begun. The head is at station +1. An acceptable method to induce labor is:
 1. IM injection of oxytocin
 2. Artificial rupture of membranes
 3. Administration of prostaglandins
 4. A tap water enema

44 Mrs. Elliot has a persistent blood show and crampy abdominal pain. The nursing intervention at this time is:
1. Typing and cross matching the patient's blood for a possible transfusion
2. Providing the patient with comfort measures used for women in labor
3. Teaching the patient how to avoid straining
4. Reviewing Lamaze breathing techniques with the patient

45 During the postpartum period it is important that Mrs. Elliot voids regularly. Retention of fluid in the bladder has no relation to the development of:
1. Atony of the bladder
2. Stasis of urine, causing infection
3. Diaphoresis following delivery
4. Postpartum bleeding

46 When Mrs. Elliot's male infant has been in the nursery for about 18 hours, the nurse caring for him notes that his breathing is below 35 per minute. No other changes are noted and, since the infant is apparently well, no record or report is made. Several hours later the infant experiences severe respiratory distress and emergency care is necessary. Legal responsibility in this instance would have to take into consideration that:
1. Any marked change in respirations is significant and should have been reported
2. Respirations in the newborn are irregular and a drop is rarely important
3. Most infants experience slow respirations during the first 24 hours
4. The respiratory tract is underdeveloped in newborns and respiratory rate is not significant

47 During the taking-hold phase, the nurse would expect Mrs. Elliot to:
1. Be concerned with her own needs
2. Touch the baby with her fingertips
3. Call the baby by name
4. Talk about the baby

48 The practice of separating parents and child immediately after birth and limiting their time with the newborn in the first few days would appear to contraindicate studies based on:
1. Rooming in
2. Bonding
3. Taking-in behaviors
4. Taking-hold behaviors

49 Research indicates that the early mother-infant relationship is vital to future mental health. Which of the following statements is true?
1. Ambivalence and anxiety about mothering are common
2. A rejected pregnancy will result in a rejected infant
3. A good mother experiences neither ambivalence nor anxiety about mothering
4. Maternal love is fully developed within the first week after birth

Situation: Mrs. Portridge has been married for 6 years and has been unable to become pregnant. Mr. and Mrs. Portridge have decided to discuss this problem with a physician, who suggests that some studies be done. Questions 50 through 53 refer to this situation.

50 A test commonly used to determine the number, motility, and activity of sperm is the:
1. Rubin test
2. Huhner test
3. Papanicolaou test
4. Friedman test

51 In the female, evaluation of all the pelvic organs of reproduction is accomplished by:
1. Cystoscopy
2. Biopsy
3. Culdoscopy
4. Hysterosalpingogram

52 After ovulation has occurred, the ovum is believed to remain viable for:
1. 1 to 6 hours
2. 12 to 18 hours
3. 24 to 36 hours
4. 48 to 72 hours

53 A factor in sterility may be related to the pH of the vaginal canal. A frequent medication that is ordered to alter the pH is:
1. Sulfur insufflations
2. Sodium bicarbonate douches
3. Lactic acid douches
4. Estrogen therapy

Situation: Mrs. Winder, age 24, complains of menstrual irregularity and infertility. Questions 54 through 56 refer to this situation.

54 A drug the physician might prescribe to treat both of Mrs. Winder's complaints is:
1. Methallenestril (Vallestril)
2. Ergonovine (Ergotrate)
3. Norethynodrel with mestranol (Enovid)
4. Relaxin (Releasin)

55 Eventually Mrs. Winder becomes pregnant. She is hospitalized when her membranes rupture during the thirty-eighth week of pregnancy. If the obstetrician decides to induce labor, which if the following drugs will probably be used?
1. Ergonovine maleate
2. Progesterone
3. Oxytocin (Pitocin)
4. Lututrin (Lutrexin)

56 During the period of induction, Mrs. Winder should be observed carefully for signs of which of the following?
1. Uterine tetany
2. Severe pain
3. Prolapse of the umbilical cord
4. Hypoglycemia

Situation: Mrs. King is a primigravida at term and is admitted to the labor room. She has attended education for childbirth classes together with her husband. When Mrs. King is admitted, she is experiencing contractions every 5 to 8 minutes, which last approximately 30 seconds. She also has a slight bloody discharge. The physician's examination reveals that the cervix is about 3 cm dilated and almost fully effaced. The vertex is presenting at a +1 station, with the occiput toward the left side of the symphysis pubis. Mrs. King is quite cheerful and at ease. Questions 57 through 64 refer to this situation.

57 Mrs. King asks the nurse if it is all right for her to get up and walk around. Based on observations of Mrs. King's contractions and knowledge of the physiology and mechanism of labor, the best action for the nurse to take would be to tell Mrs. King:
1. "Please stay in bed; walking may interfere with proper uterine contractions."
2. "I can't make a decision on that, you will have to ask the doctor."
3. "You will have to stay in bed; otherwise your contractions cannot be timed and no one can listen to the fetal heart."
4. "It is quite all right for you to be up and about as long as you feel comfortable and your membranes are intact."

58 An enema is ordered for Mrs. King. Reasons for giving enemas to patients in labor include all of the following *except:*
1. Expulsion of feces during labor predisposes the patient to infection
2. A full rectum tends to hinder the progress of labor
3. It is a routine procedure carried out for every patient in labor
4. A full lower bowel predisposes to postpartum discomfort.

59 Mrs. King's contractions gradually increase in strength and become more frequent and last longer. Her membranes rupture. The first action for the nurse to take after putting Mrs. King to bed is to:
1. Listen to the fetal heart
2. Call the physician
3. Time the contractions
4. Check blood pressure and pulse

60 The nurse observes the amniotic fluid and decides that it appears normal, since it is:
1. Clear and dark amber colored
2. Milky, greenish yellow, containing shreds of mucus
3. Clear, almost colorless, containing little white specks
4. Cloudy, greenish yellow, containing little white specks

61 An examination reveals that Mrs. King is 7 to 8 cm dilated and that the vertex is low in the midpelvis. To alleviate discomfort during contractions, the nurse would instruct Mr. King to encourage his wife in:
1. Panting
2. Abdominal breathing
3. Pelvic rocking
4. Athletic chest breathing

62 Mrs. King becomes very tense with contractions and quite irritable. She frequently states "I cannot stand this a minute longer." This kind of behavior is indicative of the fact that she:
1. Is entering the transition phase of labor
2. Needs immediate administration of an analgesic or anesthetic
3. Is developing some abnormality in terms of uterine contractions
4. Has been very poorly prepared for labor in the parents' classes

63 Mr. King is becoming very tense at this time. He asks, "Do you think it is best for me to leave, since I don't seem to do my wife much good?" The most appropriate answer to this statement would be:
1. "If you feel that way, you'd best go out and sit in the father's waiting room for awhile because you may transmit your anxiety to your wife."
2. "I know this is hard for you. Why don't you go have a cup of coffee and relax and come back later if you feel like it?"
3. "This is the time your wife needs you. Don't run out on her now."
4. "This is hard for you. Let me try to help you coach her during this difficult phase."

64 The beginning of the second stage of labor can be recognized by the patient's desire to:
1. Relax during contractions
2. Push during contractions
3. Pant during contractions
4. Blow during contractions

Situation: Mrs. Kelly is a 27-year-old gravida I para 0 with a childhood history of rheumatic fever. She has been admitted to the hospital at 35 weeks' gestation because of shortness of breath. Questions 65 through 72 refer to this situation.

65 Normal hemodynamics of pregnancy that affect the pregnant cardiac patient include the:
1. Decrease in the number of red blood cells
2. Rise in cardiac output after the thirty-fourth week
3. Gradually increasing size of the uterus
4. Cardiac acceleration in the last half of pregnancy

66 Shortly after admission, Mrs. Kelly goes into labor. To prevent cardiac decompensation during labor the nurse should:
1. Position Mrs. Kelly on her side with shoulders elevated
2. Maintain an IV infusion of potassium chloride
3. Administer sodium IV infusion
4. Administer oxytocin to strengthen contractions

67 Nursing care of a patient in premature labor includes:
1. Reassuring patient that the situation is under control
2. Explaining why pain medication is kept at a minimum
3. Encouraging the patient not to bear down
4. Keeping the patient n.p.o to prevent abdominal distention

68 During the postpartal period it is not uncommon for the new mother to have an increased cardiac output with tachycardia. The nurse should observe the patient carefully for signs of:
1. Irregular pulse
2. Respiratory distress
3. Increased vaginal bleeding
4. Hypovolemic shock

69 Mrs. Kelly's infant weighs 2062 g (4 lb, 9 oz). On admission to the nursery the nurse should routinely do all the following except:
1. Evaluate the newborn's status
2. Support body temperature
3. Administer oxygen
4. Record vital signs

70 The nurse must continuously monitor baby Kelly, since the most common complication in the preterm infant is:
1. Brain damage
2. Respiratory distress
3. Aspiration of mucus
4. Hemorrhage

71 The nurse must monitor baby Kelly's temperature and provide appropriate nursing care because the premature baby:
1. Is unable to break down glycogen to glucose
2. Has a limited ability to use shivering to produce heat
3. Has a limited supply of brown fat available to provide heat
4. Has an underdeveloped pituitary system to control internal heat

72 When meeting baby Kelly's hydration needs the nurse must consider the fact that urinary function of the premature baby:
1. Is the same as in a full-term newborn
2. Causes the loss of large amounts of urine
3. Maintains stability of acid-base and electrolyte balance
4. Tends to overconcentrate the urine

73 More than half the neonatal deaths in the United States are caused by:
1. Atelectasis
2. Prematurity
3. Respiratory distress syndrome
4. Congenital heart disease

74 The presence of multiple gestation should be detected as early as possible and the pregnancy managed with high risk in mind because:
1. Perinatal mortality is 2 to 3 times greater than in single births
2. Maternal mortality is much higher during the prenatal period in multiple gestation
3. The mother needs time to adjust psychologically and physiologically after delivery
4. Postpartum hemorrhage is an expected complication

Situation: Mrs. Kim, a 22-year-old primigravida at term, is brought to the hospital by her husband. They have attended preparation for childbirth classes and plan to be together during labor. On admission Mrs. Kim is having 3-to-5-minute contractions, she has a bloody show, and her membranes are intact. On vaginal examination the cervix is fully effaced and 6 cm dilated, the vertex presenting at a + 1 station. Vital signs are temperature 37° C (98.6° F), pulse rate 76, respirations 20, fetal heart rate 140 L.L.Q., blood pressure 118/74. Mr. Kim is coaching and supporting his wife well, and Mrs. Kim appears to be quite relaxed. Questions 75 through 80 refer to this situation.

75 According to these data, Mrs. Kim is in what phase of the first stage of labor?
1. Early phase
2. Midphase
3. Transition phase
4. Accelerated phase

76 Station + 1 indicates that the presenting part is:
1. Slightly below the ischial spines
2. Slightly above the ischial spines
3. High in the false pelvis
4. On the perineum

77 Mrs. Kim is uncomfortable and asks for medication. Demerol, 50 mg, and Phenergan, 50 mg, are ordered to be administered intramuscularly. This medication would:
1. Induce sleep until the time of delivery
2. Increase her pain threshold, resulting in relaxation
3. Act as an amnesic drug
4. Act as a preliminary to anesthesia

78 A few hours later Mrs. Kim becomes very restless, her face is flushed, and she is irritable, perspiring profusely, and feels she is going to vomit. These symptoms are indicative of:
1. Second stage
2. Late stage
3. Transition phase
4. Third stage

79 When inspecting her newborn baby girl, Mrs. Kim notices a discharge from the nipples of both breasts. The nurse should explain that this is evidence of:
1. Monilia contracted during birth
2. Congenital hormonal imbalance
3. An infection contracted in utero
4. The influence of the morther's hormones

80 During the postpartum period the nurse examines Mrs. Kim and identifies the presence of lochia serosa and a fundus 4 finger breadths below the umbilicus. This indicates that the time elapsed is:
1. 1 to 3 days post partum
2. 4 to 5 days post partum
3. 6 to 7 days post partum
4. 8 to 9 days post partum

81 During the process of gametogenesis, the male and female sex cells divide and then contain:
1. A diploid number of chromosomes in their nuclei
2. A haploid number of chromosomes in their nuclei

3. Twenty-two pairs of autosomes in their nuclei
4. Forty-six pairs of chromosomes in their nuclei

82 The production of which of the following is not an endocrine function of the placenta?
   1. Chorionic gonadotropin
   2. Follicle stimulating hormone
   3. Progesterone precursor substances
   4. Somatotropin

83 During the first 2 months of pregnancy the chief source of estrogen and progesterone is the:
   1. Anterior hypophysis
   2. Placenta
   3. Adrenal cortex
   4. Corpus luteum

Situation: Mrs. Rowan is admitted to the high-risk obstetric unit with preeclampsia. Questions 84 through 90 refer to this situation.

84 Mrs. Rowan is receiving magnesium sulfate. The nurse must be alert for the first sign of excessive blood levels, which is:
   1. Development of cardiac arrhythmia
   2. Disappearance of the knee-jerk reflex
   3. Increase in respiratory rate
   4. Disturbance of the bearing ability

85 In caring for Mrs. Rowan the nurse should:
   1. Encourage her to drink clear fluids
   2. Protect her against extraneous stimuli
   3. Isolate her in a dark room
   4. Maintain her in a supine position

86 The first sign of a convulsion in a patient with preeclampsia is frequently:
   1. Rolling of the eyes to one side with a fixed stare
   2. Spots or flashes of light before the eyes
   3. Persistent headache and blurred vision
   4. Epigastric pain, nausea, and vomiting

87 Mrs. Rowan has a convulsion. Following the convulsion she has an elevated temperature of 39° C (102° F). The nurse realizes that this may be caused by:
   1. Development of a systemic infection
   2. Dehydration caused by rapid fluid loss
   3. Disturbance of the cerebral thermal center
   4. Excessive muscular activity

88 Mrs. Rowan is afraid of having another convulsion and asks when the likelihood of convulsions will end. The nurse replies that the danger of a convulsion in a woman with eclampsia ends:
   1. After labor begins
   2. After delivery occurs
   3. 24 hours post partum
   4. 48 hours post partum

89 Mrs. Rowan's labor is long and the baby is delivered in the breech position. Since Erb-Duchenne paralysis may be seen as the result of a difficult forceps or breech delivery, the nurse would look for which of the following symptoms?

1. A flaccid arm with the elbow extended
2. A negative Moro reflex on the unaffected side
3. Loss of grasp reflex on the affected side
4. Inability to turn the head to the affected side

90 If Erb-Duchenne paralysis occurred, nursing care of the infant would include:
   1. Constant immobilization of the affected arm
   2. Immediate active ROM exercises to the affected arm
   3. Teaching the parents to manipulate the muscle
   4. Daily measurement of girth and length of the affected arm

Situation: Mrs. Jackson, 2½ months pregnant, comes to the prenatal clinic for the first time. Questions 91 through 96 refer to this situation.

91 Mrs. Jackson asks the clinic nurse whether smoking will affect the baby. The nurse's answer reflects the following knowledge:
   1. Fetal and maternal circulation are separated by the placental barrier
   2. The placenta is permeable to specific substances
   3. Smoking relieves tension and the fetus responds accordingly
   4. Vasoconstriction will affect both fetal and maternal blood vessels

92 Mrs. Jackson is concerned about the mask of pregnancy, her "dark nipples," and the "dark line" from her navel to her pubis. The nurse explains that these adaptations are caused by hyperactivity of the:
   1. Adrenal gland
   2. Thyroid gland
   3. Ovaries
   4. Pituitary gland

93 Mrs. Jackson complains of morning sickness. The nurse realizes that a predisposing factor which causes morning sickness during the first trimester of pregnancy is the adaptation to increased levels of:
   1. Estrogen
   2. Progesterone
   3. Luteinizing hormone
   4. Chorionic gonadotropin

94 The nurse can help Mrs. Jackson overcome morning sickness by suggesting she:
   1. Eat nothing until the nausea subsides
   2. Take an antacid before bedtime
   3. Request her physician to prescribe an antiemetic
   4. Eat dry toast before arising

95 Mrs. Jackson delivers a healthy baby boy. Two days post partum, after receiving a phone call from her babysitter informing her that her 2-year-old has been very upset since her admission to the hospital and is not eating, Mrs. Jackson elects to sign her baby and herself out of the hospital. Staff members have been unable to contact her physician. Mrs. Jackson arrives at the nursery ready

to leave and asks that her infant be given to her to dress and take home. Appropriate nursing action would be:

1. Explain to Mrs. Jackson that her infant must remain in hospital until signed out by the physician and that she must leave the baby in the nursery
2. Allow Mrs. Jackson time with the baby to cuddle him before she leaves, but emphasize that the baby is a minor and legally must remain until orders are received
3. Tell Mrs. Jackson that under the circumstances hospital policy prevents you from releasing the infant into her care, but she will be informed when he is discharged
4. Give the baby to Mrs. Jackson to take home, making sure that she receives information regarding care and feeding of a 2-day-old infant and any potential problems which may develop

96 When Mrs. Jackson returns to the clinic for a postpartum examination, she is very depressed. The nurse realizes that the new mother who exhibits postpartum blues is probably adapting to:
1. A decrease in progesterone levels
2. Changes in body image
3. Psychologic letdown after labor
4. Rejection of her newborn

97 In which of the fetal blood vessels is the oxygen content highest?
1. Umbilical artery
2. Ductus arteriosus
3. Ductus venosus
4. Pulmonary artery

98 The blood vessels in the umbilical cord consist of:
1. Two arteries and 1 vein
2. Two arteries and 2 veins
3. One artery and 2 veins
4. One artery and 1 vein

99 When assessing the significance of estriol studies in an antenatal patient, the nurse should understand that:
1. Elevations in estriol levels indicate fetal postmaturity
2. Estriol is the hormone used in pregnancy tests
3. The fetus contributes precursors to the synthesis of estriol
4. Elevations in estriol levels indicate fetal demise

100 Physiologic anemia during pregnancy is a result of:
1. Increased blood volume of the mother
2. Decreased dietary intake of iron
3. Decreased erythropoiesis after first trimester
4. Increased detoxification demands on the mother's liver

101 The fetus is most likely to be damaged by the pregnant woman's ingestion of drugs during the:
1. First trimester
2. Second trimester
3. Third trimester
4. Entire pregnancy

Situation: Mr. and Mrs. Singer are Rh-incompatible partners. As the pregnancy progresses, the maternal serum antibody titer continues to rise. An amniocentesis is scheduled for the twenty-eighth week of pregnancy. Questions 102 through 105 refer to this situation.

102 A common method of locating the precise position of a fetus prior to an amniocentesis is:
1. X-ray examination
2. Holography
3. Fluoroscopy
4. Sonography

103 The results of the amniocentesis indicate that the fetus is only mildly affected but does, in fact, have Down's syndrome. Mr. and Mrs. Singer elect to have the pregnancy terminated. The nurse giving postoperative care to a patient who has had her pregnancy surgically terminated should be aware that:
1. The patient is emotionally unstable at this time
2. The patient needs to express her feelings of guilt, anger, and frustration
3. Contraceptive counseling should be deferred to a later time
4. The risk of postoperative infection is high

104 After the hysterotomy, Rh_oD was administered intramuscularly to:
1. Prevent antibody formation in the mother
2. Expand the antibody pool of the mother
3. Accelerate the mother's production of immune bodies
4. Suppress the activity of Rh-negative antibodies

105 It is important for the nurse to support the decisions made by the parents of a fetus with a birth defect, since:
1. The nurse's support will relieve the pressure associated with decision making
2. Supporting them will eliminate feelings of guilt
3. The parents are legally responsible for the decision
4. It is essential for maintenance of family equilibrium

106 The most common type of ectopic pregnancy is tubal. Within a few weeks after conception the tube may rupture suddenly, causing:
1. Sudden knifelike lower quadrant abdominal pain
2. Continuous dull lower quadrant abdominal pain
3. Painless vaginal bleeding
4. Intermittent abdominal contractions

107 Which symptom would the nurse be alert for when caring for a patient with a tentative diagnosis of hydatidiform mole?
1. Painless heavy vaginal bleeding
2. Unusually rapid uterine enlargement
3. Hypertension
4. Decreased fetal heart rate

Situation: Mrs. Dowle delivers a 2811.6 g (6 lb, 3 oz) baby girl. Questions 108 through 110 refer to this situation.

108 While holding her baby, Mrs. Dowle calls the nurse and says, "My baby is sick; she sneezes a lot and look how

she breathes. Her breathing is so rapid and shallow and not regular. My neighbor's baby had to return to the hospital after she was home a week because she had pneumonia. I hope this does not happen to my baby.'' The best action for the nurse to take is to:
1. Pick up the baby and tell the mother that she will watch her closely
2. Look the baby over and tell the mother that the baby is fine, there is nothing wrong with her
3. Look the baby over and explain to the mother that sneezing is normal and helps the baby to get rid of mucus and that a baby normally has rapid, shallow, irregular respirations
4. Look the baby over, take her to the nursery immediately, and return to the mother to tell her that the physician has been called, since the baby is obviously in respiratory distress

109 The nurse's response is based on the knowledge that a normal infant's respirations are:
1. Regular, initiated by the chest wall, 40 to 60 per minute, shallow
2. Irregular, abdominal, 40 to 50 per minute, shallow
3. Regular, abdominal, 40 to 50 per minute, deep
4. Irregular, initiated by chest wall, 30 to 60 per minute, deep

110 Mrs. Dowle, who has 3 children under 5 years of age at home, comments to the nursery nurse that she cannot hold the baby for feedings once she gets home. She has just too much to do, and anyhow it spoils the baby. The best response for the nurse to make is:
1. ''That's entirely up to you, you have to do what works for you.''
2. ''Holding the baby when feeding is important for her development.''
3. ''It is most unsafe to prop a bottle. The baby could aspirate the fluid.''
4. ''You seem concerned about time. Let's talk about it.''

Situation: Mrs. Ballen is admitted to the obstetric unit in labor with contractions about 15 minutes apart. Her cervix is moderately effaced and 4 cm dilated. Questions 111 through 116 refer to this situation.

111 During labor the nurse must be aware that an early deceleration (Type I dip) is evidenced by a fetal heart rate of:
1. 140 to 160 beats per minute early in the contraction
2. 120 to 140 beats per minute early in the contraction
3. 100 to 119 beats per minute early in the contraction
4. 80 to 100 beats per minute early in the contraction

112 Mrs. Ballen's labor progresses uneventfully and she enters the transitional stage. When Mrs. Ballen is positioned on the delivery table, both legs should be placed simultaneously in the stirrups to prevent:
1. Excessive pull on the fascia
2. Pressure on the perineum

3. Trauma to the uterine ligaments
4. Venous stasis in the legs

113 During each contraction the fetal heart rate persistently drops from 140 to 110 per minute. The nurse should:
1. Continue to monitor the fetal heart rate during contractions
2. Notify the physician and prepare for immediate delivery
3. Decrease the drip rate of oxytocin to slow contractions
4. Change mother's position from back to side or side to side

114 Mrs. Ballen has decided to breast-feed her infant. When teaching breast-feeding the nurse should instruct Mrs. Ballen *not* to:
1. Try to empty the breast at each feeding
2. Use an alternate breast at each feeding
3. Wash breasts with soap and water before feeding
4. Wash breasts with water before each feeding

115 Mrs. Ballen complains of frequent leg cramps. The nurse should suspect:
1. Hypercalcemia and tell her to increase her activity
2. Hypokalemia and tell her to increase her intake of green, leafy vegetables
3. Hyperkalemia and tell her to see a physician immediately
4. Hypocalcemia and tell her to increase her intake of milk

116 Mrs. Ballen asks about the difference between cow's milk and the milk from her breasts. The nurse should respond that cow's milk differs from human milk in that it contains:
1. More protein, more calcium, and less carbohydrate
2. Less protein, less calcium, and more carbohydrate
3. Less protein, more calcium, and more carbohydrate
4. More protein, less calcium, and less carbohydrate

---

117 The pituitary hormone that stimulates the secretion of milk from the mammary gland is:
1. Prolactin
2. Oxytocin
3. Progesterone
4. Estrogen

118 Breast-feeding is always contraindicated in which of the following circumstances?
1. Pregnancy
2. Herpes genitalis
3. Inverted nipples
4. Mastitis

Situation: Baby Reisler is delivered at 29 weeks' gestation. He weighs 1619 g (3 lb, 9 oz). Questions 119 through 122 refer to this situation

119 Baby Reisler is considered to be in critical condition. According to this size and length of gestation, he would be classified as:

1. Premature
2. Immature
3. Nonviable
4. Low birth weight infant

120 Baby Reisler is being fed by gavage. This type of feeding is indicated for such infants because:
   1. The feeding can be given quickly, so handling is minimized
   2. Vomiting is prevented
   3. It conserves the baby's strength and does not depend on the swallowing reflex
   4. The amount of food given can be more accurately regulated

121 Baby Reisler is placed in an incubator to maintain his body temperature at a constant level, since the heat regulation mechanism in these infants is one of the least developed functions. Which of the following conditions is responsible for this?
   1. The surface area in these babies is smaller than in normal newborns
   2. These babies lack subcutaneous fat, which would furnish some insulation
   3. These babies perspire a great deal, thus losing heat almost constantly
   4. These babies have a limited ability to produce antibodies against infections

122 In caring for these infants, which of the following precautions should be taken against retrolental fibroplasia?
   1. Oxygen should be kept at less than 40% concentration and be discontinued as soon as feasible
   2. Temperature and humidity should be controlled very carefully
   3. A high concentration of oxygen (above 75%) should be maintained together with high humidity
   4. Phototherapy should be used to prevent jaundice and retinopathy

123 Which of the following conditions is *unrelated* to postpartal hemorrhage?
   1. Delivery of twins or hydramnios
   2. Retained placenta
   3. Toxemia of pregnancy
   4. Overdistended bladder

124 Mrs. Pattern is admitted to the emergency room with vaginal bleeding. When taking a history, the nurse learns that the patient has had 5 missed periods. Later the nurse reads the chart, which states, "stillborn delivered at 8 P.M. . . ." The nurse understands this to mean that the products of conception:
   1. Were completely expelled
   2. Were previable
   3. Weighed over 600 g
   4. Measured 13.4 cm in length

125 A decision to withhold "extraordinary care" for a newborn with severe abnormalities is actually:
   1. The same as pediatric euthanasia
   2. A decision to let the newborn die

3. Presuming that the newborn has no rights
4. Unethical and illegal medical and nursing practice

126 The earliest clinical sign in idiopathic respiratory distress syndrome in the newborn is usually:
   1. Sternal and subcostal retractions
   2. Cyanosis
   3. Rapid respiration
   4. Grunting

Situation: *After a long and difficult delivery, Baby John is admitted to the newborn nursery. Questions 127 through 132 refer to this situation.*

127 An Apgar score of 4 would most likely indicate which of the following?
   1. Body pink, extremities blue
   2. Heart rate over 100
   3. Flaccid muscle tone
   4. Respirations of 35

128 Baby John has muscle twitchings, convulsions, cyanosis, abnormal respirations, and a short shrill cry. The nurse should suspect that the infant has:
   1. Tetany
   2. Intracranial hemorrhage
   3. Spina bifida
   4. Hyperkalemia

129 When observing Baby John for signs of pathologic jaundice the nurse should be alert for:
   1. The appearance of jaundice during the first 24 hours
   2. Jaundice developing between 24 and 72 hours
   3. Neurologic signs during the first 24 hours
   4. Muscular irritability at birth

130 The nurse observes Baby John lying in a supine position with his head turned to the side, his legs and arms extended on the same side and flexed on the opposite side. This is:
   1. The Landau reflex
   2. The tonic neck reflex
   3. The Moro reflex
   4. An abnormal reflex

131 Experience has shown that parents are better able to cope with the birth of an abnormal child if informed:
   1. After the first 48 hours, when the mother's strength has returned
   2. When bringing the baby to the mother for the first time
   3. After the birth, while the mother is still in the delivery room
   4. When the parents ask if something is wrong with their baby

132 Baby John's mother has decided not to nurse her baby. The medication used to suppress lactation would include the following hormone:
   1. Testosterone
   2. Cortisone
   3. Oxytocin
   4. Estrogen

Situation: Mr. and Mrs. Light want to practice the rhythm method of contraception but do not understand how it works. Questions 133 through 136 refer to this situation.

133 The nurse's explanation is based on ovulation occurring:
1. Seven days after the completion of the menstrual period
2. Fourteen days after the completion of the menstrual period.
3. Seven days before the end of the menstrual cycle
4. Fourteen days prior to the onset of menstruation

134 The time of ovulation can be determined by taking the basal temperature. During ovulation the basal temperature:
1. Drops markedly
2. Drops slightly and then rises
3. Drops markedly and remains low
4. Rises suddenly and then falls

135 The nurse explains that the efficiency of rhythm is dependent on the basal body temperature. Which of the following factors will alter its effectiveness?
1. Frequency of intercourse
2. Age of those involved
3. Presence of stress
4. Length of abstinence

136 Mrs. Light has missed 2 periods. When she comes to the prenatal clinic, she complains of vaginal bleeding and left lower quadrant pain. The nurse suspects that Mrs. Light has:
1. An incomplete abortion
2. An ectopic pregnancy
3. Abruptio placentae
4. A rupture of the graafian follicle

Situation: Mr. and Mrs. Quinn have been married almost 7 years when the physician confirms that Mrs. Quinn is 8 to 10 weeks pregnant. Mr. and Mrs. Quinn are overjoyed. About 10 days after her visit to the physician, at the time of her normal menstrual period, Mrs. Quinn starts to stain. The physician tells her to go to bed immediately and remain on complete bed rest for at least 72 hours. Since Mr. Quinn cannot stay at home and Mrs. Quinn has no one else to care for her, she is admitted to the hospital. Questions 137 through 140 refer to this situation.

137 Mrs. Quinn is admitted because of:
1. Threatened abortion
2. Inevitable abortion
3. Ectopic pregnancy
4. Missed abortion

138 After a few hours Mrs. Quinn begins to experience bearing-down sensations and suddenly expels the fetus and placenta in bed. To give safe nursing care, the nurse should first:
1. Take her immediately to the delivery room
2. Check the fundus for firmness
3. Give her the sedation ordered
4. Immediately notify the physician

139 After delivery the nurse should observe Mrs. Quinn for:
1. Dehydration and hemorrhage
2. Hemorrhage and infection
3. Subinvolution and dehydration
4. Signs of toxemia

140 When Mrs. Quinn returns to her room, both she and her husband are visibly upset. The nurse notices that Mr. Quinn has tears in his eyes and that Mrs. Quinn has her face turned to the wall and is sobbing quietly. The best approach for the nurse to take is to go over to Mrs. Quinn and say:
1. "I know how you feel, but you should not be so upset now, it will make it more difficult for you to get well quickly."
2. "I can understand that you are upset, but be glad it happened early in your pregnancy and not after you carried the baby for the full time."
3. "I know that you are upset now, but hopefully you will become pregnant again very soon."
4. "I see that both of you are very upset. I brought you a cup of coffee and will be here if you want to talk."

---

141 Abruptio placentae is most likely to occur in a woman with the following complication of pregnancy:
1. Toxemia
2. Cardiac disease
3. Hyperthyroidism
4. Cephalopelvic disproportion

142 A predisposing factor in determining whether a woman will have a postpartum hemorrhage is the knowledge that:
1. Her uterus is overdistended
2. She has had more than 5 pregnancies
3. Her duration of labor is very short
4. She is over 40 years of age

143 Which of the following fetal and neonatal hazards is *not* associated with breech delivery?
1. Intracranial hemorrhage
2. Cephalhematoma
3. Compression of cord
4. Separation of placenta prior to delivery of head

144 Which of the following is included in the care of a patient with placenta previa?
1. Limited ambulation until the bleeding stops
2. Observation and recording of the bleeding
3. Vital signs at least once per shift
4. A tap water enema before delivery

145 The nurse would suspect an ectopic pregnancy if the patient complained of:
1. Lower abdominal cramping present over a long period of time
2. Sharp lower right or left abdominal pain radiating to the shoulder
3. Leukorrhea and dysuria a few days after the first missed period
4. An adherent painful ovarian mass

146 The most effective position for a woman in labor when the nurse notes a prolapsed cord is:
1. Sims
2. Fowler
3. Trendelenburg
4. Lithotomy

Situation: Mr. and Mrs. James are attending the infertility clinic. Questions 147 through 152 refer to this situation.

147 In dealing with a couple who have an infertility problem, the nurse should know:
1. One partner has a problem that makes them unable to have children
2. The couple has been unable to have a child after trying for a year
3. Infertility is usually psychologic in origin
4. Infertility and sterility are essentially the same problem

148 A diagnostic test used to evaluate fertility is the postcoital test. It is best timed:
1. Immediately after menses
2. Within 1 to 2 days of presumed ovulation
3. One week after ovulation
4. Just prior to the next menstrual period

149 A tubal insufflation test is done to determine whether there is a tubal obstruction. Infertility caused by a defect in the tube is usually related to a:
1. Past infection
2. Fibroid tumor
3. Congenital anomaly
4. Previous injury to a tube

150 Mrs. James returns to the clinic because she has missed her menstrual period and thinks she is pregnant. The laboratory tests for pregnancy are based on the presence of:
1. Isoimmune bodies
2. Chorionic gonadotropin
3. Estrogen
4. Progesterone

151 In assessing Mrs. James' physical condition the nurse is aware of the fact that a normal adaptation of pregnany is an increased blood supply to the pelvic region. The resulting bluish purple discoloration of the vaginal mucosa and cervix is known as:
1. Hegar's sign
2. Ladin's sign
3. Goodell's sign
4. Chadwick's sign

152 Mrs. James is concerned about gaining weight during pregnancy. The nurse explains that most of the weight gain during pregnancy is due to:
1. Metabolic alterations
2. Fluid retention
3. Increased blood volume
4. The fetus

Situation: Mrs. Page has been in labor for 18 hours and is exhausted. Questions 153 through 157 refer to this situation.

153 The most common indication for cesarean section is:
1. Cephalopelvic disproportion
2. Primary uterine inertia
3. Placenta previa
4. Vaginal atony

154 The anteroposterior diameter of the birth canal is one of the important measurements of the pelvis and is known as the:
1. Diagonal conjugate
2. Transverse conjugate
3. Conjugate vera
4. Transverse diameter

155 The most effective method of determining if there is cephalopelvic disproportion for the woman in labor is:
1. Pelvimetry
2. X-ray examination
3. Amniocentesis
4. Duration of labor

156 Mrs. Page eventually delivers her baby vaginally. The newborn has asymmetric gluteal folds, and the nurse suspects:
1. A dislocated hip
2. Peripheral nervous system damage
3. An inguinal hernia
4. Central nervous system damage

157 Mrs. Page asks the nurse why sugar is added to the baby's formula. The nurse's response would depend on the following understanding:
1. Cow's milk contains fewer calories than breast milk
2. Sugar in cow's milk is not assimilated well
3. Diluted cow's milk provides less sugar than the baby needs
4. Sugar in cow's milk is a disaccharide

158 The two most important predisposing causes of puerperal infection are:
1. Hemorrhage and trauma during labor
2. Toxemia and retention of placenta
3. Malnutrition and anemia during pregnancy
4. *Streptococcus* organism present in the birth canal and trauma during labor

Situation: Mrs. Allen is 2 weeks past her expected date of delivery. The physician has decided to perform an oxytocin challenge test (OCT), in which IV oxytocin solution is administered and the fetal heart rate and uterine contractions are recorded. Questions 159 through 164 refer to this situation.

159 Which of the following would be an indication for the oxytocin challenge test?
1. Previous abruptio placentae
2. Placenta previa
3. Premature onset of labor
4. Pregnancy of more than 40 weeks

160 Contraindications to an oxytocin challenge test would include:
1. Prematurity
2. Drug addiction
3. Hypertension
4. Uterine activity

161 Mrs. Allen responds well to the oxytocin challenge test and labor is induced. Several hours later Mrs. Allen is complaining of pain and asks for medication. A medication given to a woman in labor that might cause respiratory depression of the newborn is:
1. Meperidine (Demerol)
2. Scopolamine
3. Promazine (Sarine)
4. Promethazine (Phenergan)

162 Mrs. Allen delivers a 4260 g (9 lb, 6 oz) baby. In assessing the newborn, the nurse observes an unequal Moro reflex on one side and a flaccid arm in adduction. The nurse suspects:
1. Brachial palsy
2. Supratentorial tear
3. Fracture of the clavical
4. Crigler/Najjar syndrome

163 The evening after delivery, the nurse encourages Mrs. Allen to ambulate to:
1. Increase the tone of the bladder
2. Promote respiration
3. Increase peripheral vasomotor activity
4. Maintain tone of abdominal muscles

164 In caring for the family on a postpartum unit, the nurse must be aware that all the tasks, responsibilities, and attitdes which make up child care can be called mothering and that either parent can exhibit motherliness. A person is able to perform "mothering" because of:
1. An inborn ability based on instinct
2. Positive childhood roles and concepts
3. A good education in growth and development
4. A marriage with flexible roles

165 The most common symptom of congenital rubella syndrome that follows infection in the mother during the first trimester is:
1. Hydrocephalus
2. Phocomelia
3. Cardiac anomaly
4. Otosclerosis

166 Closure of the foramen ovale after birth is caused by:
1. A decrease in the aortic blood flow
2. An increase in the pulmonary blood flow
3. A decrease in pressure in the left atrium
4. An increase in the pressure in the right atrium

167 After birth, in a normal neonate the ductus arteriosus becomes the:
1. Ligamentum teres
2. Venous ligament
3. Ligamentum arteriosum
4. Superior vesical artery

168 An infant's intestines are sterile at birth, therefore lacking the bacteria necessary for the synthesis of:
1. Prothrombin
2. Bile salts
3. Intrinsic factor
4. Bilirubin

169 Immunity transferred to the fetus from an immune mother through the placenta is:
1. Active natural immunity
2. Active artificial immunity
3. Passive natural immunity
4. Passive artificial immunity

170 Which of the following findings would probably necessitate placing the newborn in the intensive care nursery?
1. An initial Apgar score of 5
2. A birth weight of 3500 g
3. The aspiration of 20 ml of milky-colored fluid from newborn's stomach
4. An umbilical cord that contained only 2 vessels

171 The nurse encourages continued medical supervision for the pregnant woman with pyelitis because:
1. Antibiotic therapy is given until the urine is sterile
2. Toxemia frequently occurs following pyelitis
3. Pelvic inflammatory disease occurs with untreated pyelitis
4. A low-protein diet is given until pregnancy is terminated

172 A nurse tells a pregnant woman not to wear tight clothing around her abdomen because of possible damage to the fetus. The principle responsible for the potential damage is:
1. Pascal's
2. Archimedes'
3. Newton's
4. Einstein's

173 During pregnancy, the uterine musculature hypertrophies and is greatly stretched as the fetus grows. This stretching:
1. By itself inhibits uterine contraction until oxytocin stimulates the birth process
2. Is prevented from stimulating uterine contraction by high levels of estrogen during late pregnancy
3. Inhibits uterine contraction along with the combined inhibitory effects of estrogen and progesterone
4. Would ordinarily stimulate uterine contraction but is prevented by high levels of progesterone during pregnancy

174 During pregnancy a polypeptide similar to the adrenal steroids is responsible for:
1. Symptoms of morning sickness
2. Urinary frequency
3. Linea nigra and chloasma
4. Softening of the cervix

175 A normal woman who had a hemophilic father is mated to a man with normal blood clotting. What is the probable phenotype of the offspring?
1. All children are hemophiliacs

2. Half the male children are hemophiliacs
3. All male children are hemophiliacs
4. All children are normal

176 If anemia is present with a hemoglobin level of 8 g or lower, a mother with cardiac disease probably will go into:
1. Cardiac failure
2. Heart block
3. Atrial fibrillation
4. Cardiac compensation

Situation: Mrs. Evans, a diabetic, suspects that she is pregnant because she is experiencing breast changes, has missed 2 periods, and has some early morning nausea and excessive fatigue. Despite the nausea and fatigue, her urine tests are consistently negative for sugar. Mrs. Evans seeks the advice of an obstetrician, who confirms the diagnosis of pregnancy. Mrs. Evans is taking 30 units of NPH insulin daily at this time. Questions 177 through 181 refer to this situation.

177 A diabetic mother's metabolism is significantly altered during pregnancy as a result of:
1. The increased effect of insulin during pregnancy
2. The effect of hormones produced in pregnancy on carbohydrate and lipid metabolism
3. An increase in the glucose tolerance level of the blood
4. The lower renal threshold for glucose

178 Regulation of usual insulin coverage in a pregnant diabetic woman is difficult, since:
1. Sugar can normally be found in the urine of a pregnant woman
2. Sugar is metabolized more rapidly during pregnancy
3. The basal metabolic rate is altered during pregnancy
4. Insulin is absorbed more rapidly because of increased blood volume

179 Mrs. Evans is referred to the clinic nutritionist for nutritional assessment and counseling. The dietary program worked out for her would be:
1. A low-carbohydrate, low-calorie diet to stay within her present insulin coverage and avoid hyperglycemia
2. A diet high in protein of good biologic value and decreased calories
3. Adequate balance of carbohydrate and fat to meet energy demands and prevent ketosis
4. Insulin adjusted as needed to balance increased dietary needs

180 When Mrs. Evans' newborn is admitted to the newborn nursery, the nurse should be aware that babies of diabetic mothers show symptoms of tremors, apnea, cyanosis, and poor sucking reflex because of:
1. Congenital depression of the islets of Langerhans
2. Hypoglycemia
3. Central nervous system edema
4. Hyperglycemia

181 Mrs. Evans' baby weighs 4600.8 g (10 lb, 2 oz), and she expresses concern about its size. The nurse's reply should be based upon the knowledge that babies of diabetic mothers are larger than other babies because of:

1. Increased somatotropin and lowered glucose utilization
2. Increased somatotropin and increased glucose utilization
3. Decreased somatotropin and decreased glucose utilization
4. Decreased somatotropin and increased glucose utilization

Situation: Mrs. Sawyer suspects she is pregnant when she attends the prenatal clinic for the first time. This is her first pregnancy and she is unsure whether the pregnancy should be terminated, since she and her husband depend on her salary. Questions 182 through 187 refer to this situation

182 Pregnancy and birth are called crises because:
1. They are periods of change and adjustment to change
2. There are hormonal and physiologic changes in the mother
3. There are mood changes during pregnancy
4. Narcissism in the mother affects the husband-wife relationship

183 The nurse should intervene to alleviate crisis by:
1. Involving the mother in preparation classes
2. Helping the mother express her feelings
3. Understanding the family interaction
4. Involving the father in preparation classes

184 The nurse suggests a pregnancy test. This is possible because in early pregnancy the urine contains:
1. Prolactin
2. Chorionic gonadotropin
3. Estrogen
4. Luteinizing hormone

185 At the time of her second visit to the prenatal clinic Mrs. Sawyer requests information about abortion. She is 8 weeks pregnant at this time. The nurse expresses the opinion that abortion is immoral and that many women have permanent guilt feelings after an abortion. The patient leaves the clinic in a very disturbed state. Legally the:
1. Nurse had a right to state feelings as long as they were identified as the nurse's own
2. Patient had a right to correct, unbiased information
3. Physician should have been called in, since the nurse cannot talk about it
4. Nurse's statements need not be based on scientific knowledge

186 Mrs. Sawyer returns to the clinic after deciding to continue with the pregnancy. She complains of nausea and urinary frequency. She states that she feels punished for her thoughts about abortion. The nurse explains that urinary frequency often occurs because the capacity of the bladder is diminished during pregnancy by:
1. Atony of the detrusor muscle
2. Compression by the ascending uterus
3. Constriction of the ureteral entrance at the trigone
4. Compromise of the autonomic reflexes

187 The nurse also informs her that morning sickness is not punishment but is associated with pregnancy and usually ends by the end of the:
1. Second month
2. Third month
3. Fifth month
4. Fourth month

188 The most frequent side effect associated with the use of IUDs is:
1. Rupture of the uterus
2. Excessive menstrual flow
3. Expulsion of the IUD
4. Ectopic pregnancy

189 What is the menopausal implication for women taking oral contraceptives? They:
1. Prolong menses
2. Intensify menopausal symptoms
3. Cause menorrhagia
4. Have no effect on menopause

190 An abandoned infant has been brought to the hospital. Ophthalmia neonatorum is diagnosed. You know the infant's age is:
1. One day
2. Less than 24 hours
3. At about 3 to 4 days
4. At least 2 days

Situation: Mrs. Pitis, a 28-year-old primipara, was admitted 8 hours ago, 2 cm dilated in active labor. She is now 3 or 4 cm dilated and the vertex is floating. Questions 191 through 198 refer to this situation.

191 One of the most common causes of hypotonic uterine dystocia is:
1. Toxemia
2. Maternal anemia
3. Pelvic contracture
4. Twin gestation

192 Nursing care would include a careful assessment for signs of maternal exhaustion such as:
1. Circumoral cyanosis
2. Lowered body temperature
3. Fruity odor to breath
4. Skeletal muscle irritability

193 When caring for Mrs. Pitis, who is having a prolonged labor, the nurse must be aware that the patient is very concerned when her labor deviates from what she sees as the norm. A response conveying acceptance of the patient's expressions of frustration and hostility would be:
1. "Would you like to talk about what's bothering you?"
2. "All women get weary and frustrated during labor."
3. "I'll rub your back; tell me if it helps."
4. "I'll leave so you can talk to your husband."

194 Because secondary uterine inertia has developed in Mrs. Pitis, the physician has ordered oxytocin to stimulate contractions. The most important aspect of nursing care at this time is:
1. Monitoring the fetal heart rate
2. Checking perineum for bulging
3. Timing and recording length of contractions
4. Preparing for an emergency cesarean section

195 After a trial labor with oxytocin and x-ray pelvimetry, the physician advises Mrs. Pitis that a cesarean section is necessary. In addition to the routine care given postpartum patients during the first 24 hours, the nurse should:
1. Check the fundus gently but firmly
2. Check vital signs for evidence of shock
3. Maintain IV infusion of oxytocin
4. Encourage early ambulation

196 Two-day-old Andrew Pitis, who weighs 2722 g (6 lb), is fed Enfamil every 4 hours. Newborns need about 73 ml (2 to 3 oz) of fluid per pound of body weight each day. Based on this information, the nurse knows at each feeding to give Andrew at least:
1. 2 to 3 oz
2. 1 to 2 oz
3. 3 to 4 oz
4. 4 to 5 oz

197 Andrew has begun to eat greedily and finishes the entire bottle of formula. Afterward he regurgitates and his mother is concerned. The nurse explains to the mother that this is normal and due to:
1. An underdeveloped cardiac sphincter
2. A spasm at the pyloric valve
3. Intake of air while sucking
4. His position after feeding

198 Andrew has just been circumcised. The most essential nursing action the first day is to observe for:
1. Infection
2. Decreased urinary output
3. Shrill, piercing cry
4. Hemorrhage

199 If a woman with untreated gonorrhea is allowed to deliver, the infant is in danger of being born with:
1. Ophthalmia neonatorum
2. Congenital syphilis
3. Thrush
4. Pneumonia

200 In observing the newborn infant of a mother untreated for syphilis during the second trimester, the nurse would expect to find:
1. Normal-sized liver and spleen
2. A cleft palate and harelip
3. Maculopapular lesions of the soles
4. Hypotonicity of skeletal muscles

Maternity Nursing Answers and Rationales

1. (3) The chorion is the outermost membrane that helps form the placenta. It develops villi and, through its interaction with the endometrium, becomes part of the placenta. (c)
   (1) The amnion is the innermost lining, from which amniotic fluid is secreted.
   (2) The yolk sac is part of the inner structure of the blastocyst and is lined by inner layer of cells, the entoderm; unrelated to placental formation.
   (4) The allantois is a tubular diverticulum of the posterior part of the embryo's yolk sac; fuses with the chorion to form the placenta.

2. (1) Progesterone is secreted mainly by the corpus luteum. It helps prepare the endometrium for possible implantation of a fertilized ovum. (b)
   (2) Adrenal cortex secretions contain only minute quantities of progesterone.
   (3) Endometrium is influenced by progesterone secretion but does not secrete it.
   (4) Pituitary gland secretions stimulate the target gland (e.g., corpus luteum of the ovary) to secrete progesterone.

3. (4) Gestation is divided into 3 stages—blastocyst, embryo and fetus. (b)
   (1) Known as a fetus until birth.
   (2) At the time of implantation the group of developing cells is called a blastocyst.
   (3) The fetal heart is heard between the eighteenth and twentieth weeks; known as a fetus at the end of the eighth week.

4. (4) A determination of the station (descent) of the fetus is based on the relationship of the presenting part and the spine. If too small, delivery cannot occur. (c)
   (1) The measurement of pelvic floor is not involved with the fetus' descent into the birth canal.
   (2) It is a measurement of the pelvic outlet.
   (3) It is the narrowest measurement.

5. (1) The true regular contractions of labor increase in intensity and regularity with activity. (c)
   (2) True labor, consisting of regular forceful contractions, results in descent of the baby into the birth canal.
   (3) True labor leads to progressive cervical dilation and effacement.
   (4) Pains occurring during false labor are relieved when the patient lies down.

6. (1) To allow for the larger intake of air, the normal adaptation is to increase the size of the thoracic cavity. (c)
   (2) There is no change in the height of the rib cage.

   (3) Upward displacement would decrease tidal air volume.
   (4) Blood volume is not related to tidal air volume.

7. (2) Naegle's rule is an indirect noninvasive method for estimating the date of delivery:

   E.D.C. =
        L.M.P. + 7 days − 3 months + 1 year (b)

   (1) Miscalculation.
   (3) Miscalculation.
   (4) Miscalculation.

8. (3) This response encourages further elaboration of what Mrs. Greene means by feeling very tired and sick to her stomach. It is always best to let the client explain her symptoms rather than drawing conclusions immediately. (b)
   (1) Cuts off communication; denies the patient's feelings.
   (2) True, but does not allow the patient to discuss her feelings further.
   (4) Within the scope of the nurse's information; also may cause the patient to worry that something is seriously wrong.

9. (4) A frequent change from one sitting position is important for good circulation. Walking is an excellent form of exercise to promote circulation. (b)
   (1) Elevation of the legs does not promote arterial circulation; merely fosters venous return.
   (2) Not true; patients may work until the day of delivery.
   (3) Added nourishment can be part of her regular mealtimes; in addition, nourishment will not promote circulation.

10. (1) Although pure types are unusual, the normal female pelvis is one most favorable for normal delivery. Characteristics include well-rounded inlet, straight sidewalls, well-formed sacrosciatic notches, good sacral curvature and inclination, movable coccyx, moderately sized ischial spines, and well-rounded suprapubic arches. (b)
    (2) The normal female pelvis is gynecoid; this describes an android pelvis.
    (3) The normal female pelvis is gynecoid; this is descriptive of an anthropoid pelvis.
    (4) The normal female pelvis is gynecoid; this describes a platypelloid pelvis.

11. (2) By taking a diet history, the nurse can assess the woman's level of nutritional knowledge and gain clues for appropriate methods of counseling. (a)
    (1) These foods may be too expensive and different from her normal choices, leading to noncompliance.
    (3) Salt is no longer limited in normal pregnancy.
    (4) Normal is too vague a term; the patient will need increased protein and caloric intake.

12. (3) A sudden sharp increase near the twentieth week of pregnancy may indicate water retention and the beginning of preeclampsia. (b)

(1) Untrue; weight gain is necessary to ensure adequate nutrition for the fetus.

(2) Closes off communication; does not allow the patient to ask more questions about weight gain.

(4) There is no hard-and-fast number of pounds that the patient should gain, and low-calorie diets may be harmful.

13. (4) By this time the fetus and placenta have grown, expanding the size of the uterus. The extended uterus expands into the abdominal cavity. (b)

(1) The uterus is still within the pelvic area at this time.

(2) The uterus has already risen out of the pelvis and is expanding further into the abdominal area.

(3) The uterus is still within the pelvic area.

14. (2) The saline may have gotten into the vascular system rather than into the amniotic sac. (c)

(1) A serious manifestation of water intoxication occurring when oxytocin is used in the saline abortion; not a consequence of saline administration.

(3) Bradycardia may occur with the use of spinal or regional anesthesia, not salinization.

(4) Edema may occur as a result of water intoxication when oxytocin is used in the saline abortion.

15. (4) The saline causes puffing of the placenta, fetal death, placental separation, release of fibrin, and then labor and paradoxical hemorrhaging. This takes at least 24 hours in most cases. (c)

(1) Normally labor starts 24 to 72 hours after the procedure.

(2) Too quick; it takes 24 to 72 hours for labor to begin.

(3) Too quick: usually takes 24 to 72 hours, unless oxytocin is used to hasten labor.

16. (3) Because of the irritation, the uterine lining is not receptive to the implantation of the fertilized egg. (c)

(1) A diaphragm blocks the cervical os.

(2) Mobility of the uterus is not related to contraception.

(4) The sperm can reach the fallopian tube; implantation of the fertilized egg is impaired.

17. (3) The IUD may cause irritability of the myometrium, inducing contraction of the uterus and expulsion of the device. (c)

(1) Increased vaginal infections are not reported with use of IUD.

(2) Patients do not complain of discomfort during coitus when an IUD is in place.

(4) This is a rare rather than a common occurrence.

18. (2) About 75% of all spontaneous abortions take place between 8 and 12 weeks of gestation and show embryonic defects. (b)

(1) Though possible, physical trauma rarely causes an abortion.

(3) Unresolved stress may lead to congenital defects but is rarely associated with abortion.

(4) Congenital defects are asymptomatic during pregnancy and do not usually cause abortion.

19. (4) Laminaria is a seaweed that expands in a moist environment. It is a natural and safe method of dilating the cervix. (b)

(1) Untrue; may not be as strong but certainly less traumatic.

(2) It takes 24 hours for the laminaria to expand.

(3) Anesthesia is not used in the dilation phase of abortion.

20. (1) The first trimester is the period when all major organs are being laid down. Drugs, alcohol, and tobacco may cause major defects. (a)

(2) Drugs, unless absolutely necessary, should be avoided throughout pregnancy; but the first trimester is most significant.

(3) Cutting down is insufficient; these teratogens should be eliminated.

(4) Aspirin is known to cause severe hemolysis in the fetus, and even 1 oz of alcohol is considered harmful.

21. (1) The physical principle is surface tension. Since the lung tissue of the infants lacks the group of detergents known as surfactant, water molecules strongly interact with each other by hydrogen bonding and the alveolar sacs and respiratory passages do not easily expand; the result is extremely labored, if not impossible, breathing. (b)

(2) This is related to the equal distribution of external pressure throughout a fluid in a closed vessel.

(3) This has to do with the relationship between heat and mechanical energy.

(4) This has to do with a body in water being buoyed by force equal to the weight of the fluid displaced.

22. (2) Humidity may liquefy the tenacious secretions, making gas exchange possible. (b)

(1) Side lying, rather than prone, since the babies may be too immature to raise their heads from the prone position.

(3) This is not a routine action; oxygen concentration will depend on the babies' blood gases.

(4) Actually the caloric intake will be increased; the amount, number, and type of feedings will be related to the metabolic rate.

23. (4) Bonding between parent and baby is most successful when interaction is possible right after birth. If the child is ill, contact is limited. (c)

(1) Though certainly a factor, more important is the physical condition of the twins.

(2) Relative; but most important is the physical condition of the babies.

(3) May be relative; but most important is the physical condition of the twins.

24. (3) The overdistended uterus does not contract readily. (b)

(1) This can occur in any delivery (not just twins) if careful inspection of the placental contents is not done.

(2) This is unusual and may occur with improper use of forceps; not indicated in this situation.

(4) Cause systemic responses other than hemorrhage.

25. (3) The posterior vaginal wall is pushed forward by the herniation of the rectum. This increases the intravesicular pressure, which causes incontinence. (c)

(1) This is a description of a cystocele.

(2) A rectocele is not accompanied by abdominal pain.

(4) A cystocele is associated with urinary tract infections.

26. (2) Respiratory effort rather than rate is included in the Apgar score. The rate is very erratic. Heart rate is vital. (c)

(1) Too variable; not used in Apgar scoring.

(3) May or may not be present at this time and not part of Apgar scoring.

(4) Should be assessed later, but not part of Apgar scoring.

27. (3) The rate varies with activity. Crying will increase the rate, whereas deep sleep will lower it. A rate between 120 and 140 is within normal range. (b)

(1) Rates below 120 are considered bradycardia; above 180, tachycardia.

(2) The normal rate is between 120 and 140.

(4) Below 120 is considered bradycardia.

28. (3) Rate is associated with activity and can be as rapid as 60 breaths per minute. Over 60 breaths per minute is considered tachypneic in the infant. (b)

(1) Considered to be tachypneic in the newborn.

(2) Any rate above 60 considered to be tachypneic.

(4) May go up to 60 with activity.

29. (2) Changes in equilibrium stimulate this neurologic reflex in an infant under the age of 6 months. The movements should be bilateral and symmetric. A loud noise causes the same reaction (startle reflex), but using noise as a stimulus really tests hearing. (c)

(1) Tests the baby's hearing not the Moro reflex.

(3) Tests for the Babinski reflex not the Moro.

(4) Tests for the grasp reflex not the Moro.

30. (4) The Moro reflex is a sudden extension and abduction of the arms at the shoulders and spreading of the fingers, with the index finger and thumb forming the letter c. This is followed by flexion and adduction. The legs may weakly flex, and the infant may cry vigorously. (b)

(1) Only part of the normal Moro response; should be accompanied by abduction and spreading of the fingers.

(2) Legs generally flex weakly.

(3) The reflex is abduction.

31. (3) Injury to the brachial plexus, clavicle, or humerus prevents the abductive and adductive movements of the upper extremities. (b)

(1) These injuries usually cause a symmetric loss of the Moro reflex.

(2) Not usually associated; however, if the cochlea is undeveloped or the eighth cranial (vestibulococh-

lear) nerve were injured, it would affect equilibrium and response to the test.

(4) Children with Down's syndrome exhibit a normal Moro reflex.

32. (2) The Committee on Maternal Nutrition of the National Research Council recommends a weight gain of at least 25 lb (11.3 kg) during pregnancy. Inadequate nutrition results in underweight babies. (a)

(1) Dieting is absolutely forbidden during pregnancy and can result in congenital anomalies.

(3) The cause of stillbirth is not actually known; dieting is not recommended.

(4) There is a theory that an inadequate intake of protein is related to toxemia, but it has not been totally proved.

33. (2) The nurse should become informed about the cultural eating patterns of patients so that foods containing the essential nutrients which are part of these dietary patterns will be included in the diet. (c)

(1) Pregnancy diets are not specific; merely composed of the essential nutrients.

(3) Fluid retention is only one component of weight gain; growth of the baby, placenta, breasts, etc. also contributes to weight gain.

(4) Calories and nutrients are increased during pregnancy.

34. (2) Fluids and salt should not be restricted, for they are necessary to the well-being of the mother and fetus. Elevation of the extremities several times daily is recommended to decrease the edema. (b)

(1) Salt is not limited during pregnancy.

(3) Salt is not limited during pregnancy.

(4) Diuretics can be harmful and are not used during pregnancy.

35. (3) During the painless contractions of pregnancy, the lower edge of the placenta separates from the walls of the uterus, opening placental sinuses and allowing blood to escape. (b)

(1) Abruptio placentae is usually accompanied by intense pain.

(2) Highly unlikely unless placenta previa is present.

(4) Previa, a low-implanted placenta, causes painless vaginal bleeding; alcohol ingestion does not.

36. (2) The vascular changes associated with hypertension may cause a reduction in the blood supply to the uterus, resulting in placental infarcts and separation of the placenta from the decidua. (b)

(1) There is a normal amount of amniotic fluid in patients with abruptio placentae.

(3) Rare; occurs only in patients with severe diabetes with related vascular disease.

(4) No relationship between placental separation and cardiac irregularities.

37. (1) The amnion encloses the embryo and the shock-protective amniotic fluid in which the embryo floats. (a)

(2) The yolk sac contains the stored nutrients of the ovum.

(3) The chorion is the outermost membrane; does not secrete fluid.

(4) The allantois is a component of the developing umbilical cord.

38. (4) The word originates from the Middle English word *quik,* which means alive. (c)

(1) Ballottement is the bouncing of fetus in the amniotic fluid against the examiner's hand.

(2) Engagement is when the presenting part is at the level of the ischial spine.

(3) Lightening is the descent of the fetus into the birth canal.

39. (4) This is the period in which the fetus stores deposits of fat. (b)

(1) This is the period of the blastocyst, when initial cell division takes place.

(2) The first trimester is the period of organogenesis, when cells differentiate into major organ systems.

(3) Growth is occurring, but fat deposition does not occur in this period.

40. (4) Progesterone stimulates differentiation of the endometrium into a secretory type of tissue. (b)

(1) Secondary male characteristics are influenced by testosterone.

(2) Influenced by high levels of luteinizing hormone.

(3) Influenced by estrogen.

41. (4) Polyhydramnios (excessive fluid) is associated with multiple gestation. Dehydration is generally associated with hyperemesis gravidarum. (b)

(1) Frequently high levels of chorionic gonadotropin are associated with intractable vomiting of pregnancy, especially in the presence of hydatidiform mole.

(2) This is associated with vomiting; undigested food remains in the stomach, which leads to a reflexive action and vomiting.

(3) There is a strong psychologic component related to the pernicious vomiting of pregnancy.

42. (3) Intact membranes act as a barrier against organisms that may cause an intrauterine infection. (b)

(1) Common because of increased production of mucus containing exfoliated vaginal epithelial cells; intercourse is not contraindicated.

(2) Intercourse is not contraindicated if membranes are intact; modification of sexual positions may be needed because of an enlarged abdomen after the thirtieth week.

(4) This may be occurring, but there is no literature indicating that it is harmful for the fetus.

43. (2) Transcervical amniotomy (artificial rupture of the membranes) requires that the cervix be soft, partially effaced, and slightly dilated with the presenting part engaged or engaging. This patient would meet these criteria, as demonstrated by the bloody show and the head at +1. (c)

(1) IM injection of oxytocin is extremely dangerous because of the physician's inability to control the effects of the drug; oxytocin by intravenous infusion

is considered safe as long as maternal and fetal monitoring is continuous.

(3) Prostaglandins are effective for inducing labor, but they are expensive and produce unpleasant side effects.

(4) A tap water enema would be ineffective for inducing labor.

44. (2) The patient is experiencing the expected discomforts of labor. The nurse should initiate measures that will promote relaxation. (b)

(1) There is no evidence at this time that the patient is losing excessive blood (hemorrhage).

(3) During the pushing phase, straining is unavoidable.

(4) The patient is not receptive to teaching at this time; all energy is being directed inward.

45. (3) Diaphoresis is a normal adaptation of the postpartum period and does not relate to bladder distention. It is caused by the reduction of antidiuretic hormone, leading to profuse perspiration. (b)

(1) This may follow anesthesia and cause retention.

(2) Stasis of urine and infection can occur when urinary retention is present.

(3) Postpartum bleeding may occur if the uterus is impeded from involuting because of a full bladder.

46. (1) A respiratory rate below 40 in the newborn is not within the normal range. The normal is 40 to 60 breaths per minute. A drop to 35 per minute is a significant change and should have been reported. (b)

(2) Any significant change should be reported immediately because it may be indicative of brain damage.

(3) Untrue; more likely respirations will accelerate when activity is increased.

(4) The respiratory tract is fully developed, and respiratory rate is a cardinal sign of the infant's well-being.

47. (3) The mother has completed the taking-in phase (mother's needs predominate) and has moved into the taking-hold phase (active maternal involvement with self and infant) when she calls the baby by name. (c)

(1) This is part of the taking-in phase.

(2) Initial early action of the taking-in phase.

(4) This may occur in either phase.

48. (2) There is a sensitive period in the first minutes or hours after birth during which it is necessary, for later interpersonal development to be normal, that the mother and father have close contact with their new infant. (b)

(1) Rooming-in is not immediate; it occurs once the mother is in the postpartal unit.

(3) Taking-in is a psychologic behavior described by Reva Rubin that occurs during the first 2 postpartal days.

(4) Taking-hold is a psychologic behavior described by Reva Rubin that occurs after the third postpartal day.

49. (1) Because mothering is not an inborn instinct, almost all mothers, including multiparas, report some ambivalence and anxiety about their ability to be good mothers. (a)
    (2) Untrue; very often the maternal instinct is nurtured at the sight of the infant.
    (3) Untrue; ambivalent feelings are universal in response to the infant.
    (4) Untrue; may take a much longer time.

50. (2) Determines the number and condition of sperm aspirated from the cervix within 2 hours after coitus. (b)
    (1) The Rubin test determines the patency of the fallopian tubes.
    (3) The Papanicolaou test is used for the early diagnosis of cervical cancer.
    (4) The Friedman test is done to establish the diagnosis of pregnancy.

51. (4) This test enables the examiner to visualize the uterus and fallopian tubes and the pelvic organs for reproduction. (a)
    (1) Cystoscopy is used to evaluate the urinary bladder.
    (2) Biopsy is the surgical excision of tissue for diagnostic purposes.
    (3) Culdoscopy is the direct examination of female pelvic viscera using an endoscope introduced through a perforation in the vagina.

52. (3) The ovum is capable of being fertilized for only 24 to 36 hours following ovulation. After this time it travels a variable distance between the fallopian tube and uterus, disintegrates, and is phagocytized by leukocytes. (b)
    (1) The ovum is viable for 24 to 36 hours.
    (2) It is viable a longer time.
    (4) It is not fertilizable after 48 hours.

53. (2) Sperm motility is increased at pH values near neutral or slightly alkaline. A sodium bicarbonate douche will reduce the acidity of fluids in the vagina and help optimize the pH (c)
    (1) Sulfur does not change the pH in any way.
    (3) This would increase the acid content and kill the sperm.
    (4) Estrogen does not alter the pH.

54. (3) The action of Enovid is to inhibit ovulation and establish regular menstrual cycles. This is one of the first steps in treating infertility problems. (b)
    (1) Vallestril is used for management of estrogen deficiency; no action on the ovaries.
    (2) Ergotrate is used to contract the uterus.
    (4) Relaxin is used for dysmenorrhea; causes relaxation of the symphysis pubis.

55. (3) Oxytocin is a small polypeptide hormone normally synthesized in the hypothalamus and secreted from the neurohypophysis during parturition or suckling. It promotes powerful uterine (smooth muscle) contractions and thus is used to induce labor. (c)
    (1) Ergonovine can lead to sustained contractions, which would be undesirable in labor.

(2) Progesterone builds up the endometrium; does not initiate uterine contractions.
    (4) Preludin or phenmetrazine is an appetite suppressant; not used in pregnancy.

56. (1) Since oxytocin promotes powerful uterine contractions, exogenous administration of this hormone may induce uterine tetany, which does not optimize progression of labor and may restrict fetal blood flow. (b)
    (2) Severe pain is associated with intense contractions.
    (3) Not likely to occur unless the baby is in breech position.
    (4) Unrelated to uterine contractions.

57. (4) Contractions are stronger and more regular when the woman is standing. Also, during walking the diameter of the pelvic inlet increases and allows for easier entrance of the head into the pelvis. (b)
    (1) Untrue; contractions of true labor are enhanced when the mother walks about.
    (2) Denies the nurse's understanding of the physiology of labor.
    (3) Timing can continue even if the patient walks around.

58. (3) Each patient in labor is different, with individual needs. The enema is never a routine procedure. (b)
    (1) Fecal material is considered a contaminant and may enter the vaginal canal if the membranes are ruptured.
    (2) The presence of fecal material in the rectum may impede the progress of the head into the vaginal opening.
    (4) The soreness from the episiotomy and enlarged hemorrhoids makes bowel evacuation painful.

59. (1) When the membranes rupture, there is always the possibility of a prolapsed cord leading to fetal distress, which would manifest itself in a slowed heartbeat. (b)
    (2) Unnecessary, unless there is a marked change in the fetal heart rate.
    (3) This is regularly done before and after the membranes rupture; however, fetal status takes priority.
    (4) Done routinely throughout the entire labor process; at this point, fetal status takes priority.

60. (3) By 36 weeks' gestation, normal amniotic fluid is colorless with small particles of vernix caseosa present. (a)
    (1) Dark amber suggests the presence of bilirubin, an ominous sign.
    (2) Greenish yellow may indicate the presence of meconium and suggests fetal distress.
    (4) Cloudy suggests the presence of purulent material, and greenish yellow may indicate the presence of meconium.

61. (2) This slow deep breathing expands the spaces between the ribs and raises the abdominal muscles, allowing room for the uterus to expand and preventing painful pressure of the uterus against the abdominal wall. (a)

(1) Panting is used to halt or delay the pushing out of the baby's head before complete dilation.

(3) Pelvic rocking is used during pregnancy and the puerperal period; it is not feasible during labor.

(4) Athletic chest breathing is not one of the exercises used in this stage of labor.

62. (1) The contractions become stronger, last longer, and are erratic during this stage. The intervals during the contractions are shorter than the contractions themselves. Much concentration and effort are needed by the mother to pace herself with each contraction. (b)

(2) Not true; administration of analgesic or anesthetic at this point could reduce the effectiveness of labor and depress the fetus.

(3) There is no indication that any abnormality is developing.

(4) Even patients who have been adequately prepared will experience these behaviors during the transition stage.

63. (4) Both the father and the mother need additional support during the transitional stage of labor. (b)

(1) This does not encourage him to fulfill his role in supporting the mother during labor.

(2) He should be present throughout labor to support his wife; he should be assisted in this role.

(3) Judgmental; this approach suggests that he will be failing his wife.

64. (2) The contractions in this phase of labor are expulsive in nature and cause the patient to push or bear down. (a)

(1) Contractions are now frequent and intense; the patient is anxious to complete the labor process.

(3) Panting is not a voluntary act; the patient will be pushing.

(4) Blowing is not voluntary; it is encouraged to slow down pushing.

65. (4) The heart rate increases by about 10 beats per minute in the last half of pregnancy. This increase plus the increase in total blood volume can strain a damaged heart beyond the point at which it can efficiently compensate. (c)

(1) The number of RBCs does not decrease during pregnancy; plasma volume increases, simulating lowered hemoglobin.

(2) Cardiac output begins to decrease by the thirty-fourth week of gestation.

(3) The increased size of uterus is related to growth of the fetus not to any hemodynamic change.

66. (1) The side-lying position takes the weight off large blood vessels, and blood flow to the heart is increased. Elevating the shoulders relieves pressure on the diaphragm. (c)

(2) Potassium chloride is contraindicated unless lowered potassium levels indicate the need.

(3) Sodium leads to increased fluid retention; contraindicated in the cardiac patient.

(4) Contraindicated unless some uterine inertia occurs.

67. (2) Any medication that might further depress a premature infant is given with extreme caution. (b)

(1) False reassurance; there is no absolute control of premature labor.

(3) At the proper time the patient is encouraged to bear down.

(4) If the patient is kept n.p.o., it is done to lessen the risk of aspiration should anesthesia become necessary.

68. (2) An early symptom of congestive heart failure is respiratory distress. (c)

(1) Although pulse is important, the primary observation should be for respiratory distress, which suggests impending congestive heart failure.

(3) Increased vaginal bleeding is not caused by alterations in cardiac status.

(4) Signs of congestive failure, not hypovolemic shock, might develop.

69. (3) Oxygen, as a drug, has the potential for complications (e.g., retrolental fibroplasia) when used injudiciously. The physician orders the prescribed oxygen concentration based on chemical findings and laboratory blood gas analyses. (b)

(1) All newborns are evaluated immediately.

(2) Poor thermoregulation necessitates keeping the baby warm to stabilize body temperature.

(4) This is an important part of record keeping on all newborns.

70. (2) Immaturity of the respiratory tract in preterm infants can be evidenced by a lack of functional alveoli, smaller lumina with increased possibility of collapse of the respiratory passages, weakness of respiratory musculature, and insufficient calcification of the bony thorax leading to respiratory distress. (a)

(1) Not a primary concern unless severe hypoxia occurred during labor; difficult to diagnose at this time.

(3) May be a problem, but generally the air passageway is well suctioned at birth.

(4) Not a common occurrence at the time of birth unless trauma has occurred.

71. (3) Babies are unable to shiver. They use the breakdown of brown fat to supply body heat. The premature baby has an extremely limited supply of brown fat available for this breakdown. (c)

(1) The breakdown of glycogen into glucose does not supply body heat.

(2) Newborns are unable to use shivering to supply body heat.

(4) The pituitary gland does not supply body heat.

72. (2) The premature infant has a reduced glomerular filtration rate and reduced ability to concentrate urine or conserve water. (c)

(1) Untrue; all systems of the preterm baby are less developed than in the full-term infant.

(3) The fluid and electrolyte balance of preterm infants is easily upset.

(4) The opposite occurs; urine is very dilute.

73. (2) About two thirds of neonatal deaths are caused by prematurity. There appears to be a correlation with teenage pregnancy, lack of prenatal care, nonwhite mothers, and chronic health problems. (c)
    (1) Atelectasis may occur from respiratory distress, which in turn is associated with prematurity, the leading cause of death.
    (3) Usually occurs as a result of prematurity, the leading cause of death.
    (4) Most babies with congenital heart disease die after the neonatal period.

74. (1) Perinatal morbidity and mortality are greatly increased in multiple pregnancy because the high metabolic demands increase the potential for medical and obstetric complications. (b)
    (2) Maternal mortality during the prenatal period is not increased in the presence of multiple gestation.
    (3) Multiple gestation is usually identified prior to delivery; the mother would have this time for adjustment.
    (4) Although postpartum hemorrhage does occur more frequently after multiple births, it is not a routine occurrence.

75. (2) Characteristics of the midphase of labor for the primiparous patient include regular contractions 30 to 45 seconds long and 3 to 5 minutes apart, station of the presenting part at +1 to +2, and pink to bloody show in moderate amount. (c)
    (1) Contractions are less frequent in the early phase, and dilation is not so advanced.
    (3) In this phase, dilation is 8 to 10 cm and contractions more frequent.
    (4) This terminology is not appropriate for a phase of labor.

76. (1) In reporting progress in the descent of the presenting part, the level of the tip of the ischial spines is considered to be zero and the position of the bony prominence of the fetal head is described in centimeters—minus (above the spines) or plus (below the spines). (b)
    (2) Minus (−1) would indicate that the head is above the ischial spines.
    (3) This is designated by the term "floating," meaning that the presenting part has not yet engaged.
    (4) This would be referred to as crowning and would be designated as +5.

77. (2) Meperidine (Demerol) is classified as a narcotic analgesic drug and is effective for the relief of pain. Promethazine (Phenergan) can be classified as an analgesic-potentiating drug that permits the effective use of analgesics in lower dosages. (a)
    (1) This is an undesirable effect because the mother could not participate in the delivery process.
    (3) These medications do not induce amnesia.
    (4) There is no indication that anesthesia will be used.

78. (3) The physiologic intensification of labor occurring during transition is caused by a greater energy expenditure and increased pressure on the stomach. This results in feelings of fatigue, discouragement, and nausea. (b)
    (1) This stage is from full dilation to expulsion; a heavy bloody show and pushing are evident at this time.
    (2) Unclear terminology; does not indicate the specific time of labor.
    (4) This stage is from delivery of the fetus to delivery of the placenta; the mother does not experience any physiologic symptoms.

79. (4) Some maternal oxytocin crosses the placenta and induces the secretion of fluids that have accumulated in the fetal breasts (sometimes called witch's milk). (a)
    (1) Usually manifested in the oral mucosa as thrush (white adherent patches).
    (2) An uncommon and usually undetectable occurrence in the newborn period.
    (3) Evidence of infection would not appear so rapidly after birth.

80. (2) The fundus descends 1 finger breadth per day from the day after delivery: lochia serosa begins to flow on the fifth day. (b)
    (1) The fundus would be 1 to 3 fingers below the umbilicus (1 finger breadth per day).
    (3) The fundus would be descending into the pelvis at this time.
    (4) The fundus would be within the pelvis and indiscernable at this time.

81. (2) This is the result of a reduced chromosome number, from 46 to 23, readying the sex cells for fertilization. (c)
    (1) The diploid number (46 chromosomes) is reached when fertilization occurs.
    (3) They each have 1 set of chromosomes (23).
    (4) There are only 23 pairs.

82. (2) Follicle-stimulating hormone is secreted from the anterior pituitary gland. (c)
    (1) Chorionic gonadotropin is secreted by the trophoblastic tissue, which makes up part of the placenta.
    (3) Chorionic gonadotropin is precursor of progesterone and is secreted by the trophoblastic tissue.
    (4) Produced by syncytiotrophoblastic tissue, a preplacental tissue.

83. (4) The corpus luteum supplies the estrogen and progesterone needed to sustain the pregnancy until the placenta is ready to take over (eighth week). (b)
    (1) FSH is secreted by the anterior hypophysis, but it is not secreted during pregnancy.
    (2) Placental formation is not complete until the twelfth week of pregnancy.
    (3) This is not the chief source of progesterone and estrogen; only small amounts are secreted.

84. (2) Magnesium sulfate has a CNS depressant effect; therefore toxic levels will be reflected in decreased respiration and the absence of the knee-jerk reflex. (c)

(1) May be caused by increased potassium not magnesium sulfate.

(3) There is a decrease in respirations with excessive magnesium sulfate.

(4) Unrealistic response; there is no such ability.

85. (2) Absolute bed rest, a quiet room, and minimal stimulation are essential to reducing the risk of a convulsion. (b)

(1) This would be contraindicated, since fluid retention is a problem in preeclampsia.

(3) She will need constant observation and should not be isolated.

(4) This may cause temporary supine hypotension with resultant bradycardia in the infant; could also result in aspiration should a convulsion occur.

86. (1) This is a sign of CNS involvement that the nurse can observe without obtaining subjective data from the patient. (c)

(2) This is a subjective sign and is not obvious to the nurse.

(3) These are subjective symptoms: the patient must indicate their presence.

(4) Pain and nausea are subjective symptoms and are not directly observable.

87. (3) Increased electric charges in the brain during a convulsion may disturb the cerebral thermoregulation center. (b)

(1) One elevated reading is not a conclusive sign of infection.

(2) There is no rapid fluid loss during a convulsion; actually this patient has fluid retention.

(4) Excessive muscular activity usually causes perspiration leading to a drop in body temperature.

88. (4) The danger of convulsion in a woman with eclampsia ends when postpartum diuresis has occurred, usually 48 hours after delivery. (c)

(1) Untrue; the danger of convulsion in eclampsia ends when postpartum diuresis occurs about 48 hours after delivery.

(2) Untrue; the danger of convulsion in eclampsia ends when postpartum diuresis occurs about 48 hours after delivery.

(3) Untrue; danger of convulsion in eclampsia ends when postpartum diuresis occurs about 48 hours after delivery.

89. (1) In Erb-Duchenne paralysis there is damage to spinal nerves C5 and C6, which causes paralysis of the arm. (c)

(2) There would be a negative Moro reflex on the affected side only.

(3) The grasp reflex is intact since the fingers usually are not affected; if C8 is injured, paralysis of the hand results (Klumpke's paralysis).

(4) There is no interference with turning of the head; injury usually results from excessive lateral flexion of the head during delivery of the shoulder.

90. (3) Range-of-motion exercises must be done to prevent contractures. (c)

(1) Dangerous since it would lead to permanent contractures

(2) The muscle action usually improves spontaneously when edema subsides.

(4) The length of the arm will not change on a daily basis.

91. (4) Heavy cigarette smoking or continued exposure to a smoke-filled environment causes both maternal and fetal vasoconstriction, resulting in fetal growth retardation and increased fetal and infant mortality. (a)

(1) The fetal and maternal circulations are separate; the answer is not related to the question.

(2) Smoking causes vasoconstriction; premeability of the placenta to smoke is irrelevant.

(3) There is no concrete evidence that smoking relieves tension; this is not a factor in the situation described.

92. (4) This pigmentation is caused by the anterior pituitary hormone melanotropin, which increases during pregnancy. (c)

(1) Hyperactivity of the adrenal glands is manifested by symptoms of Cushing's syndrome.

(2) Hyperthyroidism is manifested by increased temperature, pulse, and respirations and a fine hand tremor.

(3) During pregnancy ovarian activity is very quiet because of the feedback mechanism.

93. (4) Chorionic gonadotropin, secreted in large amounts by the palcenta during gestation, and the metabolic changes associated with pregnancy can precipitate nausea and vomiting in early pregnancy. (b)

(1) Estrogen is elevated throughout pregnancy; symptoms of morning sickness disappear after the first trimester.

(2) Progesterone is elevated throughout pregnancy; symptoms of morning sickness disappear after the first trimester.

(3) Luteinizing hormone is present during ovulation only.

94. (4) Nausea and vomiting of pregnancy can be relieved with small snacks of dry crackers or toast before rising, since the ingestion of carbohydrates helps settle the stomach. (a)

(1) Unsound advice, since both fetus and mother need nourishment.

(2) An antacid may affect electrolyte balance; also this will not help morning sickness.

(3) Medications in the first trimester are contraindicated; this is the period of organogenesis, and congenital anomalies could result.

95. (4) When the patient signs herself and the baby out of the hospital, she is legally responsible for her infant and must be given the baby. (c)

(1) The baby belongs to the mother and can leave with the mother when she signs them out.

(2) The mother is the baby's guardian and may take the baby with her when she leaves.

(3) The baby is under the guardianship of the mother and may leave with the mother.

96. (1) Hormone decrease causes an emotional letdown. (a)
    (2) It is more likely that changes in body image would cause adaptations during pregnancy.
    (3) After labor the mother generally has feelings of elation over a job well done rather than depression.
    (4) There is usually ambivalence toward the infant, but it does not cause postpartum blues.

97. (3) The umbilical vein carries blood high in oxygen from the placenta and empties it into the fetal vena cava by way of the ductus venosus. (a)
    (1) The blood in the umbilical artery is more deoxygenated.
    (2) Contains a mixture of arterial and venous blood.
    (4) The pulmonary artery carries only small amount of oxygenated blood since the lungs are not funtioning.

98. (1) Two umbilical arteries arise from the fetus and go to the placenta, where waste products are exchanged for oxygen and nutrients and then returned via one umbilical vein to the baby. (a)
    (2) This is an anomalous number; there are 2 arteries and 1 vein.
    (3) This is an anomalous number: there are 2 arteries and 1 vein.
    (4) This is an anomalous number; there are 2 arteries and 1 vein.

99. (3) If the fetus is in a compromised state, it does not contribute to the synthesis of estriol; consequently estriol levels fall, indicating a need for intervention. (c)
    (1) Untrue; elevated estriol levels are indicated by healthy fetal placental functioning.
    (2) Chorionic gonadotropin is the hormone used for pregnancy tests.
    (4) Fetal demise is generally preceded by lowered estriol levels.

100. (1) There is a 30% to 50% increase in maternal blood volume at the end of the first trimester, leading to a decrease in the concentration of hemoglobin and erythrocytes. (b)
    (2) This is not physiologic but is caused by lack of iron intake.
    (3) Erythropoiesis is increased.
    (4) Detoxification demands are unchanged during pregnancy.

101. (1) The greatest danger of drug-induced malformation is during the first trimester of pregnancy, since this is the period of organogenesis. (b)
    (2) May cause problems, but organogenesis has already taken place by the second trimester.
    (3) The fetus is totally formed at this time, and drug damage would not be likely.
    (4) Drugs should be avoided, but the first trimester (period of organogenesis) is the most critical.

102. (4) Sonography, based on sound wave reflection and detection, locates the position of the fetus prior to insertion of the needle in amniocentesis; this minimizes the potential for fetal damage during the procedure. (b)
    (1) X-ray examinations are contraindicated during pregnancy except at term to determine cephalopelvic disproportion.
    (2) This is not a diagnostic procedure.
    (3) Formerly done; however, now sonography is the procedure of choice.

103. (2) The patient must feel comfortable enough to verbalize her feelings of guilt if she is to be able to complete the grieving process. (b)
    (1) This is a false assumption.
    (3) Studies show that contraceptive counseling at this time is most important, since the patient may not return after the abortion.
    (4) This is a sterile procedure and should not predispose the patient to postoperative infection.

104. (1) RH$_o$D globulin attacks fetal red cells that have gained access to the maternal bloodstream at the time of delivery. It prevents antibody formation. (b)
    (2) Contraindicated, since antibody formation is undesirable; it sensitizes the mother and contributes to fetal red cell destruction in future pregnancies.
    (3) Irrelevant; there is no production of immune bodies.
    (4) RH$_o$D provides passive temporary immunity and prepares the fetal red blood cells for destruction before the mother's immune system can respond by producing antibodies against Rh-positive blood.

105. (4) Although support will help minimize guilt, it will not eliminate it. However, support will sustain family cohesion and unity. (a)
    (1) May help, but cannot completely relieve pressure.
    (2) Support may help, but in no way completely alleviates guilt feelings.
    (3) Support does not affect legal responsibility of the parents.

106. (1) A symptom of sudden rupture of the fallopian tubes is pain on the affected side, usually sudden, excruciating, and spreading over the lower abdomen. Sometimes the pain is associated with nausea, vomiting, and diarrhea. (a)
    (2) Pain is exquisite, sharp, and sudden.
    (3) There may be some vaginal bleeding with ruptured tubal pregnancy; usually severe pain is present.
    (4) There are no contractions since the pregnancy is not uterine.

107. (2) The proliferation of trophoblastic tissue filled with fluid causes the uterus to enlarge more quickly than it would with a normally growing fetus. (b)
    (1) There may be slight vaginal bleeding without pain.
    (3) Enlargement of the uterus more rapidly than expected in a normal pregnancy leads to the suspicion of a molar pregnancy; hypertension may occur later in its progress.
    (4) There is generally no living fetus with a hydatidiform mole.

108. (3) Sneezing is the way in which the newborn clears mucus from the nose. Breathing is normally rapid and irregular. (a)
 (1) This would discourage the mother from taking responsibility and slow the mothering process; it also implies that something could be wrong.
 (2) More explanation is needed, and it also shuts of communication: the mother needs to express her feelings of anxiety.
 (4) These are normal new born responses and indicate no respiratory distress.
109. (2) Normally the newborn's breathing is diaphragmatic and irregular in depth and rhythm. The rate ranges from 40 to 50 breaths per minute. (b)
 (1) Infants' respirations are irregular and abdominal in origin.
 (3) Infants' respirations are irregular.
 (4) Infants' respirations are abdominal in origin.
110. (4) Opens up an area of communication to get at what really is troubling the mother about feeding the baby. (a)
 (1) Since the nurse is aware that this is not the best method, the problem of time should be explored with the mother.
 (2) Holding can be accomplished at times other than feeding periods; does not explore the patient's feelings.
 (3) True, but the mother should not be frightened; a more gentle explanation should be used.
111. (3) Early decelerations, with onset before the peak of the contraction and low point at the peak of the contraction, are due to fetal head compression; fetal heart rates rarely drop below 100 bpm. (c)
 (1) This is not a deceleration; it is within normal limits.
 (2) This is not a deceleration; it is within normal limits.
 (4) This is marked bradycardia.
112. (3) As the uterus rises into the abdominal cavity, the uterine ligaments become elongated and hypertrophied. Raising both legs at the same time limits the tension placed on these ligaments. (b)
 (1) There is no effect on the fascia with this maneuver.
 (2) There is already pressure on the perineum from the baby's head; this maneuver places tension on the uterine ligaments.
 (4) Lifting the legs simultaneously does not affect circulation in the legs.
113. (2) Because this was an uneventful labor to this point with no prior deceleration problems and the patient just assumed the supine position on the delivery table, there is compression of the inferior vena cava reducing venous return and maternal cardiac output. The reduced fetal heart rate may indicate fetal hypoxia because of deficient perfusion. (c)
 (1) The nurse cannot assume that this is just an early deceleration (Type 1 dip); delay in intervention could lead to fetal hypoxia or death.
 (3) There is no indication that oxytocin has been infusing.

 (4) The patient is in the lithotomy position and cannot be turned on her side.
114. (3) Soap irritates, cracks, and dries breasts and nipples, making it difficult for the baby to suck. (b)
 (1) She should empty the breast at each feeding to keep milk flowing.
 (2) This is a permissible and often used technique of breast feeding.
 (4) The breasts should be washed before feeding to remove encrustations and microorganisms.
115. (4) The most likely cause is a disturbance in the ratio of calcium to phosphorus, with the amount of serum calcium reduced and the serum phosphorus increased. Milk is an excellent source of calcium. (a)
 (1) Leg cramps are usually related to low calcium intake not hypercalcemia.
 (2) A low potassium is not a usual occurrence; not improved by ingestion of leafy vegetables.
 (3) Elevated potassium levels are very serious; not manifested by leg cramps.
116. (1) Cow's milk is diluted with water and has sugar added to make it resemble human milk. (c)
 (2) Contains more protein and more calcium.
 (3) Contains more protein and less calcium.
 (4) Contains more calcium.
117. (1) Prolactin is the hormone from the anterior pituitary that stimulates mammary gland secretion. Progesterone and estrogen are ovarian hormones that influence breast development and other female sexual characteristics. (a)
 (2) Oxytocin, a posterior pituitary hormone, stimulates the uterine musculature to contract and causes the letdown reflex.
 (3) Not a pituitary hormone; secreted by the corpus luteum of the ovary.
 (4) Not a pituitary hormone; secreted by the ovaries and placenta.
118. (1) During pregnancy, secretion of milk is inhibited. It is not possible to breast-feed. (c)
 (2) Breast-feeding is not always contraindicated with this disorder.
 (3) Breast-feeding is not contraindicated with inverted nipples, since a breast shield can provide mild suction to help pull out a nipple.
 (4) Not always contraindicated; the baby already has the organism in the mouth, and nursing will decrease the mother's discomfort.
119. (1) The term "premature" describes a newborn delivered at 37 weeks' gestation or less, regardless of weight. (a)
 (2) An infant weighing less than 1136 g (2½ lb) and considerably underdeveloped at birth.
 (3) Nonviable would be before the twenty-fourth week of gestation.
 (4) Means low birth weight for related gestational age.
120. (3) Gavage feeding is preferred for immature and weak infants, those with respiratory distress or poor suck-

ing-swallowing coordination, and those who are easily fatigued. (b)

(1) Feeding the infant quickly is not desirable; vomiting with aspiration may occur.

(2) This is not a reason for instituting gavage; however, vomiting may be lessened with gavage feeding since the amount and rapidity of feeding can be controlled.

(4) The amount can be regulated with bottle-feeding as well.

121. (2) Much of a full-term infant's birth weight is gained during the last month of pregnancy (almost a third), and most of this final spurt is subcutaneous fat, which serves as insulation. The premature baby has not had the time to grow in the uterus and has a paucity of this insulating layer. (a)

(1) There is a relatively larger surface area per body weight.

(3) There is an extremely limited shivering and sweating response in the premature infant.

(4) Unrelated to the maintenance of body temperature.

122. (1) Prolonged oxygen administration at relatively high concentrations in a premature infant whose retina is incompletely differentiated and/or vascularized may result in retrolental fibroplasia. When oxygen therapy is discontinued, capillary overgrowth in the retina and vitreous body may result and include capillary hemorrhage, fibrosis, and retinal detachment. (b)

(2) Though true, temperature and humidity are not factors in the development of retrolental fibroplasia.

(3) Oxygen concentration of more than 40% is dangerous and a factor in the development of retrolental fibroplasia.

(4) Phototherapy is used to decrease hyperbilirubinemia; unrelated to retrolental fibroplasia; however, the eyes are covered to prevent ocular damage.

123. (3) Toxemia does not interfere with uterine involution, return of uterine tone, or constriction of vessels at the placental site. (c)

(1) Overdistension of the uterus may lead to delayed or poor uterine myometrial contraction at the placental site after delivery.

(2) Retained placenta inhibits uterine myometrial contractions; also manual removal of placenta may cause uterine trauma.

(4) May inhibit myometrial contraction of the uterus at the placental site.

124. (3) The term "stillborn" is used to describe a dead fetus of more than 24 weeks' gestation, weighing 600 or more grams. (c)

(1) Incomplete information given for this conclusion; only the fetus is mentioned.

(2) A fetus of 24 weeks gestation or more is considered viable.

(4) This length is indicative of a previable fetus, which is not classified as stillborn.

125. (2) Based on the family's decision, extraordinary care does not have to be employed. The child's basic needs are met, and nature is allowed to take its course. (b)

(1) Euthanasia is a deliberate intervention to cause death.

(3) If the child's physical needs are met and comfort is provided, the child's rights are not ignored; "extraordinary," not "all," care is being withheld.

(4) It is neither unethical nor illegal to withhold extraordinary treatment; once such treatment is started, it becomes a legal issue.

126. (1) Immaturity of the diaphragm and the intercostal and abdominal musculature inhibits adequate ventilation, which causes lung expansion to be inadequate. Consequently the infant must use tremendous effort. (c)

(2) Cyanosis is a later manifestation; more common with congenital heart defects.

(3) Rapid respirations are normally present in newborns.

(4) Grunting more commonly occurs when the baby is chilled or cold.

127. (3) Flaccid muscle tone is the only abnormal finding. All other choices indicate a normal newborn response and would be higher on the Apgar scale. (b)

(1) Apgar rating of 7 to 10 usually indicates this.

(2) Present with an Apgar rating of 7 to 10.

(4) Usually much slower in an infant whose Apgar score is 4.

128. (2) Intracranial bleeding may occur in the subdural, subarachnoid, or intraventricular spaces of the brain, causing pressure on vital centers. Clinical signs are related to the area and degree of cerebral involvement. (a)

(1) This is caused by hypocalcemia; manifested by exaggerated muscular twitching.

(3) This is an obvious defect of the spinal column; easily recognized.

(4) Elevated potassium causes cardiac irregularities.

129. (1) Development of jaundice in the first 24 hours indicates erythroblastosis fetalis. (c)

(2) Normal; serum bilirubin normally accumulates in the neonatal period because of the short life span of fetal erythrocytes, reaching levels of 7 mg/100 ml the second to third day, when jaundice appears.

(3) May or may not be present in first 24 hours; dependent on bilirubin level.

(4) May or may not be present during first 24 hours of life; usually develops later.

130. (2) The tonic neck reflex (fencing position) is a spontaneous postural reflex of the newborn that may or may not be present during the first days of life. Once apparent, it persists until the third month. (a)

(1) Demonstration of muscle tone while held prone and suspended in midair.

(3) This is the "startle" reflex.

(4) This is a normal, expected reflex in the neonate.

131. (3) Informing parents of the birth of an abnormal child as early as possible, and preferably in the delivery room when staff is present to support and assist them in mobilizing resources, prevents fantasizing about the problem. (b)
    (1) Crisis intervention should not be delayed; immediately informing the parents improves coping abilities.
    (2) May be too much of a shock if the mother has no awareness of the defect.
    (4) Parents may not ask.
132. (4) Androgen-estrogen preparations inhibit the release of lactogenic hormone from the pituitary. (c)
    (1) Male hormone; would not be given to suppress lactation.
    (2) Hormone of adrenal origin; not given to suppress lactation.
    (3) Pituitary hormone; initiates and enhances uterine contraction.
133. (4) Ovulation is anticipated approximately 14 days prior to menstruation. However, it is more reliable to avoid using a specific number of days and to calculate on the basis of an individual's cycle rather than an average 28-day cycle. (c)
    (1) Ovulation occurs 14 days before the onset of menstruation.
    (2) This may not be true in females with menstrual cycles longer than 28 days.
    (3) Ovulation occurs 14 days prior to the onset of menstruation.
134. (2) As ovulation approaches, there may be a drop in the basal temperature because of an increased production of estrogen. When ovulation occurs, there will be a rise in the basal temperature because of an increased production of progesterone. (b)
    (1) At ovulation the temperature drop is slight, not marked.
    (3) At ovulation the temperature drops slightly and then rises.
    (4) At ovulation the temperature rises after a slight drop.
135. (3) Stress or infection alters the body's metabolism, causing an elevation in temperature. A rise in temperature from these causes may be misinterpreted as ovulation. (b)
    (1) Frequency of intercourse may affect the volume of sperm but does not alter the female's basal temperature.
    (2) Age is not a factor concerning efficiency of the rhythm method.
    (4) This may increase sperm volume but does not affect the female's basal temperature.
136. (2) Ectopic pregnancy is one of the leading causes of first trimester bleeding. Unless an embryo and placenta happen to be located in the abdominal cavity, they cannot grow outside the uterus for more than 10 to 12 weeks without showing the classic signs of pressure and bleeding. (b)

    (1) Abdominal cramping pain is present with an incomplete abortion.
    (3) Abruptio placentae is accompanied by sharp abdominal pain with or without bleeding.
    (4) This occurs monthly during ovulation without pain or vaginal bleeding; occasionally pain occurs when the follicle ruptures (mittelschmerz), but bleeding does not.
137. (1) Staining in the first trimester may indicate that the pregnancy is in jeopardy. Bed rest, sedation, and avoidance of physical and emotional stress are recommended. Abortion is usually inevitable if the bleeding is accompanied by pain with dilation and effacement of the cervix. (a)
    (2) This can be confirmed only if vaginal examination reveals cervical dilation.
    (3) Usually accompanied by severe pain radiating to the shoulder on the affected side.
    (4) May not exhibit any outward symptoms; only the signs of pregnancy disappearing.
138. (2) After a spontaneous abortion the fundus should be checked for firmness, which would indicate effective uterine tone. If the uterus is not firm, it is hypotonic and hemorrhage may occur. Nonfirmness may also indicate retained placental tissue. (a)
    (1) Unnecessary; fetal and placental contents are small and expelled easily in bed.
    (3) The nurse would do this if necessary after checking for fundal firmness.
    (4) The priority action is to check for firmness of the fundus and possible bleeding.
139. (2) Hemorrhage may be due to retained placental tissue or uterine atony. Infection may occur from the introduction of contamination into the warm moist environment, which is favorable to microbial growth. (a)
    (1) No indication at this time that the patient has been deprived of fluids or has lost large amounts of blood.
    (3) Subinvolution usually occurs after a full term delivery and may not be obvious for several days.
    (4) Too early in pregnancy for toxemia.
140. (4) Allows the husband and wife to comfort each other while letting them know you are available and recognize and accept their feelings of loss. (b)
    (1) Telling the patient not to be upset cuts off communication and wrongly implies that it prolongs recovery.
    (2) Grieving for the unborn child will and should occur during any period of pregnancy.
    (3) An assumption that another pregnancy will ensue; also cuts off further communication.
141. (1) The association of toxemia with placental bleeding is frequent. This may be related to the hypertension during pregnancy. (c)
    (2) Generally does not affect the circulation to the placenta.

(3) May cause endocrine disturbance in the infant but does not affect the blood supply to the uterus.

(4) This may affect the delivery of the fetus but does not affect the placenta.

142. (1) Overdistention of the uterus because of a large baby, multiple gestation, or hydramnios predisposes a woman to uterine atony, which may cause postpartum hemorrhage. (b)

(2) Unless uterine atony is present, hemorrhage should not occur; a grand multipara is at risk for placenta previa.

(3) This leads to precipitous delivery (potentially harmful to the fetus) but does not affect uterine contractions after delivery.

(4) Not a factor in involution of the uterus.

143. (2) In a breech delivery the head is not the presenting part bearing the brunt of the pressure against the pelvic floor during delivery. (b)

(1) May occur if there is difficulty in delivering the head after the body is born.

(3) The cord may prolapse; and pressure of the baby can cause cord compression, resulting in fetal hypoxia.

(4) This commonly occurs in breech deliveries.

144. (2) Observation and record keeping of bleeding are independent nursing functions and necessary for implementing safe care, since hemorrhage and shock can be life threatening. (a)

(1) The patient should be restricted to complete bed rest until bleeding stops.

(3) Vital signs should be checked more often if bleeding persists.

(4) This is absolutely forbidden, since it may cause further separation of the placenta.

145. (2) A fallopian tube is unable to contain and sustain a pregnancy to term. As the fertilized ovum grows, there is excessive stretching or rupture of the fallopian tube, causing pain. (c)

(1) Pain is sudden, intense, knifelike, and usually located on one side.

(3) Leukorrhea and dysuria may be indicative of a vaginal or bladder infection.

(4) This would be difficult for the patient to identify correctly.

146. (3) A position in which the mother's head is below the level of the hips helps decrease compression of the cord and therefore increase blood supply to the infant. (a)

(1) This does not relieve the pressure of the oncoming head on the cord.

(2) This may increase the pressure of the presenting part on the cord.

(4) The pressure of the presenting part on the cord is not relieved in this position.

147. (2) Infertility is the inability of a couple to conceive after at least 1 year of adequate exposure to the possibility of pregnancy. (b)

(1) This may or may not be true; it is possible that there is a problem with both.

(3) May be; however, statistics show that physiologic problems are more often the cause.

(4) Untrue; infertility may be corrected, but sterility is irreversible.

148. (2) At this time, because of increased estrogen levels, the cervical mucus is abundant and its quality changes in such a way as to optimize sperm survival time. (b)

(1) The cervical mucus at this time is not receptive to spermatozoa.

(3) Cervical mucus at this time is still thick and not yet receptive to spermatozoa.

(4) Cervical mucus is destructive of spermatozoa at this time and sperm penetration cannot occur.

149. (1) A past infection may cause tubal occlusions, most of which are due to postinfection adhesions. (c)

(2) This is a tumor of the uterus and does not affect the tube.

(3) Rare; anomalies of the uterus are more common than those of a tube.

(4) Possible; but infections in the tube are more common.

150. (2) Human chorionic gonadotropin (HCG), an LH-like hormone, is produced by the trophoblasts of the early embryo to promote continued metabolism of the corpus luteum (source of estrogen and progesterone). HCG can be detected as early as 6 days after fertilization (by nonroutine immunofluorescent techniques) and appears in measurable amounts in the urine within about 14 days. (b)

(1) Not found in the urine of pregnant women.

(3) Estrogen is present in females all the time.

(4) Not indicative of pregnancy; found in the urine of all women, especially after ovulation.

151. (4) A bluish color results from the increased vascularity and blood vessel engorgement of the vagina. (a)

(1) Softening of the lower uterine segment.

(2) Increased vascularity and cervical softening.

(3) Softening of the cervix.

152. (4) The average weight gain during pregnancy is 9 to 11.25 kg (20 to 25 lb). Of this, the fetus accounts for 3.4 kg (7½ lb), the blood volume 0.9 to 1.8 kg (2 to 4 lb) fluid retention 2.3 kg (5 lb), amniotic fluid 0.9 kg (2 lb), uterus 1.13 kg (2½ lb), and breasts 1.36 kg (3 lb). The remainder of weight gain is fat. (c)

(1) Do not cause a weight gain.

(2) Accounts for about 20% of weight gain.

(3) Accounts for about 12% of weight gain.

153. (1) Statistically CPD (cephalopelvic disproportion) is the most common indication. (a)

(2) This may be improved by rest and hydration followed by an infusion of oxytocin (Pitocin), leading to vaginal delivery.

(3) Not done unless complete placental separation occurs before delivery.

(4) A nonexistent condition.

154. (1) The diagonal conjugate is an estimation of the true conjugate with the lower edge of the symphysis pubis used as its anterior point and the sacral promontory posteriorly. The true conjugate uses the upper ridge of the symphysis pubis anteriorly but cannot be measured on a living woman. (c)

(2) Diameter between the ischial tuberosities.

(3) Distance from the upper margin of the symphysis to the sacral promontory.

(4) Widest diameter at the inlet.

155. (2) X-ray pelvimetry is more definitive than digital pelvimetry; but because of radiation hazards it should be limited to patients in labor, in whom it is clearly essential to the outcome of pregnancy. (b)

(1) This is done by external measurement; is not an accurate assessment.

(3) This is a test of amniotic fluid; does not reveal actual size of the fetus or diameters of the pelvis.

(4) This may vary with factors other than cephalopelvic disproportion.

156. (1) Asymmetry of the gluteal dorsal surface of the thighs and inguinal folds indicates congenital dislocation of the hip. Folds on the affected side appear higher than those on the unaffected side. (a)

(2) This would be manifested by limpness or flaccidity of extremities.

(3) Evidenced by protrusion of the intestine into the inguinal sac.

(4) Impaired reflex behavior and a shrill cry, etc. would indicate CNS damage.

157. (3) Human milk contains 42% carbohydrate, and cow's milk 30% carbohydrate. The carbohydrate in cow's milk is further diluted when water is added to the formula, so additional sugar is required to supplement it. (b)

(1) The calorie content is about the same, 20 calories/ounce.

(2) It is assimilated well.

(4) It is lactose, a simple sugar.

158. (1) Blood loss depletes the normal cellular response to infection. Trauma provides an excellent medium for bacteria to grow. (c)

(2) Toxemia is generally not a predisposing cause of postpartum hemorrhage.

(3) May create problems if hemorrhage occurs since the hemoglobin and hematocrit are already low.

(4) Endogenous infection is rare; infection usually caused by outside contamination. Trauma and the denuded placental site do contribute to the development of infection.

159. (4) The oxytocin challenge test provides data concerning the circulatory-respiratory reserve of the fetoplacental unit. A positive OCT usually indicates uteroplacental insufficiency. An OCT is contrain-

dicated unless there is a specific indication of a problem. (b)

(1) This is not an indication; the OCT would be of no help in diagnosing a recurrence.

(2) An OCT would be contraindicated in placenta previa.

(3) Contraindicated; might accelerate the labor further.

160. (1) Administration of oxytocin too early in pregnancy can cause induced labor and premature delivery. (c)

(2) May be indicated to determine the fetus' response to labor.

(3) May be indicated because of hypertensive influence on the placental circulation.

(4) May be indicated to determine the fetus' response to labor.

161. (1) Respiratory depression occurs with the use of meperidine (Demerol) and produces significant depression of the infant at birth if circulating levels are high at delivery. (a)

(2) Scopolamine induces amnesia and forgetfulness in the mother but does not cause respiratory depression.

(3) Promazine (Sparine), a tranquilizer, augments the effects of Demerol, thereby lessening the amount of drug needed.

(4) Promethazine (Phenergan), a tranquilizer, does not cause respiratory depression.

162. (1) Brachial palsy results from excessive stretching of the nerve fibers that run from the neck, through the shoulder, and down toward the arm. The muscles of the upper arm are involved, and the infant holds the arm at the side with the elbow extended and the hand rotated inward. (b)

(2) Signs of CNS disturbance would be present.

(3) There would be signs of dislocation and evidence of pain with a fractured clavicle.

(4) An inborn error of metabolism relating to the body's handling of bilirubin.

163. (3) There is extensive activation of blood clotting factor after delivery. This, together with immobility, trauma, or sepsis, encourages thromboembolization, which can be limited through activity. (b)

(1) Tone would be improved by regular emptying and filling of the bladder.

(2) This can be accomplished by turning the patient from side to side and encouraging her to deep breathe and cough.

(4) Abdominal muscle tone will be improved with exercise over the next 6 weeks.

164. (2) Mothering is not an inborn instinct but rather a learned behavior based on past experiences. (c)

(1) Untrue; mothering is learned not inborn.

(3) This knowledge does not assure "motherliness."

(4) Marriage is not essential for good mothering.

165. (3) Heart development occurs between the second and eighth weeks of gestation. (b)

(1) This is a neural tube defect not associated with rubella.

(2) Associated with intake of teratogenic drugs not rubella.

(4) Generally occurs later in life; not caused by rubella. Rubella may cause nerve deafness from eighth cranial (vestibulocochlear) nerve or hearing center involvement.

166. (2) The increased pulmonary blood flow raises the pressure in the left atrium and functionally forces the septum to close the foramen ovale. (c)

(1) There is an increased aortic blood flow.

(3) Caused by increased pressure in the left atrium.

(4) There is decreased pressure in the right atrium.

167. (3) There is anatomic obliteration of the lumen by fibrous proliferation, leading to the term ''ligamentum arteriosum.'' (b)

(1) Descriptive term meaning long and round ligament.

(2) This refers to the ductus venosus.

(4) There is no such vessel.

168. (1) Bacteria, especially *Escherichia coli,* produce and synthesize prothrombin. (c)

(2) Manufactured in the liver, not synthesized by bacteria.

(3) Secreted by the gastric glands, not synthesized by bacteria.

(4) An orange bile pigment produced by the breakdown of hemoglobin.

169. (3) The immunity is that which has developed from an antigen-antibody response in the mother and is passed to the fetus. (b)

(1) Acquired by an individual in response to a disease or an infection.

(2) Acquired by an individual in response to small amounts of antigenic material (e.g., vaccination).

(4) Conferred by the injection of antibodies already prepared in another host.

170. (4) The congenital absence of a vessel in the umbilical cord is usually associated with life-threatening congenital anomalies. (b)

(1) If the Apgar score 5 minutes later showed marked improvement, there would be no need for placing the infant in the ICU.

(2) This is the average weight for a full-term newborn.

(3) The fetus may have swallowed some amniotic fluid; not unusual or dangerous.

171. (1) Medical supervision requires treatment with an appropriate antibiotic for 2 to 3 weeks until 2 negative cultures are obtained. Re-treatment may be necessary if there is a recurrence. (c)

(2) Signs of toxemia occur spontaneously; not preceded by specific infections.

(3) Pelvic inflammatory disease is associated with infections of the genital not the urinary tract.

(4) A low-protein diet would inhibit good fetal development and is contraindicated in pregnancy.

172. (1) The pressure exerted anywhere in a mass of fluid in a closed container is transmitted undiminished throughout all parts of the fluid and in all directions. (c)

(2) A principle dealing with the displacement of fluid not pressure.

(3) Laws dealing with motion not pressure.

(4) Theory dealing with relativity not pressure.

173. (4) Progesterone acts to reduce contractility of the uterine musculature and to maintain the decidual bed. (b)

(1) Elevated progesterone levels would inhibit contractility of the uterine musculature.

(2) Progesterone, not estrogen, inhibits contractions.

(3) Would tend to stimulate contractions but is inhibited by progesterone, not estrogen.

174. (3) Concentration of the polypeptide, a melanocyte-stimulating hormone, rises from the end of the second month of pregnancy until term. (a)

(1) High levels of chorionic gonadotropin, secreted by the chorion, are associated with nausea and vomiting.

(2) Related to advancing growth and pressure of the uterus on the bladder.

(4) Due to increased mucoidal secretions.

175. (2) If the woman had a hemophilic father, she must have had his X chromosome, which carries the recessive gene for hemophilia (if she had had his Y chromosome, she would have been male). Since her blood clots normally, her other X chromosome carries the dominant gene for normal blood clotting. She is represented by H_1h (the H_1 being the affected gamete). Her normal mate is represented by HY. The cross:

	Father	
	H	Y
H_1	H_1H	H_1Y
h	Hh	hY

(Mother) (c)

(1) Could happen only if both parents were hemophiliacs.

(3) Fifty percent of the male children could be normal.

(4) Fifty percent of the offspring are affected—male hemophiliacs or female carriers.

176. (1) Anemia decreases the capacity of the blood to carry oxygen and thus increases the demands on the heart. (b)

(2) This is due to disturbance in the conduction of impulses not the oxygen-carrying capacity of blood.

(3) Cardiac irregularity not associated with anemia.

(4) A diseased heart is not capable of further cardiac compensation; decompensation would result.

177. (2) The pregnant woman's increased hormones, metabolic rate, and increased blood volume place additional demands on the pancreas, thus altering carbohydrate and lipid metabolism. (b)

(1) The hormones of pregnancy act as antagonists to insulin, thus reducing its effect.

(3) The diabetic mother's glucose tolerance does not differ from that in her prepregnant state.

(4) Pregnancy lowers renal threshold for glucose in nondiabetics as well.

178. (1) Since spillage of glucose into the urine occurs in normal women who are pregnant, dietary or insulin management in a diabetic who is pregnant must be based on blood glucose levels rather than on urine glucose values. (c)

(2) Depends on body needs; pregnancy per se does not speed it up.

(3) This would be no problem if action of insulin was not antagonized by pregnancy hormones.

(4) Difficulty in regulation is unrelated to the absorption of insulin.

179. (4) Increased metabolic demands on the body during pregnancy require an increased ingestion of glucose. Appropriate levels of insulin must be administered to permit normal glucose utilization by the body. (c)

(1) This type of diet is contraindicated; would not meet the demands of pregnancy and growing fetus.

(2) The caloric content is increased, not decreased, during pregnancy.

(3) This diet would not be sufficient to prevent ketosis; insulin would be necessary to cover carbohydrate intake.

180. (2) In diabetic mothers the fetal pancreas responds to the mother's hyperglycemia by secreting more than normal amounts of insulin. This leads to infant hypoglycemia after birth. (b)

(1) To compensate for increased glucose received from the mother, the islets of Langerhans in the fetus may have become hypertrophied; are not congenitally depressed.

(3) There may be a generalized edema, but not specific to the central nervous system.

(4) Increased insulin production by the fetus diminishes the glucose content of the blood; babies are most often hypoglycemic.

181. (2) The higher-than-normal glucose levels in a fetus of a diabetic mother leads to increased fat synthesis and deposition. Increased glucose utilization is also promoted by the combined presence of pituitary growth hormone and placental somatotropin. (c)

(1) False; glucose utilization is increased, with resultant macrosomia.

(3) False; somatotropin concentration is increased and glucose utilization is increased.

(4) False; somatotropin concentration is increased during pregnancy.

182. (1) Normal periods of marked change and adjustment are called developmental crises and predispose the woman to a situational crisis. (a)

(2) These occur throughout the life cycle of a mature woman and should not now be classified as a crisis.

(3) These are transient; similar to previous mood changes and should not affect the mother's ability to cope.

(4) Becomes a crisis only if the husband withdraws support.

183. (2) The ability to express one's feelings is often a first step in the recognition and resolution of a crisis. (b)

(1) Until the mother shows a readiness for learning (e.g., accepts the pregnancy), she would not benefit from classes.

(3) Not a priority need; may come later in the nurse-patient interactions.

(4) The father, as well as the mother, must indicate a readiness for learning before beginning classes.

184. (2) Chorionic gonadotropin is present in the urine during early pregnancy and is the basis for pregnancy tests. Since this hormone appears only during early pregnancy, its presence is taken as a sure sign of pregnancy. (a)

(1) Prolactin initiates milk production and is secreted after delivery.

(3) Estrogen is secreted throughout the ovulatory cycle, not just pregnancy.

(4) Secreted into the bloodstream at the time of ovulation.

185. (2) Nurses with positive attitudes toward abortion should counsel women who are thinking of undergoing the procedure. They should know what services are available and the various methods that are used to induce abortion. (b)

(1) The nurse should give the patient only the information requested; should not state personal feelings.

(3) The nurse is capable of giving information about abortion; need not defer to the physician.

(4) Good nursing practice necessitates scientifc knowledge; statements must be based on fact, not personal feelings or beliefs.

186. (2) The uterus and bladder occupy the pelvic cavity and lie very close together. As the uterus enlarges with the growing fetus, it impinges on the space normally occupied by the bladder and thereby diminishes bladder capacity. (a)

(1) Atony would not cause frequency; more likely would lead to retention.

(3) An unlikely occurrence; the uterus would not impinge on that area.

(4) Would lead to incontinence rather than frequency.

187. (2) Because of changes in the hormone levels, morning sickness seldom persists beyond the first trimester. (a)

(1) Still present at this time; related to the high level of chorionic gonadotropin.

(3) Usually ends at end of the third month, when the chorionic gonadotropin level falls.

(4) Usually ends at end of the third month when the chorionic gonadotropin level falls.

188. (2) Subsequent to IUD insertion, menstrual periods may have an excessive flow for several cycles. This is probably because of an increase in the blood supply (inflammatory process), since the IUD is really a foreign body. (c)

(1) This may occur upon insertion but is fairly uncommon.

(3) This may occur but is not classified as a side effect.

(4) No documentation of this.

189. (1) Oral contraceptives contain varying kinds and dosages of synthetic estrogen and progestogen compounds that mimic natural cyclic hormone changes and prolong the menses. (c)

(2) Untrue; since pills contain estrogen, they will minimize menopausal symptoms that are caused by lowered estrogen content.

(3) This would be symptomatic of disease not of oral contraceptive usage.

(4) It tends to prolong menses by supplying estrogen.

190. (3) Untreated ophthalmia neonatorum becomes apparent on the third or fourth postnatal day and is evidence that the mother has gonorrhea. (b)

(1) Conjunctivitis from silver nitrate instillation develops on the first day.

(2) Ophthalmia neonatorum does not develop until the third day.

(4) The incubation period for the gonococci that cause ophthalmia neonatorum is 3 to 4 days after birth.

191. (4) Multiple pregnancy thins the uterine wall by overstretching. Thus the efficiency of contractions is reduced. (b)

(1) Toxemia may bring about premature labor; does not cause hypotonic uterine dysfunction.

(2) May cause fatigue in the mother; does not affect uterine contractility.

(3) This may lead to difficult delivery because of cephalopelvic disproportion; does not affect uterine contractions.

192. (3) A fruity odor may indicate that the patient is becoming acidotic. (c)

(1) This would be indicative of cardiac difficulties rather than exhaustion.

(2) Maternal exhaustion is usually accompanied by dehydration with a resultant temperature elevation.

(4) This would occur later if there were a severe electrolyte imbalance.

193. (3) This response provides the patient with a comfort measure while giving her an opportunity to verbalize her fears about having an abnormal labor. (b)

(1) This can be answered yes or no and leaves no further avenue for discussion.

(2) Of no help to the patient; she is concerned with what is happening to her.

(4) Closes off communication with the patient.

194. (3) The oxytocic effect of Pitocin increases the intensity and duration of contractions. Prolonged contractions will jeopardize the safety of the fetus and necessitate discontinuing the drug. (c)

(1) This is important throughout labor.

(2) Since she is only 3 to 4 cm with head floating, there will be no bulging.

(4) There is no indication at this time that a cesarean section is necessary.

195. (3) IV oxytocin (Pitocin) is used to enhance postpartum uterine contractions after cesarean sections, since palpation of the fundus is difficult and painful after surgery. The drug produces effective clamping down on the vessels. (c)

(1) This may be difficult because of the new incision.

(2) This is done routinely for all postoperative patients.

(4) This is done for all postoperative patients.

196. (1) Normal infants require about 73 ml (2 to 3 oz) or fluid per pound and 60 calories a day per pound for growth. (b)

(2) Too little; normal infants require 2 to 3 oz of fluid per pound, 18 oz/24 hr.

(3) Too much; 18 oz/24 hr is required or about 3 oz every 4 hours.

(4) Too much; 18 oz/24 hr is required or about 3 oz every 4 hours.

197. (1) The cardiac sphincter in the newborn is poorly developed. If the stomach is too full, formula backs up through the sphincter and the infant regurgitates. (b)

(2) This would be manifested by projectile vomiting, not regurgitation.

(3) This may cause cramping or colic; usually does not cause regurgitation.

(4) Nondescriptive answer; position not described; might happen if the baby were upside down.

198. (4) Clotting mechanisms are not fully effective in the infant before the eighth day of life. (a)

(1) Too soon to observe for signs of infection.

(2) If gauze is not wrapped too tightly around the penis, this should be no problem.

(3) Generally the baby is not too uncomfortable after circumcision; this may, with other signs, be indicative of central nervous system difficulty.

199. (1) Gonorrhea transmitted from the mother is usually manifested in the infant as an eye infection. It becomes apparent on the third or fourth postnatal day unless silver nitrate has been instilled into the eyes at birth. (a)

(2) Acquired transplacentally, not via the genital tract

(3) *Monilia*, not *Neisseria gonorrhoeae*, causes thrush.

(4) Usually acquired by aspiration, not exposure to gonococci.

200. (3) The spirochete *Treponema pallidum* is able to cross the placenta and cause early manifestations of syphilis after the sixteenth week of pregnancy. (c)

(1) Inflammatory the destructive changes would cause enlargement of the liver and spleen.

(2) This would have occurred in the first trimester; but not from *Treponema pallidum*, which does not infect the fetus until after the eighteenth week of gestation.

(4) Not a common finding in infants with congenital syphilis; found in infants with Down's syndrome.

5

Psychiatric Nursing

Since nursing is concerned with the basic needs of people, the nurse must be able to understand and assist the individual, being constantly aware of the many factors that influence a person's behavioral response. Individuals are constantly interacting with both the internal and the external environments and at any given moment stand as a conglomerate of their own and their forebears' experiences. The individual is continuously faced with emotional stress from the moment of birth until the moment of death. How people adapt to this stress and the problems resulting from the adaptations are the focus of psychiatric nursing. Psychiatric nursing is therefore the care of patients with emotional problems. However, the principles used in the care of psychiatric patients are applicable to all patients regardless of their diagnosis. Nursing, which is concerned with total care, must provide for the individual's physical (soma) as well as emotional (psyche) needs.

Background Information from the Behavioral Sciences

BASIC CONCEPTS FROM ANTHROPOLOGY

A. All people are influenced by the culture into which they are born
B. Cultural factors include race, nationality, and religion
C. Groups that share a common race, nationality, religion, or language are known as ethnic groups
D. Society as a whole frequently develops a fixed set of expected responses for certain ethnic groups
E. When each member of an ethnic group is expected to respond in a specific manner, the expected responses are called stereotypes
F. Cultural variability occurs in all stages of the life cycle: child rearing, marriage patterns, health maintenance, etc.

Cultural Influences

Race
A. Defined as a certain combination of physical traits that are transmitted by lineage or heredity
B. Physical traits of a race include skin color; texture and/or color of hair; eye shapes and folds; shape of nose, lips, and cheekbones; contour of the head; and body build
C. Of all the factors involved in ethnic group membership, race, which is given a great deal of emphasis, appears to be a biologic phenomenon that seems to contribute few specifics to the cultural background

Nationality
A. Defined as original or acquired membership in a particular nation

B. The culture of nationalities is passed down through generations in the form of
   1. Beliefs and superstitions
   2. Foods and national dishes
   3. Festivals and feast days
   4. Language and the meanings of certain words
C. Nationality and the culture that it imparts frequently become even more important when a group of people immigrate to a new country where the members tend to join together to form a subculture of the new national culture
D. The subculture provides its members with a sense of security by furnishing a collective identify and maintaining the familiar

Religion
A. Defined as the quest for values of the ideal life usually embodied in a particular set of beliefs practiced individually or within an organized system
B. Religious beliefs in some form have existed in every group during every period of history
C. Organized religions have been instrumental in developing an ethical and moral system that has frequently been based on a society's needs
D. Most of the world's religions have developed many rituals as part of their worship, and these rituals form the basis of the religious culture that is passed down from generation to generation
E. In contrast to traditional religion there exist numerous religious cults; persons seeking a sense of belonging and purpose join a religious cult that gives them a group identity through communal living and rigorous rituals

Culture and Health
A. General influences
   1. Cultural background influences the way in which people view both health and disease
   2. The cultural influences seem to be derived from the areas of nationality and religion rather than race
B. Specific influences
   1. National culture may influence an individual's
      a. Response to illness
      b. Response to pain and even the tolerance of pain
      c. Need for superstitions and rituals
      d. Acceptance of dietary change both in type or in consistency of food
      e. Need for support and comfort from the family
      f. Ability to communicate in understandable terms
      g. Response to loss of independence

h. Feelings about loss of privacy and exposure of parts of the body
      i. Feelings about loss of body parts
      j. Need for specific rites and rituals associated with dying
   2. Religious culture may influence an individual's
      a. Views on conception, birth, and child care
      b. Views about the meaning of pain and suffering
      c. Feelings about the meaning of death
      d. Desire for guidance from the clergy
      e. Acceptance of certain treatments such as immunizations and blood transfusions
      f. Concept of illness as a punishment
      g. Dietary restrictions including the types of food and their preparation
      h. Need for specific rites and rituals associated with dying

BASIC CONCEPTS FROM SOCIOLOGY
A. Every human society has institutions for the socialization of its members
   1. Process by which individuals are compelled or induced to conform to the customs of the group
      a. Group establishes rules and codes of conduct governing its members, and these become the norms, values, and mores of the group
      b. Role of members includes specified rights, duties, attitudes, and actions
   2. Controls established through a system of rewards and punishment
      a. Reward leads to acceptance as a member of the group
      b. Punishment for antisocial behavior leads to rejection and separation from the group
B. Development of society requires sanction of group members
   1. Growth takes place in social space
      a. Social boundaries separate one group from another
      b. Barriers to participation are established through mores and customs
   2. Leader's influence is always limited to conditions placed on it by the total group
   3. Behavioral roles are established by members of the group
C. A society is a reflection of all the functional relationships that occur between its individual members
   1. Products of group life are a major determinant in an individual's intellect, creativity, memory, thinking, and feeling
      a. Human beings have no memory, thought, or feeling that does not include society

b. Intellect and creativity can be enhanced or hampered by society

2. Members of a society have functional and rewarding social contact
   a. Members are accepted and approved and then participate in establishing rules, norms, and values
   b. The nonmembers have, at best, limited social contacts with the members; this causes a segmentation of relationships and provides few rewarding experiences for the nonmembers

D. Society or a group can change because of conflict among members

1. This conflict is greatest when there is an absence of certain members, an introduction of new members, or a change in leadership
2. Ensuing reorganization goes through 3 stages
   a. Tension—caused by the conflict
   b. Integration—during which members learn about ''the other's'' problem
   c. Resolution—during which a reconstruction of the group's norms and values takes place
3. Resolution of conflict and the restoring of equilibrium
   a. This takes place when people interact with one another and the group is dynamic
   b. Conflicts are not resolved when groups are rigid with fixed membership and ideas

E. Family is the primary group

1. Helps society to establish and maintain its code of behavior
2. Provides individual members with
   a. Strong emotional ties
      (1) Much sensory contact is present
      (2) Members learn to care about the emotional and physical well-being of each other
      (3) Members are responsive to one another's feelings, acts, and opinions
      (4) Members learn empathy by vicariously living the experiences of others
      (5) Members view selves through the eyes of others
   b. Feeling of security by meeting dependent needs
   c. System of communication
      (1) Overt—words
      (2) Covert—body language
   d. Role identification and intimacy that help to internalize the acceptable behavioral patterns of the group
   e. Spirit of cooperation and competition through sibling interaction

3. Changes that have influenced the family's ability to indoctrinate children with the norms of society
   a. The Industrial Revolution changed an agrarian society into an industrial one
      (1) Families became nuclear rather than extended
      (2) Families depended more on secondary groups for survival
      (3) New social groups were established to replace the extended family
      (4) Labor unions replaced patriarchal management
         (a) Laws enacted to protect the rights of children and other dependent people of society
         (b) Laws enacted to establish minimum wage and hour benefits
      (5) There was increased mobility of individuals
   b. Altered male and female role patterns
      (1) Changing status of women
         (a) More women go outside the home to work
         (b) Women have an increased role in decision making and are better educated
      (2) Changing status of men
         (a) More men are willing to assume homemaking responsibilities
         (b) Men share decision making with women, thus decreasing dominance
      (3) Increased partnership in home and financial management has resulted in less stereotyped sex roles
   c. Factors resulting in a reduction in the size of families
      (1) Increase in financial cost involved in raising and educating children
      (2) Emphasis on limited population growth
      (3) Wide dissemination of birth control information
      (4) Legalization of abortions
      (5) Persons choosing to marry in later adulthood

F. Peer groups help youth to establish norms of behavior and assist in the rites of passage from the family group to society

1. Youth learns about society through contact with the peer group
2. Youth develops further self-concept in contact with other youths
3. Peer group interaction can produce change in its individual members

4. Members have a strong loyalty to the peer group because of the reciprocal relationships and other rewards the group offers
5. Peer group norms may conflict with family or society's norms
G. Group membership helps individuals achieve goals that are not attainable through individual effort
1. Types of groups are task oriented, therapy, self-awareness, social
2. Group functional roles include task roles, group building or maintenance roles, individual or self-serving roles
3. Group content refers to the subject matter or task being worked on
4. Group process refers to what is happening between and to group members while working; it deals with morale, feeling tones, influence, competition, conflict
H. Type of leadership in a group depends on the needs of the group members as well as the personality of the leader
1. Authoritarian leader—rigid and uses leadership role as an instrument of power; the leader makes all the decisions, which are then handed down to the membership; little communication and interrelating between leader and group
2. Democratic leader—fair and logical, uses the leadership role to stimulate others to achieve a collective goal; the leader encourages interrelating among members by relating to all members; weaknesses as well as strengths are accepted; the contributions of all members are fostered and utilized
3. Emotional leader—reflects the feeling tones, norms, and values of the group
4. Laissez-faire leader—passive and unproductive; usually assumes the role of a participant-observer and exerts little control or guidance over group behavior
5. Bureaucratic leader—rigid and assumes a role that is determined by formal criteria or rules that are inherent in the organization and frequently unrelated to the present group; the leader is not emotionally involved and avoids interrelating with the group members
6. Charismatic leader—can assume any of the above behaviors, since the group attributes supernatural power to this person or the office and frequently follows directions without question
I. Types of roles assumed by members of the group
1. Harmonizer—brings other group members into accord while reconciling opposing positions
2. Questioner—asks questions, seeks information, and gives constructive criticism to other group members
3. Deserter—talks about irrelevant material; is indifferent and usually disruptive in some manner
4. Tension reducer—introduces levity when it is needed and appropriate
5. Encourager—contributes to the ego of others in the group; is a warm responsive member
6. Monopolizer—attempts to control and assert authority over group; does not allow others to talk
7. Clarifier—restates issues for clarification and then summarizes for rest of the group
8. Opinion giver—uses own experience to back up opinion or belief
9. Initiator—proposes ideas or topics for discussion and suggests possible solutions for group discussion
10. Listener—shows interest in the group by expressions on face or by body language while making little or no comment
11. Negativist—pessimistic, argumentative, and uncooperative
12. Energizer—pushes the group into action
13. Aggressor—hostile, aggressive; seeks attention; verbally attacks other group members
J. Community is a social organization that is considered the individual's secondary group
1. Relationships among members are usually more impersonal
2. Individuals participate in a more delimited manner or in a specific capacity
3. The group frequently functions as a means to an end
a. The group enables diversified groups to communicate
b. The group helps other groups to identify community problems and possible solutions
4. The secondary group is usually rather large and meets on an intermittent basis; contacts are usually maintained through correspondence
5. Leaders of the community facilitate group interaction
a. They have a knowledge of the community and its needs
b. They have the skill to stimulate others to act
6. Secondary groups help establish laws that are necessary to limit antisocial behavior
a. Laws provide diversified groups with a common base of acceptable behavior
b. Some laws may favor and protect the vested interests of specific groups within the society

Sociology and Health

A. Role of society
  1. Traditionally societies have placed great emphasis on caring for their members when they are ill
  2. Recently society's role in health maintenance and the prevention of disease has been given an increased priority
  3. Society's provision for health maintenance includes
     a. Protection of food, water, and drug supplies
     b. Establishment of public health agencies for the supervision, prevention, and control of disease and illness
     c. Development of public education programs
     d. Awarding scholarship grants for health education and research
     e. Development of unemployment insurance programs.
     f. Establishment of workmen's compensation insurance
     g. Establishment of Social Security and Medicare programs
     h. Establishment of social welfare services and Medicaid programs
     i. Supervision of medical and hospital insurance programs
B. Health agency as a social institution has
  1. A bureaucratic structure
  2. Policies, rules, and regulations governing behavior of its members
  3. An impersonal viewpoint
  4. A status hierarchy
  5. An increasingly specialized subculture
C. Hospital as a subculture of society
  1. Employees develop both written and unwritten hospital policies that
     a. Set standards of acceptable behavior for both patients and staff
     b. Regulate the patient's contact with the primary group by limiting visitors
     c. Force both patients and staff to relate to the secondary group
     d. Punish unacceptable behavior by any members of the group, including the patient
  2. Folklores and folkways of the hospital serve to
     a. Maintain the mystique of medicine by fostering the use of a unique language and system of symbols
     b. Attach stigmas to various social illnesses such as venereal disease, mental illness, drug addiction, and alcoholism, which are associated with certain patterns of living and acting that are not acceptable to the group

     c. Perpetuate the roles and values of the health team members and maintain the status quo
  3. Hospital has several functions
     a. Primary—to help the patient regain health and resume a role in society by providing services directed toward
        (1) Treatment of illness
        (2) Rehabilitation
        (3) Maintenance of health
        (4) Protecting the patient's legal rights
     b. Secondary—to help society by providing services directed toward
        (1) Education of health professionals
        (2) The education of the general public
        (3) Research
D. Delivery of health services—responsibility of the community
  1. Members of society become active participants in prevention of illness
  2. Community health centers care for the ill in the home rather than in the hospital
  3. Extended care facilities are established with more community and homelike atmosphere
  4. Nonmedical community leaders take an active role in establishing health policy for society
  5. Lay members of the community become involved with health agencies' policies and decisions
  6. Health maintenance and treatment are no longer considered a privilege but the right of all members of society

BASIC CONCEPTS FROM PSYCHOLOGY

A. Human beings must be able to perceive and interpret stimuli to interact with the environment
  1. Perception and cognitive functioning are influenced by
     a. The nature of the stimuli
     b. Culture, beliefs, attitudes, and age
     c. Past experiences
     d. Present physical and emotional needs
  2. Individual's personality development is influenced by the ability to perceive and interpret stimuli
     a. Through these processes the external world is internalized
     b. The external world may in turn be distorted by the individual's perceptions
B. Humans must communicate to be able to interact with the environment
  1. Communication is a behavior that is learned through the process of acculturation

2. People must communicate with others to make needs known
   a. Infant uses the cry to bring attention to needs
   b. Hearing is essential to the development of good speech, since one learns to form words by hearing the words of others
   c. Written word usually replaces the spoken word when face-to-face encounters are impractical or supplements the spoken word when further clarification is necessary
3. Productive communication depends on the consensual validation of all involved
   a. To understand the intent of the message, each person must be aware of the meaning of the spoken word as well as the inflections in the speaker's voice (verbal and nonverbal communication)
   b. Validation can best be accomplished when participants are empathetic
   c. Language and channels of communication must be adapted to the person and the purpose for which it is intended
   d. Feedback is necessary to evaluate the effectiveness of the words and guide the communication
   e. Satisfaction is enhanced for all involved when lines of communication are kept open
4. Barriers to effective communication include
   a. Variations in culture, language, and education
   b. Problems in hearing, speech, or comprehension—poor perception
   c. Refusal to listen to another point of view—inability to evaluate
   d. Use of selective inattention, which may cause an interruption or distortion of the message
5. Nonverbal behavior communicates the inner feelings of the individual performing the behavior
   a. Facial expression, posture, and body movement may express the anxiety, pain, tension, fear, happiness, joy, or satisfaction the individual is experiencing
   b. Nonverbal communication may transmit a different message than the individual's verbal communication (covert, overt messages)
   c. Confusion arises when there is a difference in the verbal and nonverbal message received
C. Psychologic experiences provide the energy that is transformed into behavior
   1. Anxiety frequently provides the push that moves people to action because it
      a. Develops when 2 goals or needs are in conflict
      b. Is a state of apprehension or tension aroused by impulses from within
      c. Prepares one for action or completely overwhelms and inhibits action
   2. Anxiety develops in stages that progress from increased alertness to panic
   3. The sympathetic nervous system prepares the body's physiologic defense for fight or flight by stimulating the adrenal medulla to secrete epinephrine and norepinephrine
      a. The heart beat is accelerated to pump more blood to the muscles
      b. The peripheral blood vessels constrict to provide more blood to the vital organs
      c. The bronchioles dilate, and breathing becomes rapid and deep to supply more oxygen to the cells
      d. The pupils dilate to provide increased vision
      e. The liver releases glucose for quick energy
      f. The prothrombin time is lowered to protect the body from loss of blood in the event of injury
   4. Selye's general adaptation syndrome (GAS) is the body's physiologic adaptation to stress (anxiety)
      a. The adrenal cortex secretes cortisone during the emergency stage
      b. When stress continues, the increased secretion of cortisone causes the body to go through a resistive stage
      c. If the process continues, the last stage is exhaustion and death
   5. Defense mechanisms serve to protect the personality by controlling anxiety and reducing emotional pressures

Development of the Personality
Factors Involved in Personality Development
A. Behavior is a learned response that develops as a result of past experiences
B. To protect the individual's emotional well-being, these experiences are organized in the psyche on 3 different levels
   1. Conscious—composed of past experiences, easily recalled, that create little if any emotional discomfort
   2. Subconscious—has been deliberately pushed out of conscious but can be recalled with some effort
   3. Unconscious—contains the largest body of material, greatly influences behavior

a. This material cannot be deliberately brought back into awareness, since it is usually unacceptable to the individual

b. If recalled, it is usually disguised or distorted, as in dreams; however, it is still capable of producing a good deal of anxiety

C. According to Freud the personality consists of 3 parts—the id, ego, and superego

1. Id contains the instincts, impulses, and urges; is totally self-centered and unconscious

2. Ego is the conscious self, the ''I'' that deals with reality; the part of the personality that is shown to the environment

3. Superego controls, inhibits, and regulates impulses and instincts whose uncontrolled expression would endanger the emotional well-being of the individual and the stability of the society

Critical Periods in the Formation of the Personality

A. Personality of an individual develops in overlapping stages that shade and merge together

1. Certain goals must be accomplished during each stage in the development from infancy to maturity

2. If these goals are not accomplished at specific periods, the basic structure of the personality will be weakened

3. Factors in each stage persist as a permanent part of the personality

4. Each stage has particular frustrations and major traumas that must be overcome

5. Successful resolution of the conflicts associated with each stage is essential to development

6. Unresolved conflicts remain in the unconscious and may, at times, result in maladaptive behavior

B. Tasks related to personality development during infancy

1. Freud: oral stage—the infant obtains gratification by taking everything in; begins to develop self-concept from the responses of others

2. Erikson: trust versus mistrust—trust develops from the inner feeling of self-worth that is transmitted through maternal care; the child learns to depend on the satisfaction that is derived from this care, and when the need is met, trust develops

3. Sullivan: need for security—the infant learns to rely on others to gratify needs and satisfy wishes; develops a sense of basic trust, security, and self-worth when this occurs

C. Tasks related to personality development during early childhood

1. Freud: anal stage—struggle of giving of self and

breaking the symbiotic ties to mother; as the ties are broken, the child learns independence

2. Erikson: autonomy versus shame and doubt—the struggle of holding on to or letting go an internal struggle for self-identity; love versus hate

3. Sullivan: learning to communicate needs through the use of words and the acceptance of delayed gratification and interference with wish fulfillment

D. Tasks related to personality development during preschool period

1. Freud: oedipal stage—love for and desire to possess parent of the opposite sex creates fear and guilt feelings; desires are repressed and role identification with parent of the same sex occurs

2. Erikson: initiative versus guilt—stage of intensive activity, play, and consuming fantasies where the child interjects parents' social consciousness

3. Sullivan: development of body image and self-perception—organizes and used experiences in terms of approval and disapproval received; begins using selective inattention and disassociating those experiences which cause physical or emotional discomfort and pain

E. Tasks related to personality development during school age or preadolescence

1. Freud: latency stage—period of low sexual activity and identification with peer groups

2. Erikson: industry versus inferiority—the child wants to learn how to make things with others and strives to achieve success

3. Sullivan: the period of learning to form satisfying relationships with peers by using competition, compromise, and cooperation—the preadolescent learns to relate to peers of the same sex

F. Tasks related to personality development during adolescence

1. Freud: genital stage—time when sexual actvity increases and sexual identity is strengthened or attacked

2. Erikson: identity versus identity diffusion—the developmental task involves integrating childhood identifications with the basic drives, native endowments, and opportunities offered in social roles

3. Sullivan: learning to be independent and to establish satisfactory relationships with members of the opposite sex

G. Tasks related to personality development during young adulthood

1. Erikson: intimacy versus isolation—developmental task involves moving from the relative

security of self-identity to the relative insecurity involved in establishing intimacy with another
2. Sullivan: becoming economically, intellectually, and emotionally self-sufficient

H. Tasks related to personality development during later adulthood
  1. Erikson: generativity versus self-absorption—the mature person is interested in establishing and guiding the next generation
  2. Sullivan: learning to be interdependent and assuming responsibility for others

I. Tasks related to personality development during senescense
  1. Erikson: the older person adapts to triumphs and disappointments with a certain ego integrity
  2. Sullivan: the older person has an acceptance of responsibility for what life is and was and of its place in the flow of history

Influence of Basic Needs on the Development of Personality

A. Humanity has certain basic needs that must be satisfied
  1. Need to communicate
    a. Through communication, humans maintain contact with reality
      (1) The individual needs to validate findings with others to correctly interpret reality
      (2) Validation is enhanced when communication conveys an understanding of feelings
    b. Through communication, the individual develops a concept of self in relation to others
  2. Need for security
    a. To feel secure as an assurance of survival is fundamental
    b. Fear emerges when survival is threatened
    c. Initially the infant's security is related to the satisfaction of physical needs
    d. Security is enhanced when the same individual meets the infant's physical needs in a consistent manner
    e. The infant must also perceive love to feel secure
    f. Security is derived from the individual's perception of self in relation to others
    g. How the individual handles these perceptions influences personality development
  3. Need to move from dependence to independence
    a. The infant is dependent on the parents but through learning acquires faculties for independence
    b. There is no real security or deep assurance of survival in being dependent on others, since

uncertainties develop if one's security is totally derived from this source
    c. The infant must feel love and security before reaching out to struggle with the problems in the environment
    d. When the need for love and security is met, the child is sustained in the failures and hurts associated with learning and independence.
    e. Denial of the opportunity to learn or frustration in the drive for independence will produce emotional problems
  4. Need to develop a self-concept
    a. Self-concept begins to develop early in infancy
    b. Determination of the self-concept develops primarily through interaction with significant persons in the environment
    c. An integral part of the self-concept is the body image
    d. First and most deeply learned perception of body image develops from the attitudes of significant others, since children view themselves as others view them
    e. Concept of the self is root of security and future developmental needs
    f. Communication enhances the development of self
    g. A person's self-concept is the basis for emotional stability or instability; a secure person has strength and capacity for independence and becomes less anxious when circumstances require the help of others
  5. Need to find relief from organic discomfort
    a. Through experience, one learns the most satisfying ways of relieving discomfort
    b. Adjustment to illness depends on how the individual adjusts to life

B. Needs of a specific individual at a given time will vary according to internal and external environmental factors.

C. To attain psychologic equilibrium and achieve need satisfaction, the individual attempts to maintain a feeling of safety and comfort in adapting to life's situations; this is often achieved by maintaining a feeling of worth and a feeling of being needed by others

Anxiety and Behavior

A. Anxiety
  1. Is a state of apprehension, tension, or uneasiness
  2. Is an internal phenomenon aroused by impulses
  3. Occurs when the ego is threatened
  4. Frequently stems from an anticipation of danger

5. May arise from known, unknown, or unrecognized sources
B. Levels of anxiety
  1. Alertness level—automatic response of the central nervous system that
    a. Prepares the body for danger by regulating internal processes
    b. Concentrates all energies for internal activity
  2. Apprehension level—response to anticipation of short-term danger that
    a. Prepares the individual for efficient performance
    b. Occurs when facing new situations
    c. Creates some conscious awareness of discomfort
  3. Free-floating level—response to generalized anxiety that
    a. Creates a feeling of impending doom
    b. Produces an acute feeling of discomfort
  4. Panic level—total response to anxiety characterized by uncontrolled, unrealistic behavior that
    a. Lessens perception of the environment to protect the ego from awareness
    b. Increases the danger to the entire system
C. Defenses
  1. Conscious—these are the first-line defenses against anxiety; used by all people in times of stress; comprise the individual's deliberate effort to maintain control, reduce tension, and limit anxiety (individual may be aware of behavior but is not always aware of underlying reason)
    a. Remove self from the source of anxiety
    b. Escape through bodily satisfactions
    c. Focus psychic energy on other, more pleasant, activities
    d. Use of substitute gratifications
    e. Consciously avoid painful subjects
    f. Give socially acceptable reasons for behavior
    g. Release tensions by acting out impulsively
  2. Unconscious—these include the second-, third-, and fourth-line defenses against anxiety; may be used by all people in extremely stressful situations; however, if used consistently, indicate that the individual is emotionally ill
    a. Second-line defenses are the personality traits developed to handle interpersonal relationships and protect the ego
      (1) Exaggerated dependency and immaturity
      (2) Passive submission
      (3) Domination of others
      (4) Aggression toward others
      (5) Withdrawal from others

      (6) Compulsive ambition
      (7) Perfectionism and grandiosity
    b. Third-line defenses are the neurotic traits developed to handle interpersonal relationships and protect the ego
      (1) Repudiation and opposition of inner drives by the use of reaction formation
      (2) Avoidance of emotional or feeling level by placing complete emphasis on intellectual reasoning
      (3) Inhibition of affective, autonomic, and visceral functions to deaden actual awareness of repressed impulses
      (4) Displacement of impulses to an external object, which is then feared and avoided
      (5) Use of compulsive rituals to magically neutralize inner impulses
    c. Fourth-line defenses are the psychotic traits developed to handle interpersonal relationships and protect the ego
      (1) Regression to dependency level of development frequently accompanied by the attitudes and behavior of the child
      (2) Denial and withdrawal from others and reality
      (3) Internalization of hostility
      (4) Excited, uncontrolled acting out
  3. As anxiety and the threat to the ego are increased or decreased, shifts in the lines of defense will occur; the individual's behavior is altered by these shifts
D. Major sources of anxiety
  1. Threat to one's biologic integrity; interference with one's basic physiologic needs
  2. Threat to one's self system—self-esteem, self-worth, self-respect

Personality Defenses

Defense Mechanisms Provide Initial Protection for the Personality

A. Commonly used normal defense mechanisms that help an individual to deal with reality are
  1. Identification—the individual internalizes the characteristics of an idealized person
  2. Substitution—the individual replaces one goal for another
  3. Compensation—the individual makes up for a perceived lack in one area by emphasizing capabilities in another
  4. Sublimation—a socially acceptable behavior is substituted for an unacceptable instinct; this mechanism is used when the expression of these instincts would prove a threat to the self

5. Compromise—reciprocal give-and-take necessary in many relationships to salvage some part of the situation or the goal

6. Rationalization—the individual makes acceptable excuses for behavior and feelings; attempts to explain behavior by logical reasoning

B. In addition to the normal defenses, all individuals may use compensatory-type defenses in times of stress; these, when used in moderation, are adaptive; if used to excess, they frequently create greater emotional problems

1. Conversion—emotional conflict is unconsciously changed into a physical symptom that can be expressed openly and without anxiety

2. Denial—emotional conflict is blocked from the conscious mind and the individual refuses to recognize its existence

3. Displacement—emotions related to an emotionally charged situation or object are shifted to a relatively safe substitute situation or object

4. Fantasy—conscious distortion of unconscious wishes and needs to obtain gratification and satisfaction

5. Projection—unconscious denial of unacceptable feelings and emotions in oneself while attributing them to others

6. Reaction formation—the individual unconsciously reverses unacceptable feelings and behaves in the exact opposite manner

7. Regression—return to an earlier stage of behavior when stress creates problems at the present stage

8. Repression—involuntary exclusion from consciousness of those ideas, feelings, and situations which are creating conflict and causing discomfort

9. Suppression—voluntary exclusion from consciousness of those ideas, feelings, and situations which are creating conflict and causing discomfort

10. Transference—positive or negative feelings and emotions that were previously present toward important figures are applied and attributed to another person in the present

11. Intellectualization—use of thinking, ideas, or intellect to avoid emotions

12. Introjection—complete acceptance of another's opinions and values as one's own

C. As the use of these compensatory defenses increases and encompasses more of the individual's life, contact with reality is interrupted and distortions begin

D. Identifiable patterns of response begin to form when individuals respond to most situations they encounter with the same type of behavior

E. These patterns of behavior are considered deviations and are usually looked on as symptoms of emotional problems

F. Although all individuals may, in times of severe emotional stress, use many of the behaviors listed, it is the repetitive use of these behaviors in most situations that is indicative of problems

Motivation, Learning, and Behavior

A. All behavior is motivated

1. Motive always implies some purpose

2. Social motives are often changed through learning

3. Symbolic rewards are the major factors in learning

4. Social approval is an important form of symbolic reward

B. Behavior and emotions

1. Emotions act as motives for behavior, since they often involve a reaction to some external situation

2. Behavior is always accompanied and often controlled by the emotions

3. Emotions may facilitate or hinder the learning process

4. Emotions exert a strong influence on the thinking process

C. Automatic behavior

1. Is the predetermined or repetitive type behavior that has been used successfully in prior situations

2. Requires little effort or thought

3. Is adapted to definite situations and can be difficult to alter if the situation changes

4. Is integrated with cognition in the functioning of a mature and independent adult

D. Life is a continually changing process, and when these changes occur in areas of significance they often produce rather distinct emotional responses; these changes include

1. Resistance to change—the individual hesitates to accept or adapt to the change and may attempt to deny its occurrence or reject its outcome

2. Regression—the individual returns to an earlier type of behavior that, at the time, provided some satisfaction and gratification and now provides an escape from the unacceptable or anxiety-producing situation

3. Acceptance and progression—the individual adapts to the change and expends energy on outside objects rather than self-centered aims

Nursing in Psychiatry

BASIC PRINCIPLES OF PSYCHIATRIC NURSING

A. These principles
   1. Are by necessity general in nature
   2. Form the guidelines for the emotional care of all patients
B. In caring for patients, the nurse should attempt to
   1. Accept and respect people as individuals regardless of their behavior
   2. Limit or reject the individual's inappropriate behavior without rejecting the individual
   3. Recognize that all behavior has meaning and is meeting the needs of the performer regardless of how distorted or meaningless it appears to others
   4. Accept the dependency needs of individuals while supporting and encouraging moves toward independence
   5. Help individuals set appropriate limits for themselves or set limits for them when they are unable to do so
   6. Encourage individuals to express their feelings in an atmosphere free of reprisal or judgment
   7. Recognize that individuals need to use their defenses until other defenses can be substituted
   8. Recognize how feelings affect behavior and influence relationships
   9. Recognize that individuals frequently respond to the behavioral expectations of others—family, peers, authority (staff)
   10. Recognize that all individuals have a potential for movement toward higher levels of emotional health

THERAPEUTIC NURSING RELATIONSHIPS

A. Phases
   1. Orientation or introductory—nurse establishes a trust relationship which the patient tests by discussing only what he or she wishes to discuss; patients are never pushed to discuss areas of concern that are upsetting to them
   2. Working—nurse and the patient discuss areas of concern and the patient is helped to plan, implement, and evaluate a course of action
   3. Termination—end of the therapeutic relationship between the nurse and the patient; the time perameters should be set early in the relationship with meetings spaced further and further apart near the end
B. Themes of communication—recurring thoughts and ideas that give insight into what an individual is feeling and tie the communication together
   1. Content—conversation may appear superficial but careful attention to the underlying theme helps the nurse identify problem areas while providing insight into the patient's self concept
   2. Mood—emotion or affect that the patient communicates to the nurse; includes personal appearance, facial expressions, and gestures that reflect the patient's mood and feelings
   3. Interaction—how the patient reacts or interacts with the nurse; includes how the patient relates and what role he or she assumes when communicating with the nurse and others
C. Fundamental requirements of a therapeutic relationship
   1. Ability to communicate therapeutically requires a basic understanding and use of interviewing techniques in developing a trusting relationship through
      a. Open-ended rather than probing questions
      b. Reflection of words and feelings and paraphrasing
      c. Acceptance of the patient's behavior
      d. Nonjudgmental objective attitude
      e. Focusing on the emotional needs of the patient
      f. Having a therapeutic goal for the interview
   2. Recognition that an individual has potential for growth
      a. Individuals need to learn about their own behavior in relation to others
      b. Exchanging experiences with others provides the reassurance that reactions are valid and feelings shared
      c. Participating with groups increases knowledge of interpersonal relationships and helps individuals to identify their strengths and resources
      d. The identification of the individual's strengths and resources helps to convey the expectation of growth
   3. Recognition that an individual needs to be accepted
      a. Acceptance is an active process designed to convey respect for another through empathetic understanding
      b. Acceptance of others implies and requires acceptance of self
      c. To be nonjudgmental, one must become aware of one's own attitudes and feelings and their effect on perception
      d. Acceptance requires that individuals be permitted and even encouraged to express their feelings and attitudes even though they may be divergent from the general viewpoint

(1) Individuals should be encouraged to express both positive and negative feelings

(2) This encouragement must occur on both the verbal and nonverbal level

e. Acceptance means showing interest in another person; interest requires

(1) Face-to-face contact and really listening to what the other person has to say

(2) Developing an awareness of the other person's likes and dislikes

(3) Attempting to understand another's point of view

(4) Using nonverbal as well as verbal expressions of acceptance

f. Acceptance requires the development of interpersonal techniques that encourage others to express problems; the listener's

(1) Reflection of feelings, attitudes, and words helps the speaker to identify feelings

(2) Open-ended questions permit the speaker to focus on problems

(3) Paraphrasing assists the speaker in clarifying statements

(4) Use of silence provides both the listener and the speaker with the necessary time for thinking over what is being discussed

g. Acceptance requires the recognition of factors that block communication, including

(1) Any overt or covert response that conveys a judgmental or superior attitude

(2) Direct questions that convey an invasive or probing attitude

(3) Ridicule that conveys a hostile attitude

(4) Talking about one's own problems and not listening, which conveys a self-serving attitude and loss of interest in the speaker

D. Recognition of behavioral changes that result from physical illness

1. Anxiety, fear, and depression occur whenever there is a health problem

a. Body image and feelings of being in control of one's body have their basis in the early developmental period

b. Anxiety develops whenever a real or imaged threat to the body image occurs

2. Signs of the anxiety, fear, and depression associated with illness are variable and include

a. Indifference to symptoms—usually related to failure to accept the occurrence of a health problem

b. Denial of reality—usually related to attempts

to maintain stability and integrity of the personality

c. Reaction formation—usually related to attempts to block the reality from consciousness and acting as if nothing is wrong

d. Failure to keep appointments and follow physician's or nurse's directions—usually related to fear of finding additional problems or admitting there is something wrong

e. Overconcern with body functions and symptoms—usually related to fear of death

f. Asking many questions and offering many complaints—usually related to attempts at keeping a staff member by the beside because of fears associated with illness; fear of abandonment

g. Opportunity to ventilate feelings

3. Emotional needs of the ill person include

a. Security of continuous relationships with friends and members of their families

b. Some way of achieving the feeling of self-worth and self-esteem

c. Assistance in accepting the dependent role of the patient

d. Assistance in resolving conflicts while maintaining security

e. Assistance in refocusing inner resources

f. Contact with the reality of the external world

4. To help the individual maintain the self-concept during illness, the nurse must understand the normal emotional stages of illness

a. Denial—the individual cannot believe it is happening

b. Anger—something has happened that one cannot control

c. Bargaining—promising to be a better person if something occurs

d. Depression—one grieves for loss or expected loss

e. Acceptance of the illness and learning how to adapt—this stage can only be reached when the individual has resolved the conflicts that develop during the earlier stages

5. Common reactions occur to the change in body image associated with many health problems

a. Attitudes toward one's body and self-concept greatly influence response

b. Fear is a universal response; individual may focus on fear of

(1) Pain

(2) Incapacitation

(3) Disfigurement

(4) Altered self-concept

(5) Rejection of loved ones

(6) Death

c. Questioning is a universal response; the individual may focus on

(1) This can't be happening to me

(2) Is this really happening to me?

(3) What did I do to deserve this?

(4) Why am I being punished?

d. Grief and mourning are universal responses; the individual may focus on

(1) What was in the past

(2) What could have been for the future

(3) Loss of missed opportunities

(4) A magnified view of the loss

(5) Avoiding interpersonal contacts

PSYCHOLOGIC FACTORS AFFECTING PHYSICAL CONDITION

A. Physical illnesses where psychogenic factors are the predominant causative agents

B. Anxiety stimulates the autonomic nervous system, and the nervous and endocrine impulses appear to center on one particular organ, creating actual physical illness and changes in the tissue structure

C. Reason a certain organ is involved with one patient and a different organ with another is still undetermined

1. Pathology—premorbid personality appears to be one of unexpressed aggression resulting from the unresolved struggle between dependent need and independent striving; may be familial

2. Symptoms

a. Skin

(1) In neurodermatitis, dermatitis factitia, pruritus, and trichotillomania, psychic factors appear to dominate

(2) There appears to be a relationship between endocrine imbalance and disturbances in the autonomic regulation of skin physiology

(3) Stress seems to lead to rash, itching, and discomfort

b. Musculoskeletal

(1) Anxiety and fear often create a tightening of muscles

(2) This becomes an aggravating factor in arthritis, backache, tension headache, or any other musculoskeletal disorder in which increased tension and spasm are involved

c. Respiratory

(1) Hyperventilation syndrome

(a) Panting occurs with tension and ex-

citement and this forced respiration can produce biochemical changes in the blood

(b) These changes can alter the cerebral circulation and cause a reduction in consciousness and syncope

(2) Bronchial asthma

(a) Stress and tension appear to create increased secretions and changes in the bronchi

(b) Individuals with asthma tend to exhibit a strong desire for protection and dependency yet fear rejection or engulfment

(c) Wheeze associated with asthma is considered by some to be a suppressed cry for this protection

d. Cardiovascular

(1) Essential hypertension

(a) Anxiety and other stresses are believed to play a role in releasing a pressor from the kidneys, which causes chronic vasoconstriction of the vessels

(b) All other primary causes for hypertension must be ruled out before this cause can be diagnosed

(c) Individuals with hypertension have difficulty handling hostile feelings, are less assertive, and have more obsessive-compulsive traits than nonhypertensive ones

(d) Hypertension may be considered a state of chronically unexpressed rage that arises from conflicts between passive/dependent longings and the struggle for independence

(2) Coronary occlusion and angina

(a) Coronary attacks frequently occur following periods of fatigue and anxiety

(b) These individuals place a high value on work and success; they become depressed when inactive

e. Hemolymphatic

(1) Certain blood dyscrasias and responses can be linked to emotional stress

(2) In some individuals the neutrophil count drops, the clotting time is decreased, both blood viscosity and erythrocyte sedimentation rate rise

(3) Nature of this response to stress is still controversial

f. Gastrointestinal
  (1) Peptic ulcer
    (a) Anxiety and other stress appear to create a condition of hyperactivity, hypersecretion, hyperacidity, and engorgement of the mucosa
    (b) Related to stresses in life, particularly those concerned with conflicts between passivity and aggression
    (c) Use reaction formation to cover the strong, somewhat irrational need to achieve security from others
  (2) Ulcerative colitis
    (a) Parasympathetic stimulation of the lower bowel produces an enzyme that interferes with the protective coating of the bowel
    (b) May occur as a reaction to a variety of stresses but most often in situations that demand accomplishment and arouse fear of not succeeding
    (c) Many patients are immature and have not gained any feelings of independence
g. Genitourinary
  (1) Disturbances in genital and urinary problems may occur under stress
  (2) Enuresis, amenorrhea, frigidity, and impotence appear to be related to psychologic factors
  (3) Depression and feelings of helplessness may be related to urinary retention
  (4) Fear may be related to urgency and frequency
h. Endocrine
  (1) Eating patterns and dependency on food for satisfaction and reduction of stress appears related to both diabetes mellitus and obesity
  (2) Feelings of insecurity and an unusual sense of responsibility appear associated with onset of hyperthyroidism
i. Organs of special sense—some evidence that certain neurologic disturbances, such as atypical facial neuralgia, are related to emotional conflict
3. Therapy—must be directed toward both the physical and emotional problems
4. Nursing approach
  a. Reduce emotional stimulation when possible
  b. Explain all procedures carefully and allow patient time for questions
  c. Provide the patient with talking time
  d. Avoid material that appears to stimulate conflict for the patient
  e. Accept the patient's behavior and encourage expression of feelings
  f. Remember that the patient is really physically ill and the symptoms have a physiologic basis

DEVIATE PATTERNS OF BEHAVIOR
Withdrawn Behavior

A. Definition—pathologic retreat from or an avoidance of people and the world of reality
B. Developmental factors
  1. Unhappy childhood caused by conflict, tension, and anxiety in the home
  2. Inconsistent relationships with parents
    a. Lack of firm standards for reward or punishment
    b. Variations between verbal and nonverbal communications
  3. Failure to develop a sense of security
  4. Failure to develop positive self-image
  5. Interpersonal relationships create a continuous source of anxiety
  6. Chronic anxiety results in loss of interest in interpersonal relationships and reality testing
  7. Extreme sensitivity, narcissism, and introversion develop
C. Compensatory mechanisms used to reduce and avoid stress include
  1. Fixation
  2. Rigidity and compulsiveness
  3. Reaction formation
  4. Sublimation
  5. Rationalization
  6. Regression
D. Effects of compensatory mechanisms on behavior
  1. Isolation and failure to test reality result in greater distortions of reality situations
  2. Behavior can progress until loss of contact with reality develops and individual retreats into the condition usually identified as schizophrenia

Projective Behavior

A. Definition—pathologic denial of one's own feelings, faults, failures, and emotions while continually attributing them to others
B. Developmental factors
  1. Parents set extremely high demands and continually raise expected standards of performance
  2. Expectations of failure are fostered, creating feelings of inadequacy and feelings of inferiority
  3. Childhood experiences continue to reinforce these feelings and, chronic insecurity, suspiciousness, and extreme sensitivity develop

4. Feelings of hostility develop and cannot be expressed
5. Inability to establish interpersonal relationships with other intereferes with reality testing
6. The individual develops a rigid, structured, narcissistic personality
7. Competitive society fosters and supports projective patterns of behavior

C. Compensatory mechanisms used to reduce and avoid stress include
 1. Displacement
 2. Projection
 3. Rigidity
 4. Denial
 5. Rationalization
 6. Delusions
 7. Ideas of reference

D. Effects of compensatory mechanisms on behavior
 1. The individual is unable to tolerate suspense, prolonged anxiety, or tension
 2. Unacceptable impulses and wishes are denied and faults and failures are disclaimed for self and attributed to others
 3. Delusional ideas develop and begin to dominate behavior
 4. Ideas of reference result in continual misinterpretation of events
 5. Delusions become more systematized and spread out
 6. Behavior can progress until loss of contact with reality is complete and the individual retreats into the condition usually identified as paranoid schizophrenia or paranoid states

Aggressive Behavior

A. Definition—pathologic anger and hostility that are turned outward onto others or inward on oneself

B. Developmental factors
 1. Security is chronically threatened, resulting in a continual struggle to maintain it
 2. Strong need for approval
 3. Failure to develop self-concept and self-esteem
 4. Chronic anxiety and tension, which are often increased by the real or imagined loss of a love object
 5. Demands and responsibilities are high

C. Compensatory mechanisms used to reduce and avoid stress include
 1. Displacement
 2. Rigidity
 3. Denial
 4. Rationalization
 5. Repression

6. Hostility that can be directed on
 a. Self
 b. Environment

D. Effects of compensatory mechanisms on behavior
 1. Need for approval results in compliance to demands
 2. Necessary compliance creates resentment
 3. Hostility develops and fosters feeling of guilt
 4. Self-doubt increases anxiety and tension
 5. Increased anxiety and tension reduce interpersonal relationships and reality testing
 6. Behavior can progress until there is a complete loss of contact with reality and the individual retreats into the condition usually identified as an affective disorder

Psychoneurotic Behavior

Includes anxiety reactions, conversion reactions, phobic reactions, and obsessive-compulsive reactions

A. Definition—maladjustive type of response, characterized by many fears, anxieties, and/or physical symptoms

B. Developmental factors
 1. Usually lack a stable family life and effective guidance
 2. Frequently overprotected and fail to acquire the necessary skills to cope with problems
 3. Experience chronic insecurity, anxiety, and tension
 4. Goals are set for them by the parents, and acceptance depends on achieving the goals
 5. Constant struggle to gain reassurance and security
 6. Gains satisfaction from behavior and substitutes this satisfaction for the satisfaction desired but not obtained through interpersonal relations

C. Compensatory mechanisms used to reduce anxiety and avoid stress include
 1. Displacement
 2. Rationalization
 3. Regression
 4. Rigidity and compulsiveness
 5. Conversion
 6. Denial

D. Effects of compensatory mechanisms on behavior
 1. Behavior is purposeful and is unconsciously resorted to when the person feels threatened
 2. Continued use of behavior can
 a. Create new problems for the individual
 b. Be out of proportion to the degree of stress, impair social effectiveness, and dominate the individual's total life
 3. When impairment of functioning occurs, the in-

dividual is usually considered to be deviating from the normal and to have an anxiety disorder

Socially Aggressive Behavior

A. Definition—maladjustive response resulting from a defect in the development of the personality that is characterized by peculiar actions or misbehavior
B. Developmental factors
1. Approval and disapproval do not appear sufficiently strong in childhood to influence the behavior along accepted patterns
2. Long history of maladjustment that creates more problems as child matures and standards for acceptable behavior are increased
3. The individual may show a history of severe emotional trauma in early life that interferes with emotional development
4. Parents frequently provide a cold, emotionally sterile environment
C. Compensatory mechanisms used to reduce anxiety and avoid stress include
1. Displacement
2. Repression
3. Denial
4. Regression
5. Hostility
6. Rejection
D. Effects of compensatory mechanisms on behavior; the individual
1. Appears competent but is usually unreliable and lacks a sense of responsibility
2. Has the potential to succeed but shows a history of repeated failure
3. Lack perseverance, honesty, and sincerity
4. Is completely egocentric and incapable of emotional investment in others
5. Experiences no remorse or shame
6. Is explosive under pressure
7. Is unable to tolerate criticism
8. Fails to profit from past experiences and care little about the consequences for present acts
9. Impairment of judgment usually creates problems and brings the individual into conflict with society; usually classified as personality disturbances

Addictive Behavior

A. Definition—repeated or chronic use of alcohol or drugs with a resulting dependency on these substances
B. Developmental factors
1. Feelings of loneliness and isolation develop

2. Chronic anxiety, fears, and low tension tolerance develop as a result of early relationships
3. Feelings of inadequacy in interpersonal relationships serve to increase anxiety
4. Inability to delay satisfaction
5. Struggle for independence yet unconscious desire to be dependent
6. Impulsiveness and resentment of responsibility
7. Peer pressure and drug availability
8. Sexual conflict
9. Family factors
C. Compensatory mechanisms used to reduce anxiety and avoid stress include
1. Denial
2. Regression
3. Rationalization
4. Addiction
5. Displacement
6. Fantasy
7. Repression
8. Intellectualization
D. Effects of compensatory mechanisms on behavior
1. Drug or alcohol reduces inhibitory self-control
2. Drug or alcohol allows for expression of inner feelings but increases the guilt and requires more of the substance to relieve the guilt.
3. Alcohol and drugs decrease feelings of inferiority and reduce anxiety
4. Alcohol and drugs increase social isolation and cause deterioration of personal habits
5. The individual becomes increasingly less efficient and devotes less energy to goals and ambitions
6. Dependency and tolerance develop and the substances are needed in increasing amounts to achieve the same dulling of reality
7. Securing the alcohol or drug becomes the main objective in life, and functioning is totally impaired; these individuals are then classified as drug addicts or alcoholics

CLASSIFICATION OF MENTAL DISORDERS*

A. Disorders evident in infancy, childhood, or adolescence
1. Mental retardation
2. Attention deficit disorders
3. Conduct disorders
4. Anxiety disorders
5. Eating disorders
6. Pervasive developmental disorders

*Adapted from Diagnostic and statistical manual of mental disorders, ed. 3, Washington, D.C., 1980, American Psychiatric Association.

7. Behavioral disorders in children as a response to illness
B. Organic mental disorders (organic brain syndromes)
 1. Delirium
 2. Dementia
C. Substance use disorders
 1. Alcohol abuse
 2. Drug dependence
D. Schizophrenic disorders
E. Paranoid disorders
F. Affective disorders
 1. Major affective disorders
  a. Bipolar disorder
  b. Major depression with psychotic features
  c. Major depression with melancholia
 2. Other affective disorders
G. Anxiety disorders
H. Somatoform disorders
I. Psychosexual disorders
 1. Paraphilias
 2. Ego-dystonic homosexuality
J. Adjustment disorders
K. Personality disorders

PATHOLOGY, SYMPTOMS, THERAPIES, AND NURSING APPROACHES FOR THE MAJOR DIAGNOSTIC ENTITIES IN PSYCHIATRY
Disorders Usually Evident in Infancy, Childhood, or Adolescence

A. Mental retardation—area of mental retardation is covered in pediatric nursing
B. Attention deficit disorders
 1. Diagnosis difficult, since the pathology must be separated from normal disturbances that occur during this period of life
 2. Evident before 7 years of age; lasting at least 6 months
 3. The child is inappropriately inattentive and demonstrates excessive impulsiveness; hyperactivity may or may not be present
 4. Nursing approach—since the nursing approach for children and adolescents is similar for all types of emotional disorders, it will be summarized at the end of this area
C. Conduct disorders
 1. The child may be socialized (evidence of social attachment) or undersocialized (little evidence of social attachment)
 2. The child may be aggressive or nonaggressive
 3. Behavior
  a. Is destructive to the child's own general aims

b. Is repeated despite rational arguments to the contrary and despite punishment
 c. Involves the discharge of affects stemming from unconscious conflicts
 d. Leads to getting caught and punished
 e. Includes stealing, truancy, running away and excessive rebelliousness
 4. Nursing approach—since the nursing approach for children and adolescents is similar for all types of emotional disorders, it will be summarized at the end of this area
D. Anxiety disorders
 1. The child demonstrates persistent and pervasive anxiety
 2. Anxiety may be specific or generalized
 3. Symptoms may include
  a. Sleeping difficulties—somnambulism and insomnia
  b. Learning difficulties—severe reading problems, underachievement and school phobias
  c. Enuresis—bedwetting
  d. Regressive reaction
  e. Physiologic disturbances
   (1) Eating problems—nausea and vomiting
   (2) Excretion problems—constipation or diarrhea
   (3) Respiratory and circulatory problems—asthma and tachycardia
   (4) Allergies—skin rashes and hives
  f. Excessive conformity
 4. Therapy
  a. Psychotherapy—in children, usually in the form of play therapy
  b. Medications—amphetamines and mild tranquilizers are quite effective with children
 5. Nursing approach—since the nursing approach for children and adolescents is similar for all types of emotional disorders, it will be summarized at the end of this area
E. Eating disorders
 See anorexia nervosa in medical-surgical nursing section
F. Pervasive developmental disorders
 1. Two basic features
  a. An alienation or withdrawal from reality
  b. A severe disturbance in the child's feeling of self-identity
 2. Pathology
  a. Many theories as to cause are being studied; however, no definitive cause has as yet been established
  b. Failure to develop satisfactory relationships with significant adults, regardless of the

cause, appears to be an underlying problem with all these children

3. Infantile autism—evident before 30 months of age; childhood onset pervasive developmental disorder evident after 30 months of age but before 12 years

4. Symptoms
   a. General
      (1) Inability to differentiate between self and environment
      (2) Confusion in self-boundaries frequently characterized by speaking of self only in the third person
      (3) A defect in ego formation or an inadequately functioning ego system
      (4) A conflict between self and reality
      (5) Defect in the adaptive, inhibitory, and steering mechanisms of the personality
      (6) Interference with intellect may be so profound, child appears to be mentally retarded
   b. Infantile autism
      (1) Lack of meaningful relationships with outside world
      (2) Use of autistic fantasy resulting in communication defects
      (3) Turning to inanimate objects and self-centered activity for security
   c. Pathologic symbiosis
      (1) Intense though morbid relationship between mother and child
      (2) The child unable to separate identity from that of mother
      (3) Lacks adequate concept of reality
      (4) Inability to relate to peers or adults
   d. Pervasive developmental disorder
      (1) Profound apathy
      (2) Looseness of association
      (3) Autistic thinking
      (4) Ambivalence
      (5) Absence of communication skills
      (6) Poor grasp of reality
      (7) Bizarre, unpredictable, uncontrolled behavior
      (8) Inability to relate to others
      (9) Total interference with intellectual functioning

5. Therapy
   a. Psychotherapy directed toward the developmental level of the child—play, group, or individual therapy
   b. Medications—tranquilizers and amphetamines provide some reduction of symptoms
   c. Removal from the home situation may be necessary, although day school situations frequently provide enough relief so that hospitalization can be avoided

6. Nursing approach—since the nursing approach for children and adolescents is similar for all types of emotional disorders, it will be summarized at the end of this area

G. Behavioral disorders in children as a response to illness
   1. Pathology
      a. Can be responses to alterations in the central nervous system cells such as those created by
         (1) Infectious disorder such as high fevers
         (2) Communicable diseases such as viral, toxic, or postinfectious encephalitis
         (3) Anemias and blood dyscrasias
         (4) Brain lesions or tumors
      b. Can be responses to organic changes in other body tissues and cells such as those created by
         (1) Thyroid, adrenal, and pituitary glands
         (2) Any change in any part of the endocrine or autonomic nervous system
      c. Can be responses to the stress of being ill
         (1) Regression to earlier levels of development occurs with any illness
         (2) Restriction in activities, pain, and separation
   2. Symptoms—depend on the cells affected as well as the child's ability to contain or integrate the experience
   3. Therapy—directed at reducing the underlying cause of the problem
   4. Nursing approach—similar for all types of emotional disorders; summarized at the end of this section

H. Nursing approach for children and adolescents with emotional problems
   1. General guidelines for the care of all children with emotional problems; care should be directed toward helping the child grow up emotionally by
      a. Establishing a favorable environment in which the child can gain or regain a favorable equilibrium
      b. Establishing a constructive relationship
      c. Helping the child to see self as a worthwhile person
      d. Recognizing that the behavior has meaning for the child
      e. Being as realistic and as truthful as possible in dealing with the child

  f. Attempting to establish trust
  g. Setting limits that are as realistic as possible but as firm as necessary
  h. Pointing out reality, but accepting the child's views of it while pointing it out
  i. Being consistent both in approach and in rules and regulations
  j. Making all explanations as clear as possible
  k. Supporting and encouraging the child's moves toward independence but allowing dependency when necessary

Organic Mental Disorders (Organic Brain Syndromes)

Associated with actual changes in the tissue of the brain

A. Delirium—syndromes from which the patient usually recovers, since the situation is often reversible and temporary
  1. Pathology
    a. Infection
      (1) Intracranial or nervous system (e.g., meningitis or encephalitis)
      (2) Systemic or toxic (e.g., pneumonia or typhoid)
    b. Trauma to the head
    c. Circulatory disturbances resulting in impairment of blood flow to the brain
    d. Metabolic disorders—electrolyte imbalance (e.g., dehydration, diarrhea, vomiting)
    e. Drug intoxication or poisoning
    f. Alcoholic intoxication
  2. Symptoms
    a. Delirium and its accompanying confusion, hallucinations, and delusions
    b. Disorientation and confusion as to time, place, identity
    c. Memory defects for both recent and remote events and facts
    d. Slurring of speech may occur along with an indistinct pronunication or use of words
    e. Tremors, incoordination, imbalance, and incontinence may develop
  3. Therapy
    a. Reduce causative agent such as fever, toxins, drugs, or alcohol
    b. Prevent further damage
    c. Provide diet high in calories, protein, and vitamins
    d. Provide mild sedative if necessary
  4. Nursing approach
    a. Provide a quiet environment, reduce stimuli

    b. Provide assurance to the patient and family
    c. Since lability of mood is common, plan care so the staff approaches these patients when they appear receptive
    d. Ensure adequate intake and output
    e. Observe for changing physiologic and neurologic symptoms
B. Dementia—syndromes from which the patient does not recover, since the damage is irreversible and permanent; there may be some improvement with treatment of the underlying cause, but disturbances in memory and judgment will remain
  1. Pathology
    a. Prenatal injury or malformation (e.g., hydrocephalus, microcephalus, neurosyphilis)
    b. Infections such as general paresis
    c. Alcohol (e.g., alcoholic encephalopathy, Korsakoff's syndrome)
    d. Trauma in which a head injury results in permanent brain damage
    e. Circulatory disturbances causing anoxia and permanent brain damage (e.g., cerebral arteriosclerosis, cerebral vascular accidents)
    f. Deterioration and death of brain cells (e.g., senility)
    g. Loss of brain tissue in presenile conditions (e.g., Alzheimer's disease, Pick's disease)
    h. Nutritional deprivation of brain cells (e.g., pellagra)
    i. Damage resulting from generalized diseases (e.g., multiple sclerosis, hepatolenticular disease, Huntington's chorea, Parkinson's disease)
    j. Damage resulting from pressures of brain tumors
  2. Symptoms—same as those resulting from delirium
  3. Therapy—same as those for delirium, with greater emphasis on preventing further damage
  4. Nursing approach
    a. Provide a safe environment
    b. Continually orient the patient to time, date, and place
    c. Keep the schedule of activities flexible to make use of the patient's lability of moods and easy distractability
    d. Provide adequate nutrition
    e. Provide exercise
    f. Provide diversional activities that the patient enjoys and can handle
    g. Provide emotional support for family

Substance Use Disorders

Alcohol Abuse

Alcohol intake that interefers with normal functioning or is necessary as a prerequisite to normal functioning

A. Pathology—premorbid personality utilizes the compensatory mechanisms of the addictive pattern of behavior

B. Patterns of drinking and symptoms
1. Intoxication—state in which coordination or speech is impaired and behavior is altered
2. Episodic excessive drinking—becoming intoxicated as infrequently as 4 times a year; episodes may vary in length from hours to days or weeks
3. Habitual excessive drinking—becoming intoxicated more than 12 times a year or is recognizably under the influence of alcohol more than once a week even though not considered intoxicated
4. Alcohol addiction—direct or strong presumptive evidence of dependence on alcohol; demonstrated by withdrawal symptoms or by the inability to go for a day without drinking; when there is a history of heavy drinking for 3 or more months, the individual is considered addicted to alcohol
5. Early symptoms of alcoholism—frequent drinking sprees, increased intake, drinking alone or in the early morning, occurrence of blackouts

C. Therapy
1. Should be multifaceted social and medical; involves psychotherapy (group, family, and individual counseling), especially with Alcoholics Anonymous
2. Negative conditioning with disulfiram (Antabuse) appears to help
3. Patients can be assisted only when they admit they need help
4. Physical needs must be cared for, since dietary needs have often been ignored for long periods

D. Nursing approach
1. Provide a well-controlled, alcohol-free environment
2. Plan a full program of activities but with adequate rest periods
3. Meet the patient's needs for a great deal of support without criticism or judgment
4. Avoid trying to talk the patient out of the problem
5. Accept the smooth facade that the patient may present while approaching the lonely and fearful individual behind it
6. Accept failures without judgment or punishment
7. Accept hostility without criticism or retaliation
8. Recognize ambivalence and limit the need for decision making by the patient
9. Maintain the patient's interest in a therapy program

Drug Dependence

Misuse of drugs, usually by self-administration

A. Pathology—premorbid personality, utilizing compensatory mechanisms of the addictive pattern of behavior

B. Definitions
1. Addiction—habituation to and tolerance of drugs other than alcohol, tobacco, and ordinary caffeine-containing beverages; medically prescribed drugs are excluded if they are taken under medical direction; addiction can occur simultaneously to 2 or more drugs or to alcohol and drugs; lately, combined addiction to a multiplicity of drugs has become more common
2. Habituation—may be both physical and psychologic dependency
3. Tolerance—physical dependency to a drug in which the presence of the drug in increasingly higher dosage is needed to achieve the same effect; tolerance can exceed the usual lethal limits of a drug

C. Symptoms
1. Needle marks on limbs along the path of a vein
2. Addicted individuals may tend to wear long-sleeved shirts, even in warm weather
3. Yawning, lacrimation, rhinorrhea, and perspiration appear 10 to 15 hours after the last opiate injection; unrealistic high; pronounced depression
4. Severe abdominal cramps if too much time has elapsed between injections
5. Physical examination may reveal an underweight, malnourished individual with multiple dental caries and depressed central nervous system functioning
6. Job or academic failure; marital conflicts; poor reality testing; personality change

D. Therapy
1. Methadone maintenance for opiate addiction—programs do not treat addiction but change the addiction from an illegal drug to a legal drug, which is administered under supervision; has proved successful only in individuals with long-standing addictions
2. High-calorie, high-protein, high-vitamin diet because of poor eating habits
3. Treatment in groups run by ex-addicts

4. Therapeutic community setting
5. Psychotherapy and family therapy on an outpatient basis
6. If the patient is to be withdrawn from drugs, decreasing amounts of methadone and/or tranquilizers must be administered to reduce the physiologic and psychologic discomfort
7. Vocational counseling

E. Nursing approach
1. Set firm controls and keep area drug free when the patient is hospitalized
2. Keep atmosphere pleasant and cheerful but not overly stimulating
3. Contribute to the patient's self-confidence, self-respect, and security in a realistic manner
4. Walk the fine line between a relatively permissive and a firm attitude
5. Expect and accept evasion, manipulative behavior, and negativism; but require the patient to shoulder certain standards of responsibility
6. Accept the patient without approving the behavior
7. Do not permit the patient to become isolated
8. Introduce the patient to group activities as soon as possible
9. Protect patients from themselves and others

Schizophrenic Disorders

Constitute the largest group of behavioral disorders in society; at the present time 1 person in 100 will spend some time in a hospital for treatment of a schizophrenic disorder, and this number is increasing

A. Pathology
1. Premorbid personality—uses the compensatory mechanisms of the withdrawal pattern of behavior; in addition, a paranoid schizophrenic uses the compensatory mechanisms of the protective pattern of behavior
2. Severe emotional problems—although unrecognized, begin early in life; however, most common age for break with reality is 18 to 34 years of age
3. Chronic insecurity and an almost total failure in interpersonal relationships
4. Etiology still unknown; however, some interesting findings in genetics, biochemistry, psychology, family therapy, and sociology present hope for a breakthrough
5. Regardless of the ultimate etiology, there appears to be a close casual relationship with the environment
6. Course of the disease—either acute or chronic; although it can stop or retrogress at any point, it

does not appear ever to permit a full restoration of integrity of the personality

B. Symptoms
1. Alterations in feeling, thinking, and relating to the external world
2. Association defects occur, and association links weaken; the individual appears incoherent, bizarre, and unpredictable
3. Distortions interfere with attention, perception, concentration, and memory
4. Affect and emotional expression are flattened
5. Ambivalence is common and frequently is so exaggerated that any action or decision becomes impossible
6. Detachment from reality results in autistic thinking and serves to further distort reality
7. Disturbance occurs in body image, since the undeveloped ego has few strengths and no boundaries; the individual frequently refers to self in the second or third person instead of using the first person
8. Secondary symptoms such as hallucinations, delusions, confusion, stupor, and catatonia may or may not be present

C. Types of schizophrenia—although historically much time and effort were directed toward identifying types of schizophrenia, it should be recognized that the classification is not static; there is a great deal of overlapping symptomatology; individuals diagnosed as being in one classification frequently are diagnosed at a later time in another classsification
1. Schizotypal personality disorder—rarely requires hospitalization; unattached, withdrawn, affectively and intellectually diminished individuals; frequently part of the vagabond or transient groups of society
2. Disorganized type—picture of severe and pronounced mental incapacity; great mental and emotional deterioration occurs; behavior is retarded, with sexual preoccupations, emotional dulling, infantile silliness; onset is usually between 12 and 25 years of age
3. Catatonic type—picture of withdrawal and distortions in reality testing, accompanied by total ambivalence, which is frequently exhibited in rather unpredictable motor activity; the ambivalence can render movement and decision making impossible, since the individual is unable to decide how or where to move; may literally be frozen in position, akinetic (stuporous)—or forced into aimless hyperkinetic fugue (excited) movements
4. Paranoid type—uses withdrawal compensatory

mechanisms to distort reality and then develops a rather intricate delusional system by using the projective pattern of behavior; is secretive and suspicious; using ideas of reference, finally develops delusions of grandeur

5. Undifferentiated type—demonstrates the primary thought, affect, and withdrawal defects of schizophrenia but cannot be classified under a specific type because of mixed symptoms

6. Schizoaffective type—demonstrates a mixture of symptoms from both schizophrenia and affective reactions; the thought processes and bizarre behavior appears schizophrenic, but there is usually marked elation or depression; often proves to be basically schizophrenic in nature

D. Therapy
1. Administration of chlorpromazine and other major tranquilizers
2. Psychotherapy (individual, family, and group counseling)
3. Motivational therapy
4. Occupational and vocational therapy
5. Electroconvulsive therapy may be useful in some instances to modify behavior
6. Day-care treatment programs in community settings
7. Pharmacologic approach—antipsychotic drugs (major tranquilizers)—control behavior when the patient's uncontrolled actions are destructive to self, others, or the environment
   a. Types of major tranquilizers
      (1) Phenothiazine derivatives
         (a) Acetophenazine maleate (Tindal)
         (b) Chlorpromazine hydrochloride (Thorazine)
         (c) Fluphenazine hydrochloride (Prolixin)
         (d) Perphenazine (Trilafon)
         (e) Prochlorperazine (Compazine)
         (f) Promazine hydrochloride (Sparine)
         (g) Thioridazine hydrochloride (Mellaril)
         (h) Trifluoperazine (Stelazine)
         (i) Triflupromazine hydrochloride (Vesprin)
      (2) Butyrophenones
         (a) Droperidol (Inapsine)
         (b) Haloperidol (Haldol)
      (3) Dihydroindolone
         (a) Molidone hydrochloride (Moban)
      (4) Thioxanthenes
         (a) Chlorprothixene (Taractan)
         (b) Thiothixene (Navane)
   b. Drug interactions—potentiate the action of

alcohol, barbiturates, antihypertensives, and anticholinergics; concomitant use should be avoided when possible; antipsychotic medications should be temporarily discontinued when spinal or epidural anesthesia is necessary
   c. Adverse effects of major tranquilizers—agranulocytosis (manifested by cold or sore throat), jaundice, signs of extrapyramidal tract irritation, drowsiness (highest incidence in initial days of therapy), orthostatic hypotension, constipation, urinary retention, anorexia, hypersensitivity reactions (tissue fluid accumulation, photoallergic reaction, impotence, cessation of menses or ovulation), cardiac toxicity
      (1) Exrapyramidal symptoms
         (a) Pseudoparkinsonism—resembles true parkinsonism (tremor, masklike facies, drooling, restlessness)
         (b) Akinesia—fatigue, weakness of arms and legs
         (c) Akathisia—motor restlessness
         (d) Persistent dyskinesia—protrusion of tongue, facial disturbances, opisthotonos; symptoms can persist even after administration of an antiparkinsonian agent and cessation of the tranquilizer; cosmetically disturbing to the patient and family
      (2) Antiparkinsonian drugs—block the extrapyramidal symptoms
         (a) Benztropine (Cogentin)
         (b) Biperiden (Akineton)
         (c) Diphenhydramine (Benadryl)
         (d) Trihexyphenidyl (Artane)
      (3) Tardive dyskinesia—symptoms seen in some patients receiving phenothiazine drugs; include linguofacial hyperkinesias and biazrre movements of the neck and trunk; can occur after drug reduction or discontinuation; antiparkinsonian drugs are most often of no benefit in alleviating these symptoms

E. Nursing approach
1. Observe the patient for adverse drug reactions whenever large doses of the major tranquilizers are being administered
2. Encourage the patient to follow a plan of organized activity and a prescribed drug regimen
3. Encourage the patient to continue medications even after symptoms abate

4. Respect the patient as a human being with both dignity and worth
5. Accept the patient at his or her present level of functioning
6. Avoid trying to argue the patient out of delusions or hallucinations
7. Accept that the patients' hallucinations and delusions are real and frightening
8. Encourage the development of interpersonal relationships between the patient and others
9. Point out reality to the patient but do not impose your concept of reality

Paranoid Disorders

Individuals who demonstrate the suspiciousness and delusions common to paranoid conditions but do not exhibit the thinking and behavioral disorganization or the personality disintegration found in the other psychoses
A. Pathology
1. Premorbid personality—uses the compensatory mechanisms of the projective pattern of behavior
2. Paranoid defenses considered by some to be a protective mechanism against unconscious homosexuality or overt hostility
3. Exact etiology unknown
B. Symptoms
1. Paranoia—exhibits a rather elaborate, highly organized paranoid delusional system while preserving other functions of the personality; in spite of this system, thinking is not interfered with and personality function usually continues without interruption
2. Involutional paranoid state—experiences an onset of delusions during the involutional period; the thought and emotional disorganization of schizophrenia are absent; the depressive overtones present lead many to believe that this state is a manifestation of the involutional psychosis
C. Therapy
1. Chemotherapy with major tranquilizers considered most helpful
2. Individual psychotherapy may provide some relief of symptoms
3. Electroconvulsive therapy may prove helpful
4. Paranoid patients are the most challenging to reach, since none of the present therapies appear to be helpful in breaking down the delusional system
D. Nursing approach
1. Provide an environment with some intellectual challenge that does not threaten security
2. Avoid counteraggression and retaliation against the patient

3. Accept and recognize the patient's need for a superior attitude
4. Meet sarcasm and ridicule in a matter-of-fact manner
5. Guard the patient's self-esteem from attack by other patients
6. Accept the patient's misinterpretations of events
7. Point out reality but do not directly challenge the patient's delusions

Affective Disorders

Major Affective Disorders
A. Bipolar disorder
1. Pathology
a. Premorbid personality—uses the compensatory mechanisms associated with aggressive patterns of behavior
b. Generally occurs between 20 and 49 years of age
2. Symptoms
a. Cyclic, periodic episodes of acute self-limiting mood swings; can be all manic, all depressed, or mixed manic and depressed; usually occurs before 40 years of age but after 20 years of age
b. Resumption of customary activities between episodes
c. Obesity a frequent precursor of attack; onset can be slowed or modified by dieting
d. Depression most common form
(1) Triad of symptoms with lowering of the mood tone—dejection, slowing of thinking and speech, decrease in psychomotor activity
(2) Insomnia—difficulty in falling asleep and staying asleep, tending to wake early
(3) Decreased appetite
(4) Feelings of guilt and worthlessness
(5) Difficulty in performing daily tasks
(6) Tearful with suicidal ruminations
(7) Speaking slowly using monosyllabic words
(8) Orientation and logic unaffected
(9) Sex drive decreased
(10) Constipation and urinary retention may occur
e. Manic phase less common
(1) Difficulty sleeping
(2) Extremely active—always in a hurry
(3) Humor good, although remarks can be caustic

(4) Monopolizing conversations; irritability only superficially covered

(5) Orientation clear, but judgment poor

(6) Always planning and scheming

(7) Increased sex drive

3. Therapy

a. Electroconvulsive therapy to reduce depression; succinylcholine chloride (Anectine), a depolarizing muscle relaxant causing paralysis, is used to reduce the intensity of muscle contractions during the convulsive stage

b. High-protein, high-carbohydrate diet is provided for energy, especially in manic phase

c. Psychotherapy

4. Pharmacologic approach in depressive phase—antidepressant drugs that increase the level of norepinephrine at subcortical neuroeffector sites

a. Norepinephrine blockers—provide elevated levels of the neurohormone by preventing reuptake and storage at the axon (tricyclic compounds)

(1) Drugs

(a) Amitriptyline hydrochloride (Elavil)

(b) Desipramine hydrochloride (Norpramin, Pertofrane)

(c) Doxepin hydrochloride (Adapin, Sinequan)

(d) Imipramine hydrochloride (Presamine, Tofranil)

(e) Nortriptyline hydrochloride (Aventyl)

(f) Protriptyline hydrochloride (Vivactil)

(2) Drug interactions—potentiate effects of anticholinergic drugs and central nervous system depressants (e.g., alcohol and sedatives)

(3) Adverse effects—orthostatic hypotension, skin rash, drowsiness, dry mouth, blurred vision, constipation, urine retention, tachycardia, CNS stimulation in elderly patients (excitement, restlessness, incoordination, fine tremor), nightmares, delusions, disorientation, insomnia

b. Monoamine oxidase inhibitors (MAOIs)—elevate norepinephrine levels in brain tissues by interfering with the enzyme MAO; act as psychic energizers

(1) Drugs

(a) Isocarboxazid (Marplan)

(b) Phenelzine sulfate (Nardil)

(c) Tranylcypromine sulfate (Parnate)

(2) Drug interactions—MAOIs potentiate the effects of alcohol, barbiturates, anesthetic agents (cocaine), antihistamines, narcotics, corticoids, anticholinergics, and sympathomimetic drugs

(3) Drug-food interactions—hypertensive crisis with vascular rupture, occipital headache, palpitation, stiffness of neck muscles, emesis, sweating, photophobia, and cardiac arrhythmias may occur when neurohormonal levels are elevated by ingestion of foods with high tyramine content (pickled herring, beer, wine, chicken livers, aged or natural cheese, chocolate)

(4) Adverse effects—CNS stimulation (headache, restlessness, insomnia), peripheral edema, orthostatic hypotension, dry mouth, constipation, urine retention, transient impotence, anorexia, nausea

5. Pharmacologic approach in manic phase—improves productivity by decreasing psychomotor activity or response to environmental stimuli

a. Norepinephrine uptake accelerator—alters sodium transport in nerve and muscle cells and affects a shift in intraneural metabolism of norepinephrine

(1) Drug—lithium carbonate (Eskalith, Lithane, Lithonate) the drug of choice

(2) Drug-food interaction—restriction of sodium intake increases drug substitution for sodium ions, which causes signs of hyponatremia (nausea, vomiting, diarrhea, muscle fasciculations, stupor, convulsions)

(3) Adverse effects—excess voiding and extreme thirst caused by drug suppression of antidiuretic hormone (ADH) function, which causes dehydration; slurred speech, disorientation, confusion, cogwheel rigidity, ataxia, renal failure, respiratory depression, and coma are toxic side effects

b. Antipsychotic agents—used when lithium is contraindicated or if symptoms persist

(1) Drug—chlorpromazine (Thorazine) or haloperidol (Haldol)

(2) Drug interaction—see pharmacologic approach under schizophrenic disorders

(3) Adverse effects—see pharmacologic approach under schizophrenic disorders

6. Nursing approach

a. Monitor the patient's intake and output

b. Keep the environment nonchallenging and nonstimulating

c. Avoid irritating routines as much as possible

d. Protect the patient against suicide during the entire episode

e. Keep activities simple, uncomplicated, and repetitive in nature; they should be of short duration and should require little concentration

f. Observe for adverse effects of drugs; monitor lithium blood levels weekly; white cell count less often

g. Encourage the patient to continue medications even after symptoms abate

h. Caution and teach the patient regarding special dietary precautions with lithium and the MAO inhibitors

i. Overactive manic patients should be
    (1) Accepted by staff even though their behavior may be rejected
    (2) Permitted to express hostility and ambivalence without reinforcement of guilt feelings
    (3) Approached in a calm, collected manner by staff members who have good self-control
    (4) Given limits for their behavior
    (5) Responded to in a nonargumentative manner, using their easy distractibility
    (6) Approached in a consistent manner by all staff members

j. Depressed patients should
    (1) Be allowed time for their slowness
    (2) Be accepted even when they are unable to carry out daily routines
    (3) Be given demands they can meet
    (4) Be helped to express hostility and have their responses accepted without rejection
    (5) Have their self-esteem realistically built up
    (6) Be presented with simple rather than complex routines and activities
    (7) Have their feelings of worthlessness accepted as real to them; their feelings should not be denied, condoned, or approved, just accepted
    (8) Be protected against suicide attempts, especially when the depression begins to lift (suicide is a real and ever-present danger)

B. Major depression with psychotic features
    1. Pathology—similar to that for bipolar disorder depressed except
        a. Usually occurs before 20 years of age or after 60 years of age
        b. Precipitating factor can always be identified

    2. Symptoms
        a. Severe depression
        b. Absence of history of repeated episodes
        c. Gross misinterpretations of reality
    3. Therapy—same as for bipolar disorder depressed
    4. Nursing approach—same as for bipolar disorder depressed
    5. Pharmacologic approach—same as for bipolar disorder depressed

C. Major depression with melancholia
    1. Pathology similar to that for bipolar disorder depressed except
        a. Depression is agitated rather than retarded
        b. Depression occurs after 40 years of age and before 60 years of age
        c. Precipitating factors such as the marriage of children, loss of a job, breakup of a marriage, death of a partner frequently is identified
        d. Depression often closely related to the menopause or climacteric; hormonal and endocrine changes are considered by many to play an important role although current thinking does not make a distinction between this depression and depressions occurring at other periods of life
        e. Usually rigid, inflexible, overassertive, overly meticulous, and worrisome
    2. Symptoms
        a. Wakes early after having had trouble falling asleep
        b. Feelings of unreality and sinfulness
        c. Complains of somatic delusions
        d. Extremely jumpy and agitated
        e. Pacing and wringing of hands as well as other increased motor activity
        f. Triad of symptoms—delusions of sin and/or poverty, obsession with death, somatic delusions especially related to the GI tract
    3. Therapy—same as for bipolar disorder depressed
    4. Nursing approach—same as for bipolar disorder depressed
    5. Pharmacologic approach—same as for bipolar disorder depressed

D. Other affective disorders
    1. Cyclothymic disorder
        a. Symptoms include alternating mood swings between elation and sadness; apparently unrelated to external environment
        b. The individual is usually warm and friendly; approaches life with an obvious enthusiasm
        c. Mood swings do not demonstrate great emotional intensity

2. Dysthymic disorder (depressive neurosis)—guilt and depression used unconsciously to relieve anxiety
   a. Symptoms of depression, insomnia, anorexia, decreased sexual drive, weight loss, constipation, fatigue; closely resembles bipolar disorder but differs in depth and awareness of reality
   b. Depression is real, and suicide can occur
3. Therapy—often unnecessary; if required, same as for bipolar disorder
4. Nursing approach—same as for bipolar disorder
5. Pharmacologic approach—often unnecessary; if required, same as for bipolar disorder

Anxiety Disorders

Common responses to emotional problems that are rarely treated in psychiatric settings; disturbances in personality, but there is no great defect in reality testing or severe antisocial behavior

A. Pathology
1. All use the compensatory mechanisms of the psychoneurotic pattern of behavior
2. Development of the symptoms usually permits some measure of social adjustment
3. Commonly begins in early 20s as a result of environmental factors in childhood
4. Early life rigid and orderly
5. Pressures of decision making regarding life-style that occur in the early adult years seem to act as precipitating factors

B. Symptoms
1. Phobic disorder—anxiety unconsciously transferred to an inanimate object or situation, which then symbolically represents the conflict and can be avoided
   a. Anxiety appears when patients find themselves in places that threaten their sense of security
   b. Attempts are made to avoid these distressing situations
   c. Depending on the phobic object, the individual's life-style is often greatly limited
   d. Common phobic disorders include
      (1) Agoraphobia—fear of being alone or in public places where help would not be immediately available if necessary; includes tunnels, bridges, crowds, buses, and trains
      (2) Social phobia—fear of public speaking or situations in which public scrutiny may occur
      (3) Simple phobia—fear of specific objects, animals, or situations
2. Anxiety states—anxiety unconsciously expressed through physical means
   a. Pervasive continuous feeling of free-floating anxiety, tension, and apprehension
   b. Episodes of dyspnea, palpitations, irritability, dizziness, insomnia, fainting, weakness, chest pain, trembling, and headaches
   c. Symptoms usually appear in relation to stress situations such as crowded rooms, public gatherings, pregnancy, military service
   d. The patient appears anxious; often mildly depressed
3. Obsessive-compulsive disorder—unconscious control of anxiety by the use of rituals and thoughts
   a. The patient complains about thoughts that persist and become repetitive and obsessive
   b. These thoughts may be turned into compulsions that are repetitive acts of irrational behavior which the individual is emotionally forced to carry out although they serve no rational purpose
   c. The patient is indecisive and demonstrates a striving for perfection and superiority
   d. Intellectual and verbal defenses are used
   e. Anxiety and depression may be present in various degrees, particularly if rituals are prevented

C. Therapy
1. Complete medical work-up to reassure the individual and rule out medical problems
2. Psychotherapy, family therapy, group therapy
3. Sedatives and minor tranquilizers if necessary
4. Pharmacologic approach—antianxiety drugs (minor tranquilizers) used when the individual is incapable of coping with environmental stresses and accomplishing daily activities
   a. Antianxiety agents
      (1) Chlordiazepoxide hydrochloride (Librium)
      (2) Clorazepate dipotassium (Tranxene)
      (3) Diazepam (Valium)
      (4) Hydroxyzine hydrochloride, hydroxyzine pamoate (Atarax, Vistaril)
      (5) Oxazepam (Serax)
   b. Sedatives and barbiturates
      (1) Phenobarbital
      (2) Secobarbital sodium (Seconal)
   c. General drug interactions—drugs potentiate depressant effects of alcohol or sedatives

d. General adverse effects of these medications—drowsiness, hypotention, muscle relaxation, decreased ability to concentrate occur frequently in initial days of therapy; hypersensitivity reactions

D. Nursing approach
1. Establish a trusting relationship
2. Accept symptoms as real to the individual
3. Attempt to limit the use of defenses, but do not stop them until the individual is ready to give them up
4. Encourage the individual to develop a balance between work and play so anxiety is lessened
5. Help the individual develop better ways of handling anxiety-producing situations through problem solving
6. Accept physical symptoms but do not emphasize or call attention to them
7. Reduce demands on the individual as much as possible

Somatoform Disorders

Conversion Disorder

Anxiety unconsciously converted to physical symptoms that are not under voluntary control; these symptoms permit the individual to avoid some unacceptable activity

A. Pathology
1. Development of symptoms usually permits some measure of social adjustment
2. Generally begins before 30 years of age
3. Early life often rigid and orderly; physical illness frequently used by the family as an excuse for problems
4. Pressures of decision making regarding life-style in the early adult years seem to be precipitating factors

B. Symptoms
1. History of lost motor or sensory function without any adequate physical cause (e.g., paralysis, blindness, deafness)
2. Noticeable lack of concern about the problem; this lack of concern has been labeled *la belle indifférence*
3. Impairment may vary over different episodes and does not follow anatomic structure; paralysis or numbness may circle the foot or arm instead of beginning at the joint and is known as stocking-and-glove anesthesia
4. The individual appears relieved by symptoms and demonstrates little anxiety when observed

C. Therapy—same as for anxiety disorders

D. Nursing approach—same as for anxiety disorders

Psychosexual Disorders

A. Paraphilias
Changing social and cultural mores have caused many of the sexual behaviors that were once considered deviations to be removed from the list of "abnormal practices." Today sexual activities are considered abnormal only if they are directed toward objects other than adults or are performed under unusual circumstances.
1. Pathology—may be symptomatic of other personality or psychiatric disorders or may occur as a behavior aberration of a disordered personality
2. Symptoms
   a. Fetishism—substitution of an inanimate object for the genitals
   b. Transvestism—wearing clothes of the opposite sex to achieve sexual pleasure
   c. Exhibitionism—sexual pleasure obtained by exposing the genitals
   d. Pedophilia—attraction to children as sex objects
   e. Voyeurism—sexual gratification obtained by watching the sexual play of others
   f. Sadism—sexual gratification obtained from cruelty to others; used as a substitute for or an accompaniment of the sex act
   g. Masochism—sexual gratification obtained from self-suffering; used as a substitute for or an accompaniment of the sex act
3. Therapy—rather unsuccessful with these individuals unless they really want to change; if change is desired, psychotherapy or psychoanalysis may be effective
4. Nursing approach
   a. Accept the individual as a person in emotional pain
   b. Avoid punitive remarks or responses
   c. Protect the individual from others
   d. Set limits on the individual's sexual acting out
   e. Provide diversional activities

B. Egodystonic homosexuality
1. Pathology—same as for paraphilias
2. Symptoms
   a. Homosexual activity that is persistent but unwanted
   b. Heterosexual arousal absent or weak although desired
   c. Homosexual activity as the preferred method of gratification between 2 consenting adults no longer considered a sexual deviation
3. Therapy—same as for paraphilias
4. Nursing approach—same as for paraphilias

Adjustment Disorders

Acute reactions to overwhelming environmental stress

A. Pathology
1. No apparent underlying mental disorder in these individuals, although present behavior may be extremely disturbed
2. The individual seems to have the capacity to adapt to the overwhelming stress when given the time to do so
3. Problems with distortions or interruptions in thinking process and decision making tend to resolve themselves

B. Symptoms of adjustment reactions
1. Infancy—extremely upset; demonstrating grief when separated from the mother
2. Childhood—regression to an earlier level of development when a new sibling arrives; intense anxiety on entering school
3. Adolescence—struggle for independence; leads to hypersensitivity and frequent episodes of heightened anxiety
4. Adult life—heightened anxiety in response to the stresses associated with marriage, pregnancy, divorce, change of employment, purchase of a house, etc.
5. Later life—menopause and climacteric, plan for retirement, ''loss'' of children to marriage, and death of a mate all serve to produce extreme stress situations

C. Therapy—determine the underlying cause of the conflict and work toward resolution

D. Nursing approach
1. Recognize and accept that a problem exists
2. Help the individual and/or parents identify the problem
3. Support and avoid humiliation of the individual
4. Provide empathic understanding

Personality Disorders

Borderline states characterized by defects in the development of the personality or by pathologic trends in its structure

A. Personality can be defined as
1. Sum of all traits that differentiate one individual from another
2. Total behavior pattern of an individual through which the inner interests are expressed
3. The individual's unique and distinctive way of behaving and interacting with others
4. Constellation of defense mechanisms for dealing with inner and outer pressures
5. A functional role within a family system

B. Manifestations of personality disorders
1. Habitual attitudes and reaction patterns in human relationships develop early in life and form the character structure of the individual
2. In most instances these behaviors create little discomfort or stress
3. Personality disturbances are, in reality, the selection and utilization of specific defense mechanisms which are used so often that they form a lifelong pattern of action that, although not normal, is neither neurotic nor psychotic
4. Premorbid personality of individuals demonstrating any of the 10 classified personality disturbances resembles the compensatory mechanisms associated with the pathologic counterpart

C. Symptoms
1. Paranoid personality disorder
   a. Frequent use of projective mechanisms
   b. Suspiciousness, fear, irritability, and stubbornness
   c. Reality testing not greatly impaired
2. Schizoid personality disorder
   a. Avoidance of meaningful interpersonal relationships
   b. Use of autistic thinking, emotional detachment, and daydreaming
   c. Introverted since childhood but maintaining fair contact with reality
3. Histrionic personality disorder
   a. Emotional instability by great excitability
   b. Extroverted and directed toward gaining attention
   c. Vain and deliberately manipulative
4. Narcissistic personality disorder
   a. Overblown sense of importance
   b. Strong need for attention and admiration
   c. Relationships marked by ambivalence
   d. Preoccupation with appearance
5. Antisocial personality disorder
   a. Chronic lifelong disturbances that conflict with society's laws and customs
   b. Unable to postpone gratification
   c. Randomly act out their aggressive egocentric impulses on society
   d. Do not profit from past experience or punishment; live only for the moment
   e. Have the ability to ingratiate themselves but ''do not wear well''
   f. Are in contact with reality but do not seem to care about it
6. Compulsive personality disorder
   a. Rigidity, overconscientiousness, inordinate capacity for work

b. Driven by obsessive concerns

c. Behavior contains many rituals

7. Passive-aggressive personality disorder

   a. Rather helpless and indecisive, demonstrating passive obstructionism while clinging and pouting

   b. Frequent outbursts and temper tantrums when frustrated

   c. Often creating problems for others

D. Therapy

1. Individual, group, and family psychotherapy

2. Crisis intervention when necessary

3. Vocational and occupational therapy

E. Nursing approach

1. Maintain consistency and concern

2. Accept the individual as is; do not retaliate if provoked

3. Protect the individual from others while protecting others from the individual

4. Place realistic limits on behavior; make known what those limits are

COMMUNITY MENTAL HEALTH SERVICES
Concepts

A. Purposes

1. To provide prevention, treatment, and rehabilitation services for individuals with emotional problems; also support for families

2. To maintain these individuals and families in the community

3. To provide hospital care within the community in those instances when the individual cannot be maintained on an outpatient basis

B. Types of settings in which services are provided

1. Outpatient services

   a. Storefront clinics

   b. Walk-in clinics in hospitals

   c. Emergency rooms

   d. Crisis intervention centers, including hot-line phone centers

   e. Day-care centers

   f. Private offices

2. Inpatient services

   a. Specialized psychiatric hospitals

   b. General hospital psychiatric units

3. Aftercare services

   a. Foster homes

   b. Halfway houses

   c. Sheltered workshops

   d. Day-care centers

C. Types of services

1. Observation and diagnosis

2. Assessment of the patient's needs

3. Crisis intervention

4. Provide direct care services to patients including

   a. Individual, family, and group therapy

   b. Medications

   c. Electroconvulsive therapy

   d. Occupational therapy

   e. Recreational therapy

5. Provide a therapeutic milieu that

   a. Supports the individual during the period of crisis

   b. Helps the individual learn new ways of coping with problems

6. Referral to proper community agencies for necessary services

7. Provide an educational setting for various professional groups in mental health concepts

8. Vocational counseling

9. Health screening

Nurse's Role

A. Case finding

B. Assessment of the individual's needs

C. Establishment of the therapeutic milieu

D. Consultation with other professionals (e.g., physicians, psychologists, social workers, school teachers, clergy)

E. Active participation with the health team, including the individual and family

F. Involvement in individual, family, and group therapy

G. Coordination of health services for the individual and family

H. Education of groups within the community

EMOTIONAL PROBLEMS ASSOCIATED WITH THE AGED
General Concepts

Feelings of loss associated with aging produce some of the behaviors often exhibited by the elderly. These behaviors are, in reality, defense mechanisms utilized to reduce anxiety and maintain self-esteem.

A. Often withdrawal when there is a felt loss or an actual change in body image or loss of a significant other; the individual turns inward, becomes unresponsive to others and the environment

B. Aggressive behavior often develops in response to feelings of guilt and anger when the individual feels helpless to control the situation; aggression may be turned inward on the self, resulting in depression, or turned outward on the environment, resulting in overt anger or hostility

C. Pattern of projective behavior may result when the individual needs to protect the self from the anxiety that feelings of blame or guilt elicit; decreased sensory perceptions associated with aging often contribute to the individual's belief that others are talking about and plotting against him or her

Nursing Approach

A. Help the patient meet physical needs
B. Allow the patient sufficient time to assume and accomplish responsibilities for self-care
C. Seek the patient out for short frequent periods of contact
D. Allow and encourage the patient's expression of feelings
E. Help the patient set realistic goals that can be achieved
F. Recognize accomplishments of the patient
G. Provide aids that will allow the patient to be more involved with the environment
H. Try to involve the patient in activities and social interactions

ADDITIONAL PHARMACOLOGY
Drugs that Produce Sedation and Sleep

A. Sedatives and hypnotics can be used in addition to tranquilizers for psychiatric and other patients; as CNS depressants they have antianxiety effects in low dosages; produce sleep in high dosages and general anesthetic-like states in very high dosages; all hypnotic drugs probably alter either the character or the duration of REM sleep
B. Types of drugs
  1. Trichloroacetic acid—produces natural sleep
    a. Drugs
      (1) Chloral betaine (Beta-Chlor)
      (2) Chloral hydrate (Felsules, Lorinal, Noctec, Somnos)
      (3) Petrichloral (Periclor)
    b. Adverse effects—gastric irritation causing diarrhea
    c. Drug interactions—potentiates the effects of alcohol taken concurrently causing sudden loss of consciousness
    d. Considerations during therapy—drug metabolites cause false positive reaction for glycosuria when Benedict's reagent is used for testing
  2. Paraldehyde—used primarily to diminish hyperactivity in alcoholics or to control convulsions; has a pungent odor and taste, and elimination from the lungs results in an environmental odor
  3. Phenothiazine derivatives—act like antihistamines; used for sleep induction in anxious patients
    a. Drugs
      (1) Methotrimeprazine hydrochloride (Levoprome)
      (2) Promazine hydrochloride (Sparine)
      (3) Propiomazine hydrochloride (Largon)
    b. Adverse effects—hypotension, dizziness, dry mouth, cardiac palpitation, pseudoparkinsonism symptoms, cholestatic jaundice, agranulocytosis
  4. Barbiturate sedatives—most frequently used hypnotics
    a. High lipoid tissue affinity—rapid response, short acting
      (1) Hexobarbital (Sombucaps, Sombulex)
      (2) Pentobarbital sodium (Nembutal)
      (3) Secobarbital sodium (Seconal)
    b. Moderate lipoid tissue affinity—moderately slow response, intermediate acting
      (1) Amobarbital (Amytal)
      (2) Aprobarbital (Alurate)
      (3) Butabarbital sodium (Bubartal Sodium, Butisol Sodium)
      (4) Probarbital calcium (Ipral)
      (5) Talbutal (Lotusate)
    c. Low lipoid tissue affinity—slow response
      (1) Barbital (Neuronidia)
      (2) Phenobarbital (Luminal)
    d. Adverse effects—morning drowsiness, hypersensitivity reactions (photosensitivity, dermatologic reactions), respiratory depression, and hypotension (most frequent with parenteral use)
    e. Fatalities from overdosage—depend on degree of lipoid tissue affinity
      (1) High lipotropic group—rapid respiratory depression, marked hypotension after ingestion of excess
      (2) Moderate lipotropic group—protracted period of sedation, but allows time-lapse for resuscitation or reconsideration
      (3) Low lipotropic group—excretion concurrent with slow action, least popular for self-induced overdosage
    f. Drug interactions—lower blood levels of orally administered griseofulvin and decrease the therapeutic effect increase activity of hepatic microsomal enzymes; the accelerated metabolism of oral anticoagulants lowers their hypoprothrombinemic effect
  5. Other sedatives and hypnotics; adverse effects
    a. Ethchlorvynol (Placidyl)—morning drowsiness, blurring vision, transient hypotension

b. Ethinamate (Valmid)—morning drowsiness
c. Flurazepam hydrochloride (Dalmane)—dizziness, tachycardia, GI disturbances
d. Methaqualone (Quaalude, Sopor)—morning drowsiness, GI disturbances
e. Methyprylon (Noludar)—morning drowsiness, GI disturbances
f. Sodium bromide (primarily for daytime sedation)—gastric irritation, generalized rash, tremors of the hands, tremulousness of the lips, and tongue, impaired mental processes, auditory and visual hallucinations, coma with long-term use
g. Glutethimide (Doriden)
   (1) Morning drowsiness, transient hypotension, and infrequently produces pharyngeal and laryngeal reflex depression
   (2) Acts synergistically with oral anticoagulants to decrease their effectiveness

C. Excess ingestion
   1. Any of the sedative-hypnotics may cause unconsciousness, coma, death
   2. Addiction to these drugs alone or in combination has increased
   3. Removal of drug from the stomach by aspiration, resuscitative measures (assisted ventilation, cardiac massage), hemodialysis of diffusible drug, vasopressor administration to counteract vascular collapse, and correction of acidosis
   4. Follow-up supervision to avoid repetition of the problem

D. Drugs are habit forming; withdrawal after long-term use may precipitate severe symptoms—anxiety, tremor, insomnia, confusion, perceptual distortions, agitation, delirium, GI disturbances, orthostatic hypotension, convulsions leading to cardiovascular collapse and death

Psychiatric Nursing Review Questions

1 Mental experiences operate on different levels of awareness. Which level best portrays one's attitudes, feelings, and desires?
  1. Foreconscious
  2. Preconscious
  3. Conscious
  4. Unconscious

2 Which level of anxiety best enhances an individual's power of perception?
  1. Mild
  2. Moderate
  3. Severe
  4. Panic

3 Sublimation is a defense mechanism that helps the individual:
  1. Act out in reverse something already done or thought
  2. Channel unacceptable sexual desires into socially approved behavior
  3. Return to an earlier, less mature stage of development
  4. Exclude from the conscious things that are psychologically disturbing

4 An example of displacement is:
  1. Ignoring unpleasant aspects of reality
  2. Imaginative activity to escape reality
  3. Pent-up emotions directed to other than the primary source
  4. Resisting any demands made by others

5 Personality is unique for every individual because it is the result of the person's:
  1. Genetic background, placement in family, and autoimmunity
  2. Biologic constitution, psychologic development, and cultural setting
  3. Childhood experiences, intellectual capacity, and socioeconomic status
  4. Intellectual capacity, race, and socioeconomic status

6 In the process of development the individual strives to maintain, protect, and enhance the integrity of the ego. This is normally accomplished through the use of:
  1. Ritualistic behavior
  2. Withdrawal patterns
  3. Defense mechanisms
  4. Affective reactions

7 Another term for the superego is:
  1. Self
  2. Ideal self
  3. Narcissism
  4. Conscience

8 Which relationship is of extreme importance in the formation of the personality?
  1. Parent-child
  2. Sibling
  3. Peer
  4. Heterosexual

9 Which part of the nervous system is primarily affected during a "fight or flight" reaction?
1. Central
2. Peripheral
3. Parasympathetic
4. Sympathetic

10 The superego is that part of the self which says:
1. I want what I want
2. I can wait for what I want
3. I should not want that
4. I like what I want

11 Groups are important in the emotional development of the individual because groups:
1. Go through the same developmental phases
2. Always protect their members
3. Are easily identified by their members
4. Identify acceptable behavior for their members

12 The family is important in the emotional development of the individual because the family:
1. Gives rewards and punishment
2. Helps one to learn identity and roles
3. Provides support for the young
4. Reflects the mores of a larger society

13 Communication ties people to their:
1. Physical surroundings
2. Environmental surroundings
3. Social surroundings
4. Materialistic surroundings

14 The primary emergence of the personality is demonstrated around the age of:
1. 6 months
2. 9 months
3. 2 years
4. 6 years

15 Problems with dependence versus independence develop during which stage of growth and development?
1. Infancy
2. Toddler
3. Preschool
4. School age

16 Strict toilet training before a child is ready will cause problems in personality development because at this age a child is learning to:
1. Identify own needs
2. Satisfy parents' needs
3. Live up to society's expectations
4. Satisfy own needs

17 The basic emotional task for the toddler is:
1. Trust
2. Independence
3. Identification
4. Industry

18 The problem of separation anxiety initially occurs during the:
1. Oral stage
2. Anal stage
3. Phallic stage
4. Latency stage

19 For an emotional balance the individual always needs:
1. Family, work, and play
2. Biologic satisfaction and social acceptance
3. Individual recognition and group acceptance
4. Security and social recognition

20 A 5-year-old boy is constantly found slapping his little sister. This behavior is probably caused by:
1. Sibling rivalry
2. Unresolved oedipal conflicts
3. Negativistic id impulses
4. Overcompensation efforts of superego

21 Since people need some gratifying communication to learn, to grow, and to function in a group, all events that significantly curtail communication will eventually produce:
1. Some degree of mental deficiency
2. Severe disturbances
3. Further attempts to increase communication
4. Withdrawal

22 In applying mental health principles to the care of any person with children, the nurse should be aware that:
1. Many parents experience feelings of resentment toward their children
2. Every parent has inborn feelings of love and acceptance for children
3. It is pathologic to feel anger and resentment toward a child
4. It is easier to adjust to the first child than to later ones

23 In which stage of growth and development should surgery be delayed, if possible, because of the effects on personality development?
1. Oral
2. Anal
3. Oedipal
4. Latency

24 A person has a mature personality if the:
1. Ego acts as a balance between the id and the superego pressures
2. Ego responds to the demands of the superego
3. Ego responds to the demands of society
4. Superego has replaced and increased all the controls of the parents

25 Play for the preschool-age child is necessary for the emotional development of:
1. Projection
2. Competition
3. Introjection
4. Independence

26 During the oedipal stage of growth and development, the child:
1. Loves the parent of the same sex and hates the parent of the opposite sex
2. Loves the parent of the same sex and the parent of the opposite sex
3. Has ambivalence toward both parents
4. Loves the parent of the opposite sex and hates the parent of the same sex

27 Which stage of growth and development is basically concerned with role identification?
1. Oral
2. Oedipal
3. Latency
4. Genital

28 Which personality factor is the main problem for patients who need props to blur reality?
1. Dependency
2. Mistrust
3. Role blurring
4. Ego ideal

29 Many persons who are "well adjusted" in ordinary daily living become dependent and demanding when physically ill and hospitalized. This is probably an example of the mechanism of:
1. Denial
2. Compensation
3. Reaction formation
4. Regression

30 The defense mechanism in which emotional conflicts are expressed through motor, sensory, or somatic disability is identified as:
1. Dissociation
2. Psychosomatic
3. Compensation
4. Conversion

31 A college boy who is smaller than average and unable to participate in sports becomes the life of the party and a mod dresser. This is an example of the mechanism of:
1. Reaction formation
2. Compensation
3. Sublimation
4. Introjection

32 A person, seeing a design on the wallpaper, perceives it as an animal. This is an example of a:
1. Delusion
2. Hallucination
3. Illusion
4. Idea of reference

33 The ability to tolerate frustration is an example of one of the functions of the:
1. Id
2. Superego
3. Ego
4. Unconscious

34 An emotional experience in childhood becomes traumatic when:
1. The ego is overwhelmed by anxiety it cannot handle
2. The superego has not been internalized
3. The child is unable to verbalize own feelings
4. The parents are harsh and restrictive

35 Resolution of the oedipal complex takes place when the child overcomes the castration complex and:
1. Rejects the parent of the same sex
2. Identifies with the parent of the opposite sex
3. Identifies with the parent of the same sex
4. Introjects behaviors of both parents

36 Which of the following is a generally accepted concept of personality development?
1. The personality is capable of change and modification throughout life
2. By the end of the first 6 years, the personality has reached its adult parameters
3. The capacity for personality change decreases rapidly after adolescence
4. The basic personality is rather firmly set by 2 years of age

37 The superego is that part of the psyche which:
1. Is the source of creative energy
2. Develops from internalizing the concepts of parents and significant others
3. Contains the instinctual drives
4. Operates on the pleasure principle and demands immediate gratification

38 Evidence of the existence of the unconscious is best demonstrated by:
1. Déjà vu experiences
2. Slips of the tongue
3. The ease of recall
4. Free-floating anxiety

39 Which one of the following is most characteristic of the emotionally disturbed child?
1. Responds to any stimulus
2. Totally involved with the environment
3. Responds to little external stimulus
4. Seems unresponsive to the environment

40 The nurse should observe the autistic child for signs of:
1. Not wanting to eat
2. Crying for attention
3. Catatonic-like rigidity
4. Enjoying being with people

41 Hyperkinesis in children is usually treated with:
1. Chlorpromazine hydrochloride (Thorazine)
2. Haloperidol (Haldol)
3. Methylphenidate hydrochloride (Ritalin)
4. Methocarbamol (Robaxin)

42 A person who deliberately pretends an illness is usually:
1. Psychotic
2. Neurotic
3. Malingering
4. Using conversion defenses

Situation: *Mrs. Avery, age 29, was a capable librarian before her marriage. However, she was always very sensitive, aloof, withdrawn, and lacking in the ability to feel warm toward others; she rarely joined any organizations and distrusted people in general. Shortly after the birth of her last child she was admitted to a psychiatric hospital for care. At this time she is convinced that the neighbors are accusing her of indiscretions and that they have her home "bugged" so that they may overhear any conversations taking place there. Since her admission she has remained aloof from the other patients, paces the floor, and believes that the hospital is a house of torture and the food poisoned. Questions 43 through 51 refer to this situation.*

43 Mrs. Avery's prepsychotic personality might be described as:
1. Suspicious and socially inadequate
2. Rigid and controlling
3. Dependent and immature
4. Schizoid and introverted

44 Nursing interventions for Mrs. Avery should appropriately be directed toward:
1. Convincing her that the hospital staff is trying to help
2. Helping her enter into group recreational activities
3. Arranging the hospital environment so that her contact with other patients is limited
4. Helping her learn to trust the staff through selected experiences

45 Mrs. Avery frequently refuses to eat because she believes that the food is poisoned. One of the most appropriate ways in which the nurse might initially handle this situation is to:
1. Simply state that the food is not poisoned
2. Suggest that food be brought in from home
3. Taste the food in her presence
4. Tell her that she will have to be tube fed if she does not eat

46 After the initial intervention the nurse should pursue the matter of Mrs. Avery's belief by saying:
1. "Why do you think the food is poisoned?"
2. "You feel someone wants to poison you?"
3. "Your feeling is a symptom of your illness."
4. "You'll be safe with me. I won't let anyone poison you."

47 Mrs. Avery has refused to eat for 36 hours. She states that the voice of her dead father has commanded her to atone for her sins by fasting for 40 days. What initial intervention on the part of the nurse might interrupt the delusional system?
1. Asking the physician to write an order for tube feeding
2. Asking Mrs. Avery exactly what the voice said
3. Telling Mrs. Avery that she has nothing to atone for
4. Suggesting other means of atonement that may be less damaging

48 Mrs. Avery remains aloof from all other patients. What might the nurse, with whom she has developed a friendly relationship, do to help her participate in some ward activity?
1. Invite another patient to take part in a joint activity with the nurse and Mrs. Avery
2. Ask the physician to speak to Mrs. Avery about entering into ward activities
3. Find solitary pursuits that Mrs. Avery can enjoy on the ward
4. Speak to Mrs. Avery about the importance of entering into activities

49 Mrs. Avery has been assigned to a 4-bed room. The night nurse reports that she has been awake for several nights. Which of the following may be the cause of her sleeplessness?
1. Fear of the other patients

2. Worry about her family
3. Trying to work out her problems
4. Watching for an opportunity to escape

50 The nurse could most appropriately begin to help Mrs. Avery with her sleep problem by saying:
1. "Don't worry, you'll sleep when you're tired."
2. "I'm going to move you to a private room."
3. "I'll get you the sedative your doctor ordered."
4. "You seem unable to sleep at night."

51 While talking with the nurse about her problem of not being able to make friends with any of the other patients, Mrs. Avery begins to cry. What action on the part of the nurse would be most therapeutic at this time?
1. Suggest that they play a game of Scrabble
2. Tell her that her crying isn't going to help
3. Sit quietly with her
4. Point out how she can change this

Situation: Mr. Frank, 21 years of age, is an only child who has never earned his own living and has always been pampered and coddled by his domineering mother and ignored by his quiet retiring father. When he started dating, his mother chose the girls he took out. Recently Mr. Frank married a woman several years older than he, even though his mother seriously disapproved of her. Despite this, he brought his wife to his home to live. Both the mother and the wife were unhappy with this arrangement. Mr. Frank had many guilt feelings about his marriage and soon began to complain of pain in his right arm, which progressed to the point of paralysis. After seeking help from competent orthopedic specialists, he was referred for psychiatric evaluation. Questions 52 through 54 refer to this situation.

52 Mr. Frank's symptoms may be an unconscious attempt to solve a conflict evolving from:
1. Hostile feelings toward his home
2. Ambivalent feelings toward his wife
3. Inadequate feelings in regard to assuming the role of husband
4. Needs to be a dependent child and an independent adult

53 What could be said about Mr. Frank's prognosis after appropriate treatment?
1. His symptoms of paralysis may spread to other parts of his body
2. Continuous psychiatric treatment will be required to maintain him as a functioning individual
3. Recovery of the use of the arm can be expected, but under stress he may utilize similar symptoms
4. It is not possible to predict what the future for this patient holds

54 In dealing with Mr. Frank, the nurse should realize that:
1. This symptom is necessary for him to cope with his present situation.
2. This symptom is an unconscious method of getting attention
3. He can get well if he is helped to focus on other things
4. His problems will be solved when he learns to deal with his mother and wife

Situation: Mrs. Sam, a 45-year-old homemaker, was recently admitted to the psychiatric hospital because of a history of hopelessness, anxiety, and suicide attempts. In the hospital she paces the halls, cries, and says that the terrible condition of the world is her fault. She believes that her insides are decayed, that her husband and children are dead, and that the food she eats is of no nutritional value to her. Mrs. Sam has 3 daughters, all of whom are away at college. Her life has always centered about her family and her meticulously kept home. She has never had any hobbies or outside interests, and her moral standards have been strict and unbending. Questions 55 through 60 refer to this situation.

55 Mrs. Sam's prepsychotic personality can best be described as:
   1. Withdrawn and seclusive, with an active fantasy life
   2. Rigid, narrow, overly conscientious
   3. Suspicious, sensitive, aloof
   4. Dependent, immature, insecure

56 One of the nurse's primary responsibilities in caring for Mrs. Sam is to:
   1. Help her realize that her children are not dead
   2. Protect her against her suicidal impulses
   3. Reassure her that she is a good woman
   4. Keep up her interest in the outside world

57 One of the nursing responsibilities is to help Mrs. Sam pace the halls less frequently, since this wears her out physically. This can best be accomplished by:
   1. Supplying her with simple monotonous tasks
   2. Restraining her in a chair so she is unable to pace
   3. Requesting a sedative order from her physician
   4. Placing her in a single room so she can pace in a smaller area

58 In reassuring Mrs. Sam concerning the many fears that are upsetting to her, it would be helpful to say:
   1. "Your daughters and your husband love you very much."
   2. "You know that you are not a bad woman."
   3. "Mrs. Sam, those ideas of yours are in your imagination."
   4. "Those ideas are part of your illness and will change as you improve."

59 The nurse continues to sit with Mrs. Sam, although there is little verbal communication. One day, Mrs. Sam asks her, "Do you think they'll ever let me out of here?" The nurse's best response is:
   1. "Why, do you think you are eady to leave?"
   2. "You have the feeling that you might not leave?"
   3. "Everyone says you're doing just fine."
   4. "Why don't you ask your doctor?"

60 Mrs. Sam confides to the nurse that she has been thinking about suicide. Which statement best explains her action?
   1. She feels safe with the nurse and can share her feelings with her
   2. She wishes to frighten the nurse
   3. She is fearful of her own impulses and is seeking protection from them
   4. She wants attention from the staff

Situation: Mrs. Jones, a 29-year-old woman, believes that doorknobs are contaminated and refuses to touch them, except with a paper tissue. Questions 61 through 63 refer to this situation.

61 What response should the nurse use in dealing with this behavior?
   1. Force her to touch doorknobs by removing all available paper tissue until she learns to deal with the situation
   2. Explain to her that her idea about doorknobs is part of her illness and is not necessary
   3. Encourage her to scrub the doorknobs with a strong antiseptic so she does not need to use tissues
   4. Supply her with paper tissues to help her function until her anxiety is reduced

62 Symptoms such as using tissues to touch doorknobs develop because the patient is:
   1. Consciously using this method of punishing herself
   2. Unconsciously controlling unacceptable impulses or feelings
   3. Listening to voices that tell her the doorknobs are unclean
   4. Fulfilling a need to punish others by carrying out an annoying procedure

63 Therapeutic treatment of Mrs. Jones should be directed toward helping her to:
   1. Forget her fears by administering antianxiety medications
   2. Understand her behavior is caused by unconscious impulses that she fears
   3. Redirect her energy into activities to help others
   4. Learn that her behavior is not serving a realistic purpose

Situation: Mrs. Smith has been admitted to a psychiatric hospital with the diagnosis of organic mental disorder. Questions 64 through 69 refer to this situation.

64 Which of the following behaviors would the nurse find atypical for a patient like Mrs. Smith?
   1. Resistance to change
   2. Tendency to dwell on the past and ignore the present
   3. Preoccupation with personal appearance
   4. Inability to concentrate on new activities or interests

65 An organic mental disorder is characterized by:
   1. Areas of brain destruction called senile plaques
   2. Periodic remissions and exacerbations
   3. Aggressive acting out behavior
   4. Hypoxia of selected areas of brain

66 Which of the following approaches would be most helpful in meeting Mrs. Smith's needs?
   1. Simplifying the environment as much as possible while eliminating need for choices
   2. Providing a nutritious diet high in carbohydrates and proteins
   3. Developing a consistent nursing plan with fixed time schedules to provide for emotional and physical needs

4. Providing an opportunity for many alternative choices in the daily schedule, to stimulate interest

67 In attempting to understand Mrs. Smith's behavior the nurse recognizes that Mrs. Smith is probably:
1. Attempting to develop new defense mechanisms to meet her current life situation
2. Not capable of using any defense mechanisms at all
3. Making exaggerated use of old familiar mechanisms
4. Using one method of defense for all situations

68 The nursing care plan for the patient with organic brain deterioration should include:
1. An extensive reeducation program
2. Details for protective and supportive care
3. The introduction of new leisure time activities
4. Plans to involve the patient in group therapy sessions

69 In planning care for Mrs. Smith the nurse should appropriately:
1. Maintain the daily routine of living with which she is familiar
2. Discuss current events to keep her in contact with reality
3. Teach her new social skills to encourage participation
4. Encourage her to talk of her youth and early experiences

Situation: Dr. Kay, a 45-year-old physician, is admitted to the psychiatric unit of a general hospital. He is restless, loud, aggressive, and resistive during the admission procedure. Questions 70 through 72 refer to this situation.

70 Dr. Kay shouts at the nurse who is trying to take his admission blood pressure, ''I'm a physician. Do you think you're more qualified than I? I'll do it myself.'' The most therapeutic response by the nurse would be:
1. ''Right now, doctor, you're just another patient.''
2. ''If you'd rather, doctor. I'm sure you'll do it OK.''
3. ''I'm sorry but I can't allow that. I must take it.''
4. ''If you won't cooperate, I'll get the attendants in to hold you down.''

71 After the admission examination a nurse is assigned to introduce Dr. Kay to the other patients. He tells her that he wishes to be introduced as Dr. Kay. The nurse's response should be:
1. ''I can't do that. It's better if they don't know you are a doctor.''
2. ''That's fine, Dr. Kay; that's how I'll introduce you.''
3. ''All the patients here call one another by their first names.''
4. ''Why do you insist on being called Doctor?''

72 By the time Dr. Kay has been a patient on the service for 3 days he has questioned everyone's authority, has advised other patients that their treatments are wrong, and has talked 4 other patients into forming their own therapy group. The staff's most appropriate response would be to:

1. Ignore him and hope he will stop trying to disrupt the ward
2. Understand that he is unable to control his actions and that limits must be set for him
3. Tell the other patients that he is just another patient and they should not pay attention to him
4. Restrict his contact with other patients until he stops bothering everyone

Situation: The nurse is assigned to care for Mr. Bishop, a 39-year-old, hyperactive, elated patient who exhibits flight of ideas. Questions 73 through 76 refer to this situation.

73 The nursing care plan for Mr. Bishop should appropriately include plans to:
1. Encourage him to talk as much as needed
2. Arouse and focus his interest in reality
3. Persuade him to complete any task that he begins
4. Provide constructive channels for redirecting his excess energy

74 In approaching Mr. Bishop during a period of great overactivity it is essential to:
1. Use a firm, warm consistent approach
2. Anticipate and physically control his hyperactivity
3. Allow the patient to choose the activities in which he will participate
4. Let him know you will not tolerate destructive behavior

75 Mr. Bishop is not eating. The nurse recognizes that this may be because he:
1. Feels that he does not deserve the food
2. Believes that he does not need the food
3. Wishes to avoid the patients in the dining room
4. Is so busy that he does not take time to eat

76 The nurse can best respond to Mr. Bishop's eating problem by:
1. Providing a tray for him in his room
2. Assuring him that he is deserving of food
3. Ordering foods that he can hold in his hand to eat while moving around
4. Pointing out that the energy he is burning up must be replaced

---

77 Two 20-year-old female patients have become very much attached to one another and were recently found in bed together. They became angry and sarcastic when the nurse asked one of them to return to her own bed. How can this situation best be handled by the nurse?
1. Ask the physician to transfer one of the patients to another unit
2. Supervise them carefully and separate them when possible throughout the day and especially at night
3. Restrict both their privileges for several days because their behavior is undesirable and immature
4. Adopt a matter-of-fact, noncondemning attitude toward these patients while setting limits on their behavior

78 Which of the following factors is a frequent finding concerning adult homosexuality?
  1. Inadequate physical development of the sexual organs
  2. Deficiency of gonadal and pituitary hormones
  3. Failure to progress normally through the stages of psychosexual development
  4. Poor adjustment due to association with homosexual companions

Situation: Mrs. Lord, 23 years old, has been married 3 months. She was admitted to a psychiatric hospital after a month of unusual behavior that included eating and sleeping very little, talking or singing constantly, charging hundreds of dollars' worth of furniture to her father-in-law, and picking up dates on the street. In the hospital, Mrs. Lord monopolizes conversation, insists on unusual privileges, and frequently becomes demanding, bossy, and sarcastic. She has periods of great overactivity and sometimes is destructive. She frequently uses vulgar and profane language. Mrs. Lord was formerly witty, gay, and the "life of the party." Questions 79 through 84 refer to this situation.

79 The symptoms that Mrs. Lord exhibits are usually found in patients experiencing:
  1. Affective disorders
  2. Schizophrenic disorders
  3. Personality disorders
  4. Major depressions
80 When Mrs. Lord's language becomes vulgar and profane, the nurse should:
  1. State: "We don't like that kind of talk around here."
  2. State: "When you can talk in an acceptable way, we will talk to you."
  3. Recognize it as part of her illness but set limits on it
  4. Ignore it, since the patient is using it only to get attention
81 During Mrs. Lord's phase of extreme elation and hyperactivity the nursing staff should consider her nutritional needs by:
  1. Following her around the dining room with her tray
  2. Providing her with frequent high-calorie feedings that can be held in the hand
  3. Accepting the fact that she will eat when she is hungry
  4. Allowing her to prepare her own meals and eat when she pleases
82 Mrs. Lord's hyperactivity might be redirected therapeutically in which one of the following ways?
  1. Give her cleaning equipment and suggest that she assist with the ward work
  2. Ask her to guide other patients as they clean their rooms
  3. Suggest that she initiate social activities on the ward for the patient group
  4. Give her a pencil and paper and encourage her to write
83 In helping Mrs. Lord with personal hygiene the nurse would:

  1. Keep makeup away from her because she will apply it too freely
  2. Suggest that she wear hospital clothing to avoid confrontations
  3. Allow her to apply makeup in whatever manner she chooses
  4. Encourage her to dress attractively and in her own clothing
84 Three new staff members are assigned to the unit on which Mrs. Lord is a patient. During their orientation tour, Mrs. Lord greets them by saying, "Welcome to the funny farm. I'm Jo-Jo the head yo-yo." This comment might mean that the patient is:
  1. Looking for attention from the new staff
  2. Unable to distinguish fantasy from reality
  3. Anxious over the arrival of the new staff members
  4. Trying to fill her role as "life of the party"

85 Projection, rationalization, denial, and distortion by hallucinations and delusions are examples of a disturbance in:
  1. Thought process
  2. Association
  3. Logic
  4. Reality testing
86 A patient expresses the belief that the F.B.I. is out to kill him. This is an example of a(n):
  1. Hallucination
  2. Self-accusatory delusion
  3. Delusion of persecution
  4. Error in judgment
87 Mr. James is withdrawn and noncommunicative; to encourage him to talk, the best plan of nursing intervention would be to:
  1. Ask simple questions that require an answer
  2. Focus on nonthreatening subjects
  3. Try to get him to discuss his feelings
  4. Sit and look through magazines with him
88 When caring for patients exhibiting withdrawn patterns of behavior, an important aspect of nursing care is to:
  1. Help the patient understand that it is harmful to withdraw from situations
  2. Involve the patient in activities throughout the day
  3. Help keep the patient oriented to reality
  4. Encourage the patient to discuss why he does not mix with the other patients
89 Observation is an important aspect of nursing care. It is especially important in the care of the withdrawn patient because it:
  1. Helps in understanding the patient's feelings
  2. Is useful in making a diagnosis
  3. Indicates the degree of psychic depression
  4. Tells the staff how ill the patient is
90 The best approach in helping a very withdrawn patient is to provide an environment with:
  1. A large variety of activities
  2. A specific routine

3. A trusting relationship
4. Group involvement

91 The most accurate definition of "depression," as used in psychiatry, is:
1. A disturbance in mood as a reaction to the loss of a love object
2. A total loss of control over emotional impulses
3. An inability to make decisions or function
4. A disturbance in mood as a result of frustration of instinctual strivings

92 Schizophrenia is considered a functional illness. This means that the:
1. Genes of the child may carry the schizophrenic factor
2. Brain itself undergoes actual physical change that produces the symptoms of schizophrenia
3. Brain itself undergoes no physical change, but the operation of the organ is disturbed, producing the symptoms of schizophrenia
4. Individual is predisposed to schizophrenia because of poor housing and living conditions during childhood

93 The affect most commonly found in the schizophrenic patient is one of:
1. Happiness and elation
2. Apathy and flatness
3. Sadness and depression
4. Anger and hostility

94 Mental illness is evidenced when an individual:
1. Has difficulty relating to others
2. Experiences frequent periods of high anxiety
3. Expresses little desire for work or social activities
4. Has difficulty completing activities

95 Carolyn Demarke has been a patient on the psychiatric unit for several days. She arouses anxiety and frustration in the ward staff and manipulates so well that she intimidates any nurse who comes near her. One morning, Carolyn yells out at the nurse, "You've worked it so that I can't go out with the group today to bowl. You're as cunning as a fox—I hate you! Get out or I'll hit you." When a nurse is threatened this way, the best response would be:
1. "You are being rude and I don't like it. Your behavior is stopping me from wanting to stay with you."
2. "Go ahead and hit me if you have a need to."
3. "Tell me what I did to hurt you."
4. "I don't really like to hear your threats and insults. Can you tell me why you feel this way?"

96 Functional mental illnesses are mainly the result of:
1. Genetic endowment
2. Social environment
3. Infection and inflammation
4. Deterioration of brain tissue

97 When there is nothing organically wrong with the organs of communication and yet the individual is unable to communicate, the condition is referred to as:
1. Organic mental disorder
2. Mental deficiency
3. Functional mental disorder
4. Chronic brain pathology

98 Mrs. Ray is hospitalized because of a severe depression. While at home she refused to eat, stayed in bed most of the time, and did not talk with family members. Finally, unable to cope with the problem, the husband took her to the hospital. Here the symptoms persist and she will not leave her room. The nurse caring for her attempts to talk to her, asking questions but receiving no answers. Finally, in exasperation, the nurse tells the patient that if she does not respond she will be left alone. The nurse:
1. Attempts to use reward and punishment to motivate the patient
2. Is really assaulting the patient and should have refrained from this
3. Recognizes that the patient has the right to make the decision
4. Should get her involved in group therapy rather than attempting one-to-one therapy

99 Mr. James, a patient on the psychiatric unit, becomes upset in the day room. In attempting to deal with the situation the nurse should:
1. Lead the patient from the room by taking him by his arm
2. Allow the patient to act out until he tires
3. Give directions in a firm low-pitched voice
4. Instruct the patient to be quiet

100 Susan is your patient. As you are talking to another patient, Susan comes up to you and yells, "I hate you. You're talking about me again," and throws a glass of juice at you. Your nursing approach would be to:
1. Remove Susan to an isolation room because she needs to have limits placed on her behavior
2. Say to yourself, "She's very sick. I must understand her behavior"; then say, "You hate me? Tell me about that."
3. Say to yourself, "She's acting this way because she's sick"; then ignore both the behavior and Susan, clean up the juice, and promise yourself you'll talk to her when she is better
4. Verbalize your own feelings of annoyance as an example to Susan that it is more acceptable to verbalize feelings than to act out

Situation: Mr. Long, age 35, has been admitted to the Mental Health Unit of a general hospital. Over the past month he has had difficulty in sleeping and has lost his appetite. Although very anxious and tense, he appears sad and has lost all initiative. He has difficulty in concentrating, and most of his thoughts center on his unworthiness and his failures. Questions 101 to 110 refer to this situation.

101 Mr. Long is being interviewed by the admitting nurse. Which question is the most appropriate at this time?
1. "Tell me what has been bothering you?"
2. "Why do you feel so bad about yourself?"
3. "Tell me how you feel about yourself."
4. "What can we do to help you during your stay with us?"

102 Which of the following behaviors best portrays Mr. Long's feelings of self-effacement?
1. Voice is quiet and monotonous
2. Lack of initiative
3. Gestures and affect are inappropriate
4. A "don't listen to me" attitude

103 The nurse needs to evaluate Mr. Long's potential for suicide. Which approach would best gain this information?
1. Ask his family if he has ever attempted suicide
2. Ask him if he has ever thought of suicide
3. In a group discussion, direct patients to talk of suicide
4. Ask him what his plans are for the future

104 Which action by the nurse would be most therapeutic when Mr. Long states, "I am no good. I'm better off dead."
1. Unobtrusively removing those articles which could be used in a suicide attempt
2. Stating, "I think you are good; you should think of living."
3. Stating, "I will stay with you until you are less depressed."
4. Alerting the staff to provide 24-hour observation of the patient

105 In making a nursing care plan for Mr. Long, which approach would be most therapeutic?
1. Allow time for his slowness when planning activities
2. Encourage the patient to perform menial tasks to meet the need for punishment
3. Help Mr. Long focus on family strengths and support systems
4. Reassure him that he is worthwhile and important

106 Mr. Long refuses to cooperate with the staff. All planned activities are rejected, since he is "just too tired." Which nursing approach best expresses an understanding of his needs?
1. Explain why the activities are therapeutic for him
2. Accept his behavior calmly, and without excessive comment set firm limits
3. Help him express his feelings of hostility toward the activities
4. Plan a rest period for him during activity time

107 The nurse understands that one of the most difficult tasks for Mr. Long is to express his:
1. Feelings of low self-esteem
2. Remorse and guilt
3. Anger toward others
4. Need for comforting

108 Mr. Long is to have electroconvulsive therapy (ECT). What information should the nurse give him about this treatment?
1. He will be put to sleep and will have no pain
2. With new methods of administration treatment is totally safe
3. Answer only those questions asked by him
4. He will have complete memory loss as a result of the treatment

109 The physician has ordered imipramine (Tofranil), 75 mg t.i.d., for Mr. Long. Which of the following is an appropriate nursing action in giving this drug?
1. Warn him not to eat cheese, fermenting products, and chicken liver
2. Do not give any barbiturates or steroids with this drug
3. Have him checked for intraocular pressure and instruct him to watch for symptoms of glaucoma
4. Observe him for increased tolerance so that therapeutic dosage is maintained

110 Mr. Long is to be discharged from the hospital. Which statement by the nurse gives the most understanding at this time?
1. "I am going to miss you; we have become good friends."
2. "Call the unit night or day if you have problems."
3. "This is my phone number; call me and let me know how your doing."
4. "I know you are going to be all right when you go home."

111 An individual with an anxiety disorder usually handles the anxiety *in all but one* of the following ways:
1. Converting anxiety into a physical symptom
2. Acting out the anxiety with antisocial behavior
3. Displacing anxiety onto less threatening objects
4. Regressing to earlier levels of adjustment

112 A phobic reaction will rarely occur unless the person:
1. Thinks about the feared object
2. Absolves the guilt of the feared object
3. Introjects the feared object into the body
4. Comes into contact with the feared object

113 School phobia is usually treated by:
1. Calmly explaining why attendance at school is necessary
2. Returning the child to school immediately
3. Allowing the parent to accompany child to classroom
4. Allowing the child to enter classroom before other children

114 The person with socially aggressive behavior needs an environment that:
1. Allows freedom of expression
2. Is mainly group oriented
3. Provides control by setting limits
4. Can be manipulated

115 The patient who has obsessive-compulsive behavior can best be treated by:
1. Calling attention to the behavior
2. Restricting his movements
3. Supporting but limiting the behavior
4. Keeping him busy to distract him

116 Many people control anxiety by ritualistic behavior. When taking care of these patients it is important to:
1. Allow time to carry out the ritual
2. Prevent patient from carrying out the ritual
3. Explain the meaning of the ritual
4. Avoid mentioning the ritual

117 Sally, age 16, is admitted to the psychiatric service. She has lost 20 pounds in 6 weeks. She is very thin but concerned about being overweight. Her daily intake is 10 cups of coffee. The most important initial nursing intervention would be to:
1. Compliment her on her lovely figure
2. Explain the value of good nutrition
3. Explore the reasons why she does not eat
4. Try to establish a relationship of trust

118 Shortly after admission, Sally falls to the floor and has tonic and clonic movements. She does not respond verbally but you note that she is still chewing gum. Which of the following is your best response?
1. Remove the chewing gum
2. Send another patient for help
3. Report and record all observations
4. Insert a tongue blade between her teeth

119 A young handsome man with a diagnosis of antisocial personality disorder is being discharged from the hospital next week. He asks you for your phone number so he can call you for a date. Your best response would be:
1. "No, you are a patient and I am a nurse."
2. "We are not permitted to date patients."
3. "I like you, but our relationship is professional."
4. "It is against my professional ethics to date patients."

120 The patient with an antisocial personality disorder:
1. Is generally unable to postpone gratification
2. Suffers from a great deal of anxiety
3. Has a great sense of responsibility toward others
4. Rapidly learns by experience and punishment

121 A person with an antisocial personality disorder has difficulty relating to others because of never having learned to:
1. Count on others
2. Be dependent on others
3. Communicate with others socially
4. Empathize with others

Situation: Mr. James has been admitted to the psychiatric unit for psychologic testing. He is a 43-year-old well-dressed man whom you find sitting with his face in his hands. He is charged with molesting a 7-year-old child. Questions 122 and 123 refer to this situation.

122 When you ask Mr. James to come to dinner, he refuses, stating "I don't want anyone to see me. Leave me alone." Your best response would be:
1. "Certainly, Mr. James. I respect your wishes."
2. "It will be easier to face other people right away."
3. "Only the staff members know why you are here."
4. "You are the hardest judge you must face, Mr. James."

123 Mr. James looks intently at you without saying anything else. You could best respond by stating:
1. "I'll be at the desk if you need me."
2. "Pull yourself together, Mr. James. I'll walk you to dinner."

3. "Tell me what you are feeling now, Mr. James."
4. "It must be difficult to be on a psychiatric unit."

Situation: Mrs. Jordon is admitted with a severe anxiety disorder. She is crying, wringing her hands, and pacing. Questions 124 through 129 refer to this situation.

124 The first nursing intervention should be to:
1. Ask the patient what is bothering her
2. Tell the patient to sit down and try to relax
3. Stay physically close to her
4. Try to get her involved in some nonthreatening activity

125 Unsatisfied needs create anxiety that motivates an individual to action. This action is brought about mainly to:
1. Relieve physical discomfort
2. Reduce tension
3. Remove the problem
4. Deny the situation

126 The nurse should teach Mrs. Jordon's family that anxiety can be recognized as:
1. Fears that are related to the total environment
2. A behavior pattern observable in ourselves and others
3. A totally unique experience and feeling
4. Consciously motivated thoughts and wishes

127 The nurse can minimize Mrs. Jordon's psychologic stress by:
1. Learning what is of particular importance to the patient
2. Explaining in fine detail all procedures and therapies
3. Confidently advising the patient that the nurse is in charge of the situation
4. Avoiding the discussion of any areas that may be emotionally charged

128 Physiologically, the nurse would expect Mrs. Jordon's anxiety to be manifested by:
1. Dilated pupils, dilated bronchioles, increased pulse rate, hyperglycemia, and peripheral vasoconstriction
2. Constricted pupils, constricted bronchioles, increased pulse rate, hypoglycemia, and peripheral vasodilation
3. Dilated pupils, constricted bronchioles, decreased pulse rate, hypoglycemia, and peripheral vasoconstriction
4. Constricted pupils, dilated bronchioles, increased pulse rate, hypoglycemia, and peripheral vasodilation

129 The most appropriate way to decrease Mrs. Jordon's anxiety is by:
1. Prolonged exposure to fearful situations
2. Introducing an element of pleasure into fearful situations
3. Avoiding unpleasant objects and events
4. Acquiring skills with which to face emergencies

Situation: Mrs. Queen, 28 years old, is admitted to the hospital with a diagnosis of conversion disorder. Questions 130 through 133 refer to this situation.

130 Mrs. Queen states that she is unable to move her legs. Which of the following behaviors would you expect to observe in her? She:
1. Appears greatly depressed
2. Exhibits free-floating anxiety
3. Appears calm and composed
4. Demonstrates anxiety when discussing symptoms

131 When caring for Mrs. Queen, a positive nursing intervention would be to:
1. Encourage her to try to walk
2. Avoid focusing on her physical symptoms
3. Tell her there is nothing wrong
4. Help her follow through with the physical therapy plan

132 In a patient such as Mrs. Queen, anxiety is:
1. Diffuse and free floating
2. Localized and relieved by the symptom
3. Consciously felt by the patient
4. Projected onto the environment

133 In planning nursing care for Mrs. Queen, the nurse recognizes that:
1. It is best to ignore her complaints
2. Her behavior indicates a lack of willpower
3. Her symptoms are evidence of a disturbed personality
4. If additional stress is added she will become psychotic

Situation: The staff and patients have just learned that, while on a weekend pass from the hospital, Sally Finn has committed suicide. A meeting is called to attempt to deal with the feelings this incident has aroused among staff and patients alike. The collective mood of the group is tense and restless. Questions 134 through 136 refer to this situation.

134 The nurse sitting beside Mrs. Smith observes that she is sobbing and rocking back and forth in a sitting position while she hugs her arms around herself and moans softly, "I'm next. Oh, my God, I'm next. They couldn't stop Sally and they can't protect me." The nurse could best respond by saying:
1. "Sally was a lot sicker than you are, Mrs. Smith."
2. "It's different, Mrs. Smith. Sally was home; you're here."
3. "You are afraid you will hurt yourself, Mrs. Smith?"
4. "Don't worry. All passes will be canceled for a while."

135 Jim May, a friend of Sally's, stands up and shouts, "Oh! I know what you're all thinking, you think that I should have known that she was going to kill herself. You think that I helped her plan this." The group leader's response should be:
1. "Oh no, Jim, we all know you liked Sally."
2. "You feel we're blaming you for Sally's death, Jim?"
3. "It'll help if you tell us the truth, Jim."
4. "Helping her plan her suicide would not be healthy."

136 During the group discussion it is learned that Sally had not shared her strong suicidal feelings and had successfully masked her depression. The group leader should be prepared primarily to deal with:
1. The guilt that the group feels because it could not prevent Sally's suicide
2. The fear and anxiety which some members of the group may have that their own suicidal urges may go unnoticed and unprotected
3. The guilt, fear, and anger of the staff, that they have failed to anticipate and prevent Sally's suicide
4. The lack of concern over Sally's suicide expressed by some of the group

Situation: Miss Hayes, 19 years of age, came to the psychiatric hospital from a girl's dormitory on a nearby college campus where she was a freshman. Throughout high school she had always been an excellent student who was interested in modern art, ballet, dancing, symphony concerts, and good literature. She played the violin very well. She had no close friends and was considered a loner. Her family states that she always has been sensitive and different from other girls. She was admitted to the psychiatric hospital when she refused to get out of bed and go to classes. Her personal appearance deteriorated steadily during the past month, and recently she did not bother to comb her hair or put on makeup. In the hospital she talks to unseen people, voids on the floor, sometimes masturbates openly, occasionally eats with her hands, and refuses to shower or wear her own clothes. Questions 137 through 145 refer to this situation.

137 The nurse's efforts should be directed especially toward which aspect of Miss Hayes' care?
1. Frequent rest periods to avoid exhaustion
2. Appropriate attempts to establish a meaningful relationship with her
3. Reduction of environmental stimuli and maintenance of dietary intake
4. Improving social relationships with her peer group

138 The most appropriate way to begin to help Miss Hayes accept the realities of daily living would be to:
1. Encourage her to join the other patients in group singing
2. Assist her to care for her own personal hygiene
3. Encourage her to take up playing the violin again
4. Leave her alone when she is disinterested in the activity at hand

139 When Miss Hayes openly masturbates, the nurse should most appropriately:
1. Restrain her hands
2. Not react to the behavior
3. Put her in seclusion
4. State that such behavior is unacceptable

140 Miss Hayes starts to repeat phrases that others have just said. This type of speech is known as:
1. Autism
2. Echopraxia
3. Echolalia
4. Neologism

141 The nurse could best handle the problem of Miss Hayes voiding on the floor by:
1. Making the patient mop the floor
2. Restricting the patient's fluids throughout the day
3. More frequent toileting with supervision
4. Withholding privileges each time the patient voids on the floor

142 When Miss Hayes eats with her hands, the nurse can handle this problem by:
1. Placing the spoon in her hand and suggesting that she use it
2. Commenting, "I thought college girls had better manners than that."
3. Removing the food and saying, "You can't have any more until you can use your spoon."
4. Saying in a joking way, "Well, fingers were made before forks."

143 While watching TV in the day room Miss Hayes suddenly screams, bursts into tears, and runs out of the room to the far end of the hallway. What would be the most therapeutic action for the nurse to take?
1. Write up the incident on the patient's chart while it is still fresh in her memory
2. Ask another patient what made Miss Hayes act as she did
3. Walk to the end of the hallway where Miss Hayes is standing
4. Accept the action as just being the impulsive behavior of a sick person

144 Miss Hayes feels that "a man on television" is responsible for her being sick. This is an example of:
1. Autistic thinking
2. Illusion
3. Hallucination
4. Delusion

145 Miss Hayes, who has been watching the nurse for a few days, suddenly walks up and shouts, "You think you're so damned perfect and good. I think you stink!" What would be the most appropriate response for the nurse to make?
1. "I can't be all that bad can I?"
2. "You seem angry with me."
3. "Stink? I don't understand."
4. "Boy, you're in a bad mood."

Situation: Mrs. Ohream is a 46-year-old woman who was admitted to the psychiatric hospital because she drank poison and slashed her wrists. She cries a great deal, refuses food, and says that she is not fit to live. The physician has ordered electroconvulsive treatment for her. Questions 146 through 151 refer to this situation.

146 Which of the following physical problems occur when succinylcholine chloride (Anectine) is administered before electroconvulsive therapy?
1. Dislocation of the jaw
2. Compression fracture of vertebrae

3. Respiratory arrest
4. Electrocution

147 Mrs. Ohream has just awakened from her first electroconvulsive therapy treatment. The most appropriate nursing intervention would be to:
1. Get Mrs. Ohream up and out of bed as soon as possible and back into her normal routine
2. Orient Mrs. Ohream to time and place and tell her that she has just had a treatment
3. Arrange for the attendant to bring Mrs. Ohream a lunch tray
4. Take Mrs. Ohream's blood pressure and pulse rate every 15 minutes until she is fully awake

148 Which of the following factors is most important in helping to evaluate the risk of suicide in a depressed patient such as Mrs. Ohream?
1. Length of time the depression has existed
2. Impending anniversary of the loss of a loved one
3. Development of plans for discharge from hospital or program
4. Presence of multiple personal problems

149 A positive nursing action in caring for Mrs. Ohream is to:
1. Allow her to make decisions for herself
2. Provide her with frequent periods of thinking time
3. Hold her hand while sitting with her
4. Playing a game of chess with her

150 You are caring for Mrs. Ohream on a day she seems more withdrawn and depressed. An appropriate nursing action would be to:
1. Ask her if you may sit with her
2. Tell her you will spend some time with her
3. Remain visible to her
4. Get her involved in group activities

151 Depressed patients such as Mrs. Ohream seem to do best in settings where they have:
1. Many varied activities
2. A great deal of stimuli
3. A simple daily schedule
4. To make only simple decisions

---

152 When pouring liquid Thorazine, the nurse should:
1. Keep it away from the face during inspiration
2. Mix it with fruit juice immediately
3. Administer immediately after pouring
4. Avoid contact with skin

153 Mrs. Somers is an elderly patient who has been taking chlorpromazine hydrochloride (Thorazine) for several months. After noticing that the patient sits rigidly in her chair, the nurse observes her closely for other evidence of adverse effects of the drug, including:
1. Inability to concentrate, excess salivation
2. Minimal use of nonverbal expression, rambling speech
3. Incoordinated movement of extremities, tremors
4. Reluctance to converse, nonverbal clues indicating fear

154 In assessing the patient for adverse effects of chlorpromazine hydrochloride (Thorazine), the nurse would also:
1. Examine her eyeballs and question her about the color of her stools
2. Assess her appetite and weigh her weekly.
3. Take her blood pressure and ask if she has frequent headaches
4. Examine her skin and ask if she has numbness or coldness of her feet

155 A patient receiving high-dosage chlorpromazine HCl (Thorazine) has developed tremors of the hands. The appropriate action of the nurse would be to:
1. Report the symptoms to the physician
2. Withhold the medication
3. Tell the patient it is transitory
4. Give the patient finger exercises

156 An extrapyramidal symptom that is a potentially irreversible side effect of chlorpromazine and other antipsychotic drugs is:
1. Pseudoparkinsonism
2. Torticollis
3. Tardive dyskinesia
4. Occulogyric crisis

157 Lithium carbonate is the drug of choice for:
1. Acute agitation of schizophrenia
2. Agitated phase of paranoid state
3. Modification of depressive phase of major depression
4. Control of manic episode of bipolar disorders

158 A common manageable side effect of the major tranquilizers is:
1. Jaundice
2. Unintentional tremors
3. Ptosis
4. Melanocytosis

159 When monoamine oxidase inhibitors (MAOIs) are prescribed, the patient should be cautioned against:
1. The use of medications with an elixir base
2. Prolonged exposure to the sun
3. Ingesting wines and cheeses
4. Engaging in active physical exercise

160 Photosensitization is a side effect associated with the use of:
1. Chlorpromazine hydrochloride
2. Thioridazine hydrochloride
3. Methylphenidate hydrochloride (Ritalin)
4. Lithium carbonate

161 The major tranquilizers are the drugs of choice to relieve symptoms of:
1. Narcotic withdrawal
2. Depression
3. Hyperkinesis
4. Psychosis

162 Drugs such as trihexyphenidyl (Artane), biperiden (Akineton), and benztropine (Cogentin) are often prescribed in conjunction with:
1. Major tranquilizers
2. Minor tranquilizers
3. Barbiturates
4. Antidepressants

163 Many psychiatric patients are given the drugs Cogentin or Artane in conjunction with the phenothiazine derivatives to:
1. Potentiate the effect of the drug
2. Reduce postural hypotension
3. Combat extrapyramidal side effects
4. Modify depression that often accompanies schizophrenia

Situation: Mr. Daniels, 19 years old and a known heroin addict, is unconscious when admitted to the emergency room with the diagnosis of narcotic (heroin) overdose. Questions 164 through 166 refer to this situation.

164 The medication used to combat an overdose of narcotics is:
1. Amphetamine sulfate (Benzedrine)
2. Naloxone hydrochloride (Narcan)
3. Dextroamphetamine (Dexedrine)
4. Caffeine sodium benzoate

165 The planned effect of this drug is to:
1. Stimulate cortical sites controlling consciousness and cardiovascular function
2. Accelerate metabolism of heroin and stimulate respiratory centers
3. Compete with narcotics for receptors controlling respiration
4. Decrease analgesia and the comatose state induced by heroin

166 Within an hour Mr. Daniels is responding. Close observation of his status is indicated because:
1. The combined action of naloxone hydrochloride and heroin causes cardiac depression
2. Naloxone hydrochloride may cause neuropathy and convulsions
3. Narcotic effect may cause return of symptoms after the naloxone chloride is metabolized
4. Hyperexcitability and amnesia may cause the patient to thrash about and become abusive

Situation: James Cote is a narcotic addict who had surgery to repair a laceration of his heart caused by a bullet. Postoperatively he is receiving methadone hydrochloride orally. Questions 167 through 172 refer to this situation.

167 Methadone hydrochloride:
1. Provides postoperative pain control without causing narcotic dependence
2. Counteracts the depressive effects of long-term opiate usage on cardiac and thoracic muscles
3. Allows symptom-free termination of narcotic addiction
4. Converts narcotic use from an illicit to a legally controlled drug

168 Drug abuse is best defined as:
1. A physiologic need for a drug
2. A psychic dependence on a drug
3. An excessive drug use inconsistent with acceptable medical practice
4. A compulsion to take a drug on either a continuous or periodic basis

169 Hard drugs easily cause dependence because of their ability to:
1. Ease pain
2. Clear sensorium
3. Blur reality
4. Decrease motor activity

170 How many hours after the last dose would the nurse expect Mr. Cote's withdrawal symptoms to reach a peak?
1. 8 to 24
2. 24 to 48
3. 48 to 72
4. 72 to 96

171 The nurse would expect Mr. Cote's basic personality to be marked by insecurity and:
1. Infantile passion for self-gratification
2. The need to delay gratification
3. The use of psychosomatic mechanisms
4. Weak id drives

172 When methadone hydrochloride dosage is lowered, Mr. Cote must be observed closely for evidence of:
1. Agitation, attempts to escape from the hospital
2. Piloerection, lack of interest in surroundings
3. Skin dryness, scratching under incisional dressing
4. Lethargy, refusal to participate in therapeutic exercise

Situation: Mr. Winford, a 42-year-old executive, is admitted for treatment of his alcoholism. Questions 173 through 178 refer to this situation.

173 Mr. Winford is suspicious of others and blames others for his difficulty. The nurse understands that the patient uses this behavior because he has problems:
1. In identifying who bothers him
2. With dependence and independence
3. In telling the truth
4. Meeting his ego ideal

174 Mr. Winford asks if you can see the bugs that are crawling on his bed. Your best reply would be:
1. "I will get rid of them for you."
2. "No, I don't see any bugs."
3. "I will stay with you until you are calmer."
4. "Those bugs are a part of your sickness."

175 Mr. Winford often makes up stories to fill in the blank spaces of his memory. This is said to be:
1. Denying
2. Confabulating
3. Lying
4. Rationalizing

176 As Mr. Winford begins to feel better, he denies excessive use of alcohol. The nurse understands that denial is meeting Mr. Winford's need to:

1. Make him look better in the eyes of others
2. Live up to other's expectations
3. Make him seem more independent
4. Reduce his feelings of guilt

177 Mr. Winford asks if it is required that he attend Alcoholics Anonymous. The nurse's best reply would be:
1. "No, it is best to wait until you feel you really need them."
2. "Yes, because you will learn how to cope with your problem."
3. "Do you have feelings about going to these meetings?"
4. "You'll find you'll need their support."

178 Groups such as Alcoholics Anonymous help people like Mr. Winford because in a group the person learns that:
1. He does not need a crutch
2. His problems are not unique
3. His problems are caused by alcohol
4. People stand stronger together

---

179 Mrs. Jane, a 45-year-old woman, is hospitalized because of chronic alcoholism. She is irritable with the nurses and seems only to wait for a friend who visits daily. After such visits Mrs. Jane seems happier and more relaxed. One day the nurse sees the visitor give her a package, which she puts away quickly. Later Mrs. Jane, obviously intoxicated, tells the staff that her friend has brought gin regularly. Mrs. Jane's husband is very upset and threatens to sue. The decision in this suit would take into consideration the fact that:
1. Patients may have gifts brought to them without prior inspection
2. Mrs. Jane's response to her friend's visit was a clue that the nurse missed
3. The nurse is responsible for observing the patient's behavior
4. Psychotic patients need close supervision

180 Chronic alcoholic patients with Wernicke encephalopathy associated with Korsakoff's syndrome are treated initially by:
1. Oral administration of paraldehyde
2. Judicious use of tranquilizers
3. Providing a high-protein diet
4. Intramuscular injections of thiamine

181 Which of the following statements regarding alcohol and drug use is correct?
1. Most polydrug abusers also abuse alcohol
2. Most alcoholics become polydrug abusers
3. An unhappy childhood is a causative factor in addictions
4. Addictive individuals tend to use hostile abusive behavior

Situation: Mr. Ray, a 32-year-old salesman, is attending his first meeting of Alcoholics Anonymous because he finally realized and admitted that he is an alcoholic. Questions 182 through 186 refer to this situation.

182 The most effective treatment of alcoholism is accomplished by:
1. Admission to an alcoholic unit in a hospital
2. Individual or group psychotherapy
3. The daily administration of disulfiram (Antabuse)
4. Active membership in Alcoholics Anonymous

183 Self-help groups such as Alcoholics Anonymous are successful because they meet the patient's need to:
1. Be trusted
2. Grow
3. Be independent
4. Belong

184 Self-help groups assist their members to:
1. Deal with present behavior and changes in behavior
2. Identify with their peers
3. Set long-term goals
4. Identify the underlying cause of their behavior

185 For patients with alcoholism, the primary rehabilitator is the:
1. Nurse
2. Physician
3. Entire health team
4. Patient

186 The most important factor in Mr. Ray's rehabilitation is:
1. His emotional or motivational readiness
2. The qualitative level of his physical state
3. His family's accepting attitude
4. The availability of community resources

Situation: Donald Raye, a 19-year-old college sophomore, has been admitted through the university health service. He had become increasingly withdrawn, unkempt, isolated, and depressed. The referring psychiatrist notes strong suicidal tendencies. A contributing factor appears to be an abrupt ending of a relationship with a 22-year-old senior. His grades have fallen to the extent that he is in danger of failing all his courses. Questions 187 through 190 refer to this situation.

187 Donald's prognosis for a reasonably rapid recovery is:
1. Poor, since he has suicidal tendencies
2. Bad, since he is failing in all sectors of his life
3. Fair, since he is intelligent enough to pull himself together
4. Good, since the onset is fairly sudden and no previous emotional problems existed

188 On the second day after his admission Donald asks the nurse why he is being observed around the clock and has his freedom of movement restricted. The nurse's most appropriate reply would be:
1. "Your doctor has ordered it. He's the one you should ask."
2. "Why do you think we are observing you?"
3. "We are concerned that you might try to harm yourself."
4. "What makes you think that, Donald?"

189 On the fourth day Donald tells the nurse, "Hey look! I was feeling pretty depressed for a while, but I'm certainly not going to kill myself." Which comment by the nurse best responds to the patient's communication?
1. "Kill yourself? I don't understand."
2. "We have to observe you until your doctor tells us to stop."
3. "Suppose we talk some more about this?"
4. "You do seem to be feeling better."

190 With treatment Donald progresses satisfactorily and is to be discharged within a day or 2. He appears to be responsible for his actions and the staff is pleased with his progress. The day before discharge the nurse leaves the door to the unit unlocked. On her return a few minutes later Donald is gone. He is found in a bathroom where he has hanged himself. In this situation:
1. Determined patients almost always succeed at suicide, even with constant supervision
2. The lifting of the depression demonstrated Donald's recovery, so supervision was unnecessary
3. Suicidal patients should be observed until all symptoms of depression have disappeared
4. Donald's actions should have been anticipated by the nurse

191 For most nurses the most difficult part of the nurse-patient relationship is:
1. Developing an awareness of self and the professional role in the relationship
2. Being able to understand and accept the patient's behavior
3. Accepting responsibility in identifying and evaluating the real needs of the patient
4. Remaining therapeutic and professional at all times

192 The goal of the therapeutic psychiatric environment is to:
1. Help the patient become popular in a controlled setting
2. Improve the patient's ability to relate to others
3. Help the staff to help the patient
4. Make the hospital atmosphere more homelike

193 During a group meeting a patient, Mr. Thomas, tells everyone of his fear of his impending discharge from the hospital. Which response by the group leader would be most appropriate?
1. "Maybe you're not ready to be discharged yet, Mr. Thomas."
2. "Maybe others in the group have similar feelings that they would share."
3. "You ought to be happy that you're leaving, Mr. Thomas."
4. "How many in the group feel that Mr. Thomas is ready to be discharged?"

194 The emotional leader of a group is one who:
1. Reflects the feeling tone of the group
2. Has an authoritarian role within the group
3. Designates the roles within the group
4. Selects those who are to be members of the group

195 Group therapy can best help those who:
1. Are emotionally ill
2. Are dependent on others
3. Feel they have a problem
4. Have no one to listen to them

196 The group setting is especially conducive to therapy, since it:
1. Creates a new learning environment
2. Fosters one-to-one relationships
3. Decreases the focus on the individual
4. Confronts individual members with their shortcomings

197 When providing group therapy, the nurse must focus on:
1. Behavior of individual members
2. Personal feelings affecting behavior
3. Jointly experienced stress
4. Confrontation between members

198 Which of the following interventions is most important in helping to resolve a crisis situation? The nurse should:
1. Meet all dependency needs
2. Encourage socialization
3. Support ego strengths
4. Involve patient in new group

199 The current trend in the treatment of the emotionally ill is to:
1. Medicate during stressful periods
2. Maintain them in the community
3. Encourage the assumption of responsibility
4. Provide occupational therapy

200 The referral of discharged psychiatric patients to a psychiatric day hospital facility in their own community is done primarily to assist them to:
1. Maintain goals attained during hospitalization
2. Increase social skills and awareness
3. Avoid direct confrontation with the community
4. Get out of the house for a few hours daily

Psychiatric Nursing Answers and Rationales

1. (4) The unconscious stores past experiences and the emotional feelings associated with them. These emotional feelings influence one's perceptions, attitudes, and behavior. (c)
   (1) There is no such thing as the foreconscious level.
   (2) Material in the preconscious can be recalled to awareness.
   (3) Material in the conscious is in a state of immediate awareness.

2. (1) Mild anxiety motivates one to action, such as learning or emotional changes. Higher levels of anxiety tend to blur the individual's perceptions and interfere with functioning. (b)
   (2) The perceptual field is narrowed.
   (3) The perceptual field is greatly reduced.
   (4) Attention is severely reduced.

3. (2) The individual using sublimation attempts to fulfill desires by selecting a socially acceptable activity rather than those which are socially unacceptable (e.g., pursuing a career in nursing as a means of giving and receiving love). (b)
   (1) This would be an example of reaction formation.
   (3) This would be regression not sublimation.
   (4) This would be an example of repression.

4. (3) When acting out against the primary source of anxiety creates even further anxiety or danger, the individual may use displacement to express feelings on a safer object. (a)
   (1) An example of denial.
   (2) This would be fantasy.
   (4) An inability to mature and accept responsibility.

5. (2) The parameters set by birth, psychologic experiences, and the environment make each individual unique. Although other factors may impinge to a slight degree, these factors form the personality. (b)
   (1) Autoimmunity plays no part in personality development.
   (3) Not inclusive; limited to only some aspects of personality development.
   (4) Not inclusive; limited to only some aspects of personality development; race plays no part.

6. (3) When the individual experiences a threat to self-esteem, anxiety increases and the normal defense mechanisms are used to protect the ego. (a)
   (1) Ritualistic behavior is not a normal aspect of the developmental process.
   (2) Withdrawal patterns are an abnormal way of coping with stress; if carried to an extreme, can become pathologic.
   (4) Affective reactions are mood disorders.

7. (4) Incorporation of parental and societal values into the superego leads to the development of a sense of right and wrong. Guilt and shame are experienced when these values are broken. Thus the superego is the conscience. (b)
   (1) The self is the total of the id, ego, and superego.
   (2) The ideal self is how a person perceives the self to be or strives to be.
   (3) Narcissism involves an excessive love of self with strong dependency needs that are impossible for others to meet.
8. (1) The child views his or her own worth by the response received from the parents. This sense of worth sets the basic ego strengths and is vital to the formation of the personality. (a)
   (2) Although important, it is not as important as the parent-child relationship.
   (3) Peer groups come later in a child's development, but the parent-child is still the most important.
   (4) This comes later in life, after the basic personality has been formed.
9. (4) The sympathetic nervous system reacts to stress by releasing epinephrine, which prepares the body to fight or flee by increasing the heart rate, constricting peripheral vessels, and increasing oxygen supply to the muscles. (b)
   (1) Although the brain responds to stress, it is the sympathetic nervous system that is primarily affected.
   (2) The sympathetic and parasympathetic nervous systems are both part of the peripheral nervous system; the sympathetic nervous system is primarily affected; the parasympathetic nervous system does not play a role in the fight or flight reaction.
   (3) This has an opposite effect on the sympathetic nervous system.
10. (3) Conscience and a sense of right and wrong are expressed in the superego, which acts to counterbalance the id's desire for immediate gratification. (b)
    (1) This is the id seeking satisfaction.
    (2) A healthy ego can delay gratification and is in balance with reality.
    (4) This does not reflect any part of the self.
11. (4) Learning from others occurs in a group setting and is reinforced by group acceptance of the norms. Group pressure is peer pressure, which is more easily accepted if the individual wants to stay in the group. (a)
    (1) Groups do not go through the same developmental phases as individuals.
    (2) One member of a group can be the target of hostility.
    (3) Not necessarily so; the group may not be easily identified by its members, and identification does not play a role in emotional development.
12. (2) Socialization, values, and role definition are learned within the famiily and help develop a sense of self. Once established in the family, the child can more easily move into society. (a)

(1) Only a very small aspect of the family's influence.
(3) This is true, but not as important as identity and roles in relation to emotional development.
(4) This is true, but not as important as identity and roles in relation to emotional development.
13. (3) Socialization occurs through communication with others. Without some form of communication there can be no socialization. (a)
    (1) People interact with other social beings not with inanimate objects.
    (2) People interact with other social beings not with inanimate objects.
    (4) People interact with other social beings not with inanimate objects.
14. (3) Before this age the infant has not developed enough ego strength to have an identity or personality. (c)
    (1) Too early; has not developed enough ego strength to have a personality.
    (2) Self-concept is nonexistent.
    (4) The primary emergence of the personality has already occurred.
15. (2) The toddler learns to say ''no'' and to express independence yet, because of human nature, is both physically and emotionally dependent on the parents. (c)
    (1) The major task during infancy is development of trust.
    (3) This stage deals with developing a sense of autonomy.
    (4) This stage deals with the task of industry and developing skills for working in and relating to the world.
16. (1) The toddler is struggling to identify his or her own needs. Too early and too strict toilet training results in ambivalence because the child's needs and physical abilities are in conflict with the parental demands. The child is faced with giving up these needs or risking parental disapproval. (b)
    (2) A child is involved from birth in satisfying the parent's needs, but toilet training is really the first time a conflict develops.
    (3) A toddler has no interest in society's expectations.
    (4) A child is involved from birth in satisfying his or her own needs.
17. (2) Testing the self both physically and psychologically occurs during the toddler stage after trust has been achieved. (c)
    (1) Trust is the task of infancy.
    (3) Between the ages of 3 and 6, a child starts to identify with the parent of the same sex.
    (4) This task is accomplished between the ages of 6 and 12.
18. (1) The infant and toddler are dependent on significant others and react strongly to separation and loss, which they view as rejection and abandonment. These needs are strongest during the ''taking in'' or oral phase of development. (c)
    (2) The child begins to exert control over the environment rather than be concerned with separation.

(3) Sexual drives for the opposite parent are dealt with and repressed; the child has already developed a sense of autonomy and is no longer as concerned with separation.

(4) The child between the ages of 6 and 12 learns a sense of self-worth through dealings with others in the environment; this age is concerned with task of industry, developing skills, and relating to the world; separation is not the major concern.

19. (3) A sense of one's self and a feeling of belonging form and basis for mental health, since it provides comfort with self and group. (c)

(1) A person could have emotional balance without all three.

(2) A person needs to have biologic needs met; does not need social acceptance; the group providing acceptance may not be socially acceptable.

(4) A person needs security but can do without social recognition.

20. (1) Rivalry between siblings is normal and arises because one child resents the care and attention given another child. One child unconsciously wishes the other would disappear and frequently acts out negatively against him or her (a)

(2) These conflicts are directed not toward siblings but toward parents.

(3) This would deal more with thoughts and desires.

(4) The superego would be involved more with making amends.

21. (2) The individual who cannot communicate cannot test reality. Without this connection to others or reality, severe emotional problems will develop. (b)

(1) Without the stimulation of communication, mental dullness or slowness will occur, not mental deficiency.

(3) There is a frustration and inability to foster communication.

(4) Lack of communication can lead to isolation and withdrawal but this response is too narrow since a variety of problems usually develop.

22. (1) Feelings of resentment toward children by parents is a normal response. To relieve feelings of guilt and shame, it is vital to help parents realize this. (a)

(2) This is an untrue generalization.

(3) These are normal feelings

(4) The first child causes the greatest amount of adjustment in one's life.

23. (3) During the oedipal stage (between 2½ and 6 years of age) the child has many fears about his or her body. Any invasive techniques done at this time can create severe emotional problems. (c)

(1) If a sense of trust has been established and a caring person is allowed to spent time with the child, no damage should occur.

(2) There will probably be some regression in motor skills, but the outcome is favorable upon return home.

(4) The child is older and better able to deal with the surgery.

24. (1) The mature personality does not respond to the immediate gratification demands of the id or the oppressive control of the superego because the ego is strong enough to maintain a balance between them. (a)

(2) There would be no healthy resolution of conflicts if the superego were always in control.

(3) With society in control there would be chaos rather than maturity.

(4) This would create a rigid personality who made impossible demands on the self.

25. (3) Values and beliefs from parents and society are expressed through the child's play world. These values become part of the child's system through the process of internalization (introjection). (c)

(1) If this happened the child would be learning to blame others for his or her own faults.

(2) This would occur at a later age.

(4) The environment and others in it, rather than play, influence independence.

26. (4) Freud's theory is that a child develops a sexualized love for the parent of the opposite sex and becomes jealous of the parent of the same sex. These thoughts result in feelings of guilt, anxiety, fear, and hate toward the parent of the same sex, which are repressed. (a)

(1) The child loves the parent of the opposite sex and hates the parent of the same sex.

(2) The child loves the parent of the opposite sex but fears and hates the parent of the same sex.

(3) In the normal stage of development, ambivalence does not occur.

27. (2) The child resolves oedipal conflicts by learning to identify with the parent of the same sex and accomplishes this by mimicking the role of this parent. (b)

(1) This is the earliest stage of development and operates solely on the pleasure principle, largely id oriented; concerned with development of trust.

(3) There is increasing sex role development; concerned with peer group identification.

(4) Interest shifts from the anal region to the genital region, and questions about sexuality arise.

28. (1) When props are needed to blur reality, the individual is not able to rely on the self to test out situations and therefore dependence on others increases. (c)

(2) The person who mistrusts has not learned to trust the environment; however, does not necessarily need props.

(3) Role blurring is not a problem requiring a prop.

(4) The person with an ego ideal would not need props to blur reality.

29. (4) During a crisis one may regress to a stage provoking less anxiety in an attempt to cope with an unacceptable situation. (b)

(1) A patient may use denial during an illness, but this would not make him or her dependent and demanding.

(2) This is a normal defense mechanism; not used specifically during times of illness.

(3) This compensatory mechanism would cause a person to try to make amends, not become more dependent and demanding.

30. (4) The defense mechanism is called conversion because the individual actually reduces emotional anxiety by converting it to a physical disability. (b)

(1) In dissociation there is separation of certain mental processes from the consciousness as though they belonged to another; a dissociative-type reaction is expressed as amnesia, fugue, multiple personality, aimless running, depersonalization, sleep walking, etc.

(2) This just identifies the term used to describe mind and body; not a defense mechanism.

(3) This is a mechanism used to make up for a lack in one area by emphazing capabilities in another.

31. (2) By developing skills in one area the individual compensates or makes up for a real or imaged deficiency, thereby maintaining a positive self-image. (a)

(1) This person is not trying to make amends for unacceptable feelings (reaction formation) but rather for a felt deficiency and a poor self-image.

(3) This would deal more with unacceptable impulses that would pose a threat.

(4) If the boy incorporated the qualities of the college athlete, that would be introjection.

32. (3) An illusion is a misperception or misinterpretation of actual external stimuli. (b)

(1) This is a false belief that cannot be changed even by evidence; a fixed false belief.

(2) This would deal with imaginary not real stimuli.

(4) A belief that others are talking about the person is not a visual distortion.

33. (3) Mediating frustration within the real world is an ego function and requires ego strengths. (b)

(1) The id is unable to tolerate frustration since it is totally involved with gratification.

(2) The superego is involved with putting pressure on the ego because of the id's not tolerating frustration.

(4) The unconscious does not deal with frustration.

34. (1) The ego develops during childhood as a result of positive experiences. When the situation in childhood is such that severe anxiety is unresolved, the ego seems to be permanently traumatized and is unable to recover totally. (b)

(2) This would have no effect.

(3) This is a normal occurrence; children are often unable to verbalize their feelings and play therapy is utilized for that reason.

(4) This in itself would not necessarily be traumatic unless abuse was also present.

35. (3) The child realizes that the parent of the same sex cannot be bested in a struggle for the affection of the parent of the opposite sex. The role and behavior of the same-sex parent are therefore assumed by the child to attract the parent of the opposite sex. (b)

(1) This would be a conflict not a resolution.

(2) This would be in conflict with heterosexual drives.

(4) Doing this would give rise to greater conflict and leave a fragmented self.

36. (1) Any behavioral therapy or learning of new methods of dealing with situations requires modifications of approach and attitudes; hence personality is always capable of change. (b)

(2) Accepting this theory would close the door on all future growth and development.

(3) The capacity for change exists throughout the life cycle.

(4) Certain personality traits are established by 2, but not the total personality.

37. (2) The superego incorporates all experiences and learning from external environments (society, family, etc.) into the internal environment. (b)

(1) The id with its drives is a source of creative energy.

(3) This is the function of the id.

(4) This is the function of the id.

38. (2) Slips of the tongue, also called "Freudian slips," are material from the unconscious that slips out in unguarded moments. (a)

(1) There is no evidence linking these experiences to the unconscious.

(3) Material in the unconscious cannot deliberately be brought back to awareness.

(4) Free-floating anxiety is linked to the unconscious, but the best evidence of the unconscious is slips of the tongue.

39. (4) Poor interpersonal relationships, inappropriate behavior and learning disabilities prevent these children from emotionally adapting or responding to the environment despite possible high level of intelligence. (b)

(1) It is the lack of response to stimulus that is the clue to a child's being emotionally disturbed.

(2) The exact opposite is true.

(3) This is true but not *most* characteristic.

40. (1) From infancy the child is nonresponsive. Not wanting to eat demonstrates a further withdrawal. (c)

(2) This is not indicative of an autistic child.

(3) This would not be characteristic of autism.

(4) An autistic child would not be labeled autistic if he or she enjoyed being with people.

41. (3) The drug of choice in this diagnosis. It appears to act by stimulating release of norepinephrine from nerve endings in the brainstem. (b)

(1) Thorazine is an antipsychotic medication.

(2) Haldol is an antipsychotic medication.

(4) This is a muscle relaxant.

42. (3) When the individual consciously pretends an illness with no physical basis it is called malingering. (c)
    (1) A psychotic person is unable to pretend an illness.
    (2) A neurotic person really believes they are sick.
    (4) Using conversion defenses is not a conscious act.
43. (1) Her stated feelings of distrust of others and her inability to mix socially can best be defined in these terms. (a)
    (2) Nothing in the situation indicates this.
    (3) Before she became sick she held a responsible job.
    (4) It was her later personality that took on schizoid qualities.
44. (4) Demonstrating that the staff can be trusted is a vital initial step in the therapy program. (b)
    (1) Even proof would not convince Mrs. Avery that her delusion is false.
    (2) Mrs. Avery is not ready to enter group activities yet and will not be until trust is established.
    (3) This would not be realistic even if it were possible; limiting contact does not develop trust.
45. (1) Patients cannot be argued out of delusions, so the best approach is a simple statement of reality. (c)
    (2) This may reinforce her delusion that the hospital food is poisoned.
    (3) This would be a form of entering into her delusions; patient would only feel that particular part was free of poison.
    (4) Threats are always poor nursing intervention no matter how exasperated the nurse feels.
46. (2) It is important to help the patient focus on her feelings and this is the only response that does so. (c)
    (1) "Why" calls for a conclusion rather than exploring the issue; the patient may not have the answer.
    (3) Although this is true, it is not something Mrs. Avery is ready to understand; it is a closed statement.
    (4) This is false reassurance and not realistic; the patient is still concerned as to what she will do when the nurse is not there.
47. (4) If patients feel a need to be punished, it is best to permit them to engage in controlled activities that expiate guilt feelings. (b)
    (1) A procedure such as this would reinforce her belief of the need to be punished.
    (2) This would do nothing to interrupt the delusional system; it would support the hallucination.
    (3) Mrs. Avery cannot be talked out of her delusion; she must believe within herself that she has nothing to atone for.
48. (1) Bringing another patient into a set situation would be the most therapeutic, least threatening approach. (b)
    (2) Transfers nursing responsibility to the physician.
    (3) At this point in time, it would not be therapeutic to allow her to remain with solitary pursuits.
    (4) Someone has already pointed this out to her, with no results.
49. (1) Since the patient has feelings that people are trying to harm her, assignment to a 4-bed room would be very threatening. (b)
    (2) This seems unlikely since it appears to have started with the transfer to a 4-bed room.
    (3) This is possible but not likely; schizophrenics have difficulty working out problems.
    (4) This is also possible but unlikely; planning an escape is not usually part of a schizophrenic pattern.
50. (2) The patient is too anxious to sleep in a 4-bed room and should simply be told she is being moved to a private room. (c)
    (1) This is false reassurance; does not get to the reason for the problem.
    (3) This would not help since she has delusions of being poisoned.
    (4) Quietly moving her to a private room would be better intervention at this time.
51. (3) Sitting quietly gives the patient the message that the nurse accepts her feelings and cares. (a)
    (1) This in effect closes the door on any further communication of feeling.
    (2) This is negating her feeling and her right to cry if she is upset.
    (4) Helping her explore the reason is more therapeutic than giving advice.
52. (4) Needing to be dependent while wanting to be independent creates a struggle that makes all movement psychologically difficult. Symptoms develop and remove psychologic choice, making movement physically impossible. (b)
    (1) It is unlikely the feelings would involve his home; rather the people in the home.
    (2) This is part but not all of it.
    (3) This is also a part of the picture but not the total picture.
53. (3) This type of defense (conversion) tends to be a learned behavioral response that the individual will use when put under stress. (b)
    (1) This is not a likely occurrence if he learns to deal with his problems.
    (2) Psychiatric treatment may be needed at different times throughout life but usually not on a continuous basis.
    (4) Based on what we know of this disorder, it usually returns when the patient is under severe stress.
54. (1) The patient is caught between two equally compelling needs, and movement is impossible. Paralysis justifies to the patient the inability to move. (b)
    (2) It is an unconscious method of solving a conflict.
    (3) It is necessary for Mr. Frank to focus on the problem causing the disorder not on other things.
    (4) It is more important that he learn how to deal with his own feelings before dealing with his wife and mother.
55. (2) From the history you can determine that the patient's contacts were limited, her schedule fixed, and her demands on self quite rigid. (b)

(1) The situation gives no evidence of this.
(3) The situation gives no evidence of this.
(4) The situation gives no evidence of this.

56. (2) Her suicidal impulses take priority, and she must be stopped from acting on them while her treatment is in progress. (b)
(1) Safety is the primary responsibility.
(3) This is an internal process; reassurance will not necessarily make it happen; safety is the priority.
(4) This has a very low order of priority.

57. (1) These patients can usually be fairly easily distracted by planned involvement in repetitious, simple tasks. (b)
(2) This would be abusive treatment for a patient with a need to pace and would reinforce her belief that she should be punished.
(3) This should be employed only if her restlessness could not be controlled with other measures.
(4) She may perceive this isolation as a punishment, and it would not allow for observation by the staff.

58. (4) Points out reality while accepting the fact that the patient believes they are real. (b)
(1) Does the nurse know this to be a fact? They may not.
(2) The opposite is true; she does believe she is a bad woman.
(3) This is reality but not supportive

59. (2) The nurse's response again urges the patient to reflect on feelings and encourages communication of feeling tones. (c)
(1) "Why" asks her to draw a conclusion, which she may not be able to do.
(3) This is not what she is asking the nurse; closes the door to further communication.
(4) This is shifting responsibility from the nurse to the doctor; is an evasion technique.

60. (3) Patients frequently report suicidal feelings so the staff will have the chance to stop them. They really ask, "Do you care enough to stop me?" (c)
(1) This may be true; but, more important, she is seeking help and protection.
(2) This could be true but is an unlikely motivation for the behavior.
(4) This could be true but is an unlikely motivation for the behavior.

61. (4) The patient is using this compulsive behavior to control anxiety. She needs to continue with it until the anxiety is reduced and more acceptable methods are developed to handle it. (b)
(1) This would greatly increase anxiety; compulsive behavior is a defense that cannot be interrupted until new defenses are learned.
(2) This would not reduce the patient's anxiety since she is aware that doorknobs are not contaminated but cannot stop the compulsive act.
(3) This would not reduce the patient's anxiety since she is aware that doorknobs are not contaminated but cannot stop the compulsive act.

62. (2) By carrying out the compulsive ritual, the patient unconsciously tries to control the situation so that unacceptable impulses and feelings will not be acted on. (b)
(1) This mechanism does not operate on a conscious level.
(3) Hallucinations are not part of a phobic disorder.
(4) They feel no need to punish others.

63. (2) Helping patients understand that a behavior is being used to control impulses usually makes them more amenable to psychotherapy. (b)
(1) This would only mask symptoms and would not get at the root of what is bothering her.
(3) Part of her treatment may be with activities to help herself not others.
(4) The patient usually understands this already.

64. (3) The patient with senile psychosis rarely expresses any concern about personal appearance. The staff must meet most of the needs in this area. (a)
(1) Resistance to change is a symptom of this disorder.
(2) The past is where they feel more comfortable as opposed to the threatening present.
(4) Typical of this disorder is a short attention span and little or no interest in new activities.

65. (1) When an elderly person's brain atrophies, some unusual deposits of iron are scattered on nerve cells. Throughout the brain, areas of deeply staining amyloid, called senile plaques, can be found; these plaques are end stages in the destruction of brain tissue. (c)
(2) It is a chronic deterioration, not one with remissions and exacerbations.
(3) This may or may not be part of the disorder.
(4) Senile psychosis may also be caused by multiple infarcts of the brain.

66. (1) Patients with senile psychosis need a simple environment. Because of brain cell destruction, they are unable to make choices. (b)
(2) A well-balanced diet is important throughout life not just during senescence; a diet high in carbohydrates and protein may be lacking other nutrients such as fats.
(3) Physical and emotional needs must be met on a continuous basis, not just at a fixed time.
(4) Mrs. Smith is incapable of making choices; this will only increase her anxiety.

67. (3) The senile patient attempts to utilize defense mechanisms that have worked in the past but uses them in an exaggerated manner. Because of brain cell destruction such patients are unable to focus on one defense mechanism or develop new ones. (b)
(1) Mrs. Smith is incapable of developing new defense mechanisms at this time.
(2) A patient like Mrs. Smith will depend on old familiar defense mechanisms.
(4) Mrs. Smith is not capable of focusing on one defense mechanism.

68. (2) Damaged brain cells do not regenerate. Care is therefore directed toward preventing further damage and providing protective and supportive care. (b)
    (1) The deterioration of the brain cells makes an extensive reeducation program unrealistic.
    (3) A patient with this disorder may not be able to grasp, understand, or enjoy new leisure activities.
    (4) It is beyond the scope of her ability to function in a group therapy session.

69. (1) The patient who has an organic mental disorder will be most comfortable with the familiar and repetitive daily routine since it creates less anxiety. (b)
    (2) Cognitive changes would make this unrealistic.
    (3) It would be beyond her capabilities to develop new skills.
    (4) The memory impairment might make this impossible.

70. (3) Simply states facts without getting involved in role conflict. (b)
    (1) Being a doctor is a big part of his self-esteem, and by her remark the nurse is threatening that self-esteem.
    (2) Firm consistent limits need to be set and the nurse-patient role established.
    (4) Threats will only make the situation worse and set the tone for future nurse-patient interactions.

71. (2) The patient has the right to decide how he will be introduced, and the staff should accept his wishes. (b)
    (1) For whom is it better—the staff, the other patients, or Dr. Kay?
    (3) It gives dignity to patients to allow them to be addressed as they wish.
    (4) The patient is a doctor, and the nurse is attacking his concept of himself.

72. (2) A patient out of control needs controls set for him. Staff must understand that the patient is not deliberately setting out to disrupt the unit. (c)
    (1) Ignoring him will not stop his disruptive behavior; the nurse has a responsibility to the other patients.
    (3) This is demeaning him in the eyes of the other patients; not dealing with the problem directly.
    (4) This may be a last resort taken to solve the problem but should not be used until other alternatives are explored.

73. (4) The hyperactive patient is usually rather easily distracted, so the excess energy can be redirected into constructive channels. (a)
    (1) Mr. Bishop will talk a great deal with no encouragement.
    (2) There is nothing to indicate at this time that he is not in touch with reality.
    (3) He will not be able to stay long enough with one thing to finish it.

74. (1) This will help reduce the patient's anxiety, thereby reducing hyperactivity. (b)
    (2) It is not possible physically to control his hyperactivity.

(3) He is not capable of choosing activities at this time.
    (4) He is not capable of controlling his overactive behavior; setting verbal limits will not be effective.

75. (4) Hyperactive patients frequently will not take the time to sit down to eat because they are overinvolved in everything that is going on. (b)
    (1) This is indicative of a depressive episode.
    (2) Mr. Bishop probably gives no thought to food; he is involved with activity in the environment.
    (3) He is unable to sit long enough with the other patients to eat a meal; this is not conscious avoidance.

76. (3) The hyperactive patient will frequently eat hand foods that do not require sitting down to eat. (b)
    (1) He will most likely ignore the tray.
    (2) Unworthy feelings are part of a depressive episode.
    (4) Unlikely that the patient would understand or care about this piece of information.

77. (4) Everyone has the right to personal sexual preference, but limits must be set on acting out behavior within the hospital. (c)
    (1) This would be a punishing attitude, especially for the patient who would be transferred.
    (2) Not a realistic approach to the situation.
    (3) Limits would need to be set, not punishment.

78. (3) Adult homosexuality is a regression to an earlier, oral and anal, stage rather than acceptance of the more mature genital heterosexual level. (b)
    (1) There is normal physical development of sexual organs in homosexuals as well as heterosexuals.
    (2) There is no proof of a deficiency of these hormones.
    (4) This has no basis in fact.

79. (1) Hyperactive behavior in individuals such as this is typical of the hypermanic flight into reality associated with affective disorders. (a)
    (2) A flat affect and apathy are more indicative of a schizophrenic disorder.
    (3) The symptoms are more indicative of an affective than a personality disorder.
    (4) Depression, loss of interest in usual activities, and poor appetite are more indicative of a major depression than of a personality disorder.

80. (3) Recognizing it as part of the illness makes it easier to tolerate, but limits must be set for the benefit of the staff and other patients. Setting limits also demonstrates to the patient that you care enough to stop her. (b)
    (1) This statement shows little understanding or tolerance of the illness.
    (2) This statement demonstrates a rejection of the patient and little understanding of the illness.
    (4) Ignoring the behavior is a form of rejection and does not set limits on the behavior.

81. (2) Hyperactive patients burn up large quantities of calories, which must be replenished. Since these patients will not take the time to sit down to eat providing them with food they can carry with them sometimes helps. (b)

(1) An exercise in futility for the nurse.

(3) Mrs. Lord will probably not be aware of any hunger and could go without food for a dangerously long time.

(4) She is not presently capable of preparing her own food.

82. (1) Physical activity will help utilize some of the excess energy without requiring her to make decisions or forcing other patients to deal with her. (c)

(2) Mrs. Lord needs guidance herself; would not be able to guide others.

(3) She would greatly disrupt the unit with her excess activity and bossiness.

(4) Her extreme activity would limit her ability to sit and write or concentrate.

83. (4) Having her wear her own clothes helps keep her more in touch with reality. (b)

(1) Mrs. Lord will need help with her makeup, since she will probably go to extremes with it.

(2) This is not helping her learn new and better ways to deal with situations.

(3) This may set her up as a target of ridicule by the other patients.

84. (3) Behavior demonstrates increased anxiety. Since it was directed toward the new staff, it was probably precipitated by their arrival. (b)

(1) This is also possible, but the remark is indicative more of increased anxiety.

(2) Mrs. Lord is aware of where she is and who she is at this time.

(4) Mrs. Lord is not filling her ''life-of-the-party'' role; is resorting to previous coping behavior in the face of extreme stress.

85. (4) When individuals use these defense mechanisms to blur the pains of reality, they are unable to test out their feelings or differentiate the real world from their personal intrapsychic perceptions. (b)

(1) The thought process is only one aspect of reality testing.

(2) Association is only one part of reality testing.

(3) Logic is only one part of reality testing.

86. (3) A delusion of persecution is a fixed and firm belief or feeling of being harassed, in danger, or at the mercy of others. (a)

(1) Hallucinations are perceived experiences that occur in the absence of actual sensory stimulation.

(2) In this instance the person blamed himself for an act that was never committed.

(4) An error in judgment can be corrected by pointing out reality, but delusion cannot.

87. (2) Nursing care must be a steady attempt to draw the patient into some response. This can best be accomplished by focusing on nonthreatening subjects that do not demand a specific reponse. (b)

(1) Questions like these do not allow a person to explore his own feelings.

(3) Mr. James is not ready yet to discuss his feelings, so the first step is to focus on nonthreatening subjects.

(4) By doing this, you are showing acceptance of him but you are doing nothing to encourage communication.

88. (3) Keeping the withdrawn patient oriented to reality prevents him from withdrawing even further into his private world. (a)

(1) This would be futile at present.

(2) A gradual involvement in selected activities would be best.

(4) The patient would be unable to tell anyone why this is so.

89. (1) By observing behavior, the nurse is able to understand the patient's feelings better. Behavior usually serves a purpose and is directed toward satisfaction of needs. (b)

(2) It is only one of the many aspects that are part of making a diagnosis; true in the care of all patients not just the withdrawn individual.

(3) It is more important to have insight into what the person may be feeling rather than the degree of depression.

(4) Observation alone is insufficient to make this judgment; however it would allow the staff to individualize the nursing care plan to suit the patient's needs.

90. (3) A one-to-one trusting relationship is essential to help the patient become more involved and interested in interpersonal relationships. (a)

(1) Selected activities, rather than a large variety of activities, are best.

(2) Specific routines are normally a part of any unit, for all patients.

(4) A very withdrawn individual needs to start with a one-to-one relationship before progressing to group involvement.

91. (1) Depression is a disturbance in the mood or affect (classified as an affective disorder) that usually develops when the ego suffers a real or imagined loss. (c)

(2) There is not a total loss of control, and the loss of control may be only part of the clinical picture.

(3) The degree of depression will determine the extent to which a person can function.

(4) This may also be true, but it is not the most accurate description.

92. (3) No organic pathology has yet been identified in schizophrenia. Behavioral responses learned in childhood cause the individual to distort events and relationships and lose the ability to relate to the world. (a)

(1) This would be an organic rather than a functional illness.

(2) This would be an organic rather than a functional illness, and there is no evidence that the brain undergoes any change.

(4) This might be a factor, but there is no proof that it is true since we do not know what causes schizophrenia.

93. (2) Disinterest in or fear of personal involvement creates distancing behavior and lack of response to the environment. (b)
    (1) This would be symptomatic more of the manic episode of a bipolar disorder.
    (3) May or may not be present.
    (4) May or may not be present.

94. (1) Mental illness is characterized by the use of abnormal defense mechanisms or the abnormal use of normal defense mechanisms. These defenses build a wall and interrupt interpersonal relationships. (a)
    (2) It is the ability or inability to handle periods of high anxiety that gives evidence of mental illness.
    (3) Possible, but may be just one factor.
    (4) Possible, but not a common factor.

95. (4) Shows acceptance for the patient yet sets firm limits on the behavior. This response also points out reality to the patient. (b)
    (1) This statement not only rejects the behavior but also attacks the patient.
    (2) The nurse accepts the patient but does not accept physical abuse from the patient.
    (3) Puts the focus on the nurse rather than on what is behind the outburst.

96. (2) Family interaction patterns and role identification and definition lay the foundations for the child's future emotional response. (b)
    (1) This, as yet, has not been proved.
    (3) This would be organic not functional.
    (4) This is a part of organic mental disorders.

97. (3) Inner psychic stress and environmental difficulties can interfere with the function of organically sound organs, resulting in a loss of ability to communicate. (a)
    (1) This would have an organic basis.
    (2) Mental deficiency has an organic basis.
    (4) This has an organic basis.

98. (2) The nurse's response really was a threat by attempting to put pressure on the patient to speak or be left alone. (b)
    (1) Reward and punishment are used in behavior modification therapy, not for severe depression.
    (3) The statement reflects an insensitivity to rather than a recognition of the patient's rights.
    (4) She is not ready yet at this stage for group involvement; she must start with a one-to-one relationship.

99. (3) Patients who are out of control are seeking control and frequently respond to simple directions stated in a firm voice. (b)
    (1) This would be done only after an attempt at calming him down had failed.
    (2) This would not be helping the patient gain control of his actions and might be frightening to other patients in the day room.

(4) "Be quiet" is an order that is nontherapeutic and is, furthermore, demeaning behavior on the part of the nurse.

100. (4) The nurse's response provides an example to the patient that feelings can be expressed by words rather than by action. This response also demonstrates that the nurse cares enough to sets limits on behavior. (b)
    (1) You are punishing Susan rather than trying to focus on what is happening at this time to cause the behavior.
    (2) You will be accepting physical abuse, which is never done.
    (3) Susan won't need you to talk to her when she is better; she needs limits set on her behavior now.

101. (3) The nurse must base nursing intervention on a patient's problems. Since major depression is due to the patient's feelings of self-rejection, it is important for the nurse to have the patient identify these feelings before a plan of action can be taken. (b)
    (1) You are asking the patient to draw a conclusion; he may be unable to do so at this time.
    (2) Asking why does not let a patient explore his feelings; usually elicits an "I don't know" response.
    (4) This is beyond the scope of his abilities at present; he would rather have you tell him how you are going to help him help himself.

102. (4) This attitude conveys to others that Mr. Long feels he is not really significant enough for anyone to listen to. (b)
    (1) Indicative of his feelings of sadness not self-effacement.
    (2) Initiative and self-effacement are two different factors.
    (3) The gestures and affect as described are appropriate to his inner feelings of depression.

103. (2) Directness is the best approach at the first interview, since this sets the focus and concern and lets you know what the patient is feeling now. (b)
    (1) This would be one resource for input; but regarding suicide, it is best to approach the patient directly.
    (3) This may be helpful during the course of treatment, but initially the direct approach with the patient is best.
    (4) At this point he is most likely unable to think past the present much less deal with future plans; too general a question.

104. (4) This is the most therapeutic approach. The staff member also provides the patient with special attention to meet his dependency needs and reduce his self-defeating attitude. (c)
    (1) This would be part of intervention; but, in addition, he will need 24-hour observation.
    (2) This is negating his feelings and cutting off further communication.
    (3) This is unrealistic since the nurse cannot be with him constantly until his depression lifts.

105. (1) Routines should be kept simple and no demands should be made that the patient cannot meet. The patient is depressed, and all his reactions will be slow. Putting pressure on him will only increase his anxiety and feelings of worthlessness. (c)
     (2) This would feed into his feelings of unworthiness and his frustration.
     (3) Mr. Long will have to focus on his own strengths, not on family strengths.
     (4) Feelings of worth must come from within the individual; the nurse must reassure the patient through actions not words.

106. (2) The patient is expressing his hostility symbolically by not being cooperative. He has a right to feel this way. If members of the staff criticize him, it will only increase his feelings of guilt. (c)
     (1) This will not change his mind about the activities; does not show an understanding of his needs.
     (3) This will only serve to increase his feelings of guilt since he is unaware of the hostility.
     (4) This would be allowing him to manipulate the environment.

107. (3) The patient is very dependent, and such individuals can never get enough attention to fill their dependence. This unfulfilled need causes anger, which he has problems expressing for fear of losing the person on whom he is dependent. (c)
     (1) He is well able to express his feelings of low self-esteem.
     (2) He is well able to express remorse and guilt.
     (4) He is expressing the need for comfort.

108. (1) Patients fear this therapy because of the expected pain. If they are reassured that they will be asleep and have no pain, there will be less anxiety and more cooperation. (b)
     (2) No treatment requiring anesthesia is totally safe.
     (3) He may not be able to realize his fears and thus not ask questions.
     (4) This is not true.

109. (3) The development of glaucoma is one of the side effects of imipramine (Tofranil), and the patient should be alerted to these symptoms. (c)
     (1) Tofranil is not an MAOI.
     (2) This is true of MAOIs.
     (4) This would be essential for a person being treated with lithium.

110. (2) This response demonstrates understanding that the newly discharged patient needs to have the support of the therapeutic unit when he goes home. He needs to feel that in a crisis he can turn to them for this support. (b)
     (1) The role of the nurse was not to become a good friend but to aid Mr. Long in becoming a functioning being again.
     (3) Unprofessional and blurs the roles of nurse and patient.
     (4) False reassurance.

111. (2) Acting out anxiety with antisocial behavior is most commonly found in individuals with personality disorders rather than anxiety disorders. (c)
     (1) An example of a conversion disorder.
     (3) An example of a phobic disorder.
     (4) Regression is an attempt during periods of stress to return to behavior that has been satisfying and is appropriate at an earlier stage of development.

112. (4) In phobias the individual transfers anxiety to a rather safe inanimate object. Therefore the anxiety and resulting feelings will only be precipitated when in direct contact with the object. (b)
     (1) It is not thinking about the feared object that causes anxiety; it is the thought of having to come into contact with it.
     (2) It is the guilt or fear within the person, not the object, that must be dealt with.
     (3) Not possible to introject the feared object within the body.

113. (2) The longer the child stays out, the more difficult it is to get him or her to return to school, since more fantasies and fears develop. (c)
     (1) This approach rarely accomplishes anything.
     (3) This will feed into the fear that the phobia is realistic.
     (4) This would increase, not decrease, the fear.

114. (3) Having poor superego control, these individuals cannot set limits for themselves and require an environment in which appropriate limits for behavior are set for them. (a)
     (1) This person has too much freedom of expression and is unable to control impulses.
     (2) This would be too stimulating for a person with socially aggressive behavior.
     (4) An environment that can be manipulated teaches the patient nothing; encourages a continuation of maladjustive behavior.

115. (3) Accepting the patient and the symptomatic behavior sets the foundation for the nurse-patient relationship. Setting limits provides external controls and helps lower anxiety. (c)
     (1) This will only increase the anxiety and increase the behavior.
     (2) Restricting a person's movements would have no effect other than to increase anxiety.
     (4) Unrealistic.

116. (1) Patients prevented from using ritualistic behavior to control anxiety will be deprived of their defense and have no way of relieving tension. (a)
     (2) Preventing such patients will only increase anxiety.
     (3) This would not decrease the ritualistic behavior.
     (4) Such patients' behavior should never be ignored; it is important to accept and support these patients during this time.

117. (4) The problem is psychologic. Therefore the initial approach by the nurse should be directed toward establishing trust. (a)

(1) She is convinced that she is overweight; telling her she has a lovely figure would not change her perception of herself.

(2) The patient is not ready for this information.

(3) This would be an initial nursing intervention after trust had been established.

118. (3) If seizures were physiologically based, the patient would not be able to continue to chew gum. This "attack" should be reported as a behavioral response, with the precipitating factors noted. (c)

(1) The chewing gum is not a danger when the patient is not having a true attack.

(2) This would probably not be necessary now.

(4) Not necessary since there is no danger of the tongue's blocking the airway as it would in a true attack.

119. (3) Accept the patient as a person of worth rather than being cold or implying rejection. However, the nurse maintains a professional rather than a social role. (a)

(1) The patient is aware that he is a patient and you are a nurse.

(2) This is shifting responsibility from the issue at hand to the institution.

(4) This is avoiding the real issue and elevates the nurse to a higher social order.

120. (1) Individuals with this personality disorder tend to be self-centered and impulsive. They lack judgment and superego controls and do not profit from their mistakes. (c)

(2) Generally, just the opposite is true.

(3) These people are too self-centered to have a sense of responsibility to anyone.

(4) These people never learn from their mistakes, experiences, and punishment.

121. (4) The lack of superego control allows the ego and the id to control the behavior. Self-motivation and self-satisfaction are of paramount concern. (c)

(1) They count on others to extricate them from the problems they find themselves faced with.

(2) These people are extremely dependent on others.

(3) These people are usually charming on the surface and can easily "con" people into doing what they want.

122. (4) The patient is in the hospital for treatment and evaluation, not judgment of behavior. Since he feels people will judge him, it is important to point out that at this time he is the only one filling this role. (c)

(1) You would be ignoring his feelings and not helping him deal with the situation.

(2) This may or may not be true and could be false reassurance.

(3) You do not know this to be a fact.

123. (4) Let the patient know that you realize he is having difficulty without asking direct questions or focusing on his specific behavior. (a)

(1) This is an avoidance technique.

(2) This would be negating his feelings.

(3) Stated more like an order rather than offering an opportunity to express his feelings.

124. (3) By staying physically close, the nurse conveys to the patient the message that someone cares enough to be there and that she is a person worth caring for. (c)

(1) Mrs. Jordan is incapable of telling anyone what is bothering her.

(2) Sitting still will increase the tension she is experiencing.

(4) This would not be an initial nursing intervention.

125. (2) When tension is reduced, anxiety diminishes and the person feels more comfortable, safe, and secure. (b)

(1) This action would have an effect on psychologic rather than physical discomfort.

(3) This is what the person hopes will happen but does not.

(4) There would be less anxiety if they were able to deny the situation.

126. (2) Anxiety is a normal human response, causing both physical and emotional changes that everyone experiences when faced with stressful situations. (b)

(1) The fear may be related to a specific aspect of rather than the total environment.

(3) Anxiety is experienced to a greater or lesser degree by every person.

(4) Anxiety does not operate from the conscious level.

127. (1) Providing support, understanding, and acceptance of feelings that the patient is experiencing is essential for reducing stress. (b)

(2) This would most likely have the effect of increasing anxiety.

(3) What would happen on the nurse's day off? Concern about this would increase anxiety.

(4) The hospital provides the patient with a safe, accepting environment in which to face problems and discuss emotionally charged areas.

128. (1) The "fight or flight" responses of the autonomic nervous system would be stimulated and result in these findings. (b)

(2) The "fight or flight" response is not aided by constricted pupils and bronchioles and hypoglycemia.

(3) The pulse rate would be increased, and blood sugar would increase not decrease.

(4) The pupils would dilate not constrict, and the blood sugar would increase not decrease.

129. (4) Learning a variety of coping mechanisms helps reduce anxiety in stressful situations. (a)

(1) Prolonged exposure would increase anxiety to possibly uncontrollable levels.

(2) Fearful situations can never be viewed as pleasurable.

(3) A person must learn to cope with unpleasant objects and events.

130. (3) The patient with a conversion disorder literally converts the anxiety to the symptom. Once the symptom develops, it acts as a defense against the anxiety and the patient is diagnostically almost anxiety free. (b)
    (1) In a conversion disorder the reactions you would expect to encounter are not in proportion to the disability; therefore she would not be greatly depressed.
    (2) The conflict is resolved by the paralysis in her legs; therefore the anxiety is under control.
    (4) Just the opposite is true.

131. (2) The physical symptoms are not the patient's major problem and therefore should not be the focus for care. This ia a psychologic problem, and the focus should be on this level. (b)
    (1) This would be focusing on the physical symptoms of her conflict; the patient is not ready to give this up.
    (3) The disorder operates on an unconscious level but is very real to the patient; denies feelings.
    (4) Psychotherapy would have to come before physical therapy.

132. (2) The patient's anxiety results from being unable to choose psychologically between 2 conflicting actions. The conversion to a physical disability removes the choice and therefore reduces the anxiety. (c)
    (1) The anxiety is put under control by the conversion to a physical disability.
    (3) The anxiety is decreased, and the conversion disorder operates on an unconscious level.
    (4) The anxiety is internalized into a physical symptom.

133. (3) The symptoms are problematic to the patient and thus have caused emotional pain that is beyond conscious control. (a)
    (1) Ignoring the patient's complaints will increase anxiety.
    (2) Willpower does not enter into it; conversion disorder operates on an unconscious level.
    (4) There is no evidence that this is so.

134. (3) Recognizes the importance of feelings and provides an opening so the patient may talk about her feelings. (b)
    (1) Mrs. Smith is not going to believe this, and it is not helping the patient express her feelings.
    (2) The nursing goal is to help people function outside the hospital environment, not be afraid to leave it.
    (4) A statement like this avoids the real issue and solves nothing.

135. (2) Puts focus on the feelings, not on a statement of what did or did not happen. (b)
    (1) This statement does not give him an opportunity to explore his feelings.
    (3) Implies that Jim may have had some part in causing Sally's death.
    (4) This statement closes the door to any further communication of feelings or fears.

136. (2) Ambivalance about life and death plus the introspection commonly found in patients with emotional problems would lead to increased anxiety and fear in the group members. (b)
    (1) This will probably be a secondary goal of the group leader.
    (3) These feelings must be handled within the support system of other staff members.
    (4) It is not a primary goal; but this lack of concern should also be explored later on to see what is behind such apparent indifference, which may be a mask to cover feelings.

137. (2) The first step in a nursing care plan should be the establishment of a meaningful relationship because it is through this relationship that the patient can be helped. (b)
    (1) The situation states that she was admitted when she refused to get out of bed; encouraging this behavior would not be therapeutic.
    (3) Reduction of stimuli may help in regard to the hallucinations, but there is no evidence she is not eating her meals.
    (4) This would be a long-term goal.

138. (2) Assisting patients with grooming keeps them in contact with reality and allows them to see that staff members care enough to help. It also places value on appearance. (a)
    (1) A one-to-one relationship would be best initially.
    (3) This would be a long-term goal.
    (4) She may withdraw even more.

139. (4) Sets limits on her behavior as well as shows the patient that staff care enough to protect her. It accepts the patient but rejects the behavior. (c)
    (1) It would be unrealistic as well as cruel to do this.
    (2) The nurse has a responsibility to the other patients to limit the behavior.
    (3) This is a punishment rather than a setting of limits.

140. (3) Echolalia is repetition of another person's remarks, words, or statements. It occurs when individuals are fearful of saying their own words and therefore just echo the words of others. (b)
    (1) This is a thought process connected with associative looseness.
    (2) Echopraxia is the reflecting of observed movements rather than of speech.
    (4) This is when words, objects, people, etc. take on private symbolic meanings.

141. (3) The patient is voiding on the floor not to express hostility but because she is confused. Taking her to the toilet frequently limits the voiding in inappropriate places. (b)
    (1) A form of punishment for something the patient cannot control.
    (2) Not realistic; will have no effect on the problem.
    (4) If the patient were doing this to express hostility, such action would be useful; but not when the patient is unable to control herself.

142. (1) The patient needs limits set. This response by the nurse sets limits and rejects the behavior but accepts the patient. (b)
    (2) A degrading remark; serves no useful purpose.
    (3) A punishing action; shows no support or acceptance of the patient.
    (4) Does not help raise the patient to a functioning level.

143. (3) Lets the patient know you are available if she needs you. It also demonstrates an acceptance of her. (b)
    (1) Although it is important to note the incident on the chart, it does not take precedence over letting the patient know you are there if she needs you.
    (2) Another patient's perception of the incident may or may not be valid.
    (4) An avoidance technique; shows a lack of acceptance of the patient as a person.

144. (4) A delusion is a fixed, false personal belief that is not founded in reality. (a)
    (1) A distortion in thought process associated with schizophrenic disorders.
    (2) This would be a misinterpretation of a sensory stimulus.
    (3) A perceived experience that occurs in the absence of an actual sensory stimulus.

145. (2) The nurse's response reflects on the patient's feelings rather than focuses on verbalization. (b)
    (1) Puts the patient on the defensive, asking for verification that the nurse is indeed a good person rather than focusing on the feeling behind the statement.
    (3) Focuses on the statement rather than on the feeling behind the statement.
    (4) Dismisses the patient's feelings.

146. (3) Succinylcholine causes paralysis of the diaphragm and the intercostal muscles as well as other muscles. This paralysis causes a cessation of respiration. (a)
    (1) Early ECT treatments sometimes had this complication, but it was not a response to Anectine.
    (2) Early ECT treatments sometimes had this complication, but it was not a result of Anectine administration.
    (4) Electrocution is not a physical problem associated with Anectine.

147. (2) Patients are confused when they awaken ᵤfter electroconvulsive therapy. They have a loss of recent memory, so it is important to orient them to time, place, and situation. (b)
    (1) This would not be appropriate for a patient who has just awakened after a treatment.
    (3) This would be a later action, if the patient asked for food.
    (4) This is not necessary.

148. (2) The anniversary frequently reemphasizes the feeling of loss and abandonment and serves to heighten the current feelings of depression and hopelessness. (c)
    (1) Length of time has less influence than the anniversary of a loss.

(3) Suicide risk may still be a factor at this time but less than at the anniversary of a loss.
    (4) This would be an important consideration, but the anniversary of the loss of a loved one would take precedence.

149. (3) Gives the patient the nonverbal message that someone cares and that she is worthy of attention and concern. (b)
    (1) She is incapable of making decisions at this time.
    (2) Depressed patients often have too much thinking time.
    (4) The concentration required for chess is too much for the patient at this time.

150. (2) Telling the patient you will spend time with her communicates that you find her worthy of your time and you care. (c)
    (1) It is unlikely that she would respond to you since she feels so unworthy and depressed.
    (3) Does not show the acceptance and care that sitting with her would.
    (4) She may be unable, at this point, to expend energy on anything outside herself.

151. (3) Depression is usually both emotional and physical, so a simple daily routine is the least stressful and least anxiety-producing. (b)
    (1) A depressed patient has limited interest in simple activities; too many may increase the anxiety.
    (2) Too many stimuli increase the anxiety in a depressed patient.
    (4) Such a patient may be incapable of making even simple decisions.

152. (4) The liquid concentrate is a highly irritating substance on contact with skin and eyes and can cause uncomfortable dermatologic conditions. (c)
    (1) No indication for this precaution.
    (2) Not necessary; and leaving it unmixed provides greater assurance that the patient will ingest the full dose of Thorazine.
    (3) Not necessary.

153. (3) Acute dystonic reactions, parkinsonian syndrome, and akathisia are observable side effects of chlorpromazine hydrochloride therapy. (b)
    (1) After the first few days of treatment, Thorazine has no effect on concentration or other mental abilities.
    (2) Not a side effect of Thorazine.
    (4) Not a side effect of Thorazine.

154. (1) This checks functioning of the liver, since liver damage may occur from use of the drug. Cholestatic hepatitis with obstructive jaundice is the most frequent form of liver disturbance and can be identified by yellow sclerae and clay-colored stools. (c)
    (2) Anorexia is not a side effect of Thorazine; the patient frequently gains weight.
    (3) Not a side effect of Thorazine.
    (4) Not a side effect of Thorazine.

155. (1) The physician is responsible for medication orders but depends on the nurse's observations in making decisions. (b)

(2) This would not be a severe enough symptom to warrant withholding the drug.

(3) It is a reaction to the Thorazine and must be treated.

(4) This would have no effect on the tremors.

156. (3) Occurs as a late and persistent extrapyramidal complication of long-term chlorpromazine therapy. Can take many forms (e.g., torsion spasm, opisthotonos, oculogyric crisis, drooping of the head, protrusion of the tongue). (c)

(1) Reversible with administration of Cogentin and Benadryl.

(2) Reversible with administration of Cogentin and Benadryl.

(4) Reversible with administration of Cogentin and Benadryl.

157. (4) Lithium carbonate does not impair intellectual activity, consciousness, or range or quality of emotional life. However, it can control the manic phase of a bipolar disorder. (b)

(1) Lithium is not used for schizophrenia.

(2) Lithium is not used for an agitated paranoid state.

(3) Lithium is not used for major depressions.

158. (2) Unintentional tremors are one of the extrapyramidal side effects of the major tranquilizers and are considered common and manageable. (a)

(1) Not a common occurrence, but periodic liver function tests should be done.

(3) Not a common side effect.

(4) Not applicable; an excessive number of melanocytes is not a side effect.

159. (3) The monoamine oxidase inhibitors can cause a hypertensive crisis if food or beverages that are rich in amines or amino acids are ingested. (b)

(1) An elixir base only makes the medications more palatable.

(2) This would be important for patients taking one of the phenothiazines.

(4) No contraindication.

160. (1) Patients taking chlorpromazine should be told to stay out of the sun. Photosensitivity makes the skin more susceptible to burning. (b)

(2) Reported as being extremely rare.

(3) Not reported with the use of Ritalin.

(4) Not a side effect of lithium.

161. (4) The major tranquilizers modify the behavior of psychotic patients so they can more effectively cope with the environment and benefit from therapy. (a)

(1) Contraindicated.

(2) Antidepressants are used for depression.

(3) The action is to decrease the severity of psychotic symptoms more than to sedate; Ritalin is used to treat hyperkinetic children.

162. (1) These drugs are used to control the extrapyramidal (parkinsonism-like) symptoms that often develop as a side effect of major tranquilizer therapy. (b)

(2) No documented use with minor tranquilizers because they do not have extrapyramidal side effects.

(3) Barbiturates do not have extrapyramidal side effects, which would respond to these drugs.

(4) Antiparkinson drugs (e.g., Cogentin) are not usually prescribed in conjunction with antidepressants; gastrointestinal tract depression can result in paralytic ileus.

163. (3) These drugs control the extrapyramidal (parkinsonism-like) symptoms associated with the major tranquilizers and are classified as antiparkinsonian drugs. (b)

(1) Does not potentiate phenothiazine derivatives.

(2) Has no effect on postural hypotension.

(4) Has no effect on depression.

164. (2) Naloxone hydrochloride (Narcan) is a narcotic antagonist that counteracts and reverses the respiratory depressive action of narcotics without causing sedation or analgesia. Nalorphine (Nalline) could also be used but can precipitate a severe withdrawal reaction. (b)

(1) A CNS stimulant with no therapeutic use for a narcotic overdose.

(3) A CNS stimulant with no therapeutic use for a narcotic overdose.

(4) A CNS stimulant with no therapeutic use for a narcotic overdose.

165. (3) Narcan is used when narcotic-induced apnea occurs. It competes for central nervous system receptor sites, thus acting as a narcotic antagonist. (c)

(1) An adverse reaction is cardiovascular irritability.

(2) Narcan does not accelerate the metabolism of heroin; competes for central nervous system receptor sites.

(4) Not the specific action of this drug; it is given to prevent respiratory arrest.

166. (3) When Narcan is metabolized and its effects are diminished, the respiratory distress caused by the original drug overdose returns. (b)

(1) Narcan counteracts the respiratory depression from heroin overdose.

(2) No known report of this.

(4) Not a known effect after use of Narcan.

167. (4) The strength of this drug is controlled and remains constant from dose to dose, which is uncertain in illicit drugs. (c)

(1) Methadone is a synthetic narcotic and can cause dependence; it is not used postoperatively.

(2) Not known to have this action.

(3) Used in the medically supervised withdrawal period to treat physical dependence on opiates; substitutes a legal for an illegal drug.

168. (3) The drug is not taken for medical reasons but for the favorable, pleasant, unusual, or desired effects it produces. It is often taken in doses that would be fatal if the individual had not established a tolerance to it. (b)

(1) True but also with psychic dependence on the drug.

(2) True but also with physiologic need for the drug.

(4) It is a physiologic and psychologic need to take the drug rather than a compulsion.

169. (3) The addict tries to avoid stress and reality. The drug produces a blurring of these feelings to the point that the addict becomes dependent on it. (a)
    (1) Later on the psychologic effect is usually more important than the ability to ease pain.
    (2) Large doses of narcotics can cause a dreamlike state.
    (4) Hard drugs such as cocaine can increase motor activity.

170. (3) The symptoms of withdrawal reach a peak on the third day. (c)
    (1) Symptoms begin within 8 hours.
    (2) Symptoms become more severe 24 hours later.
    (4) Symptoms begin to subside.

171. (1) The addictive personality is marked by low self-esteem, fear of stress, and dependence with poor self-boundaries and the need for immediate gratification. (b)
    (2) He would be operating on the pleasure principle; would be unable to delay gratification.
    (3) No evidence to support this.
    (4) He would have a strong id drive; usually the ego is weak.

172. (1) When methadone is reduced, a craving for narcotics may occur. Without narcotics anxiety will increase, agitation will occur, and the patient may try to leave the hospital to secure drugs. (b)
    (2) Not related to methadone hydrochloride reduction.
    (3) Not related to reduced methadone hydrochloride dosage.
    (4) May occur with methadone hydrochloride overdose.

173. (4) Alcoholics have a low self-image and overwhelming guilt feelings. They drink to relieve these feelings, but the drinking only adds to them. (b)
    (1) It is not with whom but with what do they have difficulty.
    (2) The problem is with low self-esteem rather than dependence/independence.
    (3) There is no evidence of this.

174. (3) Addresses the emotional impact of this hallucination. The nurse's presence can reduce anxiety and provide comfort. (c)
    (1) This would be entering into the hallucination.
    (2) This is presenting reality but not offering the comfort of your presence.
    (4) Presenting reality but not offering the comfort of your presence.

175. (2) The individual is unaware of gaps in memory, so the use of stories is an unconscious attempt to deny or cover up the gaps. (a)
    (1) Denying is blocking out of conscious awareness rather than a coverup for loss of memory.
    (3) Lying is a deliberate attempt to deceive rather than a face-saving device for loss of memory.
    (4) Rationalizing would be used to explain and justify

his behavior rather than cover up his loss of memory.

176. (4) The patient is using denial as a defense against feelings of guilt. (a)
    (1) May be part of the reason, but the bigger motivating factor is to decrease guilt feeling.
    (2) Denial would deal more with his own expectations of himself.
    (3) It would help make him seem more stable rather than independent.

177. (3) Focuses on the patient's feelings rather than the organization itself. Organization is effective only when the patient is able to discuss feelings openly. (a)
    (1) It may be too late by that time.
    (2) False reassurance; AA may give him insight but may not be able to help him cope with his problem.
    (4) This may or may not be true.

178. (2) Sharing problems with others who are also open and concerned because of similar problems can reduce guilt and shame and begin to increase ego strengths. (a)
    (1) AA is viewed by some as a crutch in itself.
    (3) His problems are caused by how he feels about himself.
    (4) AA is a support group, a self-help group.

179. (3) The nurse's failure to observe what was brought in for the patient constituted negligence. Her knowledge of the alcoholic would warrant checking to see what the patient was consuming. (b)
    (1) Not on a substance abuse unit.
    (2) This is true, except the nurse might have felt that the friend herself had a good effect on the patient.
    (4) Also true, but Mrs. Jane has no manifestation of a psychosis.

180. (4) Thiamine is a coenzyme in producing energy from glucose. If thiamine is not present in adequate amounts, nerve activity is diminished and damage or degeneration of myelin sheaths occurs. (b)
    (1) Used only in the acute phase to control delirium tremens.
    (2) Use of these has a higher risk of toxic side effects in older persons.
    (3) A diet high in the B vitamins would be included in the care plan.

181. (1) Polydrug users abuse a variety of drugs in their search for the ultimate "high." They usually will include alcohol in their search and frequently combine their abuses. (b)
    (2) Not necessarily true.
    (3) Has been mentioned as a possible causative factor but with no evidence to support it.
    (4) Not necessarily so, some become very happy and outgoing.

182. (4) Members find sympathy, patience, and understanding in the group. They are able to have their dependence needs met while helping others who are even more dependent than themselves. (a)

(1) Important for the detoxification stage not overall therapy.

(2) Helpful, but does not have the success rate of AA.

(3) Not getting at what is causing the alcohol problem.

183. (4) Self-help groups are successful because they support a basic human need for acceptance. A feeling of comfort and safety and a sense of belonging may be achieved in a nonjudgmental, supportive, sharing experience with others. (b)

(1) AA would not meet the patient's need to be trusted.

(2) If the patient had a need to grow, AA would not be able to meet this need.

(3) On the contrary, AA meets dependency needs and does little to foster independence.

184. (1) Self-help groups deal with behavior and changes in behavior rather than the underlying causes of behavior. Small steps are encouraged and when attained are reinforced by the group. (c)

(2) Help to identify with the people in the group is not necessary since they all share the same problem and identify readily.

(3) On the contrary, they deal with 1 day at a time.

(4) This is not the purpose of this group.

185. (4) According to the philosophy of Alcoholics Anonymous, the alcoholic must identify his own need to seek help and is thus the primary rehabilitator. (a)

(1) The nurse can give support but is not the primary rehabilitator.

(2) The nurse can give direction but is not the primary rehabilitator.

(3) The entire health team works for the patient, but in dealing with alcoholism the patient is the primary rehabilitator.

186. (1) Intrinsic motivation, stimulated from within the learner, is essential if rehabilitation is to be successful. Often the patient is most emotionally ready for help when he has "hit bottom." Only then is he motivationally ready to face reality and put forth the necessary energy and effort to change his behavior. (a)

(2) An important factor but not the most important one.

(3) An important factor and a helpful one but not the most important one.

(4) An important factor but not the most important one.

187. (4) Past level of success demonstrates ego strengths that can be built on. (b)

(1) This constitutes only a crisis situation, not necessarily a poor prognosis.

(2) His premorbid personality must be fairly sound since he is in his second year of college and thus has achieved some success.

(3) Intelligence has little to do with his recovery, but his ego strengths play a big part.

188. (3) Helps the patient realize that staff members care about him and that he is worthy of care. (b)

(1) An evasive tactic by the nurse.

(2) A response that places the patient on the defensive.

(4) An inappropriate response to a rather obvious situation.

189. (3) Encourages the patient to talk about feelings without really setting the focus for the discussion. (b)

(1) Would make the patient wonder where the nurse had been for 4 days.

(2) Shifts the responsibility of care to the doctor rather than deals with it directly.

(4) Cuts off any further communication of feelings; ignores what he has expressed to the nurse.

190. (4) The nurse failed to use her knowledge regarding suicidal patients and did not protect the patient from this ever-present danger. Her failure could be legally defined as negligence. (b)

(1) If the unit was left unlocked this would not be constant supervision.

(2) Patients are in more danger of suicide when they are coming out of a depression.

(3) Patients need observation even after depression has lifted, especially when plans for discharge are impending.

191. (1) The nurse's major tool in psychiatric nursing is the therapeutic use of self. Psychiatric nurses must learn to be aware of their own feelings and how they affect the situation. (c)

(2) This may be true but is not part of the nurse-patient relationship.

(3) This implies that the nurse is working alone in planning care for the patient.

(4) This may be true, but an awareness of self still seems to be the most difficult.

192. (2) The therapeutic milieu is directed toward helping the patient develop effective ways of dealing with interpersonal situations (b)

(1) This would accomplish nothing in regard to a long-term goal of functioning in society.

(3) This would be a means of achieving the goal.

(4) The hospital atmosphere should be more structured and accepting than the patient's home.

193. (2) Permits the patient to see that his feelings are not unique but are shared by others. (a)

(1) A nonsupportive remark to a fear of leaving the safety of the hospital and going back to where he had to deal with his problem.

(3) Makes Mr. Thomas worry why he does not feel happy.

(4) How the others feel about whether he is ready to be discharged is totally irrelevant.

194. (1) By sensing, supporting, and verbalizing the emotional feelings of others the individual emerges as the leader. (a)

(2) This is a role filled by many group leaders, but it doesn't permit focus on feelings.

(3) The group members do this themselves.

(4) Designation of group members may be done by many people in various ways.

195. (3) Sharing problems with others who have similar problems, thoughts, and feelings helps the individual learn new ways of coping. (b)
     (1) Emotional illness is not enough; the person must recognize that a problem exists and help is necessary.
     (2) We are all dependent on others to some degree; this would not be a criterion for group therapy.
     (4) This might be partly true, but the person should still feel he needs help in coping with a problem.

196. (1) The group setting provides the individual with the opportunity to learn that others share the same problems and needs. The group also provides an arena where new methods of relating to others can be tried. (c)
     (2) It has the opposite effect.
     (3) The focus is still on the individual, but on the individual learning how to relate to others.
     (4) This may happen from time to time with support given to the individual by the group, but it is not a main function of the group.

197. (2) Group therapy should focus on the present and how current problems and feelings are affecting current behavior. In the group setting the individual members have the opportunity to receive feedback on their behavior. (b)
     (1) The focus is the feelings behind the behavior with which others can identify.
     (3) Not the stress itself, but how to deal with the stress.
     (4) The nurse must protect the individual group members from confrontation until certain that the patient is strong enough.

198. (3) A person able to cope with life situations usually has developed fairly strong ego defenses. In a crisis situation the individual frequently just needs support to regroup strengths and reestablish the ability to cope. (b)
     (1) Not possible or realistic.
     (2) Socialization would be part of recovery, not the crisis stage.
     (4) This might have the effect of increasing anxiety, thereby making the crisis situation worse.

199. (2) The current trend in psychiatry is to treat the patient and maintain him in the community. This trend includes the family and community in the plan and has reduced the number of patients in psychiatric hospitals. (a)
     (1) This possibly would have the effect of masking the symptoms and should be used only in conjunction with psychotherapy.
     (3) This would follow when the patient was ready.
     (4) Might be part of the overall treatment plan but not the only aspect.

200. (1) The day hospital provides the patient with a therapeutic setting for a few hours daily during the transitional stage between hospital and total discharge. (b)
     (2) This would have little or no effect on social skills.
     (3) This does help during the transition stage, but it is not the primary goal of day care.
     (4) Day-care treatment would meet this goal, but that is not its primary purpose.

6

Historical and Legal Aspects of Nursing in the United States and Canada

Nursing as it is known today has had a relatively short history—only slightly over 100 years. Modern nursing is usually said to have begun with the work of Florence Nightingale. However, nursing has its roots in ancient days, and many would claim that nursing really antedates all other kinds of health and medical care. Nursing has a history, the knowledge of which should serve to make the modern nurse proud of nursing's heritage and determined to make contemporary nursing meet modern challenges.

Knowledge of nursing development and progress should help in viewing the current problems of nursing in perspective. As each generation enters the nursing field, failure to recognize what has gone before will cause that generation to repeat the mistakes of the past. As knowledge advances, as societies change, as economic situations differ, so will nursing if it is to meet society's needs. The history of nursing then reflects how the leaders in nursing have attempted to meet new demands in new ways without losing sight of the original and fundamental goals of nursing. Modern nursing is fortunate in having as its founder a woman of the stature and wisdom of Florence Nightingale. Continued study of her writings brings new insights and appreciations of her work and its influence.

In the material that follows, emphasis is placed on the modern world, particularly the twentieth century. The various movements that have occurred are treated chronologically because in this way changes and trends can be viewed more easily. Nursing cannot be seen in isolation. Since nursing acts on society and is acted on by society, it must be viewed within the context of that society.

The system of laws is a part of the fabric of a society and will affect the practice of nursing. In the United States, the system of laws has a long history and is still evolving. The influence of other legal systems, notably that of Great Britain, is obvious. All citizens are affected by the laws of the nation and the state, but some laws affect certain segments of society more than others because they specifically apply to that group. Some laws, such as those of licensure, are specific for nurses, whereas others are applied to nurses, if appropriate, such as when nurses are sued for negligence.

There are no questions following this section; the legal questions have been integrated throughout the areas and the comprehensive tests.

NURSING IN THE UNITED STATES
The Twentieth Century

Studies Affecting Nursing and Nursing Education

A. *Nursing and Nursing Education in the United States*—1923
1. Study resulted from a conference sponsored by the Rockefeller Foundation for the purpose of discussing the status of public health nursing
2. Committee for the Study of Public Health Nursing Education was formed, with C.E.A. Winslow as chairman
3. Josephine Goldmark chosen as director of the study; report popularly called the *Goldmark Report*
4. Report included recommendations relative to
   a. Desirability of establishing university schools of nursing that would be adequately financed, administered by a qualified dean, and include liberal arts in the curriculum
   b. Inadequacy of many schools and disadvantages of the apprenticeship system
   c. Need for 2 types of workers in nursing
   d. Admission requirements in hospital schools and curriculum and teaching needs
   e. Kind of training needed by nurses in public health
   f. Postgraduate courses

B. *Nursing Schools Today and Tomorrow*—1934
  1. Committee on the Grading of Nursing Schools was initiated by the National League of Nursing Education but supported by the American Nurses' Association, National Organization of Public Health Nurses, and American Medical Association; this report is popularly called the *Grading Committee Report*
  2. Recommendations included
    a. Employment of graduate nurses to replace students
    b. Closing of inadequate schools
    c. Collegiate-level education with enriched curriculum
    d. Better-prepared students
    e. Better-prepared faculty
C. *Nursing for the Future*—1948
  1. Sponsored by the National Nursing Council, the successor to the National Nursing Council for War Service
  2. Directed by Dr. Esther Lucile Brown and popularly called *The Brown Report*
  3. Included nursing service and nursing education in terms of what was best for the public, not for the profession
  4. Recommendations included
    a. Term *professional* to be used only by those graduated from professional schools or by achievement in some system of examination
    b. Both academic and professional training and basic alterations in the curriculum
    c. Requirements relative to administrative structure, facilities, faculty, and financing of nursing education
    d. Mandatory free accreditation of schools of nursing
    e. Improved training from practical nurses
D. *A Program for the Nursing Profession*—1949
  1. Committee on the Function of Nursing was formed under the aegis of the Division of Nursing Education, Teachers College, Columbia University
  2. Eli Ginsberg, economist, was chosen as chairman; the report is popularly called *The Ginsberg Report*
  3. Recommendations in many ways paralleled those of *Nursing for the Future,* which was going on concurrently
E. *Liberal Education and Nursing*—1959
  1. Study done under the aegis of the Institute of Higher Education, Teachers College, Columbia University, as part of a series covering professions that admit students directly from high school

  2. Findings included
    a. More lip service than reality to inclusion of liberal arts
    b. Some confusion as to what constitutes liberal arts
F. *Community College Education for Nursing*—1959
  1. Cooperative Research Project in Junior and Community College Education for Nursing, sponsored by the Division of Nursing Education, Teachers College, Columbia University, studied the possibility of a 2-year associate degree program to prepare for the technical practice of nursing
  2. Dr. Mildred L. Montag, whose dissertation, *The Education of Nursing Technicians,* laid the foundations for the associate degree program, was named project director
  3. Cooperated with 7 community colleges and 1 hospital school
  4. Findings included
    a. Graduates passed licensing examinations
    b. Evaluated by employers as satisfactory in practice
    c. Colleges could support these programs financially
G. *Abstract for Action*—1970
  1. National Commission for the Study of Nursing and Nursing Education established by the American Nurses' Association and National League for Nursing as a result of the recommendation of the Surgeon General's Consultant Group in Nursing
  2. Recommendations included
    a. Desirability of regional planning
    b. Necessity of research
    c. Single licensure for all in nursing occupation
    d. Academies to recognize excellence in the several specialized areas
    e. Preparation for episodic and distributive nursing
H. *The Study of Credentialing in Nursing*—1979
  1. Inaugurated by the American Nurses' Association and carried on by an independent study committee
  2. Purpose to assess adequacy of current credentialing in nursing and to recommend future directions
  3. Process included literature review, use of secondary data, and survey of certified nurses; identified issues relative to credentialing
  4. Recommendations included
    a. Licensing only one group of nurses—professional

b. Registration of qualified individuals in nursing other than professional

c. A national credentialing center

5. No decision at present as to implementation of any or all recommendations; they are significant recommendations and would require many changes in current practice

Changes in Nursing Organizations

A. American Nurses' Association
1. 1911—name changed from Nurses' Associated Alumnae of United States and Canada
2. 1952—restatement of functions following a study of various nursing organizations; all concerns of individual professional nurses retained by American Nurses' Association
3. 1962—House of Delegates of the American Nurses' Association amended the purposes of the organization
4. 1964—Study Committee appointed to recommend organizational structure to carry out functions
5. 1966—new structure adapted
   a. Three commissions formed
      (1) Economic and General Welfare
      (2) Nursing Education
      (3) Nursing Service
6. 1970—Commission on Research added
7. 1982—Federation structure adopted
   a. State associations now members of the American Nurses' Association
   b. Individual nurses hold ANA membership through membership in state associations
   c. House of Delegates is the official voting and governing body; meets annually
   d. Cabinets established with responsibilities related to functions of the ANA; they are
      (1) Nursing Education
      (2) Nursing Practice
      (3) Nursing Research
      (4) Nursing Services
      (5) Economic and General Welfare
      (6) Human Rights
   e. Councils organized with specific clinical or functional area concerns (e.g., Council on Gerontological Nursing)
8. *American Nurse,* published 10 times per year, is the official newspaper of the ANA; subscription included with membership in the ANA
9. American Nurses' Association headquarters in Kansas City, Missouri
10. Conventions held biennially
11. American Nurses' Foundation—founded in 1955 by American Nurses' Association

a. Supported by public funds as well as contributions by nurses

b. Sponsors and conducts research, disseminates research, and gives consultation

B. National League for Nursing Education
1. Name changed from American Society of Superintendents of Training Schools for Nurses in 1912
2. Membership limited to those involved in nursing education until 1943, when lay members were admitted
3. Served as the education committee of the American Nurses' Association
4. Sponsored curriculum studies and reports
   a. 1917—*Standard Curriculum for Nursing Schools*
   b. 1927—*Curriculum for Schools of Nursing*
   c. 1937—*Curriculum Guide for Schools of Nursing*
5. 1952—became part of the new organization, National League for Nursing

C. National Association for Colored Graduate Nurses
1. Organized in 1908
2. In some states black graduates were not eligible for membership in district, state, and national associations
3. Dissolved in 1951 after the American Nurses' Association (1950) absorbed its functions and responsibilities

D. National Organization of Public Health Nursing
1. Organized in 1912
2. Promotion of public health nursing—coordination and standardization of public health nursing was its major interest
3. Had nurse and lay membership even though it was primarily a nursing organization
4. 1952—became part of the new National League for Nursing

E. Association of Collegiate Schools of nursing
1. Organized in 1932
2. Membership open only to those accredited programs offering college degrees
3. Purpose was to
   a. Develop nursing on professional and collegiate level
   b. Strengthen relationships between schools of nursing and institutions of higher education
   c. Stimulate research and experimentation
4. Had a total of 37 members
5. Dissolved in 1952, becoming a part of the new National League for Nursing

F. American Association of Industrial Nurses
1. Organized in 1942

2. Growth of industry, especially in wartime, prompted greater attention to the welfare of workers and their families
3. American Nurses' Association had an industrial nurse section from 1946 to 1952
4. Was 1 of 6 national organizations that participated in a reorganization study; but withdrew in 1952, maintaining its own organization

G. National League of Nursing
   1. Organized in 1952 as a result of structure study combining the functions and activities of
      a. National League of Nursing Education
      b. National Organization of Public Health Nursing
      c. Association of Collegiate Schools of Nursing
   2. Membership included
      a. Individual members—anyone interested in nursing (registered nurses, practical nurses, nurses' aides, and lay people)
      b. Agency members—hospitals, nursing homes, public health agencies, educational programs, and public schools
   3. Functions included
      a. Identifying needs of society and fostering programs designed to meet these needs
      b. Developing and supporting services to improve nursing care and nursing service
      c. Working with American Nurses' Association for the advancement of nursing
      d. Working with governmental agencies toward the achievement of comprehensive health care
   4. Structure
      a. Membership
         (1) Individual (nurses and consumers)
         (2) Agency (nursing schools, nursing service departments)
      b. Organized in divisions
         (1) Accreditation services
         (2) Continuing education services
         (3) Consultation servces
      c. *Nursing and Health Care,* published 10 times yearly, is the official publication of the NLN
   5. Services provided
      a. Shares responsibility for recruitment with the American Nurses' Association
      b. Accreditation of nursing programs
      c. Test construction
      d. Biennial convention
      e. Headquarters at 10 Columbus Circle, New York, N.Y. 10019

H. National Student nurses' Association
   1. Organized in 1953

2. Individual membership preferred
3. Purpose is chiefly that of preparing for membership in the American Nurses association on graduation
4. Annual conventions
5. Headquarters at 10 Columbus Circle, New York, N.Y. 10019

I. National Association for Practical Nurse Education and Service, Inc.
   1. Organized in 1940
   2. Active in stimulating interest in practical nursing, accrediting programs, and seeking financial support for practical nursing

J. National Federation of Licensed Practical Nurses, Inc.
   1. Founded in 1949
   2. Membership limited to licensed practical nurses
   3. Recognized by the American Nurses' Association as official organization for practical nurses

Special Interest Organizations

A. Association of Operating Room Nurses
   1. Founded in 1957
   2. Membership includes nurses engaged in operating room work at all levels
   3. Interested in new practices and developments in operating room nursing
   4. Holds annual congress

B. American Association of Nurse Anesthetists
   1. Founded in 1931
   2. Membership open to registered nurses who have taken a 12-month course and passed a qualifying examination
   3. Purpose is to further the art of anesthesiology and develop educational standards
   4. Accredits schools of nurse anesthetists

C. American Association of Colleges of Nursing
   1. Founded in 1969
   2. Purpose is to promote university nursing programs and to take positions on issues relevant to higher education in nursing

D. Other specialty associations form as specializations increase

International Organizations

A. International Council of Nurses
   1. Founded in 1899 in Boston
   2. Federation of National Nursing Organizations, of which the American Nurses Association is a member
   3. Membership automatic for individual nurses belonging to national organizations
   4. Congress meets every 4 years—1973 in Mexico City; 1977 in Tokyo; 1981 in Los Angeles; and is scheduled for Tel Aviv in 1985

5. Purposes are to raise the worldwide standards of nursing education and promote the general welfare of nurses
6. Oldest continually functioning international council
7. Headquarters at Geneva, Switzerland

B. International Red Cross
1. Founded by Henri Dunant, a Swiss in 1863
2. Geneva Convention of 1864 confirmed Dunant's original principles
3. International Red Cross Committee coordinates national committees
4. Florence Nightingale medal authorized to be given to nurses of special distinction in 1912
5 American Red Cross—a component part of the International Red Cross
   a. Any graduate nurse may be a member of the Red Cross Nursing Service
   b. The services include
      (1) Teaching home nursing
      (2) Blood collection
      (3) Disaster nursing
      (4) Providing educational materials

C. World Health Organization
1. Organized in 1946 as an agency of the United Nations
2. Nursing recognized as integral part
3. Influential in showing nursing as an essential part of medical and health teams
4. Expert Committees on Nursing organized in 1950 and still serving
5. Reports of Expert Committees, guides for nursing surveys, reports of regional conferences, and seminars help to disseminate knowledge and recommendations about nursing

Advances in Education

A. Early developments in collegiate education
1. First nursing program in the world that was an integral part of a university was developed by the University of Minnesota in 1909
2. By 1931, there were 67 schools of nursing with some connection to a college or university
3. Collegiate programs for graduates of diploma programs were also developed
4. Curriculum influenced by publication of 3 works on curriculum—1917, 1927, 1937 plus additional works relative to faculty and other essentials required for a good school of nursing
5. Accreditation of schools of nursing began in 1939 by the National League of Nursing Education in cooperation with the North Central Association of Colleges and Secondary Schools;

first list of accredited schools was issued in 1941 and contained 70 schools
6. Nursing schools responded in 2 war crises
   a. World War I
      (1) Vassar Training Camp during the summer of 1918 prepared 400 college graduates to transfer to nursing schools in the fall
      (2) Army School of Nursing developed
   b. World War II
      (1) Authorization by Congress of the Cadet Nurse Corps (Bolton Act) in 1943 (discontinued in 1948)
      (2) Accelerated program mandated, all essential theory and practice within 2½-year period with 6 months' experience in military, federal, civilian hospitals, or public health agencies

B. Developments in the second half of the century
1. Development of the associate degree nursing program
   a. The Cooperative Research Program in Junior and Community College Education for Nurses resulted from a proposal in M. Montag's *The Education of Nursing Technicians* (1952-1957)
      (1) Purpose was to develop and test a new program preparing for those functions commonly associated with the registered nurse
      (2) Seven colleges and 1 hospital program cooperated
      (3) Results of the 5-year project published in *Community College Education for Nursing* and stated
         (a) Graduates capable of passing licensing examinations
         (b) Graduates rated by employers as good or better than other graduates of similar experience
   b. Program that developed was greatly different from existing programs in emphasis, curriculum, and length
   c. Programs have had rapid growth, totaling 753 in 1982
   d. Admissions were 61,215 in 1982, with more than half of those preparing for state licensure
2. Developments in baccalaureate degree nursing programs
   a. Designation of the baccalaureate degree as the minimal preparation for the practice of

professional nursing resulted from a recommendation in *Nursing for the Future*

  b. Graduates of diploma programs seeking a baccalaureate degree are admitted to the generic program with advanced standing (usually verified by examination)

  c. Curriculum changed to include
   (1) More emphasis on liberal arts
   (2) Reorganization of the nursing major
   (3) More selective clinical laboratory experiences
   (4) More independent study

  d. Better qualified faculties

  e. Control of the programs is now fully by the universities

  f. Federal funding of construction, special projects, grants to programs, and scholarships and loans to students have helped these programs appreciably

  g. Accreditation of programs has tended to improve quality

  h. Number of programs has increased; in 1982 there were 414

  i. Admissions totaled 36,753 in 1982.

 3. Growth of higher degree nursing programs

  a. Master's degree nursing programs
   (1) Although graduate programs existed before 1959, they have received increased attention since that date
   (2) Programs include those that
    (a) Provide functional preparation for teaching or administration in addition to clinical study
    (b) Provide only a clinical nursing specialty
   (3) Federal funding of students through traineeships has assisted in preparing nurses for careers in teaching, administration, or a clinical specialty
   (4) Programs numbered 154 in 1982, with enrollments of 17,085 (6389 full time)

  b. Doctoral degree nursing programs
   (1) Increased recognition that doctoral preparation is necessary if nursing is to develop true professional status
   (2) University faculty positions often require doctoral preparation
   (3) Research essential to a profession requires doctoral preparation
   (4) Number of nurses holding earned doctorates has increased greatly since 1950; however, the exact number holding doctorates can only be estimated because many nurses receive doctorates in areas other than nursing

 4. Diploma nursing programs

  a. Number has declined since 1955, along with a decline in admissions since that time

  b. In 1982 there were 288 programs, with admissions of 18,928

  c. Changes in curriculum have occurred as a result of the influence of college-based programs, especially the associate degree program

  d. Length has been shortened from 36 months to 27 or 24 months, often following the academic year pattern

  e. Tuition is usually charged

  f. Required living in nurses' dormitories declining, with students usually choosing their own place of residence

  g. More flexible admission requirements are common

 5. Practical nurse programs

  a. Functions stated by the American Nurses' Association and the National Federation of Licensed Practical Nurses, Inc.
   (1) Personal and environmental hygiene, comfort and safety, spiritual needs, observing and recording signs and symptoms not requiring professional judgment
   (2) Contribution to the understanding of the employing institution and staff relationships
   (3) Personal growth

  b. Most programs are now 12 months in length

  c. In 1982 there were 1319 programs, with admissions of 59,696

 6. *American Nurses' Association Position Paper on Nursing Education*—1965

  a. All nursing programs to be within the organized education system of the United States

  b. Recognized 2 types of practice
   (1) Technical—preparation in the associate degree program
   (2) Professional—preparation in the baccalaureate degree program

  c. Aides to be prepared in vocational schools or adult programs instead of on-the-job training

 7. In 1982 The American Nurses' Association House of Delegates approved a resolution describing the baccalaureate degree in nursing as the "minimum qualification for entry into professional practice"

Accreditation of Nursing Programs

A. State board of nursing approval of schools is a form of accreditation, but is mandatory rather than voluntary; no school of nursing can function without state approval under nurse practice acts

B. National League for Nursing has had responsibility for the accrediting of schools of nursing since 1952
  1. Forerunners in the voluntary accreditation of schools were
     a. National Organization of Public Health Nursing
     b. National League of Nursing Education
     c. National Nursing Accrediting Service
  2. Purpose—to improve standards and to make available to the public the names of schools meeting approved criteria
  3. Criteria are set for each type of program
  4. Period of accreditation—6 to 8 years, with reevaluation required if school is to continue on accredited list
  5. National League for Nursing recognized as the approved agency for accrediting by the National Commision on Accreditation
  6. Nurse Training Act of 1964 recognizes the National League for Nursing as the accrediting agency for programs desiring federal funds
  7. List of accredited schools published annually in *Nursing and Health Care*

Advances in Nursing Service

A. Early developments
  1. Employing graduate nurses as part of the nursing staff and thus relieving students from total responsibility for patient care began in 1930s partly as a result of
     a. Closing of small and poor schools resulting from the *Grading Committee Report*
     b. Decrease in private duty nurses as a result of the Depression
  2. Study of nursing service administration sponsored by W.K. Kellogg Foundation in 1951; 14 universities develop master's degree programs preparing for nursing service administration
  3. Introduction of team nursing
     a. Result of a combination of recommendations in *Nursing for the Future* and *A Program for the Nursing Profession*
     b. Nursing team organized to meet the needs of the patient rather than relying on acuteness of illness or techniques needed
        (1) Professional nurse—team leader plans, directs, participates in implementation and evaluates care
        (2) Other nursing personnel—practical nurses and aides contribute to planning and give such care as delegated
        (3) Daily team conference held to plan, delegate, and evaluate care
     c. Term still used, but the concept has been so misunderstood and misused that it has lost its original purpose; where properly interpreted, it can be a useful way of organizing nursing care
  4. Proliferation of workers in nursing
     a. Increased use of auxiliary workers during war years
     b. Increased development of practical nursing programs
     c. Redefinition of practical nursing makes it seem virtually like registered nursing

B. Later developments
  1. Introduction of clinical specialists
     a. Engaged in giving nursing care
     b. Assisting as consultants
  2. Changing baccalaureate curricula produced nurses who were better prepared for professional practice
  3. Increased numbers of nurses with baccalaureate degrees
  4. Introduction of college-educated graduates pointed out the obvious need for orientation of new staff and in-service education
  5. Emphasis on economic security and welfare by the American Nurses' Association
     a. Increased salaries and benefits
     b. Introduced collective bargaining
     c. Produced possibility of strikes
  6. Primary nursing—one way of organizing nursing service to permit the nurse to give total care to the patient and to be held accountable for it

Legislation Influencing Nursing

A. Works Progress Administration (1935)—economic depression of 1929 resulted in many nurses being unemployed; this act made employment possible

B. Social Security Act—1935
  1. 1951—Nurses became eligible for benefits
  2. Amendments in 1965 provided for hospital and medical care for persons 65 years of age and older (Medicare)
  3. Some funds concerned with maternal-child care, blind and crippled children, and the training and employment of nurses in this care

C. Federal Security Agency Appropriations Act—1941
  1. Administered by United States Public Health Service

2. Set aside 1.2 million dollars to assist in training nurses for national defense
3. Appropriation increased to 3.5 million dollars in 1942

D. Nurse Training Act (Bolton Act) (1943)—established the Cadet Nurse Corps
E. Hill-Burton Act (1947)—provided financial aid for construction of hospitals, nursing homes, and other health facilities
F. Health Amendments Act (1956)—provided traineeships for those preparing for teaching, supervision and administration, and public health nursing
G. Nurse Training Acts
   1. 1964—first comprehensive federal legislation to provide for increase in supply of nurses and to assist in modernizing nursing education
   2. 1968—Title II of the Health Manpower Act provided aid to students and to schools of nursing
   3. 1971—Nurse Training Act expanded and extended federal aid until 1974; continued to 1981
   4. Federal monies continue for
      a. Scholarships and loans
      b. Traineeships
      c. Construction
      d. Support for nursing schools
      e. Projects to improve nursing education and recruitment

Current Developments

A. Changes in the legal definition of nursing
   1. 1972—New York state law for the registered professional nurse was changed to include
      a. Diagnosing and treating human response to actual or potential health problems through
         (1) Case finding
         (2) Health teaching
         (3) Health counseling
      b. Providing care supportive to or restorative of life and well-being
      c. Executing the medical regimen prescribed by a licensed physician or dentist
   2. Most of the states have broadened their laws in similar fashion
   3. Current laws more nearly reflect the role nursing plays in health care
B. Many states, and the number is increasing, require continuing education for licensure; the aim is to ensure current competency
C. The American Nurses' Association has moved to organize for collective action
   1. Emphasis to be on achieving quality care
   2. Assure the public of accountability of nurses
   3. Increase accessibility of health services

4. Interest in economic welfare not abandoned but emphasis decreased
5. Commission on Education of the American Nurses' Association, after a period of relative inactivity, has become more aggressive
6. Political action committee; purpose is to promote health care of people by encouraging nurses to take a more active and effective part in government

D. Increasing numbers of professional nurses are going into private practice as individual practitioners or in groups under partnership arrangements
   1. Conduct screening
   2. Give nursing care
   3. Teach preventive health measures
E. Nursing education
   1. Career ladder
      a. Advocates of this concept desire a curriculum that begins at either the practical nurse or the associate degree level and articulates with each succeeding level up to a master's degree
      b. Opponents of this concept contend that it would virtually destroy the integrity of each program and further confuse the use of the products of each program
      c. Several programs have been designed to carry out the idea
   2. External degree program
      a Nontraditional program that does not require enrollment in or attendance at any nursing program
      b. Competency validated by both written and performance examinations
      c. Examinations include those in general education and nursing
      d. Performance examinations given in a hospital setting with actual patients
      e. Program attractiveness can be judged by the number of applicants enrolled
      f. Currently offered only by New York State
   3. Curriculum change in baccalaureate programs
      a. Focus of organization changing from the traditional ''Big 5'' to emphasis on the nursing process and nursing functions
      b. Changes necessary to implement the role of nurses as described in the new definitions of nursing
      c. Enlarging to include the expanded role of the nurse in
         (1) Health maintenance
         (2) Primary care
         (3) Screening
         (4) Community health
      d. Increasing use of independent study

4. Increasing number of practitioner programs
   a. Nurse practitioner—one skilled in assessment and management of psychosocial and developmental problems and able to function independently
   b. Specialty nurse practitioner (e.g., family nurse practitioner, pediatric nurse practitioner)
5. Increasing number of programs leading to doctorates in nursing

F. Nursing service
   1. Primary nursing
      a. Plan of organization using the nursing process whereby a nurse is responsible for total care of the patient or a group of patients
      b. Primary nurse—plans and carries out the program of care
      c. Requires greater attention to the nurse's comments regarding the patient; integrates nurses' notes with notes of other health professionals
   2. Problem-Oriented Medical Records (POMR)
      a. Increasing use of this method of categorizing the patient's problems rather than using diagnostic classification
      b. Method is criticized by some physicians and nurses
         (1) No panacea for poorly written notes by physicians or nurses
         (2) Too well-defined and categorized problems
         (3) Repetitive
   3. Peer review
      a. Nurses actively engaged in nursing appraise the quality of individual nursing care according to established standards of practice
      b. Essential if nurses are to be held accountable for care given
      c. Useful in helping individual nurses improve their own practice
      d. Useful in recommending nurses for advancement or merit increases
   4. Clinical specialist
      a. High degree of knowledge, skill, and competence in a specialized area
      b. Use is increasing as more nurses are prepared in master's degree programs

G. Institutional licensure
   1. Proposal that health care facilities would have the authority to determine proper utilization of personnel according to specific job descriptions
   2. Individual licensing laws for nurses and other health workers (except physicians and dentists) would be eliminated

3. Proponents argue that this would increase flexibility, permit better utilization of personnel, and improve health care
4. Opponents contend that, although new ways are needed in institutions, this proposal would not improve the situation
   a. Knowledge and judgment needed because the tasks rather than the mechanics of the tasks should be the controlling factor
   b. Job descriptions already present
   c. Educators cannot prepare workers unless they know what is needed
   d. Competency is an individual responsibility, not exclusively the responsibility of the employer

H. Developments related to and influencing nursing
   1. Moves toward national health insurance
      a. For several years bills have been introduced, but none has become law
      b. Believed inevitable in the future
   2. Social and economic factors
      a. Increased cost of medical care
      b. Increase in persons over 65 years of age in population
      c. Declining birth rate
      d. Family planning
      e. Need for consideration of minority groups in education and employment
      f. Housing needs
      g. Hunger and malnutrition
   3. Increase in number and types of health professionals (e.g., respiratory therapists, operating room technicians, emergency technicians)
   4. Changes in medical practice include
      a. Increased specialization
      b. Increased skill in organ transplants
      c. Improved anesthetic agents increasing safety of surgical intervention
      d. Drug research and screening—more scrutiny of drugs reaching the market
      e. Presence of physician's assistants
   5. Increase in hospital beds with concurrent emphasis on ambulatory care
   6. Proliferation of nursing homes and extended care centers
   7. Shortage of nurses—a controversial subject
      a. Largest number of registered nurses employed in history—800,000
      b. Maldistribution a factor in supply and demand
      c. Economic situation in the nation influences employment
      d. The existence of an oversupply and overuse of practical nurses is a debatable subject

8. The Patient's Bill of Rights (American Hospital Association)—a bill of particulars designed to protect patients by establishing standards governing the hospital's and professional staff's responsibility to patients and their families

NURSING IN CANADA
The Twentieth Century

Studies Affecting Nursing and Nursing Education

A. *Special Committee on Nurse Education*—1916
   1. Report presented to the Canadian National Association of Trained Nurses
   2. Recommendations included that
      a. Nurse training schools or colleges be established within the educational system of each province
      b. Nurse training schools be separated in organization from hospitals that were still to be used for practical training

B. *Survey of Nursing Education in Canada* (Weir report)—1932
   1. Study of nursing education in Canada jointly sponsored by the Canadian Nurses' Association and the Canadian Medical Association under the chairmanship of Dr. Stewart Cameron
   2. Purpose was to investigate growing criticism about nursing and its training system across the 5 main sections of Canada
   3. Report contained recommendations on
      a. Delivery of health care (e.g., the need for a comprehensive system of supervision and control of nursing personnel)
      b. Nursing as a profession (e.g., Provincial Registration Acts required amendments in areas related to nursing education)
      c. Private duty nursing (e.g., only registered graduates should be allowed to use the title *nurse*)
      d. Institutional nursing (e.g., training schools should be established within educational institutions)
      e. Student nurses (e.g., a period of internship as part of regular nurses' training may be desirable)
      f. Teachers of nursing (e.g., the number of full-time qualified teachers should be increased)
      g. Examination system (e.g., only graduates of approved training schools should be permitted to write the examination)

C. *Proposed Curriculum for Schools of Nursing*—Canadian Nurses' Association; the 1939 curriculum proposal and a 1940 supplement, *Improvement of Nursing Education in the Clinical Field,* arose from recommendations in the Weir report

D. *Evaluation of the Metropolitan School of Nursing* (Lord report)–1952
   1. Study to examine all aspects of this demonstration program (less than 3 years in length) jointly sponsored by the Canadian Nurses' Association and the Canadian Red Cross under the direction of Nettie Fidler
   2. Concluded that
      a. Average graduate of this program compared favorably with the average graduate of the control school in both bedside skills and achievement on the Registered Nurse Examination
      b. Schools with complete control of students can prepare nurses in 2 years as well as those prepared in 3 years

E. *Report on the Experiment in Nursing Education at the Atkinson School of Nursing of the Toronto Western Hospital*—1955
   1. Before the project at the Metropolitan School was completed, a project under the direction of W. Stewart Wallace was begun at the Toronto Hospital
   2. Program was to follow the same curriculum as Metropolitan School, but an "intern" third year under the control of Nursing Service was added
   3. Study showed problems developed because of the 2 plus 1 nonintegrated pattern of the program and the division of authority between the school and hospital

F. *Study of Nursing Education in New Brunswick*—1956
   1. Sponsored by the New Brunswick Department of Health and Social Service and reported by Kathleen Russell
   2. Recommendations included that
      a. Hospital schools reorganize to become independent by 1957
      b. Students be ensured more direct patient care during clinical experience
      c. Interprovincial reciprocal registration be set up
      d. A school of nursing be established at the University of New Brunswick
      e. A 3-month psychiatric affiliation be included in all nursing programs
      f. The provincial association hold 3-month institutes for the preparation of clinical instructors until postgraduate courses can be established
      g. Policies for the organization and preparation of nursing assistant groups be written

G. *Report of the Pilot Project for the Evaluation of Schools of Nursing in Canada (Spotlight on Nursing Education)*—1960
   1. Sponsored by the nursing profession through the Canadian Nurses' Association under the direction of Helen K. Mussallem to study readiness for voluntary national accreditation
   2. Recommendations included that
      a. Reexamination of nursing education in Canada be undertaken
      b. Improvement program to upgrade programs be started
      c. Quality of nursing service in clinical agencies be evaluated
      d. Accreditation program for schools be established by the Canadian Nurses' Association
H. *Royal Commission on Health Services Briefs*—1961 Projected evolvement of 2 levels of nurses: those required for leadership roles and those technically skilled for bedside nursing
I. *Report of the Royal Commission on Health Services*
   1. Suggested expansion of university schools of nursing especially at masters and doctoral levels
   2. Recommended that baccalaureate programs in nursing develop integrated curriculum
   3. Recommended establishment of a comprehensive, compulsory, universal health service program for all Canadians
   4. Specifically recommended that
      a. Schools of nursing have budgets separate from nursing service
      b. Diploma nurses be registered and graduated from 2-year nursing programs
      c. Salaries comparable with education and responsibility in other fields be paid nurses
   5. Recommendations that were implemented as a result included new patterns of nursing curricula, home care programs, health councils, and group practices
J. *Report of the Nursing Education Survey Committee for the Province of Alberta* (Scarlett report)—1961-1963
   1. Sponsored by the Department of Health in Alberta
   2. Recommendations included that
      a. A provincial council of nursing be established for licensing of all nursing personnel; licensure be mandatory for those who nurse for hire in Alberta
      b. Nursing education remain under the aegis of the University of Alberta and the program be shortened to 4 years
      c. The 2-year program as demonstrated by the Nightingale School in Toronto not be instituted in Alberta because of the costs of such a program
K. *Report on the Canadian Nurses' Association School Improvement Program* (Glenna S. Rowsell)—1961-1964
   1. Emerged from a recommendation of *The Report of the Pilot Project for the Evaluation of Schools of Nursing in Canada* in 1960; examined 168 diploma schools (98% of all such schools in Canada)
   2. Reaffirmed the impracticality of an accreditation program of schools of nursing at this time; based on task force recommendations
   3. Task force also made the following recommendations relative to the School Improvement Program:
      a. Canadian Nurses' Association create a department of nursing education to act in consultant capacity to new programs and in nursing research
      b. Canadian Nurses' Association clarify beliefs about nursing education and nurses' roles in society
   4. Indicated the need for continued study in areas of philosophy and school objectives, organization and administration, curriculum, facilities, and residence living
L. *Study of the Development of a Diploma Program in Nursing at the Ryerson Institute of Technology, Toronto*—1963
   1. Submissions made to the Royal Commission on Health Services by nursing leaders that a nursing program be conducted at a level after high school under the jurisdiction of an educational institution; program approved in 1963 by the College of Nurses of Ontario and conducted at the Ryerson Institute of Technology
   2. The 5-year experimental program had its own governing body and budget, a well-qualified teaching staff, 1 full-time teacher per 10 students, and control of student time and experience over a maximum 30-hour week
   3. 1973—success of the program evident; a provision was made for its continuance following an evaluation by Moyra Allen
M. *Plan for the Development of Nursing Education Programs Within the General Educational System of Canada*—1964
   1. Sponsored by the Canadian Nurses' Association under the direction of Helen K. Mussallem and popularly called *A Path to Quality*

2. Basic elements advocated by the project and rebuffed by the Canadian Hospital Association were that
   a. Nursing programs be developed within educational systems
   b. Two categories of nursing personnel be prepared
      (1) Professional nurse to be prepared in a 4-year university program
      (2) Technical nurse to be prepared in a 2-year program under educational auspices
   c. Two categories to be prepared in a ratio of 1 professional to 3 technical nurses
N. *Royal Commission on Health Services Nursing Education in Canada* (Dr. Helen K. Mussallem)—1964
   1. Purpose was to examine and analyze all types of formal educational programs for personnel providing nursing care with emphasis primarily on those preparing nurses for registration in the provinces
   2. Recommended that
      a. Deplorable lack of qualified teachers be remedied as soon as possible
      b. Diploma schools of nursing be part of the provinces' systems after high school
      c. Educational programs be revised to prepare 2 levels of nurses—the university and diploma nurses, with the former providing leadership in nursing practice and the latter assisting the professional nurse
      d. More graduate programs be designed to prepare nurses in research, consultation, and nursing specialties
O. *A Plan for the Education of Nurses in the Province of New Brunswick (Portrait of Nursing)*—1965
   1. Sponsored by the New Brunswick Association of Registered Nurses and directed by Katherine MacLaggan
   2. Purposes of the undertaking were
      a. To project a plan for education 2 categories of nurses
      b. To present a plan for nurse education
         (1) To those in the general educational system of the province
         (2) To those responsible for nursing education and its development
   3. Canadian Hospital Association wanted hospitals to continue operation of nursing schools even though 84 junior college programs had been initiated in the United States by this time
   4. Recommendations included that
      a. Federal, provincial, and local governments

finance nurse education at Institutes of Health Sciences
      b. Four health service groups be formed with clearly written levels of function (nurse Grades I and II, secretaries, wardkeepers)
      c. Provincial Councils on Education for Health Services be formed and be responsible to the Ministry of Education
      d. Local management boards be responsible for
         (1) Setting and receiving tuition
         (2) Approving personnel appointments
         (3) Approving all programs of education prior to submission to the Provincial Council for consideration
         (4) Contracting for clinical experience
P. Committee on the Healing Arts
   1. Established by the province of Ontario, July 1966
   2. Study investigated the role and function of nursing personnel, nature of nursing activities, supply and demand, curriculum, teaching staff requirements
   3. Recommendations included that
      a. The provincial association merge with the Ontario Association of Registered Nursing Assistants
      b. Studies be done to improve nurse resource utilization
      c. Activities representing the practice of nursing be defined
      d. The Labor Relations Act be amended according to the British Columbia model
      e. The Canadian Nurses' Association continue to develop uniform standards of registration
Q. *Report on the Project for the Evaluation of the Quality of Nursing Service* (sponsored by the Canadian Nurses' Association)—1966
   1. First attempt to evaluate the quality of nursing service, administrtion, and nursing care being provided within the concept of total patient care
   2. Recommendations were that
      a. Nursing service departments evaluate care given
      b. Roles, functions, and relationships of physicians, nurses, and administrators within patient care area be defined
      c. Standards for nursing service and hospital accreditation programs be set
      d. Nursing personnel be used more economically
      e. Individual nursing care plans be implemented

    f. More challenging clinical experiences be structured for students using problem-solving approaches

R. Ad Hoc Committee on Nursing Education, Department of Public Health, Province of Saskatchewan—1966
  1. Formed after the recommendation of the Royal Commission on Health Services that Nursing Education Planning Committees be established provincially
  2. Submitted basic guidelines for a system of educating nurses in Saskatchewan based on the belief that authority and responsibility for nurse education belonged to an agency whose primary concern was education
  3. Recommendations included that
    a. Department of Education be responsible for education of nurses including the diploma level
    b. Provincial Nurses' Association determine the minimum admission standards and standards for registration
    c. Two central schools be established by the Department of Education and hospital schools be phased into these
    d. Present 5-year university program be altered to 4-year integrated baccalaureate program and enrollment be increased by 50%
    e. University certificate courses be eventually phased out

S. *Community Colleges and Nursing Education in Ontario* (R. G. Quittendon)—1968
  1. Study initiated to provide data for optimum development of nurse training in relation to community needs
  2. Findings were that
    a. Nonuniversity, post–secondary school enrollments increased 400% between 1955 and 1966 in Canada
    b. Ontario University enrollments increased 250% between 1955 and 1965
    c. Diploma nursing enrollment in Ontario increased 35% between 1955 and 1965, whereas nursing assistant enrollment increased 100%
    d. Health science divisions were needed in community colleges for training health team members

T. *Ontario Council of Health Report*—1969
  1. Ontario Council of Health received legislative approval in 1968, becoming Senior Advisory body to Minister of Health
  2. Guidelines for study set forth by the Royal Commission on Health Services; included health care delivery, health manpower, education of health disciplines, and regional organization of health services

U. *Report of the Ontario Health Council on Health Care Delivery Systems*—1970
  1. Prepared by a subcommittee on community health and presented to the Ontario Council of Health
  2. Recommendations included
    a. Urgent need to make primary care more accessible from existing health workers
    b. Development of ambulatory care facilities
    c. Involvement of health science centers and professional faculties in primary health care delivery
    d. Examination of the role of the community health nurse in health services
    e. Establishment of health resource centers

V. *Task Force Reports on Cost of Health Services in Canada-Public Health Services*—1970
  1. Suggested that public health practice was not as effective or economically sound as it might be
  2. Recommendations included that
    a. Health services be regionalized
    b. Levels of community care be available to the public
    c. Home care programs be expanded
    d. University programs in public health be strengthened
    e. Community health centers be constructed
    f. Governments subsidize group practice by physicians
    g. Studies be done in use of physician-associates

W. *Task Force Reports on Cost of Health Service in Canada*—1970
  1. Established by the Conference of Ministers of Health of Canada in 1968 to inquire into ways of restraining escalating health services expenditures
  2. Areas of inquiry related to hospital services
  3. Recommendations included that
    a. Nursing units not be staffed for maximum nursing care loads, adding personnel as required
    b. A uniform classification of care functions be established for Canada
    c. Specialized service units be encouraged
    d. Ambulatory care facilities be developed, along with community health centers

e. Home care programs be expanded

f. Standards for nursing care be formulated and measured

g. Accreditation be mandatory for all hospitals of a national, nongovernmental nature

h. Community mental health clinics be developed

i. Further studies related to use of physician-associates be done

Changes in Nursing Organizations

A. Canadian Nurses' Association

1. 1951—*Structure Study of the Canadian Nurses' Association* undertaken by Dr. Pauline Jewett; the structure was changed in 1954

2. Structure changed again in 1962; in 1966 standing committees were reduced

3. Canadian Nurses' Association now a federation of 12 member associations (10 provinces and 2 territories); as of 1982 it represented 136,000 professional nurses

4. Affairs of the Canadian Nurses' Association are managed by a 24-member board of directors, which serves a 2-year term and is composed of 9 directors elected at a general meeting, 12 directors from association members, and 3 public-appointed representatives

5. Canadian Nurses' Association offers the following services and functions:

a. Research and advisory aid

b. Library

c. Information services

d. Labor relations

e. Testing service

f. International role

g. Liaison

6. Objectives of the Canadian Nurses' Association as stated in the constitution are to

a. Promote high standards of nursing practice

b. Promote educational programs required to achieve high standards of practice

c. Encourage understanding and unity among nurses

d. Speak for Canadian nursing and represent the Canadian Association to other organizations on national and international levels

e. Foster and participate in affairs contributing to community services

f. Promote the social and economic welfare of the nurse in the practice of the profession

g. Promote nursing research

h. Promote high standards of nursing administration

7. Canadian Nurses' Association celebrated its 50th anniversary in 1958, the year in which the first French-Canadian, Alice M. Girard, was elected president; the CNA celebrated its 75th anniversary in 1983

8. Activities included

a. 1961—establishment, with the Kellogg Foundation, of a bilingual nursing unit administration extension program

b. 1962—establishment of the Canadian Nurses' Foundation

c. 1965—first national inventory of registered nurses

d. 1967—development of the Canadian Nurses' Association Testing Service (CNATS) to be used by provincial associations for registration and for licensing purposes instead of the National League for Nursing Examinations

e. Comprehensive Examination for Registered Nurses—registration and licensing purposes (August 1980)

(1) Offered in both French and English

(2) Blueprint relates to a nursing model rather than the previously used medical model

f. Prevention of the introduction of physician's assistants

g. Support of the transfer of nursing education to the mainstream of education

h. Development of comprehensive examinations for registration based on a nursing model

i. Housing the national nurses' library

j. Development of a national data bank on collective bargaining

9. 1982—two types of membership created for organizations closely allied with the CNA

a. Associate membership for national nursing groups

b. Affiliate membership for other national groups

10. National associations with membership in the CNA include

a. Canadian Association of Neurological and Neurosurgical Nurses

b. Canadian Nurses Respiratory Society

c. National Operating Room Nurses

B. Student Nurses' Association—first organized system of student government in Canadian schools of nursing; established in 1917 at the Toronto General Hospital

C. Canadian University Nursing Student Association (CUNSA)
   1. Draws membership from 22 universities
   2. Provides a communication link, about major nursing issues, among Canadian university students
   3. Acts as a liaison with other organizations concerned with nursing
   4. Assists with or initiates nursing research
D. Canadian Association of University Schools of Nursing (CAUSN)
   1. Originally formed as the Canadian Conference of University Schools of Nursing
   2. 1971—name changed from Canadian Conference of University Schools of Nursing to allow for French translation, "Association Canadiènne des Ecoles Univérsitaires de Nursing"
   3. As of 1980, 23 university schools represented
   4. Objectives are to
      a. Develop criteria for university education in nursing
      b. Promote research in nursing
      c. Promote interchange of nursing knowledge
      d. Foster the idea that university education in nursing contributes to development of Canada's health services
   5. Assisted in the Kellogg-sponsored conference on doctoral preparation for nurses in Canada
   6. CAUSN—serves as the official accrediting agency for university nursing programs in Canada
   7. Major concerns at the 1982 annual meeting—theoretical pluralism and nursing, identification of the philosophical cutting edge of nursing, ethical imperatives of theoretical pluralism, and a conceptual model for nursing
E. Nurse Practitioners Association of Ontario
F. Canadian Council of Health Services Executives (CCHSE)—concerned with issues related to nurse administrators, including education, standards, and certification-voluntary examination for certification in 1983

Special Interest Organizations
A. Canadian Red Cross—component of the International Red Cross
B. Victorian Order of Nurses—plays an active role in health care delivery, including provincial home care programs, care of the aging, prevention of suicide among the young, and care of pregnant teenagers
C. Special interest groups
   1. Canadian Association of Practical and Nursing Assistants (CAPNA), 1972
   2. Canadian Intravenous Nurses Association (CINA), 1975
      a. Sets flexible standards for IV care
      b. Circulates *American Journal of IV Therapy* in Canada
   3. Canadian Nurses Foundation (CNF), 1962—provides scholarships for graduate studies in nursing and for nursing research
   4. Canadian Orthopedic Nurses Association (CONA)—provides continuing education in orthopedics to promote the highest standards of practice
   5. National Conference of Operating Room Nurses
      a. Concerned with continuing education and care standards for OR nurses
      b. Newest CNA affiliate
   6. Psychiatric Nurses Association of Canada, 1965
      a. Concerned with mental health and national standards of psychiatric care
      b. Publishes the *Canadian Journal of Psychiatric Nursing*
   7. Nursing Sisters Association of Canada
   8. Registered Nurses of Canadian Indian Ancestry (RNCIA), 1975
   9. National Committee of Canadian Nurse Midwives—formulation of a national association of nurse midwives; still under discussion

Advances in Education
A. Early developments in university education
   1. Several trends have strengthened the need for more advanced education for nurses
      a. Rapidly widening scope of medical practice
      b. General public concern regarding health and social welfare
      c. Increasingly critical evaluation of professional education
   2. 1919—University of British Columbia offered the first baccalaureate degree course in nursing in the British Empire; patterned on the $2+2+1$ program already established at the University of Minnesota
   3. 1920—6 universities began certificate or diploma courses of 1-year duration in public health nursing and teaching and administration with grants from the Canadian Red Cross
      a. First course in public health nursing at Dalhousie University in Halifax
      b. First course in teaching and administration established at McGill University, Montreal
   4. 1924—Grey Nuns organized first French language course in nursing education and ward administration for graduate nurses at University of Montreal
   5. 1925—first French language public health nursing course in Canada established at the University of Montreal

6. 1933—University of Toronto received a Rockefeller Grant to be utilized in establishing a 4-year, integrated basic baccalaureate degree program that would prepare graduates for varied types of nursing service (first program of this nature in Canada)
7. 1941—first joint conference of the Canadian Nurses' Association Executive Committee and directors of the Canadian University Schools of Nursing
8. Problems in establishing university programming for nurses even in the 1940s because of
   a. Ambivalent approach of many nurses
   b. Lack of qualified staff
   c. Unwillingness of hospitals to accept loss of student time and service
   d. Increased costs involved in higher education programs
9. No parallel development in graduate nursing education occurring, with the result that Canadian nurses went to the United States for postgraduate studies, a move that further delayed postgraduate programming in Canada

B. Developments in the second half of the century
   1. Esther Lucile Brown's study, *Nursing for the Future* (published in the United States in 1948)—had implications for nursing education in Canada
   2. Only 2 significant national studies in nursing education done by the Canadian Nurses' Association
   3. Hospitals own and operate 90% of schools of nursing
   4. Major development in the late 1950s—establishment of a prepaid hospital insurance program that included the cost of operating nursing schools in hospitals despite the opposition of the nursing profession
   5. Various types of nursing programs leading to the diploma rather than the baccalaureate degree exist in Canada today
      a. Traditional courses in a hospital school of nursing in Alberta, British Columbia, Manitoba, New Brunswick (phased out in 1976), Nova Scotia, and Newfoundland
      b. Community colleges in Quebec (Collèges d'Enseignement Général et Professional; the CEGEP Programs), Ontario, Alberta, Saskatchewan (Institutes of Applied Arts and Sciences), Newfoundland (started in 1975), British Columbia, and Manitoba
      c. System of Regional and Independent Schools of Nursing in Prince Edward Island and New Brunswick
      d. Programs for Psychiatric Nurses in British Columbia, Manitoba, Alberta, and Saskatchewan
   6. Nightingale School of Nursing—Toronto
      a. Begun in 1960
      b. Regional school controlling the educational program and utilizing resources within a given geographic area
      c. Supported by the Board of Governors of New Mount Sinai Hospital, Toronto
      d. Operating costs borne by the government of Ontario with monies derived from the health insurance program
      e. An alternative to the centralized school system in Alberta and the community college system in Quebec and British Columbia
   7. Quo Vadis Nursing Program
      a. Founded in Toronto in 1964 somewhat as a result of a recommendation made by Dr. Mussallem in *Nursing Education in Canada* (1962).
      b. Nursing education for women between 30 and 50 years of age, with privileges of living at home and working a regular workday 5 days per week
      c. First students graduated in 1966
      d. Program transferred to the community college system in 1973
   8. Development of diploma programs in Ontario after 1965
      a. Minister of Health challenged the pattern of diploma programs in Ontario by announcing that
         (1) Annual number of graduates doubled
         (2) Length of program reduced to 2 years within regional schools
         (3) Third internship year in a hospital nursing service required from 1965 to 1975
         (4) Schools have their own budgets with monies supplied by the Department of Health
      b. 1969—Provincial Association supported the abolition of the internship year as well as urging the financing of nurse education in the same way as other postsecondary programs
      c. 1971—internship program phased out, leaving nursing with a 2-year program pattern
      d. By 1973—all nursing education programs at the diploma level transferred to the system of Colleges of Applied Arts and Technology

e. 1980—Ministry of Colleges and Universities in Ontario decreed a change in minimum hours for diploma nursing programs from 1200 to 1625 hours of clinical practice and 750 hours of theory, not to exceed 24 months in length

9. Accelerated nursing program at Grey Nun's Hospital School of Nursing—1966
   a. Experimental 2-year nursing program in the general educational system
   b. System for which students paid tuition
   c. Students not used for hospital service
   d. Structured liberal education component included
   e. Students wrote registration examinations at the end of 2 years

10. 1966—Saskatchewan the first province in Canada to transfer authority for hospital schools of nursing from the Department of Public Health to the Department of Education

11. Collèges d'Enseignement Général et Professional (CEGEP)
    a. *Report of the Royal Commission of Inquiry on Education* (Parent report) in Quebec—nursing education should move into the general educational system, a transfer approved by the Association of Nurses for the Province of Quebec (ANPQ)
    b. Provincial legislature adopted the *Criteria for College Education* from the Parent report in 1964; among these were that
       (1) All college teachers have appropriate academic preparation
       (2) System of accreditation be established
       (3) Definite student/teacher ratio be used
    c. 1966—Concept of nursing education in Collèges d'Enseignement Général et Professional (CEGEP) introduced, with 3 colleges starting nursing options in 1967
    d. 1972—last of schools of nursing based within hospitals closed its doors, ending three fourths of a century of history

12. Diploma nursing programs in community college settings (including CEGEP programs)
    a. 1970—119 community colleges across Canada had 100,701 students enrolled in nursing programs; 32,426 in university *stream* courses, 68,275 in vocational courses
    b. 1973—of 142 diploma programs, 101 were in educational institutions; 12,882 enrolled in initial programs, and 89% of these entered at diploma level; graduations from initial programs decreased to 9514

c. A 2-year unique educational program distinct from both secondary and higher levels of education was offered by 42 Quebec CEGEP schools in 1980; at the 82nd annual assembly of the Order of Nurses of Quebec, accord was reached that the baccalaureate degree become entry to practice as recommended in the Weir report (1927)

d. 1974—brief presented to the Superior Council of Education on the advantges and perpetual deficiencies of the nursing option in the CEGEP system; recommendations include that
   (1) Information sessions on different levels of nurse training be offered by Department of Education and Order of Nurses of Quebec for vocational counselors
   (2) Professional improvement programs and incentives be established to allow employed teachers to take needed courses; in 1973 57.6% of teachers were still without a bachelor's degree
   (3) Programs of study be established to facilitate articulation between college and university programs with a minimum of upgrading
   (4) Clinical training periods be revised to improve intensity and continuity; the clinical ratio be maintained at 1:6 (theory to practice)
   (5) Hospital centers devise procedures to facilitate integration of graduates into labor market and include adequate budgets for orientation, in-service, and continuing education programs

13. Development of baccalaureate degree programs
    a. 1961—in a brief presented to the Royal Commission on Health Services in Canada, the Canadian Association of University Schools of Nursing stated that a baccalaureate degree provided generalized preparation whereas masters and doctoral programs would prepare nursing consultants, experts in the clinical fields, and researchers
    b. 1961—beginning of the Extension Course in Nursing Unit Administration at Toronto, sponsored by the Canadian Nurses' Association with the financial support of the Kellogg Foundation, to assist head nurses in upgrading their skills in administration
       (1) Sponsored jointly by the CNA and the Canadian Hospital Association (CHA); located in Ottawa, with a regional office

to oversee the French component of the program in Montreal

(2) Effective September 1982, enrollment of nurses with 3 years' current work experience permitted; requirement of an administrative position eliminated

(3) NUA program 10 months long, with a home study component and two 4-day conferences

(4) University of Montreal, Faculty of Continuing Education, now granting 9 credits to graduates of the French component of the NUA program

c. 1962—University of Montreal the first university in Canada to establish a faculty of nursing, with Alice M. Girard as Dean

d. First basic integrated degree program in the world taught in French instituted at the Institut Marguerite d'Youville, Montreal, in 1962

e. 1967—Institut Marguerite d'Youville amalgamated with the University of Montreal, becoming the first university in the world to offer both undergraduate and graduate degrees in nursing taught in French

f. Following the Royal Commission on Health Services in Canada, nursing education began a new era with the major development being the general increase in the numbers of basic integrated baccalaureate programs

(1) 1963—16 programs, 8 integrated and 8 nonintegrated

(2) 1964-1973—graduations from baccalaureate degree programs increased from 2% to 6% of total graduations

(3) 1973—ratio of basic degree graduates to diploma graduates 1:15

(4) Some 22 programs integrated, with basic baccalaureate programs having 14% of the 28,028 enrollment to initial programs

(5) 1974—nonintegrated programs phased out of universities

(6) 1982—several universities offering programs for nursing

(a) 6 French language universities offering baccalaureate degrees

(b) 19 English language universities offering baccalaureate degrees

(c) 1 polytechnical institute (Ryerson, Toronto) offering Bachelor of Applied Arts (Nursing), BAA(N)

g. 1973—University of British Columbia Program permitting students to become registered nurses on completion of first 2 years of baccalaureate program

14. Higher degree programs

a. Nurses wanting to pursue graduate study in nursing beyond baccalaureate degree until 1959 were required to do so in the United States

b. Masters programs in Canada could not evolve until sufficient numbers of baccalaureate programs and graduates had been produced; in 1982, 12 masters programs were offered, one in French at the University of Montreal and 11 in English

c. 1959—University of Western Ontario established the first Canadian masters degree program in nursing, followed by McGill University

d. 1962—Canadian Nurses' Foundation incorporated to provide monies for study at masters and doctoral levels and for research in nursing service

e. 1974—McGill University School of Nursing revised the masters program to offer 2 options: nurse clinician and nurse researcher programs

f. No doctoral programs are yet available in Canada; the Steering Committee, Operation Bootstrap, established in August, 1980, for the purpose of exploring establishment of a doctoral program was dissolved when Kellogg Foundation funding was not obtained

g. Health science centers integrated with nursing programs in at least two universities

h. Family practice nurse program offered by at least one university

15. By the year 2000—entry to nursing practice will be a baccalaureate degree

a. Implementation phase entered with appointment by the CNA of a task force in 1982

b. Chief task—to set up a comprehensive concrete national plan, including objectives, activities, and target dates for implementation; issues to be addressed will include impact of the baccalaureate degree on health care systems, educational systems, and nursing services

c. British Columbia, Alberta, Saskatchewan (degree by 1990), Quebec, and New Brunswick in agreement

d. Registered Nurses Association of Nova Scotia has agreed for the year 2001, with "grandfathering" of those registered prior to the date

e. Northwest Territories Nurses Association to discuss the issue and develop a position statement that addresses its concerns

f. Manitoba Association of Registered Nurses studying whether or not there is a need to change and the feasibility of doing so

g. Registered Nurses Association of Ontario has prepared a position paper and is developing plans of action

h. Registered Nurses Association of Prince Edward Island is working to establish a university nursing program

i. Association of Registered Nurses of Newfoundland has agreed to a degree as entry but has developed no position paper as yet

16. Nonuniversity programs for preparation of nursing personnel according to the *Canadian Hospital Directory* 1980

a. Hospital schools offering a diploma in nursing—23

b. Diploma nursing programs in provincial education systems—83

c. Diploma nursing programs in regional and independent schools—6

d. Psychiatric nurse preparation programs in British Columbia, Alberta, Saskatchewan, and Manitoba—8

e. Postdiploma programs for registered nursing assistants available in

(1) Operating room technician at Humber College, Toronto, Ontario

(2) Operating room nursing and techniques at the Wascana Institute of Applied Arts and Sciences, Regina, Saskatchewan

f. Program for registered nursing assistants certificate of achievement in the practice and supervision of care in long-term facilities at Centennial College, Scarborough, Ontario

17. Licensed practical nurse programs

a. Uncommon in Canada

b. Graduates eligible for licensure as practical nurses (LPN) are those from nursing orderly program and the Nursing Assistant Program

18. *Canadian Nurses' Association Position Paper on Nursing Education* (1960s)—supported the following:

a. All nursing education programs to be under the jurisdiction of institutes whose primary aim is education

b. Two types of nurses be prepared—university and nonuniversity

c. Graduates of diploma programs to possess a high degree of technical skill and to be prepared to assist in the assessment of nursing needs and problems

d. Merging of the roles of the diploma program–registered nurse and the registered nursing assistant to be considered

19. Canadian Testing Service Examinations

a. Established in 1970 by the Canadian Nurses' Association Testing Service (CNATS); now used in all jurisdictions

b. Operation of the testing service directed by Test Service Board

c. Master blueprint commitee constructs the overall plan for examinations

d. Blueprint subcommittees have representatives from Canada's main regions—Atlantic, Ontario, Quebec, West, and French language areas

e. 1976—all jurisdictions accept 350 as a passing score

f. 1977—*Blueprint for a Comprehensive Examination for Nurse Registration/Licensure* developed by CNATS

g. Comprehensive Nurse Registration Examination using the nursing model was implemented in August, 1980

Accreditation of Nursing Programs

A. Approval of programs

1. Nursing programs are provincially controlled within the general health category

2. Provincial associations establish minimum standards and approve nursing programs on satisfactory inspection

3. Some provinces utilize other approval channels

a. In Manitoba an accrediting committee of nurses and nonnurses establishes minimum standards that are approved by the Board of the Provincial Association

b. In Ontario the Council of Regents establishes minimum standards for diploma nursing in the CAAT system; College of Nurses continues to inspect

4. Approved nursing programs listed in the *Canadian Hospital Directory* and Canadian Nurses' Association publications

5. Association of Community Colleges in Canada is implementing a process by which National Standards for Health Science Programs will be promoted

6. Nursing programs cannot function without ap-

proval as specified under individual provincial nurses' acts

B. Accreditation
1. 1967—Executive Director of the Canadian Nurses' Association consults with the National League for Nursing on the accreditation process
2. 1972—publication of *Canadian Nurses' Association Position on Accreditation*
3. 1973—self-evaluation tools formulated on which criteria for accreditation will be based
4. 1974—optimum standards for nursing education developed by the Canadian Nurses' Association
5. Canadian nursing education programs have no national accreditation process
6. CAUSN has developed and tested in at least 3 universities an accreditation program for University Schools of Nursing
7. ACCC involved in accreditation of programs other than nursing
8. 1978—resolution passed at the CNA convention stating that the CNA with the CAUSN and ACC develop a national accreditation program for nursing education programs
9. ACCC not developing an accreditation program for diploma schools of nursing in community colleges; however, will collaborate if the CNA should proceed with development of a national voluntary accreditation program

C. *Standards for Nursing Education in Canada* (CNA, March 1978)
1. Deal with
   a. Formulation of comprehensive plans for nursing education programs
   b. Statements of beliefs about nursing
   c. Nursing philosophies and the purposes of programs
   d. Specific program activities and evaluation
2. Recommended for assessment of all existing and proposed nursing education programs in Canada and for reassessment of these programs at regular intervals

Advances in Nursing Service

A. Crisis after World War II
1. Nursing in an even greater state of chaos than after World War I because the demands for nursing care rapidly increased (as a result of newer treatment methods and social changes) whereas the number of students entering nursing programs declined
2. Nurses with leadership preparation lacking as a direct result of the economic depression following the war and the absence of educational programs above the basic level

B. 1961—Canadian Nurses' Association in cooperation with the Canadian Hospital Association sponsored an extension course in Nursing Unit Administration in Toronto; financial support for the project provided by the W.K. Kellogg Foundation

C. Development of programs for nursing assistants
1. Large group of young women needed to be absorbed from women's military forces into civilian life; government funds used to organize schools for the preparation of nursing assistants from the group of ex-service women
2. Approval and support of the nursing profession given to the proposal to initiate courses of 9- to 12-month duration in education settings
3. Title for new worker suggested by the Canadian Nurses' Association—''nursing assistant''; and with it came the thrust of the nursing assistant program across Canada
4. 1980—113 programs for nursing assistants; included are 7 that graduate LPNs and 2 that graduate nursing aides; 53 of these programs are in Quebec, 33 in Ontario

D. Problems with proliferation
1. Categories of workers in nursing became numerous in the 1960s
   a. Registered nurses (university and diploma programs)
   b. Nursing assistants
   c. Psychiatric nurses
   d. Orderlies and attendants
   e. Operating room technicians
2. Other problems
   a. Much of direct nursing care being given by nursing assistants
   b. Blurring of roles between the registered nurse and the registered nursing assistant
   c. Increasing need for nurses to spend time in teaching and supervisory functions
   d. Increasing desire of nursing assistants for advancement
3. 1968—general meeting of the Canadian Nurses' Association; the recommendation approved to phase out gradually programs from which practitioners on graduation are not eligible for licensure as registered nurses

E. In its *Statement of Delivery of Nursing Care* the Association recommended that
1. Standards of determining the levels of nursing care be formulated from within the nursing profession
2. Clear distinction be made between nursing and nonnursing activities

3. Objectives of the health agency as well as the means for achieving stated goals be defined by the nursing service

F. Team nursing
   1. See background material under American section
   2. 1968—Registered Nurses' Association of Ontario offered practical experience in team nursing in a demonstration center supported by the Ontario Hospital Services Commission, Ontario Department of Health, and Ontario Public Health Association
   3. Team nursing development project served to teach nurses how to coordinate care of patients in hospitals, but more important how to coordinate care by involving hospitals, voluntary agencies, and public health teams to promote continuity of patient care

G. Accreditation of health care facilities
   1. 1970—Canadian Council on Hospital Accreditation expanded its program to include accreditation of the 3000 extended care facilities across Canada
   2. 1974—Canadian Nurses' Association withdrew its official support for mandatory accreditation of all health agencies and joined with the Canadian Hospital Association in supporting voluntary accreditation
   3. 1977—Helen Taylor, a nurse, named Chairman of the Board of Directors of the Canadian Council on Hospital Accreditation

H. National Standards of Nursing Practice
   1. CNA definition of nursing and standards for nursing practice completed in June 1980; reflects nationwide effort to promote high-quality care
   2. Supported financially by the Health Services Promotion Branch, Health and Welfare, Canada
   3. Four standards developed, representing a step toward evaluation of care given by nurses; include a set of related behaviors
      a. Nursing practice requires that a conceptual model for nursing be the basis for the independent part of that practice
      b. Nursing practice requires the effective use of the nursing process as the method of carrying out the independent, interdependent, and dependent functions of nursing
      c. Nursing practice requires that the helping relationship be the nature of the client-nurse interaction
      d. Nursing practice requires nurses to fulfill professional responsibilities in their independent, interdependent, and dependent functions

Legislation Influencing Nursing

A. Economic security and nurse welfare
   1. Labor relations and collective bargaining
      a. 1944—Canadian Nurses' Association recognized collective bargaining as a useful process in bettering socioeconomic status of nurses
      b. 1946—British Columbia became the first province to introduce collective bargaining
      c. 1970s—nurses in British Columbia, Alberta, Manitoba, Ontario, Quebec, New Brunswick, and Nova Scotia organized and certified under provincial labor legislation
      d. "Strike right"—some Canadian nurses gained the right to strike according to provincial legislation in Quebec, Ontario (except for hospitals), Nova Scotia, and British Columbia
      e. Provincial Nurses' Association in Quebec does not bargain for nurses as a collective unit; Quebec nurses are members of professional syndicates—English chapter, which formed the United Nurses of Montreal in 1966, and La Fédération des Syndicats Professionels d'Infirmières du Quebec, which includes nurses, physiotherapists, etc.
      f. Labour Relations Department of Canadian Nurses' Association to provide services related to collection and analysis of data, information distribution, educational programs, and research activities
      g. CNA Labour Relations Services to provide computerized data bank of all collective agreements for nurses and related health care occupations in Canada
      h. 1982—collective bargaining established for all provincial territorial associations of nurses

B. National health insurance
   1. Five basic principles of the Canadian Health Care System (Charter of Health)
      a. Universal coverage
      b. Comprehensiveness
      c. Accessibility
      d. Portability
      e. Public adminstration
   2. 1966—following a recommendation from the Royal Commission on Health Services (1961), the Medical Care Act received royal assent
   3. 1971—all provinces were participants in National Health Insurance except Northwest and Yukon territories, which implemented programs by 1972
   4. 1973—Hospital Insurance and Diagnostic Services and Medical Care Directorates amalgam-

ated to administer the 2 national health insurance schemes—Hospital Insurance and Medicare

5. National Health Insurance increased the demand for medical and nursing services in agencies other than hospitals and institutions (e.g., health clinics)

6. New Canada Health Act, which is pending
   a. Incorporates the Medical Care Act and the Hospital Insurance and Diagnostic Services Act
   b. Is expected to determine the scope of nursing practice in the future
   c. The CNA will lobby for legislative changes with the Canadian Health Act to provide for
      (1) Better primary health care services
      (2) More appropriate use of health care personnel
      (3) New community-based points of entry into the health care system, especially for the elderly and chronically ill
      (4) More health maintenance and promotion programs
      (5) More extended care services
      (6) Nursing as an insured service

Current Developments

A. Need for a clear legal definition of nursing
   1. Canadian health manpower statistics show a variety of professional classifications engaged in health care, with a fragmentation of care and a clouding of roles
   2. Definition of nursing—it must
      a. Establish a well-defined role
      b. Provide for accountability
      c. Limit the number and type of health care workers
      d. Be derived from a conceptual model for nursing
   3. Standards for nursing will help clarify the nurses' areas of accountability and will influence practice, nursing education, nursing administration and nursing research
B. Mandatory versus voluntary continuing education for nurses
   1. Debate continues as to whether continuing education should be a mandatory or voluntary requirement for nurse registration and licensure
   2. Pressure for continuing education as a prerequisite for renewal of the license to practice nursing is becoming more urgent
C. Canadian Nurses' Association—continuing leadership for the present and the future, including achievement of several goals

1. Baccalaureate nursing degree for entry into practice
2. Definition of roles and functions of the nurse and identification of appropriate educational preparation for these roles and functions
3. Lobby for change in the Canada Health Act
4. National forum to consider continuing education, nursing administration, and cost-effective strategies for clinical education
5. Policy statement on social issues
6. Philosophy of nursing for the CNA
7. Committee to advise the CNA on international matters
8. Mandatory registration and licensure for all nurses employed by the federal government
9. Specialization and certification

D. Code of Ethics
   1. 1954—CNA adopted the International Council of Nurses' code of ethics (developed by the ICN in 1953); slightly revised in 1965
   2. 1980—CNA code of ethics (*An Ethical Basis for Nursing in Canada*) presented to the membership at the CNA convention and adopted
   3. Since 1980, debate and controversy have arisen over the interpretation of some of the content in the code of ethics, whose central theme is *caring*
   4. Ad hoc committee of five representatives from RNABC, RNAO, NBARN, ANPEI, and AARN appointed to make revisions and write another code of ethics
   5. Until the report and new code of ethics are submitted by the ad hoc committee, the CNA code (excluding Section III) is the one to be used in nursing practice

E. Research in nursing—Canadian Council of Nurse Researchers
   1. 1974—Third National Conference on Research in Nursing, projecting that numbers of nurse researchers would increase at all levels, appointed a task force to explore development of a Canadian Council of Nurse Researchers
   2. 1974—research unit set up by McGill University in nursing and health care to develop, study, and evaluate the nurse's expanded function, especially in primary care
   3. 1975—Fourth National Conference on Nursing Research focused on developing indicators for nursing research
   4. Canadian Nurses' Association publishes research in *Index of Canadian Nursing Studies*
   5. 1977—Canadian Nurses' Association, Canadian Nurses' Foundation, and CAUSN developed a joint approach to nursing research

6. 1980—National Nursing Research Conference approved a motion endorsing establishment of the Council of Nurse Researchers to promote development of nurse researchers and identify relevant problems for study
7. 1982—National Nursing Research Conference heard papers related to many areas such as nursing diagnoses, split-second decision making in critical care areas, the psychologic well-being of elderly and their care givers, and the practice of primary nursing compared to team nursing
8. Alberta Foundation for Nursing Research awarded 1 million dollars by the government of Alberta

F. Nursing education
1. Career ladder concept
   a. Supports a curriculum that allows articulation with succeeding levels so that one may proceed from nursing assistant level to diploma level, etc.; a program is available in Saskatchewan that allows practical nurses to become diploma graduates
   b. Report of a Royal Commission headed by Dr. Leonard Miller strongly supported the career ladder in Newfoundland
   c. Humber College of Applied Arts and Technology in Toronto developed an experimental curriculum that
      (1) Offered core courses for nurses and allied health workers
      (2) Allowed students to elect to continue toward a nursing diploma or a registered nursing assistant certificate after the common initial semester
2. Changes in curriculum
   a. Revision of baccalaureate degree programs to include increased content on community health
   b. Graduation of larger numbers of nurses from diploma (community college) and baccalaureate programs
   c. Specialization at masters level leading to the introduction of clinical specialists into health care agencies
   d. 1972—Canadian Nurses' Association issued *Statement of the Expanded Role of the Nurse,* urging modification of educational programs to allow nurses to enter a variety of health care settings
   e. 1983—entry to nursing practice being recommended as a baccalaureate degree by the year 2000
3. Nurse practitioner programs

   a. 1971—National Conference on Assistance to the Physician recommended that Canada not develop programs to produce "physician's assistants" but rather augment nursing programs to develop nurse practitioners
   b. *Report of the Committee on Nurse Practitioners* (Boudreau Report) (1972)—special Committee established by Minister of National Health and Welfare to study role of the nurse practitioner; offered description of the nurse practitioner's role and recommended that
      (1) Specific, defined tasks be delegated by physicians to appropriately prepared nurses
      (2) Nurse practitioner preparation be eventually incorporated within baccalaureate programs
      (3) Development of nurse practitioner programs become a priority
      (4) Basic preparations of nurses at diploma and university levels reflect broadened concept of nursing
      (5) Nurse practitioners receive courses in educational institutions affiliated with university health science centers; by 1972, 1 pilot project in nurse practitioner programs was operating; several universities were conducting ad hoc classes for family practice nurses; 6 universities were providing outpost nursing courses; Quebec nurses were exploring the *community nurse* concept
   c. 1973—Canadian Nurses' Association issued *Statement on Specialization in Nursing,* supporting degrees or levels of specialization in nursing after a basic diploma or baccalaureate program
   d. 1980—CNA favors compensation by provincial health care plans for independent nursing services provided by professional nurses
   e. Original focus on the nurse practitioner in a family practice setting has shifted to specialization in a variety of settings (e.g., emergency, oncology, pediatrics, Northern Health Services, independent practice, home care, occupational health)
   f. 1980—CNA promoting establishment of an occupational health nurse consultant service at the federal level
G. Nursing service
1. Expanded role
   a. Four patterns of expanding role of nurse in primary care are emerging

    (1) Physician's associate (not supported by the CNA)
    (2) Community health nurse
    (3) Northern Health Services nurse
    (4) Primary health care worker
  b. Definitions of nurse practitioner are drafted in 7 provinces; and 4 provinces (Alberta, Saskatchewan, Ontario, Manitoba) are amending their nurse practice acts to provide for the nurse's expanded role
2. Problem-oriented health records
  a. Approach to health records that requires a patient-centered focus to define presenting problems
  b. 1974—Science Council of Canada submitted a report, *Science for Health Services,* recommending that health care be organized into an integrated system using computer-based health information systems and standardized health records
  c. Canadian Nurses' Association recognized value of application of science technology to the health care system (problem-oriented medical records) but deferred endorsement of a single approach as the solution to problems in the health care system
3. Peer review
  a. Quality of nursing care given to clients is evaluated in terms of formulated standards of nursing practice
  b. Useful evaluation tool for assisting individual nurses to improve their care and in assessing nurses for advancement
  c. Essential in nurse accountability for care provided
4. Clinical specialists
  a. Definition—nurses prepared at the masters level who possess advanced knowledge, skill, and clinical competence in specialized areas
  b. Use—predicted to increase as more nurses are prepared
H. Developments related to and influencing nursing
  1. *Community Health Center Project* (Hasting report)—1972
    a. Initiated by Minister of National Health and Welfare to describe community health centers and to determine problems in health center development
    b. Recommendations included that
      (1) Provinces develop community health centers

      (2) Patient-centered, problem-solving approaches be used by all health personnel
      (3) Comprehensive system for evaluation of community health centers be instituted
      (4) Public health functions continue as a vital part of the health services system
  2. *A New Perspective on the Health of Canadians* (1974)—published by the Minister of National Health and Welfare
    a. Presented policies to be developed in the health care system within the next 10 to 15 years
    b. Study of the major causes of death and illness; identified the major health problems of the Canadian population
    c. Major focus is on the *health field concept* composed of 4 principal parts—human biology, environment, life-style, and health care organization
    d. Recommendations included that
      (1) The value system of health care organizations be revised
      (2) Programs be initiated to create safer environments and life-styles that foster good health
      (3) Programs geared to the reduction of self-imposed health risks be implemented through government involvement in public education programs
      (4) Programs directed at "neglected" areas of Canadian population be initiated (e.g., programs for the aged, mentally ill, economically deprived, chronically ill, troubled parents and children, etc.)
    e. Key proposition for nursing related to
      (1) Reduction of environmental hazards and self-imposed health risks in the population
      (2) Family counseling
      (3) Care of the mentally and chronically ill
      (4) Care of the aged population
      (5) Provision of home care
  3. Canada Health Survey, completed in 1980, reinforced the need to put "health" back into health care through health promotion programs, teaching, and counseling related to the quality of life-styles
  4. Telemedicine Projects being conducted to explore the potential of audioconferencing in the delivery of continuing education for health professionals
  5. Royal Commission of inquiry into the confiden-

tiality of health records in Ontario (Krever commission)

    a. Clarification of ownership and right to access of health records

    b. Involvement of registered nurses in the confidentiality process

    c. Establishment of policies and procedures in health care agencies to guide personnel relative to confidential information

6. Specialization in nursing

    a. 1980—CNA to study feasibility of developing examinations for certification in major nursing specialties

    b. CNA, through CNATS, assists in developing national examinations drawn up together with the Canadian Council for Occupational Health Nurses, Inc; implementation date is 1983

    c. RNABC has set up a Specialized Nursing Competencies Project in which an attempt is made to identify clinical nursing specialties and subspecialties

    d. Order of Nurses of Quebec has prepared a preliminary file on certification for specialists

    e. CNA committee has designed a 4-point plan of action that includes getting together representatives of national specialty organizations, with a view to establishing a Canadian Council on Specialty Certification; purpose would be to oversee the development and operation of a certification mechanism for specialty groups

    f. Certification of specialties is a major decision that will affect professional development for the future

NURSING PRACTICE AND THE LAW— UNITED STATES AND CANADA
Typology of Laws

A. Legal systems of modern nations influenced by both Roman civil law and English common law

B. Law arises from

  1. Statutory law (legislation)

    a. Body of law enacted by federal, provincial, state, or local government

    b. That which commands or prohibits

    c. Licensing laws belong in this category

  2. Common law (custom and precedent)

    a. Unwritten; based on customs

    b. Precedent plays large part in judge's decisions, thus giving uniformity to decisions in like situations

    c. Nurses practice under common as well as statutory law

C. The British North America Act (1867) renamed the Constitution Act (1982); incorporates existing provisions of the BNA Act with a Canadian Charter of Rights and Freedoms; establishes the political and legal foundations as well as fundamental rules for Canadians to govern Canada; also gives provincial governments power in health care activities

D. The Constitution of the United States gives states the power to police the health and welfare of its citizens

E. Military law

  1. Applies to nurses only when members of one of the military nurse corps

  2. Applies to all citizens when martial law declared

F. Private law

  1. Property law—wills, patents, copyrights, trademarks

  2. Contract law—agency, conditional sales, mortgages, bail

  3. Tort law—intentional aggression, negligence, strict liability, defamation, invasion of privacy

G. Public law

  1. Constitutional law—government structures, federal division of powers, fundamental rights

  2. Administrative law—consumer protection, social welfare

  3. Criminal law—serious offenses against the individual and society

    a. Felonies—more serious offenses against the individual and society

    b. Misdemeanors—less serious (e.g., burglary)

H. Civil law—acts contrary to a criminal statute; may result in a civil suit, since the act has violated civil law

Torts and Crimes Especially Important to Nurses

A. Torts

  1. Violations of civil law

  2. Failure to use care or failure to prevent injury

  3. Malpractice and negligence fall into this category and are unintentional torts

    a. No precise statute describes malpractice

    b. Terms often used interchangeably, but some legal experts make a distinction between them

      (1) Malpractice—professional misconduct; negligence performed in professional practice; any unreasonable lack of skill in professional duties or illegal or im-

moral conduct that results in injury or death to the client/patient/consumer
   (2) Negligence—practice without a license; measurement of negligence is "reasonableness"; involves exposure of person or property of another to unreasonable risk of injury by acts of commission or omission
4. Usual standard of conduct is that which a prudent nurse would or would not do
5. Tort different from crime, but serious tort can be tried as both civil and criminal action
6. Necessary to prove negligence—if proved, this means that the act was performed incorrectly or not at all and the nurse is responsible for injury
7. Elements essential to prove negligence
   a. Legal duty existed and a breach of duty occurred
   b. Lack of conformity to established standards
   c. Reasonable foreseeability not demonstrated, such that injury resulted
   d. Cause-effect relationship between act and injury
   e. Not dependent on a contract
8. Nurse responsible for own acts; if employed, employer may also be held responsible under the doctrine of *respondeat superior;* when responsibility shared, nursing actions must lie within the scope of employment
9. Reasonableness and prudence in actions are usually determining factors in a judgment; increasing attention is being paid to the law governing the practice of nursing
10. Examples of malpractice/negligence include leaving sponges inside a patient; causing burns from hot water bottles, heating pads, hot solutions, and electric, steam, or vapor sources; medication errors; failure to prevent falls by neglecting to raise bed or crib rails; incompetent assessment of patient situations, such as ignoring complaints of chest pain leading to subsequent inappropriate actions; improper identification of patients for operative or diagnostic procedures; and carelessness in caring for a patient's property, such as dentures, clothing, valuables
11. Intentional torts occur when a person does damage to another person in a willful, intentional way and without just cause and/or excuse; includes fraud and deceit, assault and battery, false imprisonment, exposure of person or body after death, eavesdropping, libel and slander (defamatory torts)

a. Assault—mental or physical threat
   (1) Knowingly threatening or attempting to do violence to another
   (2) Forcing a medication or treatment on a person who does not want it constitutes assault so long as touching does not occur
b. Battery—touching with or without the intent to do harm
   (1) Actually touching or wounding a person in an offensive manner
   (2) Hitting or striking a patient
c. Fraud
   (1) False presentation of facts purposefully to create deception
   (2) Presenting false credentials for purposes of entering a nursing program or gaining registration, licensure, or employment
d. Invasion of privacy
   (1) Encroachment or trespass on another's body and/or personality includes
      (a) False imprisonment—the intentional confinement without authorization by a person who physically constricts another using force, the threat of force, or confining structures and/or clothing; even without force or malicious intent, to detain another without consent in a specified area constitutes grounds for a charge of false imprisonment; the charge is not false imprisonment if it is necessary to protect an emotionally disturbed person from harming self or others or if it is necessary to confine to defend oneself, others, or property or to effect a lawful arrest
      (b) Exposure of a person—any unnecessary exposure or discussion of the patient's case is actionable unless authorized by the patient; after death, the patient's right to be unobserved, excluded from unwarranted operations, and protected from unauthorized touching of the body persists
      (c) Defamation—concerns privileged communications and privacy; law grants the right of privacy to everyone; divulgence of privileged communication whether from charts,

conversation, interview, or observation in a way that exposes the person to hatred, contempt, aversion, or a lowering of opinion; includes slander (oral) and libel (written, pictured, telecast), both of which are dependent on communication to a third party

B. Crimes
1. Criminal act—an act contrary to a criminal statute; in Canada, one contrary to the Criminal Code of Canada; violates societal law; includes felonies and misdemeanors
2. Criminal Code of Canada is determined by the Parliament of Canada, is applicable to all provinces and territories, and may be amended by Parliament to reflect society's changing values
3. Canadian Criminal Code and Death with Dignity
   a. Guidelines are needed to outline acceptable practices for nurses and physicians to follow in situations where intensive and resuscitative measures should not be applied
   b. CNA together with the CMA, CHA, and Canadian Bar Association (Law Reform Commission of Canada) are studying the issue of *do not resuscitate* orders
   c. Law Reform Commission (Report 28) recommends that cessation and refusal of treatment be given legal recognition in Canadian criminal law
   d. Law Reform Commission (Report 15) recommends that the Parliament of Canada adopt the following amendment to Section 28A of the Interpretation Act concerning Criteria of Death:
      (1) Death occurs with irreversible cessation of all brain function
      (2) Irreversible cessation of brain function can be determined by the prolonged absence of spontaneous circulatory and respiratory function
      (3) When detection of prolonged absence of spontaneous circulatory and respiratory function is made impossible by the use of artificial means of support, the irreversible cessation of brain function can be determined by any means recognized by the ordinary standards of current medical practice (Harvard criteria)
4. Crimes are wrongs punishable by the state, committed against the state, usually demon-

strate that intent was present, and are reported by the state as the complainant
5. Commission of crime requires 2 fundamental factors
   a. Committing a deed contrary to criminal law
   b. Omitting an act when there is a legal obligation to perform such an act; e.g., refraining from assistance with the birth of a child if such refusal results in injury to the newborn
6. Criminal conspiracy occurs when 2 or more persons agree to commit a crime
7. Giving aid to another in the commission of a crime makes the person equally guilty of the offense if awareness is present that a crime is being committed
8. Ignorance of the law is usually not an adequate defense when a crime or civil wrong is committed
9. Assault may be justified in instances of self-defense if only as much force as is absolutely necessary for self-protection is used
10. Search warrants are required before property can be searched
11. Administration of narcotics by a nurse is legal only when authorized by a physician who is legally registered under the Controlled Substances Act
    a. If a nurse knowingly administers a drug that causes a major disability or death, a crime may be charged
    b. Illegal possession or sale of a controlled substance makes nurse liable, as is any citizen
12. Those involved in decisions to discontinue life-support systems may be liable to charge of murder; there is a strong movement against dramatic life-saving measures in cases of terminally ill patients; these questions are as much moral as legal; nurse should know decision must be made on knowledge; nurse is accountable; "living will" aims at giving the individual the authority to say whether life-support systems should be used at all or discontinued if in use; legality of "living will" and effectiveness of legislation permitting it are under dispute

Malpractice Insurance

A. Liability can be defined as a person's legal responsibility to be accountable for wrongful acts by making financial restitution to the party wronged

B. Malpractice insurance can be purchased from nurses' associations, bargaining organizations, and private insurance companies
C. Amount of malpractice/liability insurance is dictated by factors such as
1. Type of nursing practiced (e.g., private practitioner, nursing instructor, acute care nursing)
2. Increasing inclination to sue professionals, including nurses
3. Any limits of liability established in area where nursing is practiced; e.g., in Ontario, Canada, liability of insurers is limited for each loss to 1 million dollars and further limited to 3 million dollars in total for all claims against any one insured member in any one policy period (RNAO policy)
D. Employer's insurance protects the nurse while on duty in the course of employement (concept of vicarious liability, *respondeat superior*); a nurse can, however, be personally sued and held liable for negligent or malpractice actions
E. Malpractice insurance provides monetary settlement if a suit by a client is decided in favor of the client; most policies pay legal fees and costs, as well as bond for the nurse in an appeal

Informed Consent

A. Purposes of informed consent
1. Makes possible a contract between 2 individuals with each sharing equally
2. Makes competent decision possible for patient who has the final decision
B. Consent essential for any treatment, except in an emergency where failure to institute treatment may constitute negligence
C. Major question is what constitutes informed consent
1. Elements of consent
a. Explanation of treatment to be done
b. Advantages and disadvantages
c. Possible alternatives
d. Time for decision making
e. No undue pressure
2. Problems arise in determining
a. What consitutes adequate information
b. Who should give explanation
c. Whether to give alternatives where one treatment is clearly preferable
3. The patient has a right to know, right to agree, or right to refuse
D. Nurse's responsibility is to respect rights of individual patient, thus avoiding legal action

The Nurse in the Courts

A. Nurse may be in court either as a witness if involved personally in a case or as an expert witness because of knowledge and expertise
B. Expert witness
1. Not an advocate
2. If called into court, the nurse must be
a. Informed as to standards of care that prudent, reasonable nurse would give relative to incident in question
b. Knowledgeable in the field specific to the incident
c. Without opinion unless specifically asked
3. Although a professional may elect to join in a "conspiracy of silence" when asked to testify against another professional, the basic question is ethical and concerns the willingness of the professional to deal adequately with the incompetence of another professional
4. The patient's charts, to which nurses contribute, may be used in court, therefore placing nurses in court vicariously; notes should be accurate, complete, factual, and give evidence of knowledge and judgment

The Nurse's Legal Status

A. Employee
1. Nurse acts and performs services for another and is known as *agent;* this does not eliminate the independence of the nurse in practice
2. Contract made with the employer that sets forth the nature of the services expected, the conditions of employment, and compensation
3. Elements of a written contract
a. Services to be rendered
b. Environment in which services are to be rendered
c. Duration of contract
d. Termination conditions
B. Collective bargaining increasingly involved in arranging contracts between employees and the employing agency
1. Contracts binding on both parties even though individual nurse not directly involved with the deliberations; if majority of employees agree, all are bound
2. Damages may be sought in court if contract broken
C. Independent contractor
1. A contractor who renders direct services to clients and is in control of that service, including setting fee for service

2. A small number of nurses setting up independent practices
3. Joint practice is an adaptation of the independent contractor
   a. Nurse and physician practice independently and collaboratively, each rendering service to the same group of patients
   b. The client's needs determine which professional gives the service
4. Private duty nurse is an independent contractor

The Patient's Rights

A. Patients have the legal right to refuse treatment (if mentally competent), to be given treatment in an emergency, to choose their own doctor, to have a proper standard of care, to execute voluntary and informed consent, to decide whether to be used for research or teaching, to be treated in confidentiality, to receive treatment free of discrimination, and to have protection of personal property
B. National governments of both the United States and Canada, the governments of states and provinces, and various professional associations and consumer groups have attempted to educate the public concerning their rights regarding provision and delivery of health care
C. Both governments have set stringent rules about the use of human subjects in research
D. Laws of both governments emphasize the rights of children, the mentally disadvantaged, and the elderly to health care
E. Clients/patients have the right to lodge complaints about a nurse and the care received when complaints are related to
   1. Incompetence
   2. Professional misconduct
   3. Physical or mental incapacity

Legislation Related to Nurses

A. United States
   1. Registration and licensure are used interchangeably but are not synonymous
   2. Registration—entrance of name in a registry
      a. Maintained by individual states in United States
      b. Authorizes practice as a registered nurse
      c. Protects the title of registered nurse
      d. Follows automatically after licensure
   3. Licensure—granting of a license after successful completion of the National Council Licensure Examination in the United States
      a. Protects the public and nursing practice; issued by individual states
      b. Mandatory licensure—all who practice nursing must be licensed; employees of federal government are not bound by state mandatory licensure laws
      c. Permissive licensure—protects the titles Reg N or RN, but does not protect the practice of nursing; the practice of nursing is not prohibited as long as the unlicensed person does not represent himself or herself as a registered nurse; thus anyone, licensed or not, may practice nursing so long as the title Reg N or RN is not used
      d. May be obtained by examination, waiver, or endorsement (reciprocity)
      e. American Nurses' Association, from the time of its inception, has seen the need for legislation to set standards for nursing
      f. First states with nurse licensing laws
         (1) North Carolina—1903
         (2) New York—1903
         (3) New Jersey—1903
      g. 1952—all states and territories had nurse practice acts
      h. Early laws permissive, with New York the first state to pass a mandatory licensing law in 1938 (which, because of the war, did not become effective until 1948)
      i. All but a few states now have mandatory laws
      j. Laws administered by a state board of nursing either as a department of state government or as an autonomous agency
      k. Definition of the practice of nursing is included in the law
      l. Renewal of licenses usually required every 2 or 3 years
      m. Different licensing laws and examinations required for practical nursing
      n. Licenses can be revoked for cause by the state board of nursing
         (1) Nursing's licensing body disciplines members of the profession of nursing according to the mechanisms described in nurse practice acts
         (2) Self-regulation practices are criteria of a profession, along with autonomy and expertise
   4. National Council of State Boards, Inc. (NCSBN)—separate, autonomous, nonprofit body established in 1978
      a. Membership open to any board of nursing
      b. Delegate assembly composed of one member of each board

c. National Council Licensure Examination (NCLEX) under control of this body
d. Executive director with office in Chicago
5. NCLEX, first administered in July 1982
   a. Criterion-referenced examination based on nursing behaviors that constitute safe and effective practice
   b. Comprehensive integrated examination divided into 4 sections
   c. Passing score determined by each state board
   d. Each jurisdiction agrees to adopt this examination since licensure is a state function
   e. Examination is administered by each state board of nursing 2 times yearly over a 2-day period
B. Canada
1. Registration and licensure are used interchangeably but are not synonymous
2. Registration—entrance of one's name in a registry
   a. Maintained by individual provincial professional nurses associations (except in Ontario, where it is maintained by the College of Nurses, the statutory body for nurses in Ontario)
   b. Authorizes practice as a registered nurse
   c. Protects the title of registered nurse
   d. Follows automatically after licensure
3. Licensure—granting of a license after successful completion of the Canadian Nurses' Association Testing Service Registration Examination
   a. Mandatory licensure—all who practice nursing must be licensed; employees of the federal government are not bound by provincial mandatory licensure laws
   b. CNA has publicly endorsed mandatory licensure for all nurses employed by the federal government
   c. Permissive licensure—protects the titles Reg N or RN, but does not protect the practice of nursing; the practice of nursing is not prohibited as long as the unlicensed person does not represent himself or herself as a registered nurse; thus anyone, licensed or not, may practice nursing so long as the title Reg N or RN is not used
   d. May be obtained by examination, waiver, or endorsement (reciprocity)
   e. Health Disciplines Act—Ontario
      (1) Received royal assent in 1974, but not proclaimed law until July 1975
      (2) Incorporates recommendations from the Committee on the Healing Arts and the *Royal Commission Inquiry into Civil Rights*
      (3) Allows for lay representation in the professional governing council
      (4) Creates a health disciplines board to conduct hearings related to complaints and applications for licensing
      (5) Gives the Council of the College of Nurses of Ontario authority to
         (a) Register new members and renew registration of standing members
         (b) Require nursing personnel to be currently registered with the College of Nurses
         (c) Discipline any person granted initial registration
         (d) Protect the titles Registered Nurse and Registered Nursing Assistant
         (e) Establish, maintain, and develop standards of knowledge, skill, and professional ethics
   f. Nurse practice acts
      (1) Nursing is recognized by provincial statutes (Nurses' Acts)
      (2) Purpose of registration
         (a) Registration allows for protection of the general public by distinguishing the trained nurse from the untrained nurse
         (b) Protects title of registered nurse for persons who have successfully passed registration examinations
      (3) Purposes of Nurses' Acts
         (a) In most provinces the acts do not define legal boundaries in terms of nursing functions, although there is a concerted effort by provincial associations to define nursing practice
         (b) To provide for interprovincial registration
         (c) In some provinces to provide for the registration and licensure of nursing assistants
      (4) Enactment
         (a) First in Nova Scotia (1910), followed by Manitoba (1913), New Brunswick and Alberta (1916), Ontario (1922)
         (b) Administered by provincial associations except in Ontario, where the College of Nurses registers nurses, and in Quebec, where the Order of Nurses of the Province of Quebec licenses nurses for nursing practice

(5) Control
  (a) In Ontario, with the Nurses' Act of 1961 amended, the College of Nurses of Ontario was established as the governing body of nursing with provision also for governing of nursing assistants (now titled Registered Nursing Assistant)
  (b) As of February 1974—only 1 nurses' association had the right of appeal to a legal definition of nursing written into law; this was the Order of Nurses of Quebec
  (c) Three provinces (Quebec, Prince Edward Island, and Newfoundland) protect the title nurse as well as the registered nurse
  (d) Remaining provinces and territory have permissive registration and licensure based on approval of nursing programs and successful passing of CNATS
  (e) Trend in the remaining provinces and territories is toward mandatory licensure
  (f) Order of Nurses of Quebec
    [1] February 1974—Professional Code of the Province of Quebec changed the title of Association of Nurses of the Province of Quebec (ANPQ) to Order of Nurses of Quebec (ONQ); chief purpose is protection of the public
    [2] Passage of the Professional Code created 21 professional groups—11 have exclusive rights to practice and 10 regulate only the title of the health worker
    [3] Quebec Nurses' Act now defines the profession of nursing as identification of persons' health needs, assisting with diagnosis, employing nursing interventions, and communication of health problems to clients
  (g) Northwest Territories Registered Nurses' Association (NWTRNA)
    [1] January 1975—Ordinance Respecting the Nursing Profession in the Northwest Territories approved by the Territorial Council
    [2] Gave the NWTRNA authority to
      [a] Join with the Canadian Nurses' Association
      [b] Grant and/or revoke certificates of registration to nurses practicing in the Northwest Territories
      [c] Discipline members of the nursing profession
      [d] Lay claim to being the first professional group north of the sixtieth parallel to acquire registration control over its members

Comprehensive Test 1

To simulate the comprehensive state board examination, this test should be completed within 2 hours.

Situation: *Mrs. Penny, a gravida II para 1, is admitted to the labor unit by ambulance, and delivery is imminent. She keeps bearing down, and after 2 contractions the baby's head is crowning. Questions 1 through 15 refer to this situation.*

1 The nurse should:
1. Tell her to breathe through her mouth and pant during contractions
2. Tell her to breathe through her mouth and not to bear down
3. Transfer her immediately by stretcher to the delivery room
4. Tell her to pant while supporting the perineum with her hand to prevent tearing

2 With the next contraction Mrs. Penny delivers a large baby boy spontaneously. The nurse's initial action should be to:
1. Ascertain the condition of the fundus
2. Establish an airway for the baby
3. Quickly tie and cut the umbilical cord
4. Move mother and baby to delivery room

3 The physician arrives and cares for the baby and delivers the placenta. Pitocin, an oxytocic, is administered intramuscularly. Since Mrs. Penny has had a precipitous delivery, it is important to observe for:
1. Bleeding and infection
2. Sudden chilling
3. Elevation in blood pressure
4. Respiratory insufficiency in the baby

4 If involution is progressing normally, immediately after birth the nurse would expect the fundus to be located:
1. Three centimeters above the umbilicus
2. At the level of the umbilicus
3. Two centimeters below the umbilicus
4. Two centimeters above the symphysis pubis

5 Mrs. Penny's newborn infant is taken from the delivery room to the nursery, where it is the policy for the nurse to appraise the infant. In the examination the nurse notes that the temperature, pulse, and respiration are in normal range. Other physical characteristics are also normal. The nurse records

all observations on the baby's chart. Which of the following statements is correct?
1. The nurse was making a medical diagnosis
2. Only the physician should determine the infant's physical status
3. According to the Nurse Practice Act the nurse performed correctly
4. Assessment by the nurse is not equivalent to the physician's assessment

6 Mr. and Mrs. Penny name their baby Andrew. At 10 hours of life he has a large amount of mucus and becomes slightly cyanotic. The nurse should:
1. Give the infant oxygen
2. Insert a Levin tube
3. Note the incident on the chart
4. Suction the mucus as needed

7 Baby Andrew must be observed carefully for the first 24 hours, particularly for:
1. Respiratory distress
2. Change in body temperature
3. Frequency in voiding
4. Duration of cry

8 When Andrew's mother removes his blanket and starts to examine her infant, she becomes concerned because he assumes a fencing position as she turns his head; the mother suspects neurologic damage. The nurse discusses with the mother that:
1. This is a normal response
2. The physician had been notified of this suspicious response
3. This reflex disappears around 2 months of age
4. Tonic neck reflex may indicate neurologic damage in the newborn

9 Supportive nursing care in the beginning mother-infant relationship should include:
1. Encouraging Mrs. Penny to decide between breast-feeding and bottle-feeding
2. Allowing Mrs. Penny ample time to inspect the baby
3. Requiring Mrs. Penny to assist with simple aspects of infant's care
4. Unobtrusive observation to pick up disturbed mother-infant relationship

10 Mrs. Penny has decided to breast-feed this baby. However, she has some doubts as to whether she will be successful, since her breasts are small. She is also concerned about putting on weight, since she is proud of her petite figure. Concerning Mrs. Penny's statement about the size of her breasts, the nurse's best response should be:
1. "The size of your breasts has nothing to do with the production of milk."

2. "The amount of fat and glandular tissue in the breasts determines the amount of milk produced."
3. "You seem to have some concern about breast-feeding."
4. "Everybody can be successful at breast-feeding."

11 It is now 2 days post partum and Mrs. Penny asks the nurse about cleansing the nipples. The nurse's best response would be:
1. "Thoroughly scrub the nipples with soap and water before each feeding."
2. "Cleanse the nipples with sterile water before each feeding."
3. "Cleanse the nipples with an alcohol sponge before and after each feeding."
4. "Wash the breasts and nipples daily with water."

12 On the third day following delivery Mrs. Penny states that she has a great deal of pain in her breasts and that she is afraid that the baby will hurt her when he tries to grasp the nipple. The most appropriate action for the nurse to take is to explain the reasons for the patient's discomfort and to:
1. Call the physician to obtain advice
2. Administer a medication for pain
3. Express some of the milk manually before putting the baby to breast
4. Suggest that the patient limit fluids and not try to nurse the baby for the next 2 days

13 Mrs. Penny is concerned because she heard that her neighbor's breasts suddenly dried up when she got home and she had to discontinue nursing. An appropriate comment for the nurse to make is:
1. "This commonly happens with the excitement of going home. Putting the baby to breast more frequently will reestablish lactation."
2. "This commonly happens; however, we will give you a formula to take home so the baby won't go hungry until your milk supply returns."
3. "This is not true; once lactation is established, this rarely happens."
4. "You have little to worry about, since you already have a good milk supply."

14 Mrs. Penny has heard of demand feeding and wonders how anyone ever finds time to do anything but feed the baby. The nurse's best response would be:
1. "Most mothers find babies on breast do better on demand feeding, since the amount of milk ingested varies at each feeding."

2. "Perhaps a schedule might be better, since the baby is already accustomed to hospital routine."

3. "Although the baby is on demand feedings, he will eventually set his own schedule, so there will be time for your household chores."

4. "Most mothers find that feeding the baby whenever he cries works out fine."

15 Mrs. Penny wants to know whether it is true that she will not have to use contraceptives while nursing. The nurse's most appropriate response should be:

1. "Since lactation suppresses ovulation, you probably don't have to worry about becoming pregnant."

2. As long as you have no menstrual period, you won't have to worry about using contraceptives."

3. "It is best to use contraceptive measures, since ovulation may occur without a menstrual period."

4. "It is best to delay any sexual relations until you have your first menstrual period."

Situation: Andrew Penny is now 1 month old. He has been vomiting for 1 week. Mrs. Penny explains that the vomiting has been progressively more forceful and contains undigested formula. Presently Andrew is dehydrated and has abdominal distention. A tentative diagnosis of pyloric stenosis has been made. Questions 16 through 22 refer to this situation.

16 Vomiting caused by pyloric stenosis is usually not bile stained because:

1. The obstruction is above the opening of the common bile duct

2. The bile duct is also obstructed

3. The obstruction of the cardiac sphincter prevents bile from entering the esophagus

4. The sphincter of the bile duct is connected to the hypertrophied pyloric muscle

17 While doing the physical assessment of Andrew the nurse should particularly observe for visible peristaltic waves and:

1. An olive-shaped mass in the right upper quadrant

2. Decreased bowel sounds

3. Severe cramping movements in the lower intestine

4. A boardlike abdomen

18 The physician orders a gavage tube for Andrew. How should the nurse determine the distance needed to advance the gavage tube?

1. Advance the tube until resistance is met

2. Measure the distance from the nose to the earlobe to the epigastric area of the abdomen

3. Measure from the mouth to the umbilicus and add half the distance

4. Advance the tube as far as necessary to aspirate gastric contents

19 During insertion of the tube, which sign or reaction would be considered abnormal by the nurse if demonstrated by Andrew?

1. Choking

2. Cyanosis

3. Flushing

4. Gagging

20 A Fredet-Ramstedt procedure is performed and, postoperatively, the nurse instructs Mrs. Penny regarding proper feeding techniques, such as:

1. Feed the child in the semi-Fowler position and then afterward place prone

2. Rock the child after feedings to reduce crying and ingestion of air

3. Feed the child in the supine position to reduce pressure on the sutures

4. Feed the child in an upright position and then place on the right side with the head slightly elevated

21 One month after his discharge, Mrs. Penny brings Andrew into the pediatric clinic and asks about the introduction of new foods. The nurse suggests:

1. "Mix the pureed food with the formula and give through the bottle to help him learn new tastes."

2. "Offer a new food every day until he likes one."

3. "Offer a new food after he has had some milk when he is still hungry."

4. "Offer a new food after he has had his regular feeding."

22 Mrs. Penny also asks about what foods she should begin to introduce. A likely choice would be to start with:

1. Rice cereal and fruit, then add egg yolk

2. Cereal, and add a soft-boiled egg for breakfast

3. Fruit first, then add meat and vegetables

4. Sweets, such as fruits and puddings

Situation: Mrs. Mager, age 20, is 37 weeks pregnant. She is admitted to the hospital with preeclampsia and sudden abdominal pain. Questions 23 through 35 refer to this situation.

23 On Mrs. Mager's admission to the unit the nurse should observe for:

1. Decrease in size of uterus, cessation of contractions, visible or concealed hemorrhage

2. Firm and tender uterus, concealed or external hemorrhage, shock
3. Increase in size of uterus, visible bleeding, no associated pain
4. Shock, decrease in size of uterus, absence of external bleeding

24 The nurse realizes that the abdominal pain associated with abruptio placentae is caused by:
1. Hemorrhagic shock
2. Inflammatory reactions
3. Blood in the uterine muscle
4. Concealed hemorrhage

25 Mrs. Mager is given a unit of blood. The nurse realizes that this is necessary, since the bleeding following severe abruptio placentae is usually caused by:
1. Hypofibrinogenemia
2. Hyperglobulinemia
3. Thrombocytopenia
4. Polycythemia

26 Mrs. Mager delivers a stillborn baby girl. To foster a healthy grieving response to the birth of a stillborn child, the nurse's best response to an expression of anger from Mrs. Mager would be:
1. "It's God's will; we have to have faith that it was for the best."
2. "You are young; you'll have other children."
3. "This often happens when something is wrong with the baby."
4. "You may be wondering if something you did caused this."

27 Mrs. Mager has difficulty resolving her grief and, in 6 months, appears to be increasingly anxious over her inability to conceive again. She visits her physician and after examination is admitted to the hospital with a tentative diagnosis of hyperthyroidism. The nurse would expect Mrs. Mager to exhibit:
1. Nervousness, weight loss, increased appetite
2. Protruding eyeballs, slow pulse, sluggishness
3. Increased appetite, slow pulse, dry skin
4. Loss of weight, GI disturbances, listlessness

28 When teaching Mrs. Mager about the diagnostic tests to be done, the nurse should include:
1. Radioactive iodine uptake and T_3
2. Protein-bound iodine and SMA 12
3. T_4 and x-ray films
4. Basal metabolic rate and Po_2

29 The major nursing problem in caring for Mrs. Mager would be:
1. Providing an adequate diet
2. Keeping the bed linen neat

3. Providing sufficient rest
4. Modifying hospital routines

30 The purpose of propylthiouracil, which was ordered for Mrs. Mager, is to:
1. Interfere with the synthesis of thyroid hormone
2. Produce atrophy of the thyroid gland
3. Increase the uptake of iodine
4. Decrease the secretion of thyroid-stimulating hormone

31 The physician decides that Mrs. Mager should have a subtotal thyroidectomy. In preparation for surgery, Lugol's Iodine Solution is ordered. This medication is given to:
1. Maintain the function of the parathyroid glands
2. Decrease the total basal metabolic rate
3. Block the formation of thyroxin by the thyroid gland
4. Decrease the size and vascularity of the thyroid gland

32 Mrs. Mager is concerned that the thyroidectomy will interfere with her ability to become pregnant. In replying the nurse bases the response on the following information:
1. As long as medication is taken as ordered, ovulation will occur
2. Pregnancy is not advisable for the patient with a thyroidectomy
3. Hyperthyroidism can cause abortions or fetal anomalies
4. Pregnancy will affect metabolism and will require greatly increased thyroid hormone

33 When Mrs. Mager returns to her room after surgery, the nurse should immediately:
1. Instruct her not to speak
2. Inspect the incision
3. Keep her flat in bed for 24 hours
4. Place a tracheostomy set at the bedside

34 Postoperatively the nurse should carefully observe Mrs. Mager for signs of thyroid storm. These include:
1. Hypothermia
2. Elevated serum calcium
3. Rapid heart action and tremors
4. Sudden drop in pulse rate

35 Thyroid storm is caused by:
1. Removal of the parathyroid gland
2. Increased amount of thyroid hormone in the blood
3. Increased iodine in the blood
4. A rebound increase in metabolism following anesthesia

Situation: Mrs. Kraft, a 45-year-old woman, is a severe diabetic who is admitted to the hospital for a midthigh amputation of her right leg because of a gangrenous leg ulcer. She also has a history of chronic angle closure glaucoma and has been using pilocarpine 2% eyedrops 4 times a day for the past year. Questions 36 through 45 refer to this situation.

36 The chief aim of treatment in chronic glaucoma is:
1. Controlling intraocular pressure
2. Dilating the pupil to allow for an increase in visual field
3 Resting the eye to reduce pressure
4. Preventing secondary infections that can add to the visual problem

37 Mrs. Kraft seems able to accept the amputation but appears to have difficulty dealing with the glaucoma. The nurse arranges to spend more time with her, since she realizes the patient with glaucoma needs assistance in learning to accept the disease because:
1. There is usually restriction in the use of both eyes
2. Lost vision cannot be restored
3. Total blindness is inevitable
4. Surgery will only temporarily help the problem

38 Which of the following ocular symptoms should the nurse expect Mrs. Kraft to exhibit?
1. A complete loss of central vision
2. Attacks of acute pain
3. Impairment of peripheral vision
4. Constant blurred vision

39 Before the amputation, the anesthesiologist prescribes meperidine (Demerol), 50 mg, and atropine, 0.4 mg, for Mrs. Kraft. The nurse should:
1. Withhold the atropine, since it is contraindicated
2. Give the medication as ordered
3. Administer the pilocarpine before the atropine
4. Ask the anesthesiologist to verify the order

40 Postoperatively, to prevent contractures of the hip, the nurse should:
1. Place pillows under the stump
2. Encourage Mrs. Kraft to lie in the prone position several times daily
3. Remove pillows from under the stump and elevate the head of the bed
4. Encourage Mrs. Kraft to sit in a chair as much as possible

41 To promote early and efficient ambulation when Mrs. Kraft is allowed out of bed, the nurse should encourage her to:
1. Keep hip in extension and abduction
2. Keep hip in extension and adduction
3. Keep hip in flexion and adduction
4. Keep right shoulder raised when swinging stump

42 Stump shrinkage is an important step in the healing process. There are 2 factors that contribute to stump shrinkage: one is atrophy of the muscles, and the other is:
1. Postoperative edema
2. Development of skin turgor
3. Reduction of subcutaneous fat
4. Loss of tissue and bone during operation

43 In helping Mrs. Kraft prepare her stump for a prosthesis, the nurse should encourage her to:
1. Abduct the stump when ambulating
2. Hang the stump off the bed frequently
3. Soak the stump in warm water twice a day
4. Periodically press the end of the stump against a pillow

44 When preparing Mrs. Kraft for dinner, it is the nurse's responsibility to:
1. Remove the pillow under the stump and raise the head of the bed
2. Check Mrs. Kraft's urine for sugar and acetone
3. Get Mrs. Kraft out of bed and into a chair
4. Make sure that Mrs. Kraft uses salt substitutes

45 In planning for discharge with Mrs. Kraft, the nurse discusses stump care. Because of her glaucoma, Mrs. Kraft should:
1. Use mydriatrics regularly
2. Restrict fluid intake
3. Avoid bright lights or darkness
4. Exercise in moderation

Situation: Two-year-old Tommy is brought to the pediatric clinic. His mother states he has been irritable and that she noticed swollen glands on the left side of his neck. After examination a diagnosis of otitis media is made and antibiotic eardrops ordered. Questions 46 through 51 refer to this situation.

46 To teach the correct way to administer eardrops to a small child, the nurse should instruct the parent to position the child on the right side and instill the drops while pulling the auricle:
1. Straight back
2. Up and back
3. Forward
4. Down and back

47 Physiologically the middle ear (containing the 3 ossicles) serves primarily to:
1. Communicate with the throat via the eustachian tube
2. Amplify the energy of sound waves entering the ear

3. Translate sound waves into nerve impulses
4. Maintain balance

48 Tommy's condition does not improve, and he is admitted for a myringotomy. Postoperatively the nurse would expect Tommy to have:
1. Symptoms of central nervous system irritation
2. Difficulty voiding and slight hematuria
3. Irrigations to the lacrimal glands
4. Purulent drainage into the external auditory canal

49 When Tommy is ill and has temporary dietary restrictions, the best way for the nurse to avoid any future feeding problems is to have the restrictions:
1. Limited to foods that are not essential
2. Administered by someone other than parents
3. Explained to the child by the dietitian
4. Handled in a matter-of-fact way

50 Before discharge, while his mother is talking to the nurse about his care at home, Tommy joins the other children in the playroom. You would expect him to engage in:
1. Parallel play
2. Competitive play
3. Solitary play
4. Tumbling-type play

51 While successfully learning autonomy and independence, Tommy would be learning:
1. Trust and security
2. Roles within society
3. Superego control
4. To accept external limits

Situation: May Ann Lewis, age 18, is admitted to the mental health unit of the general hospital. She has always been a shy, introverted person, but within the past few days she has retreated into a world of fantasy. She makes up her own vocabulary and talks to an imaginary person. She has taken to wearing several sets of clothing at the same time and has made up her face like a clown. The day of admission she retreats to her room, telling the family that she is wired to the television, which informed her that the family was out to kill her. Questions 52 through 59 refer to this situation.

52 Which initial action by the admitting nurse would be most therapeutic for May Ann?
1. Taking her to the day room and introducing her to the other patients
2. Telling her that the door is locked and no one can harm her here
3. Reassuring her that she will not be frightened here, away from her family
4. Introducing her to the primary nurse who will be working with her

53 When May Ann says "My lacket hss kelong mon," the nurse should respond by:
1. Trying to learn the language of the patient
2. Telling the patient she is not understood
3. Communicating in simple terms directed toward the patient
4. Recognizing that the patient needs a nurse who can understand her fantasies

54 May Ann, unprovoked, attacks another patient. A short-term plan for her would be to:
1. Protect others from her impulsive acts by secluding her
2. Keep her actively participating and in contact with reality
3. Have a staff member whom she trusts stay with her
4. Get May Ann to apologize for her behavior

55 May Ann tells you the voices have told her she is no good. She asks if you have also heard the voices. Which response is most appropriate?
1. "No, I do not hear your voices, but I believe you can hear them."
2. "The voices are coming from within you and only you can hear them."
3. "It is the voice of your conscience, which only you can control."
4. "Oh, the voices are a symptom of your illness; don't pay attention to them."

56 May Ann holds herself aloof; she ridicules and is sarcastic to other patients. She identifies with the staff. The nursing care plan at this time should be to:
1. Assign activities with the staff only
2. Accept the negative emotions; praise the positive ones
3. Explain that she should be more accepting of others
4. Encourage group participation with withdrawn patients

57 The physician has ordered chlorpromazine (Thorazine), 300 mg p.o. t.i.d. Which of the following nursing actions can alleviate the side effect May Ann might experience the first week she takes the drug?
1. Have her increase her fluid intake
2. Take her blood pressure before giving the drug
3. Give her coffee with the medication and meals
4. Give her benztropine (Cogentin) with the medication

58 The major reason for treating severe emotional disorders with tranquilizers is to:
1. Make the patient more amenable to psychotherapy

2. Prevent destructiveness by the patient
3. Reduce the neurotic symptoms
4. Prevent secondary complications

59 May Ann is much improved and, with a group of other patients, is preparing for a social evening in town. They are to go with a staff member. The purpose of visits into the community under the supervision of a professional is to:
1. Assist patients in adjusting to anxieties in the community
2. Observe a patient's ability to cope with a more complex society
3. Help the patients return to reality under controlled conditions
4. Broaden the patients' experiences by providing exposure to cultural activities

Situation: As a result of an industrial accident, Mr. Jones has suffered second-degree and third-degree burns on his left leg, left arm, and face. Questions 60 through 66 refer to this situation.

60 Burns classified as third degree involve destruction of the:
1. Epidermis layer
2. Subcutaneous tissue
3. Corium
4. Fatty layer

61 What percent of Mr. Jones' total skin surface has been burned?
1. 18%
2. 27%
3. 36%
4. 45%

62 The major objective during the early postburn phase is to:
1. Prevent infection
2. Replace blood loss
3. Restore fluid volume
4. Relieve pain

63 One difficult problem for the nurse to deal with concerning a recently admitted burned patient is:
1. Severe pain
2. Alteration in body image
3. Frequent dressing changes
4. Maintenance of sterility

64 In assessing Mr. Jones for respiratory involvement during the first 2 days, the nurse should interpret which of the following observations as indicative of this complication? Sputum that is:
1. Frothy
2. Sooty
3. Yellow
4. Tenacious

65 The nurse should assess the patient for symptoms of hypovolemic shock, which is often associated with burns because of:
1. Sodium retention as a result of the aldosterone mechanism
2. Decreased rate of glomerular filtration
3. A shift of proteins and water out of intravascular compartment
4. Excessive blood loss through the burned tissues

66 An individual with serious burns requires frequent checks of potassium levels because:
1. Damaged cells absorb potassium, causing hyperkalemia
2. Burned individuals excrete excessive potassium, resulting in hypokalemia
3. Damaged cells release potassium, causing hyperkalemia
4. Potassium loss from damaged skin may cause hypokalemia

Situation: Mr. Smith, 55, has had difficulty sleeping and eating. He has lost a great deal of time from work because he "wasn't feeling well." Lately he has just sat in his room staring at the floor with a sad look on his face. His one wish is that he would die. Questions 67 through 74 refer to this situation.

67 Mr. Smith is brought to the general hospital after taking an overdose of phenobarbital. After a lavage, Mr. Smith states, "Let me die, I'm no good." The nurse's most appropriate response would be:
1. "Of course you're good, we'll take care of you."
2. "You must have been upset to try to take your life."
3. "Do you feel like telling me why you did this?"
4. "You have been through a rough time; let me take care of you."

68 Mr. Smith has been placed on suicide precautions. A therapeutic community would provide these precautions by:
1. Removing all "cutting" objects
2. Not allowing him to leave his room
3. Giving him an opportunity to ventilate his feelings
4. Assigning a staff member to be with him at all times

69 Mr. Smith is to receive a series of electroconvulsive therapy (ECT). The nurse, in explaining this procedure to the patient, should emphasize that:
1. He will have amnesia afterward
2. The treatments will make him better

3. Someone will be with him all the time

4. He should not be afraid; it will not hurt

70 One of the side effects of ECT that Mr. Smith may experience is:

1. Loss of appetite

2. Postural hypotension

3. Confusion for a time after treatment

4. Complete loss of memory for a time

71 Mr. Smith is given a muscle relaxant just before the ECT. The major disadvantage of this drug is that it inhibits which muscles?

1. Intercostal and diaphragmatic

2. Biceps and triceps

3. Facial and thoracic

4. Sternocleidomastoid and abdominal

72 Which of the following aspects of ECT can result in the most serious complication?

1. Thiopental sodium (Pentothal) to induce sleep

2. Succinylcholine chloride to relax muscles

3. Positive pressure to inflate the alveoli

4. Electric voltage to induce convulsions

73 A treatment program is planned for Mr. Smith. The staff set specific goals directed toward helping the patient:

1. Develop trust in others

2. Express his hostile feelings

3. Set realistic life goals

4. Get involved in activities

74 Which of the following activities would be least helpful to a severely depressed patient such as Mr. Smith:

1. Allowing the patient to plan own projects

2. Specific simple instructions to be followed

3. Simple, easily completed short-term projects

4. Monotonous, repetitive projects and activities

Situation: Mr. Sill, age 45, who has smoked 3 to 4 packs of cigarettes per day for the last 25 years, was treated with irradiation of his larynx 3 months ago for squamous cell carcinoma. For the past 2 weeks he has noted recurrent hoarseness that has progressively worsened. He now enters the hospital for evaluation and further therapy. He plays the harmonica professionally. Except for findings of hoarseness and a small mass in the left vocal cord, the remainder of his physical examination in unremarkable. Total laryngectomy with block dissection of the cervical lymph nodes is performed after appropriate diagnostic studies and preparation for surgery have been carried out. Mr. Sill is discharged 14 days after surgery. Questions 75 through 81 refer to this situation.

75 An important aspect of preoperative nursing care includes

1. Adequate explanation of the nature of the surgery to be performed

2. Instruction in breathing exercises and/or equip-

ment used postoperatively to prevent complications

3. Basing instruction on those areas which Mr. Sill questions

4. Having a speech therapist visit Mr. Sill

76 Among neoplasms of the head and neck, cancer of the larynx is a major concern. Which factor would *not* predispose an individual to this disorder?

1. Heavy alcohol ingestion

2. Poor dental hygiene

3. Air pollution

4. Chronic respiratory infections

77 Immediate postoperative management for Mr. Sill would include:

1. Placing the patient in the orthopneic position

2. Removing the outer tracheostomy tube p.r.n.

3. Suctioning the tracheostomy tube at least every 10 or 15 minutes

4. Instructing the patient to whisper

78 Mr. Sill's initial feedings are by nasogastric tube. Soon afterward he begins to develop diarrhea. A possible solution to this problem would be to:

1. Increase the carbohydrate content of the formula to give it more energy value

2. Decrease the protein content to make it easier to digest

3. Dilute the formula with water to give it more volume

4. Decrease the carbohydrate content of the formula and give it more slowly

79 Mr. Sill asks how long he will have to be fed through a tube. The nurse should explain that nasogastric feedings will be required:

1. For the rest of Mr. Sill's life

2. Until healing has occurred

3. Until Mr. Sill develops the ability to belch

4. Until Mr. Sill can digest oral feedings

80 On the day Mr. Sill is being discharged he exhibits concern about the possibility that his laryngectomy tube might become dislodged. The nurse should teach him to:

1. Notify the physician at once

2. Keep calm, since there is no immediate emergency

3. Recognize that prompt closure of the tracheal opening may occur

4. Reinsert another tube immediately

81 Since Mr. Sill's tracheostomy is permanent, which of the following factors should be included in the teaching plan?

1. The sterile technique necessary for care of his tracheostomy tube

2. The establishment of a regular pattern for suctioning the tube
3. The importance of cleanliness around the site
4. The importance of covering the tube opening while bathing and swimming

Situation: Ten-year-old Marc has rheumatoid arthritis. His joints are enlarged, and he has a low-grade fever with an erythematous rash on his trunk. Questions 82 through 85 refer to this situation.

82 When planning nursing care for Marc, the nurse should know that he will most often have pain and limited movement of his joints:
1. When the latex fixation test is positive
2. When the room is cool
3. In the morning on awakening
4. After assistive exercise

83 A major difference between juvenile rheumatoid arthritis and the polyarthritis of rheumatic fever is that with rheumatoid arthritis there may be:
1. Some permanent cardiac damage
2. An exacerbation during the winter months
3. Some residual joint deformity
4. A link with the *Streptococcus* organism

84 In a patient receiving prolonged aspirin therapy, the nurse should be alert for symptoms of:
1. Urinary calculi
2. Prolonged clotting time
3. Atrophy of the liver
4. Premature erythrocyte destruction

85 When 10-year-old Marc is able to move to a two-bed room, the best suited roommate would be:
1. An 11-year-old boy with an appendectomy
2. A 10-year-old girl with a fractured femur
3. A 9-year-old boy with asthma
4. A 12-year-old girl with colitis

Situation: Mr. Leonard is an alcoholic and has cirrhosis of the liver. Questions 86 through 92 refer to this situation.

86 Mr. Leonard is brought to the emergency room in the midst of protracted clonic convulsions. He is given diazepam (Valium), which decreases central neuronal activity and:
1. Dilates the tracheobronchial structures
2. Relaxes peripheral muscles
3. Slows cardiac contractions
4. Provides amnesia for the convulsive episode

87 Mr. Leonard's serum albumin level is low, and the physician prescribes 50 ml of salt-poor albumin IV. Albumin replacement is expected to:

1. Decrease tissue fluid accumulation and the hematocrit level
2. Decrease ascites and the blood ammonia level
3. Decrease capillary perfusion and blood pressure
4. Decrease venous stasis and the blood urea nitrogen level

88 While Mr. Leonard is receiving the albumin, the planned therapeutic effect will be greater if the infusion is regulated to run:
1. Slowly, and fluid intake is restricted
2. Rapidly, and fluids are encouraged
3. Slowly, and fluids are encouraged liberally
4. Rapidly, and fluid intake is withheld

89 Mr. Leonard is having delirium tremens and is given paraldehyde (Paral) IM. Elimination of the drug can be assessed by monitoring:
1. Urination
2. Salivation
3. Diaphoresis
4. Breathing

90 Mr. Leonard is receiving neomycin sulfate (Mycifradin) orally. The purpose for administration of the drug is to:
1. Protect against infection while immune mechanisms are deficient
2. Suppress ammonia-forming bacteria in the intestinal tract
3. Increase urea digestive activity of enteric bacteria
4. Protect regenerative nodules in the liver from invading bacteria

91 Immediately before an abdominal paracentesis, the nurse should ask the patient to void because:
1. A urine specimen must be obtained at this time to check level of nonprotein nitrogen
2. A full bladder increases the danger of puncture of the bladder
3. An empty bladder will decrease the intraabdominal pressure
4. A full bladder decreases the amount of fluid in the abdominal cavity

92 Mr. Leonard, participating in an alcohol abstinence program, has a cold when he comes to the clinic. He tells the nurse he plans to use elixir of terpin hydrate for his cough. The nurse would advise him not to take it while he is taking disulfiram (Antabuse) because it will cause:
1. Abdominal cramps and muscle twitching
2. Epigastric pain and headache
3. Jitteriness and nausea
4. Dizziness and violent vomiting

Situation: Jane Bond, a 15-year-old girl, is brought into the emergency room after being found unconscious in the locker room at school. There is a strong odor of acetone to her breath and her face is flushed. Questions 93 through 99 refer to this situation.

93 After developing a relationship with the nurse, Jane admits that she has not been adhering to her diabetic regimen. As a first step in attempting to help Jane develop some understanding of the importance of a diabetic regimen, the nurse should:
  1. Give her printed material about diabetes in teenagers
  2. Impress on the parents that it is their responsibility to help and understand Jane
  3. Allow Jane to express her feelings about diabetes
  4. Assume that Jane has not been properly taught previously

94 When teaching Jane about diabetes and self-administration of insulin, the first step for the nurse should be to:
  1. Begin the teaching program at Jane's present level
  2. Find out what Jane knows about her health problem
  3. Set specific and realistic short- and long-term goals
  4. Collect all the equipment needed to demonstrate giving an injection

95 Jane exhibits a need for cognitive learning when she asks:
  1. "What is diabetes?"
  2. "How do I give myself an injection?"
  3. "When do I test my urine for S and A?"
  4. "Can I still be a cheerleader?"

96 After initial treatment to correct the acidosis, Jane is moved to the medical ward. Her height and weight are average—5 feet 3 inches, 114 pounds (160 cm tall, 51.8 kg)—and the diet ordered for her is 2200 calories, 75 g protein, 250 g carbohydrate, and 100 g fat. She is receiving NPH insulin mixed with regular insulin, according to need. In planning a menu for a juvenile diabetic such as Jane, the nurse considers a meal pattern that:
  1. Limits calories to encourage weight loss
  2. Allows for normal growth and developmetal needs
  3. Avoids using potatoes, bread and cereal
  4. Discourages substitutions on the menu pattern

97 The nurse instructs Jane and her parents to:
  1. Weigh all her food on a gram scale
  2. Eat all her meals at home
  3. Prepare her food separately from that of the rest of the family
  4. Always carry some form of sugar with her

98 The nurse plans an evening snack for Jane including milk, crackers, and cheese to provide:
  1. High-carbohydrate nourishment for immediate use
  2. Nourishment with latent effects to counteract late insulin activity
  3. Encouragment for her to stay on her diet
  4. Added calories to help her gain weight

99 A week after the nurse speaks with Jane, Mrs. Bond, whose sister died of diabetes, asks the nurse for information about the disease. The nurse should recognize that Mrs. Bond is:
  1. Too upset to learn new information
  2. Transferring attitudes about her sister to her daughter
  3. Exhibiting readiness for learning
  4. Expressing her attitudes through her behavior

Situation: Mr. Ray is admitted to the surgical unit with a diagnosis of cancer of the colon. His physician plans to do a colon resection with a permanent colostomy. During the 3 days prior to surgery, Mr. Ray is very cooperative in all preoperative procedures, responds pleasantly when approached by the nurses, and does not question staff about what is being done to him. Questions 100 through 106 refer to this situation.

100 From his behavior, the nurse recognizes that Mr. Ray most likely:
  1. Is totally denying his illness
  2. Has been fully informed by his physician about what to expect
  3. Is not verbalizing his feelings about what will happen to him
  4. Feels reassured by his frequent contacts with the nurses

101 The night before Mr. Ray's surgery the nurse notices that each time she makes rounds he is awake, despite adequate sedation. He has no requests but invites her to have a cigarette with him. Based on her understanding of Mr. Ray's behavior, the nurse's response should be to:
  1. Send in a nurse's aide to keep him company while he smokes
  2. Point out to him that nurses cannot smoke in patients' rooms
  3. Light his cigarette and tell him to call her again if he still can't sleep
  4. Light his cigarette and indicate that she has noticed his inability to sleep

102 After surgery the most effective way of helping Mr. Ray accept his colostomy would be to:
  1. Give him literature containing factual data about colostomies

2. Point out to him the number of important people who have had colostomies
3. Begin to teach him self-care of his colostomy immediately
4. Contact a member of Colostomies, Inc. to speak with him

103 Mr. Ray's postoperative diet order reads "diet as tolerated." Principles that should guide food choices include:
1. A low-residue diet should be followed indefinitely to avoid overstimulating the intestine
2. A return to a regular diet as soon as possible gives psychologic support and more rapid physical rehabilitation
3. Many foods will cause all individuals with a colostomy the same discomfort
4. More rigid dietary rules limiting food choices are needed to provide security

104 During a colostomy irrigation, if Mr. Ray complains of abdominal cramps, the nurse should:
1. Raise the irrigating can so the irrigation can be completed quickly
2. Reassure him and continue the irrigation
3. Pinch the tubing so that less fluid enters the colon
4. Clamp the tubing and allow Mr. Ray to rest

105 Mr. Ray's colostomy is located on the left side of the abdomen. What type of stools would the nurse expect Mr. Ray to expel?
1. Moist, formed
2. Pencil shaped
3. Liquid
4. Mucus coated

106 During the rehabilitation period, when discussing with Mr. Ray the regaining of some measure of bowel control, the nurse should emphasize:
1. Having a set time each day for his colostomy irrigation
2. The importance of a soft low-residue diet
3. The importance of managing his fluid intake
4. The necessity for a high-protein diet

Situation: *Mr. Gold, a 42-year-old insurance broker, is admitted to the hospital with a diagnosis of coronary occlusion and is experiencing pain and distress. Questions 107 through 114 refer to this situation.*

107 The nurse realizes that the pain associated with coronary occlusion is caused primarily by:
1. Arterial spasm
2. Irritation of nerve endings in the cardiac plexus
3. Ischemia of the heart muscle
4. Blocking of the coronary veins

108 On Mr. Gold's admission the nurse immediately gives him oxygen to:
1. Prevent dyspnea
2. Prevent cyanosis
3. Increase oxygen concentration to heart cells
4. Increase oxygen tension in the circulating blood

109 During the acute period of Mr. Gold's illness the nurse should make the bed by:
1. Changing the top linen and only the necessary bottom linen
2. Changing the linen from top to bottom without lowering the head of the bed
3. Sliding him onto a stretcher, remaking the bed, then sliding him back to the bed
4. Lifting rather than rolling him from side to side while changing the linen

110 Mr. Gold's orders include strict bed rest and a clear liquid diet. The nurse should explain to the patient that the primary reason for this diet is to reduce:
1. Gastric acidity
2. The metabolic work load associated with digestion
3. His weight
4. The amount of fecal elimination

111 Two days after admission Mr. Gold's temperature rises to 38.3° C (101° F). The nurse should realize that this elevation indicates:
1. Possible infection
2. Tissue necrosis
3. Pulmonary infarction
4. Pneumonia

112 In creating a therapeutic environment for Mr. Gold the nurse should provide for:
1. Daily papers in the morning
2. Telephone communication
3. Short family visits
4. Television for short periods

113 The monitor shows a PQRST wave for each beat and indicates a rate of 120. The rhythm is regular. The nurse should note that the patient is experiencing:
1. Atrial fibrillation
2. Ventricular fibrillation
3. Sinus tachycardia
4. First-degree heart block

114 Mr. Gold complains of severe nausea, and his heartbeat is irregular and slow. The nurse should recognize these symptoms as toxic effects of:
1. Lanoxin
2. Lidocaine
3. Morphine sulfate
4. Meperidine hydrochloride

Situation: Johnny has been attending a day care center for autistic children. Questions 115 through 120 refer to this situation.

115 Autism can usually be diagnosed when the child is about:
1. 6 months of age
2. 1 to 3 months of age
3. 2 years of age
4. 6 years of age

116 In planning activities for Johnny the nurse must remember that autistic children respond best to:
1. Loud cheerful music
2. Own self-stimulating acts
3. Individuals in small groups
4. Large group activity

117 Since autistic children withdraw into their own world, relationships are difficult to establish. The nurse may be able to reach Johnny by:
1. Body contact, such as cuddling
2. Encouraging his participation in group activities
3. Imitating and participating in his activities
4. Providing a quiet, safe place for rocking

118 The nurse would expect Johnny to demonstrate:
1. Sad, blank facial expressions
2. Flapping of hands and rocking
3. Inappropriate smiling with flat emotions
4. Lack of response to any stimulus

119 When using play as therapy with Johnny the nurse should:
1. Play music and dance with Johnny
2. Provide mechanical and inanimate objects for him to play with
3. Talk with Johnny while touching his hands
4. Provide brightly colored toys and blocks that he can handle

120 Given a choice, the autistic child would usually enjoy playing with a:
1. Cuddly toy
2. Large red block
3. Small yellow block
4. Playground merry-go-round

How to Use Worksheet 1: Errors in Processing Information

Common errors in processing information are listed in the left hand column of this worksheet. At the top of the worksheet is a row of blank spaces for inserting the number of the question missed. Directly below each number, check any errors you made in answering that question. You may have made more than one type of error in an answer.

Worksheet 1: Errors in Processing Information

Question no.																							
Did not read situation/question carefully																							
Missed important details																							
Confused major and minor points																							
Defined problem incorrectly																							
Could not remember terms/facts/concepts/ principles																							
Defined terms incorrectly																							
Focused on incomplete/incorrect data in assessing situation																							
Interpreted data incorrectly																							
Applied wrong concepts/principles in situation																							
Drew incorrect conclusions																							
Identified wrong goals																							
Identified priorities incorrectly																							
Carried out plan incorrectly/incompletely																							
Was unclear about criteria for evaluating success in achieving goals																							

How to Use Worksheet 2: Knowledge Gaps

Types of common knowledge gaps are listed along the top of this worksheet. Write a brief description of topics you want to review in the spaces provided. For example, if you missed a question on administration of a particular drug, write the drug name and problem (e.g., dosage) in the appropriate space under the column labeled Pharmacology.

Worksheet 2: Knowledge Gaps

Basic science	Skills/ procedures	Basic human needs	Growth & develop- ment	Normal nutrition	Psycho- social factors	Clinical area/ topic	Stressors/ coping mechanisms	Patho- physiology	Pharma- cology	Therapeutic nutrition	Legal implications	Other

Answers and Rationales

1. (4) Gentle pressure is applied against the baby's head as it emerges so it is not delivered too rapidly. The head is never held back, and it should be supported as it emerges so there will be no vaginal lacerations. (b); IM; AP; SH; OB*
   (1) It is impossible to breathe and pant at the same time.
   (2) Unless she pants and blows breath out, she will push involuntarily.
   (3) Unless she pants to slow the pushing, she will deliver on the stretcher.

2. (2) Position the baby wth head lower than chest and rub the infant's back to stimulate crying so he can oxygenate his lungs. (a); IM; AP; NU; OB
   (1) This is not the priority at the present moment; the uterus still contains placenta and will not contract.
   (3) There is no need for haste in cutting the cord; a clear airway is the priority.
   (4) There is no time, and the mother will not be able to cooperate with a move to the stretcher.

3. (1) Precipitate delivery may be injurious to both mother and infant. The maternal morbidity rate is increased by infection and/or hemorrhage resulting from the trauma of a rapid forceful delivery in a contaminated field. (b); EV; AN; NU; OB
   (2) This is common to all patients after all types of delivery; due to the change in blood volume.
   (3) This may be due to the use of oxytocin or to impending toxemia, not to a precipitous delivery.
   (4) Unless there is some airway obstruction, a precipitous delivery will not have any influence on the baby's respirations.

4. (2) The first hour after delivery is called the fourth stage of labor. During this time the uterus is at the level of the umbilicus, and each day after delivery it descends one finger breadth. (c); AS; CP; NU; OB
   (1) The uterus descends below the umbilicus, rising above it only if the bladder is full.
   (3) This will happen on the second day post partum; the uterus descends one finger breadth each day.
   (4) This will happen on the fourth or fifth day post partum; the uterus descends one finger breadth per day.

5. (3) The Nurse Practice Act requires nurses to diagnose human responses. (b); AS; KN; NU; OB
   (1) This is physical assessment, not medical diagnosis, and is within the nurse's role
   (2) Fortunately not true, since the physician may not be present; the nurse is capable of making physical assessment.
   (4) Assessment should not differ if done by the nurse.

6. (4) To maintain a patent airway and promote respiration and gaseous exchange, mucus must be removed from the respiratory tract. (b); IM; AN; NU; OB
   (1) If the airway is obstructed, oxygen will be of no use; therefore suctioning is a priority.
   (2) This is for aspirating the stomach contents not for airway clearance.
   (3) Documentation is important but secondary to clearing a passageway for air.

7. (1) Respiratory distress is a frequent response indicative of possible immaturity of the infant's respiratory tract—such as a small lumen, weakness of the respiratory musculature, paucity of functional alveoli, or insufficient calcification of the bony thorax. (b); AS; KN; NU; OB
   (2) Temperature generally stabilizes after 8 hours, unless the baby is premature.
   (3) This would not yet be important since the baby's intake is limited in the first 24 hours.
   (4) Tone (i.e., high, shrill) would be more pertinent than duration.

8. (1) The tonic neck reflex is normal in the newborn and disappears within 3 to 6 months. (b); IM; AN; SH; OB
   (2) This is a normal newborn response and does not need medical attention.
   (3) This response disappears between 3 and 4 months.
   (4) Lack of this reflex may indicate neurologic impairment.

9. (2) Allowing the mother time to inspect the child permits viewing, touching, and holding, promoting bonding. (b); PL; AP; SH; OB
   (1) The mother should have made this decision before delivery.
   (3) Mrs. Penny will proceed at her own rate; requiring her to do things is not supportive.
   (4) This can be done only by allowing the mother ample time to inspect and interact with her baby.

10. (3) Some mothers will respond to mores and pressures by trying to nurse in spite of the fact that they would prefer to give the baby a bottle. The nurse should elicit more information before responding. (b); IM; AP; SH; OB
    (1) Although true, the mother's statement indicates some reluctance to breast-feed and should be further explored.
    (2) The baby's suckling and emptying the breasts will determine the amount of milk.
    (4) Untrue; successful breast-feeding requires mastery, and many women are unable to do this.

*The letters following the rationales represent an analysis of each question. The letter in parentheses refers to the level of difficulty. The first set of capital letters refers to steps in the nursing process: AS, assessing; AN, analyzing; PL, planning; IM, implementing; EV, evaluating. The second set of capital letters represents the cognitive level of the question: KN, knowledge; CP, comprehension; AP, application; AN, analysis. The third set refers to the locus of decision making: NU, nurse; SH, shared; CL, client. The last set refers to the clinical area: ME, medical; SU, surgical; OB, obstetrical; PS, psychiatric; PE, pediatric.

11. (4) Daily washing of the breasts and nipples with water is sufficient for cleanliness; soap may be drying. (b); IM; AP; SH; OB

    (1) Scrubbing as well as the use of soap may irritate and dry nipples, which may already be tender.

    (2) Unnecessary to use sterile water; the inside of the baby's mouth is not sterile.

    (3) Alcohol is drying; may leave a taste that causes the infant to reject the nipple.

12. (3) The pressure and tenderness resulting from accumulated milk can be relieved by manually expressing some of the fluid. (b); IM; AP; SH; OB

    (1) The nurse is capable of independent action that involves patient teaching.

    (2) Pain medications would be offered only if other measures were unsuccessful; limits transfer of medication to the infant through breast milk.

    (4) Very unsound advice; the mother needs to drink fluid and keep nursing to ensure the flow of breast milk.

13. (1) Frequently the emotional excitement of going home will diminish lactation and/or the letdown reflex for a brief period. When the mother has knowledge that this may happen and how to cope with it, the problem is apt to be a minor one and easily overcome. (b); IM; AP; SH; OB

    (2) Lacks an explanation of why it happens as well as concrete instructions for remedying the situation.

    (3) Many factors (stress) inhibit lactation, and the patient should be aware of this; false reassurance.

    (4) This supply may diminish or stop under stress factors; false reassurance.

14. (3) Most average-sized babies regulate themselves on an approximate 4-hour schedule. However, wide variation does exist. (b); IM; AP; SH; OB

    (1) Although true, this does not answer the mother's question concerning the time for doing things.

    (2) It is best to allow the baby to set his own schedule; usually close to hospital routine.

    (4) Some of the episodes of crying do not indicate that the baby is hungry; the mother will learn difference.

15. (3) Anovulation occurs in nursing mothers for varying periods. Lactation does affect the degree of infertility, but it is generally not a reliable method of birth control. (a); IM; AP; SH; OB

    (1) Untrue; lactation may delay menses but does not suppress ovulation.

    (2) Ovulation can occur without menstruation.

    (4) Menstrual periods may not occur for several months; this would put undue strain on marital relationships.

16. (1) The common bile duct enters the duodenum. The pyloric sphincter is located between the end of the stomach and the beginning of the duodenum; therefore, when it is hypertrophied, the tight sphincter prevents any mixing of formula with bile. (b); AS; CP; NU; PE

    (2) Pyloric stenosis involves hypertrophy and hyperplasia of the muscle of the pyloric sphincter, causing a severe narrowing between the stomach and the duodenal canal.

    (3) The area obstructed in pyloric stenosis is the pyloric sphincter, between the stomach and duodenum.

    (4) The bile duct enters the duodeum at a site different from the pyloric sphincter and is uninvolved in pyloric stenosis.

17. (1) The hypertrophied muscle becomes elongated and is palpable as an olive-shaped mass. Because of its normal anatomic location, it is felt in the upper right quadrant of the abdomen. (b); AS; CP; NU; PE

    (2) Normal transmission of ingested food is interrupted, but normal digestive processes are intact.

    (3) Food does not reach the lower GI tract.

    (4) The upper abdomen may be distended since food is unable to leave the stomach and progress through the remainder of the GI tract.

18. (2) Prior to inserting the tube the nurse measures the anatomic pathway the tube will follow—i.e., from the nose to the earlobe (corresponding to the nasopharynx) to the epigastric area of the abdomen (lower end of stomach). It is then marked and inserted to this point. (b); IM; AN; NU; PE

    (1) Resistance to the passage of a gavage tube may be felt, and rotation of the tube often changes placement enough to continue insertion to the point marked by measurement.

    (3) This distance would be much too long.

    (4) This distance might not place the tube well into the stomach and would increase the risk of aspiration.

19. (2) If the nasogastric tube is accidently passed into the trachea rather than the esophagus, it will occlude the airway, causing cyanosis. (b); EV; AN; NU; PE

    (1) Choking may occur as the tube passes through the back of the throat.

    (3) Flushing may result if the infant attempts to fight the passage of the tube.

    (4) Gagging may occur as the tube passes from the nasal passage through the pharynx.

20. (4) During and after feeding, the position most favoring gravity is employed to promote retention of fluid and prevent vomiting. (c); IM; AP; SH; PE

    (1) Postoperative positioning with the head elevated helps to assist food passage; the prone position would promote vomiting.

    (2) Vomiting may continue postoperatively, so limited movement of the child after feedings is suggested.

    (3) Feeding any child in the supine position greatly increases the risk of aspiration.

21. (3) Offering a new food after giving formula associates this activity with eating and takes advantage of the child's unsatisfied hunger. (b); IM; AP; SH; PE

    (1) Solid food should be introduced by spoon to acquaint the child to new tastes and textures as well as the use of the spoon.

(2) New foods should be initiated one at a time and continued for 4 or 5 days to assess for allergy.

(4) Offering food after the regular feeding decreases the chance of success since the infant's hunger is already satisfied.

22. (1) The first solid foods added to the infant's diet should be easily digestible, such as fruits and cereals, and rich sources of iron, such as cereals and egg yolk. (b); IM; AP; CL; PE

(2) Egg white is added very late because of the allergic reactions associated with it.

(3) Meats are more difficult to digest and so are added later.

(4) Sweets have less nutritional value and may make an infant less accepting of other foods later.

23. (2) Signs of mild to moderate placental separation include uterine discomfort and tenderness because of concealed bleeding. Visible bleeding may be scant, moderate, or heavy. (b); AS; AN; NU; OB

(1) Uterine size may increase because of accumulated blood at the placental site.

(3) There is a great deal of pain because of accumulated blood in the uterine cavity.

(4) Uterine size increases from accumulated blood; vaginal bleeding may be present.

24. (4) The blood cannot escape from behind the placenta. Thus the abdomen becomes boardlike and painful because of the entrapment. (b); AN; CP; NU; OB

(1) Symptoms of hemorrhagic shock do not include pain.

(2) This is not an immediate response; may occur later if the patient's resistance is lessened.

(3) Blood may be at the site of placental separation but not in the uterine muscle.

25. (1) Clotting defects are common in moderate and severe abruptio placentae because of the loss of fibrinogen from severe internal bleeding. (b); AN; CP; NU; OB

(2) Excessive globulin in the bood; unrelated to clotting.

(3) Decrease in the number of platelets; bleeding of abruptio is caused by depletion of fibrinogen.

(4) Excessive amount of red blood cells; not related to the depletion of fibrinogen.

26. (4) Parents must be helped to identify their feelings. (a); IM; AP; SH; PS

(1) Answer based on the nurse's religious belief; no indication that the patient has the same belief; closes off communication.

(2) Unpredictable; does not encourage the patient to explore her feelings.

(3) Many stillborn children are apparently free of any defects.

27. (1) Excessive thyroid hormones increase the metabolic rate, causing nervousness, weight loss, increased appetite, heat intolerance, and tachycardia. (a); AS; CP; SH; ME

(2) Exophthalmos is common in hyperthyroidism; how-

ever, the pulse rate is rapid and the patient is nervous and hyperactive.

(3) Although the appetite is increased, moist skin and rapid pulse rate are associated with hyperthyroidism; a slow pulse rate and dry skin accompany hypothyroidism because of a decreased metabolic rate.

(4) Although loss of weight is associated with hyperthyroidism, GI disturbances and listlessness occur with hypothyroidism because of a decreased metabolic rate.

28. (1) The radioactive iodine uptake test involves administering trace amounts of ^{131}I and subsequently evaluating its uptake. In hyperthyroidism, blood levels of both ^{131}I and T_3 (triiodothyronine) are increased. (b); IM; AP; SH; ME

(2) The results with the sequential multichannel autoanalyzer (SMA 12) are not specific to thyroid disease; the protein bound iodine test is not definitive because it is influenced by the intake of exogenous iodine.

(3) X-ray results would not indicate thyroid disease, and elevation of T_4 (thyroxine) might indicate hyperthyroidism; however, this would be a false reading because of the presence of thyroid-binding globulin (TBG).

(4) P_{O_2} is not specific to thyroid disease, and the basal metabolic rate is a measure of energy expenditure, not thyroid function (for which it is inaccurate); results of the BMR would be readily altered by CHF, anemia, caffeine, obesity, and adrenal disease.

29. (3) Promotion of rest to reduce metabolic demands is a challenging but essential task with a patient who has hyperthyroidism. (b); PL; CP; SH; ME

(1) Diet can be increased to meet metabolic demands; the patient usually has an excellent appetite.

(2) The neatness of linen is not an important aspect of the patient's care; the patient is usually hyperactive, and it is difficult to promote rest.

(4) Hospital routines should not be considered a nursing problem; routines should always be flexible to meet patient needs.

30. (1) Propylthiouracil (Propacil), used in the treatment of hyperthyroidism, blocks the synthesis of thyroid hormones by preventing iodination of tyrosine. (b); IM; CP; NU; ME

(2) Iodine solutions reduce the size and vascularity of the thyroid gland.

(3) Propylthiouracil does not increase the uptake of iodine.

(4) Thyroid-stimulating hormone (TSH), secreted by the anterior pituitary, is not affected by propylthiouracil.

31. (4) Lugol's solution provides iodine, which aids in decreasing the vascularity of the thyroid gland, decreasing the risk of hemorrhage. (b); IM; CP; NU; SU

(1) Calcium is needed to maintain parathyroid function.

(2) Thyroid hormone substitutes will regulate the body's metabolism.

(3) Antithyroid drugs, not iodine, prevent the formation of thyroxine.

32. (1) Medication is regulated to maintain the normal blood levels of thyroxin; therefore ovulation is not affected, and future pregnancy is possible. (c); IM; AN; SH; OB

(2) Pregnancy is not contraindicated after a thyroidectomy.

(3) The patient will no longer be hyperthyroid after surgery because the overactive tissue is excised.

(4) Thyroid hormones may have to be increased; however, the alterations in dosage are based on individual needs.

33. (4) Thyroid surgery sometimes results in accidental removal of the parathyroid glands. A resultant hypocalcemia may lead to contraction of the glottis, causing airway obstruction; edema also causes obstruction. (b); IM; AP; NU; SU

(1) Speaking is important in determining the status of the glottis.

(2) Although inspection of the dressing is important, the incision cannot normally be visualized without removal of the dressing; the physician usually changes the first dressing 24 to 48 hours after surgery; the airway takes priority.

(3) The patient should be maintained in a semi-Fowler position to maximize respiratory excursion.

34. (3) Thyroid storm refers to a sudden and excessive release of thyroid hormones, which cause pyrexia, tachycardia, and exaggerated symptoms of thyrotoxicosis. Surgery or infection will generally precipitate this life-threatening condition. (b); AS; AN; NU; SU

(1) Temperature would be elevated in thyroid storm because of the sudden excessive release of thyroid hormones, which elevate the basal metabolic rate.

(2) Hypercalcemia is not related to thyroid storm; hypocalcemia may result from accidental removal of the parathyroid glands.

(4) Pulse rate would be rapid in thyroid storm because of the sudden excessive release of thyroid hormones, which elevate the basal metabolic rate.

35. (2) Thyroid trauma, thyroid surgery, or psychologic stress in a patient with hyperthyroidism may lead to the release of abnormally high levels of thyroid hormones. This intensifies all symptoms of hyperthyroidism—thyroid storm (increased pulse, elevated temperature, restlessness, vomiting, and often death). (b); AN; CP; NU; SU

(1) Tetany occurs from this inadvertent surgical excision.

(3) Iodine would bind with thyroxin, decreasing the potential storm.

(4) Anesthesia would depress metabolism, not increase it.

36. (1) Glaucoma is a disease in which there is increased intraocular pressure resulting from narrowing of the aqueous outflow channel (canal of Schlemm). This can lead to blindness caused by compression of the nutritive blood vessels supplying the rods and cones. (a); AN; CP; SH; ME

(2) Pupil dilation increases intraocular pressure because it narrows the canal of Schlemm.

(3) Intraocular pressure is not affected by activity of the eye.

(4) Increased intraocular pressure can result in blindness and, therefore, must be reduced; although secondary infection are not desirable, the priority is to maintain vision.

37. (2) Retinal damage caused by the increased intraocular pressure of glaucoma is permanent and is progressive if the disease is not controlled. (b); PL; CP; SH; PS

(1) One eye may be affected, and there is no restriction in the use of the eyes.

(3) Blindness may be prevented if treatment is early.

(4) Surgery can open up drainage and permanently reduce pressure.

38. (3) In chronic glaucoma there is a loss of peripheral vision long before the central vision is affected. The patient may also complain of seeing halos around lights. (b); AS; CP; SH; ME

(1) This occurs when there is damage to the central retina; peripheral vision is affected in glaucoma.

(2) Acute glaucoma causes pain; chronic glaucoma is usually insidious.

(4) Blurred vision may be due to a refractive error; peripheral vision is affected in glaucoma.

39. (4) Atropine causes the pupils to dilate, leading to increased intraocular pressure in the patient with glaucoma. Any such order must be questioned because permanent damage might result. (b); IM; AP; NU; SU

(1) Administration of medication is a dependent function; the drug may not be withheld but must be changed by the physician.

(2) The nurse cannot give a medication knowing its effect will harm the patient; would be an act of negligence.

(3) Pilocarpine is often used when preoperative atropine is indicated but must be ordered by the physician; administration of medication is a dependent function.

40. (2) The prone position stretches the flexor muscles, thus preventing hip flexion contractures. (b); IM; AP; SH; SU

(1) Elevating the stump would cause hip flexion, which could result in a hip flexion contracture.

(3) The stump should be elevated during the first 24 hours; elevating the head of the bed would cause hip flexion, which could result in a hip flexion contracture.

(4) Sitting flexes the hips, which could result in a hip flexion contracture.

41. (2) Muscles that originate at the vertebrae or pelvic girdle and insert on the femur act to abduct, adduct, flex, extend, and rotate the femur. Normal body alignment should be maintained because it facilitates the safe and efficient use of muscle groups for balance and stability. (b); IM; AP; SH; SU

(1) This position does not approximate normal body alignment; abduction of the stump will alter the center of gravity.

(3) This position does not approximate normal body alignment; hip flexion will alter the center of gravity and promte the development of a hip flexion contracture.

(4) This will interfere with the development of a normal gait; muscles that originate at the vertebrae and pelvic girdle should be used to move the stump.

42. (3) Subcutaneous fat is reduced by the pressure of the initial constricitve bandage and the socket of the prosthesis. (c); AN; KN; NU; SU

(1) Edema is limited and contributes minimally to the size of the postoperative stump.

(2) Restoration of skin turgor does not affect stump size.

(4) Tissue and bone excised remain constant; after surgery there is no additional loss.

43. (4) The patient is usually instructed to push forcefully yet gently over the bone to toughen the limb for weight bearing. This process is begun by pushing the stump against increasingly harder surfaces. (a); IM; AP; SH; SU

(1) Abduction of the stump does not maintain normal alignment and should be avoided; does not prepare the stump end for a prosthesis.

(2) Dangling the stump does not help prepare it for a prosthesis and may impede venous return, which would prolong healing.

(3) This procedure would soften the stump, impeding its potential for weight bearing.

44. (2) Since Mrs. Kraft has severe diabetes, it is essential that her urine be tested before meals for sugar and ketones to evaluate the success of control of diabetes and the possible need for insulin coverage. (c); IM; AP; NU; ME

(1) Raising the head of the bed flexes the hips, which could result in hip flexion contractures.

(3) To prevent flexion contractures of the hip, the patient should not sit in a chair for a prolonged time.

(4) Salt restriction is not indicated for this patient.

45. (4) Exercise should not include bending and the Valsalva maneuver, which might increase intraocular pressure. (b); PL; AP; CL; ME

(1) Mydriatics are contraindicated in glaucoma because they dilate the pupil, which increases intraocular pressure.

(2) Fluids may be taken as desired because they have no effect on intraocular pressure.

(3) Lighting conditions have no effect on intraocular pressure.

46. (4) In small children the eustachian tube is shorter, wider, and straighter. Pulling the auricle down and back facilitates passage of fluid to the drum. (b); IM; AP; SH; PE

(1) Pulling the auricle down and back helps straighten the canal for passage of the drops.

(2) Pulling the auricle up and back is used for older children and adults.

(3) Pulling the auricle down and back facilitates passage of the eardrops.

47. (2) The middle ear contains the 3 ossicles—malleus, incus, and stapes—which, with the tympanic membrane and oval window, form an amplifying system. (b); AN; KN; NU; PE

(1) Normally the eustacian tube, which connects the middle ear and nasopharynx, is closed and flat to prevent organisms from entering the middle ear; however, it allows air into the middle ear and thus equalizes pressure on both sides of the eardrum.

(3) The pressure of sound waves is amplified in the middle ear and transmitted to the cochlea (inner ear), where it is detected by the organ of Corti and transmitted along the acoustic nerve.

(4) The inner ear contains both the organ of hearing (the cochlea) and the organ of balance (the vestibule).

48. (4) Myringotomy relieves pressure and prevents spontaneous rupture of the eardrum by allowing pus and fluid to escape from the middle ear into the external auditory canal, from which the exudate drains. (b); AS; CP; NU; SU

(1) Miringotomy involves drainage of the middle ear through an incision made in the eardrum; the CNS is not involved.

(2) These symptoms might be expected after surgery involving some part of the urinary tract.

(3) The lacrimal glands are the tear-producing glands.

49. (4) Toddlers are ritualistic and do not tolerate change well. Any change in diet should be done matter-of-factly. Because of their characteristic struggle for independence, toddlers should not be forced to eat. (b); AS; KN; CL; PE

(1) This is not always possible in dietary restrictions.

(2) The toddler is still dependent on the parents and therefore responds better to them than to strangers.

(3) The toddler does not have the cognitive capacity to understand reasons for behavior.

50. (1) The toddler is still dependent on the mother, is narcissistic, and still plays alone but is aware of others playing next to him. (a); AS; KN; CL; PE

(2) Competitive play would be seen in school-age children.

(3) Solitary play or onlookers' play is characteristic of the 1-to-2-year-old.

(4) Tumbling-type play is not a commonly accepted

term used to refer to how play incorporates other children.

51. (4) Appropriate limit setting and discipline are necessary for children to develop self-control while learning the boundaries of their abilities. (c); AN; KN; CL; PE
    (1) Trust and security are tasks that the infant learns.
    (2) Roles within society are learned by the school-age child.
    (3) Superego control begins in the preschooler.

52. (4) Introducing May Ann to the nurse who will be primarily working with her on a one-to-one basis is extremely important because the withdrawn patient can be assisted back to reality by a caring individual (nurse) who is interested in everything that happens to her. (b); IM; AP; SH; PS
    (1) This would be a later action.
    (2) Would have no effect, since she is involved with a strong delusional pattern.
    (3) How does the nurse know she will not be frightened: False reassurance.

53. (2) A simple statement that the patient is not understood provides feedback to the patient and points out reality. (b); IM; AN; SH; PS
    (1) Neologisms have only symbolic meaning for the patient.
    (3) This will be of limited help and does not present reality.
    (4) There is no one other than herself who can understand the fantasies.

54. (3) May Ann needs someone who has been working with her and whom she trusts to stay with her until she is calmer. She has lost control and needs the protection of another person who will observe her, anticipate her actions, and prevent her from acting out her destructive impulses. (c); PL; AP; NU; PS
    (1) It may still be necessary to do this, but staying with her is a better immediate action.
    (2) She may not be ready for participation though she does need to be kept in touch with reality.
    (4) At this time she cannot be held responsible for her behavior.

55. (1) The nurse demonstrates knowledge of her own perceptions and can accept the patient's, even though they are hallucinatory. (b); IM; AP; SH; PS
    (2) The patient would be unable to accept this; it would only increase her fear
    (3) This would increase the patient's guilt and fear.
    (4) Presents reality but negates the patient's feelings and asks for unrealistic responses.

56. (2) Once May Ann realizes that the staff members do not recognize her negative behavior (which is a defense against feelings of inferiority) but praise her for real accomplishments, she will no longer need the superior attitude. She will have gained recognition and self-esteem for socially acceptable behavior. (b); PL; AN; SH; PS

(1) Unrealistic, since a goal is to function again in society.
(3) This is expecting too much of her at present.
(4) The withdrawn patients must be protected from her ridicule and sarcasm just as she must be protected.

57. (3) The caffeine in coffee acts as a stimulant to counteract the drowsiness she may experience during the first week of treatment. After the first week, drowsiness may be replaced by a feeling of calmness. (c); IM; AN; NU; PS
    (1) Rinsing her mouth would help alleviate the dryness, but increasing her fluid intake would have little effect.
    (2) Postural hypotension is a possible side effect, so patient teaching is important; but blood pressure should be checked after giving the drug.
    (4) Not necessary to give Cogentin unless she starts exhibiting extrapyramidal effects.

58. (1) Tranquilizers reduce anxiety levels and make patients more amenable to looking at new approaches to handling stress. (b); AN; KN; NU; PS
    (2) The major tranquilizers are used to treat psychotic symptoms, which may include destructive behavior; however, not the major reason for administration.
    (3) They are used to treat severe emotional illness, not neurotic symptoms.
    (4) They cannot prevent any secondary complications.

59. (2) Maladaptive behavior that may be accepted in the hospital will not be approved in the community. The nurse's observations can help determine which patients are ready to cope with life's realities and which need further help. The nurse can report the observations to the medical team, and appropriate actions can be taken. (c); AN; CP; SH; PS
    (1) A social evening in town would not accomplish this.
    (3) A social evening in town would not by itself constitute reality.
    (4) There is nothing to indicate that any of these patients needed broadening cultural experiences.

60. (2) Third-degree burns are those extending into the subcutaneous tissue. They are not painful, because of nerve destruction. (c); AS; KN; NU; SU
    (1) Burns affecting the outer layer of skin are first degree.
    (3) Burns extending through the epidermis and involving the corium (the fiberous inner layer of skin just below the epidermis) are second degree.
    (4) Burns affecting the underlying fat, muscles, tendons, and bones are fourth degree.

61. (3) By the rule of nines: each arm is 9%, each leg is 18%, and the head is 9%. Therefore the total percentage of burned area on Mr. Jones is 36%. (a); AS; KN; NU; SU
    (1) This figure reflects a miscalculation of the rule of nines.
    (2) This figure reflects a miscalculation of the rule of nines.

(4) This figure reflects a miscalculation of the rule of nines.

62. (3) In the first 48 hours after a severe burn, fluid moves into the tissues surrounding the injured area. Fluid is also lost in drainage and from evaporation. This results in a decreased blood volume and could lead to shock. (a); PL; AN; NU; SU

  (1) The burn wound is generally considered sterile for the first 24 hours; if fluid losses are not replaced immediately, the patient may die before infection can set in.

  (2) Blood loss is usually minimal; the loss of fluid, colloids, and electrolytes is what causes the hypovolemia.

  (4) Although pain relief is an important aspect in the care of patients with burns, the immediate priority is to replace fluid losses to prevent death.

63. (1) The severe pain experienced by the patient during debridement of burns places an emotional strain on the nurse. (a); AN; AN; SH; SU

  (2) According to Maslow, basic needs of survival and safety take precedence over higher-level needs. Pain becomes all encompassing, and the nurse must help the patient cope with it.

  (3) This answer is not complete. The frequency with which the nurse must perform tasks is not the problem; rather it is the pain associated with debridement and the nurse's inability to eliminate the pain.

  (4) Maintaining sterility is not a problem if the nurse understands surgical asepsis.

64. (2) The mucous membranes of the respiratory tract may be charred after inhalation burns. This is evidenced by the production of sooty sputum. (c); AN; CP; NU; ME

  (1) Frothy sputum is usually indicative of pulmonary edema.

  (3) This finding may indicate respiratory infection.

  (4) This finding may indicate respiratory infection.

65. (3) The shift of plasma proteins into the burned area increases the tissue colloid osmotic pressure (TCOP). This results in fluid diffusion from the intravascular to the interstitial fluid compartment. The result is decreased blood volume and hypovolemic shock. (c); AS; CP; NU; SU

  (1) Sodium passes to the burned area and helps cause blister formation.

  (2) Decreased glomerular filtration may occur because of hypovolemia; it is not involved in the etiology of hypovolemia.

  (4) Extracellular fluid is lost through burned tissue.

66. (3) Cellular catabolism, as in burns, results in the loss of potassium from cells, this raises the K^+ level in the extracellular fluid (normal range, 3.5 to 5.5 mEq/L). Such hyperkalemia may lead to arrhythmias (peaked T wave at 6 mEq) and, as a terminal event, cardiac arrest. (c); AS; CP; NU; SU

  (1) Hypokalemia may result on the fourth or fifth post-

burn day as potassium shifts from the extracellular fluid into the intracellular compartment.

  (2) The shift of potassium from the intracellular to the extracellular compartment results in hyperkalemia. In addition, *to excrete* means to eliminate waste matter by a normal discharge; the loss of fluids and electrolytes through a damaged integument is not a normal discharge.

  (4) Potassium loss from damaged tissues results in hyperkalemia as the potassium shifts from the intracellular to the extracellular spaces.

67. (2) Showing understanding of and identifying the patient's feelings by giving feedback helps in establishing a therapeutic relationship. (b); IM; AN; SH; PS

  (1) Negates the person's feelings and cuts off any further communication of feelings.

  (3) Too direct; does not allow the patient time to reflect and explore feelings.

  (4) Encourages dependence; does not allow for exploration of feelings.

68. (4) Emotional support and close surveillance can demonstrate the staff's caring and their attempt to prevent acting out of suicidal ideation. (b); IM; AP; SH; PS

  (1) This would be routinely done; by itself not necessarily therapeutic.

  (2) This would be punishment for him; he could still find a way to kill himself in his room.

  (3) This is not a suicide precaution.

69. (3) The staff's presence provides continued emotional support and helps relieve anxiety. (b); IM; AP; SH; PS

  (1) He may not, and if he does it will pass; emphasis on amnesia will increase fear.

  (2) They may not make him better; would be false reassurance.

  (4) This will be part of explaining the treatments; does not need the emphasis that being with someone should have.

70. (3) The relatively massive electrical energy passing through the cerebral cortex during ECT results in a temporary state of confusion after treatment. (b); EV; AP; NU; PS

  (1) Not a usual side effect.

  (2) Not a side effect.

  (4) Not an expected side effect.

71. (1) Succinylcholine chloride (Anectine) causes paralysis of muscles, including the intercostals and diaphragm, so artificial support of respirations is required to sustain life. (a); AN; KN; NU; PS

  (2) This is the purpose of the drug; not a disadvantage.

  (3) This is the purpose of the drug; not a disadvantage.

  (4) This is the purpose of the drug; not a disadvantage.

72. (2) Succinylcholine chloride temporarily paralyzes the muscles, including those of respiration. Therefore some artificial means of respiration is necessary un-

til the drug is metabolized and excreted. (b); AN; KN; NU; PS

(1) Pentothal decreases the possibility of nausea.

(3) This is necessary to prevent respiratory acidosis.

(4) The most significant therapeutic factor in ECT is the convulsion itself.

73. (2) Depressed patients find it difficult to express anger and hostility because they have internalized these feelings and turned them on themselves. (b); PL; AP; SH; PS

(1) This would develop in time; not really a goal of therapy.

(3) There is nothing to indicate that Mr Smith has unrealistic goals.

(4) This would be part of the intervention, not a goal.

74. (1) Severely depressed patients are not motivated to take action or to plan ahead. They are unable to direct their energy on the enviornment. (c); PL; AP; SH; PS

(2) This would be helpful to a severely depressed patient, whose attention span is limited.

(3) This would be helpful to a severely depressed patient, since it requires little thought and provides gratification and satisfaction.

(4) This would be helpful for a person with mental retardation rather than a severe depression.

75. (3) Before teaching, the nurse must determine the patient's areas of concern. Learning increases when anxiety decreases, and it is hoped that knowledge will reduce anxiety. (c); IM; AN; SH; SU

(1) Although this may be part of the information included in preoperative teaching, the teaching should begin at the patient's level.

(2) The patient will be dependent on a respirator postoperatively; breathing exercises are not required.

(4) This is not beneficial for all preoperative patients.

76. (2) Poor dental hygiene may predispose a person to oral infections but would be only remotely involved in laryngeal neoplasms. (c); AS; KN; NU; SU

(1) Alcohol is an irritant which may initiate a tissue change that results in a malignant neoplasm.

(3) The irritation of air polutants may initiate a tissue change that can lead to malignancy.

(4) Tissue alterations caused by repeated microbiologic stress may result in a malignant neoplasm.

77. (3) Secretions are increased because of alterations in structure and function. A patent airway must be maintained. (b); IM; AP; NU; SU

(1) The orthopneic position may cause neck flexion and block the airway.

(2) The outer tube is not removed because the stoma may close.

(4) Whispering can put tension on the suture line; initially nonverbal and written forms of communication should be encouraged.

78. (4) Slow feeding of foods with reduced carbohydrate content helps to prevent rapid peristalsis and subsequent diarrhea. (c); PL; AP; NU; SU

(1) The energy value of food is not related to its effect on intestinal peristalsis; carbohydrates should be reduced to prevent rapid emptying of the stomach and a shift of fluid into the intestinal lumen.

(2) The diarrhea is unrelated to the digestibility of the feedings.

(3) High fluid content shortens the time the feeding will remain in the stomach, leading to increased peristalsis and diarrhea.

79. (2) Food should be avoided until the area is totally healed. This will keep the area from becoming irritated and contaminated and will generally promote healing. (c); IM; AP; SH; SU

(1) Tube feedings are usually required for the first 2 weeks after surgery.

(3) The ability to belch has no bearing on the decision to resume oral feedings.

(4) The ability to tolerate oral feedings is not necessarily lost; such feedings are withheld to prevent irritation to the surgical site.

80. (2) The patient's concerns will be reduced if he knows the stoma will stay open long enough that another tube can easily be inserted. (b); IM; AN; SH; SU

(1) The patient is in no immediate danger, and it is not imperative to notify the physician at once.

(3) A permanent opening into the trachea is formed after 2 to 3 weeks and will not close quickly.

(4) A permanent opening into the trachea is formed after 2 to 3 weeks, and a tube need not be promptly reinserted.

81. (3) The procedure should be explained so the patient understands that the tracheostomy can serve as an entrance for bacteria and that cleanliness is imperative. (b); PL; AP; SH; SU

(1) Sterile technique is not required; medical aseptic technique is adequate and realistic.

(2) Suctioning must be performed only as needed; a pattern is not necessary.

(4) Laryngectomy patients may no longer swim, since water will flood the lungs.

82. (3) Inactivity over an extended time increases stiffness and pain in joints. (a); PL; CP; SH; PE

(1) The latex fixation test is positive when the rheumatoid factor is found in blood serum; this factor is present in many conditions, including rheumatoid arthritis, aging, narcotic addiction, and SLE.

(2) Application of moist heat or cold packs may decrease joint discomfort.

(4) Assistive exercises help maintain joint mobility.

83. (3) Polyarthritis of rheumatic fever is transitory and does not cause deformity. Rheumatoid arthritis is chronic and causes changes in joints. (a); AN; CP; NU; PE

(1) Cardiac damage is often associated with rheumatic fever.

(2) Juvenile rheumatoid arthritis involves chronic inflammation of the joints; exacerbations are most often related to stress.

(4) The etiology of rheumatic fever is related to a previous occurrence of strep throat; rheumatoid arthritis is unrelated.

84. (2) Aspirin interferes with platelet aggregation, thereby lengthening bleeding time. (b); EV; CP; NU; ME
   (1) Urate excretion is enhanced by high doses of aspirin.
   (3) Aspirin is readily broken down in the GI tract and liver.
   (4) Aspirin inhibits platelet aggregations.

85. (1) Ten-year-old boys prefer the company of the same sex and age group. Also, Marc needs to avoid stressful situations that would tend to increase exacerbations. (b); IM; AN; NU; PE
   (2) Same-sex roomates are desirable for companionship and to maintain privacy needs.
   (3) Asthmatic children may have severe respiratory difficulties; this may be too stressful for Marc, who needs rest.
   (4) Same-sex roomates are desirable for companionship and to maintain boy/girl separateness of this age group.

86. (2) Valium is a tranquilizer and anticonvulsant used to relax smooth muscles during seizures. (a); EV; CP; NU; ME
   (1) This is not an effect of Valium.
   (3) This is not an effect of Valium.
   (4) This is not an effect of Valium.

87. (1) Serum albumin is administered to maintain serum levels and normal oncotic pressures. It does this by pulling fluid from the interstitial spaces into the intravascular compartment, thus decreasing the hematocrit level. (c); EV; CP; NU; ME
   (2) Serum albumin will not affect blood ammonia levels; fluid accumulated in the abdominal cavity is best removed via paracentesis.
   (3) The administration of albumin results in a shift of fluid from the interstitial to the intravascular compartment; this will probably increase the blood pressure.
   (4) Albumin administration does not affect venous stasis or blood urea nitrogen.

88. (1) Albumin acts to elevate the blood pressure to normal levels when it is administered slowly and oral fluid intake is restricted. It causes fluid to move from the interstitial spaces into the circulatory system. (b); IM; AN; NU; ME
   (2) Rapid administration could cause circulatory overload; high fluid intake would limit the shift of fluid from the interstitial to the intravascular compartment, interfering with the optimal effects of the drug.
   (3) Fluids are restricted to facilitate the optimal effects of the drug, which shifts fluids from the interstitial tissues to the intravascular compartment.
   (4) Rapid administration could cause circulatory overload; fluid is restricted, not withheld.

89. (4) Paraldehyde is excreted through the lungs and gives off a specific identifiable odor. (c); EV; AP; NU; ME
   (1) This drug is eliminated through the lungs and kidneys, not the gastrointestinal tract.
   (2) This drug is eliminated through the lungs and kidneys, not excreted in saliva.
   (3) This drug is eliminated through the lungs and kidneys, not through the skin.

90. (2) Neomycin aids in reducing the intestinal flora that act on protein substances, causing the production of ammonia. Ammonia is detoxified in the liver. When the liver is unable to perform this function adequately, blood ammonia levels rise, causing encephalopathy. (c); IM; AP; NU; ME
   (1) Although immune mechanisms may be limited in alcoholism and cirrhosis, the neomycin is administered to limit ammonia levels.
   (3) Bacteria in the intestines do not digest urea.
   (4) This does not occur; neomycin controls protein metabolism, a severe problem in liver disease.

91. (2) When the bladder contains large amounts of urine, it becomes distended and may push upward into the abdominal cavity, where it can be punctured. (a); IM; CP; SH; SU
   (1) A urine specimen is not necessary; an empty bladder prevents accidental trauma to the bladder during a paracentesis.
   (3) This is not the rationale for wanting the bladder to be empty.
   (4) The amount of fluid in the bladder has no relationship to ascites.

92. (4) Elixir of terpin hydrate should be avoided because it contains alcohol and will promote an Antabuse reaction. (a); IM; AN; CL; ME
   (1) These symptoms do not occur if the patient ingests both Antabuse and alcohol.
   (2) These are not symptoms of an Antabuse reaction.
   (3) The patient will not only be nauseated but also experience violent vomiting.

93. (3) Psychoemotional factors related to chronic illness often affect the individual's compliance with a medical regimen. These feelings must be explored and worked out for acceptance of the treatment plan. (b); IM; AP; SH; PE
   (1) This may be helpful later, but Jane needs an opportunity now to share her feelings about the disease.
   (2) Adolescents need control but are capable of handling most of their health care needs.
   (4) Jane's knowledge and feelings should be explored.

94. (2) Before planning and instituting a teaching plan, the nurse must assess the patient's attitudes, experience, knowledge, and understanding of the health problem. (b); IM; AN; SH; PE
   (1) Before teaching can begin, assessment of the present level of the knowledge is necessary.
   (3) Before goals can be set, assessment must be carried out.

(4) Before teaching begins, assessment and planning must occur.

95. (1) The acquiring of knowledge or understanding aids in developing concepts rather than skills or attitudes and is a basic learning task in the cognitive domain. (b); AN; CP; CL; PE

    (2) The acquiring of skills and tasks is psychomotor learning.

    (3) The acquiring of skills and tasks is psychomotor learning.

    (4) The acquiring of values and attitudes is in the affective domain.

96. (2) As a result of hormones involved in growth and development, patients with juvenile diabetes have different and changing needs regarding nutrition and exogenous insulin. (a); PL; CP; SH; PE

    (1) Adequate caloric intake is needed by the average-sized adolescent since adolescence is a time of growth.

    (3) Potatoes, bread, and cereals contain necessary fiber and nutrients.

    (4) Some flexibility is needed to promote adherence to any dietary regimen.

97. (4) An insulin-dependent diabetic patient must carry sugar or candy as a ready source of carbohydrate in the event of signs of hypoglycemia. (a); IM; AP; SH; PE

    (1) This is an unnecessary and time-consuming procedure.

    (2) This is an unrealistic and unnatural pattern for an adolescent.

    (3) Jane should be made to feel a part of the family; the diabetic diet will have foods that will be nutritious for the entire family.

98. (2) The protein in milk and cheese may be slowly converted to carbohydrate (gluconeogenesis), providing the body with some glucose during sleep while the NPH is still acting. (b); PL; AP; SH; PE

    (1) The foods chosen are rich in protein and will be utilized slowly.

    (3) The purpose of an evening snack is to cover for NPH activity during sleep.

    (4) Jane's physical size does not indicate a need to gain weight.

99. (3) In the later stages of adaptation an individual is better able to understand and integrate information. When a patient or family member asks for information, this is a clue identifying readiness for learning. (b); AN; AP; SH; PE

    (1) Asking this question indicates readiness to learn.

    (2) Data are not evident to indicate this.

    (4) The question indicates a desire for more information.

100. (3) A diagnosis of cancer and a colostomy both drastically alter a person's self-image and body image. People react differently to this stress, often finding it difficult to express their concerns verbally; however, their actions may demonstrate an awareness of the situation. (b); AN; AN; SH; PS

    (1) Not enough information to determine this.

    (2) Not enough information to determine this.

    (4) Not enough information to determine this.

101. (4) Insomnia is often caused by anxiety. By stating an observation about the patient's activity, the nurse communicates both concern and a recognition that the patient may have more covert problems that he wishes to verbalize. (a); IM; AP; SH; PS

    (1) Denies the patient's request and serves to cut off communication.

    (2) Denies the patient's request and serves to cut off communication.

    (3) Denies the patient's request and serves to cut off communication.

102. (4) Patients who have radical changes in their body image as a result of surgery are usually best able to relate to someone who has faced the same stress and successfully adapted. (b); IM; AN; SH; PS

    (1) Would provide information but do little to aid acceptance.

    (2) Would do little to aid acceptance.

    (3) The patient cannot learn to do colostomy care until he psychologically accepts its presence.

103. (2) A diet as close as possible to normal after a colostomy is recommended for the stated reason that individuals will discover their own food intolerances and should eat accordingly. (b); PL; CP; SH; SU

    (1) A low-residue diet is not necessary; once healing occurs, a diet with adequate residue promotes peristalsis and colostomy functioning.

    (3) Each person is an individual and reacts differently to foods.

    (4) Rigid dietary regulations usually increase anxiety; return to normally tolerated foods provides security.

104. (4) Rapid instillation of fluid into the colon may cause abdominal cramps. By clamping off the tubing, the nurse allows the cramps to subside so the enema can be continued. (b); IM; AP; SH; SU

    (1) Contraindicated; this will increase the force of flow, which will increase the abdominal cramps.

    (2) Emotional support will not interrupt the physical adaptation of abdominal cramps; the irrigation must be temporarily discontinued.

    (3) Although this may reduce the force of the fluid, it will not eliminate the flow of fluid completely; the irrigation should be temporarily discontinued.

105. (1) A colostomy located on the left side of the abdomen would be in the descending colon. Since most but not all of the fluid would be absorbed, the stool would be moist and formed. (c); AS; KN; NU; SU

    (2) This would be associated with conditions that narrow the intestinal lumen; not usually associated with a colostomy.

    (3) This would be associated with a colostomy involving the ascending colon.

(4) Stools are not usually covered with mucus; they may be moist but not mucoid.

106. (1) Colostomy irrigations done daily at the same time help establish normal patterns of bowel evacuation. The diet should be as close as possible to normal. (b); IM; AP; SH; SU

(2) A soft low-residue diet is not necessary; it should be as close to normal as possible.

(3) Although fluid is important to prevent hard stools, it will not help the patient regain bowel control; a daily regimen is the priority.

(4) Initially after surgery, protein promotes healing; protein intake has no relationship to bowel control.

107. (3) Ischemia causes tissue injury and the release of chemicals, such as bradykinin, that stimulate sensory nerves and produce pain. (b); AN; CP; NU; ME

(1) Arterial spasm, resulting in tissue hypoxia and pain, is associated with angina pectoris.

(2) Tissue injury and pain occur in the myocardium.

(4) Arteries, not veins, are involved in the etiology of a myocardial infarction.

108. (3) Administration of oxygen increases the transalveolar O_2 gradient, which improves the efficiency of the cardiopulmonary system. This increases the oxygen supply to the heart. (b); AN; CP; NU; ME

(1) This is not a specific or inclusive answer; increased oxygen to the heart cells will improve cardiac output, which may or may not prevent dyspnea.

(2) Pallor is usually associated with myocardial infarction.

(4) Although this may be true, it is not specific to heart cells, which are hypoxic when there has been a myocardial infarction.

109. (1) Until the patient's condition has reached some degree of stability after myocardial infarction, routine activities such as changing sheets are avoided so the patient's movements will be minimized and the cardiac workload reduced. (b); IM; AP; NU; ME

(2) Changing all the linen causes unnecessary movement, which increases oxygen demands and makes the heart work harder.

(3) Activity is contraindicated because it increases oxygen consumption and cardiac workload.

(4) Any activity is counterproductive to rest; rest must take precedence so the cardiac workload will be reduced.

110. (2) Acute care of the patient with a myocardial infarction is aimed at reducing the cardiac workload. Foods that are easily digested help reduce this workload. Sympathetic nervous system involvement causes decreased peristalsis and gastric secretion, so limiting food intake will help prevent gastric distention. (b); AN; CP; SH; ME

(1) Gastric acidity is not reduced by a clear liquid diet.

(3) Weight control is not a concern immediately following coronary occlusion.

(4) Feces are in the intestine generally 4 days after the ingestion of foods. The patient's desire to have a bowel movement will be the result of pre-hospitalization meals; the liquid diet will affect future elimination.

111. (2) The body's general inflammatory response to myocardial necrosis causes an elevation of temperature as well as leukocytosis within 24 to 48 hours. (b); AN; CP; NU; ME

(1) This is not an expected finding after tissue damage associated with an infarction

(3) This is not a common complication after myocardial infarction; it is usually associated with phlebitis or multiple fractures.

(4) This is not an expected complication after myocardial infarction.

112. (3) Visits by family members can allay anxiety and consequently reduce emotional stress, an important risk factor in cardiovascular disease. (a); PL; AP; SH; PS

(1) The patient may be disturbed by current news. This would raise the metabolic rate, increasing oxygen demands on the heart.

(2) Family, community, or work problems conveyed by phone may cause anxiety; only vital communications with family should be permitted.

(4) Television programs can cause anxiety or excitement, which would increase the metabolic rate and cardiac output.

113. (3) The presence of a P wave before each QRS complex indicates a sinus rhythm. A heat rate of over 100 beats per minute is referred to as tachycardia. (a); AN; CP; NU; ME

(1) Atrial fibrillation causes irregular rhythm.

(2) Ventricular fibrillation is irregular and shows no PQRST configurations.

(4) Heart block pattern is irregular and slow.

114. (1) Signs of digitalis toxicity include cardiac arrhythmias, anorexia, nausea, vomiting, and visual disturbances. Cardiac arrhythmias result from the inhibition, by digitalis, of myocardial Na^+, K^+, and ATP. Extracardiac effects may be due to CNS or local disturbances. (a); EV; AN: NU; ME

(2) Although nausea and heartblock may occur with lidocaine, these symptoms are rarely seen; drowsiness and CNS disturbances are more common side effects of lidocaine.

(3) Toxic effects of morphine sulfate are slow deep respirations, stupor, and constricted pupils; nausea is a side effect, not a toxic effect.

(4) Nausea is a side effect of meperidine hydrochloride (Demerol); toxic effects include dilated pupils, tremor, confusion, and respiratory depression.

115. (3) By 2 years of age the child should demonstrate an interest in others, communicate verbally, and possess the ability to learn from the environment. Before these skills develop, autism is difficult to diagnose. (b); AS; KN; NU; PS

(1) Infantile autism can occur at this age but is difficult to diagnose.

(2) Infantile autism can occur at this age but is difficult to diagnose.

(4) The autism can be diagnosed long before this age.

116. (2) Autistic behavior turns inward. These children do not respond to the environment but attempt to maintain emotional equilibrium by rubbing and manipulating themselves and displaying a compulsive need for behavioral repetition. (a); PL; AP; NU; PS

(1) These children do seem to respond to music, but not necessarily loud cheerful music.

(3) Part of the autistic pattern is the inability to interact with others in the environment.

(4) Large group (or small group) activity would have little effect on the autistic child's response.

117. (3) One begins by trying to enter the world where the child's attention is currently focused; this is a way of making human contact, since the child's usual contacts are inanimate objects. (b); IM; AP; NU; PS

(1) Autistic children generally cannot tolerate cuddling and will become rigid when anyone attempts to do so.

(2) The autistic child is unable to participate in group activities.

(4) This would have no effect on the nurse's ability to reach Johnny; rather it would reinforce his withdrawal.

118. (2) Isolated unrelated activities predominate. The child's behavior reflects withdrawal or feelings of destructive rage. (b); AS; KN; NU; PS

(1) The facial expression is blank; sadness would be a response to the external world, from which the child has withdrawn.

(3) The autistic child rarely if ever smiles.

(4) The autistic child seems to overrespond to stimuli in the environment.

119. (2) Self-isolation and disinterest in interpersonal relationships lead the autistic child to find security in nonthreatening, impersonal objects. (c); IM; AP; SH; PS

(1) This would be too threatening to an autistic child.

(3) Touching him might prove to be too threatening.

(4) These children do not respond to bright-colored toys and blocks as other children do unless there is movement involved.

120. (4) The rhythmic movement of the merry-go-round provides soothing and nonthreatening comfort to the autistic child who cannot reach out to his environment. (c) IM; KN; CL; PS

(1) The autistic child rejects cuddling and anything that feels cuddly.

(2) The child would prefer a mechanical object over a colored block.

(3) The child would prefer a mechanical object over a colored block.

Comprehensive Test 2

To simulate the comprehensive state board examination, this test should be completed within 2 hours.

Situation: Mrs. Wyer, 21 years old, is 6 months pregnant with her second child and is being visited at home by a community health nurse as part of her prenatal care. Her first child is 15 months old. While in the kitchen with Mrs. Wyer, the nurse notes that her lunch includes salami, cheese, and a cola drink. During assessment the nurse notes increased edema in Mrs. Wyer's ankles. Questions 1 through 13 refer to this situation.

1 Besides advising rest with legs elevated, the nurse discusses the foods Mrs. Wyer has been eating and gives instructions concerning her diet. In this instance:
   1. Dietary preferences must influence the food that is eaten
   2. The food selected should have a low salt content
   3. The nutritionist should be brought in to plan a diet
   4. The patient should be advised to attend the prenatal clinic to see the physician

2 Mrs. Wyer complains of constipation. The nurse should explain that constipation frequently occurs during pregnancy because of:
   1. Pressure of the growing uterus on the anus
   2. Increased intake of milk as recommended during pregnancy
   3. The slowing of peristalsis in the gastrointestinal tract
   4. Changes in the metabolic rate

3 Mrs. Wyer begins labor close to her expected date of delivery and is admitted to the hospital. The nurse notices a gush of fluid from the patient's vagina. After checking the fetal heart rate the nurse should:
   1. Notify the physician immediately about the gush of fluid from the vagina
   2. Place the patient in a modified lithotomy position and inspect the perineum
   3. Keep the patient flat in bed and elevate her legs
   4. Place the patient on her side and obtain her blood pressure

4 After several hours of labor the physician orders oxytocin (Pitocin). When a patient in labor is

being infused with oxytocin, it is the nurse's responsibility to:
1. Obtain a physician's order to slow the IV in the presence of hypertonic contractions
2. Flush the IV tubing if the flow slows
3. Shut off the IV in the presence of hypertonic contractions
4. Monitor fetal heart tones every 2 hours

5 The nurse knows that Mrs. Wyer has begun the transitional phase of labor when she:
1. Complains of pains in the back
2. States that the pain has lessened
3. Perspires and her face flushes
4. Assumes the lithotomy position

6 Shortly following delivery Mrs. Wyer says she feels as if she is bleeding. On checking the fundus the nurse finds a steady trickling of blood from the vagina. The first action should be to:
1. Call the physician immediately
2. Hold the fundus firmly and gently massage it
3. Check Mrs. Wyer's blood pressure and pulse
4. Take no action, since this is a common occurrence

7 While checking Mrs. Wyer's fundus 2 days post partum the nurse observes that it is at the umbilicus and displaced to the right. This means that the patient probably has:
1. A full, overdistended bladder
2. Overstretched uterine ligaments
3. A slow rate of involution
4. Retained placental fragments

8 Mrs. Wyer is discharged 5 days after delivery and is referred for home care follow-up. The initial visit to Mrs. Wyer will be more productive if scheduled when:
1. The nurse has more time to expend
2. She is feeding the children
3. Her husband is at work
4. It is convenient for the family

9 The role most likely to foster sound interpersonal relationships during the first visit to the Wyer home is that of:
1. Stranger
2. Teacher
3. Counselor
4. Surrogate

10 When the nurse first talks with Mrs. Wyer, the type of interview that is likely to be most productive is:
1. Information-giving
2. Problem-solving
3. Exploratory
4. Directive

11 On arrival for the first visit at 10 A.M., the nurse find Mr. Wyer at home. He is temporarily collecting unemployment benefits, and the family is on welfare. Mrs. Wyer is worried and ill at ease in the situation. The infant is due for bottle-feeding and the toddler is playing on the floor. At this time the nurse's best action would be to ask Mr Wyer if he would mind:
1. Giving the baby a bottle
2. Taking the toddler for a walk
3. Leaving you and Mrs. Wyer alone
4. Participating in the discussion

12 The 15-month-old child has had no inoculations. Mr. Wyer says he does not believe in them. The nurse's best response to this statement would be:
1. "Scientific evidence proves you wrong."
2. "Have you discussed this with a doctor?"
3. "How can you risk the life of your child?"
4. "You feel they may be harmful?"

13 After discussion with the nurse, Mr. and Mrs. Wyer agree to have their 15-month-old immunized. The initial immunizations on the first visit to the health clinic are:
1. Diphtheria and tetanus toxoids and pertussis vaccine (DTP) and trivalent oral poliovirus vaccine (TOPV)
2. Measles, rubella, and mumps combined vaccines
3. Diphtheria and tetanus toxoids and pertussis vaccine (DTP), trivalent oral poliovirus vaccine, and tuberculin test
4. Combined tetanus and diphtheria toxoid (Td), trivalent oral poliovirus vaccine, and tuberculin test

Situation: *Julie Syms, a 12-month-old girl, is admitted to the hospital with a diagnosis of failure to thrive. Her weight is below the third percentile, her development is retarded, and she shows signs of neglect. Questions 14 through 18 refer to this situation.*

14 Based on this assessment, what behaviors might also support the possibility of parental deprivation?
1. Julie is cuddly, responsive to touch, and wants to be held
2. Julie is stiff, unpliable, and uncomforted by touch
3. Julie is a poor eater, sleeps soundly, and is easily satisfied
4. Julie is responsive to adults, rarely cries but shows no interest in her environment

15 A plan of care that would best meet the needs of this child should include:
1. A vigorous schedule of stimulation geared to the infant's present level of development

2. A plan to have all staff members pick her up and play with her whenever they can

3. A schedule of care that allows the infant stimulation and physical contact by several staff members

4. As consistent a caregiver as possible, with stimulation that is moderate and purposeful

16 During the nurse's assessment of Julie, she observes that the child has good head control, can roll over, but cannot sit up without support or transfer an object from one hand to the other. Based on these facts, the nurse concludes that Julie is developmentally at age:
1. 2 to 3 months
2. 3 to 4 months
3. 4 to 6 months
4. 6 to 8 months

17 Which toys would be unsuited for Julie based on her present developmental age?
1. Brightly colored mobiles
2. Soft stuffed animals that she can hold
3. Small rattle that she can hold
4. Snap toys, large snap beads

18 The nurse who has been caring for Julie decides on a plan of care for the mother as well. The plan calls for:
1. Setting up a schedule for teaching the mother how to care for her baby
2. Discussing the matter with her in a nonthreatening manner
3. Showing by example how to care for the infant and satisfy her own needs
4. Supplying emotional support to the mother and encouraging her dependence

Situation: John Gray, a 21-year-old physical education major in college, sustained a crushing fracture of the third and fourth lumbar vertebrae with severance of the cord while practicing on the trampoline. Three days after the injury the physician explained to him that he was a paraplegic and what this diagnosis entailed. Questions 19 through 30 refer to this situation.

19 The nurse understands that paraplegia involves:
1. Paresis of both lower extremities
2. Paralysis of one side of the body
3. Paralysis of upper and lower extremities
4. Paralysis of both lower extremities

20 When caring for John, the initial responsibility of the nurse is to:
1. Prevent contractures and atrophy
2. Avoid flexion or hyperextension of the spine
3. Prevent urinary tract infections
4. Prepare the patient for vocational rehabilitation

21 Considering the diagnosis, the nurse knows that John must be encouraged to drink a lot of fluids to prevent:
1. Urinary tract infections
2. Fluid and electrolyte imbalance
3. Dehydration
4. Constipation

22 John was placed on a CircOlectric bed primarily to:
1. Promote mobility
2. Prevent calcium loss from long bones
3. Prevent pressure sores
4. Promote orthostatic hypotension

23 Two weeks after the accident John begins vomiting thick coffee-ground material and appears restless and apprehensive. The nurse should:
1. Change the patient's diet to bland
2. Prepare for insertion of a nasogastric tube
3. Check laboratory reports for hemoglobin level
4. Collect a stool specimen and check for occult blood

24 While caring for John the nurse would immediately report which of the following observations?
1. Tachycardia, diaphoresis, and cold extremities
2. Complaints of thirst and warm flushed skin
3. Nausea, weakness, and headache
4. Dyspepsia, distention, and diarrhea

25 Perforation has occurred, so a gastrectomy is performed. In the immediate postoperative period John's nasogastric tube is draining a bright red liquid. The nurse should expect this drainage for:
1. 1 to 2 hours
2. 3 to 4 hours
3. 10 to 12 hours
4. 24 to 48 hours

26 John is returned to his room on the second postoperative day. An IV of 1000 ml of 5% glucose in water containing 40 mEq potassium chloride is running. Parenteral preparations of potassium are administered slowly and cautiously to prevent which of the following complications?
1. Acidosis
2. Cardiac arrest
3. Edema of the extremities
4. Psychotic-like reactions

27 John's IV stopped and was restarted by the IV team in his other arm. The nurse coming on duty checked the IV bottle, noting that it was practically full and seemed to be dripping adequately. She did not count the drip rate or check the site of infusion. Later in the morning it was noted that a large infiltrated area had developed, and the needle had

to be removed. The area of infiltration became reddened, and ultimately sloughing of tissue occurred. In situations such as this:
1. The staff nurse is not responsible for IVs when the hospital has an IV team
2. The rate of flow should have been regulated and maintained at a slow rate
3. Sloughing of tissue is a frequent complication of IV therapy
4. The rate of flow is unrelated to the problem of infiltration

28 After the nasogastric tube is removed, John is placed on a gradually increasing diet, which he tolerates fairly well. As the diet is increased, John develops the dumping syndrome. Dumping syndrome refers to:
1. Buildup of feces and gas within the large intestine
2. Rapid passage of osmotic fluid into the jejunum
3. Reflux of intestinal contents into the esophagus
4. Nausea due to a full stomach

29 Management of the dumping syndrome is best accomplished by planning to maintain the patient on:
1. Low-protein, high-carbohydrate diet
2. Low-residue, bland diet
3. Fluid intake below 500 ml
4. Small frequent feedings

30 Three weeks after his injury, John explains to the nurse that he must get out of the hospital soon to practice for the upcoming intercollegiate gymnastic tournament. In light of what the patient is saying, the nurse should realize that John is:
1. No longer able to adapt
2. Extremely motivated to get well
3. Verbalizing a fantasy
4. Exhibiting denial

Situation: *Baby Ginger Little is admitted to the newborn nursery. The nurse weighs her and performs a newborn evaluation. Questions 31 through 41 refer to this situation.*

31 The most important weak or absent reflex for the nurse to report in her initial evaluation of the newborn is:
1. Moro
2. Tonic neck
3. Gag
4. Babinski

32 Baby Ginger has small, whitish, pinpoint spots over her nose, which the nurse knows are caused by retained sebaceous secretions. When charting this observation, the nurse identifies it as:

1. Lanugo
2. Milia
3. Whiteheads
4. Mongolian spots

33 When changing Baby Ginger, the nurse notices a brick red stain on the diaper. This is:
1. A normal but uncommon occurrence
2. A symptom of low iron stores
3. Due to medication given to the mother
4. To be expected in female babies

34 Three days after birth, Ginger is slightly jaundiced. The nurse knows that this is due primarily to her:
1. Immature liver function
2. Mother's high hemoglobin level
3. High hemoglobin and low hematocrit levels
4. Inability to synthesize bile

35 The physician orders phototherapy. During the therapy the nurse should apply eye patches to Ginger's eyes to:
1. Be sure the eyes are closed
2. Prevent injury to conjunctiva and retina
3. Reduce overstimulation from bright lights
4. Limit excessive rapid eye movements and anxiety

36 At 3 months Ginger is admitted to the hospital because of increasing head size and a possible diagnosis of hydrocephalus. In performing a developmental appraisal, what clue would be most important to the nurse in light of the diagnosis?
1. Absence of Moro, tonic neck, and grasp reflexes
2. Presence of the Babinski reflex
3. Head lag
4. Inability to sit unsupported

37 Because of the diagnosis, the nurse is especially alert to signs of increasing intracranial pressure, such as:
1. Bulging fontanel, "sunset" eyes, projectile vomiting not associated with feeding
2. Depressed fontanel, bulging eyes, irritability
3. Dilated scalp veins, depressed and sunken eyeballs, decreased blood pressure
4. High shrill cry, decreased skin turgor, elevated fontanels

38 Proper positioning of Ginger is essential to prevent breakdown of the scalp. A suitable position would be:
1. Prone, with her legs elevated about 30 degrees
2. Prone or supine, with her head elevated about 45 degrees

3. Positioned on either side and flat
4. Supine and Trendelenburg

39 Hydrocephalus, if untreated, can cause mental retardation because:
  1. Hypertonic CSF disturbs normal plasma concentration, depriving nerve cells of vital nutrients
  2. CSF dilutes blood supply, causing cells to atrophy
  3. Increasing head size necessitates more oxygen and nutrients than normal blood flow can supply
  4. Gradually increasing size of ventricles presses the brain against the bony cranium: anoxia and decreased blood supply result

40 After several tests have been performed, the diagnosis of noncommunicating hydrocephalus is confirmed and a ventriculoperitoneal shunt is performed. Postoperative care of Ginger includes all the following *except:*
  1. Positioning her flat for about 48 hours
  2. Administering sedatives and analgesics to keep her quiet
  3. Encouraging the parents not to pick up Ginger even to prevent crying
  4. Checking the valve frequently and pumping it as ordered

41 Mr. and Mrs. Little have been very anxious during their child's admission and especially concerned about the prognosis. The nurse should explain that:
  1. The prognosis is excellent and the valve is permanent
  2. The shunt may need to be revised as the child grows older
  3. If any brain damage has occurred, it is reversible during the first year of life
  4. Hydrocephalus usually is self-limiting by 2 years of age and then the shunt is removed

Situation: Mrs. Hanson is an obese 59-year-old secretary with a long history of asthma dating back to her childhood. She has varicosed veins and has been admitted to the hospital for surgery. Questions 42 through 56 refer to this situation.

42 Varicosed veins are usually the result of:
  1. Atherosclerotic plaques along the veins
  2. External compression of the muscles of the legs
  3. Defective valves within the veins
  4. The formation of thrombophlebitis

43 The nurse should expect Mrs. Hanson to complain of:
  1. Continued edema of the affected extremity

2. A positive Homans' sign
3. Coolness and pallor of the affected extremity
4. Cramping sensations in the calf muscle

44 A simple test for varicose veins is the:
  1. Trendelenburg test
  2. Babinski reflex
  3. Romberg's sign
  4. Arteriography

45 Mrs. Hanson is going to have a vein ligation and stripping. The nurse explains that prior to surgery the physician must be certain:
  1. She understands the need to lose weight
  2. The deep veins of the leg are not occluded
  3. The saphenous vein has no sign of aneurysms
  4. She is aware of the need for several weeks of bed rest

46 The nurse should base preoperative teaching on the fact that Mrs. Hanson:
  1. Can control and limit her asthmatic attacks if she wants
  2. Should try to limit coughing, since this causes distention of the chest
  3. Can control her anxiety and decrease the severity of postoperative asthma attacks
  4. Will be quite prone to respiratory tract infections

47 When Mrs. Hanson returns from the recovery room, the nurse should position her:
  1. Supine with legs elevated 30 degrees
  2. Flat with the knee gatch engaged
  3. In a semi-Fowler position with knees slightly flexed
  4. Head elevated, feet tight against the footboard

48 The evening of surgery, after Mrs. Hanson is fully reacted, the nurse should:
  1. Apply a binder for support
  2. Assist her out of bed to a chair
  3. Perform passive range of motion exercises to legs
  4. Ambulate her in the room

49 Five days postoperatively Mrs. Hanson develops an acute episode of bronchial asthma. Mrs. Hanson is experiencing difficulty in breathing due to:
  1. Spasms of the bronchi, which trap the air
  2. A too rapid expulsion of air
  3. An increase in the vital capacity of the lungs
  4. Hyperventilation due to an anxiety reaction

50 Nursing management of Mrs. Hanson is now directed toward:
  1. Raising mucus secretions from the chest
  2. Limiting pulmonary secretions by decreasing fluid intake

3. Curing the condition permanently
4. Convincing the patient that her condition is emotionally based

51 The nurse administers aminophylline via suppository to Mrs. Hanson as ordered. The effect of this therapy is:
1. Rest and relaxation
2. Evacuation of the lower bowel
3. Relaxation of bronchial muscles
4. Reduction of intestinal bacteria

52 Mrs. Hanson has an IV infusion to keep the vein open for emergency medications. What should the nurse initially do when the IV infusion infiltrates?
1. Attempt to flush the tube
2. Elevate the IV site
3. Discontinue the infusion
4. Apply warm, moist soaks

53 The physician orders daily sputum specimens to be collected from Mrs. Hanson. When is the most appropriate time for the nurse to collect this specimen?
1. On awakening
2. Before meals
3. Before an IPPB treatment
4. After activity

54 The nurse understands that Mrs. Hanson's asthmatic wheeze is thought to be:
1. An impairment of cardiovascular function
2. An unexpressed rejection of independence
3. A dilation of the bronchi
4. An expression of hypochondriasis

55 Mrs. Hanson is found to be allergic to dust. The teaching plan for her should include the fact that:
1. She will probably be unable to do her own housework in the future
2. It is imperative that her entire house be redecorated, since she must live in a dust-free environment
3. Damp-dusting her house will help limit dust particles in the air
4. She may as well accept her condition, since dust cannot be avoided

56 Before discharge Mrs. Hanson is instructed on the use of elastic stockings. Which of the following instructions would be most appropriate concerning the stockings? They should be:
1. Left in place until the physician advises otherwise
2. Worn only at night when she is less active
3. Put on before getting out of bed in the morning
4. Alternately kept on 2 hours and off 2 hours

Situation: Maria Lory, a 12-year-old girl, is admitted to the hospital with the diagnosis of acute lymphocytic leukemia. Questions 57 through 64 refer to this situation.

57 Which signs and symptoms would the nurse consider unusual with this diagnosis?
1. Multiple bruises, petechiae
2. Marked fatigue, pallor
3. Enlarged lymph nodes, spleen, and liver
4. Marked jaundice and generalized edema

58 A pathophysiologic change underlying the production of symptoms in leukemia is:
1. Progressive replacement of bone marrow with fibrous tissue
2. Destruction of red blood cells and platelets by overproduction of white blood cells
3. Proliferation and release of immature white blood cells into the circulating blood
4. Excessive destruction of blood cells in the liver and spleen

59 To induce a remission, Maria is started on a drug regimen that includes prednisone, vincristine, and L-asparaginase. Which of the following side effects of these drugs requires the greatest preparation of this patient?
1. Constipation
2. Generalized, short-term paralysis
3. Retarded growth in height
4. Alopecia

60 A major objective of nursing care related to Maria's disease and drug regimen is to:
1. Maintain reverse isolation
2. Reduce unnecessary stimuli
3. Check her vital signs every 2 hours
4. Prevent all physical activity

61 Understanding the side effects of vincristine, the nurse plans a diet for Maria that is:
1. Low in residue with increased fluids
2. High in iron with decreased fluids
3. High in both roughage and fluids
4. Low in fat with regular fluids

62 Because Maria's platelet count is very low, the nurse plans to observe her urine for the presence of:
1. Erythrocytes
2. Leukocytes
3. Casts
4. Lymphocytes

63 Maria's physician also plans a program of irradiation of the spine and skull. The nurse explains that this treatment is used mainly because:
1. Leukemia cells invade the nervous system more slowly, but the usual drugs are ineffective in the brain

2. Radiation will retard growth of cells in bone marrow of the cranium
3. Neoplastic drug therapy without radiation is effective in most cases, but this is a precautionary treatment
4. Radiation will decrease cerebral edema and prevent increased intracranial pressure

64 One day Mr. Lory asks the nurse whether he should tell his son, who is 7 years old, the truth about Maria. The nurse should reply:
1. "A child of his age cannot comprehend the real meaning of death, so don't tell him until the last moment."
2. "Your son probably fears separation most and wants to know that you will care for him, rather than what will happen to his sister."
3. "Your son probably doesn't understand death as we do but fears it just the same. He should be told the truth to let him prepare for his sister's possible death."
4. "Why don't you talk this over with your doctor, who probably knows best what is happening in terms of Maria's prognosis?"

Situation: David King is a 34-year-old sales manager. He frequently experiences weakness and difficulty in moving his right hand. A thorough medical examination reveals no physical pathologic condition. The physician now believes the symptoms are the result of a somatoform disorder. Questions 65 through 71 refer to this situation.

65 A somatoform disorder is:
1. A psychosomatic reaction to stress
2. An unconscious means to control conflict
3. A psychologic defense against stress
4. A conscious defense against anxiety

66 A person who habitually expresses anxiety through physical symptoms is displaying which of the following defense mechanisms?
1. Psychoneurotic
2. Psychosomatic
3. Regressive
4. Projective

67 Conversion disorder is the term used to describe the phenomenon whereby anxiety associated with stress or conflict has been repressed and converted into specific physical manifestations. One of the characteristics of the patient's reaction to the physical symptom is:
1. Agitation
2. Indifference
3. Anger
4. Anxiety

68 The basic difference between psychosomatic illness and hypochondria is that in psychosomatic illness there is:
1. An emotional cause
2. A feeling of illness
3. An actual tissue change
4. A restriction of activities

69 David is scheduled for an occupational therapy group. While listening to instructions for the group project, he experiences the feeling of weakness and is unable to move his right arm. After a check of pulse and respirations, the nurse's best response would be:
1. "Exactly when did the weakness begin?"
2. "Is this similar to what you usually experience?"
3. "What emotion were you feeling before you felt the weakness?"
4. "Would you like to leave the group for a while?"

70 The occurrence of this pattern of behavior can be reduced if the nurse:
1. Decreases anxiety by limiting discussion of problems with the patient
2. Provides patient teaching regarding medical care
3. Teaches the family how to decrease stress at home
4. Assists the patient in developing altered life patterns

71 During group therapy other members accuse David of intellectualizing and avoiding his feelings. He asks if the nurse agrees with the others. The nurse's best answer would be:
1. "It seems that way to me, too."
2. "I'd rather not give my personal opinion."
3. "What is your perception of my behavior?"
4. "You seem to need my opinion."

Situation: Mr. Dime, age 39, an unmarried executive producer for one of the major television networks, was in a serious auto accident. He is admitted with multiple fractures and deep lacerations with hemorrhage. He is in severe shock and is rushed to the operating room. A blood transfusion proves incompatible with his blood type. Questions 72 through 83 refer to this situation.

72 The initial sign of such a transfusion reaction, which the nurse should observe for, is:
1. Dyspnea
2. Backache
3. Cyanosis
4. Bradycardia

73 As a result of this transfusion reaction, Mr. Dime suffers kidney damage. In determining kidney damage, the most significant clinical response that the nurse should assess is:
1. Acute pain over kidney area
2. Decreased urinary output
3. Hematuria
4. Polyuria

74 Although Mr. Dime does not request an analgesic, the nurse should be alert for a sign of an involuntary reaction to pain, which is:
1. Perspiration
2. Crying
3. Pulling knees up to the abdomen
4. Grimacing

75 Mr. Dime's kidney function has not returned and is currently about 10% of normal. Peritoneal dialysis is ordered when his BUN begins to rise. Once instituted, peritoneal dialysis:
1. Is largely a nursing responsibility
2. May be maintained from 12 to 48 hours
3. Requires checking of vital signs every 15 minutes
4. Should be discontinued if the patient complains of abdominal pain

76 The purpose of peritoneal dialysis is to:
1. Reestablish kidney function
2. Clean the peritoneal membrane
3. Remove toxins and metabolic wastes
4. Provide fluid for intracellular spaces

77 Mr. Dime complains of nausea, pain in the abdomen, diarrhea, and muscular weakness. The nurse notes an irregularity in pulse and signs of pulmonary edema. These are probably manifestations of:
1. Calcium deficiency
2. Calcium excess
3. Sodium deficiency
4. Potassium excess

78 Between dialysis treatments, Mr. Dime is maintained on a modified Giordano-Giovannetti diet. Which of the following statements is *not* true of this dietary regimen?
1. Protein is low, which causes use of excess urea nitrogen to synthesize amino acids for tissue synthesis
2. Potassium is high to replace losses
3. Sodium is allowed according to need
4. Calories are allowed as needed within designated food lists

79 In caring for Mr. Dime when he is being dialyzed, the nurse should:
1. Maintain the patient in a flat, supine position during the entire procedure

2. Notify the physician if there is a deficit of 200 ml in the drainage fluid
3. Apply firm manual pressure on the lower abdomen if fluid is not draining properly
4. Remove the cannula at the end of the procedure and apply a dry, sterile dressing

80 If Mr. Dime is observed to have severe respiratory difficulty, the most immediate nursing action would be to:
1. Change the patient's position
2. Drain fluid from the peritoneal cavity
3. Notify the physician
4. Discontinue the treatment

81 Mr. Dime has been immobilized in traction for 3 weeks. The nurse realizes that he may develop renal calculi as a complication because:
1. He has more difficulty urinating in a supine position
2. His dietary patterns have changed
3. Lack of muscle action and normal tension cause calcium withdrawal from the bone
4. Fracture healing requires more calcium and thus increases total calcium metabolism

82 Mr. Dime's leg is set in a long leg cast. The nurse should observe for which of the following signs that indicates compromised circulation in a patient with a long leg cast?
1. Foul odor
2. Swelling of the toes
3. Increased temperature
4. Drainage on the cast

83 Mr. Dime is waiting for a renal transplant. In teaching Mr. Dime, the nurse informs him that:
1. He will require immunosuppressive drugs daily for the rest of his life
2. He will be unable to follow a full program of work and recreation, including sports
3. Symptoms of rejection include fever, hypotension, and edema
4. Urine production will be delayed after surgery

Situation: Mrs. Loft, 42 years of age, is admitted to the hospital with a tentative diagnosis of chronic adrenal insufficiency. Questions 84 through 91 refer to this situation.

84 A room assignment contraindicated for Mrs. Loft would be one:
1. With an elderly CVA patient
2. With a middle-aged woman who has pneumonia
3. That is private and away from the nurses' station
4. Next to a 17-year-old girl with a fractured leg

85 Mrs. Loft complains of weakness and dizziness on arising from bed in the morning. The nurse realizes that this is most probably caused by:
1. Postural hypertension
2. A hypoglycemic reaction
3. A lack of potassium
4. Increased extracellular fluid volume

86 After a Thorn test shows an increased eosinophil count, Mrs. Loft is advised that she has Addison's disease. It is most important that the nurse discuss with her the need for:
1. Frequent visits to the physician
2. Restriction of physical activity
3. A special low-salt diet
4. Hormone replacement therapy

87 In teaching Mrs. Loft about her diet, the nurse should tell her to:
1. Add a little extra salt to her food
2. Limit intake to 1200 calories
3. Omit protein foods at each meal
4. Restrict her daily intake of fluids

88 In the event Mrs. Loft neglects to continue the cortisone therapy, an adrenal crisis may occur. The predominant symptom she should be advised to report is:
1. Hypertension
2. A high body temperature
3. Muscle spasms
4. Diarrhea

89 Patients on prolonged cortisone therapy may exhibit adaptations caused by its glucocorticoid and mineralocorticoid actions. The nurse should teach Mrs. Loft and her family to observe for:
1. Hypoglycemia and anuria
2. Weight gain and moon face
3. Anorexia and hyperkalemia
4. Hypotension and fluid loss

90 When Mrs. Loft shows concern about the fact that she is developing signs of masculinity, the nurse should tell her:
1. It is a further sign of the illness
2. That this is due to the therapy
3. Not to worry, since it will disappear with therapy
4. That this is not important, so long as she gets better

91 In observing Mrs. Loft for cortisone overdose, the nurse should be particularly alert for:
1. Behavioral changes
2. Severe anorexia
3. Hypoglycemia
4. Anaphylactic shock

Situation: Gail, 17 years old, has a history of being a loner. She made excellent grades in school, but often her thinking was highly symbolic. During her senior year in high school she refused to get out of bed, experienced loss of appetite, and displayed disorganized speech. She was hospitalized at a community hospital. Questions 92 through 99 refer to this situation.

92 One of the primary goals in providing a therapeutic environment for Gail is to:
1. Get her involved in a group with her peers
2. Remove her from the home
3. Foster a trusting relationship
4. Give her medication on time

93 While in the hospital Gail still refuses to get out of bed and becomes very hostile with the staff when approached. The most immediate therapeutic nursing approach would be:
1. Require that she get out of bed at once
2. Stay with her until she calms down
3. Give her the p.r.n. tranquilizer that is ordered
4. Allow her to stay in bed for now but leave her alone

94 Gail sits huddled in a chair and seldom leaves it. She occasionally lets out a scream and runs to the end of the hallway and crouches in a corner. The nurse realizes that this type of behavior is classified as:
1. Reactive
2. Regressive
3. Disassociative
4. Hallucinatory

95 To begin to establish a therapeutic relationship with Gail, the nurse must:
1. Obtain a complete history from her family
2. Ascertain what topics are of interest to her
3. Protect her from herself
4. Plan to keep her anxiety at a minimum

96 The priority goal is for Gail to develop:
1. A sense of identity
2. Ego strengths
3. Trust
4. An ability to socialize

97 Gail is taking chlorpromazine (Thorazine), 2000 mg, every day. She comes to the nurse complaining that her fingers are twitching. The best reply would be:
1. "This is a temporary situation until your body adjusts to the medication."
2. "I will get the doctor to order a medication that will help overcome this. It is a side effect of the drug you are taking."
3. "You need the medication that we are giving you. You will soon get used to the side effects."

4. "Let's wait a few days and see whether the side effects of the drug you are taking go away."

98 Which of the following symptoms would cause the nurse to stop giving chlorpromazine to Gail until further laboratory work was done?
1. Photosensitivity
2. Shuffling gait
3. Yellow sclerae
4. Grimacing

99 On being discharged Gail should be encouraged to:
1. Go back to her regular activities
2. Continue in the aftercare clinic
3. Call the unit whenever upset
4. Find a group that has similar problems

Situation: Mrs. Sims is returned to her room after a radical neck dissection for a malignant tumor. Questions 100 through 106 refer to this situation.

100 Mrs. Sims has an endotracheal tube still in place. The nurse should:
1. Change the dressing to observe for covert bleeding
2. Irrigate the tube to maintain patency
3. Reposition the endotracheal tube when the gag reflex returns
4. Have a tracheostomy set at the bedside

101 When Mrs. Sims' color improves and she is able to breathe on her own, the anesthesiologist removes the endotracheal tube. That evening the nurse decides Mrs. Sims is showing signs of respiratory embarrassment and notifies the physician immediately. Which of the following signs might the nurse have observed?
1. Decreased pulse and respirations
2. Restlessness and confusion
3. Cyanosis and clubbing of the fingers
4. Anxiety and constricted pupils

102 A tracheostomy is performed and Mrs. Sims is placed on a mechanical ventilator. For a patient on a ventilator, the nurse must be sure to check the cuff of the tracheostomy tube, which:
1. Must be inflated during suctioning
2. Must remain deflated for 10 minutes every hour
3. Should allow only a slight air leak at the height of inspiration
4. Should create a tight seal between the trachea and the tube

103 When doing deep tracheal suction for a patient after a tracheostomy, the nurse hould:
1. Be sure the cuff of the tracheostomy is inflated during suctioning

2. Instill acetylcysteine (Mucomyst) into the tracheostomy prior to suctioning to loosen secretions
3. Apply negative pressure as the catheter is being inserted
4. Suction the patient with the head turned to either side

104 When doing tracheostomy care for Mrs. Sims, the nurse must:
1. Monitor her temperature after the procedure
2. Use sterile gloves during the procedure
3. Use Betadine to clean the inner cannula when it is removed
4. Place Mrs. Sims in the semi-Fowler position

105 As a result of the tracheostomy the nurse is aware that which one of the following drugs would be contraindicated for Mrs. Sims?
1. Pyrvinium pamoate (Povan)
2. Atropine
3. Chloral hydrate
4. Nalorphine (Nalline)

106 Mrs. Sims' tracheostomy tube has an inner cannula. In providing tracheostomy care the nurse should plan to remove the inner cannula:
1. And use sterile applicators to cleanse the outer cannula
2. Only after the cuff is deflated
3. And cleanse it with peroxide
4. Only when the obturator is in place

Situation: Mrs. Simon, a 72-year-old with congestive heart failure, is having difficulty breathing as a result of pulmonary edema. She is being treated with digitalis and diuretic therapy and also with a 1 g sodium diet. Questions 107 through 113 refer to this situation.

107 At 9 P.M. Mrs. Simon asks for a glass of juice. Since the only kinds of juice on the ward are pear nectar, apple, and tomato, the nurse should:
1. Explain to Mrs. Simon that she should not have juice between meals but she may have a glass of water
2. Ask her which she prefers, the apple juice or the pear nectar
3. Explain to her that the only kind she can have is tomato juice
4. Tell her that she cannot have any kind of juice because she is on a low-sodium diet

108 Mrs. Simon is to receive 0.2 mg of digoxin IM. The ampule is labeled 0.5 mg = 2 ml. How many milliliters should be administered?
1. 8 ml
2. 0.8 ml

3. 1 ml
4. 1.2 ml

109 Mrs. Simon's ankles are swollen on admission. The nurse should prepare to:
1. Restrict fluids
2. Elevate the legs
3. Apply elastic bandages
4. Do range-of-motion exercises

110 Assuming all the food involved is cooked without salt, which of the following meal plans would the nurse *not* order for Mrs. Simon, who is on a 1-gram sodium diet?
1. Baked chicken, boiled potatoes, broccoli, coffee
2. Mixed fruit salad bowl with cottage cheese; crackers, relish dish (celery, carrot, olives, sweet pickles), tea
3. Soft cooked egg, salt free toast, jelly, skim milk
4. Fillet of sole, baked potato, lettuce and tomato salad, fresh fruit cup, milk

111 To help monitor Mrs. Simon's physical status, a central venous catheter is inserted. The nurse can take a correct central venous pressure reading when the water level in the manometer:
1. Drops and then rises
2. Synchronizes with the blood pressure
3. Rises and stops at a specific plateau
4. Fluctuates with respirations

112 Mrs. Simon is receiving hydrochlorothiazide (Diuril) and furosemide (Lasix) to relieve edema. The nurse should observe for evidence of:
1. Excessive loss of potassium ions
2. Elevation of the urine specific gravity
3. Negative nitrogen balance
4. Excessive retention of sodium ions

113 Mrs. Simon will be taking digitalis at home. She asks the nurse why this is necessary. The nurse bases the answer on the fact that digitalis:
1. Slows and strengthens cardiac contractions
2. Lengthens the refractory phase of the cardiac cycle
3. Reduces edema in extracellular spaces
4. Increases ventricular contractions

Situation: Mr. Norman, a husky 6-foot man, 30 years of age, hospitalized with a diagnosis of bipolar disorder, is active and sometimes combative. Since his admission he has been alone in a room. A 45-year-old man is admitted and placed in the room with Mr. Norman. Mr. Norman seems to accept the newcomer and the nurse pays little attention to them for the rest of the afternoon. Questions 114 through 120 refer to this situation.

114 Suddenly a commotion is heard, and Mr. Norman is found beating the other patient. Legally:
1. The admitting office should not have put the patient in with Mr. Norman
2. Knowing that Mr. Norman was frequently combative, close observation was indicated
3. Patients who are combative should never be left unsupervised
4. A combative patient like Mr. Norman should have been sedated with tranquilizers

115 Mr. Norman is receiving lithium carbonate. While the medication is being administered, it is important that the nurse:
1. Restrict the patient's sodium intake
2. Test the patient's urine weekly
3. Withhold other medications for the first week
4. Monitor the patient's blood level regularly

116 While the nurse is talking with Mr. Norman in his room, the patient's conversation becomes embarrassingly vulgar. The nurse should respond to his behavior by:
1. Restricting Mr. Norman's contact with staff until this symptom passes
2. Tactfully teasing him about the use of such vulgarity
3. Asking him to limit his vulgarity and continuing the conversation with him
4. Discreetly refusing to talk to him when he is speaking in this manner

117 Activities that would be most therapeutic for Mr. Norman and that the nurse should encourage include:
1. Carving figures out of wood
2. Sanding and varnishing wooden bookends
3. Stenciling designs on copper sheeting
4. Lacing tooled leather wallets

118 Mr. Norman is noisy, loud, and disruptive. The nurse informs him that, unless he is more quiet, he will be isolated and put in restraints, if necessary. Legally:
1. Restraint of Mr. Norman is justified for his own protection
2. The information given Mr. Norman is actually a threat
3. Patients like Mr. Norman cannot be expected to understand instructions.
4. Mr. Norman's behavior is to be expected and should be ignored

119 During a period of hyperactivity, Mr. Norman demands to be allowed to go downtown to do his shopping. He has no privileges at the present time.

Which of the following responses would be the best response?
1. "I'm sorry, Mr. Norman, you can't go. Let's look through this new catalog."
2. "You cannot leave the ward, Mr. Norman."
3. "You'll have to ask your doctor, Mr. Norman."
4. "Not right now, Mr. Norman. I don't have a staff member to go with you."

120 One day while the nurse is staying with Mr. Norman, who is shaving, he states, "I have hidden a razor blade and tonight I am going to kill myself." The nurse's best reply is:
1. "You're going to kill yourself?"
2. "You'd better finish shaving, since it's time for lunch."
3. "I'm sure you don't really mean that."
4. "Things can't really be that bad."

How to Use Worksheet 1: Errors in Processing Information

Common errors in processing information are listed in the left hand column of this worksheet. At the top of the worksheet is a row of blank spaces for inserting the number of the question missed. Directly below each number, check any errors you made in answering that question. You may have made more than one type of error in an answer.

Worksheet 1: Errors in Processing Information

Question no.																							
Did not read situation/question carefully																							
Missed important details																							
Confused major and minor points																							
Defined problem incorrectly																							
Could not remember terms/facts/concepts/ principles																							
Defined terms incorrectly																							
Focused on incomplete/incorrect data in assessing situation																							
Interpreted data incorrectly																							
Applied wrong concepts/principles in situation																							
Drew incorrect conclusions																							
Identified wrong goals																							
Identified priorities incorrectly																							
Carried out plan incorrectly/incompletely																							
Was unclear about criteria for evaluating success in achieving goals																							

How to Use Worksheet 2: Knowledge Gaps

Types of common knowledge gaps are listed along the top of this worksheet. Write a brief description of topics you want to review in the spaces provided. For example, if you missed a question on administration of a particular drug, write the drug name and problem (e.g., dosage) in the appropriate space under the column labeled Pharmacology.

Worksheet 2: Knowledge Gaps

Basic science	Skills/ procedures	Basic human needs	Growth & develop-ment	Normal nutrition	Psycho-social factors	Clinical area/ topic	Stressors/ coping mechanisms	Patho-physiology	Pharma-cology	Therapeutic nutrition	Legal implications	Other

Answers and Rationales

1. (2) The nurse fulfilled the expectation set forth in the Nurse Practice Act, which includes teaching. In this case she had knowledge of dietary needs and their relation to the patient's well-being during pregnancy. (b); IM; AP; SH; OB
   (1) False; low-salt foods would be recommended if a diagnosis of preeclampsia was made.
   (3) Immediate planning based on the nurse's knowledge of proper diet is better intervention.
   (4) Unless the nurse thought there was a need for medical intervention, she could supervise prenatal care.

2. (3) The longer matter remains in the GI tract, the more water is reabsorbed; and constipation results. (b); AN; CP; SH; OB
   (1) The growing uterus tends to exert pressure on the bladder; it is way above the anus.
   (2) Milk is not constipating.
   (4) The metabolism increases but does not affect the bowel.

3. (2) Rupture of the membranes and the gush of fluid can carry the umbilical cord downward. Immediate placement in the lithotomy position and inspection may lead to identification of prolapse and prevention of fetal distress. (b); IM; AN; NU; OB
   (1) Fluid is due to rupture of membranes; unless it is meconium stained or followed by the cord, this is normal and needs no medical intervention.
   (3) Keeping the patient flat in bed may decrease blood flow, and cause hypoxia in the fetus as well as hypotension in the mother.
   (4) This is done routinely in labor, not just after membrane rupture.

4. (3) Hypertonic contractions of the uterus, if allowed to continue, can lead to uterine rupture. Therefore the infusion should be discontinued so the hypertonic contractions cease. (b); IM; AP; NU; OB
   (1) The resulting delay could lead to uterine rupture; the nurse should discontinue the IV.
   (2) The IV should be carefully monitored with a Harvard pump or IVAC to ensure a regulated and continuous flow.
   (4) Fetal heart tones should be monitored more frequently (q. 15 min.) if a fetal monitor is not used.

5. (3) As cervical dilation nears completion, labor is intensified with an increase in pain and energy expenditure. (b); AN; CP; NU; OB
   (1) Back pain usually indicates a posterior-lying position of the infant.
   (2) Pain is increased since contractions are more frequent and intense and they last longer.
   (4) The patient is usually very restless and thrashes about, assuming no particular position.

6. (2) A relaxed uterus is the most frequent cause of bleeding in the early postpartum period. The uterus can be returned to a state of firmness by intermittent gentle fundal massage. (a); IM; AN; SH; OB
   (1) Immediate action is directed toward the patient's safety; the physician is called if uterine massage does not control bleeding.
   (3) Assessment of the uterus and massage take priority; then the vital signs are checked.
   (4) Steady bleeding is neither common nor normal and must be attended to immediately.

7. (1) A distended bladder will easily displace the fundus upward and laterally. (a); AN; CP; NU; OB
   (2) From this assessment the nurse can make no judgment about overstretched uterine ligaments.
   (3) This would be manifested by slow contractions and uterine descent into the pelvis.
   (4) If this were true, in addition to being displaced the uterus would be soft and boggy and vaginal bleeding would be present.

8. (4) Forcing the family to be involved at the nurse's convenience will interfere with the development of a productive relationship and affect cooperation of the family. (a); PL; AP; SH; OB
   (1) May be at a time that would be inconvenient for the family and thus interfere with productivity.
   (2) This would be an inconvenient time for the mother and interfere with productivity.
   (3) The father should be included in the visit if at all possible.

9. (1) The role of stranger is the initial role in any relationship. (a); PL; KN; SH; PS
   (2) If the nurse moves in too quickly, future relationships may be severely hampered.
   (3) If the nurse moves in too quickly, future relationships may be severely hampered.
   (4) If the nurse moves in too quickly, future relationships may be severely hampered.

10. (3) The first step in the problem-solving process would be exploration so family needs could be identified. (b); AS; CP; SH; PS
    (1) Without exploring family needs first, the nurse would not know what information was needed.
    (2) Without exploring family needs first, the nurse would not know the problems that needed solving.
    (4) Without exploring family needs first, the nurse would not know what direction the family needed.

11. (4) Inclusion in the interview will avoid a feeling of ostracism by Mr. Wyer and will foster his cooperation. (b); IM; AN; SH; PS
    (1) Observing Mrs. Wyer feed the baby provides the nurse a valuable opportunity to assess interaction.
    (2) Removing Mr. Wyer from the situation decreases his participation.
    (3) Mr. Wyer is part of the family and his feelings will affect Mrs. Wyer as well.

12. (4) This allows Mr. Wyer to express his feelings and is nonjudgmental (a); IM; AP; SH; PE

(1) Direct contradiction often causes defensive reactions and decreases future cooperation.

(2) Mr. Wyer, as the parent, has a right to make his own decisions; this question will place him on the defensive.

(3) This value-laden statement will place him on the defensive.

13. (3) The schedule for immunization of children not immunized in early infancy is altered and adapted from the schedule followed for infants. The tuberculin test normally given at 1 year is added to the first of the DTP and TOPV series. (c); PL; KN; NU; PE

(1) The TB test usually given at 1 year will be added to the first series of immunizations

(2) MMR is never given before 15 months; this will be given 1 month after the initial series is begun.

(4) The Td toxoid is given to children 6 years and older.

14. (2) These children have difficulty reaching out to the environment and tend to be withdrawn. They get little response from parents and do not learn how to respond to others. (b); AS; CP; NU; PE

(1) The infant suffering from maternal deprivation is nonresponsive or only poorly responsive to human contact.

(3) These children are very difficult to comfort; show little satisfaction.

(4) These children do not respond readily to human contact.

15. (4) A consistent caregiver enhances the formation of a trusting and mutually satisfying relationship between child and nurse. (b); PL; AP; NU; PE

(1) Stimulation should proceed gradually and be geared to the present level of development.

(2) Overstimulation should be avoided.

(3) A consistent caregiver enhances the development of trust.

16. (3) Head control and rolling over are achieved at 4 and 5 months respectively. Transferring objects from one hand to another and sitting unsupported are achieved at 7 and 8 months. (b); AS; CP; NU; PE

(1) The ability to roll over is achieved by approximately 5 months of age.

(2) The ability to roll over is achieved by approximately 5 months of age.

(4) Transferring objects from hand to hand is usually achieved at 6 to 7 months.

17. (4) Fine motor coordination is inadequately developed to manipulate snap toys. (a); PL; CP; SH; PE

(1) These are appropriate to stimulate visual attention.

(2) These provide the sense of touch; and since voluntary grasp appears at about 3 to 4 months, they would be handled satisfactorily.

(3) Voluntary grasp will allow her to hold this, and the rattling sound will stimulate the auditory system.

18. (3) Teaching them by example is a nonthreatening approach that allows them to proceed at their own pace. (b); PL; AN; SH; PE

(1) Mothers of failure-to-thrive children are usually insecure and easily threatened.

(2) Mothers need demonstration of appropriate mothering skills.

(4) Satisfying the mother's needs will allow her to develop reserves to give the child; promotes security in her role and facilitates more independent caretaking.

19. (4) Paraplegia is the paralysis of both lower extremities and the lower trunk resulting from damage to the spinal cord from the thoracic to the lumbar segments. (b); AN; KN; NU; SU

(1) Paresis is a slight or partial paralysis; paraplegia is paralysis of both lower extremities.

(2) This is hemiplegia.

(3) This is quadriplegia.

20. (2) The priority of care at this time is to protect the spinal area from strain to prevent additional damage to the traumatized area while it heals. (c); IM; AP; NU; SU

(1) Although an important aspect of care, it is not the priority item in the immediate postinjury period.

(3) This usually results from prolonged immobility; although important, it is not the immediate priority.

(4) Survival and safety take priority; vocational rehabilitation will assume greater importance after the patient's condition stabilizes.

21. (1) Patients with early spinal cord damage experience an atonic bladder, which is characterized by the absence of muscle tone, an enlarged capacity, no feeling of discomfort with distention, and overflow with a large residual. This leads to urinary stasis and infection. High fluid intake limits urinary stasis and infection by diluting the urine and increasing urinary output. (b); IM; CP; SH; ME

(2) A fluid and electrolyte imbalance is not a major problem after spinal cord injury.

(3) Dehydration is not a major problem after spinal cord injury.

(4) Constipation may occur because of the lack of neural stimulation not decreased fluids.

22. (3) The CircOLectric bed facilitates frequent vertical turning of the patient to prevent decubiti, which can form within 24 hours because of pressure. (b); IM; CP; NU; ME

(1) The patient with paraplegia is immobile, and the special bed does not increase mobility.

(2) Because of the lack of weight bearing on bones, calcium is generally lost in patients confined to bed; the special bed does not prevent this from occurring.

(4) Orthostatic hypotension is not desired; the movement of the bed may allow for gradual changes of position that would prevent it from developing.

23. (2) The patient should have a nasogastric tube inserted to prevent aspiration and keep the stomach decompressed. (b); AN; AN; NU; SU

(1) Diet change requires a physician's order; patients who are vomiting may have food withheld.

(3) This information is important; however, prevention of aspiration takes priority.

(4) This would be indicated at the next bowel movement; however, maintenance of vital functions is most important.

24. (1) These signs could be indicative of hemorrhage from perforation and require immediate surgical intervention. (a); AN; AN; NU; SU

(2) These complaints should be noted since they may indicate early signs of diabetes mellitus; however, the nurse's primary observation should be for symptoms of perforation and shock.

(3) These complaints should be noted; however, they are not indicative of potential priority problems.

(4) These complaints should be noted but they do not indicate an emergency situation that would threaten life.

25. (3) The trauma of surgery results in some seeping or oozing of blood into the remaining gastric area, which is being immediately suctioned out of the body via the nasogastric tube. (c); AN; AP; NU; SU

(1) The trauma of surgery will result in some blood loss, which will continue until coagulation takes place; this is too short a time for this to occur.

(2) The trauma of surgery will result in some blood loss, which will continue until coagulation takes place; this is too short a time for this to occur.

(4) If bright red liquid is still draining 24 to 48 hours after surgery, it is abnormal; the physician should be notified.

26. (2) Too rapid administration can result in hyperkalemia, which can cause a long refractory period in the cardiac cycle and result in cardiac arrhythmias and arrest. (c); IM; AP; NU; SU

(1) This statement is too general; no indication of whether it is respiratory acidosis or metabolic acidosis. Metabolic acidosis can cause hyperkalemia.

(3) Hyperkalemia usually causes nausea, vomiting, and diarrhea, which may result in dehydration; in this instance fluid would shift from interstitial spaces to the intravascular compartment. With edema the fluid shift is in the opposite direction.

(4) This reaction does not occur in hyperkalemia.

27. (4) The nurse should not only count the rate but also inspect the infusion site, no matter who started the IV. Failure to do so constitutes negligence. (c); EV; AN; NU; SU

(1) The staff nurse is always responsible for meeting the patient's nursing needs regardless of whether other members of the health team are available; the nurse was negligent.

(2) The rate of flow should have been maintained at the rate ordered by the physician; the infusion site should also be monitored routinely.

(3) This is untrue; it occurred because the nurse was negligent.

28. (2) When high-osmotic fluid passes rapidly into the small intestine, it causes hypovolemia. This results in a sympathetic response with tachycardia, diaphoresis, and dizziness. The symptoms are also attributed to a sudden rise and subsequent fall in blood sugar. (b); AN; CP; NU; SU

(1) This is usually associated with paralytic ileus; dumping syndrome leads to increased intestinal motility.

(3) This could occur with intestinal obstruction; dumping syndrome is associated with increased motility originating in the jejunum. Reflux would need reverse peristalsis.

(4) The stomach is not full; its contents rapidly empty into the jejunum.

29. (4) Small feedings reduce the amount of bulk passing into the jejunum and therefore reduce the fluid shifting into the jejunum. (b); PL; AP; SH; SU

(1) Concentrated sweets pass rapidly out of the stomach and increase fluid shifts; consequently the diet should be low in carbohydrates. Protein is needed to promote tissue repair.

(2) Although a diet high in roughage may be avoided, a low-residue bland diet is not necessary.

(3) Total fluid intake does not have to be restricted; however, liquids should not be taken immediately before, during, or after a meal because they promote rapid stomach emptying.

30. (4) John's denial is a pattern of defense often demonstrated in the self-protective stage of adaptation to illness. His thoughts and feelings are so painful and provoke such anxiety that he rejects the existence of his paraplegia. (b); AS; AN; SH; PS

(1) Denial is a method of psychologic adaptation.

(2) Motivation must have realistic goals in mind; the patient is in denial.

(3) From information available, one cannot assume that the patient is fantasizing; a fantasy is the transformation of undesirable experiences into imagined events to fulfill an unconscious wish or need.

31. (3) Absent or diminished gag reflex could be life threatening. The infant might aspirate mucus or formula. (b); AN; KN; NU; OB

(1) Important but may be delayed because the mother has been anesthetized; the gag reflex is of primary importance.

(2) Important but may be delayed because the mother has been anesthetized; the gag reflex is of primary importance.

(4) Important but may be delayed because the mother has been anesthetized; the gag reflex is of primary importance.

32. (2) Milia occur commonly, are not indicative of any illness, and eventually disappear. (a); AN; KN; NU; OB

(1) Lanugo is fine dark hair.

(3) This is a lay term for milia.

(4) These are bluish black spots on the buttocks that present on darkly pigmented infants.

33. (1) The brick-red color is caused by albumin and urates that are concentrated because of dehydration, which is normal in the first 10 days. (c); AN; CP; NU; OB
    (2) Iron is eliminated via the gastrointestinal tract.
    (3) No medication used in delivery would cause this discoloration.
    (4) If bile is not synthesized, it will color neither the stool nor the urine.

34. (1) Jaundice occurs because of the normal physiologic breakdown of fetal red blood cells and the immaturity of the infant's liver. (a); AN; CP; NU; OB
    (2) Unrelated to the infant hemoglobin level; the mother and baby have separate circulations
    (3) The baby has high hemoglobin and high hematocrit levels.
    (4) Conjugation and excretion, not synthesis of bile, are compromised because of the immature liver.

35. (2) Eye patches are applied to prevent drying of the conjunctiva, injury to the retina, and alterations in biorhythms. (c); IM; CP; NU; OB
    (1) The baby will automatically close the eyes in response to bright lights and application of a patch.
    (3) The baby should be exposed to bright lights periodically so normal rhythms will become established.
    (4) These are automatic during sleep phases and will not be affected by eye patches.

36. (3) Head lag in an infant 6 months old is abnormal and is frequently a sign of cerebral damage. (c); AS; AN; NU; PE
    (1) The tonic reflex and grasp reflex usually disappear at 2 and 3 months respectively.
    (2) The Babinski reflex is normally present until 2 years of age.
    (4) The ability to sit unsupported is achieved at 7 to 8 months.

37. (1) Increased intracranial pressure results in pressure exerted against the cranium. This is especially evident in areas with less confinement, such as the fontanelles (which bulge), the orbits (which are pushed foward so the eyelids are pulled taut and upper lids are above the irides [sunset eyes]), and the brain (vomiting center stimulated regardless of activity of eating). (b); AS; CP; NU; PE
    (2) The fontanelles will show signs of increased fluid volume in the skull and therefore bulge.
    (3) The eyeballs will show signs of increased fluid volume in the skull and be pushed forward, pulling the lids taut; systolic pressure is elevated and diastolic the same or lower, creating a widening pulse pressure.
    (4) A high shrill cry and decreased skin turgor are not signs associated with increased intracranial pressure.

38. (2) The child can be positioned on the back or abdomen to allow for a routine change of head position. The head is elevated to decrease the intracranial pressure by gravity. (b); IM; AP; NU; PE

(1) The head is elevated to decrease the intracranial pressure by gravity.
(3) The head is elevated to minimize the increased pressure through gravity
(4) Trendelenburg positioning would be contraindicated since it might aggravate the ICP.

39. (4) Cellular destruction occurs as the brain is pressed against the unyielding skull. This occludes blood vessels and deprives the cells of oxygen. (a); AN; CP; NU; PE
    (1) Hydrocephalus results when CSF is produced in too great quantities or is not adequately circulated or absorbed; no change in the fluid itself.
    (2) Pressure may cause occlusion of the blood supply in hydrocephalus.
    (3) Oxygen deprivation occurs when blood vessels are occluded secondary to the pressure in the skull caused by hydrocephalus.

40. (2) Sedatives and analgesics are avoided. They can mask signs of impending loss of consciousness. (c); IM; AN; NU; PE
    (1) A flat position helps prevent problems associated with too rapid reduction of intracranial fluid.
    (3) Initially, positioning flat is important to preventing serious complications.
    (4) Checking and pumping the valve provide a means of assessing and promoting function of the shunt.

41. (2) Shunts need to be revised; as child grows, the length of tubing needs to be changed. The shunts are also prone to malfunction and may need revision. (a); IM; AP; SH; PE
    (1) Although treatment of hydrocephalus by shunt replacement is quite successful, there is danger of malfunction and infection of the shunt.
    (3) Damage to brain cells is irreversible.
    (4) Hydrocephalus necessitates treatment for the life of the child.

42. (3) Varicosed veins are dilated veins that occur as a result of incompetent valves. Varicosities may be due to numerous factors, including heredity, prolonged standing (which puts strain on the valves), and abdominal pressure on the large veins of the lower abdomen. (b); AN; CP; NU; ME
    (1) Atherosclerotic plaques usually occur in arteries not veins.
    (2) This is the rationale for elastic stockings; their action limits venous pooling.
    (4) Thrombophlebitis is usually a sequela of varicosed veins.

43. (4) Because of the dilation in the veins and concomitant decrease in arterial flow, the patient may experience heaviness or muscle cramps in the legs. Edema, if present, can be relieved by elevating the legs. (b); AS; CP; SH; ME
    (1) Edema may be decreased when the extremity is elevated.

(2) Homan's sign is present in deep vein thrombosis.

(3) These signs may indicate early arterial occlusion.

44. (1) The Trendelenburg test evaluates the backflow of blood through defective valves. If, after raising the legs to empty the veins, the patient stands and the veins fill from above the site of the suspected varicosity, the diagnosis is supported. (c); AS; CP; SH; ME

(2) This test is used to determine injury of the pyramidal tract in adults; if present, it is obtained by firmly stroking the lateral aspect of the sole of the foot.

(3) This is present in alcoholic neuritis; the patient loses balance when standing erect with feet together and eyes closed.

(4) This is not a simple test that the nurse can perform.

45. (2) Since the superficial vein (saphenous) will be ligated, it is first necessary to determine whether the deep veins will be capable of supporting the return circulation. (a); AS; CP; SH; SU

(1) Weight loss is desired; however, it is not a prerequisite for surgery.

(3) This vein is generally ligated in surgery.

(4) Bed rest would promote stasis and thrombus formation.

46. (4) Hypersecretion of the mucous glands provides an excellent, warm, moist medium for microorganisms. (b); PL; AP; SH; SU.

(1) Asthma is not a disease that is voluntarily controlled

(2) Coughing must be encouraged; prevents retention of mucus, which is an excellent medium for microorganisms. Excessive secretions also limit gaseous exchange.

(3) Anxiety is not willfully controlled.

47. (1) The legs should be elevated to promote venous return by gravity. (a); IM; AP; SH; SU

(2) This position increases pressure on the popliteal space, which may interfere with venous return from the legs.

(3) Flexion of the knees and hips with the legs lower than the heart interferes with venous return.

(4) Dorsiflexion of the feet places tension on the suture line and should be avoided; placing the legs lower than the level of the heart will not promote venous return.

48. (4) Muscle contraction of the legs promotes venous return and prevents thrombus formation (c); PL; AP; NU; SU

(1) Binders are used after abdominal surgery.

(2) Sitting in a chair is generally avoided; flexes the hip and keeps the legs dependent, which diminishes venous return.

(3) Active exercises a more beneficial after vein ligation.

49. (1) Asthma involves spasms of the bronchi and bronchioles as well as an increased mucus production. This decreases the size of the lumina, interfering

with inhalation and exhalation. (b); AN; CP; SH; ME

(2) Not a mechanism involved in asthma, in which there is interference with both inhalation and exhalation.

(3) There will be a decrease in the vital capacity.

(4) The patient cannot hyperventilate because of mucosal edema, bronchoconstriction, and secretions, all of which cause airway obstruction. Emotional stress is only one precipitating factor that has been identified; allergens, temperature changes, odors, chemicals, and other irritants may also be causative factors.

50. (1) In addition to dilation of bronchi, treatment is aimed at expectoration of mucus. Mucus interferes with gas exchange in the lungs. (a); PL; AP; SH; ME

(2) Increased fluid intake helps liquefy secretions.

(3) This is an unrealistic goal; asthma is a chronic illness.

(4) Asthma is psychosomatic, which does not imply that emotions are the only etiologic factor; there is an interaction between the psyche and the soma.

51. (3) Aminophylline relaxes the smooth muscles, causing bronchodilation and thereby relieving respiratory distress and promoting rest. (a); EV; CP; NU; ME

(1) Aminophylline is not a skeletal muscle relaxant.

(2) Aminophylline is not a cathartic.

(4) Aminophylline is not an antibiotic.

52. (3) When an IV infusion is infiltrated, it should be removed to prevent swelling of the tissues and pain. (b); IM; AP; NU: ME

(1) This would add to the infiltration of fluid.

(2) Elevation does not change the position of the IV cannula; the infusion must be discontinued.

(4) Soaks may be applied, if ordered, after the IV is removed.

53. (1) During sleep mucus secretions in the respiratory tract move more slowly toward the throat. On awakening, increased ciliary motion raises such secretions more vigorously; this facilitates expectoration and the collection of sputum specimens. (a); PL; AP; SH; ME

(2) Sputum may leave an unpleasant taste in the mouth, which could interfere with eating.

(3) Sputum would more likely be collected after an IPPB treatment because this mobilizes secretions due to positive pressure.

(4) Although activity mobilizes secretions, there may not be any secretions present at the time of activity; sputum is most plentiful upon arising.

54. (2) Individuals who have difficulty asking for help may "cry for help" through a psychosomatic illness. (b); AN; CP; NU; ME

(1) A wheeze is related to the respiratory system, not the cardiovascular system.

(3) It is due to a constriction of the bronchi.

(4) Hypochondriasis is a chronic abnormal concern about one's health; not part of the psychopathology of asthma.

55. (3) Although dust cannot be avoided completely, use of a damp cloth helps eliminate the amount of airborne particles that might be inhaled. (a); PL; AP; CL; ME
   (1) This is unrealistic.
   (2) Redecorating will not eliminate dust; it is a part of our environment.
   (4) Untrue; there are ways to limit the amount of airborne particles.

56. (3) The purpose of the support hose is to apply external pressure on the veins, preventing the retrograde pressure or flow that may occur in standing or sitting positions. When the stockings are put on before arising, the veins do not have the chance to become engorged. (a); IM; AP; CL; ME
   (1) Stockings must be removed so the legs can be washed and dried at least daily. They usually do not need to be worn while in bed with the feet elevated because gravity prevents venous pooling.
   (2) Since they promote venous return, they do not need to be worn when the legs are elevated when sleeping.
   (4) If feet are permitted to be dependent before stockings are put on, venous pooling and edema may occur; application of elastic stockings at this time can cause tissue trauma.

57. (4) Marked jaundice generally indicates liver damage or excessive hemolysis and is not a sign of leukemia, unless hepatic damage from late effects of the disease or drugs has occurred. Edema is not a manifestation of the disease, since the pathophysiology does not involve transport of fluids. (a); AS; CP; NU; PE
   (1) Multiple bruises and petechiae are due to thrombocytopenia associated with leukemia.
   (2) Marked fatigue and pallor are the result of anemia associated with leukemia.
   (3) Enlarged lymph nodes, spleen, and liver are due to the infiltration of these organs with leukemic cells.

58. (3) Acute leukemia is an excessive uncontrolled production of immature white blood cells that compete for nutrients and eventually crowd the bone marrow, preventing formation of other blood cells. (b); AN; CP; NU; PE
   (1) Proliferating cells depress bone marrow production of the formed elements of blood.
   (2) RBCs and platelets are crowded out by proliferation of leukemic cells.
   (4) The liver and spleen are invaded by leukemic cells.

59. (4) A side effect of vincristine is alopecia. To adolescents, who are very concerned with identity, this represents a tremendous threat to their self-image. (a); PL; AN; SH; PE
   (1) Constipation, though possibly uncomfortable, can be minimized with medication and diet.

(2) This is very temporary and therefore not as much of a concern as alopecia.
   (3) This will not be immediately obvious.

60. (1) Infection from lowered resistance is a constant threat from the disease and from the immunosuppressant drugs, both of which affect white blood cells. (b); IM; AN; NU; PE
   (2) Maria needs normal stimuli for a 12-year-old except when acutely ill from drug therapy.
   (3) Although vital signs need to be checked to assess for changes in pulse or blood pressure changes, unless there is other clinical evidence of bleeding, q. 2 hour frequencies are not needed.
   (4) Maria needs to maintain the physical activity she can tolerate.

61. (3) Constipation from adynamic ileus can be prevented with high-fiber foods and liberal fluids. These will keep the stool bulky and soft, promoting evacuation. (c); PL; AP; SH; PE
   (1) Vincristine causes constipation; roughage and fluids are needed.
   (2) Treatment of constipation, a common side effect of vincristine, calls for roughage and fluids.
   (4) Roughage and fluids are recommended; help minimize the constipation associated with vincristine.

62. (1) Low platelet count predisposes to bleeding, which may be evident in the urine. Red blood cells are seen microscopically in the sediment. (b); PL; CP; NU; PE
   (2) White blood cells occur in the urine when there is a urinary tract infection.
   (3) Casts are seen in the urine in some kidney disorders.
   (4) Lymphocytes are not normally found in the urine.

63. (1) The protective blood-brain barrier initially screens leukemic cells from the CNS. However, in advanced stages leukemic infiltration occurs. The chemotherapeutic agents, also screened out by the blood-brain barrier, are ineffective. (c); IM; CP; SH; PE
   (2) Radiation destroys leukemic cells.
   (3) Radiation to the cranium is needed because chemotherapy does not pass the blood-brain barrier.
   (4) Radiation affects the leukemic infiltrates into the CNS.

64. (3) Children at early school age are not yet able to comprehend death's universality and inevitability but fear it, often personifying death as a bogey-man or death-angel. They need an opportunity to prepare for this. (b); IM; AP; SH; PE
   (1) A child this age needs to know the seriousness of the illness and that recovery may not be possible.
   (2) Children of this age interpret death as separation and punishment; they fear this in addition to death itself.
   (4) This response only avoids the question.

65. (2) The individual cannot resolve the conflict consciously because of emotional pressure pulling him

in both directions. As anxiety increases, the unconscious seeks a solution. The conversion selected usually resolves the initial conflict by making action impossible, thus removing the need to select one or the other choice. (c); AN; KN; NU; PS
(1) This is the body's response to stress, not an unconscious resolution of a conflict.
(3) It is a psychologic response to stress, not a defense against it.
(4) The conversion to physical symptoms operates on an unconscious level.

66. (1) The development of physical symptoms without a physical cause is an anxiety-reducing mechanism specific to the psychoneurotic pattern of behavior. (b); AN; KN; NU; PS
(2) This would be the body's response to stress.
(3) Going back to an earlier state when one felt safer and more secure is not converting anxiety into physical symptoms.
(4) Blaming others in the environment for failure and mistakes is not converting anxiety into physical symptoms.

67. (2) The development of the symptom is the unconscious method of reducing the anxiety. Because the symptom is meeting this need, it does not create anxiety itself but is passively accepted. (b); AN; CP; NU; PS
(1) There is no agitation; symptoms are passively accepted.
(3) There is no anger; symptoms are passively accepted.
(4) There is no anxiety; the conflict is resolved by the physical symptom.

68. (3) The psychosomatic response (hyperfunction or hypofunction) creates actual tissue change. Hypochondria is an exaggerated body concern unrelated to organic changes. (b); AN; CP; NU; PS
(1) There is an emotional component in both instances.
(2) There is a feeling of illness in both instances.
(4) There may be a restriction of activities in both instances.

69. (3) This response focuses the patient on the relationship between emotion and physical symptoms in a nonthreatening accepting manner. (b); AS; AN; SH; PS
(1) The nurse knows when the weakness began; redundant to ask.
(2) This does not help pinpoint what the person was feeling when the weakness happened.
(4) This would be a secondary gain since he elicits sympathy and gets out of doing something that he apparently does not wish to do.

70. (4) Until the patient learns new ways of dealing with anxiety, he will continue to use this pattern of behavior. Learning new ways to operate will break the pattern. (b); IM; AN; SH; PS
(1) This would be unrealistic since the patient must learn to cope with problems.
(2) This would reinforce the sick role.
(3) There is a certain amount of stress in everyday fam-

ily situations and the patient, not the family, must learn new coping mechanics.

71. (4) Helps the patient identify behavior and feelings in a nonthreatening manner. (c); IM; AP; SH; PS
(1) This would be ganging up on the patient.
(2) This evasion and refusal to answer would have the psychologic effect of removing the nurse from the group.
(3) The nurse's behavior is not the issue; the situation should be turned back to the patient's behavior.

72. (2) The mismatched blood cells are attacked by antibodies, and the hemoglobin released from the ruptured erythrocytes plugs the kidney tubules; such kidney involvement results in backache. (c); AS; CP; NU; ME
(1) This symptom is not common to transfusion reactions.
(3) This symptom is not common to transfusion reactions.
(4) This symptom is not common to transfusion reactions.

73. (2) The cessation of renal function is usually evidenced by a decrease in output to less than 400 ml/24 hr. (b); AS: AP; NU; ME
(1) Although this symptom is related to the renal system, its presence does not indicate kidney damage.
(3) Although this symptom is related to the renal system, its presence does not indicate kidney damage.
(4) Although this symptom is related to the renal system, its presence does not indicate kidney damage.

74. (1) Perspiration is an involuntary physiologic response. It is mediated by the autonomic nervous system under a variety of circumstances, such as rising ambient temperature, high humidity, stress, and pain. (a); AS; CP; NU; SU
(2) This is a voluntary emotional response.
(3) This is a voluntary action that may limit tension on the abdomen, reducing pain.
(4) This is a result of voluntary contraction of the facial muscles, a common response to pain.

75. (1) The patient is assessed and observed. Then the dialysis solutions are instilled, equilibrated, and drained by the nurse. (b); PL; KN; NU; SU
(2) Dialysis may be maintained for longer than 48 hours.
(3) Vital signs may be checked less frequently unless complications occur.
(4) Abdominal discomfort may be relieved by repositioning the patient.

76. (3) Peritoneal dialysis uses the peritoneum as a selectively permeable membrane for diffusion of toxins and wastes from the blood into the dialyzing solution. (a); AN; KN; NU; SU
(1) Substitute for kidney function; toxins and wastes pass from the blood into the dialyzing solution by diffusion.
(2) The dialysate does not clean the peritoneal mem-

brane; the semipermeable membrane allows toxins and wastes to pass into the dialysate within the abdominal cavity.

(4) Fluid in the abdominal cavity does not enter the intracellular compartment.

77. (4) Hyperkalemia occurs in renal failure. Because the kidneys are damaged, the body does not excrete K^+. (b); AN; AP; SH; ME

(1) Calcium deficiency would be manifested by tingling of the nose, ears, and fingertips along with muscle spasms and tetany.

(2) Calcium excess would produce renal calculi and pathologic fractures.

(3) Hyponatremia would cause headache, muscle weakness, apathy, and abdominal cramps.

78. (2) Potassium is always low to prevent hyperkalemia. (c); AN; CP; SH; ME

(1) Protein is low, but as high in essential amino acids as possible, forcing synthesis of nonessential amino acids from excess urea nitrogen; this prevents muscle wasting and decreases the production of protein catabolites and azotemia.

(3) Sodium is the most abundant extracellular cation and is needed to maintain life.

(4) Calories are needed to meet metabolic needs and prevent a negative nitrogen balance.

79. (3) If fluid is not draining properly, the patient should be positioned from side to side or with the head raised; or manual pressure should be applied to the lower abdomen to facilitate drainage by the use of external pressure and gravity. (c); IM; AP; NU; SU

(1) The patient's position may be changed p.r.n.; a supine position does not facilitate drainage by the use of gravity.

(2) This deficit is not enough to require notifying the physician.

(4) The physician removes the cannula.

80. (2) When respiratory embarrassment occurs, possibly from pressure of the dialysate on the diaphragm, fluid should be removed and the patient's vital signs and status observed. (c); EV; AP; NU; SU

(1) This may be indicated after the solution is drained and the diaphragmatic pressure decreased.

(3) The physician should be notified after immediate action is taken.

(4) Treatment is discontinued only if ordered.

81. (3) All patients who are confined to bed for any considerable period risk losing calcium from bones. This is precipitated in the urine and causes calculi. (b); AN; AP; NU; SU

(1) Although this may occur from inability to assume a normal anatomic position and the emotional impact of using a urinal, it usually does not predispose a patient to the development of renal calculi unless fluid intake is low and stasis occurs.

(2) There is no indication that his diet has changed.

(4) The presence of a healing fracture does not increase

total calcium metabolism; however, there will be increased deposition of bone at the fracture site.

82. (2) Constriction of circulation decreases venous return and increases pressure within the vessels. Fluid then moves into the interstitial spaces, causing edema. (a); AS; AP; NU; SU

(1) This would indicate infection.

(3) This would indicate infection.

(4) This would indicate infection.

83. (1) Immunosuppressive agents are administered to decrease the immune system's tendency to reject the transplanted organ. (b); IM; AP; SH; ME

(2) Untrue; recreation and exercise are encouraged. Only contact sports should be avoided.

(3) Although fever and edema would occur, hypotension would not; an increased blood pressure would usually be due to fluid retention.

(4) Urine production occurs almost immediately.

84. (2) Exposure to infection, cold, or overexertion in a patient with chronic adrenocortical insufficiency (Addison's disease) can cause circulatory collapse. (b); PL; AN; NU; ME

(1) This would be an appropriate room assignment.

(3) This would be an appropriate room assignment.

(4) This would be an appropriate room assignment.

85. (2) Deficiency of the glucocorticoids causes hypoglycemia in the patient with Addison's disease. Signs of hypoglycemia include weakness, dizziness, cool moist skin, hunger, tremors, and nervousness. (c); AN; CP; SH; ME

(1) Weakness with dizziness on arising is called postural hypotension.

(3) Hypokalemia is evidenced by nausea, vomiting, muscle weakness, and arrhythmias.

(4) This would be evidenced by edema, increased blood pressure, and moist rales in the lungs.

86. (4) Patients with Addison's disease must take glucocorticoids regularly to enable them to adapt physiologically to stress and prevent an addisonian crisis, a medical emergency similar to shock. (b); PL; AN; SH; ME

(1) Frequent visits are not indicated after control is established.

(2) Activity is permitted as tolerated.

(3) Sodium should be taken as desired since hyponatremia frequently occurs from diminished mineral corticoid secretion.

87. (1) Because of diminished mineralocorticoid secretion, patients with Addison's disease are prone to development of hyponatremia. Therefore the addition of salt to the diet is advised. (c); IM; AP; CL; ME

(2) Caloric intake is determined on an individual basis; diet is not necessarily restricted to 1200 calories.

(3) Protein is not omitted from the diet; ingestion of essential amino acids is necessary for normal metabolism.

(4) Fluids are not restricted in Addison's disease.

88. (2) When there are not enough circulating glucocorticoids and mineralocorticoids to sustain normal functioning of the body, the following symptoms occur: hypotension, fever, pallor, tachycardia, cyanosis (an addisonian crisis). (b); EV; AP; CL; ME
    (1) This is not a sign of an addisonian crisis; hypotension occurs.
    (3) Muscle spasms do not occur in an addisonian crisis; the patient usually progresses into a coma.
    (4) This does not occur in an addisonian crisis.
89. (2) Prolonged steroid therapy may produce Cushing's syndrome. Signs include slow wound healing, buffalo hump, hirsutism, weight gain, hypertension, acne, moon face, thin arms and legs, and behavioral disturbances. (c); IM; AP; CL; ME
    (1) Cortisone therapy has a glucocorticoid action, which increases blood glucose levels.
    (3) Hyperkalemia occurs with Addison's disease; cortisone therapy helps correct fluid and electrolyte imbalances.
    (4) Hypertension and fluid retention occur.
90. (2) Some cortisol derivatives possess 17-ketosteroid (androgenic) properties, which result in masculinization. (c); IM; AP; SH; ME
    (1) Masculinization is not part of the disease, it results from the androgens present in cortisol.
    (3) Saying not to worry denies the patient her concerns; masculinization results from the therapy and will not go away.
    (4) Denies the patient's feelings.
91. (1) Development of mood swings and psychosis is possible from overdose of glucocorticoids as a result of fluid and electrolyte alterations. (b); EV; CP; NU; ME
    (2) This is not a sign of glucocorticoid overdose.
    (3) This is not a sign of glucocorticoid overdose.
    (4) This is not a sign of glucocorticoid overdose.
92. (3) An interpersonal relationship based on trust must be established before patients can be helped back to reality. (a); PL; AP; SH; PS
    (1) Socialization would come at a later time in her therapy.
    (2) There is nothing to indicate an urgency to remove her from her home.
    (4) An important part of her treatment and care, but of lesser importance than a trusting relationship.
93. (2) Provides support and security without rejecting the patient or placing value judgments on behavior. (b); IM; AP; SH; PS
    (1) Limits will have to be set in Gail's care, but staying with her and showing acceptance are an immediate nursing action.
    (3) This would only calm her down; does not try to deal with the problem.
    (4) This would be ignoring the problem; isolation would imply punishment.
94. (2) This behavior reflects the early fetal position. The

individual curls up for both protection and security. (c); AN; CP; NU; PS
    (1) Does not seem to be in response to an observable stimulus.
    (3) Behavior does not indicate dissociation or depersonalization.
    (4) Gail gives no indication of a hallucinatory pattern.
95. (4) When the patient who is out of control feels that someone is assuming control, it promotes a feeling of security. As this continues, a sense of trust in this individual is established. (c); IM; AN; SH; PS
    (1) This would be important in planning care but not in establishing a therapeutic relationship.
    (2) Less important in the beginning phase of a relationship.
    (3) She exhibits no self-destructive tendencies at this time.
96. (3) Trust is basic to all other therapy. Without it a therapeutic relationship cannot be established. (b); PL; AN; CL; PS
    (1) There is nothing to indicate that Gail does not have a sense of identity.
    (2) Part of treatment is to build on present ego strengths; not a priority goal.
    (4) Helping her relate to others is a part of her treatment, not a priority goal.
97. (2) This response reassures the patient that the staff member is able to help and that the patient's feelings are accurate. (b); EV; AP; SH; PS
    (1) It is a reversible condition that can be treated with benztropine mesylate (Cogentin) or diphenhydramine hydrochloride (Benadryl).
    (3) It is not a symptom that requires adjusting to; rather one that must be treated.
    (4) Early treatment to reverse the symptoms is important.
98. (3) Yellow sclerae are a sign of jaundice, indicating liver damage, which can be irreversible if drug therapy is continued. (b); EV; AN; NU; PS
    (1) Photosensitivity is not a problem as long as the patient is cautioned to stay out of the sun.
    (2) This is Parkinson's syndrome, which can be reversed with treatment; continuation of medication is permitted.
    (4) A usually irreversible side effect even when medication is stopped.
99. (2) Close follow-up and continued monitoring of medication, behavior, and emotional state are necessary to enable the patient to maintain a positive behavioral change. (a); PL; AP; CL; PS
    (1) It would depend on what her regular activities were.
    (3) Would encourage dependence.
    (4) A self-help group might or might not be effective.
100. (4) If a tracheostomy is not performed with radical neck surgery, tracheal edema may cause obstruction of the airway after the endotracheal tube is removed. (a); IM; AP; NU; SU

(1) Fresh postoperative dressings should be removed by the surgeon.

(2) An endotracheal tube is not irrigated to maintain patency, as is a nasogastric tube; the endotracheal tube is in the trachea, leading to the lungs.

(3) It is not necessary to reposition the endotracheal tube if the gag reflex returns; when the patient is able to breathe on her own, the anesthesiologist will remove the tube.

101. (2) Inadequate oxygenation of the brain may produce restlessness or behavioral changes. The pulse and respiration rates increase as a compensatory mechanism for hypoxia. (b); AS; CP; NU; SU

(1) The pulse and respiration rates increase with hypoxia.

(3) Clubbing of the fingers, the result of increased vascularization, is an adaptation to prolonged hypoxia.

(4) The pupils dilate with cerebral hypoxia.

102. (3) The cuff should be inflated to the minimum occlusive volume, which allows the desired volume to be achieved but does not press against the trachea, constricting circulation. This can be judged by using a stethoscope to listen for a slight air leak at the back of the throat. (c); IM; AP; NU; SU

(1) The cuff is usually deflated during suctioning to prevent tracheal necrosis; secretions just above the cuff drop by gravity and can also be removed by suctioning.

(2) Several minutes per hour is recommended; some high-volume, low-pressure cuffs need minimal deflation.

(4) The seal should be minimally occlusive; a tight seal could result in tracheal necrosis.

103. (4) To facilitate entry of the suction catheter into the bronchi, the patient's head should be turned from side to side. For entry into the left bronchus the head should be turned to the right; for entry into the right bronchus, to the left. (c); IM; AP; NU; SU

(1) The cuff should be deflated during suctioning.

(2) When ordered, this drug is usually given by inhalation not instillation.

(3) Negative pressure is applied as the catheter is withdrawn.

104. (2) The tracheostomy site is a portal of entry for microorganisms. Sterile technique must be used. (c); IM; AP; NU; SU

(1) Body temperature is not related to the suctioning procedure.

(3) The cannula is generally cleaned with peroxide and saline.

(4) The Fowler position promotes maximum aeration of the lungs.

105. (2) Drugs such as atropine and opiates are contraindicated because the effects of drying secretions and depressing the cough reflex are undesirable. (c); AN; AN; NU; SU

(1) Pyrvinum pamoate (Povan), a drug for pinworms, is not contraindicated in persons with a tracheostomy.

(3) Chloral hydrate, a hypnotic, is not contraindicated in persons with a tracheostomy.

(4) Nalorphine (Nalline), a synthetic narcotic analgesic antagonist, is not contraindicated in persons with a tracheostomy.

106. (3) The inner cannula must be removed, cleaned with peroxide, and rinsed with saline to prevent mucus accumulation and occlusion of the tube. (b); IM; AP; NU; SU

(1) The outer cannula is left in place, its patency maintained through suctioning.

(2) The status of the cuff has no effect on tracheostomy care.

(4) This is used only for inserting the outer cannula.

107. (2) Apple juice and pear nectar have low sodium content and are therefore the better choices for this patient. (b); IM; AP; SH; ME

(1) The patient is permitted juice between meals.

(3) Tomato juice has a high sodium content; should be avoided to prevent fluid retention.

(4) Low-sodium juices are not contraindicated.

108. (2) $\dfrac{0.2 \text{ mg}}{0.5 \text{ mg}} \times \dfrac{x}{2 \text{ ml}}$ $0.2 \text{ mg}:x = 0.5 \text{ mg}:2 \text{ ml}$
$0.5x = 0.4 \text{ ml}$ $0.5x = 0.4$
$x = 0.8 \text{ ml}$ $x = 0.8 \text{ ml}$

(a); IM; AN; NU; ME

(1) This would be an overdose.

(3) This would be an overdose.

(4) This would be an overdose.

109. (2) Elevation of an extremity promotes venous and lymphatic drainage by gravity. (a); PL; AP; NU; ME

(1) This is a dependent function of the nurse.

(3) This is a dependent function of the nurse.

(4) This procedure will have little effect on edema.

110. (2) This combination of foods has the highest sodium content. (b); PL; AP; NU; ME

(1) This meal is low in sodium.

(3) This meal is low in sodium

(4) This meal is low in sodium

111. (4) Fluctuation of IV fluid in the manometer with respirations is due to alteration of intrathoracic pressure during inhalation and exhalation. (c); IM; AP; NU; ME

(1) The fluid in the manometer must be allowed to rise above the expected reading before the line to the patient is opened to permit the fluid in the manometer to drop; when the fluid level stops dropping, it reflects the patient's venous pressure.

(2) CVP is a measure of venous, not arterial, pressure.

(4) The fluid in the manometer must be allowed to rise above the expected reading before the line to the patient is opened to permit the fluid in the manometer to drop; when the fluid level stops dropping, it reflects the patient's venous pressure.

112. (1) Furosemide (Lasix) inhibits sodium reabsorption in the ascending loop of Henle, whereas chlorothiazide (Diuril) inhibits the reabsorption of sodium and

chloride. Water and potassium are not reabsorbed by the distal renal tubules, and dehydration and hypokalemia may result. (b); EV; CP; NU; ME

(2) With an increased fluid loss the specific gravity would more likely be lowered.

(3) These drugs do not affect protein metabolism.

(4) These drugs inhibit the reabsorption of sodium.

113. (1) Digitalis increases the strength of the myocardial contractions (positive inotropic effect) and, by altering the electrophysiologic properties of the heart, slows the heart rate (positive chronotropic effect). (a); AN; AP; NU; ME

(2) The PR interval is prolonged.

(3) Although this may result from the increased blood supply to the kidneys, it is not the primary reason for administering digitalis.

(4) Too general; digitalis increases the strength of the contractions but decreases the heart rate.

114. (2) The nurse was negligent in not providing close supervision, since she knew Mr. Norman was combative. A reasonable, prudent nurse would have closely observed Mr. Norman to protect him from himself as well as to protect others. (a); EV; AP; NU; PS

(1) The admitting office may have had no knowledge of the situation; therefore it was the nurse's responsibility.

(3) This is true of all patients, not only those who are combative.

(4) It would be unrealistic to keep him sedated at all times.

115. (4) Lithium carbonate alters sodium transport in nerve and muscle cells and causes a shift toward intraneuronal metabolism of catecholamines. Since the range between therapeutic and toxic levels is very small, the patient's serum lithium level should be monitored closely. (b); IM; AN; NU; PS

(1) Restricting sodium intake for patients receiving lithium may cause an electrolyte imbalance.

(2) Not necessary or useful.

(3) Not necessary; would depend on what the patient was receiving.

116. (3) This sets appropriate limits for the patient who cannot set them for himself. It rejects the behavior but accepts the patient. (b); IM; AP; SH; PS

(1) This does not show acceptance of the patient or help him control his behavior.

(2) May have the effect of reinforcing behavior rather than decreasing it.

(4) Does not deal with the problem directly; can confuse the patient, since he may be unaware of why the nurse refuses to talk to him.

117. (2) Activities that release tension and use up energy can decrease anxiety. (b); PL; AP; SH; PS

(1) Requires too much concentration, and he may hurt himself in the process.

(3) Requires too much concentration.

(4) Requires sitting still and a dexterity that he would probably find impossible at this time.

118. (2) A threat is a type of assault that is an intentional tort. (c); EV; AN; NU; PS

(1) Restraints would be cruel, illegal, and unnecessary for Mr. Norman.

(3) This draws a conclusion that may not be true.

(4) The behavior can be expected but should not be ignored; behavior should be dealt with directly.

119. (1) Patients who are hyperactive are easily diverted. It is best to use this characteristic behavior rather than precipitate a confrontation. (a); IM; AP; SH; PS

(2) Shows no consideration of how he may feel.

(3) Shifts responsibility to the physician; the nurse should know that a shopping trip is unrealistic at this time.

(4) Only postpones having to deal directly with the problem; does not deal with reality.

120. (1) The patient is asking for help to prevent suicide. This response focuses on feelings and does not challenge or deny them. (a); IM; AN; SH; PS

(2) The nurse is ignoring a cry for help and not following through on what he is expressing.

(3) The nurse is denying what the patient is telling her.

(4) The nurse is negating his feelings and putting her own interpretation on his situation.

Comprehensive Test 3

To simulate the comprehensive licensing examinations, this test should be completed within 2 hours.

Situation: *Mrs. Winet, a 32-year-old gravida III, para 2, spontaneously delivers a 4082.3 g (9 pound) baby boy en route to the hospital after a brief labor. Questions 1 through 13 refer to this situation.*

1 The nurse should be aware that the chief hazard to a child in precipitate delivery is:
   1. Brachial palsy
   2. Intracranial hemorrhage
   3. Dislocated hip
   4. Fractured clavicle

2 Perineal laceration is a common complication of precipitate delivery. In addition to regular perineal care, Mrs. Winet's nursing care would include:
   1. Encouraging early and frequent ambulation
   2. Encouraging perineal exercises to strengthen muscles
   3. Telling the patient to expect slower healing
   4. Providing a high-protein, high-roughage diet

3 Baby Winet has sustained an intracranial hemorrhage because of a tear in the tentorial membrane. The nurse would expect the baby to display which one of the following symptoms?
   1. Extreme lethargy
   2. Weak, timorous cry
   3. Anormal respirations
   4. Generalized purpura

4 The nurse checks Baby Winet's Babinski reflex and finds it to be positive. A positive Babinski sign in a newborn infant is due to:
   1. Immaturity of the central nervous system
   2. Hypoxia during labor and delivery
   3. Hyperreflexia of the muscular system
   4. Neurologic impairment

5 Nursing care of Baby Winet would include:
   1. Stimulating frequently to monitor level of consciousness
   2. Elevating his head higher than his hips
   3. Checking reflexes every 15 minutes
   4. Weighing him daily before feeding

6 A diagnosis of cerebral palsy (CP) is suggested in the nursery and confirmed when Baby Jimmy Winet visits the health clinic at 6 weeks. Mrs. Winet

cries, "What did we do to deserve this?" The nurse responds:

1. "Why do you feel you are being punished?"
2. "You didn't do anything; let me tell you about this disorder."
3. "Let's sit down and have a cup of coffee."
4. "I know you must be upset, but it's too early to tell."

7. As Jimmy Winet develops, his vision, hearing, and speech are fine but he does have a slight general sensory loss in position, pain, and temperature in both legs. He uses braces and special appliances to provide self-care. He is admitted to the hospital at the age of 7 years for a tendon-lengthening procedure. While in bed after surgery, he must wear his braces and shoes for at least 8 hours a day. This is to:

1. Continue his acceptance of physical restraints
2. Maintain hip and knee alignment and prevent footdrop
3. Stretch his ligaments and strengthen muscle tone
4. Encourage ambulation as soon as possible

8 The orthopedic surgeon is anxious to get Jimmy onto crutches. In preparing Jimmy for crutch walking the nurse must determine:

1. The weight-bearing ability of Jimmy's upper and lower extremities
2. Whether Jimmy has the power in his trunk to drag his legs forward when erect
3. When Jimmy's circulation can tolerate an erect position
4. The ability of Jimmy's shoulder girdle to support his body weight when it leaves the floor

9 It is decided that Jimmy be taught the 4-point alternate crutch gait. This gait was probably chosen because:

1. There are always 2 points of support on the floor
2. Jimmy has more power in the upper extremities than in the lower extremities
3. It provides for equal but partial weight bearing on each limb
4. Jimmy has no power or step ability in the lower extremities

10 In view of his slight sensory loss in the legs, Jimmy and his parents should be taught to:

1. Keep the braces in good repair and pad them well
2. Check alignment of the braces (brace joints should coincide with body joints)
3. Select shoes which have heels that are wide and low

4. Examine the skin for evidence of pressure points

11 When teaching Jimmy to ambulate with crutches, the nurse should remember that:

1. Learning progresses on a line forward and upwark
2. Because of his age, Jimmy's experiential background is limited
3. Learning is a result of adequate teaching
4. Jimmy must first understand normal walking patterns

12 Because of the diminished sensation in Jimmy's legs, he should be taught the following safety precautions:

1. Test the temperature of water in any water-related activity
2. Set the clock 2 times during the night to awaken and change position
3. Tighten straps and buckles more than usual on braces when ambulating
4. Look down at the lower extremities when crutch walking to determine proper positioning of the legs

13 When planning long-term care for Jimmy, it is important for the nurse to recognize that:

1. Cerebral palsy is unstable and unpredictable
2. Jimmy should have genetic counseling before planning a family
3. His illness is not progressively degenerative
4. Jimmy probably has some degree of mental retardation

Situation: *Mrs. White, a 73-year-old widow, lives with her daughter. While picketing for senior citizens' rights at the state legislature, she fell and fractured her right hip. Mrs. White is admitted to the hospital for reduction of the fracture and insertion of a pin. On admission her blood pressure is 180/102 with some dependent edema. Questions 14 through 24 refer to this situation.*

14 During the day the nurse puts Mrs. White's side rails up specifically:

1. As a safety measure because of the patient's age
2. Because all patients over 65 years of age should use side rails
3. Because elderly people are often disoriented for several days after anesthesia
4. To be used as handholds and to facilitate the patient's mobility

15 Mrs. White is apprehensive about being hospitalized. The nurse realizes that one of the stresses of hospitalization is the strangeness of the environ-

ment and activity. Extension of this stress can best be limited by:
1. Listening to what Mrs. White has to say
2. Calling the patient by her first name
3. Visiting Mrs. White frequently
4. Explaining to Mrs. White what is expected of her

16 A 1-gram sodium diet and furosemide (Lasix) IM are prescribed for Mrs. White. She does not like her diet and tells the nurse that her sister is bringing in some "good home-cooked food." The initial, most effective, nursing action should be to:
1. Call in the dietitian for patient teaching
2. Tell Mrs. White that she cannot have salt, since it will raise her blood pressure
3. Wait for Mrs. White's sister and discuss the diet with both of them
4. Catch Mrs. White's sister before she goes into the room and tell her about the diet

17 Since sodium is the major cation controlling fluid outside the cells, diet therapy in congestive heart failure with subsequent cardiac edema is aimed at reducing the sodium intake. In teaching Mrs. White about her diet, the nurse should encourage her to exclude which group of foods?
1. Fruits
2. Vegetables
3. Grains
4. Processed foods

18 The nurse should explain to Mrs. White that sodium restriction is an effective therapeutic tool in the treatment of congestive heart failure because its restriction:
1. Helps to prevent the potassium accumulation that occurs when sodium intake is higher
2. Helps to control food intake and thus weight
3. Causes excess tissue fluid to be withdrawn and excreted
4. Aids the weakened heart muscle to contract and improves cardiac output

19 Since Mrs. White has gluteal edema in the unaffected hip, the nurse should use the deltoid muscle for administration of drugs IM, mainly because at edematous sites:
1. Deposition of an injected drug causes pain
2. Blood supply is insufficient for drug adsorption
3. Fluid leaks from the site for long periods after injection
4. Tissue fluid dilutes the drug before it enters the circulation

20 An independent nursing action that could be used to prevent thrombus formation in the unaffected leg would be:

1. Gentle massage
2. Passive range-of-motion exercises
3. Encouraging fluids
4. Elastic stockings

21 While assisting Mrs. White to transfer from the bed to a wheelchair, the nurse should remember that:
1. During a weight-bearing transfer the patient's knees should be slightly bent
2. Transfers to and from the wheelchair will be easier if the bed is higher than the wheelchair
3. The transfer can be accomplished by pivoting while bearing weight on both upper extremities and not on the legs
4. The appropriate proximity and visual relationship of wheelchair to bed must be maintained

22 To prepare Mrs. White for crutch walking, the nurse should encourage the patient to:
1. Sit up straight in a chair to develop the back muscles
2. Keep the affected limb in extension and abduction
3. Do exercises in bed to strengthen her upper extremities
4. Use the trapeze to strengthen the biceps muscles

23 When assisting Mrs. White to ambulate, the nurse should be standing:
1. In front of the patient
2. Behind the patient
3. On the left side of the patient
4. On the right side of the patient

24 Mrs. White is being discharged from the hospital; however, she needs assistance with activities of daily living and needs to learn how to use a cane, since her daughter works full time and cannot care for her. The most appropriate place for Mrs. White to convalesce would be:
1. Her own home, with visits from the public health nurse
2. A nursing home
3. An adult facility
4. An extended care facility

Situation: Mrs. Malone, 48 years old, has discovered a lump in her breast on self-examination. It is fixed, and the physician can aspirate no fluid. She is admitted for a possible right radical mastectomy. Questions 25 through 35 refer to this situation.

25 A priority of nursing intervention for Mrs. Malone in the preoperative period would be to:
1. Teach isometric arm exercises
2. Ascertain how the patient will adjust to radical mastectomy

3. Cleanse the operative site with Betadine several times
4. Have a representative from Reach to Recovery visit her

26 During her morning care Mrs. Malone tells the nurse that she is worried about what she will look like after the surgery. The nurse's most appropriate *initial* response is:
1. "Try not to think about the surgery now."
2. "Why don't you discuss this with your husband?"
3. "I can understand that you'd be concerned."
4. "Everyone having this surgery feels the same way."

27 After the surgery the nurse should position Mrs. Malone's right arm:
1. In abduction surrounded by sandbags
2. Lower than the level of the right atrium on pillows
3. In adduction supported by sandbags
4. With the hand higher than the arm on pillows

28 When teaching Mrs. Malone postmastectomy arm exercises, it is important for the nurse to:
1. Exercise both arms simultaneously
2. Exercise the right arm only
3. Have Mrs. Malone wear a sling in between exercises
4. Wait until the incision has healed

29 Mrs. Malone's physician plans chemotherapy 2 weeks after the surgery. The delay in instituting the plan for drug therapy is because the drugs:
1. Interfere with cell growth and delay wound healing
2. Cause vomiting, which endangers the integrity of the large incisional area
3. Decrease red blood cell production, and the resultant anemia would add to postoperative fatigue
4. Increase edema in areas distal to the incision by blocking lymph channels with destroyed lymphocytes

30 Mrs. Malone has been symptom free for 3 years. At her 6-month visit she complains of headaches and difficulty with her embroidery. Her blood pressure is elevated and her pupils react sluggishly. She is admitted to the hospital for further evaluation. Which of the following findings should the nurse question in doing an assessment of Mrs. Malone for increased intracranial pressure?
1. Jacksonian seizures
2. Rapid pulse
3. Psychotic behavior
4. Nausea and vomiting

31 Which of the following orders written by Mrs. Malone's physician should the nurse question?
1. Administer osmotic diuretic as ordered
2. Place the patient in a reverse Trendelenburg position
3. Administer steroids as ordered
4. Apply rotating tourniquets

32 The nurse assists the physician in performing a lumbar puncture. When pressure is placed on the jugular vein during a lumbar puncture, there is normally a rise in the spinal fluid pressure. This is referred to as:
1. Chvostek's sign
2. Romberg's sign
3. Queckenstedt's sign
4. Homans' sign

33 Mrs. Malone has a tumor of the cerebellum. In view of the functions of this organ, what symptom should the nurse expect to observe?
1. Absence of the knee-jerk and other reflexes
2. Inability to execute smooth, precise movements
3. Inability to execute voluntary movements
4. Unconsciousness

34 Before preparing Mrs. Malone for cranial surgery, the nurse should:
1. Wash the patient's hair with pHisoHex
2. Help the patient choose a wig
3. Obtain consent for shaving the head
4. Wait to shave the head until the patient is anesthetized

35 In caring for Mrs. Malone postoperatively, the nurse should:
1. Take only axillary temperatures
2. Encourage coughing but discourage deep breathing
3. Report yellow drainage on dressing to the physician immediately
4. Administer narcotics and sedatives at the first sign of irritability

Situation: Mrs. Janeway is 36 weeks pregnant and is attending a class in preparation for childbirth with her husband. Questions 36 through 48 refer to this situation.

36 Mrs. Janeway verbalizes, "I am sick and tired of wearing these same old clothes; how I wish all this would be done and over with." The nurse's best response would be:
1. "Is there something bothering you? You sound discouraged."
2. "Most women feel the same way you do at this time."
3. "I understand how you feel; what do you know about labor?"

4. "Yes, this is the most uncomfortable time during pregnancy."

37 In the prepration for childbirth class the nurse would teach that labor:
   1. Should be painless and uneventful
   2. May be uncomfortable, but medication is available when needed
   3. Will be painful, but patients will be taught how to tolerate it
   4. Will be uncomfortable; however, medication will not be needed.

38 Mrs. Janeway is admitted to the labor and delivery unit in extreme discomfort with contractions occurring 3 minutes apart. The nurse realizes that the greatest influence on the perception of pain for a woman in labor is the:
   1. Difficulty of the labor
   2. Length of the labor
   3. Tension of the patient
   4. Parity of the patient

39 The nurse takes the fetal heart rate during a contraction and finds it is 115 per minute. The next nursing action should be to:
   1. Notify the physician immediately
   2. Take a second reading during decrement
   3. Take a second reading during the acme of the next contraction
   4. Administer oxygen immediately

40 The nurse knows that Mrs. Janeway has begun the advanced stage of labor when:
   1. She feels the need to move her bowels
   2. She complains of sudden intense back pain
   3. The cervix is dilated to 6 cm
   4. Restlessness and thrashing increase

41 One hour following delivery the nurse finds that Mrs. Janeway's uterus has become boggy. The initial response should be to:
   1. Notify the physician
   2. Check the blood pressure
   3. Massage it until firm
   4. Observe the amount of bleeding

42 Mrs. Janeway's baby girl has a unilateral cleft lip and palate. The physician recommends that the lip be repaired as soon as possible after birth because the baby is in otherwise good physical condition. Cleft lip is usually repaired early because of:
   1. Emotional impact on the parents
   2. Feeding difficulty
   3. Infection
   4. Obstruction of breathing

43 Mr. and Mrs. Janeway are very concerned about the defect and ask the nurse, "What caused our baby to be born deformed?" The nurse should reply:
   1. "I don't know, but you don't need to worry because surgery can correct it."
   2. "I am glad that you are able to ask these kinds of questions."
   3. "Are you feeling guilty?"
   4. "It sounds as if you are wondering what you might have done to cause this situation."

44 While informing the parents about the significance and etiology of cleft lip and palate, the nurse should:
   1. Assess the family history for presence of the defect in other siblings or relatives
   2. Emphasize that the 2 defects follow laws of mendelian genetics
   3. Prepare the parents for the likelihood of mental and psychologic problems in the child
   4. Stress that the defect is rare and will probably never happen twice in the same family

45 Before Baby Sarah was born, Mrs. Janeway had wanted to breast-feed. Now feeding will probably be:
   1. With a rubber-tipped syringe or medicine dropper
   2. Too difficult because of breathing problems
   3. With a soft, large-holed nipple
   4. IV fluids

46 Sarah's cleft lip predisposes her to infection primarily because of:
   1. Poor nutrition from disturbed feeding
   2. Poor circulation to the defective area
   3. Mouth breathing, which dries the oropharyngeal mucous membranes
   4. Waste products that accumulate along the defect

47 Mrs. Janeway has walked to the nursery numerous times to see Sarah each day. Three days post partum she complains of pain in her right leg. The nurse's initial response should be to:
   1. Encourage ambulation and exercise
   2. Massage the affected area
   3. Apply hot soaks
   4. Maintain bed rest and notify the physician

48 Baby Sarah's lip is repaired 4 days after birth. Which of the following would be *contraindicated* during postoperative care?
   1. Observe for swelling of the tongue, lips, and mucous membranes
   2. Place her on her abdomen to prevent aspiration
   3. Keep the suture line clean and free of crusting
   4. Encourage the parents to visit as much as possible to prevent the infant from crying

Situation: Mrs. Jones, a 35-year-old mother of 4 children, is di-agnosed as having Cushing's syndrome. Questions 49 through 60 refer to this situation.

49 In planning her care the nurse should take into consideration the fact that Mrs. Jones would have:
1. Hypotension and sodium loss
2. Hyperkalemia and edema
3. Muscle weakness and frequent urination
4. Muscle wasting and hypoglycemia

50 Mrs. Jones would probably demonstrate which of the following symptoms?
1. Lability of mood
2. Decrease in the growth of hair
3. Ectomorphism with a moon face
4. Increased resistance to bruising

51 Prior to Mrs. Jones' undergoing an adrenalectomy the nurse should:
1. Withhold all medications for 48 hours
2. Administer steroids IM or IV
3. Provide a high-protein diet
4. Collect a 24-hour urine specimen

52 Postoperatively, prior to maintenance steroid ther-apy, the nurse would expect to see signs of:
1. Hyperglycemia
2. Sodium retention
3. Potassium excretion
4. Hypotension

53 In teaching Mrs. Jones about her medications, the nurse should plan to emphasize the fact that:
1. Once she is regulated, her dosage will remain the same for life
2. Taking her medications late in the evening may cause sleeplessness
3. While she is taking medications, her salt intake may have to be restricted
4. Steroid therapy will be given in conjunction with insulin

54 Mrs. Jones is very upset after visiting hours. She tearfully tells the nurse that her 2-year-old son Alex is being admitted to the hospital in the morn-ing for a circumcision because of phimosis. After quieting Mrs. Jones, the nurse notifies the physi-cian, since Mrs. Jones:
1. Will probably require mild sedation to ensure her rest
2. Should have her steroid medication dosage re-duced
3. Has a decreased ability to handle stress despite steroid therapy
4. Will have feelings of exhaustion and lethargy as a result of stress

55 Alex is admitted in the morning for the circumci-sion and is now ready to go to the OR in 1 hour.

As the nurse enters his room with a preoperative injection, he begins to scream and flail about the bed. His father is sitting at his bedside and gets up to leave. The nurse's best reponse to this situation is to:
1. Leave the room and ask another nurse to come in to hold Alex during the injection
2. Allow Alex to say goodbye to his father before giving the injection
3. Tell Mr. Jones he can return to comfort Alex after the injection is given
4. Ask Mr. Jones to stay to comfort and hold Alex while the injection is given

56 Attendance of parents during painful procedures on their children should be:
1. Based on the type of procedure to be performed
2. Encouraged and permitted if the child desires their presence
3. Based on individual assessment of the parents
4. Discouraged for the benefit of the parents and the child

57 The gluteal muscle is generally not used when giv-ing IM injections to infants and young children be-cause they:
1. Fear intrusive procedures
2. Are able to wiggle and change position when placed on their abdomen
3. Have an undeveloped muscle mass in this area
4. Associate this area with punishment

58 A major nursing responsibility in caring for Alex postoperatively is to:
1. Limit oral fluids
2. Monitor IV fluids carefully
3. Apply ice packs to the penis
4. Observe for bleeding at the operative site

59 Mrs. Jones and Alex are being discharged to-gether. In response to her question the nurse ex-plains to Mrs. Jones that her therapy includes a low-sodium, high-potassium diet because:
1. Excessive secretions of aldosterone and corti-sone cause renal retention of sodium and loss of potassium
2. Her use of salt had probably contributed to her disease
3. She is losing excess salt in her urine and re-quires less renal stimulation
4. She will gain excessive weight if sodium is not limited

60 After discharge Mrs. Jones begins to manifest signs of diabetes mellitus. The nurse recognizes that diabetes mellitus may develop because:
1. The cortical hormones created a too rapid weight loss

2. The excessive glucocorticoids secreted by the adrenal gland caused excessive tissue catabolism and gluconeogenesis
3. A negative nitrogen balance resulted from the tissue catabolism
4. The excessive ACTH damaged pancreatic tissue

Situation: Mr. Burn, 55, is admitted to the hospital with benign prostatic hypertrophy. Surgery is scheduled for the next day. Questions 61 through 67 refer to this situation.

61 The night nurse reports that Mr. Burn is complaining of inability to void. On making the morning rounds it is noted that his bladder is distended. Nursing intervention should be to:
1. Force fluids to induce voiding
2. Encourage use of a urinal
3. Apply pressure over the pubic area
4. Assist him into a warm tub bath

62 Mr. Burn has undergone a suprapubic prostatectomy. In addition to a Foley catheter, the nurse should expect the patient to have:
1. A rectal incision and a ureteral catheter
2. A ureterostomy with gravity drainage
3. A nephrostomy tube with tidal drainage
4. An abdominal incision and a cystostomy tube

63 The most significant complication immediately after this surgery is:
1. Hemorrhage
2. Impotence
3. Urinary incontinence
4. Spasms

64 Mr. Burn has just returned from the recovery room after the suprapubic prostatectomy. He accidently pulls out the urethral catheter. The nurse should:
1. Check for bleeding by irrigating the suprapubic tube
2. Reinsert a new catheter
3. Notify the physician immediately
4. Take no immediate action if the suprapubic tube is draining

65 In the postoperative care of Mr. Burn an important action to prevent secondary bladder infection is to:
1. Observe for signs of uremia
2. Attach the catheter to suction
3. Clamp off the connecting tubing
4. Change the dressings frequently

66 Mr. Burn complains of pain in the area operated upon. The initial response of the nurse should be to:
1. Administer the prescribed analgesic
2. Measure and record the vital signs before administering an analgesic

3. Inspect the drainage tubing for occlusion
4. Encourage intake of fluids to dilute urine

67 After a prostatectomy the nurse should:
1. Have the patient stand to void
2. Aspirate the catheter with a bulb syringe
3. Discourage straining for a bowel movement
4. Notify the physician if the patient does not void in 12 hours

Situation: Mr. Jay is admitted to the psychiatric service by his parents, who can no longer deal with him. He is a handsome, smooth-talking bright young man who as been married 3 times and has a child by each wife. He states he has never loved any of his wives, does not intend to support his children, and has no reason to be sorry for anything he has ever done. Questions 68 through 74 refer to this situation.

68 The nurse would expect Mr. Jay's behavior to demonstrate a defect in:
1. Id development
2. Ego development
3. Superego development
4. Sexual development

69 In working with Mr. Jay the nurse should be which of the following?
1. Sincere, cautious, and consistent
2. Strict, punishing, and restrictive
3. Accepting, supportive, and friendly
4. Sympathetic, motherly, and encouraging

70 Mrs. Jones, one of the nurses, is taking a new patient on an orientation tour of the unit when Mr. Jay rushes down the hallway and asks her to sit and talk to him. Which would be the most appropriate action by the nurse?
1. Excuse herself from the new patient and speak with Mr. Jay
2. Suggest to Mr. Jay that he talk with another staff member
3. Introduce Mr. Jay and suggest that he join them on the tour
4. Tell Mr. Jay that she will speak with him later

71 Mr. Jay responds by smiling broadly and saying, "Mrs. Jones you sure do look messy today." Which would be the most appropriate response by the nurse?
1. "That's not a nice thing to say, Mr. Jay."
2. "Don't you feel well today, Mr. Jay?"
3. "I didn't get a chance to set my hair last night."
4. "You're angry with me, Mr. Jay."

72 Mr. Jay takes Mrs. Jones by the shoulder, suddenly kisses her, and shouts "I like you." Which would be the most appropriate response for the nurse to make?

1. "I like you too but please don't do that again."
2. "I wish you wouldn't do that."
3. "Don't ever touch me like that again."
4. "Thank you, I like you too."

73 Mr. Jay has just been given his first day pass from the hospital. He is due to return at 6 P.M. At 5 P.M. Mr. Jay telephones the nurse in charge of the ward and says "Six o'clock is too early. I feel like coming back at 7:30." Which approach by the nurse would be most therapeutic at this time? Tell him to:
1. Return immediately, to demonstrate control
2. Return on time or he will be restricted
3. Come back by 6:45, as a compromise to set limits
4. Come back as soon as he can or you'll have to send police

74 Mrs. Jones is leaving in 2 weeks and tells Mr. Jay. Which response would indicate that he is progressing in his ability to maintain more mature relationships? He:
1. Tells her that he must get well enough by then so that he may also leave
2. Wishes her good luck and thanks her for helping him
3. Tells her that her leaving is just another loss he must adjust to
4. Informs her that, since she is leaving, this should be their last meeting

Situation: Mr. Brown, a 48-year-old man with a long history of chronic obstructive lung disease, is admitted to the hospital for a segmental resection of the right lower lobe. Questions 75 through 82 refer to this situation.

75 Intermittent positive pressure breathing is given preoperatively to:
1. Encourage respiration at a faster rate than that established by respiratory center control
2. Provide more adequate lung expansion than could be achieved by unassisted breathing
3. Force air through the infected secretions that accumulated in the lung bases
4. Remove air and fluid from the pleural cavity

76 Because of Mr. Brown's history of COPD, the nurse should be aware of complications involving:
1. Kidney function
2. Peripheral neuropathy
3. Cardiac function
4. Joint inflammation

77 When scheduling intermittent positive pressure breathing treatments, the nurse should realize that the *least* appropriate time of day to receive an IPPB treatment is:

1. On awakening
2. Before a meal
3. At bedtime
4. After a meal

78 Immediately after Mr. Brown's arrival in the recovery room, the nurse should undertake which of the following measures concerning the closed chest drainage apparatus?
1. Secure the chest catheter to the wound dressing with a sterile safety pin
2. Mark the time and the fluid level on the side of the drainage bottle
3. Raise the drainage bottle to bed level to check patency of the system
4. Add 3 to 5 ml of sterile saline to the water seal

79 The purpose of the water in the closed chest drainage bottle is to:
1. Facilitate emptying bloody drainage from the chest
2. Foster removal of chest secretions by capillarity
3. Prevent entrance of air into the pleural cavity
4. Decrease the danger of sudden change in pressure in the tube

80 Mr. Brown has a large amount of respiratory secretions. Independent nursing care should include:
1. Turning and positioning
2. Cupping
3. Clapping
4. Postural drainage

81 Mr. Brown requires oxygen. All of the following are factors to consider when determining the method of oxygen administration to be used for a specific patient. Which is of *major* concern?
1. Facial anatomy
2. Pathologic condition
3. Age and mental capacity
4. Level of activity

82 A preventive measure to be taken by the nurse regarding the untoward effects of oxygen therapy is:
1. Padding elastic bands of the face mask
2. Humidifying the gas
3. Taking the apical pulse before starting therapy
4. Placing the patient in the orthopneic position

Situation: Mr. Paley, a 56-year-old plumber, is hospitalized with a recent myocardial infarction. Questions 83 through 90 refer to this situation.

83 The nurse goes to Mr. Paley's bedside to administer his 10 A.M. dose of digoxin (Lanoxin). He has a lidocaine hydrochloride (Xylocaine) IV drip running at 3 mg/minute for control of premature ventricular contractions. The cardiac monitor

shows 20 PVCs per minute, and his heart rate is 78. The nurse's first actions should be to:
1. Increase the lidocaine flow rate and check for sources of excess neural stimuli
2. Check the availability of the defibrillator and run an ECG rhythm strip
3. Administer the digoxin and increase the lidocaine flow rate
4. Run an ECG rhythm strip and administer the digitalis

84 The nurse should recognize that the greatest danger of premature ventricular contractions is that they can lead to ventricular fibrillation if they strike on the:
1. P wave
2. PR interval
3. R wave
4. T wave

85 Three days after admission Mr. Paley has a cardiac arrest and is successfully defibrillated. The nurse is aware that the use of electric currents to defibrillate the heart during cardiac arrest depends on the body fluids:
1. Containing electrolytes
2. Containing base elements
3. Being a colloidally dispersed medium
4. Resembling pure water

86 After the arrest Mr. Paley is receiving dopamine hydrochloride (Intropin) intravenously for regulation of blood pressure. The planned effect of the drug is based on the fact that it:
1. Exerts an inotropic effect on the myocardium
2. Constricts the renal vasculature
3. Depresses cholinergic receptors in the arteries
4. Increases adrenal output of epinephrine

87 The nurse should administer a dopamine hydrochloride drip via an infusion control device because:
1. The drug must be infused slowly, since it is irritating to the vein
2. Administration of the drug above the established rate may cause generalized arterial constriction
3. Extravasation of the drug into subcutaneous tissues causes sloughing
4. Hypotension and renal shutown occur when the infusion runs rapidly

88 Mr. Paley is receiving digoxin (Lanoxin) at 10 A.M. daily. At 9 A.M. he states that he has been nauseated since awaking. He has a p.r.n. order for trimethobenzamide (Tigan) and receives aluminum hydroxide gel (Amphojel) every 2 hours. The nurse should:

1. Give the Amphojel now and the Lanoxin at 10 A.M.
2. Give the Tigan now and the Amphojel at 10 A.M. and withhold the Lanoxin
3. Hold the Lanoxin for 1 hour and give the Amphojel now
4. Give the Amphojel and Tigan now and the Lanoxin at 10 A.M.

89 Mr. Paley questions the nurse about the length of time it takes the heart to heal. The nurse replies that myocardial tissue usually heals within:
1. 3 to 4 weeks
2. 6 to 8 weeks
3. 10 to 14 weeks
4. 20 to 24 weeks

90 Mr. Paley is being discharged from the hospital. He has a prescription for procainamide hydrochloride (Pronestyl) which he is to take for control of ventricular irritability. He should be taught that:
1. His heart rate will be slower and he may experience fatigue
2. The drug must be taken at exact time intervals prescribed to maintain the therapeutic effect
3. He should plan a schedule for taking the drug during highest periods of activity
4. The total daily dosage of drug must be maintained, but the schedule may be adjusted to avoid taking the drug with meals

Situation: *Mrs. Grite, who is 35 weeks pregnant and a diabetic, is admitted to the hospital to await delivery. Questions 91 through 95 refer to this situation.*

91 Mrs. Grite's questions about why she is being hospitalized can be answered best if the nurse understands that in diabetic pregnant women:
1. Complete rest prior to the work of delivery is essential
2. Fetal death usually occurs after the thirty-sixth week of gestation
3. Fetal development is completed and should be monitored
4. Insulin needs to be administered intravenously before labor begins

92 The nurse should be aware that diabetic pregnant women such as Mrs. Grite require:
1. Increased dosage of insulin
2. Administration of estrogenic hormones
3. Decreased caloric intake
4. Administration of pancreatic enzymes

93 Mrs. Grite asks why she cannot take the oral hypoglycemic pills she used for her diabetes. The nurse's response should be based on the fact that

oral hypoglycemics are not used during pregnancy because:

1. The fetal pancreas compensates for the mother's inability to secrete adequate insulin
2. The effect of exogenous insulin on the fetus is uncertain
3. They may produce deformities in the fetus
4. During the latter part of pregnancy, diabetes can usually be controlled by diet alone

94 Mrs. Grite's delivery is induced and she delivers a baby girl. A sign of hypoglycemia in Baby Grite for which the nurse should be alert is:

1. Excessive birth weight
2. Excessive body movement
3. Pallor of the skin and mucosa
4. Poor sucking reflex

95 In caring for Baby Grite the nurse should provide:

1. A decreased glucose intake
2. Routine newbon care
3. For administration of insulin
4. Special high-risk care

Situation: Mr. Osgood is admitted to the hospital for surgery for an incarcerated hernia. Questions 96 through 100 refer to this situation.

96 The nurse recognizes the diagnosis of incarcerated hernia to mean that:

1. The blood supply to the intestine has been cut off
2. The protruding hernia cannot be reduced
3. An erosion of the involved intestine has occurred
4. The bowel has twisted on itself

97 Prior to Mr. Osgood's hernia repair the nurse should:

1. Place the patient in the supine position
2. Periodically check the patient's vital signs
3. Observe the patient's bowel movements
4. Monitor the patient's serum enzyme levels

98 The physician returns the incarcerated tissue to the abdominal cavity and uses a stainless steel mesh to reinforce the muscle wall, thereby preventing a future recurrence. This procedure is referred to as a:

1. Herniorrhaphy
2. Herniotomy
3. Herniectomy
4. Hernioplasty

99 After Mr. Osgood's surgery to help limit a common complication of this surgery, the nurse should:

1 Place a rolled towel under the scrotum
2. Encourage a high-carbohydrate diet

3. Have Mr. Osgood cough and deep breathe frequently
4. Apply a Scultetus binder

100 An important part of discharge planning is educating Mr. Osgood about body mechanics. Which of the following statements is an important concept in body mechanics?

1. Bending at the waist reduces tension on the inguinal muscles
2. Keeping the body straight when lifting reduces pressure on the abdomen
3. Placing the feet apart will increase the stability of the body
4. Relaxing the abdominal muscles and using the extremities prevent strain

Situation: Mr. Walter is admitted to the psychiatric unit with a diagnosis of paranoid schizophrenia. Questions 101 through 108 refer to this situation.

101 During the admission procedure Mr. Walter appears to be responding to voices. He cries out at intervals, "No, no, I didn't kill him," and states, "You know the truth, tell that policeman. Please help me!" The nurse should:

1. Respond by saying, "Mr. Walter, I want to help you and I realize you must be very frightened."
2. Sit there quietly and not respond at all to his statements
3. Respond by saying, "Whom are they saying you killed, Mr. Walter?"
4. Respond by saying, "Mr. Walter, do not become so upset. No one is talking to you; we are alone. This is part of your illness."

102 Mr. Walter has delusions that his food is poisoned and he refuses to eat. The nurse tells him that it is foolish for him to believe that, since his food comes from the same kitchen as for all other patients. The nurse states "Unless you eat, you will have to be fed by other means." This response indicated that:

1. Mr. Walter needed nourishment and therefore had to eat
2. Mr. Walter's misinterpretations had to be corrected
3. Mr. Walter had to be reminded about needing to eat
4. The nurse really did not know how to handle the situation

103 One evening the nurse finds Mr. Walter trying to leave the unit. He says, "Please let me go. I trust

you. The Mafia are going to kill me tonight.'' The nurse should respond:

1. ''Nobody here wants to harm you, you know that. I'll come with you to your room.''
2. ''Mr. Walter, you are frightened. Come with me to your room and we can talk about it.''
3. ''Thank you for trusting me, Mr. Walter. Maybe you can trust me when I tell you no one can kill you while you're here.''
4. ''Come with me to your room. I'll lock the door and no one will get to you to hurt you.''

104 In caring for Mr Walter, whose behavior is characterized by pathologic suspicion, one of the goals of nursing care should be to:

1. Help him realize suspicions are unrealistic
2. Remove as much environmental stress as possible
3. Help him to feel accepted
4. Ask him to explain the reasons for his feelings

105 The nurse has been observing Mr. Walter for some time. He is quite delusional, talking about people who are out to get him. Staff notices he is pacing more than usual. One afternoon the nurse decides that Mr. Walter is beginning to lose control of himself. The best nursing intervention would be to:

1. Allow him to use a punching bag
2. Move him to a quiet place on the unit
3. Allow him to continue pacing
4. Suggest that he sit down for a while

106 Mr. Walter is receiving large doses of chlorpromazine (Thorazine) and the nurse is concerned, since the phenothiazine derivatives produce a wide variety of untoward side effects. The presence of which side effect should signal the nurse to withhold the drug?

1. Masklike facies
2. Blurred vision
3. Edema
4. Jaundice

107 Mr. Walter tells the nurse that he used to believe that he was God, but now he knows that this is not true. The nurse's best response would be:

1. ''You really believed that?''
2. ''You must be getting well.''
3. ''What caused you to think you were God?''
4. ''Many people have this delusion.''

108 Mr. Walter is to be discharged with orders for chlorpromazine therapy. In developing a teaching plan for discharge the nurse should include cautioning Mr. Walter against:

1. Taking medications containing aspirin
2. Staying in the sun

3. Driving at night
4. Ingesting wines and cheeses

Situation: Mrs. Garvin, age 38, has cancer of the cervix. She is hospitalized for internal radiation therapy with radium. Questions 109 through 113 refer to this situation.

109 When Mrs. Garvin returns to her room, after the insertion of radium, the nurse should:

1. Immediately place her in a high Fowler position to prevent dislodging of the radium
2. Check her voiding and catheterize her if necessary, since a distended bladder can interrupt the path of radiation
3. Check that a low-residue diet has been ordered to prevent bowel movements and the possibility of dislodging the radium
4. Stay with her for half an hour to watch for symptoms of radiation sickness

110 Six months later Mrs. Garvin is readmitted for an abdominal hysterectomy. During her preoperative care she asks how the surgery will affect her periods. The nurse should respond:

1. ''Initially your periods will increase.''
2. ''You will no longer menstruate.''
3. ''Your monthly periods will be more regular.''
4. ''Your monthly periods will be lighter.''

111 Mrs. Garvin is admitted to the recovery room after surgery. Which of the following observations should be reported to the physician immediately?

1. Increased drainage from the Levin tube
2. Serosanguinous drainage on the perineal pad
3. Decreased urinary output
4. Apical pulse of 90

112 Abdominal distention develops in Mrs. Garvin. Which of the following measures would most likely provide immediate relief?

1. Restriction of oral intake and frequent change of position
2. Ambulation and carbonated drinks
3. Insertion of a rectal tube and application of heat to the abdomen
4. Nasogastric intubation and administration of cholinergic agents

113 Mrs. Garvin's physician has ordered that she wear a girdle while out of bed. The nurse should explain that this is to:

1. Prevent pooling of blood in the pelvic area
2. Increase wound healing
3. Prevent feelings of nausea
4. Support abdominal muscles

Situation: Virginia Wills, age 36, visits her gynecologist to confirm a suspected pregnancy. Questions 114 through 117 refer to this situation.

114 During the nursing history Mrs. Wills states that her last menstrual period began on April 11. She experienced some spotting on May 8. The nurse calculates Mrs. Wills' due date as:
1. January 10
2. January 18
3. February 12
4. February 15

115 Which change in the hematologic system is expected during the first trimester of pregnancy?
1. A decrease in sedimentation rate
2. An increase in blood volume
3. A decrease in WBCs
4. An increase in hematocrit

116 Mrs. Wills is concerned about Down's syndrome. An amniocentesis is performed during the sixteenth week of gestation. Examination of the amniotic fluid will also provide information regarding which of the following:
1. Fetal lung maturity
2. Cardiac anomalies
3. Development of anencephaly
4. Fetal diabetes

117 During the fifth month Mrs. Wills arrives for her appointment and begins to cry as she tells the nurse that her husband wants to have intercourse at least three times per week. The nurse's most appropriate response would be:
1. "Intercourse is permitted during your pregnancy."
2. "Have you talked with your husband about this?"
3. "I can see you're concerned; what's bothering you the most?"
4. "Have you and your husband spoken about this to the physician?"

Situation: George Brown, 4 years old, is admitted to the hospital with multiple bruises and a dislocated shoulder. Child abuse is suspected. Questions 118 through 120 refer to this situation.

118 In many states, failure by the nurse to report a suspected case of child abuse is punishable by law. Child abuse is one of the major causes of death in young children. When a child is admitted to the hospital with traumatic injuries, a common clue that the child was battered is that he:
1. Cries for longer periods and has large hematomas
2. Ignores offers of toys and favors and cries when picked up
3. Shows no expectation of being comforted
4. Does not cry during painful procedures

119 There are many common reactions of parents who batter their children. One reaction the nurse should be aware of is that the parents:
1. Seldom touch or look at the child
2. Show signs of guilt about the child's injury
3. Are quick to inquire about the discharge date
4. Are very concerned about their own physical health

120 Another behavior that is most typical of the parents of the battered child is that they:
1. Present many details related to how the trauma occurred
2. Show concern about the child's medical condition.
3. Become irritable about having the history taken
4. Give contradictory explanations about what happened

How to Use Worksheet 1: Errors in Processing Information

Common errors in processing information are listed in the left hand column of this worksheet. At the top of the worksheet is a row of blank spaces for inserting the number of the question missed. Directly below each number, check any errors you made in answering that question. You may have made more than one type of error in an answer.

Worksheet 1: Errors in Processing Information

Question no.																							
Did not read situation/question carefully																							
Missed important details																							
Confused major and minor points																							
Defined problem incorrectly																							
Could not remember terms/facts/concepts/ principles																							
Defined terms incorrectly																							
Focused on incomplete/incorrect data in assessing situation																							
Interpreted data incorrectly																							
Applied wrong concepts/principles in situation																							
Drew incorrect conclusions																							
Identified wrong goals																							
Identified priorities incorrectly																							
Carried out plan incorrectly/incompletely																							
Was unclear about criteria for evaluating success in achieving goals																							

How to Use Worksheet 2: Knowledge Gaps

Types of common knowledge gaps are listed along the top of this worksheet. Write a brief description of topics you want to review in the spaces provided. For example, if you missed a question on administration of a particular drug, write the drug name and problem (e.g., dosage) in the appropriate space under the column labeled Pharmacology.

Worksheet 2: Knowledge Gaps

Basic science	Skills/ procedures	Basic human needs	Growth & develop-ment	Normal nutrition	Psycho-social factors	Clinical area/ topic	Stressors/ coping mechanisms	Patho-physiology	Pharma-cology	Therapeutic nutrition	Legal implications	Other

Answers and Rationales

1. (2) A rapid delivery does not give the fetal head adequate time for molding, so pressure against the head is increased. (b); AN; CP; NU; OB
   (1) This is due to excessive pulling on the head and shoulders during delivery: certainly not incurred in precipitous delivery.
   (3) Likely to occur in footling breech delivery.
   (4) May occur with pull on the shoulders during delivery; not likely to occur with precipitous delivery.

2. (3) Lacerated tissue does not heal as quickly as a smooth, closely approximated surgical incision. (c); PL; AN; SH; OB
   (1) This is a routine postpartum intervention, not specific for patients with perineal lacerations.
   (2) The perineum at this time is too sore to be contracted as part of perineal exercise.
   (4) High protein would be acceptable, but high roughage would cause large stools and pain on defecation.

3. (3) Tears in the tentorial membrane cause bleeding into the cerebellum, pons, or medulla oblongata. The respiratory regulation centers are located in the medulla and pons. (c); AN; CP; NU; OB
   (1) Lethargy would be more indicative of cerebellar injury.
   (2) A weak timorous cry would be more indicative of cardiac or respiratory difficulty; a high-pitched shrill cry is usually present with CNS difficulty.
   (4) Purpura is unrelated to tentorial or other CNS injuries.

4. (1) The newborn's immature neuromuscular development normally causes dorsiflexion of the big toe and fanning of the remaining toes, a positive Babinski sign. (b); AN; CP; NU; OB
   (2) CNS damage from hypoxia can result in a negative Babinski sign, an abnormal finding in an infant.
   (3) Hyperreflexia is an abnormal increase in reflexes; a positive Babinski is a normal response in the infant.
   (4) A positive Babinski is a normal response in an infant; its absence may demonstrate neural impairment.

5. (2) Elevation of the head helps decrease intracranial pressure by gravity. (c); IM; AP; NU; OB
   (1) Frequent stimulation may cause further irritability to an already traumatized CNS.
   (3) This may be disturbing to the infant and impair his ability to rest.
   (4) This is done routinely on all neonates; not specific for this injury.

6. (3) Sitting down shows the patient that the nurse cares enough to spend time. It also opens up channels of communication. (a); IM; AP; SH; PS
   (1) The nurse sets dimensons on the mother's feelings; does not promote free expression of feelings.

(2) This statement ignores the mother's need to express feelings; takes a cognitive approach to the problem.
(4) This statement provides false hope; the diagnosis has been made.

7. (2) Braces are used to enable the spastic child to control motions. They also prevent deformities from poor alignment. (a); AN; CP; CL; PE
   (1) Since Jimmy is at the age when self-reliance is important (Erickson's stage of industry vs. inferiority) and dependent on his braces for self-care, it is unlikely that he would reject them.
   (3) Exercises are used to stretch ligaments and improve muscle strength and tone.
   (4) Early ambulation is promoted by maintaining muscle strength and tone.

8. (1) The choice of gait is based on the weight-bearing capabilities of each of the 4 extremities. (b); AS; CP; SH; PE
   (2) The cerebral palsied child uses upper extremity strength for crutch control and lower extremity strength to facilitate some movement.
   (3) Under normal circumstances orthostatic circulatory impairment is unlikely in the child with cerebral palsy.
   (4) Because of the decreased muscle control in CP, Jimmy will not likely be able to utilize a gait involving complete support of body weight off the floor.

9. (3) The 4-point alternate crutch gait is a simple, slow, but stable gait because there are always 3 points of support on the floor with equal but partial weight bearing on each limb. (b); AN; AN; SH; PE
   (1) The 4-point gait provides for 3 points of support.
   (2) A 4-point gait divides weight bearing equally among the limbs.
   (4) Jimmy has uncoordinated movement in the lower extremities because of the CP

10. (4) When sensory perceptions are impaired, with resultant lack of effective specific motor responses, an individual will be more vulnerable to skin irritation and trauma. (a); IM; AP; CL; PE
    (1) Jimmy's lack of sensation makes him more vulnerable to skin irritation from braces; observation of the skin takes priority in sensory loss.
    (2) Alignment of brace joints to body joints is important to facilitate joint mobility; observation of the skin takes priority in sensory loss.
    (3) A wide flat shoe will facilitate balance; observation of the skin takes priority in sensory loss.

11. (2) Many behaviors require a background of knowledge, skills, and attitudes (experiential readiness). If this background is not available, then more learning must take place before the individual can function. (c); AN; CP; SH; PE
    (1) Learning progress varies according to the individual; there are both progressive and regressive periods.
    (3) Although teaching may facilitate learning, other fac-

tors related to readiness for learning and willingness to learn affect whether learning occurs.

(4) Jimmy will be able to learn the 4-point gait without understanding normal walking.

12. (1) Patients whose thermoreceptive senses are impaired are unable to detect changes or degrees of temperature. They must be taught to test the temperature in any water-related activity to prevent scalding and burning. (a); IM; AP; CL; PE

(2) The cerebral palsied child normally has uncontrolled movement of voluntary muscles; makes it unnecessary to reposition on a schedule.

(3) Overtightening straps and buckles may lead to circulatory impairment and/or skin breakdown.

(4) After some practice, Jimmy will be able to place his legs in appropriate positions for walking without looking down.

13. (3) The damage is fixed. It does not become progressively greater. (c); AN; CP; NU; PE

(1) Cerebral palsy is a nonprogressive chronic condition.

(2) The etiology of cerebral palsy is related to anoxia in the prenatal, perinatal, or postnatal periods.

(4) Although mental retardation may be present in some children with CP, Jimmy cannot be assumed to be mentally retarded.

14. (4) Devices such as side rails can help patients increase their mobility by facilitating movement in bed. Side rails are an immovable object and provide a handhold for leverage when changing positions. (c); IM; AP; SH; ME

(1) The need to use side rails for safety must be evaluated for each individual based on his mental and physical status.

(2) The need to use side rails for safety must be evaluated for each inividual based on his mental and physical status.

(3) The need to use side rails for safety must be evaluated for each individual based on his mental and physical status.

15. (4) Explaining procedures and routines decreases the patient's anxiety about the unknown. (a); IM; AP; SH; PS

(1) Although therapeutic, this does not change the fact that the hospital environment is strange to her.

(2) The nurse should not confuse the role of professional with that of being a friend; the patient should be called Mrs. White unless she requests use of her first name.

(3) The nurse should not confuse the role of professional with that of being a friend; ''visiting'' has a social connotation.

16. (3) Patients and their families should be included in dietary teaching. (a); PL; AP; SH; ME

(1) The dietician is a resource person who can give specific information about diet and food preparation that is more practical once the patient has a basic understanding of the reasons for the diet.

(2) Foods high in sodium are not always salty tasting; this teaching is inadequate.

(4) The patient shoud be included in her own care; she will ultimately assume the responsibility.

17. (4) Processed foods generally have sodium (usually in the form of sodium chloride) added to enhance the taste and help preserve the food. (a); PL; AP; CL; ME

(1) Most fruits have a low sodium content.

(2) Most vegtables have a low sodium content; carrots and celery should be avoided.

(3) Although grain products contain sodium, the content is much less than in processed food.

18. (3) A lowered concentration of extracellular sodium brings about a decrease in the release of ADH. This leads to increased excretion of urine. (b); AN; CP; NU; ME

(1) Potassium is inefficiently retained by the body; an adequate intake of potassium is needed.

(2) The sodium restriction does not control the volume of food intake; weight is controlled by a low-calorie diet and by prevention of fluid retention.

(4) The resulting elimination of excess fluid reduces the workload of the heart but does not improve contractility.

19. (2) Fluid in the interstitial spaces impairs circulation, leading to poor absorption of drugs as well as predisposing to skin breakdown. (b); AN; CP; NU; ME

(1) The pain caused by injection is influenced by the type and volume of the drug, not the site.

(3) Interstitial fluid may leak from edematous tissue, but this is not the rationale for altering sites.

(4) The dilution of the drug does not significantly affect absorption.

20. (2) Range-of-motion exercises keep muscles in good tone and prevent venous statis through physical compresson of veins; such compression propels venous blood toward the heart, facilitated by venous one-way valves. (b); IM; AP; NU; ME

(1) Massage may dislodge a thrombus causing a fatal embolus.

(3) Fluids do not effect venous return and thus do not prevent thrombi.

(4) Application of elastic stockings is a dependent funtion.

21. (4) The wheelchair should be angled close to the bed so the patient will have to make only a simple pivot on the stronger leg. When the wheelchair is within the patient's visual field, the patient will be aware of the distance and direction that the body must navigate to transfer safely and avoid falling. (c); IM; CP; SH; SU

(1) If the patient's knees are flexed she may be unable to support her weight on her unaffected leg.

(2) Moving a patient back to bed in this situation would encompass moving against gravity.

(3) The large muscles of the legs rather than the arms should be used to prevent muscle strain.

22. (3) In crutch walking the patient uses the triceps, trapezius, and latissimus muscles. A patient who has been in bed may need to implement an exercise program to strengthen these shoulder and upper arm muscles before initiating crutch walking. (a); IM; AP; CL; ME
    (1) Back muscles are not used in crutch walking.
    (2) Keeping the leg in abduction alters the center of gravity which impedes ambulation.
    (4) This activty does not strengthen muscles used in crutch walking.

23. (3) When ambulating a patient, the nurse walks on the patient's stronger or unaffected side. This provides a wide base of support and therefore increases stability during the phase of ambulation that calls for weight-bearing on the affected side as the unaffected limb moves forward. (c); IM; AP; SH; ME
    (1) This tends to change the center of gravity from directly above the feet and may cause instability.
    (2) This tends to change the center of gravity from directly above the feet and may cause instability.
    (4) The nurse should stand on the patient's stronger or unaffected side (left side).

24. (4) An extended care facility would best meet the patient's convalescent needs, since a wide range of services beyond acute care are provided at a lower cost than hospital care. Its health services are more appropriate for this patient because they are greater than those provided in an adult facility but less than those provided in a nursing home. (a); PL; AN; CL; ME
    (1) This would be appropriate only if the patient were capable of some activities of daily living and did not require continuous supervision.
    (2) A nursing home provides skilled nursing care which this patient does not require.
    (3) Residents in an adult facility are generally responsible for their own activities of daily living.

25. (3) Preoperative skin preparation includes washing the operative site with an antiseptic agent several times to reduce the number of microorganisms on the skin. (c); PL; AN; SH; PS
    (1) Although the patient should be informed in advance of the care she is to expect, learning specific exercises would be impeded by high preoperative anxiety level.
    (2) It is impossible to ascertain how an individual will react to a situation that has not occurred; efforts should be made to establish a therapeutic relationship so that feelings can be ventilated.
    (4) The patient may not require a mastectomy; these arrangement are made postoperatively.

26. (3) Women facing breast surgery often have many feelings relating to their sexuality, change in body image, etc. The nurse plays a vital role in helping the patient to verbalize feelings and this response keeps channels of communication open. (a); IM; AN; SH; PS

(1) The patient's concerns are real and such a statement will only block further communication.
(2) This can be interpreted as the nurse's reluctance to listen; patient may not be able to talk with husband about this.
(4) Does not focus on the importance of the patient as an individual; each person feels differently.

27. (4) Postoperatively the arm on the operated side is elevated on pillows with the hand higher than the arm to prevent muscle strain and edema. (b); IM; AP; SH; SU
    (1) Although the arm is slightly abducted, sand bags are not utilized because complete immobility should be prevented.
    (2) This would impair venous return and increase edema.
    (3) Total immobilization should be avoided, and adduction may put undue pressure on the operative site.

28. (1) Postmastectomy exercises should be bilateral, using both arms simultaneously to prevent shortening of muscles and contracture of joints. (b); IM; AP; SH; SU
    (2) Both arms should be exercised to maintain symmetry of muscle tone and strength.
    (3) A sling immobilizes the arm creating joint stiffness and loss of muscle tone.
    (4) Exercises of the affected arm are usually started within 24 hours to prevent contractures and muscle atony.

29. (1) Chemotherapeutic agents are not specific for malignant cells. They generally interfere with protein synthesis and cell division in all rapidly dividing cells, including those regenerating traumatized tissue (as in wound healing), bone marrow, and cutaneous and alimentary tract epithelial tissue. (b); AN; CP; SH; SU
    (2) The muscles underlying the incision are not primarily involved in vomiting so the integrity of the area is not endangered.
    (3) Decreased RBC levels caused by bone marrow depression can be corrected with transfusions.
    (4) Chemotherapy would not increase edema.

30. (2) When there is increased pressure within the cranial cavity, the body adapts by increasing the blood pressure and decreasing the pulse. (c); EV; CP; NU; ME
    (1) Signs and symptoms reflect the part of brain upon which pressure is exerted, so that changes in behavior, judgment, consciousness and motor function may occur as well as autonomic changes, such as pupil size and reactivity, vital signs, and vomiting.
    (3) Signs and symptoms reflect the part of brain upon which pressure is exerted, so that changes in behavior, judgment, consciousness and motor function may occur as well as autonomic changes, such as pupil size and reactivity, vital signs, and vomiting.
    (4) Signs and symptoms reflect the part of brain upon

which pressure is exerted. Thus changes in behavior, judgment, consciousness, and motor function may occur as well as autonomic changes, such as pupil size and reactivity, vital signs, and vomiting.

31. (4) Rotating tourniquets are used to decrease venous return to the heart and would have no value in the treatment of increased intracranial pressure. (b); AN; AN; NU; ME
    (1) Osmotic diuretics such as mannitol may be used to draw fluid from the cerebral tissue into the vascular space to decrease cerebral edema and intracranial pressure.
    (2) Elevation of the head helps reduce edema because of gravitational force on the fluid.
    (3) Steroids inhibit the inflammatory response, preventing increased edema.

32. (3) If there is no obstruction, pressure on the jugular vein causes increased intracranial pressure. This, in turn, causes an increase in spinal fluid pressure. (b); AS; KN; NU; ME
    (1) Chvostek's sign is twitching elicited by tapping the angle of the jaw if hypocalcemia is present.
    (2) Romberg's sign is failure to maintain balance when the eyes are closed; indicates cerebellar pathology.
    (4) Homan's sign is calf pain elicited by dorsiflexion of the foot if thrombophlebitis is present.

33. (2) The cerebellum is involved in the synergistic control of muscle action. Below the level of consciousness it functions to produce smooth, steady, coordinated, and efficient movements. (b); AS; CP; NU; ME
    (1) The brain is not involved in a simple reflex arc.
    (3) The cerebrum is responsible for motor function.
    (4) The cerebrum is responsible for the level of consciousness.

34. (3) Because of cosmetic concerns, consent must be obtained before a patient's head may be shaved. (b); IM; AP; SH; SU
    (1) Usually unnecessary; the hair will be shaved to help prevent contamination of surgical site.
    (2) The patient will not be able to wear a wig until healing occurs; by this time the hair will begin to regrow.
    (4) Shaving is usually performed before the patient is taken to the surgical suite.

35. (3) Yellow drainage may be CSF and should be reported immediately. (a); AN; AN; NU; SU
    (1) Temperature evaluation must be accurate; axillary temperatures are influenced by environmental conditions and are lower than oral or rectal temperature.
    (2) Deep breathing expands the lungs and mobilizes secretions to prevent respiratory complications; secretions may be removed by suctioning to avoid increased intracranial pressure associated with coughing.
    (4) Administration of narcotics makes accurate neurologic assessment impossible; narcotics depress the central nervous system.

36. (2) Near term, most mothers are tired of the pregnant state and anxious for labor to begin. It is helpful to know that this is a common reaction. (c); IM; AP; SH; OB
    (1) The patient has just told the nurse what is bothering her; this response does not encourage the patient to discuss her feelings further.
    (3) Narrows the patient's verbalization to what the nurse sees as the patient's area of concern.
    (4) Does not encourage further verbalization, merely closes off communication.

37. (2) Preparation for parenthood classes should help couples develop realistic expectations of the laboring process, including associated discomfort and ways of dealing with it. (b); IM; AP; SH; OB
    (1) Untrue and unpredictable; contractions are uncomfortable, but childbirth preparation helps the patient cope with discomfort.
    (3) Patients are taught what to expect and the proper exercises to expedite labor.
    (4) There is no way of predicting whether medication will be needed; however, the patient should be assured of its availability.

38. (3) Tension in the woman prevents relaxation and has the greatest influence on how she will progress through labor and on her perception of pain. Tension is related to the expectation of pain, which is based on cultural norms and past experiences. (a); AN; CP; CL; OB
    (1) Although the difficulty of labor affects the amount of pain, it does not play a major role in the woman's perception of pain.
    (2) Although the woman frequently becomes more uncomfortable and tired near the end of labor, the length of labor does not play a major role in her perception of pain.
    (4) Parity does not play a major role in the woman's perception of pain.

39. (2) It is important to listen to the fetal heart rate (FHR) during contractions even though it may be difficult to hear. If the FHR slows during contraction and then resumes the normal rate within 30 seconds after acme, it is not serious. (c); EV; AP; NU; OB
    (1) Data are incomplete; during a contraction the FHR may be inaudible or slowed; should be retaken at the end of the contraction to see whether it remains decelerated.
    (2) The FHR should not be taken at the height of a contraction; wait until the contraction subsides to obtain the FHR.
    (4) Unless the FHR remains decelerated, there is no sign of hypoxia and oxygen is not necessary.

40. (1) In the advanced stage of labor the presenting part is low in the birth canal and may cause strong sensations of pressure on the rectum. (c); AN; CP; SH; OB
    (2) This may occur with persistent posterior pressure; usually not sudden and not a sign of advanced labor.

(3) Transitional or advanced labor begins when the cervix is 8 to 10 cm dilated.

(4) Restlessness and thrashing are generally not present in the early or middle phases of labor; begin during the transitional phase.

41. (3) Immediate action to prevent excessive bleeding is to massage the fundus until it is firm. This stimulates uterine muscle contraction. (a); IM; AP; NU; OB

(1) Not necessary unless bleeding persists after massaging of the uterus.

(2) The immediate action is to promote uterine contraction; obtaining the blood pressure would be indicated if a large amount of bleeding occurred or bleeding persisted.

(4) If the uterus does not contract after massage, the nurse should notify the physician; not just observe the bleeding.

42. (1) The tremendous visual impact of cleft lip on parents may significantly affect the parent-child attachment process and is often considered a reason for early surgical intervention. (c); AN; CP; SH; PE

(2) Feeding can be accomplished by use of special equipment; not an indication for early surgery by itself.

(3) Precautions may be taken to prevent ear and upper respiratory tract infections.

(4) The baby uses the mouth to facilitate breathing.

43. (4) An almost universal reaction to birth of an imperfect child is guilt. Encouraging the parents to discuss such feelings, without actually asking whether they feel guilty, allows them an opportunity to express such thoughts. (b); IM; AN; SH; PS

(1) This statement cuts off the parents' expression of feelings.

(2) This statement does not show recognition of the concern the parents are expressing.

(3) This statement lacks sensitivity in dealing with the parents' feelings.

44. (1) Cleft lip and palate demonstrate a familial pattern of inheritance that is significantly increased when a close relative is similarly affected. (b); AS; CP; SH; PE

(2) Mendelian laws of inheritance do not apply to these defects.

(3) The way the child responds to these defects is dependent on the parental response.

(4) The defects are hereditary; however, no exact pathogenesis has been found.

45. (1) Because the infant with a cleft lip and palate is unable to form the vacuum needed for sucking, a rubber-tipped syringe or dropper is used. This allows formula to flow along the sides and back of the mouth, minimizing the danger of aspiration. (a); AN; AN; SH; PE

(2) Feeding can be accomplished with the child in an upright position to facilitate swallowing and prevent choking; impaired sucking prevents breast-feeding in most situations.

(3) A soft crosscut nipple may be used with some infants but rapid flow can cause aspiration.

(4) Feeding can be accomplished with special equipment; IV feedings do not supply ample calories.

46. (3) Infants with cleft lip breathe through their mouth, bypassing the natural humidification provided by the nose. As a result, the mucous membranes become dry and cracked and are easily infected. (b); AN; AN; NU; PE

(1) Feeding can be adequate with special equipment and a slow approach.

(2) Circulation to the area is unimpaired.

(4) The area may be kept clean by washing with water after feeding.

47. (4) Although thrombophlebitis is suspected, prior to a definitive diagnosis the patient should be confined to bed so further complications will be avoided. (a); IM; AN; SH; OB

(1) Assessment of the leg may indicate thrombophlebitis; the patient should be put to bed.

(2) If a thrombus is present, massage may dislodge it and lead to pulmonary embolism.

(3) May cause extreme vasodilation, which would allow a thrombus to dislodge and circulate freely.

48. (2) After cleft lip repair, children are always placed supine or slightly on their side to prevent damage to the suture line. (b); IM; AP; NU; PE

(1) Swelling in or near the area traumatized by surgery is a complication that may occur postoperatively.

(3) For maximum healing and minimal scarring, a clean suture line is essential.

(4) Crying may disturb the suture line; the parents should be encouraged to hold the infant to reduce crying.

49. (3) Increased gluconeogenesis may lead to hyperglycemia and glycosuria, which can produce urinary frequency. Protein catabolism will cause muscle weakness (c); AS; AN; NU; ME

(1) These are symptoms of Addison's syndrome; in this case sodium and fluid retention leads to hypervolemia and hypertension.

(2) As sodium ions are retained, potassium is excreted; the result is hypokalemia. Edema occurs because of sodium retention.

(4) Muscle wasting results from increased protein catabolism; however, hyperglycemia rather than hypoglycemia will result from increased gluconeogenesis.

50. (1) Excess adrenocorticoids cause emotional lability, euphoria, and psychosis. (c); AS; CP; SH; ME

(2) Increased secretion of androgens result in hirsutism.

(3) As a result of tissue wasting and deamination, the extremities appear thin; but abnormal fat distribution and edema cause the development of a moon face, buffalo hump, and protruding abdomen.

(4) Capillary fragility results in multiple ecchymotic areas.

51. (2) Steroid therapy is usually instituted preoperatively and continued intraoperatively to prepare for the acute adrenal insufficiency that follows surgery. (b); IM; AP; NU; SU
    (1) Glucocorticoids must be administered preoperatively to prevent adrenal insufficiency during surgery.
    (3) The diet must supply ample protein and potassium; however, must be low in calories, carbohydrates, and sodium to promote weight loss and reduce fluid retention.
    (4) Urine is routinely tested for sugar and acetone, but 24-hour urine is unnecessary.
52. (4) Because of instability of the vascular system and the lability of circulating adrenal hormones after adrenalectomy, hypotension frequently occurs until the hormonal level is controlled by replacement therapy. (c); AS; CP; NU; SU
    (1) This is a sign of excessive adrenal hormones; after an adrenalectomy, adrenal hormones are not secreted.
    (2) This is a sign of hyperadrenalism; does not occur after the adrenals are removed.
    (3) This is an adaptation to excessive adrenal hormones; after an adrenalectomy, adrenal hormones are lowered until replacement therapy is regulated.
53. (3) Administration of adrenocortical hormones causes sodium retention by the kidneys. Dietary intake of salt must therefore be limited. (b); PL; AP; CL; SU
    (1) Since there is normally an increased secretion of glucocorticoids under stressful situations, dosage must be adjusted accordingly.
    (2) Insomnia is not an adverse effect of adrenocortical hormones.
    (4) Since pancreatic function is unimpaired, insulin therapy is not normally indicated.
54. (3) Patients with adrenocortical insufficiency who are receiving steroid therapy usually require increased amounts of medication during periods of stress, since they are unable to produce the excess needed by the body. (c); AN; CP; NU; SU
    (1) Although sedation may be prescribed, the major concern is the regulation of glucocorticoids in the presence of emotional or physiological stress.
    (2) Increased stress requires increased glucocorticoids.
    (4) Although these symptoms may occur and may be minimized by an increase in glucocorticoids, the primary reason for an adjustment in dosage is to assist the body's ability to adapt to stress.
55. (4) The 2-year-old child is extremely fearful of separation as well as intrusive procedures. If parents are present, they should be encouraged to stay and give comfort. (b); IM; AP; CL; PE
    (1) Two-year-olds are still dependent on their parents; the parent should be encouraged to participate in care.
    (2) Two-year-olds still depend on their parents for comfort and control.

(3) Mr. Jones may provide comfort to Alex during the procedure as well.
56. (3) If able to handle personal anxiety and give comfort to the child, parents can be a real help to the staff as well as the child. If the parents are extremely anxious, their anxiety can be transmitted, making the child even more anxious. (b); AN; CP; SH; PE
    (1) It is how the parents cope with the situation, rather than the situation itself, that helps determine how helpful their presence may be.
    (2) Two-year-olds are cognitively unable to make decisions of this nature.
    (4) Parents can be helpful to the child and the staff; they often want to participate in the child's care.
57. (3) Infants and small children have small buttocks with a very proximal sciatic nerve. (b); AN; CP; NU; PE
    (1) This age of children fears the procedure no matter what site is chosen.
    (2) Children properly restrained can be held still in this position.
    (4) Preschoolers tend to associate many treatments, and illness itself, with punishment.
58. (4) It is difficult to apply adequate pressure to this vascular site. Therefore observation for early signs of bleeding is imperative. (b); IM; AP; NU; PE
    (1) Fluids should be encouraged as soon as Alex tolerates them.
    (2) This simple procedure usually requires minimal or no IV fluid therapy.
    (3) Ice packs are not necessary.
59. (1) Patients with Cushing's syndrome or who are receiving cortical hormones must limit their intake of salt and increase their potassium intake. The kidneys are retaining sodium and excreting potassium. (b); IM; AN; CL; ME
    (2) Excessive secretion of adrenocortical hormones in Cushing's syndrome causes sodium retention; therefore sodium should be restricted.
    (3) Because of steroid therapy, excess sodium may be retained rather than excreted.
    (4) Although sodium retention causes fluid retention and weight gain, the need for increased potassium must also be considered.
60. (2) Excess glucocorticoids cause hyperglycemia. Signs of diabetes mellitus may develop. (c); AN; CP; NU; ME
    (1) Adrenocortical hormones cause sodium retention and subsequent weight gain.
    (3) Although muscle wasting is associated with excessive corticoid production, this will not cause diabetes mellitus.
    (4) ACTH affects the adrenal cortex, not the pancreas.
61. (4) Warm water will often relax the urinary sphincter, enabling a patient to void. (b); IM; AP; SH; SU
    (1) Since the bladder is already distended, increased fluid intake will only increase pressure and may result in hydronephrosis.

(2) The patient has already indicated that he was unable to void.

(3) Pressure over a distended bladder induces pain, which causes muscular contraction of the urinary sphincters.

62. (4) A suprapubic prostatectomy involves an abdominal incision to gain access to the prostate through the bladder. Postoperatively the patient has a suprapubic cystotomy tube to drain urine as well as a Foley catheter to limit bleeding, maintain patency, and drain urine. (b); PL; KN; NU; SU

(1) An incision is made into the lower abdomen; a ureteral catherter is not used.

(2) The ureters are not involved in this surgery.

(3) The kidneys are not involved in this surgery.

63. (1) Because of the vascularity of the involved tissue, hemorrhage and shock constitute the immediate postoperative danger after a prostatectomy. (a); AN; CP; NU; SU

(2) Impotence is a relatively rare complication.

(3) Incontinence is relatively rare; leakage of urine may occur for a few days after the Foley is removed due to sphincter trauma.

(4) Bladder spasms may occur but are not potentially life threatening; observing for hemorrhage is a priority.

64. (3) The catheter must be reinserted by the physician to ensure bladder emptying, maintain pressure at the operative site, and prevent hemorrhage. (a); IM; AP; NU; SU

(1) Irrigations require a physician's approval.

(2) Because of the danger of further trauma to the urethra and surgical site, the surgeon should insert the catheter.

(4) In addition to urinary drainage, the balloon of the urethral catheter exerts pressure against the prostate to help control bleeding and should be reinserted.

65. (4) After a suprapubic prostatectomy there is generally leakage of urine around the suprapubic tube, creating an environment in which bacteria can flourish if the dressing is not changed frequently. (b); PL; CP; NU; SU

(1) Uremia is caused by inadequate kidney function; not directly related to bladder infection.

(2) Negative pressure on the bladder may traumatize the delicate tissue; urine should flow by gravity.

(3) Clamping off the tube causes urinary stasis, which increases the risk of infection.

66. (3) Pain after a suprapubic prostatectomy may denote retention of urine as a result of blocked drainage tubes or infection, or it may be a normal response to surgery. The possibility of any complication must first be investigated. (a); EV; AP; NU; SU

(1) Analgesics can be administered after the cause of pain has been investigated; assessment should occur before implementation.

(2) The need for vital signs is dependent upon the an-

algesic ordered; assessing the cause of pain takes priority.

(4) Encouraging fluids without a patent drainage tube will increase pressure and discomfort; assessment should occur before implementation.

67. (3) Straining applies pressure to the operative site. (c); IM; AN; SH; SU

(1) A retention catheter is routinely in place.

(2) To prevent trauma, negative pressure should not be exerted on the bladder.

(4) A retention catheter is routinely in place.

68. (3) Superego development reflects the internalized norms of the family and society; the sociopath has never achieved this internalization. (b); AN; CP; NU; PS

(1) A person with this behavior has an overdeveloped need to seek pleasure.

(2) The ego is not balanced; the defect is in the superego.

(4) There may be a defect in sexual attitudes but not in sexual development.

69. (1) A sincere, cautious, and consistent attitude limits the sociopath's ability to manipulate both situations and staff members. (b); PL; AN; NU; PS

(2) An attitude such as this would allow Mr. Jay to rationalize his manipulative behavior to deal with the response he received.

(3) In accepting the person, the nurse should not support negative behavior; a friendly attitude may encourage further problem behavior.

(4) This would only encourage Mr. Jay to continue in his lifestyle rather than learn better ways to relate to his environment.

70. (4) Sets realistic limits on behavior without rejecting the patient. (b); IM; AP; SH; PS

(1) This would encourage further manipulation of the staff by Mr. Jay.

(2) This would be rejecting the person rather than the behavior.

(3) The other patient is entitled to a special time with the nurse; this is inconsistent limit setting on the part of the nurse.

71. (4) Helps the patient focus on feelings rather than just points out that current behavior is unacceptable. (b); IM; AP; SH; PS

(1) Points out the behavior in front of another patient.

(2) Give Mr. Jay an alibi for unacceptable behavior.

(3) The nurse is becoming defensive rather than dealing with the problem directly

72. (1) Accepts the patient while rejecting and setting limits on the behavior the patient is using. (b); IM; AP; SH; PS

(2) A confusing message is sent to the patient since it is unclear what the nurse did not like.

(3) A rejection of the patient instead of the behavior.

(4) Encourages this type of behavior instead of setting limits.

73. (2) Sets limits, points out reality, and places responsibility for behavior on the patient. (b); IM; AN; CL; PS
    (1) This is a punishing response and endangers the trust relationship.
    (3) People such as Mr. Jay need limits set; changing the time shows inconsistency.
    (4) The nurse using this response is showing inconsistency, endangering the trust relationship, and using a threat to gain control.

74. (2) Demonstrates the patient's acceptance of the professional role of the nurse as well as the ability to end dependent relationships. (b); EV; AN; CL; PS
    (1) Shows an inability to relate to other staff members involved with his care.
    (3) This still shows the existence of manipulation on his part.
    (4) Shows a childish need to punish the nurse for leaving.

75. (2) Intermittent positive pressure breathing (IPPB) is used to provide full expansion of the lungs, to loosen secretions, and to administer medication. (a); AN; CP; NU; SU
    (1) By improving the efficiency of respiration, IPPB should ultimately decrease the respiratory rate.
    (3) IPPB is used prophylactically before infection occurs.
    (4) Positive pressure forces air into the lungs; negative pressure or suction is not involved.

76. (3) As a result of chronic obstructive pulmonary disease, there is increased pressure in the pulmonary circulation. The right side of the heart hypertrophies (called cor pulmonale), and congestive heart failure may ensue. (b); AN; CP; NU; SU
    (1) This system is not as closely related to the pulmonary system as the cardiac system is; kidney problems do not usually occur.
    (2) Peripheral nerves are not as closely related to the pulmonary system as the cardiac system is; peripheral neuropathy does not occur.
    (4) The skeletal system is not truly related to the pulmonary system; joint inflammation does not occur.

77. (4) Productive coughing induced by IPPB can cause nausea and vomiting. (b); PL; CP; SH; ME
    (1) Upon awakening, mucus secretions are plentiful and tenacious; an IPPB treatment at this time would be most beneficial.
    (2) Approximately 1 hour before meals is a preferred time for IPPB; the resulting cough and mucus production will be less likely to affect dietary intake.
    (3) Since coughing must be encouraged after treatment, sleep is postponed; but as breathing is facilitated, sleep may then be more restful.

78. (2) The fluid level and time must be marked so the amount of drainage in a closed drainage system (e.g., with chest tubes) can be evaluated. (a); IM; AP; NU; SU
    (1) The catheter is secured by sutures and the dressing itself.

(3) The drainage system must be kept below chest level to promote drainage of the pleural space so the lung can expand.
(4) The amount of sterile water used to create a water seal depends on the drainage system used and is usually more than 3 to 5 ml; once the water seal is created, the nurse does not add additional water.

79. (3) Atmospheric pressure is greater than the pressure inside the pleural space. If a chest tube were not attached to underwater seal drainage, air would enter the pleural space and collapse the lung (pneumothorax). (b); AN; AP; NU; SU
    (1) The water seal does not affect the amount of suction used.
    (2) Capillarity is the tendency of cohesive liquid molecules to rise in a tube; not the purpose of water in a closed chest drainage system.
    (4) The concern is not primarily for pressure within the tube itself but to prevent atmospheric pressure from collapsing the lung.

80. (1) Turning and positioning prevent pooling of secretions in lungs as well as maximize lung expansion. (c); IM; AP; SH; SU
    (2) Cupping is a dependent nursing function.
    (3) Clapping is a dependent nursing function.
    (4) Postural drainage is a dependent nursing function.

81. (2) There are several modes for the administration of oxygen. Selection is based upon the disease and the patient's adaptations. (b); AN; CP; NU; ME
    (1) Although comfort may be one factor considered, selection depends on the therapeutic effect relative to the patient's disease and needs.
    (3) Although these will be taken into consideration, the ultimate decision is based on the pathologic condition and therapeutic needs.
    (4) Although consideration may be given to activity, selection is based on the pathologic condition and therapeutic needs.

82. (2) Oxygen can dry the mucous membranes of the respiratory tract and must be humidified for administration. Drying of mucous membranes can predispose to infection. (a); IM; CP; NU; ME
    (1) Padding is required because of irritation by some equipment; not related to the untoward effects of oxygen therapy.
    (3) Although vital signs should be assessed so the effect of treatment can be evaluated, an apical pulse is not necessary.
    (4) The orthopneic position promotes lung expansion and is often used in conjunction with oxygen therapy; not an untoward effect.

83. (2) Any arrhythmia should be documented by an ECG strip. Frequent PVCs indicate ventricular irritability, which may progress to ventricular filbrillation requiring emergency precordial shock. (c); IM; AN; NU; ME
    (1) Ventricular irritability rather than neural stimuli is

responsible for PVCs; adjusting the rate of lidocaine hydrochloride (Xylocaine) would be based on established protocol, once documentation had been made (normal IV infusion is 1 to 4 mg/min).

(3) Digoxin (Lanoxin) is not used to control ventricular arrhythmias; PVCs may indicate digitalis toxicity.

(4) Lanoxin is not used to control ventricular arrhythmias; PVCs may indicate digitalis toxicity.

84. (4) The T wave is the period of repolarization of the ventricles. Stimulation of the ventricles during this vulnerable period often causes ventricular fibrillation. (c); AN; KN; NU; ME

(1) The P wave represents atrial contraction.

(2) The PR interval represents transmission of impulses from the SA to the AV node.

(3) The R wave represents initiation of ventricular contraction.

85. (1) A defibrillator delivers a massive electric charge to the myocardium, simultaneously depolarizing and then throwing into refraction all heart regions. Rhythmic contractions resulting from SA node depolarization may then restore normal heart action. The defibrillating current reaches the heart from the body surface through the electric conductivity of the body fluids, which contain many ions. (b); AN; KN; NU; ME

(2) Base elements do not affect electrical activity.

(3) A colloidally dispersed medium does not affect electrical activity.

(4) Body fluid is not similar to pure water.

86. (1) Dopamine hydrochloride acts on beta$_1$ receptors of the heart (which increase heart contractility, elevating cardiac output) and on alpha adrenergic receptors (which constrict arterioles, increasing the blood pressure). (c); AN; CP; NU; ME

(2) It dilates the renal vasculature.

(3) It affects alpha adrenergic receptors in the arterioles.

(4) Not an action of dopamine.

87. (2) Because of potential hypertension from arteriolar constriction, administration of dopamine hydrochloride (Intropin) must be monitored carefully. The flow rate must be exact, and an infusion control device should be used as a safeguard to prevent inaccurate infusion rates. (b); IM; CP; NU; ME

(1) The infusion rate is based on continuous assessment of blood pressure; does not significantly irritate the vein

(3) Although extravasation causes necrosis, an infusion control device will not prevent infiltration; flowrates must be accurate, and an infusion control device helps.

(4) Overdosage may cause vasoconstriction, resulting in hypertension.

88. (2) Knowing that nausea and vomiting are possible signs of digitalis toxicity, the nurse should withhold the drug and call the physician. (c); IM; AN; NU; ME

(1) Digoxin (Lanoxin) should not be administered until digitalis toxicity has been ruled out; antacids may reduce the absorption of digitalis.

(3) Lanoxin should not be administered until digitalis toxicity has been ruled out; antacids may reduce the absorption of digitalis.

(4) Lanoxin should not be administered until digitalis toxicity has been ruled out; antacids may reduce the absorption of digitalis.

89. (2) After a myocardial infarction it generally takes 6 to 8 weeks for replacement of necrotic tissue by scar tissue. (c); IM; KN; SH; ME

(1) Healing of myocardial tissue does not occur in such a short time.

(3) This is too long a time; scar tissue usually replaces myocardial tissue by 8 weeks.

(4) Myocardial tissue destruction is usually replaced by scar tissue in 8 weeks; collateral circulation is generally well established by this time.

90. (2) Procainamide hydrochloride (Pronestyl) is rapidly absorbed from the GI tract and excreted in the urine. To maintain a therapeutic blood level, it must be taken at prescribed intervals. (b); IM; CP; CL; ME

(1) Has little effect on cardiac output; however, may cause tachycardia because of anticholinergic effect.

(3) Since the aim is to maintain a certain blood level, the intervals between administration should be considered rather than the Pronestyl taken only with increased activity.

(4) The drug may be administered with meals to prevent GI upset.

91. (2) Fetal death usually occurs in diabetic mothers after 36 weeks of gestation. It results from acidosis and placental dysfunction. The fetus may be delivered by cesarean section or induction as necessary. (c); AN; KN; NU; OB

(1) Exercise and ambulation are needed to promote adequate circulation and prevent thromboembolism.

(3) Fetal growth continues as long as placental functioning is still intact.

(4) This is not a routine procedure; insulin is administered according to the patient's needs.

92. (1) Usually, as pregnancy progresses, there are alterations in glucose tolerance and in the metabolism and utilization of insulin. The result is an increased need for exogenous insulin. (a); PL; CP; NU; OB

(2) Estrogenic hormones are not administered during pregnancy.

(3) Caloric intake is increased to meet demands of the growing fetus.

(4) Pancreatic enzymes or hormones other than insulin are not affected by pregnancy.

93. (3) The effects of insulin on the fetus are known since the fetal pancreas secretes insulin. However, the effects of oral hypoglycemics are not well known; such agents may be teratogenic. (b); AN; CP; SH; OB

(1) The fetal pancreas does not compensate for the mother's diabetes but hypertrophies because of increased insulin secretion to cover increased circulating glucose.

(2) Hypoglycemics are not insulin; also they may have a teratogenic effect on the fetus.

(4) There is often a need for larger amounts of insulin in the latter part of pregnancy.

94. (4) Feeding difficulties are due to hypoglycemic effects on the fetal CNS. (c); AS; AP; NU; OB

(1) Excessive birthweight is common but does not indicate hypoglycemia.

(2) May be related to hypoxia not lowered blood sugar.

(3) May be related to prematurity; generally not related to hypoglycemia.

95. (4) The infant of a diabetic mother is a newborn at risk because of the interplay between the maternal disease and the developing fetus. (b); IM; AP; NU; OB

(1) The baby may be prone to hypoglycemia and will need increased glucose.

(2) Infants of diabetic mothers are high risk and are admitted to intensive care nurseries.

(3) Babies are generally hypoglycemic because of oversecretion of insulin by their hypertrophied pancreas.

96. (2) When the intestine cannot be returned to the body cavity, the hernia is incarcerated. (c); AN; CP; NU; SU

(1) This is a strangulated hernia.

(3) Erosion of intestinal tissue may be caused by a variety of conditions; usually results in perforation.

(4) This is a volvulus.

97. (3) A possible complication of hernias is intestinal obstruction. If an obstruction occurs, there will be no passage of flatus or normal bowel movements. (b); IM; AP; SH; SU

(1) The supine position would have no effect on an incarcerated hernia.

(2) This is done for all patients; not specific for a patient with a hernia. Observation of signs of intestinal obstruction takes priority.

(4) This would not assist in the definitive diagnosis of a hernia and its complications.

98. (4) Hernioplasty involves not only the reduction of a hernia but also an attempt to change or strengthen the structure to prevent recurrence. (b); AN; KN; NU; SU

(1) Herniorrhaphy is surgical repair of a hernia.

(2) Analysis of the word shows that it means an opening cut into the hernia; does not refer to repair of a hernia.

(3) There is no such word; hernias are not cut out. They are reduced and/or reinforced to prevent recurrence.

99. (1) After inguinal hernia repair, the scrotum frequently becomes edematous and painful. Drainage is facilitated by elevating the scrotum on a rolled towel or using a scrotal support. (c); IM; AP; SH; SU

(2) Obesity is a factor in the development of hernias; high-carbohydrate diets should not be encouraged.

(3) Coughing increases intraabdominal pressure and may strain the operative site.

(4) An abdominal binder would not support the operative site; the incision is too low.

100. (3) Placing the feet apart creates a wider base of support and brings the center of gravity closer to the ground. This improves stability. (b); IM; CP; CL; SU

(1) Bending at the waist should be avoided; strains the lower back muscles.

(2) Pressure on the abdomen is prevented by tightening the abdominal and gluteal muscles to form an internal girdle; keeping the body straight does not reduce strain on the abdominal musculature.

(4) Relaxing the abdominal muscles with physical activity increases strain on the abdomen.

101. (1) This response demonstrates an understanding of the patient's feelings and encourages the patient to share feelings, which is an immediate need at the moment. (b); IM; AP; SH; PS

(2) This would have the effect of only increasing the fears.

(3) The nurse is entering into the hallucination, thereby reinforcing it.

(4) This response argues with the patient, making him defensive and reinforcing the hallucination.

102. (4) You cannot argue a patient out of a delusion. Statements made by the nurse show a lack of knowledge and constitute a threat, which is a form of assault. (c); EV; AN; NU, PS

(1) Everyone needs nourishment, but threats accomplish little.

(2) A person cannot be argued out of a delusion.

(3) There is no indication that he needed a reminder to eat.

103. (2) This response recognizes the patient's feelings and provides assurance that the staff member will stay with him. (a); IM; AP; SH; PS

(1) Mr. Walter does not know this; if he did, he would not have a delusion.

(3) The patient is not ready to accept this; he really believes he is going to be killed.

(4) Locking the patient in a room by himself will only increase the fear and delusion.

104. (3) Delusions are protective and can be abandoned only when the individual feels secure and adequate. This response is the only one directed at building the patient's security and reducing anxiety. (b); AN; AP; SH; PS

(1) This would be a nursing action to help him develop trust; the goal is to have trust.

(2) This is helpful more in regard to hallucinations than delusions.

(4) He is unable to explain the reason for his feelings.

105. (2) Patients losing control feel frightened and threatened. They need external controls and a reduction in external stimuli. (b); IM; AP; NU; PS

(1) This is helpful for pent-up aggressive behavior but not for agitation associated with delusions.

(3) He may get completely out of control if he is allowed to continue pacing.

(4) He would be unable, at this time, to sit in one place; his agitation is building.

106. (4) Jaundice signifies liver cell damage, a side effect of the phenothiazine drugs, which can be irreversible and life threatening. The nurse should immediately stop the medication if this side effect is noted. (b); EV; CP; NU; PS

(1) A reversible side effect with treatments using benztropine mesylate (Cogentin) or diphenhydramine (Benadryl).

(2) A common anticholinergic effect that will pass.

(3) Not a known side effect.

107. (2) This response supports reality and self-awareness while helping the patient to look to the future rather than focus on the past. (c); IM; AP; SH; PS

(1) May be taken as ridicule of the patient; focuses on the past.

(3) What made him have this delusion is unimportant at the moment; still focuses on the past.

(4) This may or may not be so; the statement dismisses an opportunity for validating how he feels at the present time.

108. (2) The phenothiazine drugs cause photosensitivity. Severe burning can occur on exposure to the sun. (b); PL; CP; CL; PS

(1) No contraindication with aspirin.

(3) No known side effect that would affect night driving.

(4) This would be true if the patient were taking a MAO inhibitor.

109. (3) Patients with internal radiation for cervical cancer are given low residue diets and often medications to suppress peristalsis and prevent pressure from bowel movements. (c); IM; AN; NU; ME

(1) The head of the bed can be only slightly elevated to prevent the implant from being dislodged by gravity.

(2) A catheter is routinely inserted to prevent bladder distention and possible radiation damage or alteration of implant position.

(4) Since the patient is the source of radiation, the nurse must limit the time spent with her to avoid excessive exposure.

110. (2) A total abdominal hysterectomy in the premenopausal woman produces artificial onset of menopause. (a); IM; CP; SH; SU

(1) Untrue; because the uterus was removed, there will be no uterine endometrial proliferation and no desquamation.

(3) Untrue; because the uterus was removed, there will be no uterine endometrial proliferation and no desquamation.

(4) Untrue; because the uterus was removed, there will

be no uterine endometrial proliferation and no desquamation.

111. (3) Accidental ligation of a ureter is a serious complication of a total abdominal hysterectomy. A decrease in urine output should be reported immediately to the surgeon. (c); AS; CP; NU; SU

(1) A nasogastric tube is not routinely inserted.

(2) Serosanguineous vaginal drainage is to be expected.

(4) An apical rate of 90 falls within normal limits but should be evaluated in relation to the patient's previous vital signs.

112. (3) Abdominal distention, caused by retention of flatus, is a frequent postoperative problem. A rectal tube will usually accomplish expulsion of flatus in 20 to 30 minutes. Application of heat, in addition to its vasodilating effect, will relax tensed muscles. (b); IM; AP; SH; SU

(1) Although position changes may promote peristalsis, restriction of oral intake will not.

(2) Carbonated drinks increase flatulence.

(4) Distention usually occurs as a result of flatus in the intestines and would not be alleviated by gastric decompression.

113. (4) Postoperatively a patient may wear a girdle to provide abdominal support and/or do exercises to strengthen the abdominal muscles. (a); IM; CP; SH; SU

(1) Constriction may actually impair venous return if not fitted accurately.

(2) Since pressure is being applied to the incision, healing is not directly facilitated.

(3) Abdominal binders do not prevent nausea; may actually induce it if applied too tightly.

114. (2) Using Naegele's rule, subtract 3 months and add 7 days to the first day of the last menstrual period, April 11. (b); AN; CP; SH; OB

(1) To have an EDC of January 10, Mrs. Wills' last menstrual period would have been April 3.

(3) To have an EDC of February 12, Mrs. Wills' last menstrual period would have begun on May 5.

(4) Even though Mrs. Wills had some spotting on May 8, her last normal menstrual period was April 11.

115. (2) Blood volume increases by approximately 50% during pregnancy. Peak blood volume occurs between 30 and 34 weeks of gestation. (b); AN; CP; NU; OB

(1) The sedimentation rate increases because of a decrease in plasma proteins.

(3) White blood cell values remain stable during the antepartum period.

(4) The hematocrit decreases as a result of hemodilution.

116. (1) Fetal lung maturity can be estimated by the L/S ratio (lecithins:sphingomyelins) in the amniotic fluid. (c); AS; CP; SH; OB

(2) Cardiac disorders cannot be detected.

(3) Anencephaly can be only suspected.

(4) Fetal diabetes cannot be detected.

117. (3) This response shows empathy and gives the patient an opportunity to ventilate her feelings. (b); IM; AP; SH; OB

(1) Closes off any opportunity for real discussion.

(2) Important question but may close off communication between the nurse and patient.

(4) Ignores the patient's feelings; focuses on the husband's desires.

118. (3) Children who have been abused quickly learn that attention-seeking behavior such as crying for comforting provokes more abuse. Therefore they learn to accept the battering silently. (c); AS; AN; SH; PE

(1) Battered children seldom cry.

(2) Battered children rarely cry; tend to seek the approval of strangers.

(4) This may or may not be true.

119. (1) Typically, abusing parents have difficulty showing concern for their child. They are unable to comfort him, such as through touch, and give little indication of realizing how he feels. (b); AS; AN; SH; PE

(2) Rather than guilt, battering parents tend to feel angry at the child for the injury.

(3) Battering parents rarely show concern about the child's care or progress.

(4) This is not particularly a characteristic reaction of abusive parents.

120. (4) In an attempt to block the hospital staff from discovering what happened, abusing parents frequently provide inconsistent accounts. (c); AS; AN; SH; PE

(1) Battering parents tend to be vague about the details of the accident but maintain the child injured himself.

(2) Battering parents tend to show more concern about how the child's condition affects them than about how the child is affected.

(3) This may or may not occur.

Comprehensive Test 4

To simulate the comprehensive licensing examinations, this test should be completed within 2 hours

Situation: Mr. Wilson, a 57-year-old man with a history of myocardial infarction, is admitted to the hospital for a hemorrhoidectomy. Question 1 through 3 refer to this situation.

1 The nurse should expect Mr. Wilson's preoperative diet to be:
   1. High protein
   2. Low residue
   3. Bland
   4. Clear liquid

2 Mr. Wilson is in pain on the second postoperative day. A method usually ordered to relieve pain, which the nurse uses, is:
   1. A medicated suppository
   2. Water-soluble jelly
   3. Sitz baths
   4. Ice packs

3 Mr. Wilson is having his first postoperative bowel movement. When cleaning the anus, Mr. Wilson should be instructed to use:
   1. Moist cotton swabs
   2. Betadine pads
   3. Sterile 4 × 4–inch gauze pads
   4. Soft facial tissue

Situation: Roy Brown, an 18-month-old boy, is admitted to the hospital with an upper respiratory tract infection. It is his first hospitalization and prolonged separation from his mother. Questions 4 through 9 refer to this situation.

4 Based on this information, the nurse may expect to see which type of behavior during the initial admission?
   1. Generally crying when people enter the room, but does respond with a smile after a few minutes
   2. Crying relentlessly, consoled by no one except his mother or father
   3. Withdrawn, sitting quietly, not interested in playing
   4. Initially unhappy and crying, but contented after meeting his roommates

5 After a prolonged period of hospitalization, Roy becomes depressed, withdrawn, and apathetic to-

ward his mother. Eventually, he begins playing with toys and relating to others, even strangers. The nurse should realize that he has:

1. Accepted his hospitalization well and has matured because of this experience
2. Grown out of the stage of separation and realizes that he has to depend on others
3. Probably become somewhat detached because of this traumatic separation
4. Finally recognized that the staff is not out to hurt him

6 Studies of young children institutionalized for some time indicate that they show signs of retarded development. Not all aspects of development are equally affected. The nurse should be aware that the least affected is:

1. Neuromuscular development
2. Hearing
3. Ability to understand
4. Ability to express himself

7 The major depriving factor in long-term hospitalization of which the nurse should be aware is usually the:

1. Absence of interaction with a mother figure
2. Lack of multisensory inputs
3. Care provided only by a mother substitute
4. Lack of play objects

8 The nurse should be aware that studies of histories of children who have suffered prolonged maternal deprivation early in life indicate that these children:

1. Are unable to love
2. Establish warm relationships with a mother substitute
3. Recall past experiences vividly
4. Are particularly conscious of time

9 When Roy's mother is getting ready to take him home, she asks the nurse what kind of behavior she should expect Roy to display. The nurse informs her that Roy will probably be:

1. Hostile toward her
2. Making excessive demands on both parents
3. Cheerful but have a shallow attachment to all adults
4. Apathetic and withdrawn from all emotional ties to her

Situation: John and Mary June are a young married couple. He is 24 and has a history of colitis; she is 21. John is the first of his family to attend college. Mary is supporting the family by working as a keypunch operator at a large insurance company. They have decided to postpone starting a family until John finishes his education in 2 years. Mary has therefore been taking oral contracep-

tives since shortly before the marriage. She has always had a regular menstrual cycle. Understandably then she is concerned when she misses her regular menstrual period. After 3 weeks pass she decides to go to a physician for a check-up. She tells the nurse interviewing her that she suspected she might be pregnant because she missed taking her contraceptive pills for more than a week when she had the flu. Questions 10 through 24 refer to this situation.

10 Concerning the patient's statement about her possible pregnancy, the best response for the nurse to make is:

1. "Contraceptive pills are very unpredictable anyhow. You probably would have become pregnant even if you had taken them regularly as prescribed."
2. "You may well be correct; one of the reasons for prescribing an exact schedule is that the effect of contraceptive drugs depends on the regularity with which they are taken."
3. "Don't think about that now. It's too late to worry anyhow. First find out whether you really are pregnant. If you are, you may want to consider having an abortion."
4. "That's the trouble with using contraceptive pills. People become too careless and don't use proper restraint. If you had used the rhythm method, this probably would not have happened."

11 While Mrs. June is being prepared for the examination, she complains of feeling very tired and being sick to her stomach, particularly in the morning. The best response for the nurse to make is:

1. "This is a common occurrence during the early part of pregnancy and you need not worry.
2. "This is a common occurrence due to all the changes going on in your body."
3. "These are common occurrences. You say your sick feelings bother you most often in the morning?"
4. "Perhaps you might discuss this with the doctor when he arrives."

12 Mrs June asks, "Is it true the doctor will do an internal examination today?" The nurse should answer:

1. "Yes, an internal is done on all mothers on the first visit."
2. "Yes, an internal is done on all mothers, but it is only sligtly uncomfortable."
3. "Are you fearful of having an internal examination done?"
4. "Yes, he will; have you ever had an internal examaination done before?"

13 Mrs June asks when she may expect her baby. She states that her last menstrual period was April 14. Her expected date of delivery most likely is:
1. December 21
2. January 7
3. January 21
4. February 1

14 Mrs. June is concerned because she had read that nutrition during pregnancy is important for proper growth and development of the baby. She wants to know something about the foods she should be eating. The nurse should proceed by:
1. Giving her a list of foods to refer to in planning meals
2. Asking her what she usually eats at each meal
3. Emphasizing the importance of limiting salt and highly seasoned foods
4. Instructing her to continue eating a normal diet

15 Mrs. June's work as a keypunch operator would necessarily have implications for her plan of care during pregnancy. The nurse should recommend that Mrs. June:
1. Ask for time in the morning and afternoon to elevate her legs
2. Tell her employer she cannot work beyond the second trimester
3. Ask for time in the morning and afternoon to obtain nourishment
4. Try to walk about every few hours during the workday

16 Since Mrs. June is a primigravida, she should be told to come to the hospital when:
1. Contractions are 2 to 3 minutes apart and she cannot walk about
2. Contractions are 10 to 15 minutes apart
3. She has a bloody show and back pressure
4. Membranes rupture or contractions are 5 to 8 minutes apart

17 During the examination the nurse asks Mrs. June if she would like to listen to her baby's heartbeat. She is delighted and after listening comments on how rapid it is. She appears frightened and asks if this is normal. The nurse should respond:
1. "The baby's heart rate is usually twice the mother's pulse rate."
2. "The baby's heartbeat is rapid to accommodate the nutritional needs."
3. "The baby's heart rate is normally rapid, so you needn't worry."
4. "It is far better that the heart rate is rapid; when it is slow, there is need to worry."

18 Mrs. June spontaneously delivers a 2953.6 g (6 lb 8 oz) baby daughter. Although Mr. June expresses

delight, he appears anxious and tends to avoid physical contact with the baby. One evening he says to the nurse, "My wife seems so wrapped up with the baby, I hope she has time for me when she gets home." The nurse should respond by saying:
1. "Do you think your parents will be able to help out, Mr. June?"
2. "I can understand your concern about the changes you'll have to make."
3. "You seem to feel you'll have to fend for yourself."
4. "You'll both be so busy you won't even miss her attention."

19 When the baby is 2 months old, Mr. June, pale, thin, and dehydrated, is admitted to the hospital with an exacerbation of colitis. He is placed on a residue-free, bland, high-protein diet, and vitamins B, C, and K parenterally. An IV solution containing electrolytes is also started. The type of person who most frequently develops ulcerative colitis is:
1. Hard driving and immature
2. Sensitive and dependent
3. Quick tempered and hostile
4. Unassuming and secure

20 The nurse administers vitamins parenterally because:
1. More rapid action results
2. They are ineffective orally
3. They decrease colon irritability
4. Intestinal absorption may be inadequate

21 Mr. June is to receive 2000 ml of IV fluid in 12 hours. The drop factor is 10 gtt/1 ml. The nurse should regulate the flow so the number of drops per minute is approximately:
1. 27 to 29
2. 30 to 32
3. 40 to 42
4. 48 to 50

22 Which of these food combinations should be included on his residue-free diet?
1. Lean roast beef, buttered white rice with egg slices, white bread with butter and jelly, tea with sugar
2. Creamed soup and crackers, omlet, mashed potatoes, bran muffin, orange juice, coffee
3. Stewed chicken, baked potato with butter, strained peas, white bread, plain cake, milk
4. Baked fish, macaroni with cheese, strained carrots, fruit gelatin, milk

23 Mr. June's diet is designed to reduce:
1. Gastric acidity
2. Colonic irritation

3. Electrolyte depletion
4. Intestinal absorption

24 In addition, the nurse encourages a high-protein diet to:
1. Correct anemia
2. Slow peristalsis
3. Improve muscle tone
4. Repair tissues

Situation: Mrs. O'Hanlon, a childless widow, born in Ireland, is employed as a cook in the sandwich shop of the local department store. She has been an outpatient in the medical clinic for 6 months, under treatment for diabetes and hypertension. Her regimen includes tolbutamide (Orinase), a low-sodium, diabetic diet, and reserpine (Serpasil) b.i.d. On the occasion of a regular visit her urine sample shows sugar 3+ and a trace of acetone. Questions 25 through 37 refer to this situation.

25 The nurse interviewing Mrs. O'Hanlon would be most concerned to find out about any changes in her:
1. Eating habits
2. Blood pressure
3. Weight range
4. Serum glucose

26 In discussing the patient's present metabolic state, the nurse should mention that people taking oral antidiabetic agents:
1. Should not work where food is readily accessible
2. Consciously or unconsciously may tend to relax dietary rules
3. Are not as threatened by their disease as those taking insulin
4. Need not be concerned about serious complications

27 Mrs. O'Hanlon tells the nurse that she cannot eat big meals and prefers to snack throughout the day. The nurse should carefully explain that:
1. Small, frequent meals are better for digestion
2. Large meals can contribute to a weight problem
3. Salt and sugar restriction is her main concern
4. Regulated food intake is basic to her control

28 When promoting affective learning (developing attitudes), the nurse must first consider the influence of the:
1. Patient's pesonal resources
2. Type of onset of the disease
3. Physical and emotional stress of the situation
4. Patient's past experiences

29 Mrs. O'Hanlon complains that she finds the low-salt food very tasteless. The nurse's best response is:
1. "Salt can be very harmful to your health."

2. "I know how difficult it is for you."
3. "You miss your ham and cabbage?"
4. "Ask the doctor if you can splurge occasionally."

30 Mrs. O'Hanlon is scheduled to have a serum glucose test the following morning. To ensure accuracy in the result, the nurse should instruct her to:
1. Take her regular dose of tolbutamide
2. Abstain from food and fluid
3. Have clear fluids for breakfast
4. Eat her usual diet

31 Mrs. O'Hanlon has a cough. She tells the nurse that she takes Robitussin (glyceryl guaiacolate) cough syrup about every 2 hours when she has a cold. The nurse should tell her that she:
1. May take the cough syrup if her urine test remains negative
2. Must calculate the sugar in her daily carbohydrate allowance
3. Can substitute an elixir for the syrup
4. Can increase her fluid intake and humidify her bedroom to control the cough

32 Mrs. O'Hanlon complains of difficulty seeing at night. The nurse knows this frequently occurs in diabetes because of:
1. Poor glucose supply to rods and cones
2. Lack of glucose in the retina
3. The effect of ketones on retinal metabolism
4. Atherosclerotic changes in blood vessels within the eyes

33 Mrs. O'Hanlon is admitted to the hospital with a cerebral vascular accident. Three weeks later she still has left-sided paresis but is able to ambulate fairly well with a cane. She is very frustrated and angry because of her expressive aphasia. The nurse anticipates she will have difficulty with:
1. Following specific instructions
2. Recognizing words for familiar objects
3. Speaking and/or writing
4. Understanding speech and/or writing

34 Mrs. O'Hanlon gets frustrated and upset when she tries to communicate with the nurse. To help alleviate this frustration the nurse should:
1. Face the patient and raise her voice so Mrs. O'Hanlon can see and hear her better
2. Limit Mrs O'Hanlon's contact with other patients to limit the frustration
3. Anticipate Mrs. O'Hanlon's needs so she does not have to ask for help
4. Gives Mrs O'Hanlon plenty of time to speak and respond so she does not have to formulate a response under pressure

35 Although Mrs. O'Hanlon has regained control of her bowel movements, she is still incontinent of urine. To help her reestablish bladder function, the nurse should encourage her to:
1. Assume her normal position for voiding
2. Void every 4 hours and attempt to hold urine between set times
3. Drink a minimum of 4000 ml of fluid equally divided among the hours she is awake
4. Attempt to void more frequently in the afternoon than in the morning

36 Mrs. O'Hanlon is using a cane specifically to:
1. Prevent further injury to weakened muscles
2. Maintain balance and improve stability
3. Relieve pressure on weight-bearing joints
4. Aid in controlling involuntary muscle movements

37 When teaching Mrs. O'Hanlon to ambulate with a cane, the nurse should instruct her to:
1. Hold it in the hand on the same side as the affected lower extremity
2. Lean the body toward the cane when ambulating
3. Advance the cane and the affected extremity simultaneously
4. Shorten the stride of the unaffected extremity

Situation: Mrs. Lobinski, a 52-year-old Polish woman, is admitted for diagnostic evaluation for arteriosclerotic heart disease. In the year since her husband's death she has lived with her son and daughter-in-law. Currently she is not physically distressed but is apprehensive and alienated. Questions 38 through 48 refer to this situation.

38 Nursing care that may help Mrs. Lobinski to feel more at ease includes:
1. Telling her that everything is all right
2. Giving her a copy of hospital regulations
3. Reassuring her that staff will be available if she becomes upset
4. Orienting her to the environment and unit personnel

39 In understanding Mrs. Lobinski's diagnosis, the nurse knows that atherosclerosis is:
1. A loss of elasticity in and thickening and hardening of the arteries
2. Development of atheromas within the myocardium
3. A mobilization of free fatty acid from adipose tissue
4. Development of fatty deposits within the intima of the arteries

40 The nurse's initial approach to creating a therapeutic environment for Mrs. Lobinski should give priority to:
1. Accepting her individuality
2. Promoting her independence
3. Providing for her safety
4. Explaining everything that is being done for her

41 On one occasion after her family has been visiting, the patient is angry and says to the nurse, "My daughter-in-law says they can't take me home until the doctor lets me go. She doesn't understand; she isn't Polish." The nurse should best:
1. Ignore the statement for the present
2. State, "The physician makes decisions about discharge."
3. Reflect on the patient's feelings about the present situation
4. State, "You feel she doesn't want you home."

42 Mrs. Lobinski is placed on nitroglycerine therapy for angina. In administering nitroglycerine the nurse should:
1. Make certain the medication is stored in a dark container
2. Discontinue the medication if the patient complains of a headache
3. Limit the number of tablets to 4 daily
4. Replace the tablets if the patient complains of a sublingual tingling sensation

43 Mrs Lobinski demonstrates an increasing lability of mood and forgetfulness. She becomes disoriented to both time and place. A diagnosis of Alzheimer's disease is made. The nurse knows that Alzheimer's disease is characterized by:
1. Slowly progressive deficits in intellect, which may not be noted for a long time
2. Transient ischemic attacks
3. Remissions and exacerbations
4. Rapid deterioration of mental functioning because of arteriosclerosis

44 Mrs. Lobinski frequently switches from being pleasant and happy to being hostile and sad without apparent external cause. The nurse can best care for Mrs. Lobinski by:
1. Avoiding her when she is angry and sad
2. Attempting to give nursing care when she is in a pleasant mood
3. Encouraging her to talk about her feelings
4. Trying to point out reality to her

45 The nurse should provide Mrs. Lobinski with an environment that is:
1. Challenging
2. Nonstimulating

3. Variable
4. Familiar

46 It is important for a team working with patients who have a diagnosis of organic mental disorder to adapt a common approach of care because the patients need to:
1. Learn that the staff cannot be manipulatd
2. Relate in a consistent manner to staff
3. Accept external controls that are fairly applied
4. Have sameness and consistency in their environment

47 Patients who have an organic mental disorder need assistance in maintaining contact with society for as long as possible. Which one of the following groups might help Mrs. Lobinski achieve this goal?
1. Psychodrama
2. Recreation therapy
3. Remotivation therapy
4. Occupational therapy

48 The objective of remotivational therapy in psychiatry is to stimulate:
1. Face-to-face contact with other patients
2. Diminished psychologic faculties
3. Interaction with environment
4. Participation in educational activities

Situation: Melanie, a 21-year-old heroin addict, delivers a 2268 g (5 lb) baby boy. On the third day after delivery she leaves the hospital because the person caring for her 3-year-old Mary can no longer do this. She assures the staff she can care for both Mary and Baby Jesse. Questions 49 through 57 refer to this situation.

49 The nurse administers vitamin K intramuscularly to Jesse immediately after birth to:
1. Prevent increased levels of serum bilirubin
2. Promote the synthesis of prothrombin
3. Substitute for normal bacterial flora
4. Decrease calciferol until renal clearance can take over

50 Typical signs of drug dependence in babies are due to withdrawal and usually begin within 24 hours after birth. The nurse should observe for:
1. Prolonged periods of sleep
2. Hyperactivity
3. Dehydration and constipation
4. Hypotonicity of muscles

51 Nursing care of Jesse should include:
1. Increasing environmental stimuli
2. Reducing elevated body temperature
3. Offering small frequent feedings
4. Administering methadone

52 When preparing Melanie prior to her discharge the nurse should:

1. Keep Melanie and the baby separated until Melanie is drug free
2. Refer Melanie to a drug rehabilitation program
3. Support Melanie's positive maternal responses
4. Help Melanie understand that Jesse's problems are due to her drug intake

53 Two weeks after Melanie and Baby Jesse are discharged, 3-year-old Mary is admitted with second- and third-degree burns over 30% of her body. She is placed in a warm isolation room with a humidifier, and strict sterile technique is instituted. The physician orders a Foley cather to be inserted and IV therapy to begin immediately. One nurse is asigned to care for Mary each shift for the first 48 hours. Nursing observations in the first 48 hours of hospitalization are directed primarily toward preventing:
1. Pneumonia
2. Contractures
3. Dehydration
4. Shock

54 Despite Mary's physical distress and discomfort, her weight must be accurately taken because it provides a:
1. Baseline for future growth
2. Measure of the burned surface area
3. Basis for fluid replacment and medications
4. Guideline for dietary and fluid management

55 On the second day of hospitalization Mary has decreased urinary output with edema. The nurse, recognizing this as one sign of possible complications that commonly occur in the first 2 days, should watch for other signs of complications, which are:
1. Vomiting, bradycardia
2. Subnormal temperature, slow pulse
3. High fever, disorientation
4. Rapid pulse, low blood pressure

56 The nurse must accurately measure Mary's urinary output each hour to evaluate kidney function. The minimum safe output of urine per hour is:
1. 10 to 20 ml
2. 25 to 50 ml
3. 40 to 60 ml
4. 75 to 100 ml

57 As Mary's burns begin to heal, the nurse attempts to involve her in therapeutic play to give her the opportunity to:
1. Learn to accept the hospital situation
2. Know the other children on the unit
3. Forget the reality of the situation for a while
4. Work out ways of coping with her fears

Situation: Mrs. Felton is admitted after an argument with her daughter, during which she incurred a sucking stab wound of the left thorax. Questions 58 through 72 refer to this situation.

58 In the emergency room the nurse should position Mrs. Felton:
   1. On her back with her feet elevated
   2. On her left side with head elevated
   3. In a high Fowler position with her left side supported
   4. On her right side flat in bed with a pillow supporting her left arm

59 When assessing Mrs. Felton the nurse should be concerned primarily with the:
   1. Quality and depth of respirations
   2. Blood pressure and pupillary response
   3. Amount of serosanguineous drainage
   4. Degree and level of pain

60 Mrs. Felton has a large pressure dressing over the stab wound. The nurse recognizes that the purpose of this dressing is to:
   1. Seal off major vessels
   2. Prevent additional contamination
   3. Protect the pleura
   4. Maintain negative intrathoracic pressure

61 Twenty-four hour IV fluids are ordered for Mrs. Felton. The fluid orders read: Bottle 1: 1000 ml 5% D/W; bottle 2: 1000 ml 5% D/0.9% NaCl; bottle 3: 1000 ml 5% D/0.33% NaCl. What is the approximate flow rate in drops per minute (IV tubing = 20 gtt/ml)?
   1. 22
   2. 27
   3. 36
   4. 42

62 The nurse should encourage Mrs. Felton to perform deep breathing exercises. The reason for this is that deep breathing exercises help to:
   1. Counteract respiratory acidosis
   2. Expand the residual volume
   3. Increase blood volume
   4. Decrease partial pressure of oxygen

63 Mrs. Felton has chest tubes attached to a Pleurevac suction. When caring for Mrs. Felton, the nurse should:
   1. Change the dressing daily using aseptic technique
   2. Palpate the surrounding area for crepitus
   3. Empty the drainage bottles at the end of the shift
   4. Clamp the chest tubes when suctioning the patient

64 Mrs. Felton complains of severe pain 2 days following surgical repair of the wound. Initially the nurse should:

   1. Have the patient rest
   2. Take vital signs
   3. Administer p.r.n. analgesic
   4. Check time of patient's last medication

65 Arlene Felton, the 23-year-old daughter of Mrs. Felton, is arrested and is admitted to the psychiatric service for observation. On admission she has delusions of persecution and auditory hallucinations. The nurse greets Ms. Felton by saying "Good evening, Arlene. How are you?" Ms. Felton answers, "Arlene is bad." This is an example of:
   1. Dissociation
   2. Reaction formation
   3. Displacement
   4. Transference

66 Which of the following factors is most important in planning care for a confused or delusional patient such as Arlene?
   1. Maintain quiet, dim surroundings to minimize stimuli
   2. Encourage realistic activity considering the patient's ability
   3. Recognize she is completely unable to differentiate fantasy from reality
   4. Provide physical hygiene and comfort to demonstrate she's worthy of receiving care

67 That evening Arlene appears quite upset. As the nurse approaches, Arlene states, "I am hearing voices that are saying bad things about me." The nurse should:
   1. Tell her she does not hear the voices
   2. Encourage her not to listen to what the voices are saying
   3. Suggest she join other patients playing cards
   4. Let her know the staff understands she is frightened and stay with her

68 One day the nurse and Arlene sit together and draw. Arlene draws a face with horns on top of the head and says, "This is Arlene. She is a devil." The nurse should respond:
   1. "Arlene, you are not a devil. Don't talk about yourself like that."
   2. "Let's go to the mirror, Arlene, and see what you look like."
   3. "Arlene, when I look at you, I see a young woman not a devil."
   4. "I don't see a devil. Why do you see a devil?"

69 Arlene is receiving a major tranquilizer b.i.d. Two thirds of the daily dose is given in the evening, one third in the morning. This is done to:
   1. Help her sleep at night
   2. Reduce sedation during the daytime

3. Maintain diurnal rhythms

4. Reduce increased assaultiveness in the evening

70 After 2 weeks of drug therapy the nurse notices that Arlene has become jaundiced, but she continues to give the tranquilizers until the psychiatrist can be consulted. In situations such as this:

1. Jaundice is sufficient reason to discontinue the tranquilizers

2. The psychiatrist's order for tranquilizers should be reduced by the nurse

3. Jaundice is a benign side effect and has little significance

4. The blood level of tranquilizers must be maintained once established

71 Arlene describes her delusions to the nurse. The nurse should:

1. Change the topic as soon as she begins to discuss her delusions

2. Encourage Arlene to discuss her delusions

3. Get Arlene involved in a repetitive project

4. Accept this as Arlene's reality without argument

72 After a couple of weeks in the hospital the nurse notices Arlene's hair is dirty and asks if she would like to wash it. Arlene answers, "Yes and I'd like to set it, too." The nurse uses this information to assess that Arlene:

1. Has some feelings of self-worth

2. Has a need for social reassurance and approval

3. Is quite open to suggestions

4. May be entering a hyperactive phase

Situation: Eight-year-old Kim is admitted to the hospital for the first time with a diagnosis of diabetes. Questions 73 through 77 refer to this situation.

73 Juvenile (Type I) diabetes:

1. Has a more rapid onset than adult diabetes

2. Occurs more often in obese children

3. Does not always require insulin

4. Involves early vascular changes

74 The nurse plans to include the entire family in Kim's care and is especially concerned that:

1. The parents receive immediate instruction about urine testing

2. Kim is taught to give injections before being discharged

3. The parents and child be helped to understand their feelings about diabetes

4. Kim's activity be limited and the parents understand the need for this

75 The physician orders 12 units of NPH insulin daily for Kim. The vial reads 1 ml = 40 units of NPH.

The nurse does not have an insulin syringe so, using a regular syringe, gives:

1. 6 minims

2. 4.5 minims

3. 4 minims

4. 3.5 minims

76 A night feeding planned for a juvenile diabetic includes milk, crackers, and cheese. This will provide:

1. High-carbohydrate nourishment for immediate utilization

2. Nourishment with latent effect to counteract late insulin activity

3. Encouragement for the child to stay on a diet

4. Added calories to help the child gain weight

77 Before Kim goes home, the nurse reviews with the family the importance of their knowing that Kim's insulin needs will be decreased when:

1. There is an emotional upset

2. An infectious process is present

3. She reaches puberty

4. She participates in active exercise

Situation: Mrs. Donira is a 29-year-old obstetric patient with a history of 3 spontaneous abortions. Questions 78 through 85 refer to this situation.

78 Mrs. Donira is being observed in the high-risk clinic and has expressed anxiety about remaining at home during this pregnancy. The nurse should question Mrs. Donira to determine her knowledge of the:

1. Signs and symptoms of impending labor

2. Causes of spontaneous abortion

3. Mechanisms of early labor

4. Interrelationship between rest, normal delivery, and diet

79 Mrs. Donira complains of heartburn. When counseling her, the nurse explains that during pregnancy:

1. The pyloric sphincter relaxes and acid is regurgitated

2. The cardiac sphincter relaxes and acid is regurgitated

3. Gastric acidity and motility are increased

4. There is increased gastric motility, which causes acid to be regurgitated

80 When involved in prenatal teaching, the nurse should also inform the patient that an increase in vaginal secretions during pregnancy is called leukorrhea and is caused by increased:

1. Metabolic rate

2. Functioning of the Bartholin glands
3. Production of estrogen
4. Supply of sodium chloride to the cells of the vagina

81 Mrs. Donira is trying to decide whether she should breast-feed or bottle-feed her expected baby. She asks the nurse what advantage breast-feeding has over bottle-feeding. The nurse replies that one major group of substances in human milk that are of special importance to the newborn and cannot be redproduced in any bottle formula is:
1. Gamma globulins
2. Complex carbohydrates
3. Amino acids
4. Essential ions (electrolytes)

82 During labor Mrs. Donira states that she does not want "eyedrops or ointment" placed in her baby's eyes immediately after delivery. Which of the following is the most appropriate response by the nurse?
1. "Mrs. Wills, they are required and should be administered right after delivery."
2. "Mrs. Wills, the medication protects the infant, and that's why it's used."
3. "Mrs. Wills, is there a reason why you don't want the medication instilled?"
4. "Mrs. Wills, you'll have to check with your doctor regarding this."

83 During labor Mrs. Donira receives continuous caudal anesthesia. When she has a sudden episode of severe nausea and her skin becomes pale and clammy, the nurse's immediate reaction is to:
1. Notify the physician
2. Elevate the patient's legs
3. Monitor the fetal heart rate every 3 minutes
4. Check for vaginal bleeding

84 During delivery the physician performs an episiotomy. The nurse explains to Mrs. Donira that this is most commonly done to:
1. Prevent lacerations during birth
2. Limit postpartal discomfort
3. Stretch the perineum
4. Reduce trauma to the fetus

85 Mrs. Donira delivers a normal baby boy. When assessing the newborn's respiratory status, the nurse should expect respirations to be:
1. Shallow and thoracic
2. Deep and retracting
3. Abdominal and irregular
4. Stertorous and regular

Situation: *Mrs. Ryan, 82 years of age, is hard of hearing and has severe painful rheumatoid arthritis. She was admitted to a nursing home when she became incontinent and her family could no longer care for her. Questions 86 through 91 refer to this situation.*

86 Mrs. Ryan's condition indicates that a primary consideration in her care should be her need for:
1. Immobilization of joints
2. Bladder control reeducation
3. Control of pain
4. Motivation and teaching

87 The nurse should be aware that the drug of choice in rheumatoid arthritis is:
1. Methocarbamol (Robaxin)
2. Aspirin
3. Cortisone
4. Gold salts

88 As to bed position, the nurse should encourage Mrs. Ryan to:
1. Assume a position that is most comfortable
2. Place pillows beneath her knees
3. Assume the Fowler position
4. Maintain the limbs in extension

89 Since Mrs. Ryan's admission to the nursing home she has not been incontinent. While discussing her past and present elimination patterns the patient told the nurse of her anger at being bedridden and inability to go anywhere or see anyone. The nurse deduced that the patient's incontinence at home was:
1. An unconscious expression of hostility
2. A method to determine her family's love for her
3. A physiologic response expected with the elderly
4. A way of maintaining control

90 When caring for Mrs. Ryan, the nurse should:
1. Frequently ask if she needs the bedpan to void
2. Create an environment that prevents sensory monotony
3. Limit her fluid intake in the evening
4. Provide television or radio when the patient is alone

91 Mrs. Ryan uses an air-conduction hearing aid. This increases hearing sensitivity in instances of:
1. Diminished sensitivity of the cochlea
2. Perforation of the tympanic membrane
3. Immobilization of the auditory ossicles
4. Destruction of the auditory nerve

Situation: *Mrs. Cole brings her son Johnny to the emergency room with severe gastrointestinal distress symptoms. Johnny is a normal infant who weighed 7.2 kg (16 lb) on his 6-month checkup last week. Questions 92 through 98 refer to this situation.*

92 The nurse immediately prepares for:
1. Type and cross match
2. Intestinal intubation with continuous suction
3. Placement in an Isolette
4. Insertion of an IV line

93 Johnny is admitted to the hospital. The most important clinical manifestation of the degree of dehydration would be:
1. Sunken fontanel
2. Weight loss
3 Decreased urine output
4. Dry skin

94 When observing Johnny's laboratory reports, the nurse should be especially concerned about a decrease in sodium and:
1. Potassium
2. Chlorides
3. Calcium
4. Phosphates

95 Johnny is receiving parenteral therapy. His IV orders are 400 ml of 5% D/W to run in 8 hours. How many drops per minute should the IV run? (A minidropper is not available, so the nurse selects an IV set with a drop factor of 20 gtt per milliliter)
1. 10 to 11 drops
2. 14 to 15 drops
3. 16 to 17 drops
4. 18 to 19 drops

96 Johnny may be given liquids in small amounts. Which of the following liquids would be most beneficial for the nurse to give?
1. Cranberry juice
2. Liquefied gelatin
3. Ginger ale
4. Skim milk

97 An essential nursing action when caring for the small child with severe diarrhea is to:
1. Force fluids orally
2. Take daily weights
3. Replace lost calories
4. Keep body temperature below 37.7° C (100° F)

98 Johnny improves, and prior to discharge the nurse discusses Johnny's diet with Mrs. Cole. Mrs. Cole asks when Johnny should be able to drink from a cup. The nurse responds:
1. Five months
2. Seven months
3. Twelve months
4. Eighteen months

Situation: Mrs. Palecek, a 33-year-old housewife, is admitted to the hospital with a diagnosis of acute cholecystitis, biliary colic, and possible obstructive jaundice. She has a history of a bipolar-type affective disorder, which is currently under control. Questions 99 through 110 refer to this situation.

99 In addition to pain in the right upper quadrant, what other manifestations should the nurse expect Mrs. Palecek to have?
1 Intolerance of foods high in lipids
2. Vomiting of coffee-ground emesis
3. Gnawing pain when the stomach is empty
4. Melena and diarrhea

100 A cholecystectomy is scheduled. Vitamin K is administered to Mrs. Palecek prior to surgery, since it is used in the formation of:
1. Bilirubin
2. Prothrombin
3. Thromboplastin
4. Cholecystokinin

101 After surgery Mrs. Palecek is transferred to the recovery room with a nasogastric tube in place. She vomits 30 ml of bile-colored fluid. The nurse should:
1 Administer an antiemetic
2. Check the patency of the tube
3. Elevate the head of the bed
4. Encourage the patient to breathe deeply

102 Once Mrs. Palecek is returned to her unit, the nurse continues to make frequent checks of the wound area to note any tendencies toward excess bleeding or hemorrhage. These observations are made because:
1. Diaphragmatic excursion places pressure on the suture line
2. Mrs. Palecek's temperature is slightly elevated
3. Blood clotting may be hindered by lack of vitamin K absorption
4. Mrs. Palecek is complaining of much pain

103 Mrs. Palecek is prone to upper respiratory tract complications because of the:
1. Proximity of the incision to the diaphragm
2. Length of time required for surgery
3. Lowered resistance caused by bile in the blood
4. Transfer of bacteria from the biliary tract to the blood

104 Three days after the cholecystectomy Mrs. Palecek begins a full fluid diet. When the breakfast tray arrives, it has whole milk and cream for cereal. The luncheon tray includes whole milk and ice cream. When the surgeon visits at lunchtime, he notes the tray's contents and, disturbed that the

diet is not low in fat, takes the tray away. In situations such as this the:
1. Dietitian should check the diet that the patient receives
2. Physician orders the diet, and the order should be carried out as written
3. Nurse shares responsibility, since the physician's order was not questioned
4. Patient should have followed the physician's directions

105 When Mrs. Palecek is ready to be discharged, the dietitian instructs her to remain on her prescribed diet for several more weeks, Afterward she asks her nurse, ''Will I have to stay away from fat for the rest of my life?'' Which of the following responses would be most appropriate?
1. ''You'll have to remain on a fat-free diet from now on to avoid problems.''
2. ''It's too early to say. Later, when we see whether your operation is successful, we'll know the answer.''
3. ''Only the doctor can answer that. Why don't you ask him about it before your discharge from the hospital?''
4. ''After you have fully recovered from surgery, you'll probably be able to eat a normal diet, avoiding excessive fat.''

106 Six months later Mrs. Palecek is readmitted to the hospital. She has been eating and sleeping very little and has charged hundreds of dollars worth of purchases to her husband. The symptoms that the nurse should expect Mrs. Palecek to exhibit in the hospital would include:
1. Decreased psychomotor activity
2. Increased interest in the environment
3. Depressed mood and crying
4. Increased insight into her behavior

107 In view of Mrs. Palecek's elated state, the nurse should arrange for her to be in a room:
1. That will provide a great deal of stimuli
2. With as little furniture as possible
3. With a patient scheduled for a cholecystectomy
4. With another patient who is very quiet

108 Mrs. Palecek becomes loud and insulting and says to a staff member, ''Get lost you old buzzard!'' The nurse should say:
1. ''Now, Mrs. Palecek, he isn't an old buzzard.''
2. ''Don't be so rude, Mrs. Palecek, it isn't necessary.''
3. ''Here is something I feel you might be interested in, Mrs. Palecek.''
4. ''Could you tell me why you are angry, Mrs. Palecek?''

109 Mrs. Palecek leaves group therapy in the middle of the session. She is obviously upset and crying when she meets the nurse. She tells the nurse that the group's discussion is too much for her. The most therapeutic nursing action would be to:
1. Suggest kindly but firmly that she return to the group to work out the conflict
2. Suggest that she accompany you to her room so that the two of you can talk about it
3. Respect her right to decline therapy at this time and simply report the incident to the rest of the health team
4. Ask the group leader what happened in the group and base your intervention on this additional information

110 Mrs. Palecek is to receive lithium carbonate. Which of the following studies should the nurse ensure is done prior to drug administration?
1. Neurologic studies
2. Fluid and electrolye studies
3. Enzyme studies
4. Renal studies

Situation: *Mrs. Wallace is a 22-year-old primigravida who is 6½ months pregnant. Questions 111 through 116 refer to this situation.*

111 When she is seen by the physician Mrs. Wallace's blood pressure is 135/85 and she has gained 2.27 kg (5 lb) in the last 2 weeks. The nurse should:
1. Give Mrs. Wallace an appointment for 2 weeks hence
2. Prepare Mrs. Wallace for a vaginal examination
3. Take Mrs. Wallace's temperature and pulse
4. Prepare the equipment for testing Mrs. Wallace's urine

112 Preeclampsia is first suspected in a pregnant woman when there is:
1. An excessive weight gain
2. Fluctuation of the blood pressure
3. Progressive ankle edema
4. Presence of albuminuria

113 Mrs. Wallace has been diagnosed as having preeclampsia. When counseling Mrs. Wallace, the nurse instructs her to follow a diet that includes:
1. Normal sodium with ample calories and protein
2. High sodium and calories and low protein
3. Moderate sodium, low calories, and ample protein
4. Low sodium and calories and high protein

114 Mrs. Wallace is receiving magnesium sulfate (MgSO$_4$) 10 mg IM, every 4 hours. The nurse

should check which of the following before giving the drug?
1. Respirations and patellar reflex
2. Blood pressure and apical pulse
3. Urinary output equal to fluid intake
4. Temperature and pulse rate

115 When giving MgSO₄ IM, the nurse should:
1. Add 1% normal saline to maximize the dispersion of the drug
2. Add 1% procaine to minimize the pain caused by the drug
3. Use a large-gauge needle to expedite the dispersion of the drug
4. Give the injection in the outer aspect of the thigh

116 In severe preeclampsia, changes in blood values include an elevation of the hematocrit. This results from:
1. Hemodilution of pregnancy caused by increases in blood volume
2. Vasodilation caused by an alteration in circulating fluid
3. Agglutination of red cells caused by membrane fragility
4. Hemoconcentration caused by a decrease in plasma volume

Situation: Sallie Gerraghty, a 36-year-old primigravida with a history of endometriosis, is admitted to labor and delivery. Her husband accompanies her as her labor coach. A fetal monitor is being used. Questions 117 through 120 refer to this situation

117 When caring for Sallie while her fetus is being monitored, the nurse must realize that:
1. The machinery can be very frightening to the laboring couple
2. The mother may need a mild sedative every 4 hours for comfort
3. Internal monitoring is usually employed when severe complications are suspected
4. Older primigravidas have more complications than younger women

118 Sallie, who has been successfully treated for endometriosis, completes this much-desired pregnancy with the delivery of a 4082.4 g (9 pound) baby girl. During the pregnancy the symptoms caused by endometriosis were alleviated. Sallie expresses concern that her symptoms will return now that the pregnancy is over. Which response by the nurse is most appropriate?
1. "A hysterectomy will be necessary if the symptoms recur."
2. "Breast-feeding your baby will delay the return of menstruation."
3. "Pregnancy usually cures the endometriosis."
4. "Endometriosis will usually cause an early menopause."

119 Four hours after delivery Sallie still has not voided. The nurse's initial action should be to:
1. Encourage voiding by placing Sallie on a bedpan frequently.
2. Inform the physician of Sallie's inability to void and await orders
3. Palpate Sallie's subrapubic area for distention
4. Place Sallie's hands in warm water to encourage micturition

120 The public health nurse visits Sallie at home for the first time. She is breast-feeding her infant and complains that her breasts are swollen and painful. In teaching her about breast-feeding, the nurse can give what information to assist her in preventing engorgement in the future?
1. "Feed the baby 4 times a day. This will prevent rapid filling of the breast."
2. "Use a bottle for feeding when you are experiencing discomfort."
3. "Nurse the baby frequently and for at least 10 minutes on each breast."
4. "Limit nursing to 4 to 6 minutes on each breast, 4 times a day."

How to Use Worksheet 1: Errors in Processing Information

Common errors in processing information are listed in the left hand column of this worksheet. At the top of the worksheet is a row of blank spaces for inserting the number of the question missed. Directly below each number, check any errors you made in answering that question. You may have made more than one type of error in an answer.

Worksheet 1: Errors in Processing Information

Question no.																								
Did not read situation/question carefully																								
Missed important details																								
Confused major and minor points																								
Defined problem incorrectly																								
Could not remember terms/facts/concepts/ principles																								
Defined terms incorrectly																								
Focused on incomplete/incorrect data in assessing situation																								
Interpreted data incorrectly																								
Applied wrong concepts/principles in situation																								
Drew incorrect conclusions																								
Identified wrong goals																								
Identified priorities incorrectly																								
Carried out plan incorrectly/incompletely																								
Was unclear about criteria for evaluating success in achieving goals																								

How to Use Worksheet 2: Knowledge Gaps

Types of common knowledge gaps are listed along the top of this worksheet. Write a brief description of topics you want to review in the spaces provided. For example, if you missed a question on administration of a particular drug, write the drug name and problem (e.g., dosage) in the appropriate space under the column labeled Pharmacology.

Worksheet 2: Knowledge Gaps

Basic science	Skills/ procedures	Basic human needs	Growth & develop- ment	Normal nutrition	Psycho- social factors	Clinical area/ topic	Stressors/ coping mechanisms	Patho- physiology	Pharma- cology	Therapeutic nutrition	Legal implications	Other

Answers and Rationales

1. (2) A low-residue diet limits stool formation. (a); PL; CP; SH; SU
   (1) A high-protein diet is indicated postoperatively to promote healing.
   (3) Bland diets are usually employed in the management of upper, not lower, GI disturbances.
   (4) Although a clear diet is low in residue, it does not meet normal nutritional needs; a poor nutritional status increases the risk of postoperative complications.

2. (3) Sitz baths provide moist heat, which dilates the blood vessels and promotes circulation. It also relieves local inflammation and itching. (b); IM; AP; SH; SU
   (1) Medicated suppositories are used preoperatively but not after surgery because of the possibility of causing bleeding.
   (2) This would not alleviate pain.
   (4) Ice may alleviate pain; but it also causes vasoconstriction, which can impair healing.

3. (1) Moist cotton is not irritating and is the most soothing to the anal mucosa. (b); IM; AP; CL; SU
   (2) Betadine may cause excessive drying and irritation; the rectum is normally contaminated; external cleansing with Betadine will not appreciably affect the bacteria present.
   (3) Sterile gauze pads are not needed; the rectal area is considered contaminated.
   (4) Moist cotton is softer and more effective in removing feces than is dry facial tissue, which is irritating and can cause trauma.

4. (2) The first phase of separation anxiety is protest, which is characterized by loud crying, rejection of all strangers, and inconsolable grief. (a); AS; AP; SH; PE
   (1) An 18-month-old is not so easily consoled when separated from parents.
   (3) This would be indicative of despair, a more advanced stage of separation anxiety.
   (4) Toddlers do not socialize well with peers.

5. (3) The child has progressed to the third phase, detachment, in which he resigns himself to the loss of his mother and superficially appears adjusted to his environment. (c); AN; AP; NU; PE
   (1) This is often the mistaken interpretation of such behavior.
   (2) Eighteen-month-olds have not outgrown separation anxiety.
   (4) Staff members are usually viewed by toddlers as unfamiliar, frightening, and often threatening.

6. (2) Hearing is a sense that is not greatly influenced by emotional response in the young child. (b); AN; CP; NU; PE

(1) Institutionalized children often manifest delays in neuromuscular development.
(3) The emotional trauma of institutionalization will influence the child's cognitive development.
(4) The trauma of institutionalization may also result in speech and other expressive delays.

7. (1) The child experiencing long-term hospitalization is forced to relate to a variety of significant adults instead of to a single figure providing mothering. The lack of continuity creates anxiety. (a); AN; CP; NU; PE
   (2) Even with sufficient sensory stimulation, the young child will still suffer from the lack of a mother figure.
   (3) Although mother surrogates are helpful, they do not replace the other figure.
   (4) Even with sufficient play objects, the child will still suffer from the lack of a mother figure.

8. (1) The child learns to love others by the love he receives. When he receives love, he feels he is worthy of being loved and can share this feeling with others (a); AN; CP; NU; PE
   (2) These children have difficulties forming attachments to people.
   (3) Studies do not address this issue.
   (4) Studies do not address this issue.

9. (4) Until trust has been reestablished, the child will be unable to develop an emotional tie to his mother. (b); IM; AP; SH; PE
   (1) At this stage of separation anxiety, the child would be too detached to be hostile.
   (2) In extreme cases of separation, the child will be withdrawn from his parents.
   (3) The child will be despairing and withdrawn.

10. (2) An oral contraceptive program requires taking 1 tablet daily from the fifth day of the cycle and continuing for 20 or 21 days. Interrupting the monthly dosage program may permit release of luteinizing hormone, then ovulation, and then possible pregnancy. (b); IM; AP; SH; OB
    (1) Untrue; there is a very high rate of success if the oral contraceptive is taken regularly and correctly.
    (3) Too much information being given; also telling the patient not to worry may close off communication.
    (4) Judgmental; a value statement on the part of the nurse. Contraceptive practice is the patient's choice.

11. (3) Knowing that others share the same problems may be comforting. The second part of the nurse's statement is open ended and allows the patient to describe her physical and emotional feelings. (a); AN; AP; SH; OB
    (1) Telling the patient not to worry closes off communication; does not allow exploration of avenues for further discussion.
    (2) Too factual; closes off communication. The patient needs to explore with the nurse the means for feeling better.

(4) Within the nursing purvue; should be handled at this time.

12. (4) Before health teaching is instituted, the nurse should ascertain the patient's past experiences. They will influence the teaching plan. (b); AS; AP; SH; OB

(1) This answer does not give the patient a chance to discuss her feelings about the examination.

(2) This answer does not give the patient a chance to discuss her feelings about the examination; the nurse can only assume that the patient's concerns are related to discomfort.

(3) Presupposes a yes or no answer; does not really give the patient an opportunity to discuss it further.

13. (3) In calculating the expected date of delivery, subtract 3 months and add 7 days to the date of the last menstrual period. (b); AS; KN; SH; OB

(1) Incorrect; count back 3 months and add 7 days.

(2) Incorrect; count back 3 months and add 7 days.

(4) Incorrect; count back 3 months and add 7 days.

14. (2) Successful dietary teaching usually incorporates, as much as possible, the patient's food preferences and dietary patterns. (c); AS; AP; SH; OB

(1) This does not take into considerations the patient's likes and dislikes or cultural preferences; would not foster patient compliance.

(3) Salt is not limited during pregnancy unless a disease process is present or develops; seasoned foods are permissible if the patient does not experience discomfort from them.

(4) This presupposes that the patient has been eating a normal diet; does not provide for additional caloric or protein requirements of pregnancy.

15. (4) Maintaining the sitting position for prolonged periods may constrict the vessels of the legs, particularly in the popliteal spaces, as well as diminish venous return. Walking contracts the muscles of the legs, which apply gentle pressure to the veins in the legs, and promotes venous return. (b); AN; AP; CL; OB

(1) A better means of improving circulation would be to walk about several times each morning and afternoon; she could also keep her legs elevated while sitting at her desk.

(2) If she is feeling well, there are no contraindications to working until her due date.

(3) Adequate nourishment can be obtained during meal times; she does not require extra nutrition breaks.

16. (4) When the membranes rupture, the potential for infection is increased; and when the contractions are 5 to 8 minutes apart, they are usually of sufficient force to warrant medical supervision. Therefore, for the safety of the mother and fetus, the mother should go to the hospital. (b); PL; AP; CL; OB

(1) This is indicative of advanced labor, and the patient may have difficulty getting to the hospital at this time.

(2) Too early; the patient still has a great deal of time and would be better off with her family and moving about at home.

(3) These may be early signs of labor or signs of posterior labor; need further evaluation by the physician.

17. (3) The fetal heart rate is usually between 120 and 160 beats per minute. This is to be expected normally, and the mother should be made aware of this fact. (a); IM; AP; SH; OB

(1) This is too variable; the normal heart rate for a fetus is 120 to 160 beats per minute.

(2) To accommodate to the oxygen needs of the fetus, the heart rate is rapid.

(4) Unnecessary information; the mother should be informed only of that which is normal.

18. (2) Lets him know that the nurse understands adjustments will have to be made. It also is open ended enough to let him talk about feelings. (b); IM; AP; CL; PS

(1) Has not expressed his feelings enough for the nurse to offer any specific suggestions for help.

(3) Not open ended enough to foster expression of feelings about what is bothering him.

(4) This may compound his anxiety; also does not let him explore feelings.

19. (2) The sensitive and dependent individual who has a conflict accepting the need for dependence frequently develops ulcerative colitis. The exact neural mechanism resulting in colonic inflammation is unknown. (c); AN; CP; NU; ME

(1) These characteristics are associated with peptic ulcer disease.

(3) Since the individual directs hostility outward, visceral changes may not occur.

(4) An individual who is secure is not predisposed to developing visceral disorders as the result of psychologic stress.

20. (4) Since the mucosa of the intestinal tract is damaged, its ability to absorb vitamins taken orally is greatly impaired. (a); IM; CP; NU; ME

(1) Although this is true, the risks associated with IV administration will outweigh the benefits unless other factors are considered.

(2) Vitamins are effective orally unless there is disease involving the GI tract that hampers absorption.

(3) IV vitamins do not decrease colonic irritability.

21. (1) $\dfrac{\text{Amount to be infused} \times \text{Drop factor}}{\text{Amount of time (in minutes)}}$

$$\frac{2000 \times 10}{12 \times 60} = \frac{20,000}{720} = 27.77 \text{ drops/min}$$

(b); IM; AP; NU; ME

(2) Incorrect calculation; would result in excessive fluid administration.

(3) Incorrect calculation; would result in excessive fluid administration.

(4) Incorrect calculation; would result in excessive fluid administration.

22. (1) This grouping of foods does not contain high-residue fruits, vegetables, or whole grains, which are irritating to the intestinal mucosa, cause bulk, and increase peristalsis. (c); PL; AN; SH; ME
    (2) Includes whole grain foods, which leave increased residue.
    (3) Includes vegetables and grain, which leave increased residue.
    (4) Includes vegetables and grain, which leave increased residue.

23. (2) The key in treatment of this disease is to prevent spastic intestinal activity. (a); AN; CP; NU; ME
    (1) Reduction of gastric acidity is the aim of bland diets used in the treatment of peptic ulcers.
    (3) Electrolyte depletion may be prevented by reducing colonic irritation, but this is a secondary benefit.
    (4) By reducing colonic irritation, motility, and spasticity, it is hoped that absorption will increase.

24. (4) The affected areas of the intestine are in need of repair. Protein is required in the building and repairing of tissues. (a); PL; CP; SH; ME
    (1) Anemia may result from chronic bleeding; it usually is corrected, however, with increased iron and normal intake of protein.
    (2) Increased protein will not significantly affect peristalsis.
    (3) Protein is given to promote healing; once tissues are repaired, muscle tone may improve.

25. (1) Since her diabetes appears to be out of control, dietary indiscretions or changes should be ruled out. Information about habits can be elicited only during a patient interview. (b); AS; AN; SH; ME
    (2) This information can be objectively assessed by examination of past and present medical records, which should serve as the primary source for these types of data.
    (3) This information can be objectively assessed by examination of past and present medical records, which should serve as the primary source for these types of data.
    (4) This information can be objectively assessed by examination of past and present medical records, which should serve as the primary source for these types of data.

26. (2) Taking a pill may give the patient a false sense that the disease is under control, and this can lead to dietary indiscretions. (b); IM; CP; SH; ME
    (1) A person's ability to follow dietary restrictions is highly individual; the employment setting is not a universal factor in such behaviors.
    (3) Individuals receiving insulin may also believe that their diabetes is under control and may not adhere to their prescribed diet; having to take medication every day can be threatening to some people.
    (4) Diabetes is a chronic disease; and its complications can affect all individuals with the disease, particularly those who do not comply with the prescribed regimen.

27. (4) An understanding of the diet is imperative for compliance. A balance of carbohydrates, proteins, and fats usually apportioned over 3 main meals and 2 between-meal snacks needs to be tailored to the patient's specific needs, with due regard for activity, diet, and insulin therapy. (b); IM; CP; SH; ME
    (1) True; however, indigestion is not the basis for the patient's problems.
    (2) Total caloric intake, rather than the distribution of meals, is the major factor in weight gain.
    (3) Although restriction of calories and sodium is essential, a total dietary regimen must be followed to ensure adequate nutrition and control of the disease.

28. (4) Past experiences have the most meaningful influence on present learning. (b); PL; CP; SH; PS
    (1) Although this consideration affects learning, its influence is not as great as that of all past experiences.
    (2) Although this consideration affects learning, its influence is not as great as that of all past experiences.
    (3) Although this consideration affects learning, its influence is not as great as that of all past experiences.

29. (2) Nonjudgmentally identifying the patient's feelings encourages further verbalization about those feelings and the diet. (a); IM; CP; SH; PS
    (1) The nurse should first acknowledge the patient's feelings and then assess the patient's level of knowledge before imparting such information.
    (3) This response is inappropriate; no mention of specific foods.
    (4) Suggests that adherence to the prescribed medical regimen is unnecessary.

30. (2) Fasting prior to the test is indicated for accurate and reliable results. Food will elevate the blood glucose levels through metabolism of the nutrients. (b); IM; AP; CL; ME
    (1) Medications are withheld because of their influence on blood sugar.
    (3) Clear fluids contain carbohydrates, which will increase the blood glucose levels.
    (4) Food should not be ingested; it will raise the serum glucose levels, negating the accuracy of the test.

31. (2) Cough syrup contains a sugar base. This must be taken into account by diabetic patients. (b); IM; AN; CL; ME
    (1) Additional glucose may increase serum glucose levels without altering sugar and acetone results; once control is achieved, it is unwise to alter dietary intake or medication without supervision.
    (3) Elixirs have an alcohol base and also contain sweeteners.
    (4) Although this will loosen secretions, it will not suppress a cough when rest is desired.

32. (4) In diabetes mellitus, progressive thickening of the capillary basement membranes and medial sclerosis of small arteries leading to the eyes gradually occlude the vessel lumina. This significantly reduces retinal perfusion and leads to blindness. (b); AN; AP; NU; ME

(1) There is usually an increase in serum glucose with diabetes mellitus; thickening of the capillary basement membranes often occurs, even if the glucose level is maintained within normal limits.

(2) There is usually an increase in serum glucose with diabetes mellitus; thickening of capillary basement membranes often occurs, even if the glucose level is maintained within normal limits.

(3) Ketones do not usually affect retinal metabolism; retinopathy is due to vascular changes, retinal detachment, and hemorrhage within the eye.

33. (3) Damage to Broca's area, located in the posterior frontal region of the dominant hemisphere, causes problems in the motor aspect of speech. (a); AN; CP; SH; ME

(1) This would be associated with receptive aphasia, not expressive aphasia; receptive aphasia is associated with disease of Wernicke's area.

(2) This would be associated with receptive aphasia not expressive aphasia, receptive aphasia is associated with disease of Wernicke's area.

(4) Although difficulty writing may be associated with expressive aphasia, understanding speech would be associated with receptive aphasia.

34. (4) Giving the patient adequate time to respond and employing a calm, accepting, deliberate, and interested manner will reduce the patient's anxiety and tension as well as increase her self-esteem. (a); IM; AP; SH; ME

(1) The patient's sensory pathways are unaffected; she can see, hear, and understand.

(2) Isolation is not therapeutic; the patient must be encouraged to remain in contact with others.

(3) The patient should continue to speak so she can develop new pathways and gradually improve her speech.

35. (1) Assuming a normal position for voiding reduces tension (physical and psychologic), facilitates the movement of urine into the lower portion of the bladder, and relaxes the external sphincter (increasing pressure and initiating the micturition reflex). (c); IM; AP; CL; ME

(2) Bladder training should be instituted by encouraging voiding every 1 to 2 hours and progressively increasing the time between voiding.

(3) This is an extremely large fluid intake and will result in a large volume of urine, probably increasing the frequency of incontinence.

(4) Voiding should be encouraged at regular and frequent intervals during waking hours, not just in the afternoon.

36. (2) Left-sided paresis creates instability. Using a cane provides a wider base of support and, therefore, greater stability. (a); AN; CP; CL; ME

(1) Activity should not injure but strengthen weakened muscles.

(3) Since inflammation of these joints is not mentioned, this is unnecessary.

(4) The use of a cane will not prevent involuntary movements if they were present.

37. (3) The body is supported partially on the affected limb and partially on the cane as the unaffected limb moves forward. (b); IM; AP; SH; ME

(1) The cane is held on the unaffected side and advanced at the same time as the affected extremity to increase the base of support and provide stability.

(2) Leaning the body will change the center of gravity and cause instability.

(4) Normal ambulation should be approximated; this would produce an awkward gait and instability.

38. (4) Orienting the patient to the hospital provides knowledge that may reduce the strangeness of the environment, whereas introducing staff members lets the patient know who will be caring for her as well as provides a personal touch. (b); IM; AP; SH; PS

(1) This may be false reassurance since no one can guarantee that everything will be all right.

(2) This would be part of orienting her to the unit.

(3) This implies that staff members are available to her only if she becomes upset.

39. (4) Atherosclerosis begins with the accumulation of fatty deposits (plaques) within the inner lining (intima) of the arteries, leading to a narrowing of the lumen. Later the plaques enlarge, cause greater occlusion, and harden by deposition of calcium (atheroarteriosclerosis), eventually increasing the work of the heart. (b); AN; KN; NU; ME

(1) This is arteriosclerosis.

(2) Atheromas develop within the intima of arteries, not in the cardiac muscle.

(3) Although atheromas or plaques are deposited from circulating fat, mobilization from adipose storage is not a prerequisite.

40. (1) Each person is unique. The nurse should avoid making the patient feel dehumanized. (b); PL; AP; SH; PS

(2) This would be a later nursing action.

(3) The patient is in the hospital for tests: although safety is important, it is not a priority need.

(4) It is important that the patient understand what is happening to her; however, her individuality must be considered first.

41. (4) Identifying and accepting feelings helps to open lines of communication with the patient. (b); IM; AP; SH; PS

(1) This does not allow the patient to explore her feelings with an accepting person.

(2) This is avoiding the real issue.

(3) Focuses on only one aspect of the statement; does not allow her to explore her real feelings.

42. (1) Nitroglycerine is sensitive to light and moisture and must be stored in a dark airtight container. (b); IM; AP; NU; ME

(2) This may be an expected side effect.

(3) This medication is usually taken p.r.n. The daily number may be as high as 12 to 15 tablets; if more

than 3 are necessary in a 15 minute period, the doctor should be notified.

(4) Expected response; if it does not occur, tablets should be replaced.

43. (1) Alzheimer's disease is an insidious atrophy of the brain. The individual maintains the ability to make socially correct comments, but the intellect is diminished. (c); AN; KN; NU; PS

(2) TIAs may precede a cerebral vascular accident; unrelated to Alzheimer's disease.

(3) Alzheimer's is a progressive, deteriorating disease.

(4) It is a slow chronic deterioration.

44. (2) Since these patients do experience a lability of mood, it is best to attempt to establish a relationship and give care when they are feeling receptive. (c); PL; AN; SH; PS

(1) This rejects the patient when she needs the nurse most.

(3) This may be of limited help; she may be unable to do it.

(4) Patients with this disorder have limited contact with reality.

45. (4) Sameness provides security and safety and reduces stress for the patient. (b); IM; AP; SH; PS

(1) A challenging environment would increase anxiety and frustration.

(2) A nonstimulating environment would add to her diminishing intellect.

(3) Patients with this disease do not do well in a constantly changing environment.

46. (4) A consistent approach and consistent communication from all members of the health team help the patient who has a chronic brain syndrome remain a bit more reality oriented. (b); PL; AP; NU; PS

(1) Patients who have this disorder do not attempt to manipulate the staff.

(2) It is the staff members who need to be consistent.

(3) Not needed in working with patients who have this disorder; consistency is most important.

47. (3) Patients with long-term psychiatric problems who have limited contact with reality can usually still become involved with a remotivation therapy group. The demands of this type of group are limited and self-confining. (c); AN; CP; SH; PS

(1) This is suitable for working through emotional problems; these patients are unable to follow the dramatization of emotions.

(2) The object of such therapy is to develop social skills; these goals are inappropriate for patients with this disorder.

(4) The object of such therapy is to develop social skills; these goals are inappropriate for patients with this disorder.

48. (3) Remotivation therapy is designed to encourage patients to interact with their environment by focusing their attention on some common ''emotionally safe'' article that most patients can recognize and talk about. (b); AN; CP; SH; PS

(1) They do have face-to-face contact with other patients, but that is not the objective of the group.

(2) More appropriate for patients who have a schizophrenic disorder than for those with an organic brain disorder.

(4) The focus is on interpersonal skills and becoming competent in the activities of daily living.

49. (2) Vitamin K stores are almost absent in the newborn because the intestinal flora that produces this vitamin is not present. Vitamin K is an essential precursor of prothrombin, which supports the clotting mechanism. (b); IM; CP; NU; OB

(1) Increased bilirubin in the blood occurs in newborns because of the rapid breakdown of RBCs and the liver's difficulty in conjugating such large amounts; not influenced by vitamin K.

(3) The normal flora develops as the newborn is exposed to extraneous living conditions.

(4) The young kidneys operate at a functional level appropriate to the needs of a healthy infant; not influenced by vitamin K.

50. (2) Drug dependence in the newborn is physiologic. As the drug is cleared from the body, symptoms of drug withdrawal become evident. Tremors, irritability, difficulty sleeping, twitching, and convulsions may result. (b); AS; CP; NU; OB

(1) Symptoms of drug withdrawal involve signs of excessive stimulation.

(3) Dehydration is secondary to poor feeding; not a result of withdrawal per se.

(4) Hypertonicity of muscles would be seen.

51. (3) Drug-dependent newborns are poor feeders because of hyperactivity, nausea, vomiting, respiratory distress, excessive mucus, and pyrexia. Small frequent feedings should be given to prevent dehydration. (c); PL; AP; NU; OB

(1) To minimize extraneous stimulation, environmental stimuli should be decreased.

(2) Infants of drug-addicted mothers are prone to hypothermia, not hyperthermia.

(4) Infants need supportive care during the time the drug is leaving their systems; methadone only modifies withdrawal, does not prevent it.

52. (3) The nurse should attempt to support the mother-child relationship. The mother is experiencing a developmental crisis while having to deal with drug addiction and possibly guilt. (a); IM; AP; SH; PS

(1) Melanie needs contact with her new infant to facilitate bonding.

(2) The timing for this is after adjustment to the present situation has begun.

(4) This will make Melanie feel guilty and not facilitate positive action at this point.

53. (4) The immediate postburn period is marked by dramatic alterations in circulation because of large fluid losses through the denuded skin, vasodilation, edema formation, and a direct response on the con-

tractility of the heart muscle. The precipitious drop in cardiac output causes shock. (a); AN; AN; NU; PE

(1) In Mary's case, pneumonia would be a later complication associated with immobility.

(2) Contractures are a later complication associated with scarring and aggravated by improper positioning and splinting.

(3) Fluid dynamics are drastically altered; dehydration is a concern closely following shock in importance.

54. (3) Body weight is used in the calculation of body surface area. It is the main criterion in determining drug dosage and fluid requirements. (b); AN; CP; NU; PE

(1) It is inappropriate to be concerned about growth in the face of an acute situation.

(2) Measurement of the burned surface is determined by parts of the body involved.

(4) Dietary management is a later consideration.

55. (3) High fever and disorientation may be initial indications of infection and/or early signs of hypoxia from respiratory complications. (c); AS; AN; NU; PE

(1) Tachycardia is normally associated with the early phases of burn injury; vomiting may be a sign of circulatory collapse or paralytic ileus or may be nonspecific.

(2) High temperatures and increased basal metabolic rate are seen with burns.

(4) Decreased blood pressure is rarely seen unless the patient is in severe shock.

56. (2) The minimum urine volume is 10 to 20 ml per hour in children under 2 years and 20 to 30 ml per hour in children over 2 years of age. (b); AS; KN; NU; PE

(1) This is the minimum safe output in children under 2 years.

(3) This volume is higher than minimum.

(4) This volume is higher than minimum.

57. (4) Because their verbal ability is limited, children act out their feelings via play. (a); IM; CP; SH; PE

(1) Acceptance of the hospital situation is not as important as dealing with her own feelings.

(2) Therapeutic play does not necessarily involve other children.

(3) Mary needs to cope with her feelings rather than forget them.

58. (2) By the patient's lying on her affected side, the unaffected lung can expand to its fullest potential. Elevation of the head facilitates respirations by reducing the pressure of the abdominal organs on the diaphragm and allowing the diaphragm to descend with gravity. (c); IM; AN; NU; SU

(1) Maximum lung expansion is inhibited when the head is not elevated.

(3) Not a specific answer. What does "left side supported" mean? Although it facilitates diaphragmatic movement, it does not assist expansion of the right lung.

(4) Pressure against the right thorax limits right intercostal expansion and gaseous exchange in the right lung; the supine position allows the abdominal viscera to restrict contraction of the diaphragm and does not permit the diaphragm to drop by gravity.

59. (1) The rate and characteristics of respiration should be assessed so the amount of exertion required for breathing can be determined. The nurse should also evaluate signs such as unilateral chest movements that may indicate pneumothorax and tachypnea, which are associated with hypercapnea and acidosis. (b); AS; AN; NU; SU

(2) Excessive blood loss might affect blood pressure, but such bleeding would be indicated first by respiratory changes because the blood would accumulate in the pleural space; pupillary response would be unaffected.

(3) Drainage may accumulate in the pleural space, which is inaccessible for direct assessment.

(4) Although important, it is not a life-threatening symptom.

60. (4) Maintains negative intrathoracic pressure by limiting the amount of air rushing in from the outside. This can result in total pneumothorax and mediastinal shift, severely embarrassing respiration. (b); AN; CP; NU; SU

(1) Major blood vessels are not occluded by a thoracic pressure dressing.

(2) A sterile dressing without pressure would suffice in preventing contamination.

(3) The dressing does not prevent injury to the pleura.

61. (4) $\dfrac{\text{Total amount to be infused} \times \text{Drop factor}}{\text{Total time for infusion (in minutes)}}$

$\dfrac{3000 \times 20}{24 \times 60} = 41.66 \text{ drops/min}$

(b); IM; AP; NU; SU

(1) Inaccurate calculation; would not deliver an adequate amount of fluid.

(2) Inaccurate calculation; would not deliver an adequate amount of fluid.

(3) Inaccurate calculation; would not deliver an adequate amount of fluid.

62. (1) Retention of carbon dioxide in the blood lowers the pH, causing respiratory acidosis. Deep breathing maximizes gaseous exchange, ridding the body of excess carbon dioxide. (b); IM; CP; CL; SU

(2) Although regular deep breathing improves the vital capacity, residual volume is unaffected.

(3) Deep breathing improves oxygenation of the blood, but it does not affect volume.

(4) Deep breathing increases the partial pressure of oxygen.

63. (2) Leakage of air into the subcutaneous tissue is evidenced by a crackling sound when the area is gently palpated. This is referred to as crepitus. (c); EV; AN; NU; SU

(1) To minimize the risk of pneumothorax, the dressing is not routinely changed.

(3) The system is kept closed to prevent the pressure of the atmosphere from causing a pneumothrorax; drainage levels are marked on the bottles to measure output.

(4) Although hemostats should be readily available for any patient with chest tubes in the event of a break in the drainage system, clamping the tube would not be otherwise necessary.

64. (2) Immediately prior to administration, an assessment of vital signs is necessary to determine whether any contraindications to analgesia exist (e.g., hypotension, a respiratory rate of 12 or less). (c); AS; AP; NU; SU

(1) Pain prevents both psychologic and physiologic rest.

(3) Before administration, the nurse must check the physician's orders, the time of the last administration, and the patient's vital signs.

(4) Prior to determining the time of the last dose, the nurse should record the patient's vital signs; assessment is the first step of the nursing process.

65. (1) Talking in the third person reflects poor ego boundaries and a dissociation from the real self. (a); AN; CP; NU; PS

(2) Reaction formation is the expression of an emotion opposite the one really felt.

(3) Displacement is the attempt to reduce anxiety by transferring the emotions associated with one object or person to another.

(4) Transference is the movement of emotional energy and feelings from one person to another.

66. (2) These patients need sensory stimulation to maintain orientation and should be encouraged to do as much as possible for themselves, depending on their ability. (c); PL; AP; SH; PS

(1) Surroundings should be bright to minimize confusion of stimuli.

(3) Patients are usually not completely out of contact with reality; it is important to differentiate fantasy from reality, but this would not take top priority in care.

(4) Although it is important to make certain that patients receive physical hygiene and comfort, they should be encouraged to help themselves as much as possible.

67. (4) When the patient's perceptions are especially frightening, the nurse must let her know that her fears are recognized as real and frightening to her even if the nurse does not share her perceptions. Staying with the patient will convey concern as well as reduce her fears. (b); IM; AP; SH; PS

(1) Nontherapeutic; the voices are real to the patient.

(2) Nontherapeutic; the patient is unable to separate the voices from reality.

(3) The patient will be unable to play cards because she cannot concentrate when the voices are speaking to her.

68. (3) This response points out reality while attempting to let the patient understand that the nurse sees her as a person of worth. (c); IM; AN; SH; PS

(1) This is a somewhat punitive response; cuts off communication.

(2) Nontherapeutic; the patient may indeed see herself as a devil.

(4) Asks the patient to explain feelings, an unrealistic goal.

69. (2) Major tranquilizers tend to make the patient listless or drowsy and can interfere with the ability to participate in the therapeutic regimen. (b); AN; CP; NU; PS

(1) Major tranquilizers do not really induce sleep; just listlessness.

(3) Major tranquilizers do not appreciably affect diurnal rhythms.

(4) Assaultiveness is associated with increased anxiety rather than time.

70. (1) Liver damage is a well-documented toxic side effect of the major tranquilizers. By continuing to administer the drug, the nurse failed to use professional knowledge in the performance of responsibilities as outlined in the Nurse Practice Act. (b); EV; AP; NU; PS

(2) The tranquilizer should be stopped not reduced; liver damage is a well-documented toxic side effect.

(3) False; liver damage, indicated by jaundice, is a well-documented side effect.

(4) False; blood levels must be reduced when signs of liver damage are present.

71. (4) The delusional patient can never be argued out of a delusion, since it serves as a defense against reality and is the patient's reality. It is best to accept the delusion without discussion. (c); IM; AP; SH; PS

(1) This action can lead to increased feelings of guilt about the delusion since the patient will not understand why the nurse is changing the topic.

(2) Encouraging discussion gives credulence to the delusion rather than points out reality to the patient.

(3) The patient would have difficulty getting involved in a repetitive activity, and the activity would not stop the delusion.

72. (1) When an individual expresses interest in physical appearance, it demonstrates a rebuilding of the self-image and the return of feelings of worth and concern for how others see them. (a); AS; CP; SH; PS

(2) The information provided does not demonstrate a need for social reassurance or approval.

(3) The patient's response goes further than the nurse's implied suggestion; she is expressing her own needs.

(4) The patient's response is well within the normal range; does not indicate the beginning of a hyperactive phase.

73. (1) One of the characteristic differences between juvenile and adult diabetes is the rapid onset of the dis-

ease in children. Diabetes is often first diagnosed during acute ketoacidosis. (a); AS; KN; NY; PE

(2) Although adult-onset diabetes often occurs in obese individuals, juvenile diabetes occurs in children of thin or normal build.

(3) Juvenile diabetics are insulin dependent.

(4) Vascular changes are a complication associated with long-standing diabetes.

74. (3) Helping families understand their feelings about juvenile diabetes is essential in assisting them to develop positive attitudes for optimal control of the disease and promotion of a normal life for the child. (a); PL; AP; SH; PE

(1) Instruction in specific psychomotor tasks should be preceded by an assessment of the family's acceptance of the diagnosis and knowledge about the disease.

(2) Important; however, if feelings are not dealt with first, compliance with insulin injections is less likely.

(4) Kim should participate in the activities normal for her and her age group. Adequate exercise is an important part of the treatment regimen for diabetes.

75. (2) Equation no. 1

$$40 \text{ units} : 1 \text{ ml} = 12 \text{ units} : x$$
$$40x = 12$$
$$x = 0.3 \text{ ml}$$

Equation no. 2

$$1 \text{ ml} = 15 \text{ minims}$$
$$0.3 \text{ ml} \times 15 \text{ minims/ml} = 4.5 \text{ minims}$$

(b); IM; AP; NU; PE

(1) Too large.

(3) Not exact.

(4) Too small.

76. (2) A bedtime snack is needed for the evening. NPH insulin lasts for 24 to 28 hours. Protein and carbohydrate ingestion prior to sleep prevents hypoglycemia during the night, when the action of NPH insulin will still be high. (a); PL; AN; NU; PE

(1) The snack contains mainly protein-rich foods to help cover the long-acting insulin during sleep.

(3) The snack is important for diet insulin balance during the night.

(4) There are no data to indicate such a need; a bedtime snack is routinely provided to help cover long-acting insulin during sleep.

77. (4) Exercise reduces the body's need for insulin. Increased muscle activity accelerates the transport of glucose into the muscle cells, thus producing an insulin-like effect. (b); PL; AN; CL; PE

(1) An emotional upset is a stress that requires insulin.

(2) An infectious process, if severe enough, may require increased insulin.

(3) With increasing growth and associated dietary intake, the need for insulin increases.

78. (1) If the patient is to remain at home, she must be aware of when to notify the physician of her symptoms. (b); AS; AN; SH; OB

(2) The actual causes of spontaneous abortion are not known.

(3) This is factual information; will not alleviate anxiety concerning a possible abortion.

(4) Too broad an explanation; unrelated to the worry about imminent abortion.

79. (2) Tension may be the precipitating cause of gastroesophageal reflux early in pregnancy. Displacement of the stomach and delayed emptying of stomach contents because of uterine enlargement may be the cause of heartburn later in pregnancy. (c); IM; AP; SH; OB

(1) This would allow acid to pass into the small intestine.

(3) Gastric motility and acidity are generally decreased in pregnancy.

(4) Increased motility would utilize acid, leaving little or none to be regurgitated.

80. (3) The increase of estrogen during pregnancy causes hyperplasia of the vaginal mucosa, which leads to increased production of mucus by the endocervical glands. The mucus contains exfoliated epithelial cells. (b); IM; AP; SH; OB

(1) Increased metabolism leads to many systemic changes but does not increase vaginal discharge.

(2) Normal functioning of the glands, which lubricate the vagina during intercourse, remains unchanged during pregnancy.

(4) There is no additional supply of sodium chloride to the cells during pregnancy.

81. (1) The antibodies in human milk provide the newborn infant with immunity against all or most of the pathogens that the mother has encountered. (b); IM; CP; CL; OB

(2) Complex carbohydrates are not required by the infant.

(3) Present in commercial formulas.

(4) Present in commercial formulas.

82. (3) Provides the mother an opportunity to express her concerns regarding prophylactic eye medication. (b); IM; AP; CL; OB

(1) Blocks communication; instillation can be delayed for an hour.

(2) Does not respond to the mother's statement.

(4) Does not respond to the mother's statement.

83. (2) Maternal hypotension is a common complication of conduction anesthesia for labor, and nausea is one of the first clues that this has occurred. Elevating the extremities restores blood to the central circulation. (c); EV; AN; NU; OB

(1) If signs and symptoms do not abate after elevation of the legs, the physician should be notified.

(3) If the fetal heart rate is being monitored, it is a constant process; if not, the FHR should be monitored every 15 minutes.

(4) This is not a specific observation after caudal anesthesia; it is part of the general nursing care during labor.

84. (1) A neat surgical incision is easier to repair and quicker to heal than an irregular laceration. (a); IM; CP; SH; OB
    (2) An episiotomy will contribute to rather than limit postpartal discomfort.
    (3) Contrariwise; upon healing it will tighten up the perineum.
    (4) May or may not influence birth trauma to the fetus; usually reduces trauma to the mother.

85. (3) Respirations are normally abdominal, diaphragmatic, and irregular. The rate is 30 to 50 per minute. (b); AS; CP; NU; OB
    (1) The newborn's respirations are abdominal not thoracic.
    (2) Retractions are a sign of respiratory distress.
    (4) Stertorous breathing may indicate respiratory distress.

86. (3) After the need to survive (air, food, water) the need for comfort and freedom from pain closely follow. Care should be given in order of the patient's needs. (b); PL; AN; NU; ME
    (1) Joints must be exercised to prevent stiffness, contractures, and muscle atony.
    (2) Although bladder training should be included in care, it is not a priority item when the patient is in pain.
    (4) Motivation and learning will not occur unless basic needs, such as freedom from pain, are met.

87. (2) The antiinflammatory action of acetylsalicylic acid (A.S.A) is effective in reducing the discomfort and pain associated with rheumatoid arthritis. (b); AN; KN; NU; ME
    (1) Methocarbamol is a muscle relaxant; it does not reduce the inflammation associated with arthritis.
    (3) Cortisone is employed when more conservative treatment fails; its use is avoided because of associated adverse effects (e.g., osteoporosis, gastric ulceration, psychosis, decreased resistance, hirsutism, hyperglycemia, edema, hypertension).
    (4) Gold salts are employed if more conservative treatment fails; they must be administered intramuscularly and are highly toxic.

88. (4) Maintenance of joints in extension offsets the deformity often seen in rheumatoid arthritis. It also frequently prevents potentially deforming contractures. (b); PL; AN; CL; ME
    (1) Patients often assume a fetal position, which results in flexion contractures of all extremities; this should be avoided.
    (2) Pressure on the popliteal space can impede venous return, increasing the risk of thrombus formation; it can also promote knee flexion contractures.
    (3) The Fowler position is not required; respiratory function is unimpaired.

89. (1) Incontinence without a physiologic basis is an act of hostility that the individual uses to deal with anxiety-producing situations. (a); AN; AN; SH; PS
    (2) Incontinence is rarely the result of conscious effort.
    (3) Incontinence is not a necessary complication of age and inactivity; can be prevented by a bladder-training program.
    (4) Incontinence is often seen as a symbol of regression and loss of control.

90. (2) For psychologic equilibrium Mrs. Ryan's environment must be one of novel and changing stimuli, promoting physical activity and effective interaction with others. (b); PL; AP; SH; PS
    (1) Since the patient has been able to regain control of elimination, frequent toileting is unnecessary.
    (3) To prevent urinary stasis and dehydration, fluid intake should be encouraged.
    (4) Although stimulation is important, it should be varied and the patient's preferences taken into consideration; radio and television do not promote interaction.

91. (1) Since air-conduction hearing aids utilize the person's own middle ear, they increase hearing acuity in cases of diminished sensitivity of the cochlea. The amplified signal from the hearing aid gives the cochlea greater stimulation and promotes hearing. (b); AN; KN; SH; ME
    (2) Perforation of the tympanic membrane prevents ossicular conduction, which involves transmission of resonant vibrations from the tympanic membrane to the ossicles to the cochlea; hearing aids will not correct this.
    (3) Immobilization of the ossicles prevents conduction of resonant vibrations from the tympanic membrane to the cochlea; air-conduction hearing aids will not correct this problem.
    (4) Destruction of the auditory nerve results in deafness because impulses cannot be transmitted to the brain's auditory center.

92. (4) GI distress causes disturbance in intestinal motility and absorption, accelerating excretion. IV fluids are necessary, since severe dehydration and fluid and electrolyte imbalance occur rapidly and can lead to death in infancy because of the infant's large fluid content. (b); IM; AP; NU; PE
    (1) This test is used to determine blood type when a transfusion is indicated.
    (2) Intestinal intubation with suction is utilized to remove stomach contents when there is blockage or it is necessary to have the GI tract clear of contents.
    (3) Isolettes serve to isolate, warm, and if necessary oxygenate small infants and newborns.

93. (2) Loss of fluid as a result of dehydration is most objectively assessed by measuring the child's weight, since total body water accounts for approximately 60% of body weight. (c); AS; CP; NU; PE
    (1) This is a clinical sign of dehydration but not an accurate way to measure hydration.

COMPREHENSIVE TEST 4 **725**

(3) Decreased urine output is hard to measure in non-toilet-trained individuals.

(4) Dry skin may be indicative of conditions other than dehydration.

94. (1) Sodium, potassium, and bicarbonate are the electrolytes most often lost because of diarrhea. They are excreted before they can be absorbed. (b); AS; CP; NU; PE

(2) Chloride serves to maintain electrolyte neutrality and accompanies sodium losses or excesses.

(3) Calcium serum levels are indicators of parathyroid function and calcium metabolism.

(4) Phosphorus levels are determined by calcium metabolism, parathormone, and to a lesser degree intestinal absorption.

95. (3) $\dfrac{\text{Total amount} \times \text{Drop factor}}{\text{Total time (in minutes)}}$

$$\frac{400 \times 20}{8 \times 60} = \frac{8000}{480} = 16.6 \text{ gtt}$$

(a); IM; AP; NU; PE

(1) Too slow to achieve fluid ordered.
(2) Too slow to achieve fluid ordered.
(4) Will provide more fluid than ordered.

96. (2) Clear liquids with sugar added provide glucose without bulk. (c); PL; AN; SH; PE

(1) Fruit juices may cause fermentation, which can stimulate peristalsis.

(3) Ginger ale adds a great deal of unnecessary carbonation.

(4) Clear liquids are best tolerated after a gastric upset.

97. (2) Weight is the best indicator of fluid loss if measured each day at the same time, on the same scale, and with the same amount of clothes. (b); IM; AN; NU; PE

(1) In cases of severe diarrhea, an IV is usually employed until this is better controlled; fluids are gradually added as tolerated.

(3) Because of the diarrhea, food will not be properly absorbed.

(4) This temperature is not unusual in infants.

98. (3) By 12 months of age a child can usually drink from a cup, although fluid may spill and a bottle may be preferred at times. (c); AN; CP; SH; PE

(1) The child is just beginning lip control at 5 months and cannot handle a cup.

(2) At 7 months a child can handle a bottle but not a cup.

(4) Since this skill is present at 12 months, by 18 months most children are quite proficient.

99. (1) An interference with bile flow into the intestine will lead to increasing inability to tolerate fatty foods. The unemulsified fat remains in the intestine for prolonged periods, and the result is inhibition of stomach emptying with possible gas formation. (a); AS; CP; SH; ME

(2) Coffee ground emesis is usually indicative of gastric bleeding; it is not associated with cholecystitis.

(3) Associated with peptic ulcers.

(4) Melena is tarry stools associated with upper GI bleeding; diarrhea would be associated with increased intestinal motility, and clay-colored stools with obstructive jaundice.

100. (2) Vitamin K is necessary in the formation of prothrombin to prevent bleeding. It is a fat-soluble vitamin and is not absorbed from the GI tract in the absence of bile. (a); AN; KN; NU; SU

(1) Bilirubin is the bile pigment formed by the breakdown of erythrocytes.

(3) Thromboplastin converts prothrombin to thrombin in the normal coagulation process.

(4) Cholecystokinin is the hormone that stimulates pancreatic secretion and contraction of the gallbladder.

101. (2) A nasogastric tube attached to suction removes gastric secretions and prevents vomiting. However, if it becomes clogged, secretions may accumulate, leading to distension, nausea, and vomiting. (b); EV; AN; NU; SU

(1) An antiemetic should be administered if nausea persists after the patency of the nasogastric tube is established.

(3) To promote drainage of vomitus and prevent aspiration, the patient should be initially turned on her side.

(4) Deep breathing will not prevent vomiting if the nasogastric tube is not patent.

102. (3) Bleeding disorders are common when bile does not flow through the intestine. Vitamin K, a fat-soluble vitamin requiring bile salts for its absorption, is needed by the liver to synthesize prothrombin. (a); AS; AN; NU; SU

(1) Diaphragmatic excursion itself does not put pressure on the suture line; deep breathing does result in pain.

(2) Temperature elevation is associated with infection, not with bleeding.

(4) Pain is expected because of the location of the incision near the diaphragm.

103. (1) An incision close to the diaphragm (as in surgery of the biliary tract) causes a great deal of pain when the patient coughs and deep breathes. These patients tend to take shallow breaths, which leads to inadequate expansion of the lungs, the accumulation of secretions, and infection. (a); AN; AN; NU; SU

(2) Cholecystectomy does not require more time than other uncomplicated abdominal surgery.

(3) Elevation of serum bilirubin does not affect the immune mechanisms.

(4) There is no evidence of an infection present.

104. (3) A full fluid diet ordered by the physician after a cholecystectomy should be verified by the nurse, since there are different schools of thought concerning the use of creamed fluids. Providing a correct

diet is the shared responsibility of the physician and the nurse. (b); EV; AP; NU; SU

(1) The meal was consistent with the physician's orders; the dietician is not at fault.

(2) The nurse is responsible for transcribing the orders and notifying the appropriate departments; unreasonable orders should not be carried out but should be questioned.

(4) The patient may not be aware of the orders or the significance of such a diet.

105. (4) Although the gallbladder has been removed, the liver will continue to produce and secrete the bile necessary for emulsification of fatty foods. As soon as any inflammation affecting the common bile duct subsides, the bile will flow into the duodenum, but not in concentrated form. (a); IM; AP; CL; SU

(1) Since bile is still produced by the liver, a low-fat diet is not continued indefinitely.

(2) This is an evasive answer; the surgery was performed to remove an inflamed gallbladder and was successful.

(3) This is an evasive answer; the nurse is a resource person and shares the responsibility for patient education.

106. (2) In an attempt to ward off anxiety, the manic patient runs headlong into it, becoming totally involved in everything that goes on in the environment. (b); AS; AN; SH; PS

(1) Just the opposite is true; psychomotor activity is greatly increased.

(3) This would be more indicative of the depressive episode.

(4) During this phase there is no insight into behavior.

107. (2) Overactive individuals are stimulated by environmental factors. A responsibility of the nurse is to simplify their surroundings as much as possible. (c); IM; AP; NU; PS

(1) During this phase the patient needs a decrease in stimuli.

(3) A patient scheduled for surgery needs rest; this would be impossible in a room with a hyperactive patient because she would become the target of the overactivity.

(4) A quiet patient may become the target of her overactivity.

108. (3) Patients in the manic phase of a bipolar disorder are easily distracted. Rather than placing emphasis on their behavior, staff members should use the easy distractability of these patients to redirect this behavior to more constructive channels. (a); IM; AN; SH; PS

(1) Encourages the patient to defend the statement rather than what is behind the statement; does not foster communications about feelings.

(2) Focuses on the behavior; a punitive response does not foster communications.

(4) She would be unable to tell the nurse why she was angry.

109. (2) This approach incorporates the principles of starting where the patient is and helping the patient verbalize feelings. It also provides for more data collection to carry out the nursing process. (b); IM; AN; SH; PS

(1) The patient is obviously not ready to do this.

(3) She should not be forced back to the group; rather another nursing intervention should be attempted at this time.

(4) This would be a second step, after the initial nursing action, to plan future intervention.

110. (4) Because of the severity of side effects and the stress it places on the renal as well as the cardiovascular system, its administration is contraindicated in patients with renal or cardiovascular diseases. (b); AS; AN; NU; PS

(1) Not necessary; lithium does not alter neurologic functions.

(2) Necessary after the start of lithium administration.

(3) Necessary after the start of lithium administration.

111. (4) Albumin in the urine is a sign of toxemia, as are an elevated blood pressure and a weight gain of more than 2 pounds per week. (c); AN; AN; NU; OB

(1) Blood pressure indicates that pregnancy-induced hypertension is present; the patient must be seen more frequently than every 2 weeks.

(2) These signs indicate pregnancy-induced hypertension; treatment of this does not require vaginal examination.

(3) Blood pressure and weight are more relative; changes in the pulse rate and temperature are not associated with pregnancy-induced hypertension.

112. (1) Weight gain caused by fluid retention is the earliest objective sign of mild preeclampsia. (c); AS; CP; NU; OB

(2) Continued elevations are significant; emotional upset, anxiety, and other factors may cause fluctuations or variations in blood pressure.

(3) Edema progresses as the signs of preeclampsia worsen due to abnormal retention of fluid.

(4) May occur; however, it usually becomes evident after weight gain and a progressive increase in blood pressure.

113. (1) The latest concept concerning preeclampsia or eclampsia is that this condition is a consequence of salt loss during pregnancy and poor protein intake. The recommendations therefore call for a diet containing normal sodium, high protein, and a sufficient number of calories. (c); IM; AP; CL; OB

(2) Low protein is contraindicated for normal fetal growth; no indication for increasing sodium.

(3) There is an additional daily requirement of 500 calories during pregnancy.

(4) Lowering the intake of calories and sodium is detrimental to both fetus and mother.

114. (1) The cumulative effects of magnesium sulfate include depressed respirations and an absent or weak knee-jerk reflex. (b); EV; AN; NU; OB

(2) Blood pressure is monitored after administration of MgSO$_4$; apical pulse is not relative.

(3) Urinary output is increased after administration of MgSO$_4$.

(4) Temperature and pulse are not affected by administration of MgSO$_4$.

115. (2) Magnesium sulfate given by deep IM injection is very painful. One percent procaine hydrochloride may be mixed with the drug by physician's order or as established hospital protocol. (c); IM; AN; NU; OB

(1) One percent procaine hydrochloride, not 1% normal saline, is added to the fluid to be injected; normal saline would not maximize dispersion of the drug.

(3) May be additionally traumatic; the drug is dispersed by turning the needle.

(4) Tissue in this area may not be deep enough for the injection of MgSO$_4$.

116. (4) In severe preeclampsia, fluid is drawn from the plasma into the tissues and the blood becomes more concentrated. This is reflected in the elevated hematocrit level. (b); AN; CP; NU; OB

(1) The hemodilution results in a reduced hematocrit since there is more blood volume than there are cells.

(2) Vasodilation would not alter the ratio of cells to fluid volume.

(3) MgSO$_4$ does not cause agglutination of cells.

117. (1) Nurses can become very blasé about the equipment used in labor and forget that it may be frightening for the lay person. (b); AP; AN; SH; OB

(2) Sedation is never given on a routine basis to the patient in labor.

(3) External monitoring is now being used with much greater frequency, even on low-risk patients.

(4) Not universally true; older primigravidas may have totally uncomplicated labors.

118. (2) Lactation delays ovarian function after delivery. It will also therefore delay the symptoms of endometriosis. (b); IM; CP; CL; OB

(1) Conservative medical therapy will be used first; a hysterectomy is only a last resort.

(3) Pregnancy temporarily suppresses ovarian function; the aberrant endometrial tissue is still present.

(4) Endometriosis may lead to sterility; does not cause menopause.

119. (3) Physical assessment is a form of data collection. It is the first step in planning care. (a); AS; AP; SH; OB

(1) Implementation is not the initial action.

(2) Too soon for medical intervention; other nursing measures should be tried first.

(4) Implementation is not an initial action.

120. (3) Frequent nursing reduces the possibility of engorgement. A 10-minute period provides for complete emptying of the breast. (a); PL; AP; CL; OB

(1) Will not decrease engorgement.

(2) A relief bottle will prevent emptying of the breast; will increase pain and swelling.

(4) Does not provide for complete emptying of the breasts.

Comprehensive Test 5

To simulate the comprehensive licensing examinations, this test should be completed within 2 hours

Situation: Mr. Manning, a 48-year-old photographer, has developed fatigue and dyspnea on exertion. His ECG shows atrial fibrillation. The physician suspects mitral stenosis. Questions 1 through 8 refer to this situation.

1 The nurse is doing a physical assessment of Mr. Manning. Which one of the following facts elicited in his health history is the most significant?
   1. Rubella, age 6
   2. Streptococcal throat infection, age 12
   3. Pleurisy, age 20
   4. Cystitis, age 28

2 After the initial workup, the physician orders a cardiac catheterization for Mr. Manning. In caring for the patient after the procedure, the nurse should:
   1. Provide for rest
   2. Check pulse in the area distal to the cutdown
   3. Check the ECG every 30 minutes
   4. Administer oxygen

3 Mr. Manning requires surgery due to mitral incompetence. He is admitted to the hospital and states, "I need a new valve—and do an oil change too!!" The nurse replies, "Welcome to our unit, Mr. Manning. . . .
   1. "I'm glad to see you're handling the situation so well."
   2. "I'm sure you have a great deal to ask about this procedure."
   3. "You really don't need to hide your anxieties."
   4. "You sure came to the right place for a valve job."

4 Mr. Manning undergoes a mitral replacement. Postoperatively his peripheral pulses must be checked frequently. The chief purpose of this is to detect:
   1. The existence of emboli
   2. Arteriovenous shunting
   3. Postsurgical bleeding
   4. Atrial fibrillation

5 Mr. Manning develops a temperature of 39° C (102.8° F). The nurse notifies the physician, because elevated temperatures:

1. May indicate cerebral edema
2. May be a forerunner of hemorrhage
3. Increase the cardiac output
4. Cause diaphoresis and possible chilling

6 During the first 24 hours after surgery, 1000 ml of serosanguineous fluid drains from the chest tube. The expected drainage during this period is:
1. 800 to 1000 ml
2. 100 to 300 ml
3. 750 to 900 ml
4. 400 to 500 ml

7 During a blood transfusion Mr. Manning develops chills and headache. The nurse's best action is to:
1. Stop the transfusion immediately
2. Lightly cover the patient
3. Notify the physician STAT
4. Slow the blood flow to keep vein open

8 Mr. Manning's fever does not respond to A.S.A. He is placed on a hypothermia blanket. One reaction to hypothermia that should be prevented is:
1. Venous stasis
2. Hypotension
3. Shivering
4. Dehydration

Situation: Mrs. Ivy is a 35-year-old woman who compulsively washes her hands. Her ritual includes 4 separate scrubs, which are carried out methodically. Questions 9 through 12 refer to this situation.

9 Although the nurse becomes tense as the ritual is carried out, it should be recognized that a compulsive act is one which:
1. A person performs willingly
2. Is performed after long urging
3. Is purposeful but useless
4. Seems absurd but is necessary to the person

10 Mrs. Ivy's basic personality is probably characterized by:
1. Marked emotional maturity
2. Elaborate delusional system
3. Doubts, fears, and indecisiveness
4. Rapid, frequent mood swings

11 In caring for Mrs. Ivy it is most important that the nurse:
1. Promote reality by showing that the ritual serves little purpose
2. Try to ascertain the meaning of the ritual by discussing it with the patient
3. Interrupt the ritual to demonstrate that the ritual does not control what happens.
4. Allow the patient sufficient time to carry out the ritual

12 If interrupted in the performance of the ritual, Mrs. Ivy would most likely react with:
1. Aggression
2. Anxiety
3. Withdrawal
4. Hostility

Situation: An incision and drainage of a rectal abscess was performed 2 days ago on Mr. Silson, 48 years of age. He is receiving meperidine hydrochloride (Demerol) for pain and sitz baths t.i.d. to promote comfort and drainage. Questions 13 through 18 refer to this situation.

13 The nurse turns from preparing Mr. Silson's sitz bath and discovers he is lying on the floor. After ascertaining that the patient is unconscious, the nurse should:
1. Help him back to bed
2. Check the blood pressure
3. Check the carotid pulse
4. Call for assistance

14 The nurse sends the nurse's aide for help and begins CPR. When there is only one person to perform cardiopulmonary resuscitation, the ratio of ventilation(s) to cardiac compressions is:
1. 1:5
2. 1:10
3. 2:15
4. 4:15

15 In performing external cardiac compression on Mr. Silson the nurse should exert downward vertical pressure on the lower sternum by placing:
1. The heels of each hand side by side, extending the fingers over the chest
2. The heel of one hand on the sternum and the heel of the other on top of it, interlocking the fingers
3. The fingers of one hand on the sternum and the fingers of the other hand on top of them
4. The fleshy part of the clenched fist on the lower sternum

16 The cardiac arrest team arrives and places Mr. Silson on a monitor. To prepare the skin area for placement of the electrodes for cardiac monitoring, the nurse:
1. Uses a scrubbing motion while cleansing the skin
2. Scrubs the area with povidone iodine solution
3. Makes certain the area is moistened with normal saline before applying the electrodes
4. Applies electrode paste only if the skin becomes excoriated

17 The cardiac monitor shows ventricular fibrillation. The nurse from the coronary care unit should prepare for:
 1. An IM injection of digoxin (Lanoxin)
 2. An IV line for emergency medications
 3. Immediate defibrillation
 4. Elective cardioversion

18 Because the cells are deprived of oxygen in the patient with cardiac arrest, metabolic acidosis develops. The nurse should be prepared to administer:
 1. Potassium chloride
 2. Calcium gluconate
 3. Sodium bicarbonate
 4. Regular insulin

Situation: Mrs. Carpenter enters the hospital with esophageal strictures. She has been unable to eat solid food for many weeks. Nutritional edema does not mask the emaciation and malnourishment present. Questions 19 through 24 refer to this situation.

19 The nurse is aware that Mrs. Carpenter's nutritional edema is a result of the following primary homeostatic mechanism:
 1. The capillary fluid shift mechanism
 2. The aldosterone mechanism
 3. The ADH mechanism
 4. Nitrogen balance

20 The nurse can prevent a major reaction to hyperalimentation infusions by:
 1. The slow administration of the fluid
 2. Checking vital signs every 4 hours
 3. Changing site every 24 hours
 4. Recording intake and output

21 Later, a gastrostomy tube is inserted and Mrs. Carpenter is to be discharged with the tube in place. An advantage of gastrostomy tube feeding over nasogastric tube feeding is that:
 1. More tube feeding mixture can be given each time
 2. The procedure does not require gravity
 3. There is less chance of aspiration
 4. The patient can self-administer the feeding

22 The nurse administers the initial tube feeding. What observation indicates that the patient is unable to tolerate further tube feeding?
 1. Passage of flatus
 2. Rapid flow of feeding
 3. Epigastric tenderness
 4. Rise of formula in the tube

23 In teaching the tube feeding procedure to Mrs. Carpenter, the nurse advises her that she should:
 1. Heat the feeding 10° above body temperature

 2. Finish the feeding with water
 3. Maintain a supine position the entire time
 4. Instill fluid prior to feeding to ensure that the tube is in the stomach

24 Mrs. Carpenter must utilize a gastrostomy tube as her only route of ingestion. To maintain the pleasure of eating, the nurse may advise her to:
 1. Chew the food prior to using it for feeding
 2. Use the blender to puree favorite foods
 3. Feed via the tube at normal mealtimes
 4. Chew gum during gastrostomy tube feeding

Situation: Mrs. Gold is a 50-year-old woman with a history of an affective disorder. She is diagnosed as having a bipolar disorder/depressed. She is agitated, paces in her room almost continuously, and has difficulty sleeping at night. Questions 25 through 31 refer to this situation.

25 Mrs. Gold frequently states that she will die. The nurse tells her this is not true and she should not dwell on the subject. The nurse urges Mrs. Gold to go to the day room to talk with the other patients. Mrs. Gold becomes more agitated and ultimately has to be sedated. In instances such as this:
 1. The nurse must be accepting and should not try to talk a patient out of a delusion
 2. The sleeplessness and agitation should have been treated as a symptom
 3. Mrs. Gold has to be encouraged to relate to the other patients
 4. Mrs. Gold should have been given a tranquilizer before this incident developed

26 The treatment plan for Mrs. Gold would probably include:
 1. High doses of mood elevators
 2. Psychoanalysis
 3. Electroconvulsive therapy
 4. Nondirective psychotherapy

27 In caring for Mrs. Gold the nurse should keep in mind that:
 1. Patients with simple depressions rarely attempt suicide
 2. Once the severe depression begins to lift, the danger of suicide is no longer a problem
 3. Depressed patients are potentially suicidal during the entire course of their illness
 4. Opportunities to attempt suicide are practically absent on a closed psychiatric ward

28 Mrs. Gold appears preoccupied. She remains seated when it is time for the patients to go to eat. The nurse's best approach would be to:
 1. Overlook her not eating and leave snacks in the room

2. Tell her she must eat now, since no food will be served later
3. Ask her whether she would like to eat in her room instead of the dining room
4. Take her by the hand and accompany her to the dining room

29 Mrs. Gold is eating very little at this time. A part of the nursing care plan should be to assist her with her meals. Besides encouraging nourishment, this action also:
1. Shows her she is a worthwhile individual
2. Gets her out of the dining room with the rest of the patients
3. Proves to her that she can tolerate food
4. Provides her with some special attention

30 Mrs. Gold is taking lithium carbonate. It is vital that the nurse carefully monitor her
1. Daily weight
2. Toxicology reports
3. Psychomotor activity
4. Leukocyte count

31 Mrs. Gold is much improved and is permitted passes to leave the hospital. She is going home for a 3-day weekend. The nurse should advise her to:
1. Adjust her lithium dosage if her mood changes
3. Have a snack with milk before going to bed
2. Avoid participation in controversial discussions
4. Maintain her sodium intake

Situation: Eighteen-month-old Molly Brown is admitted with croup. She is clinging to her mother crying and responds negatively to all suggestions. Questions 32 through 38 refer to this situation.

32 In assessing Molly, the nurse would expect to find:
1. Bronchospasm, whooping cough
2. Expiratory stridor, rales
3. Laryngospasm, barking cough
4. Productive cough, inspiratory stridor

33 Mr. and Mrs. Brown ask the nurse what they should do if Molly has another attack of croup at home. The nurse suggests that Molly's parents interrupt the croup attack by administering:
1. Cheracol syrup
2. Syrup of ipecac
3. Hydrocortisone succinate (Solu-Cortef)
4. Epinephrine

34 The nurse's teaching is based on the action of this drug, which results in:
1. Dilation of the bronchi
2. Reduction of the inflammation
3. Interruption of the spasm
4. Depression of the cough center

35 When Mrs. Brown returns with Molly to the physician's office for medical follow-up, she tells the nurse that Molly has been "driving her crazy", by saying no to everything she suggests. She asks the nurse for help in handling her. The nurse explains to Mrs. Brown that Molly's negativism is normal for her age and that it is helping her meet her need for:
1. Discipline
2. Independence
3. Attention
4. Trust

36 Mrs. Brown states, "This morning I gave Molly her juice and she said 'no' and I get angry, but she needs her fluids. What shall I do?" The nurse suggests that she:
1. Be firm and hand her the glass
2. Distract her with some food
3. Let her see that she is making her mother angry
4. Offer her a choice of 2 things to drink

37 The nurse plans to talk to Mrs. Brown about toilet training Molly, knowing that the most important factor in the process of toilet training is the:
1. Child's desire to be dry
2. Approach and attitude of the parent
3. Ability of the child to sit still
4. Parent's willingness to work at it

38 Before Mrs. Brown leaves the clinic, the nurse tells her that she can best help her daughter learn to control her own behavior by:
1. Rewarding her for good behavior
2. Allowing her to learn by her mistakes
3. Punishing her when she deserves it
4. Setting limits and being consistent

Situation: Mrs. Allen, a gravida III, para 2, has an uneventful labor and delivery. After a 7-hour labor she delivers a 3692 g (8 lb 2 oz) baby girl spontaneously. Questions 39 through 44 refer to this situation.

39 Two hours after delivery, the nurse finds that Mrs. Allen's fundus is firm, shifted to the right, and 2 fingers above the umbilicus. This would indicate:
1. A normal process
2. Retained secundinae
3. A full bladder
4. Impending bleeding

40 After delivery, when checking Mrs. Allen's vital signs, the nurse should normally find:
1. An elevated basal temperature with a decrease in respirations
2. A decided bradycardia with no change in respirations

3. A slight lowering of basal temperature with an increase in respirations
4. A decided tachycardia with a decrease in respirations

41 Eight hours after delivery the nurse notices that Mrs. Allen is voiding frequently in small amounts. Intake and output are important in the early postpartal period, since small amounts of output:
1. Are commonly voided and should cause no alarm
2. May be indicative of beginning glomerulonephritis
3. May indicate retention of urine with overflow
4. Are common because less fluid is excreted following delivery

42 In helping Mrs. Allen develop her parenting role, the nurse should:
1. Do things for the baby in the mother's presence
2. Find out what she knows about babies and proceed from there
3. Demonstrate baby bathing and care before discharge
4. Provide enough time for her and the baby to be together

43 Mrs. Allen's infant develops a cephalhematoma. The nurse should plan to explain to Mrs. Allen that:
1. This usually does not occur with natural delivery
2. It will resolve spontaneously in 3 to 6 weeks
3. The swelling may cross a suture line
4. The soft sac will bulge when the infant cries

44 Nursing care of baby Allen is directed primarily toward:
1. Supporting the parents
2. Applying ice packs to the hematoma
3. Recording neurologic signs
4. Protecting the infant's head

Situation: *Mr. Boise, a 45-year-old tunnel guard, is diagnosed as having emphysema and is waiting for the examining physician. He has cyanosis of his lips and fingernails and is short of breath. Questions 45 through 52 refer to this situation.*

45 Mr. Boise's difficulty in breathing is caused by:
1. Spasm of the bronchi that traps the air
2. A too rapid expulsion of the air from the alveoli
3. An increase in the vital capacity of the lungs
4. Difficulty in expelling the air trapped in the alveoli

46 In which position should the nurse place Mr. Boise?
1. Moderate Fowler supported with pillows

2. Semirecumbent with one pillow
3. Sitting on the edge of the bed
4. Supine with his head slightly elevated

47 The nurse administers epinephrine hydrochloride (Adrenalin) immediately. The therapeutic respiratory effect of the drug is an outcome of action at:
1. Beta-adrenergic receptors in the bronchi and heart
2. Alpha-adrenergic receptors in the arteries and veins
3. Beta-adrenergic receptors in the arteries and veins
4. Alpha-adrenergic receptors in the bronchi and heart

48 The physician orders oxygen given in low concentration and intermittently, rather than in high concentration and continuously, to prevent:
1. Depression of the respiratory center
2. Decrease in red cell formation
3. Rupture of emphysematous bullae
4. Excessive drying of the respiratory mucosa

49 Mr. Boise has been advised to use an isoproterenol hydrochloride (Isuprel) inhaler for intermittent periods of bronchial constriction. The nurse should tell him he might have:
1. Slow pulse, headache, and muscle tension
2. Facial flushing, tingling in his fingers, and dizziness
3. Rapid pulse, dizziness, and pounding of his heart
4. Coldness of his fingers and toes, muscle cramps, and headache

50 When teaching the method of inhalation to Mr. Boise, the nurse explains that he should:
1. Inhale the vapors until all the drug has been nebulized
2. Stop inhaling the vapors as soon as he obtains relief
3. Never inhale more than 0.3 ml during any 20-minute period
4. Not repeat the dose more frequently than every 2 hours

51 The nurse also tells Mr. Boise that problems occurring with use of the inhaler can be lessened by following a few simple instructions:
1. Limit use of the drug to the time required for relief of dyspnea
2. Use rapid, shallow (panting) respirations while breathing through the inhaler
3. Interrupt the spray of inhalant while continuing normal breathing patterns
4. Gradually decrease pressure on the spray control after initial relief is obtained

52 Mr. Boise, who also has asthma, had been taking aminophylline at home. The planned effect of the drug is to:
1. Increase the ventilation perfusion ratio of the bronchioles
2. Stimulate chemoreceptor control of bronchial dilation
3. Dilate the bronchial and coronary arteries
4. Dilate the smooth muscles of the bronchi

Situation: *Mrs. Coan, 9 months pregnant, is admitted to the hospital with bleeding caused by possible placenta previa. The laboratory technician takes blood samples and IV fluids are begun. Questions 53 through 57 refer to this situation.*

53 The nurse, following the physician's orders, begins administering oxygen by mask. The patient's apprehension is increasing and she asks the nurse what is happening. The nurse tells her not to worry, that she is going to be all right and everything is under control. The nurse's statements are:
1. Correct, since only the physician should explain why treatments are being done
2. Proper, since the patient's anxieties would be increased if she knew the dangers
3. Adequate, since all preparations are routine and need no explanation
4. Questionable, since the patient has the right to know what treatment is being given and why

54 Nursing care of Mrs. Coan includes:
1. Withholding food and fluids
2. Encouraging ambulation with supervision
3. Inspecting the bed for hemorrhage
4. Avoiding all extraneous stimuli

55 If a vaginal examination is to be performed on Mrs. Coan, the nurse must be prepared for an immediate:
1. Induction of labor
2. Cesarean section
3. Forceps delivery
4. X-ray examination

56 Which of the following should Baby Coan, weighing 2840 g (6 lb 4 oz), have daily?
1. 740 ml (25 oz) of fluid and 450 calories
2. 592 ml (20 oz) of fluid and 400 calories
3. 532.8 ml (18 oz) of fluid and 375 calories
4. 888 ml (30 oz) of fluid and 500 calories

57 While working in the newborn nursery, the nurse observes a yellowish color in the skin of Baby Coan. The immediate nursing action should be to:
1. Cover the baby's eyes with a blindfold and put the baby under the ultraviolet light
2. Notify the physician of the development

3. Take a heel blood sample and send it to the laboratory
4. Ascertain the age of the infant

Situation: *Baby boy Charles Brown, 7 days old, is admitted to the pediatric unit from the nursery with a diagnosis of Down's syndrome. Questions 58 through 64 refer to this situation.*

58 Which of the following problems can be expected in caring for Baby Brown?
1. Slowed development as the child reaches 1 or 2 years of age
2. High incidence of circulatory problems.
3. Proneness to respiratory tract infections
4. Difficulty in hearing

59 The symptom of Down's syndrome most evident to the nursery nurse during the initial newborn assessment would be:
1. Asymmetric gluteal folds
2. Hypertonicity of the skeletal muscles
3. A rounded occiput
4. A transverse palmar (simian) crease

60 Special nursing care for Baby Brown should include:
1. Frequent handling and rocking to keep him from crying
2. Helping parents learn about their child
3. Teaching infant to nipple-feed
4. Preventing aspiration of formula by frequent bubbling

61 When observing a newborn with Down's syndrome, the nurse should be aware that a common defect associated with the condition is:
1. Deafness
2. Congenital heart defect
3. Hydrocephaly
4. Muscular hypertonicity

62 Which one of the following factors would probably be most significant for the nurse working with the Brown family? Mr. and Mrs. Brown's:
1. Response to family's and friends' reactions to their infant
2. Ability to give physical care to their infant
3. Ability to talk about changing plans they had made for their infant
4. Understanding of the factors causing Down's syndrome

63 As Charles grows, his development lags and it is found that he is moderately retarded. Which of the following suggestions would be most helpful to his parents? They should:
1. Offer challenging, competitive situations
2. Offer simple, repetitive tasks

3. Concentrate on teaching detailed tasks
4. Offer complete directions at the beginning of the task to be accomplished

64 The handicapped child has the same needs as the normal child, although his means of satisfying these needs are limited. This limitation frequently causes:
1. Emotional disability
2. Overcompensation
3. Frustration
4. Rejection

Situation: Mrs. Lamb is 39 years of age and has 3 children, aged 12, 9, and 5 years. She was admitted to the hospital with the diagnosis of severe metrorrhagia and menorrhagia of 1-year duration. She was found to have a submucous myoma that had grown over the past 6 months. Mrs. Lamb was told that a hysterectomy was necessary. Questions 65 through 69 refer to this situation.

65 The term *metrorrhagia* refers to:
1. Episodes of bleeding between menstrual periods
2. Severe bleeding during each menstrual period
3. Presence of blood in the vaginal discharge
4. Painful intercourse

66 To provide preoperative teaching the nurse should know that after a hysterectomy:
1. Ovarian hormone secretion ceases, but the hypophysis continues secretion of gonadotrophic hormones
2. The cyclical oscillation of hormones between the hypophysis and ovaries continues
3. Menstruation ceases and ovarian hormone secretion decreases
4. Menopause begins immediately with the cessation of ovarian hormone production

67 Mrs. Lamb is recovering from the hysterectomy. Which of the following signs would be indicative of a developing thrombophlebitis?
1. A reddened area at the ankle
2. Pruritus on the calf and thigh
3. Pitting edema of the ankle
4. A tender, painful area on the leg

68 As the nurse walks into Mrs. Lamb's room on the fifth postoperative day, the patient asks for sanitary pads because she feels as if she is going to menstruate. The nurse's response is based on knowledge of which of the following statements?
1. Mrs. Lamb will have a surgical menopause
2. It will take several weeks before Mrs. Lamb has a normal menstrual flow
3. Mrs. Lamb is showing signs of psychosomatic responses

4. The postoperative appearance of frank vaginal bleeding is expected

69 Mrs. Lamb's roommate has undergone a hysterectomy and oophorectomy. Her therapy differs from Mrs. Lamb's in that she is receiving estrogen therapy to suppress:
1. Heat intolerance
2. Flushing of the face
3. Premature aging
4. Dysmenorrhea

Situation: Miss Daley, a 24-year-old secretary, is pregnant for the first time. She discussed the pregnancy with her boyfriend, who told her everything would work out fine. Two days later she received a letter from him with $500 and the news that he had left town. Miss Daley is very upset, feels at the end of her rope, and calls the crisis intervention center for help. Questions 70 through 74 refer to this situation.

70 The nurse recognizes that Miss Daley is experiencing a crisis because:
1. She is under a great deal of stress
2. Her boyfriend left her when she was pregnant
3. She is going to have to raise her child alone
4. Her past methods of adapting are ineffective for this situation

71 The nurse suggests a crisis intervention group. These groups are successful because the:
1. Client is encouraged to talk about herself
2. Client is assisted to investigate alternative approaches to solving the identified problem
3. Crisis intervention worker is a psychologist and understands behavior patterns
4. Client is supplied with a workable solution to her problems

72 When talking with Miss Daley, the crisis intervention nurse should:
1. Respect her and involve her in deciding what she will do and how she will do it
2. Restate the problem, putting it in the proper perspective
3. Explain to her that the center has helped many other people with the same problem
4. Explore her religious and cultural beliefs so the instructions are within her value system

73 Miss Daley has decided to go through with the pregnancy and keep the baby. Now the crisis intervention nurse's primary responsiblity is to:
1. Support her for making a wise decision
2. Make an appointment for her to see a physician for prenatal care
3. Explore other problems she may be experiencing

4. Provide information about other health resources where she may receive additional assistance

74 Miss Daley is now excited and looking forward to caring for her baby. The nurse recognizes her decision to attend prenatal child care classes is an example of:
1. Extrinsic motivation
2. Operant conditioning
3. Intrinsic motivation
4. Behavior modification

Situation: After an uneventful labor and delivery Mrs. Handler delivers a 3181 g (7 lb) boy with a bilateral cleft lip and palate. She does not see the baby in the delivery room. Mr. Handler has been told of the defect and has seen the baby. He is very upset, but his major concern is for his wife and her reaction. Questions 75 through 78 refer to this situation.

75 While looking at the baby, Mr. Handler says to the nursery nurse, "Oh, what am I going to do, how could this happen to us, what is my wife going to do? It would have been better if she had never become pregnant." The most appropriate response for the nurse to make is:
1. "How can you say that? You have a lovely healthy baby; the cleft lip can be fixed and then the baby will be fine."
2. "I know how hard this must be for you. But believe me, you will love the baby so much, you won't even notice that he is disfigured."
3. "This must be very hard on you. Would it help if I went with you when the doctor talks to your wife?"
4. "I know that this is very difficult for you. But you can't think of yourself now. Your wife needs you. You must be strong."

76 After the physician talks to Mrs. Handler, she seems quite composed and asks to see the baby. To assess Mrs. Handler's reaction, the nurse should:
1. Bring the baby to her immediately
2. Tell her exactly what the baby looks like before bringing him to her
3. Encourage her to express and explore her feelings; bring the baby to her and stay with her during this time
4. Show her some pictures and give her some literature on harelip and cleft palate and discuss the treatment with her before bringing the baby to her

77 When Mrs. Handler sees the baby, she becomes very disturbed, pushes him away, and says, "Oh, take him away, I never want to see him again."

This reaction would indicate to the nurse that Mrs. Handler is:
1. Unable to cope with the situation and that arrangements will have to be made to place the baby in a foster home, at least for the first few months
2. Responding as most normal new mothers, who find it difficult to accept that their baby is less than perfect
3. Severely emotionally disturbed and is in immediate need of psychiatric help
4. Rejecting the baby and he will have to be placed for adoption

78 Afterward Mrs. Handler asks how she is going to feed the baby if his mouth is deformed and he cannot suck properly. The nurse teaches her carefully and gently how feedings are to be given and states:
1. "Try using a soft nipple with an enlarged opening so that he can get the milk through a chewing motion"
2. "Since he tires easily, it is best to have him lying in bed while he is being fed"
3. "He should be held in a horizontal position and fed slowly to avoid aspiration"
4. "Give him brief rest periods and frequent burpings during feedings to expel swallowed air"

Situation: Mrs. Heath is scheduled for electromyography (EMG) after being admitted to the hospital for paresis and pain of the left leg. Questions 79 through 83 refer to this situation.

79 Before the electromyography the nurse should explain that:
1. Needles will be inserted into the affected muscles during the test
2. Mrs. Heath will be kept in a recumbent position after the procedure
3. Mrs. Heath's heart rate and rhythm will be frequently monitored
4. The involved area will be shaved immediately before testing

80 After further testing, Mrs. Heath is diagnosed as having a herniated intervertebral disc. She is complaining of pain. The nurse recognizes that the pain is caused by the:
1. Increased pressure of cerebrospinal fluid within the vertebral column
2. Compression of the spinal cord by the extruded nucleus pulposus
3. Shifting of two adjacent vertebral bodies out of alignment
4. The inflammation of the lamina of the involved vertebrae

81 The nurse should teach Mrs. Heath that the pain will most likely increase if she:
1. Sits for long periods
2. Flexes her knees
3. Coughs excessively
4. Lies on her side

82 To limit Mrs. Heath's pain, the nurse should anticipate the need for:
1. Maintenance doses of narcotic analgesics
2. Prolonged application of heat
3. Maintenance of a prone position
4. Use of a lumbar supportive device

83 Mrs. Heath requests the bedpan. The nurse should:
1. Slide the bedpan into place while Mrs. Heath pulls up on the trapeze
2. Assist her to roll first to her side and then back onto a fracture pan
3. Tell Mrs. Heath to first flex her knees and then raise her hips
4. Enlist the aid of another nurse to lift Mrs. Heath onto the bedpan

Situation: After a car accident Ed, an 18-year-old high school senior, is taken to the local hospital with a back injury. He did not lose consciousness and remembers that he was unable to move his legs following the accident. Questions 84 through 89 refer to this situation.

84 After an accident in which there is a questionable back injury, the individual involved:
1. May be transported in sitting position, if necessary, to secure immediate medical care
2. May be transported in any position because position is not important, since damage to the cord has already occurred
3. Should be protected from flexion and hyperextension of the spine
4. May be transported best when placed in the side-lying position

85 After the examination the physician indicates that Ed is paraplegic. His family asks the nurse what this means. The nurse explains that:
1. Both lower and upper extremities are paralyzed
2. Upper extremities are paralyzed
3. One side of the body is paralyzed
4. Lower extremities are paralyzed

86 When caring for Ed, the nurse should plan to provide a high intake of fluid to help:
1. Prevent elevation of temperature
2. Maintain electrolyte balance
3. Prevent dehydration
4. Prevent urinary tract infection

87 Teaching Ed to care for himself while in the hospital is:
1. Unnecessary; he will be back to normal when he leaves the hospital
2. Avoided; it is too complicated to be undertaken by a layperson
3. Unnecessary; his family will be able to care for him at home
4. An essential part of his nursing care plan

88 The paraplegic patient frequently loses calcium from the skeletal system. Which of the following factors contributes to this condition?
1. Decreased activity
2. Decreased calcium intake
3. Inadequate kidney function
4. Inadequate fluid intake

89 Sympathetic hyperreflexia is a syndrome seen in patients with spinal cord injuries. The signs and symptoms include diaphoresis, pulsating headaches, and goose bumps. This syndrome may occur when:
1. The bowel and/or sheath is deteriorating
2. The myelin sheath is deteriorating
3. The patient is upright on a tilt table
4. The spinal cord is crushed rather than severed

Situation: Mrs. Virginia Rose, a 39-year-old married woman, is admitted to the psychiatric service with the diagnosis of anxiety disorder. Questions 90 through 94 refer to this situation.

90 The nurse and Mrs. Rose walk to a quiet corner of the unit. Mrs. Rose's anxiety mounts. She becomes increasingly restless, moving rapidly from one foot to the other, and wringing her hands. Her face is contorted as though she is in pain. The nurse suddenly feels uncomfortable and experiences a strong desire to leave. The probable reason for feeling is the:
1. Empathic communication of anxiety
2. Desire to go off duty after a busy day
3. Inability to tolerate any more bizarre behavior
4. Fear of the patient's becoming assaultive

91 Mrs. Rose is crying and states that she has never been in the hospital except to have children. The nurse realizes that an environment conducive to reducing emotional stress and providing psychologic safety is one in which:
1. Needs are a primary concern
2. All the patient's needs are met
3. Realistic limits and controls are set
4. The physical environment is kept in order

92 Mrs. Rose attempts to manipulate the staff and control situations. Just before the nurse is to go off

duty she is confronted by Mrs. Rose, who says, "That feeling, it may come back. I'm so afraid that the evening staff won't like me like this. They'll seclude me." The nurse can best assist the patient by saying:

1. "Don't worry, I told you that you'd be all right."
2. "Mrs. Rose, you know I leave at this time. Can we talk about this in the morning?"
3. "Tell me more about what you're feeling now."
4. "I'll ask the staff not to lock you up."

93 The next afternoon Mrs. Rose meets the nurse in the hallway. She says, "That was a terrible feeling I had yesterday. I'm so afraid to talk about it." The nurse's most useful response would be:

1. "Okay, let's not talk about it."
2. "It's best that you try to talk about it."
3. "What were you doing yesterday when you first noticed the feeling?"
4. "Don't worry; that feeling probably won't come back."

94 Mrs. Rose cries bitterly after a conference with her psychiatrist. She pounds the bed in frustration and threatens to kill herself. What response by the nurse would be most helpful?

1. Pat her reassuringly on the back and say, "I know it is hard to bear."
2. Sit beside her and listen attentively if she wishes to talk about the situation
3. Ask her to talk about her troubles and point out that other people also have problems
4. Leave her for a short period until she regains control

Situation: Mrs. Clare, a 49-year-old woman with scleroderma, comes to the physician's office for a routine checkup. Questions 95 through 99 refer to this situation.

95 Mrs. Clare complains that she has been having difficulty chewing and swallowing. In counseling her about her diet, the nurse should advise her to:

1. Liquefy her food in a high-speed blender
2. Take frequent sips of water with her meals
3. Use a local anesthetic mouthwash before eating
4. Puree all foods to reduce chewing

96 Mrs. Clare tells the nurse that she frequently has numbness and tingling in her hands followed by blanching of her fingers. The nurse recognizes that she has Raynaud's phenomenon, a condition frequently associated with scleroderma. The proper advice for Mrs. Clare is to:

1. Take anticoagulants that will be prescribed to prevent attacks
2. Bathe her hands frequently in hot water
3. Briskly rub her hands to increase circulation
4. Keep her hands warm by wearing gloves

97 As part of the teaching plan, Mrs. Clare is informed of the need for special skin care. The nurse should advise her to:

1. Keep her skin well lubricated with oil
2. Take frequent baths to remove scaly lesions
3. Use calamine lotion for pruritus
4. Apply warm soaks to the inflamed areas

98 The physician orders a regimen of daily exercises for Mrs. Clare. The nurse understands that exercises are performed to:

1. Preserve muscle strength
2. Prevent spread of the disease
3. Promote a sense of well-being
4. Promote tissue regeneration

99 Mrs. Clare complains of heartburn in her epigastric area after eating. Which of the following recommendations by the nurse is most appropriate?

1. Lie down for about an hour after eating
2. Take an antacid before eating
3. Eat small, frequent meals
4. Avoid eating large amounts of carbohydrates

Situation: Carrie Walsh, a 39-year-old primigravida, is admitted to labor and delivery for sonography to determine fetal age, since she appears to be large for her expected date of delivery. She is 36 weeks pregnant, but her uterus is the size expected at 40 weeks. Questions 100 through 102 refer to this situation.

100 Before the test begins, Mrs. Walsh complains of severe abdominal pain. Her blood pressure drops from 128/80 to 102/60, and her pulse rate increases from 80 to 104. Heavy vaginal bleeding begins with the onset of the pain. The nurse should suspect that Mrs. Walsh has a:

1. Marginal placenta previa
2. Complete abruptio placentae
3. Vena caval syndrome
4. Hydatidiform mole

101 The nurse notifies the physician of Mrs. Walsh's condition and prepares for:

1. A high forceps delivery
2. An immediate cesarean section
3. The insertion of a fetal monitor
4. The administration of oxytocin (Pitocin)

102 Mrs. Walsh is prepared for delivery. Nursing care for this patient should include:

1. An abdominal prep and administration of a Fleet enema

2. Inserting a Foley catheter and administration of a tap water enema
3. Obtaining an informed consent and assessment for drug allergies
4. Teaching coughing and deep-breathing techniques

Situation: Jason Agnew, 6 months old, is brought to the emergency room with a fever of unknown origin and projectile vomiting. Because meningitis is suspected, he is admitted to the pediatric unit. Questions 103 through 105 refer to this situation.

103 Which one of the following tests would be done immediately to confirm the diagnosis of meningitis?
1. Meningomyelogram
2. Peripheral skin smears
3. Lumbar puncture
4. Blood cultures

104 Jason is receiving 500 ml of IV fluid per 24 hours. Using an IV set with a drop rate of 60 drops/ml, the nurse should plan to regulate the IV at:
1. 8 drops per minute
2. 13 drops per minute
3. 21 drops per minute
4. 24 drops per minute

105 According to Piaget's theory of cognitive development, which of the following should Jason be demonstrating?
1. Beginning of object permanence
2. Repetitious use of reflexes
3. Early traces of memory
4. Beginning sense of time

Situation: After trying for several years, Mr. and Mrs. Gosney have succeeded in becoming parents. He is a successful lawyer, and she teaches at the local community college. Questions 106 through 113 refer to this situation.

106 When Mrs. Gosney is 10 weeks pregnant, she calls the gynecologist's office and complains of morning sickness, which interferes with her job. What might the nurse suggest to promote relief?
1. Increasing her protein intake before bedtime
2. Eating dry crackers before arising
3. Having two small meals daily and a snack at noon
4. Drinking more high-carbohydrate fluids with meals.

107 Mrs. Gosney complains of feeling tired. The nurse recognizes that this is probably related to which of the following cardiovascular changes?
1. Decrease in cardiac output

2. Increase in hematocrit
3. Increase in blood volume
4. Increase in blood pressure

108 When Mrs. Gosney is 36 weeks pregnant, her membranes rupture spontaneously. The physician calls and informs the delivery room that her cervix is 2 cm dilated and 75% effaced and that she is being admitted. When Mr. and Mrs. Gosney arrive, the nurse should:
1. Immediately attach an external fetal monitor to evaluate the fetal heart
2. Have them wait in the admission room while the nurse notifies the physician that they have arrived
3. Send Mrs. Gosney to the admission room to undress while the nurse takes her history from Mr. Gosney.
4. Introduce self to Mr. and Mrs. Gosney and try to make them feel welcome.

109 Mrs. Gosney's labor progresses. She should be moved to the delivery room when the nurses observes:
1. An increase in the amount of bloody discharge from the perineum
2. That she is becoming irritable and does not follow instructions
3. That her perineum is beginning to bulge with each contraction
4. That her contractions are occurring every 2 to 3 minutes and lasting 60 seconds

110 Mrs. Gosney delivers a 2953.6 g (6½ lb) baby boy. She becomes extremely upset that her newborn son has a nevus vasculosus on the midthigh. The nurse can best respond by telling her:
1. "This is a superficial area that will fade in a few days."
2. "This mark will not grow or fade, but will be covered by clothes."
3. "The area will spread rapidly and then regress."
4. "Surgical removal will be necessary as soon as the infant is older."

111 Mrs. Gosney plans to breast-feed her baby. The nurse helps Mrs. Gosney understand the advantages of breast-feeding by explaining that:
1. Allergic responses are diminished in breast-fed infants
2. Breast milk has a larger concentration of protein than does cow's milk
3. Breast-fed infants adhere more easily to a 4-hour schedule
4. Breast-feeding inhibits ovulation in the mother

112 Mrs. Gosney is being discharged. In teaching her to care for her newborn who, has just been circumcised, the nurse should instruct her to:
1. Observe for fussy behavior
2. Observe for yellow exudate
3. Apply petrolatum gauze to the penis
4. Leave the infant undiapered

113 After 6 months, Mrs. Gosney returns to work. Shortly thereafter, she is appointed Dean of Students. Mr. and Mrs. Gosney decide to postpone adding to their family, and Mrs. Gosney has an IUD inserted. Immediately following insertion, the nurse explains, it is important that she observe for:
1. Nausea, rash, and bleeding
2. Lethargy, syncope, and tachycardia
3. Syncope, diaphoresis, and bradycardia
4. Bradycardia, visual changes, and hypertension

Situation: *Miss Jean Bradley is admitted to the hospital for a thyroidectomy. She is 27 years old, and the physical assessment reveals no other health problems. Questions 114 through 116 refer to this situation.*

114 Immediately after Miss Bradley's surgery the nurse should be especially observant for:
1. Signs of restlessness
2. Increased blood pressure
3. Urinary retention
4. Signs of respiratory obstruction

115 Nerve injury can occur as a result of the trauma of surgery. When assessing for this complication, the nurse should evaluate Miss Bradley's ability to:
1. Swallow
2. Purse her lips
3. Turn her head
4. Speak

116 On the first postoperative day Miss Bradley tolerates a full fluid diet. This is changed to soft on the second postoperative day. She then complains of a sore throat when swallowing. The nurse should:
1. Reorder the full fluid diet
2. Notify the physician immediately
3. Administer analgesics as prescribed prior to meals
4. Provide a humidifer to moisten the mucous membranes

Situation: *Miss Abigal Jones, age 17 years, is admitted to the obstetric unit in labor. She is 41 weeks pregnant and experiencing mild contractions every 15 minutes, lasting 10 seconds each. Vaginal examination reveals the cervix to be 1 cm dilated, membranes intact, and vertex at station − 1. A fetal monitor is used. Questions 117 through 120 refer to this situation.*

117 One problem that confronts the client when an external indirect fetal monitor is being used is the:
1. Restriction of movement
2. Interference with Lamaze techniques
3. Increased frequency of vaginal examinations
4. Inability to take sedatives

118 The nurse asks about Abigail's marital status. Abigal refuses to answer and becomes very agitated, telling the nurse to leave. The nurse should:
1. Have restricted questions to those relevant to the situation
2. Have this information to complete the patient's history
3. Question the family about the marital status of the patient
4. Refer the patient to a social service organization for help

119 After an 8-hour uneventful labor Miss Jones delivers a baby boy spontaneously under epidural block anesthesia. As the nurse places the baby in her arms immediately following delivery, she asks, "Is he normal?" The most appropriate answer would be:
1. "Of course he is; your pregnancy and labor were so normal."
2. "Shall we unwrap him so you can look him over for yourself?"
3. "He must be all right, he has such a good strong cry."
4. "Most babies are normal; of course he is."

120 The major concern for a pregnant out-of-wedlock teenager is that she is:
1. Socially ostracized
2. Diabetogenic
3. Financially dependent
4. Prone to toxemia

How to Use Worksheet 1: Errors in Processing Information

Common errors in processing information are listed in the left hand column of this worksheet. At the top of the worksheet is a row of blank spaces for inserting the number of the question missed. Directly below each number, check any errors you made in answering that question. You may have made more than one type of error in an answer.

Worksheet 1: Errors in Processing Information

Question no.																							
Did not read situation/question carefully																							
Missed important details																							
Confused major and minor points																							
Defined problem incorrectly																							
Could not remember terms/facts/concepts/ principles																							
Defined terms incorrectly																							
Focused on incomplete/incorrect data in assessing situation																							
Interpreted data incorrectly																							
Applied wrong concepts/principles in situation																							
Drew incorrect conclusions																							
Identified wrong goals																							
Identified priorities incorrectly																							
Carried out plan incorrectly/incompletely																							
Was unclear about criteria for evaluating success in achieving goals																							

How to Use Worksheet 2: Knowledge Gaps

Types of common knowledge gaps are listed along the top of this worksheet. Write a brief description of topics you want to review in the spaces provided. For example, if you missed a question on administration of a particular drug, write the drug name and problem (e.g., dosage) in the appropriate space under the column labeled Pharmacology.

Worksheet 2: Knowledge Gaps

Basic science	Skills/ procedures	Basic human needs	Growth & develop- ment	Normal nutrition	Psycho- social factors	Clinical area/ topic	Stressors/ coping mechanisms	Patho- physiology	Pharma- cology	Therapeutic nutrition	Legal implications	Other

Answers and Rationales

1. (2) Streptococcal infections occurring in childhood may result in damage to the heart valves. An autoimmune reaction occurs between antibodies made against the bacteria and the heart valves, particularly the mitral. (b); AS; AN; SH; ME
   (1) Rubella virus would not affect the vales of the heart.
   (3) Pleurisy usually follows pulmonary problems unrelated to streptococcal infection; would not result in damage to the heart valve.
   (4) Cystitis is usually caused by *Escherichia coli,* which would not affect the heart valves.

2. (2) The pulse should be assessed, since a cutdown may interfere with venous flow distal to the site. There is also a danger of phlebitis in the area. (a); IM; AP; SH; SU
   (1) The patient does not usually require additional rest after catheterization.
   (3) It is not necessary to check the ECG every 30 minutes following the procedure.
   (4) This would be determined on an individual basis; not routine.

3. (2) The nurse should foster open lines of communication with the patient. (a); IM; AP; SH; PS
   (1) Cuts off further communication.
   (3) Blocks additional verbalization; puts the patient on the defensive.
   (4) Cuts off further communication; does not recognize the patient's concern.

4. (1) Because blood pools in the extremities, there is an increased hazard of peripheral emboli in patients who have received a mitral replacement. (c); IM; AP; SH; SU
   (2) This is not a danger after mitral replacement.
   (3) Bleeding is detected by checking the wound dressing and observing for signs of shock (e.g., lowered blood pressure, tachycardia, restlessness).
   (4) Peripheral pulses alone will not reveal atrial fibrillation; to detect the presence of a pulse deficit, one must compare them with the apical pulses.

5. (3) Temperatures over 38.9° C (102.2° F) lead to increased metabolism and cardiac workload. (a); AN; AN; NU; SU
   (1) Elevated temperature is not an early sign of developing cerebral edema, although the temperature may rise eventually because of medullary compression.
   (2) Fever is unrelated to hemorrhage; in hemorrhage with shock, the temperature decreases.
   (4) These symptoms are caused by an elevated temperature, which is the primary reason for increased metabolism and cardiac workload.

6. (4) Fluid will accumulate in the intrapleural space after thoracic surgery because of trauma and the inflammatory response. During the first 24 hours 500 ml of fluid is not uncommon. Gradually this amount will decrease. (c); AS; AP; NU; SU
   (1) Excessive amount; may indicate complications.
   (2) When no air leak is noted and less than 150 ml of fluid is aspirated in 24 hours, the tube may be removed.
   (3) Excessive amount; may indicate complications.

7. (1) Chills, headache, nausea, and vomiting are all signs of a transfusion reaction. (a); IM; AN; NU; SU
   (2) The infusion must be stopped before treatment of the symptoms begins.
   (3) The physician should be notified after the transfusion is stopped.
   (4) Slowing the infusion will continue the reaction; may lead to kidney damage.

8. (3) Shivering should be prevented. Peripheral vasoconstriction increases the temperature, the circulatory rate, and oxygen consumption. (b); IM; CP; NU; SU
   (1) Not a response to treatment with hypothermia.
   (2) Not a response to treatment with hypothermia.
   (4) Not a response to treatment with hypothermia.

9. (4) The patient's exact compliance in carrying out the compulsive ritual relieves anxiety, at least temporarily. Furthermore, it meets a need and is necessary to the patient. (a); AN; CP; SH; PS
   (1) The person cannot stop the activity; it is not under voluntary control.
   (2) Urging has no effect on trying to have the patient start or stop the ritualistic behavior.
   (3) The compulsive act is purposeless repetition and useful only in that it decreases anxiety for the patient.

10. (3) The anxiety disorders are characterized by anxiety and minor distortions of reality. The anxiety results in an inability to reach a decision, since all alternatives are threatening. (a); AS; CP; NU; PS
    (1) Just the opposite is true; part of emotional maturity is the ability to relate to people, and these people have difficulties in this area.
    (2) Would be indicative of severe emotional illness, not an anxiety disorder.
    (4) Would be indicative of an affective disorder.

11. (4) Rituals are a means for the individual to control anxiety. If not permitted to carry out ritual, the patient will probably experience unbearable anxiety. (c); IM; AP; SH; PS
    (1) Mrs. Ivy understands this already but is unable to stop the activity.
    (2) She has no idea what the ritual means; only that she must continue with it.
    (3) This would have the effect of increasing anxiety in Mrs. Ivy, possibly to panic levels.

12. (2) Since the compulsive ritual is used to control anxiety, any attempt to prevent the action would greatly increase the anxiety. (c); EV; CP; CL; PS

(1) Possible only if the anxiety reached panic levels and caused the person overtly to express anger.

(3) Not a pattern of behavior associated with this disorder.

(4) Underlying hostility is considered to be part of the disorder itself; not a reaction to an interruption of the ritual.

13. (3) Because of its proximity to the heart, the carotid pulse is used to determine whether the ventricles are contracting effectively. The absence of a carotid pulse, in the absence of other vascular problems, indicates ventricular fibrillation or standstill, and immediate cardiopulmonary resuscitation is required to prevent death. (a); AS; AN; NU; ME

(1) If the patient has had a cardiac arrest, CPR should be instituted immediately to prevent irreversible brain damage.

(2) If the pulse is absent, there is no blood pressure to be measured.

(4) The presence or absence of the carotid pulse will determine the nature of assistance needed.

14. (3) CPR carried out by 1 person is less efficient than that performed by 2. Approximately 80 compressions per minute are needed to provide adequate tissue perfusion. (b); IM; KN; NU; ME

(1) This ratio would be used when 2 people were administering CPR.

(2) Ineffective; would result in the circulation of unoxygenated blood.

(4) Ineffective; blood would not be circulated while four breaths were being administered, and thus hypoxia would result.

15. (2) This provides the best leverage for depressing the sternum. Thus the heart is adequately compressed, and blood is forced into the arteries. Grasping the fingers keeps them off the chest and concentrates the energy expended in the heel of the hand while minimizing the possibility of fracturing ribs. (a); IM; AP; NU; ME

(1) Pressure spread over 2 hands may inadequately compress the heart and fracture the ribs.

(3) Application of pressure by the fingers is less effective; inadequate cardiac compression.

(4) Both hands must be utilized; pressure on the lower portion of the sternum may fracture the xiphoid process, which can injure vital underlying organs.

16. (1) Hair and oils in the skin may interfere with conduction of electric impulses. Therefore the chest hair immediately around the site may need to be shaved; the area must be scrubbed to remove oils and debris. (c); IM; AP; NU; ME

(2) The use of an antimicrobial agent is unnecessary since there will be no break in the skin.

(3) Moisture will prevent adherence of the electrodes and thus interfere with impulse conduction.

(4) Electrode paste facilitates conduction of electrical impulses and is used regardless of excoriation.

17. (3) When ventricular fibrillation is verified, the first intervention is defibrillation. It is the only measure that will terminate this lethal arrhythmia. (b); PL; AN; NU; ME

(1) Digitalis preparations are not used in the treatment of ventricular arrhythmias.

(2) If not already in place, an IV line should be inserted as soon as the patient is defibrillated.

(4) Electric cardioversion delivers a shock during the R wave; since there is no R wave in ventricular fibrillation, the arrhythmia would continue and death would result.

18. (3) In the absence of oxygen, the body derives its energy anaerobically. This results in a buildup of lactic acid. Sodium bicarbonate, an alkaline drug, will help neutralize the acid, raising the pH back to normal. (a); PL; AP; NU; ME

(1) Although potassium is essential for cardiac function, it will not correct acidosis.

(2) Calcium gluconate is used primarily in the treatment of hypocalcemia, but its inotropic effect may be utilized in the management of cardiac arrest.

(4) Insulin is used in the treatment of diabetes mellitus; it lowers blood sugar by facilitating the transport of glucose across cell membranes.

19. (1) When protein intake is inadequate, the liver is unable to manufacture albumin, the major plasma protein. There is a drop in intravascular collodial osmotic pressure, with a resulting fluid shift to the interstitial spaces. (c); AN; CP; NU; ME

(2) The renin/aldosterone mechanism is not directly linked to inadequate nutrition

(3) ADH is secreted when the intravascular osmotic pressure increases, not decreases.

(4) Nitrogen balance is the relationship between intake and output of nitrogen; linked only indirectly to fluid shifts.

20. (1) Hyperalimentation should be infused at a slow, constant rate. This will prevent both cellular dehydration from too rapid infusion of hypertonic solutions and hyperglycemia. (b); PL; AP; NU; SU

(2) Monitoring vital signs may indicate a complication such as infection; will not prevent it.

(3) Generally a major vein is selected for administration of hyperalimentation; the site is not changed every 24 hours.

(4) Recording intake and output is essential because of the danger of fluid overload; however, will not prevent the complication.

21. (3) A gastrostomy is an opening made directly through the abdominal wall into the stomach. When tube feedings are given via this route, they bypass the upper GI tract and reduce the risk of tracheal aspiration. (b); PL; CP; SH; SU

(1) The amount of feeding is not affected.

(2) Both methods utilize gravity.

(4) Patients can be taught to feed themselves with either method.

22. (4) A rise in the level of formula within the tube indicates a full stomach. (a); EV; AP; NU; SU
   (1) Passage of flatus reflects intestinal motility, which does not pose a potential problem.
   (2) A rapid inflow is the result of holding the container too high or using a feeding tube with too large a lumen.
   (3) Epigastric tenderness is not necessarily caused by a full stomach.

23. (2) Water is administered after the tube feeding to prevent the thicker feeding solution from obstructing the lumen of the tube. (b); IM; AP; CL; SU
   (1) Tube feedings are best tolerated at body temperature.
   (3) To prevent regurgitation and aspiration, a Fowler position is recommended.
   (4) If the feeding tube is incorrectly situated in the trachea, administration of fluid may cause aspiration pneumonia.

24. (1) Since mastication of food is a psychologically satisfying activity, patients are advised to chew their food before putting it in the blender. (c); IM; AP; CL; SU
   (2) The texture as well as the taste of food provides a source of satisfaction; not experienced when food enters the stomach directly through a feeding tube.
   (3) The texture as well as the taste of food provides a source of satisfaction; not experienced when food enters the stomach directly through a feeding tube.
   (4) The texture as well as the taste of food provides a source of satisfaction; not experienced when food enters the stomach directly through a feeding tube.

25. (1) Patients use delusions as a defense and cannot be argued out of them. The nurse's response did not demonstrate acceptance of the patient and only added to her anxiety and agitation. (b); EV; AP; SH; PS
   (2) There is nothing to indicate that treatment has not been started toward relieving these symptoms.
   (3) Mrs. Gold should have a one-to-one relationship before attempting to relate to other patients on the unit.
   (4) That would be masking the problem rather than planning more suitable intervention.

26. (3) Electroconvulsive therapy helps relieve severe depression by interrupting established patterns of behavior, thereby limiting possible suicide attempts. (a); EV; AP; SH; PS
   (1) This would be used if the patient showed little or no response to the antidepressants.
   (2) Psychotherapy combined with antidepressants is the treatment of choice; not psychoanalysis.
   (4) Psychotherapy is helping the person learn new coping mechanisms and better ways of dealing with problems; the depressed patient needs direction to accomplish this.

27. (3) Feelings of hopelessness, helplessness, and isolation dominate the emotional state of the depressed patient. The ability to attempt to act out suicide ideation frequently does not occur until psychomotor depression begins to lift. (a); AN; CP; NU; PS
   (1) This is not true; they frequently attempt suicide.
   (2) This is when the danger is greatest; more energy at this time to follow through on a plan.
   (4) A person intent on self-destruction will find a way on any type of unit.

28. (4) Preoccupied patients are usually not aware of events in the environment. The patient has not refused to eat but has simply not responded to external stimuli. Taking her by the hand to the dining hall simply puts her where she needs to be. (c); IM; AP; SH; PS
   (1) She may be too preoccupied to eat anything; part of intervention is aimed at her nutritional needs.
   (2) She probably would not care and will not respond.
   (3) This would allow a withdrawal pattern to continue.

29. (1) Spending time with patients communicates to them that the staff members feel they are worthy of their attention and that someone cares. (b); IM; CP; SH; PS
   (2) The goal is eventually to have her relate to the other patients not get away from them.
   (3) Nothing indicates that she has a delusion regarding food.
   (4) It does give her some special attention, but the goal is to increase her self-esteem and have her believe she is a worthwhile person.

30. (2) The therapeutic level of lithium carbonate is very close to the toxic level. Therefore it is vital that blood levels of the drug be monitored twice a week during the acute phase and bimonthly once the patient is on maintenance dosage. (c); EV; AP; NU; PS
   (1) Lithium does not affect fluid retention; monitoring daily weights is not necessary.
   (3) Psychomotor activity should decrease once the maintenance dosage is achieved; careful monitoring, though, is not a major priority.
   (4) Lithium does not affect the leukocyte levels; monitoring the leukocyte count is unnecessary.

31. (4) Lithium decreases sodium reabsorption by the renal tubules. If sodium intake is decreased, sodium depletion can occur. In addition, lithium retention is increased when sodium intake is decreased; a low-sodium intake can lead to lithium toxicity. (c); IM; AP; CL; PS
   (1) Patients should never adjust the dosage of prescribed medication without the physician's approval.
   (2) This would not have any effect on the lithium therapy.
   (3) If the patient were well enough to go home for 3 days, participation in controversial discussions would not be contraindicated.

32. (3) A predominant clinical sign of croup is reactive spasm of the laryngeal muscles, which produces partial respiratory obstruction. Cough is tight, with a barking metallic sound. (b); AS; CP; NU; PE
    (1) Children with croup experience spasm of the larynx rather than the bronchi; whooping cough (pertussis) is a separate communicable disease.
    (2) Children with croup experience inspiratory rather than expiratory stridor.
    (4) The cough of croup is tight and nonproductive.
33. (2) Syrup of ipecac is a nonprescription emetic causing vomiting. It helps interrupt the laryngospasm characteristic of croup. (c); IM; AN; CL; PE
    (1) This does not interrupt the laryngospasm associated with croup.
    (3) This is a prescription drug; not something parents can give to interrupt the attack.
    (4) This too is a prescription drug; although it will cause bronchodilation, it will not help laryngospasm.
34. (3) Ipecac causes forceful vomiting. The reversal of peristalsis puts pressure on the glottis and interrupts the spasm. (b); AN; AP; NU; PE
    (1) Ipecac does not cause bronchodilation.
    (2) Ipecac does not reduce inflammation.
    (4) Ipecac does not influence the cough center.
35. (2) The toddler is in Erikson's stage of acquiring a sense of autonomy. The negativism is the result of Molly's need to express her will and test out her environment. (a); AN; AP; SH; PE
    (1) She does not assert herself to obtain discipline.
    (3) Although this is a factor, toddlers assert themselves in an attempt to attain more autonomy.
    (4) This is the development task achieved in infancy.
36. (4) Children who are expressing negativism need to have a feeling of control. One way of achieving this within reasonable limits is for the parent or care giver to provide a choice of 2 items, rather than force one on the child. (a); IM; AN; CL; PE
    (1) Will probably not be successful with a toddler; will probably end in disaster.
    (2) Will not achieve the goal of giving her fluids.
    (3) Will only complicate the situation and further inhibit the child's willingness to take fluids.
37. (2) The parents' attitude, approach, and understanding of the child's physical and psychologic readiness are essential to letting the child proceed at his own pace with appropriate interventions by the parent. (a); PL; CP; SH; PE
    (1) This will not be the major motivation for toilet training.
    (3) Although this will definitely be a factor, it is not a major one.
    (4) This, of course, is a factor; but the major factor is the child herself, who is strongly influenced by the parents' attitudes and approach.
38. (4) Children learn socially acceptable behavior when consistent reasonable limits that provide guidelines are established. (b); IM; AP; CL; PE
    (1) Rewards should not always be necessary for good behavior; will become expected.
    (2) Not always safe or reasonable for very young children.
    (3) Authorities vary on their attitudes about punishment; it should not, however, become the major means of teaching children to control their behavior.
39. (3) A distended bladder usually displaces the fundus upward and toward the right. (a); AN; CP; NU; OB
    (1) The normal position of the fundus is at the level of the umbilicus, or below, in the midline rather than shifted to the right.
    (2) If parts of the placenta and/or membranes were retained, bleeding would be present.
    (4) The fundus is firm; therefore bleeding at this time is not a problem.
40. (2) In the immediate postpartum period a slower than normal pulse rate can be anticipated as a result of a combination of factors—horizontal position, emotional relief and satisfaction, enforced rest after labor and delivery. (c); AS; AP; SH; OB
    (1) The temperature may rise slightly, but respirations generally are unchanged.
    (3) The temperature may rise, but respirations generally are unchanged.
    (4) Bradycardia more likely; respirations generally are unchanged.
41. (3) Retention of urine with overflow will be manifested in small, frequent voidings. The bladder should be palpated for distention. (a); AN; CP; NU; OB
    (1) There should be large amounts of urine voided because of the increased fluid volume at this time.
    (2) An elevated temperature with urinary symptoms would be indicative of impending infection.
    (4) Untrue; more circulating fluid is present, causing an increased output.
42. (4) Parenting can begin only when the baby and mother get to know each other. To promote normal development, the nurse should provide time for parent-child interaction. (b); PL; AP; CL; OB
    (1) This may make the mother feel incompetent and retard her mothering.
    (2) Ineffective; knowledge does not ensure good mothering. Time with the infant is more important.
    (3) Time must be provided for the mother with baby to return demonstrations and ask questions.
43. (2) Cephalhematoma is a collection of blood between the skull bone and its periosteum as the result of trauma. It resolves spontaneously in 3 to 6 weeks. (c); PL; CP; NU; PE
    (1) That is trauma caused by pressure of the head against the birth canal; can occur in natural delivery.
    (3) Caput succedaneum, rather than cephalhematoma, crosses the suture line.
    (4) This is a hard indurated area; remains immobile even when the infant cries.

44. (1) Parents need support and reassurance that their child is not permanently damaged. (c); AN; CP; NU; PE
    (2) Cephalhematomas resolve spontaneously; no ice is applied.
    (3) Cephalhematomas do not cause impaired neurologic functioning.
    (4) No special protection of the head is required; routine safety measures are adequate.

45. (4) Emphysema involves destructive changes in the alveolar walls, leading to dilation of the air sacs. There is subsequent air trapping and difficulty with expiration. (a); AN; CP; NU; ME
    (1) Bronchospasm is characteristic of asthma; causes narrowing of airways.
    (2) Although slow expiration tends to keep the airways open so there is less air trapping, rapid expulsion of air is not the primary problem.
    (3) Vital capacity is increased to compensate for inefficient gaseous exchange; however, this is a secondary adaptation.

46. (3) The sitting position permits the diaphragm to lower by gravity, allowing for greatest lung expansion. (b); IM; AP; SH; ME
    (1) A moderate Fowler position does not permit full lung expansion.
    (2) This is the semi-Fowler position; does not allow the diaphragm to drop fully by gravity.
    (4) The supine position permits the abdominal viscera to press against the diaphragm; limits lung expansion and gaseous exchange.

47. (1) Epinephrine acts on both alpha and beta receptors. However, the stimulation of the beta receptors is what causes bronchial relaxation and increased heart rate and contractility. (c); AN; KN; NU; ME
    (2) Stimulation of these alpha receptors causes vasoconstriction; produces a hypertensive effect.
    (3) Stimulation of these beta receptors causes dilation of the skeletal blood vessels.
    (4) There are no alpha receptors in the bronchioles.

48. (1) Patients with chronic obstructive pulmonary disease (COPD) must be given only low concentrations of oxygen. A decreased O_2 blood level is their only stimulus for breathing. (b); AN; CP; NU; ME
    (2) Prolonged hypoxia will stimulate erythrocyte production; the goal of therapy is to relieve hypoxia.
    (3) The pressure, rather than the concentration, at which oxygen is administered increases this risk.
    (4) To prevent its drying effects on secretions and the mucosa, all oxygen is humidified.

49. (3) Isoproterenol (Isuperel) is a catecholamine. It acts on the beta receptors, leading to increased heart rate and contractility as well as dilation of the arteries of the skeletal muscles. (b); EV; AP; CL; ME
    (1) Isuprel will cause tachycardia.
    (2) Isuprel may cause pallor from peripheral vasoconstriction.
    (4) Isuprel generally relaxes nonvascular smooth muscles.

50. (2) Isoproterenol is a potent bronchodilator used in the treatment of asthmatic attacks. Indiscriminant use leads to heart palpitations, nausea, tremors, and precordial pain. (c); IM; AP; CL; ME
    (1) Inhalation of vapors once relief is obtained increases the risk of serious complications; also the effectiveness of the vapors decreases with their increased use.
    (3) Represents overdosage; a 15 ml vial provides a minimum of 300 inhalations. The normal dose is 1 to 2 inhalations.
    (4) To prevent excessive cardiac stimulation, the dose should should not be taken more often than at 3-to-4-hour intervals.

51. (1) In addition to the desired effect of bronchodilation, isoproterenol inhalation can lead to tachycardia and palpitations. Therefore use of the drug should be limited to periods of dyspnea. (b); PL; AP; CL; ME
    (2) To use the inhaler, one closes the lips around the mouthpiece; and then, after maximum exhalation, inhales deeply while activating the spray.
    (3) The lips are sealed around the mouthpiece during the spray of the inhalant; to obtain maximum relief, it is necessary to hold one's breath briefly.
    (4) If relief is obtained, the spray should be terminated.

52. (4) Aminophylline, a theophylline derivative, causes relaxation of the smooth muscles of the bronchi, interrupting spasms and constriction. (b); AN; CP; SH; ME
    (1) Does not directly affect the ventilation/perfusion ratio.
    (2) Does not affect chemoreceptors; bronchodilation is achieved by preventing the breakdown of cyclic adenosine monophosphate (cAMP) so the smooth muscles of the bronchioles relax.
    (3) Although an action of aminophylline, it is not the reason for the drug's being given to Mr. Boise; relaxation of constricted bronchi and bronchioles is.

53. (4) The patient's rights were violated. Mrs. Coan has the right to a complete and accurate explanation of treatment. (a); AN; AP; SH; OB
    (1) When administering treatment, the nurse is responsible for explaining to the patient what and why the treatment is being done.
    (2) The Patient's Bill of Rights states that the patient should be informed.
    (3) All preparations or procedures should be explained since they are not routine to the patient.

54. (3) To prevent further maternal and fetal complications, patients must be continuously observed for blood loss by the monitoring of external bleeding and the counting and weighing of pads. (b); AS; AP; SH; OB
    (1) This would be necessary only if bleeding were continuous and profuse; a cesarean section might be necessary.
    (2) To minimize further placental separation, the patient would be confined to complete bed rest.

(4) Unnecessary; no indication that the patient is toxemic or that cerebral irritation is present.

55. (2) A vaginal examination might precipitate severe bleeding, which would be life threatening to the mother and infant and necessitate an immediate cesarean section. (b); PL; AP; SH; OB

 (1) The vaginal examination might precipitate severe bleeding; there would be no time for induction of labor.

 (3) This might lead to further placental separation and severe bleeding before the fetus could be delivered.

 (4) Not a priority item after a vaginal examination, which can precipitate severe bleeding; x-ray examination would not reveal placental separation, only fetal size and position.

56. (3) An infant should receive 60 calories and 88.8 ml (3 oz) of fluid per pound daily. (b); PL; AN; NU; OB

 (1) Too much; 74 ml (2 to 3 oz) fluid and 60 calories per pound per day required.

 (2) Too much; 74 ml (2 to 3 oz) fluid and 60 calories per pound per day required.

 (4) Too much; 74 ml (2 to 3 oz) fluid and 60 calories per pound per day required.

57. (4) Development of jaundice before 48 hours after birth may indicate a blood dyscrasia, requiring immediate medical investigation. Jaundice occurring between 48 and 72 hours after birth is a consequence of the normal physiologic breakdown of fetal red cells and immaturity of the liver. (c); EV; AN; NU; PE

 (1) Bilirubin studies would be done first to determine whether the amount of bilirubin present warranted phototherapy.

 (2) Unless pathologic (occurring in the first 24 hours of life), this is not necessary.

 (3) First, the age of the infant must be ascertained to see whether this is physiologic; then, the nurse can do a "heel-stick" to determine the amount of bilirubin.

58. (3) Babies with Down's syndrome have decreased muscle tone, which compromises respiratory expansion as well as the adequate drainage of mucus. These factors contribute to increased susceptibility to upper respiratory tract infections. (b); AN; AP; NU; PE

 (1) Slowed development is usually apparent at birth or soon after.

 (2) Cardiac, but not circulatory, problems are common in these children.

 (4) Impaired hearing is not an expected problem in Down's syndrome.

59. (4) A simian crease is a common clinical manifestation. It is readily observable when present. (a); AS; KN; NU; PE

 (1) Not a characteristic of children with Down's syndrome, but of children with congenital hip dislocation.

(2) Children with Down's syndrome usually manifest hypotonicity of skeletal muscles.

(3) Many normal children also have rounded occiputs.

60. (2) Parents' responses to their child may greatly influence decisions regarding future care. Learning about their child and Down's syndrome can help lessen guilt feelings. (a); PL; AP; SH; PE

 (1) Frequent handling and rocking are essential for all babies.

 (3) Important for all babies.

 (4) Not particularly necessary for infants with Down's syndrome.

61. (2) Babies with Down's syndrome have a high incidence of congenital heart disease, especially atrial defects. (b); PL; AP; NU; PE

 (1) Deafness is not usually a problem in Down's syndrome.

 (3) Infants with Down's syndrome usually have normal-sized heads.

 (4) The muscles of infants with Down's syndrome are usually hypotonic.

62. (3) When the parents can verbalize the need to change plans they have made for their infant, it usually signifies that they are beginning to face reality. (a); EV; AN; SH; PE

 (1) Probably not critically significant to the nurse.

 (2) Not usually a problem; is therefore not the most significant factor to the nurse.

 (4) Would be after the fact; is not the most significant factor to be considered by the nurse.

63. (2) For a child who is moderately retarded, simple repetitive tasks provide all the challenge needed. (b); IM; AP; CL; PE

 (1) Asking too much of a moderately retarded child.

 (3) Asking too much of a moderately retarded child.

 (4) Moderately retarded children will not be able to follow many instructions given at a single time.

64. (3) When one's efforts toward meeting a goal are blocked or thwarted, frustration results. The child with Down's syndrome may be constantly thwarted in trying to meet his needs, especially in an environment where certain achievements beyond his ability are expected. (a); AN; CP; NU; PE

 (1) Does not occur frequently.

 (2) Does not occur.

 (4) An external factor that has little to do with the child's ability to deal with his limitations.

65. (1) Metrorrhagia is uterine bleeding at any time other than during the menstrual period. (a); AN; KN; NU; SU

 (2) Severe menstrual bleeding is menorrhagia.

 (3) This is menstruation when it occurs in a cyclic pattern after menarche.

 (4) This is dyspareunia.

66. (2) In a hysterectomy the uterus is removed, but no other female organs. Consequently menstruation

ceases but the hypophyseal and ovarian hormone cycles continue. (a); PL; CP; SH; SU

(1) An oophorectomy was not performed; ovarian hormones continue to be secreted.

(3) Removal of the uterus does not affect the secretion of ovarian hormones.

(4) Normally menopause begins gradually; after an oophorectomy it begins immediately. However, an oophorectomy was not performed.

67. (4) Thrombophlebitis, common after pelvic surgery, is inflammation of a vein. The signs include pain, redness, swelling, and heat. It is associated with the formation of a clot (thrombosis). (a); AS; AP; NU; SU

(1) Classically thrombophlebitis is usually located in the area of the calf; however, may occur elsewhere.

(2) Itching is not a symptom of phlebitis.

(3) Although swelling accompanies thrombophlebitis, it is not a pitting edema.

68. (1) Menstruation is the shedding of the endometrial lining of the uterus. A patient who has undergone hysterectomy has had her uterus removed and will no longer menstruate. (b); AN; AN; NU; SU

(2) After a hysterectomy there is no endometrial lining to shed.

(3) Not a psychosomatic reaction, which would imply the presence of both physical and mental components; there is no uterus.

(4) Frank bleeding is not expected postoperatively.

69. (2) Flushing of the head and neck with accompanying diaphoresis is known as hot flashes. It is a symptom of estrogen deprivation. (c); AN; CP; NU; SU

(1) Heat intolerance is not a symptom associated with estrogen deprivation.

(3) Aging is not accelerated through lack of estrogen.

(4) There is no menstruation after this surgery.

70. (4) A crisis is defined as a situation in which the client's previous methods of adaptation are inadequate to meet present needs. (b); AN; AN; NU; PS

(1) A crisis is not necessarily related to the degree of stress; it occurs when past coping mechanisms are ineffective.

(2) This is not causing the crisis; her lack of coping mechanisms is.

(3) This is not the immediate stress for which she has no coping mechanism.

71. (2) A crisis intervention group helps clients reestablish psychologic equilibrium by assisting them to explore new alternatives to coping. It considers realistic situations using rational and flexible problem-solving methods. (a); IM; CP; SH; PS

(1) This is not an immediate goal of crisis intervention.

(3) It is not necessary for crisis intervention workers to be psychologists.

(4) Clients are never given a solution; they are assisted in arriving at their own acceptable, workable solutions.

72. (1) Behavior that reflects the recognition of the intrinsic worth of each individual is essential in all supportive relationships. Problem-solving potential is increased when clients are involved in exploring alternatives that will affect the direction of their own lives. (a); PL; AP; SH; PS

(2) The client, not the worker, is encouraged to identify the problem.

(3) Useless; the patient is unable to empathize with others at this time.

(4) Impossible during immediate intervention; the client needs to find direction immediately.

73. (4) The crisis center nurse's main responsibility is to assist the client in utilizing the problem-solving process. Miss Daley will be helped in exploring alternative solutions to a situation and will be given information regarding other agencies, facilities, and services. (b); PL; AP; SH; PS

(1) This is part of the general interaction with the patient; not a specific primary responsibility.

(2) Part of many instructions for which the patient must take primary responsibility.

(3) Not part of the immediate goal after the crisis; the patient may be encouraged to seek help for other problems.

74. (3) Intrinsic motivation is motivation that is stimulated from within the learner. It is most effective because the learner recognizes the need to know, is self-directed, and is ready to learn. (b); EV; AN; CL; PS

(1) This is stimulation from without and is very often ineffective; desire must come from within.

(2) There is no external reward for attending classes.

(4) This is a new behavior based on a new situation; there is no external reward for attending classes.

75. (3) Identifying feelings and providing support during stressful times are both ways of demonstrating concern during a crisis. (a); IM; AN; SH; PS

(1) Not a supportive or insightful reply.

(2) Lacks insight and supportiveness.

(4) Inappropriate reply that may instill guilt feelings; the father as well as the mother needs support through this crisis.

76. (3) Allowing the patient time to talk about her feelings and staying with her when she sees the baby for the first time provide support, acceptance, and understanding. (c); AS; AP; SH; PS

(1) This does not give the nurse a chance to assess the mother's feelings.

(2) This does not give the nurse a chance to assess the mother's feelings; anomalies are difficult to describe accurately in words.

(4) Showing pictures may not be helpful, and discussing treatment is premature.

77. (2) The usual initial response to a crisis situation such as this is denial that it could occur and that she and her husband could produce a less than normal child.

Mrs. Handler's reponse is her way of dealing with the reality of the situation. (a); EV; AN; SH; PS
(1) First reactions to a child with a congenital anomaly cannot be judged as final.
(3) The mother's reaction is a normal part of the grief response.
(4) Although the mother initially rejected her baby, time, coping, and love will help her accept his anomaly.

78. (4) The congenital defect prevents the infant from creating a tight seal with his lips to promote sucking. As a result he swallows large amounts of air when feeding. The mother should be taught to provide frequent rest periods and to bubble the infant often to expel the excess air in the stomach. (b); IM; AP; CL; PE
(1) Newborn infants cannot chew.
(2) Infants with cleft lip and palate should be held upright during feedings.
(3) Infants with cleft lip and palate should be held upright during feedings.

79. (1) Done to assess electrical activity and determine whether symptoms are primarily musculoskeletal or neurologic. (a); IM; CP; SH; ME
(2) No special care required after the procedure.
(3) No special care required after the procedure.
(4) No special preparation required.

80. (2) Herniation of a disc into the spinal column irritates the spinal cord or the roots of spinal nerves. (a); AN; CP; NU; ME
(1) Circulation of cerebrospinal fluid is not affected.
(3) The vertebral bodies themselves are not shifting.
(4) The lamina is that portion of the vertebrae which is removed during surgery to gain access to the disc.

81. (3) Coughing places strain on the lumbar area, increasing the herniation of the disc. (b); IM; AP; CL; ME
(1) Will not increase pressure or cause pain.
(2) Will not increase pressure or cause pain; flexed knees are usually a more comfortable position.
(4) Does not increase intervertebral pressure.

82. (4) Supportive devices provide temporary relief of pain by reducing strain on the lumbar area. (b); PL; AP; SH; ME
(1) Risk addiction; narcotics should not be ordered in maintenance doses.
(2) Increases congestion; short application may be helpful.
(3) Causes hyperextension of the lumbar vertebrae and increased pressure of the disc on the cord.

83. (2) Log rolling maintains alignment and avoids torsion with its increasing intervertebral pressure. (a); IM; AP; SH; ME
(1) Use of the trapeze increases lumbosacral strain.
(3) Causes hyperextension of the lumbar vertebrae, increasing pressure of the disc on the cord.
(4) Causes hyperextension of the lumbar vertebrae, increasing pressure of the disc on the cord.

84. (3) In transfer, the suspected back-injured patient should be positioned to keep the vertebral column in perfect alignment (back straight) to prevent further spinal cord damage by vertebral (bone) movments. (a); IM; AP; NU; SU
(1) To prevent additional damage to the spinal cord, the vertebral column should be kept in alignment.
(2) To prevent additional damage to the spinal cord, the vertebral column should be kept in alignment.
(4) To prevent additional damage to the spinal cord, the vertebral column should be kept in alignment.

85. (4) Both legs and generally the lower part of the body are paralyzed in paraplegia. (a); IM; KN; SH; SU
(1) This is quadriplegia.
(2) There is no term to describe this condition; all parts below an injury are affected.
(3) This is hemiplegia.

86. (4) Lack of or reduced body movement predisposes the paraplegic or quadriplegic patient to urinary tract infection and stone formation. (a); PL; AP; SH; SU
(1) Fluids do not prevent temperature elevation, unless it is elevated because of dehydration.
(2) Administration of fluids does not maintain electrolyte "balance."
(3) All individuals require fluid to prevent dehydration; not why fluids are encouraged for this patient.

87. (4) Care should be aimed at encouraging independence. (a); PL; AP; CL; SU
(1) A patient with this type of injury will never return to previous function.
(2) Lay persons may be taught to care for patients with a spinal cord injury.
(3) Independence should be encouraged in patients with a chronic disability; they should not rely totally on others for care.

88. (1) The bones respond to the stress of activity (walking, running, etc.) by laying down new bone substance along the lines of stress. Inactivity leads to reduced bone deposition and actual bone decalcification. (b); AN; CP; NU; SU
(2) Calcium intake does not alter bone demineralization in the bedridden patient.
(3) Kidney function may be altered as bone decalcification occurs and stones are formed in the kidneys.
(4) Fluid intake has no effect on bone decalcification.

89. (1) Bowel or bladder distention causes autonomic nerve impulses to ascend in the cord to the point of injury. Here the reflex is completed, and autonomic outflow causes piloerection (goosebumps), sweating, and splanchnic vasoconstriction. The last causes hypertension and a pounding headache. (c); AN; AN; NU; SU
(2) Not involved in the sympathetic hyperreflexia mechanism.
(3) Not involved in the sympathetic hyperreflexia mechanism.
(4) Not involved in the sympathetic hyperreflexia mechanism.

90. (1) Anxiety is communicable. Because it can be an interpersonal experience, it is contagious; the nurse has a strong urge to get away. (b); AN; AN; NU; PS
    (2) The desire to go off duty would not suddenly make the nurse uncomfortable.
    (3) There is no indication that this or any other behavior encountered has been bizarre.
    (4) Possible but not probable; the patient is exhibiting anxiety, not hostility, at this time.

91. (3) These actions make the environment as emotionally unthreatening as realistically possible. (b); AN; AP; NU; PS
    (1) The person must learn how to deal with delaying gratification.
    (2) It is not possible or realistic to meet all of a person's needs.
    (4) Order in the environment is of less importance; providing a nonthreatening environment is the priority action.

92. (2) This response demonstrates acceptance of the patient but does set limits on the patient's behavior. (c); IM; AP; SH; PS
    (1) False reassurance; the nurse can not make everything all right.
    (3) The nurse would be allowing further manipulation by Mrs. Rose in not leaving when the shift was over.
    (4) False reassurance; adds to attempts at further manipulation of the next shift.

93. (3) Helps the patient focus on situations that precipitate feelings. (b); IM; AP; SH; PS
    (1) The nurse would not be helping Mrs. Rose focus on her feelings.
    (2) Not a specific focus; the nurse cannot be certain what the patient means.
    (4) False reassurance; the nurse cannot guarantee that feelings will not come back.

94. (2) Sitting with her indicates acceptance and demonstrates that the nurse feels she is worthy of spending time with. (b); IM; AN; SH; PS
    (1) Would have the effect of closing off further communication and denying the patient's feelings.
    (3) Would be of little comfort.
    (4) It would be better to stay with her quietly until she regained control; also prevents a follow-through on her threat.

95. (4) In neuromotor disorders such as scleroderma it is equally difficult to swallow solids and liquids. A pureed diet is given. (b); IM; AP; CL; ME
    (1) Liquefied foods are difficult to swallow; there is decreased esophageal peristalsis, and they are easily aspirated.
    (2) Will not help; it is equally difficult to swallow solids and liquids.
    (3) Ineffective; no oral pain is associated with scleroderma.

96. (4) Raynaud's phenomenon is caused by vasospasm, precipitated by exposure to cold. (a); IM; AP; CL; ME
    (1) Vasodilators, not anticoagulants, are prescribed to counteract vasospasm and increase blood flow.
    (2) Decreased blood flow would interfere with perception of temperature and increase the risk of burns.
    (3) Trauma to the hands must be avoided; nerve endings are affected by diminished blood supply.

97. (1) In scleroderma the skin becomes dry because of interference with the underlying sweat glands. (c); PL; AP; CL; ME
    (2) There are no skin lesions associated with scleroderma.
    (3) There are no pruritic scabs associated with scleroderma.
    (4) There are no inflamed areas associated with scleroderma.

98. (1) Changes in connective tissue lead to muscle weakness. Optimal function must be preserved. (b); AN; CP; SH; ME
    (2) Prevention of spread is not possible in this systemic disease, which involves a number of organs.
    (3) Exercise of stiff and painful joints causes pain, not a sense of well-being.
    (4) Tissue regeneration will not occur; this is a progressive degenerative disorder.

99. (3) Small meals reduce secretion of gastric juices. Eating frequently provides food to mix with gastric juices. (a); IM; AP; CL; ME
    (1) This would interfere with gravity drainage of the esophagus and cause gastric reflux.
    (2) Antacids are given postcibally to neutralize and/or bind gastric juices released during a meal.
    (4) Restriction of carbohydrates is a recommendation to prevent the dumping syndrome, not heartburn.

100. (2) Severe pain accompanied by bleeding at term or close to it is symptomatic of complete premature detachment of the placenta. (b); AS; CP; SH; OB
    (1) Bleeding caused by marginal placenta previa should not be painful.
    (3) There is no bleeding with vena caval syndrome.
    (4) Hydatidiform mole does not usually last until 36 weeks; no severe pain accompanies it.

101. (2) Immediate cesarean section is the treatment of choice for complete placental separation. The risk of fetal death is too high. (a); IM; CP; NU; OB
    (1) Too slow; besides, a high forceps delivery is rarely used because the forceps may further complicate the situation by tearing the cervix.
    (3) The fetus would probably expire if this course of action were taken.
    (4) The fetus would probably expire if this course of action were taken.

102. (3) In an emergency surgical situation when invasive techniques may be necessary, it is important to have a consent signed as well as a history of the patient's known allergies. (a); IM; AP; SH; OB

(1) An enema is not given to a bleeding patient; may stimulate contractions and further bleeding.

(2) An enema is not given to a bleeding patient; may stimulate contractions and further bleeding.

(4) Not a priority item in an emergency such as this.

103. (3) A lumbar puncture would reveal the presence of a causative organism (e.g., the pneumococcus, tubercle bacillus, meningococcus, or streptococcus). (b); AN; CP; NU; PE

(1) Used to detect the presence of abnormalities by the injection of a contrast medium into the subarachnoid space; does not identify the organism.

(2) Would demonstrate the presence of bacteria on the skin, not identify organisms in the cerebrospinal fluid.

(4) Not a definitive test, although advisable; occasionally will prove positive when a CSF culture is negative.

104. (3) $\dfrac{\text{Amount of fluid} \times \text{Drop rate}}{\text{Time (in minutes)}}$

$\dfrac{500 \times 60}{24 \times 60} = 21$ drops

(a); PL; AN; NU; PE

(1) Too slow to infuse the desired amount.

(2) Too slow to infuse the desired amount.

(4) Too rapid; the fluid would run out before 24 hours had elapsed.

105. (1) The concept of object permanence begins to develop around 6 months of age. (c); AS; CP; SH; PE

(2) Occurs during the first several months of life.

(3) Occurs between 13 and 24 months.

(4) Occurs between 13 and 24 months.

106. (2) Nausea and vomiting in the morning occur in almost 50% of all pregnancies. Eating dry crackers before getting out of bed in the morning is a simple remedy that may provide relief. (a); IM; AP; CL; OB

(1) Increasing protein intake does not relieve the nausea.

(3) Two small meals and a snack at noon would not meet the nutritional needs of a pregnant woman; nor would it relieve nausea. Some women find that eating 5 or 6 small meals daily instead of 3 large ones is helpful.

(4) This is not helpful; separating fluids from solids at mealtime is more advisable.

107. (3) The nurse should expect to see an increase in blood volume by as much as 40% above prepregnant levels. During pregnancy, fluid in all body compartments increases. (c); AN; AN; SH; OB

(1) An increase in cardiac output is seen as early as the end of the first trimester; due to increased blood volume.

(2) The hematocrit decreases as a result of the hemodilution of pregnancy.

(4) Blood pressure remains essentially unchanged throughout pregnancy.

108. (4) Mrs. Gosney is in early labor, and the first priority of care is to establish a trusting relationship with her and her husband. This will help to allay their anxiety. (a); IM; AP; SH; OB

(1) May be necessary later; however, not of the first priority.

(2) Also not an initial priority item; the physician knows she is on her way.

(3) The history should be taken from the patient as long as she is capable of providing it.

109. (3) The bulging perineum indicates that the fetal head is on the pelvic floor and birth is imminent. (a); AS; CP; NU; OB

(1) This is a sign that occurs during transition or the beginning of the second stage; the second stage lasts approximately 1 hour in a primipara, and Mrs. Gosney would be more comfortable in the labor room then.

(2) This is a sign that occurs during transition or the beginning of the second stage; the second stage lasts approximately 1 hour in a primipara, and Mrs. Gosney would be more comfortable in the labor room then.

(4) This is a sign that occurs during transition or the beginning of the second stage; the second stage lasts approximately 1 hour in a primipara, and Mrs. Gosney would be more comfortable in the labor room then.

110. (3) This is the usual pattern that a nevus vasculosus follows. (b); IM; CP; SH; OB

(1) False; a nevus vasculosus involves the dermal and subdermal layers.

(2) False; a nevus vasculosus grows and fades. Saying it will be covered by clothes gives little reassurance.

(4) Surgical removal is not recommended.

111. (1) The antibody system is not functioning in neonates. Antibodies are transferred from the mother in the milk. (a); IM; CP; SH; OB

(2) Breast milk has 1.1 g protein/100 ml; cow's milk has 3.5 g/100 ml.

(3) Because of the higher carbohydrate content of breast milk, infants wake more easily; carbohydrate is digested more rapidly.

(4) Lactating mothers rarely ovulate for the first 9 weeks post partum; however, they may any time after that.

112. (3) Vaseline gauze helps control bleeding and prevent adherence of the diaper. (b); IM; AP; CL; PE

(1) Fussy behavior is normal for a few hours after the procedure.

(2) Yellow exudate is normal; not part of an infectious process.

(4) Not too realistic with a male infant.

113. (3) The woman must be watched closely for symptoms associated with stimulation of the vagus nerve. This response is manifested by syncope, pallor, diaphoresis, weakness, lethargy, and bradycardia. (c); AS; AP; CP; OB

(1) Nausea and rash are not associated with insertion of an intrauterine device; since IUDs are inserted during the menstrual period, most women do not notice the small amount of bleeding that may occur after insertion.

(2) Lethargy and syncope are associated with a vagal response; tachycardia is not.

(4) Bradycardia is seen with vagal stimulation; visual changes and hypertension are not.

114. (4) The first and most important observation should be for respiratory obstruction. If this occurs, treatment must be instituted immediately. (a); AS; CP; NU; SU

(1) Can be due to the anesthesia; however, it is not life threatening and usually passes.

(2) Blood pressure is not significantly affected by this type of surgery; however, surgery itself can have an influence on it. If the blood pressure had significantly dropped, other symptoms would be present.

(3) A later concern; not in the immediate postoperative period.

115. (4) The laryngeal nerve is close to the operative site and can be inadvertently damaged. (b); AS; AN; SH; SU

(1) Loss of the gag reflex occurs with all surgery; the ability to swallow signifies its return.

(2) This might test the seventh cranial (facial) nerve, which would not be affected in thyroid surgery.

(3) Muscles and nerves involved in turning the head are not near the thyroid gland.

116. (3) Soreness is to be expected. A progression to a soft diet will provide nutrients needed for healing and energy and will stimulate the return of bowel activity. Analgesics as ordered will reduce soreness during meals. (c); IM; AN; SH; SU

(1) This is not a nursing function.

(2) Soreness is to be expected; is not an emergency necessitating medical action.

(4) The soreness is not due to drying; a humidifer might help reduce soreness but would not help the patient eat the soft diet.

117. (1) Because the patient is attached to a machine and movement may alter the tracings, movement is discouraged. (b); AN; CP; SH; OB

(2) Lamaze techniques work well with a monitor.

(3) An external monitor does not necessitate more frequent vaginal examinations.

(4) Placement of the monitor leads does not interfere with the administration of sedatives.

118. (1) Any other action would be an invasion of privacy. The marital status has little bearing on the needs of the patient at this time. (b); AS; CP; SH; PS

(2) Marital status has no bearing on the course of labor.

(3) This is an invasion of privacy.

(4) No indication at this time that the patient requires this referral.

119. (2) Mothers need to explore their infants visually and tactilely to assure themselves that the infant is normal in all respects. (a); AS; CP; SH; PE

(1) Pregnancy and labor have no relationship to "normalcy" of the infant.

(3) Crying is not indicative of congenital defects; a strong cry does not assure "normalcy."

(4) Assumption; closing off communication with the mother at a very opportune moment.

120. (4) The pregnant teenager is more prone to toxemia because of age, poor diet, and often poor prenatal care. (c); AN; AN; NU; PE

(1) False assumption; societal mores vary, and an unwed pregnancy may be totally acceptable.

(2) Unrelated; no proof that teenagers are more diabetogenic than other pregnant women.

(3) May or may not be true.

Comprehensive Test 6

To simulate the comprehensive licensure examination, this test should be completed within 2 hours.

Situation: Robert Dorn, 5 weeks old, is admitted to the hospital with a tentative diagnosis of congenital heart defect. His mother states that he tires easily and has difficulty breathing and feeding. Questions 1 through 5 refer to this situation.

1 Part of the nursing care for Robert would include proper positioning. The best position in which to place Robert would be:
   1. Supine with the knees flexed
   2. Orthopneic with pillows for support
   3. Side-lying with the head and chest elevated
   4. Prone with the head supported by pillows

2 A cardiac catheterization is performed. Postoperatively Robert is brought back to the pediatric unit for observation. The leg used for the procedure is mottled. The nurse should immediately:
   1. Check the pulse in the extremity
   2. Notify the physician of the situation
   3. Cover the baby with a blanket
   4. Elevate the leg

3 Baby Robert is in the pediatric recovery room after open heart surgery for the repair of a ventricular septal defect. A nursing priority should be to:
   1. Determine the status of the operative site
   2. Ascertain Robert's pulmonary status
   3. Check the patency of the intravenous catheter
   4. Monitor Robert's urinary output

4 The Dorns are informed that Robert is in the recovery room and is stable. Mrs. Dorn is crying and extremely worried. The nurse can best help allay her anxiety by:
   1. Bringing her and her husband to the recovery room for several minutes.
   2. Reassuring them that Robert is doing well
   3. Allowing her to continue to express her feelings
   4. Encouraging them to go have a cup of coffee and return in 2 hours

5 When Robert is ready to go home, Mrs. Dorn asks the nurse, "Shall I continue to boil my baby's formula?" Prior to replying, the nurse should remember that during early infancy:
   1. The gastric acidity is low and unable to provide bacteriostatic protection

2. The absence of hydrochloric acid renders the stomach vulnerable to infection
3. *Escherichia coli*, the bacterium normally found in the stomach, does not act on milk
4. Infants are almost completely lacking in immunity and need sterile fluids

Situation: Miss Louise Monroe, age 62, has a hiatal hernia. She tells the nurse that she wakes up frequently at night with heartburn. Questions 6 through 9 refer to this situation.

6 Which suggestion by the nurse would be most likely to reduce the symptoms of heartburn?
1. Having a light snack of orange juice and crackers at bedtime
2. Elevating the head of the bed on 6-inch blocks
3. Eating her largest meal at noontime
4. Taking an intestinal sedative, such as hyoscyamine sulfate (Donnatal), at night

7 The physician prescribes a bland diet for Miss Monroe. She asks the nurse about foods that must be avoided on a bland diet. Which of the following should the nurse instruct her to exclude from her diet?
1. Poached eggs
2. Roast beef
3. Whole wheat bread
4. Green beans or peas

8 Miss Monroe tells the nurse that she takes one-half teaspoon of baking soda in a glass of water for heartburn. The nurse suggests that she use an antacid preparation such as aluminum hydroxide (Maalox). This response is based on the fact that antacids:
1. Cause few side effects such as diarrhea or constipation
2. Are readily absorbed by the stomach mucosa
3. Have no direct effect on systemic acid-base balance
4. Contain little if any sodium

9 Which of the following factors should the nurse plan to include when teaching Miss Monroe about antacid therapy?
1. Antacids should be taken only at 4-hour intervals
2. Tablets are equally as effective as the liquid forms
3. Antacids interfere with the absorption of other drugs
4. Antacids should be taken 1 hour before meals

Situation: John McNabb has been feeling very tired and has developed anorexia and jaundice. After a diagnostic workup at the clinic, he is diagnosed as having infectious hepatitis type A. Questions 10 through 12 refer to this situation.

10 His wife asks about gamma globulin for herself and other family members. The most appropriate response by the nurse would be:
1. "Don't be concerned. Your husband's type of hepatitis is no longer communicable."
2. "A vaccine has not yet been developed for this type of hepatitis."
3. "You should contact your physician immediately about getting gamma globulin."
4. Gamma globulin provides passive immunity for serum hepatitis."

11 John's wife explains that he likes seafood. She asks about preparing seafood to avoid infection with hepatitis virus type A. Which of the following cooked foods is most likely to remain contaminated by the virus that causes infectious hepatitis?
1. Broiled shrimp
2. Baked haddock
3. Canned tuna
4. Steamed lobster

12 John asks when he will be able to go back to work. The best response by the nurse is:
1. "As soon as you're feeling less tired, you may go back to work."
2. "Unfortunately, few people fully recover from hepatitis in less than 6 months."
3. "You cannot return to work for 6 months, since the virus will still be present in your stools for this period."
4. "Gradually increase your activities. Relapses are very common in people who return to full activity too soon."

Situation: Mrs. Evad, with a history of upper abdominal pain, nausea, and vomiting, is admitted to the hospital for a diagnostic workup of cancer of the pancreas. She has a history of hypertension and is taking antihypertensive medication. Questions 13 through 19 refer to this situation.

13 As Mrs. Evad is admitted to her room, she asks the nurse, "Do you think I have anything serious—like cancer?" The nurse's best reply would be:
1. "Why don't you discuss this with your doctor?"
2. "Don't worry, we won't know until all the test results are back."
3. "What makes you think you have cancer?"
4. "I don't know if you do, but let's talk about it."

14 A complete blood count, urinalysis, and x-ray examination of the chest are ordered for Mrs. Evad prior to surgery. She asks why these tests are done. The nurse's best answer would be:
1. "Don't worry, these tests are strictly routine."
2. "They are ordered for all patients undergoing surgery."
3. "I don't know; the doctor ordered them."
4. "They determine whether it's safe to proceed with surgery."

15 An abdominal resection is to be performed on Mrs. Evad. The first priority of preoperative nursing care is directed toward:
1. Teaching and answering all questions
2. Maintaining proper nutritional status
3. Recording accurate vital signs
4. Alleviating the patient's anxiety

16 The most significant influence on Mrs. Evad's perception of pain is her:
1. Overall physical status
2. Intelligence and economic status
3. Previous experience and cultural values
4. Age and sex

17 A progressive ambulation schedule is to be instituted for Mrs. Evad the morning after surgery. Morphine sulfate, 10 mg, has been ordered q. 4 h. p.r.n. for pain. When the nurse helps her out of bed, she should first sit on the edge of the bed with her feet dangling because her expected adaptation will be:
1. Postural hypotension
2. Respiratory distress
3. Initial hypertension
4. Abdominal pain

18 Early symptoms of morphine overdose are:
1. Profuse sweating, pinpoint pupils, and deep sleep
2. Slow respirations, dilated pupils, restlessness
3. Slow pulse, slow respirations, sedation
4. Slow respirations, constricted pupils, and deep sleep

19 On the second postoperative day Mrs. Evad complains of pain in her right calf. The nurse should first:
1. Elevate the extremity
2. Apply warm soaks
3. Notify the physician
4. Chart the symptoms

Situation: Indira Mohamet, age 33, has difficulty becoming pregnant. She visits her gynecologist and is diagnosed as having endometriosis. Questions 20 through 22 refer to this situation.

20 Endometriosis is characterized by:
1. Amenorrhea and insomnia
2. Ecchymoses and petechiae
3. Painful menstruation and backache
4. Early osteoporosis and pelvic inflammation

21 When obtaining a health history, the nurse would eliminate which of the following conditions as a possible complication of endometriosis?
1. Menopause
2. Metrorrhagia
3. Bowel stricture
4. Voiding difficulties

22 An antiovulatory medication of combined progestogen and estrogen is prescribed for Mrs. Mohamet. The nurse, instructing her about the medication, should include the need to:
1. Have a bimonthly Pap smears
2. Report any vaginal bleeding
3. Temporarily restrict sexual activity
4. Increase her intake of calcium

Situation: Mr. Ryan is admitted to the hospital with GI bleeding and a burning epigastric pain. The initial diagnosis is peptic ulcer or gastric carcinoma. Questions 23 through 29 refer to this situation.

23 The emotional response that most frequently contributes to psychosomatic illness is:
1. Anxiety
2. Depression
3. Fear
4. Rage

24 To differentiate between a gastric ulcer and gastric carcinoma, which one of the following diagnostic tests would provide conclusive evidence?
1. Gastric analysis
2. GI series
3. Gastroscopy
4. Stool examination

25 Mr. Ryan is placed on a stretcher and restrained with Velcro straps for his transport to the x-ray department for an upper GI examination. While coming out of the elevator, he shifts his position, the Velcro strap breaks, and he falls to the floor, sustaining a fractured arm. He later comments that "the Velco strap was worn, just at the very spot where the strap snapped." The nurse is:
1. Completely exonerated, since only the hospital, as principal employer, is primarily responsible for the quality and maintenance of equipment
2. Exempt from any law suit because of the doctrine of *respondeat superior*
3. Normally liable, along with the employer, for

misapplication of equipment or use of defective equipment that harms the patient

   4. Totally and singly responsible for the obvious negligence because of her failure to report defective equipment

26 Barium salts in the GI series and barium enemas serve to:
   1. Give off visible light and illuminate the alimentary tract
   2. Fluoresce and thus illuminate the alimentary tract
   3. Dye the alimentary tract and thus give it color contrast
   4. Absorb x rays and thus give contrast to the soft tissues of the alimentary tract

27 Peptic ulcer is diagnosed. This is considered to be a psychosomatic disorder about which it is believed that:
   1. Structural changes have occurred as a result of psychologic conflicts
   2. Illness is a defense against psychologic conflicts
   3. Structural changes have occurred as a result of physiologic changes caused by psychologic conflict
   4. Physiologic changes stimulated psychologic changes

28 The nurse should be aware that the most common complication of peptic ulcer is:
   1. Perforation
   2. Hemorrhage
   3. Pyloric obstruction
   4. Esophageal varices

29 Which of the following foods would be served to Mr. Ryan?
   1. Sliced oranges, pancakes with syrup, coffee
   2. Applesauce, Cream of Wheat, milk
   3. Orange juice, fried eggs, sausage
   4. Tomato juice, raisin bran cereal, tea

Situation: Mrs. Smith is admitted to the hospital with a diagnosis of possible bronchogenic carcinoma. Questions 30 through 34 refer to this situation.

30 When Mrs. Smith returns to the room following a bronchoscopy and biopsy, she is fully awake. The nurse should:
   1. Advise her to stay flat in bed for 2 hours
   2. Provide ice chips to reduce swelling
   3. Encourage her to cough frequently
   4. Evaluate the presence of a gag reflex

31 Mrs. Smith's diagnosis of bronchogenic carcinoma is confirmed and a right pneumonectomy is per-

formed. During the surgery the phrenic nerve is severed to:
   1. Produce an atonic diaphragm
   2. Limit the postoperative pain considerably
   3. Allow the diaphragm to rise and partially fill the space
   4. Permit greater excursion of the thoracic cavity

32 Mrs. Smith returns from surgery to the intensive care unit with an endotracheal tube in place. Which of the following would be the most effective way for the nurse to loosen Mrs. Smith's secretions?
   1. Administration of fluids
   2. Pulmonary toileting
   3. Administration of humidified oxygen
   4. Instillation of a saturated solution of potassium iodide into the endotracheal tube

33 Immediately postoperatively, which position would be most beneficial for Mrs. Smith?
   1. Right side with head slightly elevated
   2. Left Sims with the head of the bed elevated 45 degrees
   3. High Fowler
   4. Flat in bed with knees flexed slightly

34 The nurse should palpate Mrs. Smith's trachea at least once a day because:
   1. Tracheal edema may lead to an obstructed airway
   2. The position may indicate mediastinal shift
   3. Nodular lesions may demonstrate metastasis
   4. The cuff of the endotracheal tube may be overinflated

Situation: Mr. and Mrs. Monrow, a couple in their late twenties, happily receive the news that Mrs. Monrow is pregnant. A year before, Mrs. Monrow had spontaneously aborted in the sixteenth week. It is determined that she is about 8 weeks pregnant and healthy. Questions 35 through 39 refer to this situation

35 While in the office for a prenatal checkup during the twelfth week of her pregnancy, Mrs. Monrow says to the nurse, "Everyday I wonder if I'll ever have this child." The nurse's best response would be:
   1. "You have the best doctors possible. What was the problem with your previous pregnancy?"
   2. "I can understand why you're worried. You will have other chances in the future."
   3. "Just do exactly what the doctors tell you to do. I can understand why you're worried, though."
   4. "It's understandable for you to feel concerned that you may not carry this pregnancy to term."

36 Sixteen weeks into her pregnancy, Mrs. Monrow begins to experience heavy bleeding and severe abdominal cramping. She is admitted to the hospital with an incomplete abortion. Her doctor orders a dilation and curettage. She says to the nurse, ''We wanted this baby so badly.'' The nurses's best response would be:
1. ''You must be disappointed, but don't feel guilty. These things sometimes happen.''
2. ''It's not your fault. This is nature's way of dealing with babies that may have problems.''
3. ''It must be difficult to lose something that was important to you both.''
4. ''The D & C will give you a new start. I bet you'll become pregnant again soon.''

37 Mrs. Monrow tells the nurse that her doctor explained to her that she has had an incomplete abortion but she does not understand what was said. The nurse's best response would be:
1. ''I think it would be best if you asked your doctor for the answer to that question.''
2. ''An incomplete abortion is when the fetus is expelled but part of the placenta and membranes are not.''
3. ''I really don't think you should focus on what happened right now.''
4. ''An incomplete abortion is when the fetus dies but remains attached to the uterine wall.''

38 The evening after the D & C, Mrs. Monrow says, ''We've always wanted this pregnancy. How come this happened to us again?'' The nurse is aware that Mrs. Monrow is exhibiting the usual initial reaction to a loss, which is:
1. Apathy and sadness
2. Shock and denial
3. Despair and anger
4. Dissociation and rationalization

39 When making rounds during the night, the nurse enters Mrs. Monrow's room and finds her crying. The most appropriate action would be to:
1. Document on the chart that Mrs. Monrow is having difficulty accepting the loss of her baby.
2. Pull the curtain to provide privacy for Mrs. Monrow.
3. Sit down and stay with Mrs. Monrow, allowing her to cry.
4. Explain to Mrs. Monrow that her feelings are normal and will pass with time.

Situation: Mrs. Johnson, a 47-year-old obese housewife, is admitted to the hospital with a diagnosis of Ménière's disease. Questions 40 through 42 refer to this situation.

40 When assessing Mrs. Johnson during an attack, the nurse should expect her to experience:
1. Nystagmus
2. An increase in temperature
3. Diarrhea
4. A declrease in pulse rate

41 To control the disease, Mrs. Johnson is given a salt-restricted diet to reduce endolymphatic fluid. When discussing her diet with the nurse, she states that she has four favorite foods. Which of these may she still eat?
1. Baked clams
2. Grilled cheese
3. Carrot cake
4. Macaroni

42 When discussing weight loss with Mrs. Johnson, the nurse should make which suggestion that would be most therapeutic?
1. Get involved in diversionary activities when there is an urge to eat
2. Enroll in an exercise class at the local high school
3. Limit intake to 900 calories a day
4. Keep a diary of all foods eaten each day, making certain to list everything

Situation: Four-year-old Ted Corleone is admitted to the hospital with a hemoglobin count of 7 g/100 ml and a red blood cell count of 2,500,000/100 ml. Questions 43 through 50 refer to this situation.

43 In addition to weakness and fatigue, what symptom should the nurse expect Ted to exhibit?
1. Cold, clammy skin
2. Cyanosis of the nail beds
3. Increased pulse rate
4. Elevated blood pressure

44 Ted has never been separated from his parents. His parents must be encouraged to:
1. Stay with him throughout the hospitalization
2. Bring a favorite toy to the hospital for him
3. Visit as often as possible during visiting hours
4. Allow the nurse to be the major care giver

45 While Ted is playing in the hall, he complains of feeling ''woozy.'' The nurse's best initial response would be to:
1. Check his pulse and blood pressure
2. Assist him back to his room and place him supine in bed
3. Use spirits of ammonia to prevent fainting
4. Have him sit until the dizziness subsides

46 The nurse should recognize that the most probable cause of Ted's dizziness was:
1. Decreased levels of serum glucose
2. A sudden drop in blood pressure
3. Insufficient cerebral oxygenation
4. An inflammation of the inner ear

47 The physician orders a liquid iron preparation for Ted. The nurse should:
1. Administer this at least an hour before meals
2. Caution Ted's mother to avoid orange juice or other citrus juice
3. Have Ted use a straw to take the medication
4. Explain that loose stools are common with iron

48 When Ted develops gastrointestinal discomfort, the physician prescribes a daily parenteral iron preparation. In administering this medication, the nurse should:
1. Rotate injections among the four extremities
2. Firmly massage the site after withdrawal of the needle
3. Change needles after drawing the drug into the syringe
4. Apply ice packs to the site after the injection

49 The nurse attempts to meet Ted's emotional needs. The most appropriate method would be to:
1. Encourage Ted to draw pictures of what he is feeling
2. Explain the procedures to Ted in simple terms at least an hour before they are scheduled
3. Allow Ted to play with a needle and syringe
4. Provide Ted with a doll and other equipment and observe his behavior

50 Ted requires multiple transfusions. Because of his anemia, he has an increased risk of developing what complication?
1. Pulmonary edema
2. Allergic response
3. Hemolytic reaction
4. Serum hepatitis

Situation: *Susan Langham, a 19-year-old single parent, gives birth to a 2268 g (5 lb) baby boy with severe cleft palate. The nurse brings the baby to Susan. Questions 51 through 54 refer to this situation.*

51 Which response by Susan to her deformed baby would represent a fairly typical reaction?
1. "No, you must have brought me the wrong baby."
2. "I'm unhappy and I guess I'm being punished."
3. "I shouldn't have had this baby. Now John will never marry me."

4. "What will my parents say? What could have happened?"

52 Susan refuses to look at her baby. Which nursing approach would be most therapeutic?
1. Gently tell Susan that she should stop blaming herself for the child's handicap
2. Explain the problem to Susan's family and encourage them to help comfort her
3. Reinforce the physician's explanation of the handicap and allow Susan time to discuss her fears
4. Wait until Susan has sufficiently recovered from the stress of delivery before bringing her the baby again

53 Susan brings her son, Steve, who is now 18 months old, to the clinic. In discussing him with the nurse, she asks why Steve is so difficult to please, has temper tantrums, and annoys her by throwing food from the table. The nurse should explain that:
1. Steve is learning to assert his independence, and his behavior is considered normal for his age
2. Steve needs to be disciplined at this stage to prevent development of antisocial behaviors
3. It is best to leave Steve alone in his crib after calmly telling him why his behavior is unacceptable
4. This is the usual way for a toddler to express his needs during the initiative stage of development

54 The nurse asks Susan what she does when Steve has a tantrum. Which of Susan's actions demonstrates that she understands the information she received in the well-baby classes at the clinic?
1. Ignoring and isolating Steve until he behaves properly
2. Disciplining Steve by restricting a favorite food or activity
3. Partially giving in to Steve before his tantrums become excessive
4. Allowing Steve to choose between two reasonable alternatives

Situation: *Twenty-year-old Jimmy Barbino is involved in a motorcycle accident and sustains a cervical fracture. To maintain cervical immobilization, he is placed in Crutchfield tongs and on a Circ-Olectric bed. Questions 55 through 59 refer to this situation.*

55 In providing care the nurse should:
1. Keep a roll behind the patient's neck to provide support
2. Provide for urinary elimination when in the prone position

3. Keep sandbags on each side of the head to keep it immobilie

4. Monitor the vital signs before and after turning the patient

56 The plan for Jimmy's care is based on the nurse's awareness that:

1. Two people must be present when turning the bed

2. The patient is rotated from side to side to prevent decubiti

3. A receptacle for elimination is easily accessible

4. Postpural hypotension after prolonged bed rest can be prevented

57 In caring for Jimmy, the nurse should:

1. Avoid the cervical spine area when administering back care

2. Clean the area around the tongs daily and apply antibiotic ointment

3. Relieve tension on the tongs for 5 minutes every hour

4. Remove the weights from tongs prior to rotating the CircOlectric bed

58 Jimmy asks the nurse how long it will take before he can walk out of the hospital. The nurse's reply is based on her knowledge that destroyed nerve fibers in the brain or spinal cord do not regenerate because they lack:

1. A myelin sheath

2. A neurilemma

3. Nissl bodies

4. Nuclei

59 Crushing of the spinal cord above the level of phrenic nerve origin will have significance for the nurse because it will result in:

1. Ventricular fibrillation

2. Dysfunction of the vagus nerve

3. Retention of sensation but paralysis of the lower extremities

4. Respiratory paralysis and cessation of diaphragmatic contractions

Situation: Mrs. Acker has missed her second menstrual period and attends the prenatal clinic. Questions 60 through 67 refer to this situation.

60 Mrs. Acker asks the nurse why menstruation ceases once pregnancy occurs. The nurse's best reponse would be that this occurs because of the:

1. "Production of estrogen and progesterone by the ovaries."

2. "Secretion of luteinizing hormone produced by the pituitary."

3. "Secretion of follicle-stimulating hormone produced by the pituitary."

4. "Reduction in the secretion of hormones by the ovaries."

61 When Mrs. Acker returns for her fourth-month checkup, she is very upset and indicates that her husband was recently diagnosed as having genital herpes. Which of the following statements concerning sexual activity should the nurse include when providing health teaching to Mrs. Acker?

1. It will be necessary to refrain from all sexual contact during pregnancy

2. Meticulous cleaning of her hands and vaginal area after intercourse is essential

3. Use of condoms by her husband during sexual activity will be required

4. Sexual abstinence should be practiced during the last 6 weeks of pregnancy

62 In the fifth month, ultrasonography is performed. The results indicate that the fetus is small for gestational age and there is evidence of a low-lying placenta. In the last trimester the nurse should use this information and assess Mrs. Acker for signs of possible:

1. Precipitate delivery

2. Abruptio placentae

3. Placenta previa

4. Premature labor

63 Three weeks prior to her expected date of delivery, Mrs. Acker experiences painless vaginal bleeding and is admitted to the hospital. The nurse's care plan for the patient should include:

1. Administering vitamin K to promote clotting

2. Administering an enema to prevent contamination during delivery

3. Performing a rectal examination to determine cervical dilation

4. Placing her in a semi-Fowler position to increase cervical pressure

64 Mrs. Acker's bleeding increases and the physician decides to perform a cesarean section. A premature male infant is delivered. One of the criteria the nurse should use in assessing the gestational age of Mrs. Acker's baby is:

1. The presence of reflex stability

2. Breast bud size

3. The presence of simian creases

4. Finger nail length

65 The initial nursing action after the birth of the baby should be to:

1. Clamp and cut the umbilical cord

2. Quickly dry the baby and place him in a thermometrically controlled warm environment

3. Obtain a footprint and apply an identification band
4. Assist the physician with resuscitative measures

66 About 1 hour after delivery the nurse can expect Baby Acker to be:
1. Relaxed and sleeping quietly
2. Hyperresponsive to stimuli
3. Intensely alert with eyes wide open
4. Crying and cranky

67 Mrs. Acker is moved to the recovery room after delivery. When her dressing is examined for signs of drainage, a nursing priority should be to:
1. Note the color and consistency of the drainage
2. Circle the drainage on the bandage and note the date and time
3. Observe behind the small of the back for drainage
4. Reinforce the dressing if drainage is excessive

Situation: David Brown, 5½ years old, is admitted with a diagnosis of lead poisoning. He is listless and has had two convulsions within the last 48 hours. Questions 68 through 70 refer to this situation.

68 The nurse should suspect lead-induced renal damage to the proximal tubules when a urinalysis demonstrates the presence of:
1. Albumin, glucose, amino acids, and phosphate
2. Protein, calcium, glucose, and amino acids
3. Glucose, amino acids, potassium, and calcium
4. Protein, calcium, phosphate, and glucose

69 David is started on a regimen of chelation therapy that consists of intramuscular injections of calcium disodium edetate (EDTA) and dimercaprol (BAL) q. 4 h. for 5 days. The nurse understands that a combination of these drugs is preferred because it:
1. Removes lead from the blood more rapidly and decreases deposition in the bones.
2. Has fewer side effects and removes lead from the brain more effectively
3. Eliminates lead from the body more rapidly through the urine
4. Removes lead from the bone marrow more efficiently

70 Recognizing that David's mother shares characteristics in common with other mothers whose children chronically ingest lead, the nurse could help her prevent a recurrence by:
1. Discussing with her ways to renovate her home to remove sources of lead and teaching her measures to improve her parenting.
2. Educating her about the dangers of lead ingestion and the type of treatment and medical care required

3. Helping her recognize factors in her maternal-child interactions and in the home environment that predispose her son to pica
4. Initiating referrals to appropriate social and public health service agencies for the total management of her problem

Situation: Mrs. Owens, a 72-year-old woman with congestive heart failure, is often troubled by edematous feet and ankles. She comes to the clinic for evaluation. Questions 71 through 74 refer to this situation.

71 Mrs. Owens admits to you that she has not been following her salt-restricted diet and now is experiencing markedly increased ankle edema, orthopnea, and dyspnea on exertion. Which of the following might also accompany her apparent overhydration?
1. Dizziness on rising
2. Weak and thready pulse
3. Rhinitis and headache
4. Decreased hemoglobin count and hematocrit

72 Mrs. Owens also has osteoporosis. This is best described as:
1. A decrease in bone substance
2. Hyperplasia of osteoblasts
3. Pathologic fractures
4. Avascular necrosis

73 Mrs. Owens' care plan for osteoporosis includes active and passive exercises, calcium supplements, and daily vitamins. The desired effect of therapy would be noted by the nurse if Mrs. Owens:
1. Had fewer bruises than on admission
2. Increased her mobility
3. Developed fewer cardiac irregularities
4. Developed fewer muscular spasms

74 Two weeks after discharge Mrs. Owens experiences mild epigastric pain and is returned to the hospital by her daughter, who is very concerned. Mrs. Owens is admitted to the coronary care unit for observation. She states, ''I know I'm sick but I could really take care of myself at home.'' The nurse recognizes that Mrs. Owens is attempting to:
1. Deny her illness
2. Suppress her fears
3. Reassure her daughter
4. Maintain her independence

Situation: Mrs. Bartin, 46 years old, has a history of alcohol abuse. She is admitted to an alcohol rehabilitation center, where she is being detoxified. Questions 75 through 78 refer to this situation.

75 A nursing assessment of Mrs. Bartin would probably reveal:
   1. Nausea, hypertension, and loss of appetite
   2. Hypotension and agitation
   3. Hypertension, bradycardia, and hyperactivity
   4. Lethargy and hypotension

76 In the initial interview with Mrs. Bartin the nurse should plan to include:
   1. An explanation of the unit's routines
   2. An explanation of the client's role on the unit
   3. A complete list of the unit's rules and regulations
   4. A description of acceptable behavior on the unit

77 Mrs. Bartin should be assigned to a:
   1. Room that is well lit and away from areas of activity
   2. Room without windows and close to the nurse's station
   3. Room with adequate lighting from the corridor
   4. Room with dim lights shared by a quiet, withdrawn patient

78 Which of the following plans would best gain Mrs. Bartin's involvement in her own hygienic care?
   1. Give her a schedule and require her to bathe and dress herself each morning
   2. Draw up a schedule with her and make certain that she adheres to it
   3. Bathe and dress her each morning until she is willing to do it for herself
   4. Assist her in bathing and dressing by giving her clear, simple directions

Situation: Mr. Rudolph is admitted to the burn unit with second- and third-degree burns. Questions 79 through 84 refer to this situation.

79 Fluid shifts are a great danger to the patient with burns. Which of the following would be expected to occur?
   1. Increased fluid shifts and irreversible shock after 2 hours
   2. Loss of sodium and increase in blood potassium
   3. Decreased capillary permeability
   4. Rise in blood volume

80 IV fluid replacement therapy is important. Which of the following would the nurse expect in the first 24 hours?
   1. Intake, 8000 ml; output, 480 ml
   2. Intake, 12,000 ml; output, 4500 ml
   3. Intake, 3000 ml; output, 2400 ml
   4. Intake, 6000 ml; output, 1200 ml

81 The rate of fluid replacement for a patient with severe burns during the first 48 hours is considered satisfactory if the urinary output is approximately:
   1. Half the intake
   2. One tenth the intake
   3. One third the intake
   4. Equal to the intake

82 To maintain Mr. Rudolph's nutrition during convalescence, which of the following measures would be most important?
   1. Reduce protein intake to avoid overtaxing the kidneys
   2. Limit caloric intake to decrease the work of the body
   3. Encourage the drinking of orange juice or other fluids containing vitamin C
   4. Encourage increased intake of sodium

83 Which of the following statements, true of the recovery and convalescent periods, should be considered when planning Mr. Rudolph's care?
   1. Death may still occur from septicemia
   2. The danger of physical complications is past
   3. Because of the patient's need for rest, diversional therapy must be delayed
   4. To decrease the patient's anxiety about appearance, mirrors should be removed

84 Mr. Rudolph asks why he is being given an antacid. The nurse explains that it is prophylactic and is used to prevent which condition that tends to occur 2 weeks after the burn?
   1. Curling's ulcer
   2. Gastric ulcer
   3. Colitis
   4. Gastritis

Situation: Mr. and Mrs. Halloway are expecting their first child after 10 years of marriage. In the thirty-eighth week of pregnancy Mrs. Halloway is scheduled for a nonstress test. Questions 85 through 89 refer to this situation.

85 Mrs. Halloway asks if the nurse thinks the nonstress test is necessary. The nurse's best reply would be:
   1. Certainly; you have had problems and we want to reduce the risks.''
   2. Your physician feels it is necessary so I think you should have it done.''
   3. "You still have doubts about this test, don't you.''
   4. "It is a fast procedure and totally harmless.''

86 Two weeks later Mrs. Halloway is admitted to the labor and delivery unit in active labor. When as-

sessing her, the nurse recognizes true labor by the occurrence of:
1. Regular contractions
2. Cervical dilation
3. Leakage of fluid from the vagina
4. Rectal pressure

87 Mrs. Halloway's labor progresses, and she complains of low back pain. Which comfort measure should the nurse recommend that Mr. Halloway use to relieve her discomfort? He should:
1. Place her in the supine position
2. Instruct her to flex her knees
3. Apply back pressure during contractions
4. Help her perform neuromuscular control exercises

88 The nurse withholds food and limits fluids as the second stage approaches because:
1. The mechanical and chemical digestive process requires energy that is needed for labor
2. Undigested food and fluid may cause nausea and vomiting and limit the choice of anesthesia
3. Food will further aggravate gastric peristalsis, which is already increased due to the tension of labor
4. The gastric phase of digestion stimulates the release of hydrochloric acid and may cause dyspepsia

89 Mrs. Halloway delivers a 2721.6 g (6 lb) baby girl. As part of the physical assessment of this baby the nurse observes for the presence of an umbilical hernia. This assessment can best be accomplished when the baby is:
1. Crying
2. Sucking
3. Inhaling
4. Sleeping

Situation: Ann Julio, a newborn, is admitted to the neonatal intensive care unit immediately after birth. Questions 90 through 94 refer to this situation.

90 When assessing Ann, the nurse should suspect the possibility of hydrocephalus if:
1. The infant's cry sounds high pitched
2. The head circumference is 2 to 3 cm greater than the chest circumference
3. The infant's Apgar score was less than 5
4. The infant has a lumbosacral meningomyelocele

91 Ann is diagnosed as having communicating hydrocephalus. In explaining communicating hydrocephalus to the parents, the nurse should state:

1. "Too much cerebrospinal fluid is produced within the ventricles of the brain."
2. "The cerebrospinal fluid is prevented from proper absorption by a blockage in the ventricles of the brain."
3. "The part of the brain surface that normally absorbs cerebrospinal fluid after its production is not functioning adequately"
4. "There is a flow of cerebrospinal fluid between the brain cells and the ventricles, which do not empty properly into the spinal cord."

92 Several days later a ventriculoperitoneal shunt is inserted. In discharge planning, the nurse should teach the parents to observe for the most common complications after this type surgery—which include:
1. Eyes with sclerae that are visible above the irises
2. Fever, irritability, and decreased responsiveness
3. Violent involuntary muscle contractions
4. Excessive fluid accumulation in the abdomen

93 In teaching Ann's parents to pump the valve of the ventriculoperitoneal shunt, the nurse explains to them that the primary purpose of this procedure is to:
1. Drain excessive cerebrospinal fluid rapidly
2. Increase absorption of cerebrospinal fluid
3. Keep the tubing of the shunt patent
4. Divert the cerebrospinal fluid from the ventricles

94 Ann demonstrates urinary incontinence and flaccidity of the lower extremities. The teaching plan for her parents would include that:
1. She will probably wear diapers for a lifetime since bladder training is impossible.
2. An ileal bladder will be necessary once she is of school age.
3. She will probably be a candidate for an intermittent straight catheterization program
4. An indwelling Foley catheter offers the best hope for bladder management

Situation: Mrs. Jane Donnley, a 32-year-old woman with a history of mild rheumatic heart disease, is in the first trimester of her first pregnancy. Questions 95 through 104 refer to this situation.

95 During the seventh week of her pregnancy, Mrs. Donnley complains of dependent edema in her ankles. The nurse advises her to:
1. Limit her fluid intake during the day
2. Stop using salt for the next 3 months

3. Elevate her legs more frequently during the day
4. Call her physician immediately for a mild diuretic

96 Nutritional management is most important for the pregnant woman with cardiac problems. The nurse should advise Mrs. Donnley to eat a diet with:
1. Increased fats
2. Increased sodium
3. Decreased protein
4. Decreased calories

97 In the eighth month Mrs. Donnley is scheduled for an oxytocin challenge test (OCT). The nurse caring for her understands that the OCT is used in evaluating the:
1. High-risk mother's ability to tolerate a vaginal delivery
2. Fetal heart rate
3. Contractibility of the pregnant uterus prior to delivery
4. Uteroplacental function

98 One important instruction for Mrs. Donnley prior to the oxytocin challenge test is that she should:
1. Take diazepam (Valium) 5 mg p.o. ½ hour before the test
2. Empty her bladder before the test
3. Eat nothing for 2 hours before the test and 6 hours after the test
4. Be prepared to be in the hospital for 12 hours after the test

99 Prior to the start of the oxytocin challenge test (OCT) the nurse explains to Mrs. Donnley that:
1. The fetal heart rate will be monitored for 30 minutes prior to actual testing
2. She will be placed in a right lateral position, which must be maintained throughout testing
3. At least 6 contractions must be observed before the test is discontinued
4. A double-voided urine specimen will be collected prior to the test

100 Mrs. Donnley gives birth to a 3124 g (6 lb 14 oz) baby boy, and the nurse is performing a newborn assessment. In what order should Baby Donnley's vital signs be measured?
1. Respirations, temperature, pulse
2. Temperature, pulse, respirations
3. Respirations, pulse, temperature
4. The sequence of measurement is unimportant

101 Mrs. Donnley is breast-feeding her son. One day when the nurse brings him to be fed, Mrs. Donnley mentions that she cannot believe her newborn wants to breast-feed again since she just fed him

2½ hours ago. The nurse should plan to teach Mrs. Donnley that a newborn usually should be nursed:
1. Every hour
2. Every 2 hours
3. Every 4 hours
4. Every 5 hours

102 Mrs. Donnley is afraid that her heart condition will prevent her from being able to care for her baby and her home properly when she is discharged. The most appropriate nursing intervention is to:
1. Speak to her husband alone and explain how he can assist
2. Ask Mrs. Donnley to explain more fully why she feels this way
3. Tell Mrs. Donnley to speak to her physician about her concerns
4. Suggest that Mrs. Donnley's husband arrange for help at home

103 Mr. Donnley tells the nurse that he is anxious about feeling like a father. The priority in planning to meet the father's needs would be to:
1. Provide a demonstration on diapering, feeding, and bathing the baby.
2. Provide the opportunity to ask questions after viewing the film *Our New Baby*.
3. Provide time for the father to be alone with and get to know the baby.
4. Encourage the father's participation in a fathering class

104 On her 6-week postpartum visit, Mrs. Donnley tells the nurse she wants to feed her baby a whole milk (cow's milk) formula after 2 months since she will be returning to work. The nurse should plan to teach her that whole milk does not meet the infant's nutritional requirements because it is low in:
1. Thiamin and sodium
2. Protein and carbohydrates
3. Fat and calcium
4. Vitamin C and iron

Situation: Mary Jane Lee, age 33, is admitted from the emergency room to the neurologic service with a diagnosis of myasthenia gravis. Questions 105 through 111 refer to this situation.

105 Because of the involvement of the ocular muscles, a common early symptom the nurse should observe for is:
1. Nystagmus
2. Diplopia
3. Blurring
4. Tearing

106 A test that might be performed on Ms. Lee in diagnosing this condition involves the use of which drug?
1. EDTA
2. Edrophonium (Tensilon)
3. Prednisolone
4. Phenytoin (Dilantin)

107 The prognosis of myasthenia gravis is most likely to be:
1. Poor, with termination in a few months
2. Chronic, with exacerbations and remissions
3. Slowly progressive without remissions
4. Excellent with proper treatment

108 The sex and age most frequently affected are:
1. Males ages 15 to 35
2. Females ages 10 to 30
3. Both sexes ages 20 to 40
4. Children ages 5 to 15

109 Ms. Lee is receiving neostigmine bromide (Prostigmin) for control of myasthenia gravis. In the middle of the night the nurse finds her weak, unable to move, and barely breathing. Signs that would identify the problems as being related to overactivity of neostigmine bromide are:
1. High-pitched, gurgling bowel sounds
2. Rapid pulse with occasional ectopic beats
3. Distention of the bladder
4. Fine tremor of the fingers and eyelids

110 Ms. Lee's husband asks the nurse whether his wife will be an invalid. Recognizing the individuality of responses to disease, the best answer would be:
1. "The progression is slow, so she will spend her young life with few problems."
2. "Deformities will occur, but she will not be an invalid."
3. "With continuous treatment the disease progression can be controlled."
4. "There will be periods when she is confined to bed rest and times when she can have fairly normal activity."

111 Which one of the following diversional activities would meet the nursing objectives for Ms. Lee during remissions?
1. Watching selected television shows
2. Swimming with the family
3. Teaching sewing classes
4. Short hikes with the family

Situation: Mrs. Clara Reed, 72 years of age, is admitted to the psychiatric unit with a tentative diagnosis of primary degenerative dementia. Questions 112 through 115 refer to this situation.

112 The nurse understands that primary degenerative dementia results from:

1. Cerebral atrophy specifically involving the frontal lobes
2. A delayed response to severe trauma in early adulthood
3. Anatomic changes in the brain that produce acute but transient symptoms
4. A long history of poor nutrition and associated avitaminosis

113 Mrs. Reed tells the nurse, "I am useless to everyone, even myself." The nurse recognizes that Mrs. Reed has probably not successfully accomplished which of Erickson's developmental tasks?
1. Ego integrity versus despair
2. Autonomy versus shame and doubt
3. Identity versus role diffusion
4. Generativity versus stagnation

114 A nurse's aide complains to the nurse that Mrs. Reed will do things, but only when she feels like doing them, and wonders how one can deal with this. The nurse's response to the aide should be based on the understanding that the elderly:
1. Lose their ability to cooperate
2. Are ambivalent toward authority
3. Lose ego flexibility
4. Utilize strong superego control

115 Mrs. Reed has difficulty following simple directions and selecting her clothes for the day. The nurse recognizes that these problems are the results of:
1. Clouding of consciousness
2. Impaired judgment
3. Loss of abstract thinking ability
4. Decreased attention span

Situation: Mr. Bunger, age 45, has been aware of a mass in his right cheek and upper neck for several years. Although the mass had become increasingly noticeable, he did not seek medical attention. As a result of an extensive campaign in his community, he made an appointment at a local hospital for a cancer detection examination. He was informed by the physician that he should be hospitalized for surgery immediately for a tumor involving the parotid gland. Questions 116 through 120 refer to this situation.

116 Although the physician has explained the possible extent of surgery, the patient is still quite anxious. Nursing intervention should be aimed at:
1. Attempting to discover what is bothering the patient
2. Elaborating on what the physician has already told the patient
3. Planning for postoperative communication, since a tracheostomy is likely to be performed
4. Teaching the patient to use the suction equipment preoperatively

117 At surgical intervention the tumor proves to be malignant, and right total parotidectomy is performed. A complication, distressing to the patient, for which the nurse should be alert is:
1. Tracheostomy
2. Facial nerve dysfunction
3. Frey's syndrome
4. Salivation

118 Postoperatively Mr. Bunger is kept in a high Fowler position to:
1. Promote drainage of the wound
2. Prevent venous oozing from the incision
3. Prevent strain on the incision
4. Provide stimulation for the patient

119 When Mr. Bunger complains that his dressing is tight, the nurse should plan to:
1. Check it for signs of bleeding
2. Check it for signs of constriction
3. Inform the patient that a tight dressing is necessary
4. Alter it to relieve the sensation

120 Mr. Bunger's condition deteriorates, and he is in the terminal stage. The nurse must understand that in dealing with terminally ill patients perhaps the most important factor relative to therapeutic nurse-patient relationships is:
1. How the nurse feels about the situation
2. The nurse's recognition of the family's ability to cope
3. The nurse's knowledge of the grieving process
4. Previous experiences with terminally ill patients

How to Use Worksheet 1: Errors in Processing Information

Common errors in processing information are listed in the left hand column of this worksheet. At the top of the worksheet is a row of blank spaces for inserting the number of the question missed. Directly below each number, check any errors you made in answering that question. You may have made more than one type of error in an answer.

Worksheet 1: Errors in Processing Information

Question no.																					
Did not read situation/question carefully																					
Missed important details																					
Confused major and minor points																					
Defined problem incorrectly																					
Could not remember terms/facts/concepts/ principles																					
Defined terms incorrectly																					
Focused on incomplete/incorrect data in assessing situation																					
Interpreted data incorrectly																					
Applied wrong concepts/principles in situation																					
Drew incorrect conclusions																					
Identified wrong goals																					
Identified priorities incorrectly																					
Carried out plan incorrectly/incompletely																					
Was unclear about criteria for evaluating success in achieving goals																					

How to Use Worksheet 2: Knowledge Gaps

Types of common knowledge gaps are listed along the top of this worksheet. Write a brief description of topics you want to review in the spaces provided. For example, if you missed a question on administration of a particular drug, write the drug name and problem (e.g., dosage) in the appropriate space under the column labeled Pharmacology.

Worksheet 2: Knowledge Gaps

Basic science	Skills/ procedures	Basic human needs	Growth & develop-ment	Normal nutrition	Psycho-social factors	Clinical area/ topic	Stressors/ coping mechanisms	Patho-physiology	Pharma-cology	Therapeutic nutrition	Legal implications	Other

Answers and Rationales

1. (3) With the head and chest elevated, gravity promotes respiratory excursion; alternating side-lying positions allows for pulmonary drainage and expansion. (b); PL; AP; NU; PE
   (1) Would permit the abdominal viscera to impinge on the diaphragm, impeding lung expansion.
   (2) Difficult to maintain a 5-week-old infant in this position; also would not promote rest.
   (4) Would make it difficult for the lungs to expand, causing difficulty in breathing.

2. (1) Some mottling is expected because of the circulatory disruption and arterial spasm. Further assessment (e.g., palpation of the pedal pulse) is done to rule out total occlusion. (a); IM; AP; NU; PE
   (2) Other observations should be made before the physician is notified.
   (3) Mottling would occur all over if due to the external temperature; a blanket would interfere with observation.
   (4) Elevation of leg would be contraindicated; might support bleeding from the puncture site.

3. (2) A patent airway and adequate pulmonary ventilation are always priorities after surgery. (a); AS; AP; NU; PE
   (1) This is important, but adequate ventilation is the priority.
   (3) IV lines would be checked once the airway, breathing, and circulation are determined to be functioning well.
   (4) Too soon to be a priority; however, it certainly must be assessed later.

4. (1) This provides the best reassurance as long as they know what to expect in the recovery room. (b); IM; AP; SH; PE
   (2) If recovery room visit were not possible, this would be the next best action.
   (3) This might increase Mrs. Dorn's anxiety; seeing her child would be more therapeutic.
   (4) There is an immediate need to reduce anxiety; having coffee will not meet this need.

5. (1) The formula should be boiled until the baby is about 6 months old. Before then gastric acidity is low and incapable of exerting bactericidal action. (c); AN; CP; SH; PE
   (2) There is hydrochloric acid, but not enough to protect the infant.
   (3) *E. coli* is the normal intestinal bacterium; not found in the stomach.
   (4) The infant is born with passive immunity from maternal antibodies.

6. (2) Elevating the head of the bed will prevent reflux of gastric contents into the esophagus. (b); IM; AP; CL; ME

(1) Eating at bedtime and drinking orange juice would stimulate gastric secretions.
   (3) Small frequent meals would relieve symptoms of fullness and prevent gastric stimulation.
   (4) Would delay emptying of the stomach, which would increase gastric secretions and the feeling of fullness.

7. (3) Whole grain cereals and breads are irritating, provide bulk, and should be excluded from a bland diet. (a); IM; KN; CL; ME
   (1) Eggs are permitted except when fried.
   (2) Meats are permitted except pork.
   (4) All cooked vegetables are permitted; raw vegetables should be avoided.

8. (3) Sodium bicarbonate is absorbed and can alter the acid-base balance. Antacids are not absorbed, so they do not alter acid-base balance. (c); AN; CP; SH; ME
   (1) False; these are side effects of nonsystemic antacids.
   (2) False; nonsystemic antacids are insoluble and not readily absorbed.
   (4) False; aluminum hydroxide preparations contain sodium and should be used only with caution.

9. (3) Antacids interfere with absorption of drugs such as anticholinergics, barbituates, tetracycline, and digoxin. (b); PL; CP; CL; ME
   (1) May be taken as frequently as every 1 to 2 hours without adverse effects.
   (2) Liquid antacids are faster acting and more effective.
   (4) False; antacids should be given 1 or 2 hours *after* meals and at bedtime.

10. (3) Gamma globulin provides passive immunity in infectious hepatitis. It is given to all individuals who come into direct contact with the patient. (b); PL; CP; CL; ME
    (1) Infectious hepatitis virus is found in the stools of infected patients before the onset of symptoms and during the first few days of illness.
    (2) Gamma globulin is available; it is given 2 to 7 days after exposure with a second dose later.
    (4) Gamma globulin provides passive immunity in infectious hepatitis.

11. (4) Temperature during steaming is never high enough or sustained long enough to kill organisms. (b); IM; CP; CL; ME
    (1) Because of the extremely high temperature, broiling sufficiently destroys the virus.
    (2) Not a shellfish; baking would destroy the organisms.
    (3) Processing destroys the organisms.

12. (4) Relapses are common. They occur after too early ambulation and too much physical activity. (b); PL; CP; CL; ME
    (1) Fatigue is a cardinal symptom; if the patient is tired at rest, he should not return to work.
    (2) The majority of patients recover in 3 to 16 weeks with no further problems.
    (3) Hepatitis is most communicable before the onset of symptoms and during the first few days of fever.

13. (4) The nurse should demonstrate to the patient a recognition of her concern and a willingness to listen.
(c); IM; AP; SH; PS

(1) Avoiding the question indicates that the nurse is unwilling to listen.

(2) Could increase anxiety and would not reduce worry;
furthermore, it cuts off communication and denies
feelings.

(3) The patient did not state that she thought she had
cancer; this response forces her to defend her feelings.

14. (2) Certain diagnostic tests (e.g., CBC, urinalysis,
chest x-ray examination) are done preoperatively to
rule out the existence of other health problems that
could increase the risks involved with surgery. (c);
IM; AP; SH; SU

(1) Feelings would not be dispelled by this response;
also blocks further communication.

(3) Lack of knowledge without a statement of plans to
obtain the information suggests incompetence on the
part of the nurse.

(4) False information; surgery poses a risk despite test
results.

15. (4) Anxiety experienced by a preoperative patient can
be a disruptive force affecting the patient's ability
to adapt psychologically and physiologically. For
other nursing measures to be effective, it must be
alleviated. (b); PL; AP; NU; SU

(1) Learning is hampered by high anxiety levels.

(2) Diet is limited prior to surgery so residue in the intestines will be decreased.

(3) Vital signs must be recorded, for they will serve as
a baseline in postoperative assessment; however, reduction of anxiety is the first priority.

16. (3) Interpretation of pain sensations by each patient is
highly individual and is based on the patient's past
experiences, which include cultural values. (b); AN;
CP; CL; SU

(1) Overall physical condition may affect one's ability
to cope with stress; but unless the nervous system
were involved, it would not greatly affect perception.

(2) Intelligence is a factor in understanding pain, so it
can be better tolerated, but does not affect the perception of intensity; economic status has no affect
on pain perception.

(4) Age and sex affect pain perception only indirectly
because they generally account for past experience
to some degree.

17. (1) After confinement to bed for a time or administration of certain antihypertensives, the patient's neu-
rocirculatory reflexes may have some difficulty adjusting to the force of gravity in an upright position.
Postural or orthostatic hypotension occurs, and there
is a temporarily decreased blood supply to the brain.
(a); PL; AP; SH; SU

(2) Respiratory distress is an adverse effect of morphine
but is not prevented by the intervention described.

(3) Hypertension does not occur.

(4) Abdominal pain will not be prevented by the intervention described.

18. (4) Used for its analgesic effects, morphine is a central
nervous system depressant. Its major adverse effect
is respiratory depression; but it can also cause lethargy, pupillary constriction, and depressed reflexes,
and it could lead to coma and death. (b); EV; KN;
NU; SU

(1) Although diaphoresis may accompany hypotension,
it is only indirectly related to the drug and is not
profuse.

(2) Overdose causes miosis rather than dilated pupils.

(3) These occur to some extent with therapeutic doses
because of their effect on the CNS; however, not
symptoms of an overdose.

19. (3) Pain in the calf may be a sign of thrombophlebitis,
a possible postoperative complication. If the thrombus becomes dislodged, it may lead to pulmonary
embolism. Any patient with this complaint should
immediately be confined to bed, and the physician
notified. (a); AN; AN; NU; SU

(1) The leg should not be elevated above heart level
without a physician's order; gravity may dislodge
the thrombus, creating an embolism.

(2) Application of heat is a dependent nursing function.

(4) Charting does not take precedence over notifying
the physician of a potentially serious complication.

20. (3) Endometriosis is the presence of aberrant endometrial tissue outside the uterus. The tissue responds to
ovarian stimulation, bleeds during menstruation,
and causes severe pain. (a); AS; KN; NU; OB

(1) Incorrect by definition.

(2) Ecchymoses and petechiae are not characteristic of
this disorder.

(4) Osteoporosis may be a complication of menopause
due to the decreased estrogen levels; pelvic inflammation usually results from infection.

21. (1) Menopause is a normal developmental adaptation. It
is not caused by endometriosis, the abnormal bleeding of aberrant tissue outside the uterus. (c); AS;
AP; SH; OB

(2) Bleeding between periods is due to the bleeding of
endometrial tissue outside the uterus.

(3) Excessive tissue may impinge on the colon and
cause ribbonlike stools.

(4) Excessive tissue may impinge on the bladder and
ureter; can cause voiding difficulties.

22. (2) Antiovulatory drugs suppress menstruation. Breakthrough bleeding is abnormal and will lead to recurrence of symptoms. (b); PL; CP; CL; OB

(1) There is no indication for increased Pap smears;
once a year is sufficient.

(3) No restriction of sexual activity is indicated when
one is taking oral contraceptives.

(4) Increased calcium to counteract osteoporosis from
menopause is not indicated for this patient.

23. (1) Anxiety causes an increase in body secretions, which stimulates tissue changes. (c); AN; KN: NU; PS
(2) This emotional response does not cause an alteration in tissue.
(3) Fear is usually not a prolonged emotional response; would not cause an alteration in tissue.
(4) Fear is usually not a prolonged emotional response; would not cause an alteration in tissue.
24. (3) This test allows the physician to perform a biopsy of the gastric mucosa. (c); AS; CP; NU; ME
(1) Done to determine the response of gastric secretion after an intravenous injection of secretin; normally there should be a decrease. This will not confirm the presence of malignant cells.
(2) Will outline structural changes; however, it will not identify the presence of malignant cells.
(4) Not a tissue study; will not confirm the diagnosis of cancer.
25. (3) The nurse was negligent in using a stretcher with worn straps. Such oversight did not reflect the actions of a reasonably prudent nurse. (b); EV; AP; NU; ME
(1) The nurse is responsible for determining the safety of hospital equipment.
(2) The nurse is responsible for own actions and must ascertain the adequate functioning of equipment.
(4) The hospital shares responsibility for safe equipment functioning.
26. (4) Barium salts used in a GI series and barium enemas coat the inner lining of the GI tract and then absorb x rays passing through. They thus outline the surface features of the tract on a photographic plate. (a); IM; AP; SH; ME
(1) Barium has no light-emitting properties.
(2) Barium does not fluoresce.
(3) Barium has no properties of a dye.
27. (3) Anxiety or stress causes a hypersecretion of hydrochloric acid. This produces actual physiologic changes in the tissue itself. (a); AN; CP; NU; ME
(1) The changes are the result of psychologic conflicts that cause physiologic changes.
(2) Illness may result from psychologic conflicts but is not a defense mechanism.
(4) Physiologic changes do not cause psychologic changes.
28. (2) Hemorrhage after erosion of blood vessel walls is often the first symptom that leads the patients to seek medical assistance. (b); AS; KN; NU; ME
(1) Perforation would occur well after hemorrhage, and treatment would have been sought at the time of hemorrhage.
(3) Not a common complication.
(4) Occur because of portal hypertension not peptic ulcers.
29. (2) Applesauce, Cream of Wheat, and milk are bland foods that do not irritate the gastric mucosa. (c); IM; AP; NU; ME

(1) Not considered bland; may be irritating to the mucosal lining.
(3) Not considered bland; may be irritating to the mucosal lining.
(4) Not considered bland; may be irritating to the mucosal lining.
30. (4) After administration of a local anesthetic during a bronchoscopy, fluids and food should be withheld until the gag reflex returns. (a); IM; AP; SH; SU
(1) To allow drainage and maximize respiratory status, the patient should be kept in a semi-Fowler position.
(2) Ice chips must not be given until the gag reflex returns.
(3) Coughing should not be encouraged; it might initiate bleeding from the site of the biopsy.
31. (3) The phrenic nerve stimulates the diaphragm. After destruction of the nerve on the operative side, the diaphragm will move upward, decreasing the size of the empty space and helping prevent mediastinal shift. (c); AN; KN; NU; SU
(1) Would occur if both nerves were severed.
(2) Since the phrenic nerve stimulates the diaphragm, its effect on postoperative pain would be negligable.
(4) There is less excursion because the nerve has been severed.
32. (3) Because Mrs. Smith has just undergone major surgery, she has an endotracheal tube in place. Secretions can be loosened by the administration of humidified air and by frequent turning and coughing. (b); PL; AN; NU; SU
(1) A patient with an endotracheal tube in place is not permitted fluids by mouth.
(2) Would be too vigorous for a patient in the immediate postoperative state.
(4) Potassium is never instilled into the lungs.
33. (1) To maintain normal expansion of the remaining lung after a pneumonectomy, the patient should be positioned on the operative side or the back. (c); IM; AP; SH; SU
(2) The patient should not be placed on the unaffected side; will impede lung expansion.
(3) A high Fowler position may cause the patient to slip down in the bed, diminishing thoracic excursion.
(4) Keeping the patient flat will decrease lung expansion; gatching a bed may cause peripheral circulatory complications.
34. (2) After a pneumonectomy the mediastinum may shift toward the remaining lung, or the remaining lung could shift toward the empty space, depending on the pressure within the empty space. Either of these shifts would cause the trachea to move from its normal midline position. (The trachea is palpated above the suprasternal notch.) (c); IM; AP; NU; SU
(1) Tracheal edema cannot be assessed through palpation; edema is not a concern when the endotracheal tube is in place
(3) Metastatic lesions would not appear rapidly.

(4) The cuff of the endotracheal tube cannot be assessed through palpation of the trachea.

35. (4) This response recognizes fearful feelings. It also permits further communication. (a); IM; AP; SH; PS
 (1) Does not recognize feelings of fear; changes the focus of the conversation.
 (2) Does not recognize feelings; instills fear by implying that this pregnancy may not go to term, for which there is no evidence.
 (3) Closes off communication and may increase anxiety.

36. (3) This response acknowledges the loss and the grieving process. It also encourages ventilation through acceptance. (a); IM; AP; SH; PS
 (1) Guilt feelings were never expressed by the patient; this response may reflect the nurse's feelings.
 (2) Minimizes the loss; may reflect the nurse's feelings. It also plants thoughts of a less than perfect fetus.
 (4) Does not recognize the loss; cuts off communication.

37. (2) A correct and simple definition answers the question and fulfills the patient's need to know. (b); IM; AP; SH; OB
 (1) The nurse can independently reinforce and clear misconceptions.
 (3) Denies the patient's right to know.
 (4) This is the definition of a missed abortion.

38. (2) Initial disbelief and denial help protect the ego from the pain of reality in a stressful situation. (c); AS; AN; SH; PS
 (1) Once the initial shock is over, these are the usual results as the self realizes the loss.
 (3) May result from guilt or feelings of inadequacy because of the loss; but occurs later.
 (4) There is no evidence of either dissociation or rationalization.

39. (3) This action demonstrates recognition of the patient's behavior as a normal response to the situation. (a); IM; AN; SH; PS
 (1) May be done later; the need to respond to the patient's feelings is the priority at this time.
 (2) May make her feel that she is doing something wrong or is annoying others.
 (4) Closes off communication; does not allow the patient to talk about her feelings.

40. (1) Jerky lateral eye movement, particularly toward the involved ear. (b); AS; AN; NU; ME
 (2) Not usually associated with Ménière's disease.
 (3) Not usually associated with Ménière's disease.
 (4) Not usually associated with Ménière's disease.

41. (4) Prepared without salt, this food has the least sodium. (a); PL; AP; CL; ME
 (1) Have a high sodium content, which promotes fluid retention and increases endolymphatic fluid in the cochlea.
 (2) Has a high sodium content.
 (3) Has a high sodium content.

42. (4) Keeping a record of what one eats helps limit unconscious and nervous eating by making the individual aware of food intake. (b); PL; AP; CL; ME
 (1) Not always practical and is difficult to implement; assessment of dietary habits is the priority.
 (2) Exercise causes rapid head movements, which may precipitate an attack.
 (3) Limiting calories to 900 per day requires a physician's order.

43. (3) Inadequate oxygenation increases demands on the heart. This leads to tachycardia as the body tries to compensate. (a); AS; AP; NU; PE
 (1) RBC levels are close to normal; suggests anemia caused by iron deficiency rather than by blood loss. This could cause cold clammy skin.
 (2) Results from excess carboxyhemoglobin; pallor is more common with anemia.
 (4) Not generally an adaptation associated with decreased hemoglobin.

44. (3) The 4-year-old child has developed trust but still needs frequent support from his parents. (a); IM; AP; CL; PS
 (1) Appropriate for an infant who is just developing trust in his parents; hospitalization should not interfere with this important aspect of personality development.
 (2) The parents may bring a toy; but their presence to provide support and reinforce trust is more important.
 (4) The parents should participate in their son's care as much as possible, so there will be no interference with the trust relationship and to provide support.

45. (4) Immediate physical safety takes priority. The patient must sit down before he falls down. Follow with the supine position. (b); IM; AP; SH; PE
 (1) Immediate physical safety takes priority over further assessment.
 (2) Gravity promotes cerebral blood flow in this position; however, immediate physical safety takes priority.
 (3) Subjective symptoms of dizziness alone do not warrant this; immediate physical safety takes priority.

46. (3) Decreased oxygen-carrying capacity of the blood may lead to hypoxia during exercise, when oxygen demand is greater. (b); AN; CP; NU; PE
 (1) Although this may be a cause of the symptom, it is not directly related to anemia.
 (2) Although this may be a cause of the symptom, it is not directly related to anemia.
 (4) Although this may be a cause of the symptom, it is not directly related to anemia.

47. (3) Liquid iron preparations may stain tooth enamel, so they should be diluted and administered through a straw. (a); IM; AP; SH; PE
 (1) To avoid gastric irritation, iron should be given with food.

(2) To improve absorption, iron may be given with orange juice.

(4) Constipation, rather than loose stools, often results.

48. (3) Residual medication on the needle may stain the skin during penetration. (a); IM; AP; NU; PE

(1) Deep penetration is necessary; only the gluteal muscles should be used because of their size and the decreased visibility of staining.

(2) Should be avoided; might cause seepage of drug through the needle track, with subsequent tissue irritation and staining.

(4) Would constrict blood vessels and impair absorption.

49. (4) The 4-year-old can express himself better through play than with words. (b); IM; AP; SH; PE

(1) This may help the nurse understand emotional problems; however, it is not as helpful as play therapy in meeting the child's emotional needs.

(2) Understanding explanations requires abstract thinking; 4-year-olds think in a concrete manner.

(3) A needle is dangerous; even a play syringe would focus the child's attention on one aspect of treatment, without eliciting broader feelings.

50. (1) The added cardiac workload of individuals with anemia increases the risk of heart failure, leading to pulmonary edema. (b); AN; AN; NU; PE

(2) Untrue; not increased by anemia.

(3) Untrue; not increased by anemia.

(4) Untrue; not increased by anemia.

51. (1) Denial or disbelief and shock are considered initial responses of grieving. There is a feeling of guilt and inadequacy when a child is born with a defect or abnormality. (a); AS; CP; SH; PS

(2) It would be unusual for a patient initially to verbalize feelings of punishment or guilt so directly.

(3) It would be unusual for a patient to use rationalization and voice it so obviously.

(4) A sense of shame and guilt is voiced later; after denial, disbelief, and shock.

52. (3) This approach allows for ventilation of feelings and clarifies explanations that probably were not heard or understood because of anxiety. (b); IM; AP; SH; PS

(1) Closes off communication by not allowing free expression of grief.

(2) Excludes the client from facing the problem, thereby increasing her feeling of loss of control.

(4) Supports avoidance of the reality of the situation; does not help the problem.

53. (1) The psychosocial need during the early toddler age is the development of autonomy. The toddler objects very strongly to discipline. (b); AN; CP; SH.; PE

(2) Untrue; excessive discipline leads to feelings of shame and self doubt, the major crisis at this stage of development.

(3) It is frightening for a child to be left alone; leaves

him with feelings of rejection, isolation, and insecurity.

(4) The sense of initiative is attained during the preschool age, not during the toddler age.

54. (4) This action of Susan's gives her child more control by allowing him to make a decision. It also shows an understanding of what the toddler can and cannot do safely. (c); EV; CP; CL; PS

(1) Although tantrums as attention-getting devices largely must be ignored, ignoring the child will produce feelings of isolation and insecurity.

(2) Boredom, hunger, and insecurity can lead to additional frustration and anger.

(3) This could lead to the development of more manipulative tactics, since the action brought a degree of success initially.

55. (4) This action determines the patient's tolerance of turning. Orthostatic hypotension can occur, and the physician should be alerted if the vital signs do not stabilize in 5 to 10 minutes. (b); PL; AP; NU; SU

(1) The neck should be maintained in a neutral position; a roll under the neck causes hyperextension.

(2) The patient is maintained in a supine position unless the physician indicates otherwise; a retention catheter is usually inserted.

(3) Sandbags are generally unnecessary; constant pressure is being exerted by skull traction to reduce the fracture.

56. (4) The CircOlectric bed turns patients from a horizontal supine position vertically to a horizontal prone position. It can also remain stationary in a vertical position. The change of position alters the body pressures periodically while the patient is confined to the bed. (c); PL; KN; NU; SU

(1) It is possible for one nurse to turn a patient in a CircOlectric bed.

(2) Lateral turning is not possible with a CircOlectric bed.

(3) Although in some mattresses a pad can be removed so that a bed pan may be inserted, a receptacle itself would be impractical since the entire bed turns.

57. (2) Asepsis around the site of insertion must be maintained, since it is a break in the first line of defense. (b); IM; AP; NU; SU

(1) Skin care is essential in preventing breakdown; however, it must be administered carefully.

(3) Constant traction must be maintained to reduce the fracture.

(4) The weights must be guided, but not removed during position changes.

58. (2) The Schwann cells that compose the neurilemma of peripheral nerve fibers (dendrites and axons) are capable of supporting nerve fiber regeneration. (b); AN; KN; SH; SU

(1) The myelin sheath, produced peripherally by the Schwann cells and centrally by the oligodenrocytes, is not involved directly in the regenerative process.

(3) Found in all neurons.

(4) Found in all neurons.

59. (4) The phrenic nerves innervate the diaphragm. Therefore a crushing spinal cord injury above the level of phrenic origin would stop diaphragmatic contractions and result in respiratory paralysis. (b); AN; CP; NU; SU

(1) Cardiac activity would not be affected; the heart is regulated by the autonomic nervous system from fibers originating in the medulla.

(2) Activities regulated by the vagus nerve would be unaffected; the vagi originate in the medulla, which is superior to the cervical region (the phrenic nerves originate from the cervical plexuses).

(3) In a crushing spinal injury both motor and sensory conduction would be affected.

60. (4) Menstruation during pregnancy is interrupted because secretion of the ovarian hormones ceases. This response answers the patient's question in understandable terms. (b); IM; CP; SH; OB

(1) These hormones are needed to rebuild the layers of cells lining the uterus that are sloughed off during menstruation.

(2) LH stimulates the maturation of a primitive follicle into a vesicular graafian follicle; also promotes secretion of estrogen by the ovary.

(3) This brings about the development of the ova.

61. (4) Abstinence 4 to 6 weeks prior to delivery is the best way to avoid contracting the virus and having an outbreak prior to delivery. (c); AN; AP; CL; OB

(1) Abstinence is necessary only when disease symptoms are present in the partner and during the last 4 to 6 weeks.

(2) Washing is not enough to prevent contraction of this virus; contact has already been made.

(3) Since the herpesvirus is smaller than the pores of a condom, this kind of protection is not effective.

62. (3) Placenta previa is defined as an abnormally implanted placenta (i.e., low lying or covering the cervical os). (a); AN; AN; SH; OB

(1) Can occur without a low-lying placenta; factors such as poor muscular tone of the uterus and excessive oxytocin during induction may cause this to occur.

(2) Premature separation of the placenta can occur with normally implanted placentas

(4) Can occur at any time; not specific to low-lying placentas.

63. (4) Placing the expectant mother in a semi-Fowler position forces the heavy uterus to put temporary pressure on the blood vessels at the site of the separating placenta. This controls bleeding to some extent. (b); PL; AN; NU; OB

(1) No indication that the clotting mechanism is disturbed.

(2) Contraindicated in any patient admitted with vaginal bleeding.

(3) Contraindicated when placenta previa is suspected; may further dislodge the placenta.

64. (2) The size of the breast bud is an indication of gestational age. Small undeveloped nipples reflect prematurity. (c); AS; KN; NU; OB

(1) Not a good indication of gestational age; reflexes may be impaired in full-term infants also.

(3) Not present in normal newborns; a clinical manifestation of Down's syndrome.

(4) Not related to gestational age.

65. (2) Cold stress produces hypoxia and acidemia. Because of physiologic factors, the premature infant is most vulnerable to cool temperatures. (b); IM; AP; NU; OB

(1) Not a priority; keeping the baby warm is more important.

(3) Not a priority; keeping the baby warm is more important.

(4) No indication that this is necessary.

66. (3) This is the first period of reactivity. The newborn is alert and awake. (c); AN; AP; NU; OB

(1) First sleep usually occurs more than 1 hour after delivery.

(2) This occurs after the first sleep.

(4) Untrue; after the initial cry, the baby will settle down and become quiet and alert.

67. (3) Excessive drainage flows down the sides of the abdomen to the small of the back by gravity. Observing for hemorrhage is the priority. (b); IM; CP; NU; OB

(1) Color and consistency should also be noted; however, for patient safety, recording the amount takes precedence.

(2) This might also be done, but assessing the total amount of drainage would be the priority.

(4) If drainage is excessive, the physician should be notified first.

68. (1) These substances are not normally excreted in the urine. When found, they indicate renal disease. (b); AN; AN; NU.; PE

(2) Excess calcium is normally excreted.

(3) Potassium is normally excreted by the kidneys to maintain electrolyte balance.

(4) Excess calcium is normally excreted.

69. (2) Fewer side effects mean better elimination of the lead, which means that further irreversible damage can be prevented. (b); EV; CP; NU; PE

(1) Each drug is able to accomplish this, but singly given each can cause more side effects; may be fatal if rapidly infused.

(3) No marked difference in the rate of elimination when these agents are used together.

(4) The combination is preferred because it removes lead more effectively from the brain rather than from bone marrow.

70. (1) Active sharing of responsibility will prove most helpful. It will contribute to the success of the mother's efforts to overcome dependency and passivity and assure that lead sources are removed. (c); IM; AP; SH; PE

(2) Will not resolve etiologic factors or accomplish prevention.

(3) Omits the need to remove lead from the environment; therefore will not assure prevention.

(4) A good idea, but does not guarantee action; concrete action should be taken first.

71. (4) An increase in the extracellular fluid volume can cause a relative decrease in the hemoglobin and hematocrit by dilution of the blood. (c); AS; AN; NU; ME

(1) Occurs when pooling of blood in the peripheral vessels causes hypotension; rarely occurs with hypervolemia.

(2) The increased fluid volume in the intravascular compartment (overhydration) will cause the pulse to feel full and bounding.

(3) Headache might accompany overhydration, but rhinitis would not.

72. (1) This defect in bone matrix formation weakens the bones, making them unable to withstand normal stresses. (a); AN; KN; NU; ME

(2) Incorrect; not related to osteoporosis. This occurs during bone healing.

(3) Occurs during normal activity or after minimal injury in bones weakened by disease.

(4) This is death of bone tissue; results from reduced circulation to bone.

73. (2) This regimen limits bone demineralization. It also reduces osteoporitic pain, which promotes increased activity. (c); EV; AN; SH; ME

(1) Would be expected if the patient were receiving vitamin C and calcium for capillary fragility.

(3) Not related to osteoporosis or the rationale for therapy.

(4) Would be expected if the patient were receiving calcium for hypocalcemia.

74. (4) The patient's statement is really saying, "I can manage this myself. I am capable." (c); AS; AN; SH; PS

(1) Nothing in her statement can be interpreted as denial; she has stated, "I know I'm sick."

(2) None of the information given would lead to this conclusion.

(3) Her statement would not be reassuring to the daughter who brought her to the hospital and probably is more reassured having her there.

75. (1) It has been medically proved that during the first stage of detoxification, nausea, anorexia, and hypertension are experienced. (c); AS; CP; SH; PS

(2) Hypertension (not hypotension) and agitation are experienced during this stage.

(3) Hypertension, hyperactivity, and tachycardia (not bradycardia) are experienced during this stage.

(4) Psychomotor hyperactivity (not lethargy) and hypertension (not hypotension) are experienced during this stage.

76. (1) This would provide some security since the patient would know what to expect at different periods during the day. (b); PL; AP; SH; PS

(2) Inappropriate; would probably increase anxiety, and there is no one prototype of a patient's role.

(3) Inappropriate; would be somewhat overwhelming. Many of the regulations would not even apply to Mrs. Bartin.

(4) Inappropriate; would increase anxiety and serve little purpose. Necessary limits should be individual, not set by regulation.

77. (1) A well-lit and quiet room helps reduce the fears and illusional experiences of the patient experiencing alcoholic withdrawal. (c); PL; AN; NU; PS

(2) The nurses' station is usually a busy place; a room nearby is not the ideal location for the alcoholic patient experiencing delirium. Noises can be frightening and may stimulate hallucinations or illusions.

(3) Bright lights from corridors can cast shadows on the walls and ceiling of a darkened room, increasing stimulation and illusions of frightening objects.

(4) Dim lights in the room increase stimulation, producing illusions and hallucinations; strangers may increase the patient's fear, restlessness, and confusion.

78. (4) This action would provide the disorganized patient with the necessary structure to encourage participation and support of self-image. (b); PL; AP; SH; PS

(1) Would increase her anxiety and withdrawal and decrease her level of function.

(2) Would increase her anxiety and withdrawal and decrease her level of function.

(3) Would increase dependency and add to her self-doubt.

79. (2) Because of tissue destruction, sodium ions are lost in the interstitial fluid whereas potassium ions are liberated from the injured cells. The result is hyperkalemia. (c); AN; CP; NU: SU

(1) Fluid shifts may cause shock but it is reversible with therapy.

(3) Capillary permeability is increased in burns.

(4) Blood volume decreases, and hypovolemic shock may occur.

80. (4) Because of fluid loss and sodium retention, urinary output is diminished. However, output of less than 30 ml per hour is considered a sign of shock. (c); PL; AP; NU; SU

(1) This amount would overload the patient; output is less than 30 ml per hour.

(2) This intake is excessive, as is the output; would not be expected in the newly burned patient.

(3) This amount of fluid replacement would be inadequate, and fluid loss excessive, in the newly burned patient; very little fluid is left to replace losses during the first few days.

81. (3) Since a great deal of intravascular fluid is lost during the first 48 hours through evaporation and in the exudate and edema, urinary output is not expected to equal the intake but increases from that of the

first day. An output of less than 30 ml per hour is an indication of shock. (c); EV; CP; NU; SU

(1) If half the intake is excreted, insufficient fluid is left to replace losses.

(2) This would probably indicate inadequate kidney perfusion, shock, or kidney damage.

(4) This would not allow for replacement of fluid lost due to burns.

82. (3) Vitamin C is essential for wound healing. It provides a component of intercellular ground substance that develops into collagen and is necessary to build supportive tissue. (a); IM; AP; CL; SU

(1) To help in repairing damaged tissue, protein intake should be increased.

(2) Decreasing calories could increase the work of the body; would promote catabolism of body tissue.

(4) To prevent excess fluid retention, which would increase the cardiovascular workload, sodium intake should be regulated.

83. (1) The skin is the first line of defense against infection. When much of it is destroyed, the individual is left vulnerable to infection. (a); PL; CP; SH; SU

(2) Complications such as infection may also occur during the convalescent phase.

(3) Diversional therapy as tolerated may be helpful physically and psychologically.

(4) Removing mirrors can increase anxiety about body image and lead the patient to conclude that the situation is even worse than it is.

84. (1) Curling's ulcer (an ulcer of the upper GI tract) is related to the excessive secretion of stress-related hormones. These increase hydrochloric acid production. (a); IM; KN; SH; SU

(2) Not a complication of burns.

(3) Not a complication of burns.

(4) Not a complication of burns.

85. (3) This reply encourages the patient to discuss fears and anxieties. (a); IM; AP; SH; PS

(1) Does not encourage the patient to discuss the situation further; mention of risk may frighten the patient.

(2) Opinions or value judgments should not be expressed by the nurse; should deal only with the patient's feelings.

(4) Cuts off communication; does not allow the patient to express her fears and anxiety.

86. (2) False labor does not produce cervical dilation. Only true labor does. (b); AS; CP; SH; OB

(1) Braxton Hicks contractions may have some regularity.

(3) Urine may appear to leak from the vaginal orifice.

(4) Some women have diarrhea prior to labor.

87. (3) The application of back pressure combined with frequent positional changes will help alleviate the discomfort. (a); IM; AP; CL; OB

(1) The supine position places increased pressure on the back; aggravates the pain.

(2) Although this may be comfortable for some individuals, rubbing the back and alternating positions are more universally effective.

(4) Neuromuscular control exercises are used to teach selective relaxation in childbirth classes; not utilized in labor.

88. (2) Gastric peristalsis often ceases during periods of stress. Abdominal contractions put pressure on the stomach and can cause nausea and vomiting, increasing the risk of aspiration. (a); IM; CP; NU; OB

(1) Gastric activity and digestion cease during periods of tension.

(3) Gastric activity and digestion cease during periods of tension.

(4) Although food may cause dyspepsia, the primary reason for withholding it is to prevent aspiration.

89. (1) Increased intraabdominal pressure associated with crying, coughing, or straining will cause protrusion of the hernia. (a); AS; AP; NU; OB

(2) Does not increase intraabdominal pressure.

(3) The lowering of the diaphragm may increase intraabdominal pressure slightly but not enough to cause protrusion of the hernia.

(4) Does not increase intraabdominal pressure.

90. (4) Hydrocephalus complicates approximately 90% of lumbosacral meningomyeloceles. (b); AS; CP; NU; PE

(1) A shrill high-pitched cry often accompanies progressive hydrocephalus; however, may also indicate other neurologic problems.

(2) Normal for a newborn.

(3) Hydrocephalic infants may or may not have a low Apgar score.

91. (3) This is what occurs in communicating hydrocephalus. (c); IM; AP; SH; PE

(1) This is often caused by a choroid plexus tumor and does not interfere with the flow of cerebrospinal fluid through the ventricles.

(2) This reflects the pathophysiologic process of noncommunicating hydrocephalus.

(4) Inaccurate answer; brain cells and the spinal cord are not involved.

92. (2) These are associated with infection, the greatest postoperative hazard for children with shunts for hydrocephalus. (b); PL; AN; SH; PE

(1) Occur with progressively increasing intracranial pressure, usually before shunt insertion; considered a sign, not a complication.

(3) May be a complication, sometimes as a result of an infected shunt; however, not the most common complication.

(4) The peritoneum absorbs cerebrospinal fluid adequately; ascites is not a problem.

93. (3) Periodic pumping of the valve ensures the patency of the tubing and allows the fluid to move through. (b); IM; AN; CL; PE

(1) Bleeding results if cerebrospinal fluid is drained too

rapidly; the pump may be used for this purpose, but this is not its primary function.

(2) Pumping the shunt does not affect the absorption of cerebrospinal fluid.

(4) This is the purpose of the shunt itself; pumping the valve only keeps the tubing patent.

94. (3) Most children with spinal cord damage from communicating hydrocephalus can be managed successfully with this approach. (b); PL; AP; SH; PE

(1) This is a devastating and inaccurate statement to make to any young infant's parents.

(2) Most children with spinal cord damage from this defect can be managed successfully with intermittent straight catheterization.

(4) Inaccurate statement, and the least desirable approach because of recurrent urinary tract infections.

95. (3) This is normal. It results from the increased pressure of the uterus on venous return. Elevating the legs encourages venous return. (a); IM; AN; SH; OB

(1) Can be harmful; increased circulating blood volume during pregnancy must be maintained.

(2) Contraindicated; salt is necessary to retain fluid for increased circulating blood volume during pregnancy.

(4) Diuretics are not used during pregnancy; may decrease the circulating blood volume.

96. (4) This is recommended to keep weight gain in balance and to control blood pressure. (c); PL; CP; CL; OB

(1) Increasing fats could cause accumulation of unwanted adipose tissue.

(2) Increasing sodium intake is not advised for patients with cardiac problems.

(3) Decreasing protein intake is not advised for patients with cardiac problems.

97. (4) Uteroplacental insufficiency correlates well with a positive OCT (potential fetal distress). Prompt intervention is indicated. (c); AN; CP; SH; OB

(1) The OCT is unrelated to the mother; it is concerned only with the ability of the fetus to tolerate labor.

(2) An incomplete statement; the occurrence of decelerations and accelerations is also evaluated.

(3) The small dose of oxytocin is too small to test completely the ability of the uterus to contract.

98. (2) The OCT will take 1 to 2 hours, during which time the patient is confined to bed. Movement on and off a bedpan should be avoided. (a); IM; AP; SH; OB

(1) Valium could interfere with the results of the OCT since the baby would be sedated.

(3) No food restrictions are indicated.

(4) She may go home 1 hour after the test.

99. (1) This is done to measure baseline variability of the FHR and to observe any alteration in the FHR without oxytocin-induced stress. (c); IM; AP; SH.; OB

(2) The semi-Fowler position with a left-sided tilt is the position of choice.

(3) False; the test involves monitoring the fetal heart during 3 uterine contractions within a 10-minute period.

(4) There is no indication for this; the test is concerned only with observing the FHR.

100. (3) Touching for pulse and inserting the thermometer increase anxiety and cause elevated vital signs. This sequence is least disturbing. (a); AS; AP; NU; PE

(1) Respirations should be measured first, but temperature should be measured after the pulse rate.

(2) Temperature should be measured last.

(4) Sequence *is* important, since the baby's vital signs will change when touched.

101. (2) Breast milk is digested faster than formula. Breast-fed infants therefore become hungry sooner. (c); PL; CP; CL; OB

(1) An infant may want to nurse hourly if irritable, but this is not a usual feeding pattern.

(3) A breast-fed newborn must be fed more often than this.

(4) All infants must be fed more often than this.

102. (2) Information seeking is the first step in problem solving. (b); IM; AP; SH; PS

(1) The nurse assumes that the husband will solve the problem; violates the confidence between nurse and patient.

(3) Shifts the responsibility to the physician.

(4) Presumptuous and expensive; makes the decision for the patient.

103. (3) This provides the opportunity for paternal-infant bonding. Handling the infant may reduce some of his anxiety. (c); PL; AP; CL; OB

(1) Does not recognize his anxiety; also he may not be ready to absorb this information.

(2) A simplistic approach to his emotional needs; does not deal with the real situation.

(4) Although helpful, does not meet the need for paternal-infant bonding.

104. (4) Whole milk does not meet the infant's need for vitamin C and iron. Also, it contains high amounts of protein and sodium, which may be harmful. (c); PL; CP; SH; PE

(1) Whole milk contains adequate thiamin; the sodium content is 3 times that found in human milk.

(2) Whole milk contains adequate carbohydrates; the protein content is 3 times that found in human milk.

(3) Whole milk contains adequate fats; the calcium content is 3½ times that found in human milk.

105. (2) In myasthenia gravis the effectiveness of acetylcholine is reduced, interfering with muscle contraction. Inadequate contraction of the ocular muscles results in double vision (diplopia). (b); AS; AP; SH; ME

(1) Nystagmus is a common symptom of multiple sclerosis.

(3) Not a symptom of myasthenia gravis.

(4) Not a symptom of myasthenia gravis.

106. (2) Tensilon is an anticholinesterase compound that drastically increases muscle strength when administered to an individual with myasthenia gravis. (c); AS; CP; SH; ME

(1) EDTA is a calcium chelating agent sometimes used in the treatment of digitalis intoxication.

(3) Prednisolone is a steroid; not used to diagnose this disease.

(4) Dilantin is an anticonvulsant; not used to test for myasthenia.

107. (2) Myasthenia gravis is a chronic degenerative disorder with exacerbations that are precipitated by emotional stress, ingestion of alcohol, and physical stress such as infection. (a); AN; CP; NU; ME

(1) The disease is chronic; death does not occur within a short period but usually after the muscles of respiration are affected.

(3) The disease is characterized by exacerbations and remissions.

(4) The prognosis is not excellent; there is no cure.

108. (3) Myasthenia gravis is a degenerative disease that occurs equally in both sexes during adulthood. (b); AN; KN; NU; ME

(1) Occurs equally in both sexes.

(2) Occurs equally in both sexes.

(4) Not a disease common in childhood.

109. (1) Neostigmine bromide (Prostigmin) is an anticholinergic that increases the peristaltic activity of the intestines. The result is hyperactive bowel sounds. (b); EV; AP; SH; ME

(2) Bradycardia and hypotension may occur with neostigmine.

(3) Bladder distension is not associated with neostigmine.

(4) These are not side effects associated with neostigmine.

110. (4) The response should be kept as optimistic as possible while still being realistic. (b); IM; CP; SH; ME

(1) The individual response varies; gives false reassurance.

(2) False reassurance; her status will depend on her individual response.

(3) Medication does not affect progression; only treats the symptoms.

111. (2) Swimming would help keep the muscles supple, without requiring fine motor activity. (b); AN; AP; CL; ME

(1) Sedentary activities are not helpful in maintaining muscle tone.

(3) Sewing requires fine motor activity; would be difficult for the patient.

(4) Might prove too rigorous for the patient.

112. (1) The gross pathology in primary degenerative dementia is brain tissue degeneration with loss of brain neurons. (c); AS; CP; NU; PS

(2) Severe emotional trauma may contribute to but does not necessarily cause primary degenerative dementia.

(3) False; nerve cells do not have the capacity to regenerate. Neural degeneration leads to permanent, not transient, changes.

(4) Poor nutrition may be one of the factors that bring about a general decline of health; however, no direct evidence that avitaminosis causes primary degenerative dementia.

113. (1) The sense of ego integrity comes from satisfaction with life and acceptance of what has been and what is. Despair is due to guilt or remorse over what might have been. (c); AS; AP; NU; PS

(2) Autonomy is developed during the toddler period and corresponds to the child's ability to control his body and environment; doubt can result when he is made to feel ashamed or embarrassed.

(3) During puberty the adolescent attempts to find himself and integrate his values with those of society; inability to solve conflict results in confusion and hinders mastery of future roles.

(4) During early and middle adulthood the individual is concerned with his ability to produce and to care for that which is produced or created; failure during this stage leads to self-absorption or stagnation.

114. (3) Fears and anxieties about themselves and their possesions are common in aging because of decreased self-concept and altered body image. (c); AN; CP; NU; PS

(1) Aging need not necessarily bring about losing one's ability to cooperate.

(2) The attitude of elderly persons about authority or others in their environment is set; indecision about life situations may be due to insecurity.

(4) The elderly fear the loss they must face in almost every aspect of their lives; this leads to lowering of their self-esteem and faulty reality testing.

115. (3) Impairment of abstract thinking interferes with interpretation and defining of words. Skill in abstract thinking is required to follow directions and select clothes. (c); AN; AH; SH; PS

(1) Primary degenerative dementia does not cause a clouding of consciousness.

(2) Following directions does not require skill in judgment or decision making.

(4) The selection of clothes does not require an intact attention span.

116. (1) Various aspects of hospitalization and diagnosis could cause the patient anxiety. The nurse should determine what factor(s) disturbs the patient most. (b); PL; AP; SH; SU

(2) An anxious patient will not be receptive to learning.

(3) A tracheostomy may not be performed, depending on the extent of the surgery and edema.

(4) This may cause the patient unnecessary anxiety.

117. (2) The facial nerve may be damaged during surgery. Drooping of the area results from loss of muscle tone. (b); AS; AN; NU; SU

(1) A tracheostomy may not be performed; it is not a complication but rather a preventive measure.

(3) This is also called auriculotemporal syndrome; may follow infection and suppuration of the parotid gland. It produces pain and erythema of the cheek.

(4) The parotid is a salivary gland; its removal would decrease salivation.

118. (2) This position minimizes the discomfort associated with venous engorgement. It also promotes venous drainage by gravity. (c); IM; AP; NU; SU

    (1) Drainage from the wound would not be affected.

    (3) This position would neither increase nor decrease strain on the suture line.

    (4) Providing stimulation would not be a priority item; this position would not affect the degree of stimulation.

119. (2) If the dressing is too tight, impaired cerebral circulation may result. (b); PL; AP; SH; SU

    (1) Bleeding would not cause the patient to complain of tightness.

    (3) Untrue; impaired cerebral circulation may result from a tight dressing.

(4) The dressing may be removed only if indicated by the physician.

120. (1) To be truly effective in the relationship with the patient, the nurse must know and understand personal feelings about terminal illness and death. (b); AN; CP; SH; PS

    (2) Although the family is an important part of the patient's support system, the patient's feelings are more important to the relationship.

    (3) In dealing with terminal illness, knowledge alone is not enough to assure a good nurse-patient relationship.

    (4) Previous experiences could be positive or negative and would not guarantee an effective nurse-patient relationship.

Bibliography

Medical-Surgical Nursing

Andreoli, K.G.: Comprehensive cardiac care: a text for nurses, physicians, and other health practitioners, ed. 5, St. Louis, 1983, The C.V. Mosby Co.

Anthony, C.P., and Thibodeau, G.A.: Textbook of anatomy and physiology, ed. 11, St. Louis, 1983, The C.V. Mosby Co.

Axnick, K., and Yarbrough, M.: Infection control: an integrated approach, St. Louis, 1983, The C.V. Mosby Co.

Berne, R.M.: Physiology, St. Louis, 1983, The C.V. Mosby Co.

Berne, R.M., and Levy, M.N.: Cardiovascular physiology, ed, 4, St. Louis, 1981, The C.V. Mosby Co.

Billings, D.M., and Stokes, L.G.: Medical surgical approaches throughout the life cycle, St. Louis, 1982, The C.V. Mosby Co.

Broadwell, D.C., and Jackson, B.S.: Principles of ostomy care, St. Louis, 1981, The C.V. mosby Co.

Brooks, S.M.: Instrumentation for the operating room: a manual, ed. 2, St. Louis, 1982, The C.V. Mosby Co.

Budassi, S.A., and Barber, J.: Mosby's manual of emergency care: practices and procedures, ed. 2, St. Louis, 1984, The C.V. Mosby Co.

Collins, M.: Communication in health care: the human connection in the life cycle, ed. 2, St. Louis, 1982, The C.V. Mosby Co.

Conover, M.B.: Understanding electrocardiography, ed. 4, St. Louis, 1984, The C.V. Mosby Co.

Conway-Rutkowski, B.L.: Carini and Owens neurological and neurosurgical nursing, ed. 8, St. Louis, 1982, The C.V. Mosby Co.

Daily, E.K., and Schroeder, J.S.: Hemodynamic waveforms: exercises in indentification and analysis, St. Louis, 1983, The C.V. Mosby Co.

Douglass, L.M.: Nursing management and leadership in action, ed. 4, St. Louis, 1983, The C.V. Mosby Co.

Douglass, L.M.: The effective nurse: leader and manager, ed. 2, St. Louis, 1984, The C.V. Mosby Co.

Ebersole, P., and Hess, P.: Toward healthy aging: human needs and nursing response, St. Louis, 1981, The C.V. Mosby Co.

Estes, N.J., and Heinemann, M.E.: Alcoholism: development, consetuqnces and interventions, ed. 2, St. Louis, 1981, The C.V. Mosby Co.

Forbes, V.J., and Fitzsimons, V.M.: The older adult: a process for wellness, St. Louis, 1981, The C.V. Mosby Co.

Gahart, B.L.: Intravenous medications, ed. 3, St. Louis, 1981, The C.V. Mosby Co.

Given, B.A., and Simmons, S.J.: Gastroenterology in clinical nursing, ed. 4, St. Louis, 1983, The C.V. Mosby Co.

Godow, A.G.: Human sexuality, St. Louis, 1982, The C.V. Mosby Co.

Goth, A.: Medical pharmacology: principles and concepts, ed. 10, St. Louis, 1981, The C.V. Mosby Co.

Gress, L., and Bahr, R.T.: The aging person: a holistic perspective, St. Louis, 1984, The C.V. Mosby Co.

Griffith, J.W., and Christensen, P.J.: The nursing process: application of theories, St. Louis, 1982, The C.V. Mosby Co.

Groer, M.E., and Shekleton, M.E.: Basic pathophysiology: a conceptual approach, ed. 2, St. Louis, 1983, The C.V. Mosby Co.

Gruendemann, B.J., and Meeker, M.H.: Alexanders care of the patient in surgery, ed. 7, St. Louis, 1983, The C.V. Mosby Co.

Guthrie, D.W., and Guthrie, R.A.: Nursing management of diabetes mellitus, ed. 2, St. Louis, 1982, The C.V. Mosby Co.

Hahn, A.B., et al.: Pharmacology in nursing, ed. 15, St. Louis, 1982, The C.V. Mosby Co.

Holloway, N.M.: Nursing the critically ill adult, Menlo Park, Calif., 1979, Addison-Wesley Publishing Co., Inc.

Johanson, B.C., et al.: Standards for critical care, St. Louis, 1984, The C.V. Mosby.

Kozier, B.B., and Erb, G.L.: Fundamentals of nursing: concepts and procedures, ed. 2, Menlo Park, Calif., 1983, Addison-Wesley Publishing Co., Inc.

Luckmann, J., and Sorensen, K.C.: Medical surgical nursing: a psychophysiologic approach, ed. 2, Philadelphia, 1980, W.B. Saunders Co.

Malasanos, L., et al.: Health assessment, ed. 2, St. Louis, 1981, The C.V. Mosby Co.

Marriott, H.J.L., and Conover, M.H.B.: Advanced concepts in arrhythmias, St. Louis, 1982, The C.V. Mosby Co.

Pagana, K.D., and Pagana, T.J.: diagnostic testing and nursing implications: a case study approach, St. Louis, 1982, The C.V. Mosby Co.

Phipps, W.J., et al.: Shafer's medical-surgical nursing, ed. 7, St. Louis, 1980, The C.V. Mosby Co.

Phipps, W.J., et al.: Medical-surgical nursing: concepts and clinical practice, ed. 2, St. Louis, 1983, The C.V. Mosby Co.

Ray, O.S.: Drugs, socity, and human behavior, ed. 3, St. Louis, 1983, The C.V. Mosby Co.

Redman, B.K.: The process of patient education, ed. 5, St. Louis, 1984, The C.V. Mosby Co.

Saxton, D.F., et al.: Programmed instruction in arithmetic, dosages, and solutions, ed. 5, St. Louis, 1982, The C.V. Mosby Co.

Saxton, D.F., and Hyland, P.A.: Planning and implementing nursing intervention: stress and adaptation applied to patient care, ed. 2, St. Louis, 1979, The C.V. Mosby Co.

Saxton, D.F., Pelikan, P.K., Nugent, P.M., and Hyland, P.A.: Addison-Wesley's manual of nursing practice, Menlo Park, Calif., 1983, Addison-Wesley Publishing Co., Inc.

Smith, S.F., and Duell, D.: Nursing skills and evaluation, St. Louis, 1982, The C.V. Mosby Co.

Strauss, A.M.L., et al.: Chronic illness and the quality of life, ed. 2, St. Louis, 1984, The C.V. Mosby Co.

Sundeen, S.J., et al.: Nurse-client interaction: implementing the nursing process, ed. 2, St. Louis, 1981, The C.V. Mosby Co.

Thompson, J.M., and Bowers, A.C.: Clinical manual of health assessment, ed. 2, St. Louis, 1984, The C.V. Mosby Co.

Tilkian, S.M., et al.: Clinical implications of laboratory tests, ed. 3, St. Louis, 1983, The C.V. Mosby Co.

Tucker, S.M., et al.: Patient care standards, ed. 3, St. Louis, 1984, The C.V. Mosby Co.

Vinsant, M.O., and Spence, M.I.: Commonsense approach to coronary care, ed. 3, St. Louis, 1980, The C.V. Mosby Co.

Wade, J.F.: Comprehensive respiratory care: physiology and technique, ed. 3, St. Louis, 1982, The C.V. Mosby Co.

Weldy, N.J.: Body fluids and electrolytes, ed. 4, St. Louis, 1984, The C.V. Mosby Co.

Williams, S.R.: Nutrition and diet therapy, ed. 4, St. Louis, 1981, The C.V. Mosby Co.

Woods, N.F.: Human sexuality in health and illness, ed. 3, St. Louis, 1984, The C.V. Mosby Co.

Psychiatric Nursing

Aguilera, D.C., and Messick, J.M.: Crisis intervention: theory and methodology, ed. 4, St. Louis, 1981, The C.V. Mosby Co.

American Psychiatric Assocation: Diganostic and statistical manual of mental disorders, ed. 3, Washington, D.C., 1980, The Association.

Beck, C.M., et al.: Mental health-psychiatric nursing: a holistic life-cycle approach, St. Louis, 1984, The C.V. Mosby Co.

Burgess, A.W., and Lazare, A.: Psychiatric nursing in the hospital and the community, ed. 3, Englewood Cliffs, N.J., 1980, Prentice-Hall, inc.

Burnside, I.M.: Psychosocial nursing care of the aged, ed. 2, New York, 1980, McGraw-Hill Book Co., Inc.

Estes, N.J., and Heinemann, E.: Alcoholism: development, consequences, and interventions, ed. 2, St. Louis, 1981, The C.V. Mosby Co.

Foley, T., and Davies, M.: Rape: nursing care of victims, St. Louis, 1983, The C.V. Mosby Co.

Gorton, J., and Partridge, R.: Practice and management of psychiatric emergency care, St. Louis, 1982, The C.V. Mosby Co.

Haber, J., et al.: Comprehensive psychiatric nursing, ed. 2, New York, 1983, McGraw-Hill Book Co., Inc.

Hagerty, B.M.: Psychiatric-mental health assessment, St. Louis, 1984, The C.V. Mosby Co.

Kyes, J., and Hofling, C.K.: Basic psychiatric concepts in nursing, ed. 4, Philadelphia, 1980, J.B. Lippincott Co.

Lancaster, J.: Community mental health nursing: an ecological perspective, St. Louis, 1980, The C.V. Mosby Co.

Lofstedt, C.R.: Mereness' essentials of psychiatric nursing: learning and activity guide, St. Louis, 1981, The C.V. Mosby Co.

Murray, R.B., and Huelskoetter, M.M.W.: Psychiatric-mental health nursing: giving emotional care, Englewood Cliffs, N.J., 1983, Prentice-Hall, Inc.

Pasquali, E.A., et al.: Mental health nursing: a bio-psycho-cultural approach, St. Louis, 1981, The C.V. Mosby Co.

Physician's desk reference, ed. 36, Oradell, N.J., 1982, Medical Economics Co., Inc.

Saxton, D.F., and Haring, P.W.: Care of patients with emotional problems, ed. 4, St. Louis, 1984, The C.V. Mosby Co.

Sedgwick, R.: Family mental health: theory and practice, St. Louis, 1981, The C.V. Mosby Co.

Stuart, G.W., and Sundeen, S.J.: Principles and practice of psychiatric nursing, ed. 2, St. Louis, 1983, The C.V. Mosby Co.

Sundeen, S.J., et al.: Nurse-client interaction, ed. 2, St. Louis, 1981, The C.V. Mosby Co.

Taylor, C.M.: Mereness' essentials of psychiatric nursing, ed. 11, St. Louis, 1982, The C.V. Mosby Co.

Van Servellen, G.M.: Group and family therapy: a model psychotherapeutic nursing practice, St. Louis, 1984, The C.V. Mosby Co.

Wilson, H.S., and Kneisl, C.R.: Psychiatric nursing, ed. 2, Menlo Park, Calif., 1983, Addison-Wesley Publishing Co., Inc.

Maternity Nursing

Bobak, I.M., and Jensen, M.D.: Essentials of maternity nursing, St. Louis, 1984, The C.V. Mosby Co.

Butnarescu, G.F., and Tillotson, D.M.: Maternity nursing: theory to practice, New York, 1983, JohnWiley & Sons, Inc.

Clark, A.L., and Affonso, D.: Childbearing: a nursing perspective, ed. 2, Philadelphia, 1979, F.A. Davis Co.

Clausen, J.P., Flook, M., and Ford, B.: Maternity nursing today, ed. 2, New York, 1977, McGraw-Hill Book Co., Inc.

Friedman, E.A.: Obstetrical decision making, Chicago, 1982, B.C. Decker

Hamilton. P.M.: Basic maternity nursing, ed. 5, St. Louis, 1984, The C.V. Mosby Co.

Hawkins, J.W., and Higgins, L.P.: Maternity and gynecological nursing, Philadelphia, 1981, J.B. Lippincott Co.

Ingalls, A.J., and Salerno, M.C.: Maternal and child health nursing, ed. 5, St. Louis, 1983, The C.V. Mosby Co.

Jensen, M.D., Benson, R.C., and Bobak, I.M.: Maternity care: the nurse and the family, ed. 2, St. Louis, 1981, The C.V. Mosby Co.

Jensen, M.D., and Bobak, I.M.: Handbook of maternity care: a guide for nursing practice, St. Louis, 1980, The C.V. Mosby Co.

Klaus, M.H., and Kennell, J.H.: Parent infant bonding, ed, 2, St. Louis, 1982, The C.V. Mosby Co.

Moore, M.L.: Realities in childbearing, ed. 2, Philadelphia, 1983, W.B. Saunders Co.

Olds, S.B., et al.: Obstetric nursing, Menlo Park, Calif., 1980, Addison-Wesley Publishing Co., Inc.

Phillips, C.R.: Family-centered maternity-newborn care: a basic text, St. Louis, The C.V. Mosby Co.

Phillips, C.R., and Anzalone, J.T.: Fathering: participation in labor and birth, ed. 2, St. Louis, 1982, The C.V. Mosby Co.

Reeder, S.R., Mastroianni, M.L., and Fitzpatrick, E.: Maternity nursing, ed. 15, Philadelphia, 1983, J.B. Lippincott Co.

Riordan, J.: A practical guide to breastfeeding, St. Louis, 1983, The C.V. Mosby Co.

Varney, H.: Nurse midwifery, Boston, 1980, Blackwell Scientific Publishers, Inc.

Wiggins, J.D.: Childbearing: physiology, experiences, needs, St. Louis, 1979, The C.V. Mosby Co.

Woods, N.F.: Human sexuality in health and illness, ed. 3, St. Louis, 1984, The C.V. Mosby Co.

Worthington, B.S., et al.: Nutrition in pregnancy and lactation, ed. 2, St. Louis, 1981, The C.V. Mosby Co.

Pediatric Nursing

Chinn, P.L.: Child health maintenance: concepts in family-centered care, ed. 2, St. Louis, 1979, The C.V. Mosby Co.

Chinn, P.L., and Leitch, C.J.: Child health maintenance: a guide to clinical assessment, ed. 2, St. Louis, 1979, The C.V. Mosby Co.

Endres, J.B., and Rockwell, R.E.: Food, nutrition, and the young child, St. Louis, 1980, The C.V. Mosby Co.

Endres, J.B., and Rockwell, R.E.: A parent's guide to kids' nutrition, St. Louis, 1983, the C.V. Mosby Co.

Hamilton, P.M.: Basic pediatric nursing, ed. 4, St. Louis, 1982, The C.V. Mosby Co.

Hazinski, M.F.: Pediatric critical care: a nursing perspective, St. Louis, 1984, The C.V. Mosby Co.

Ingalls, A.J., and Salerno, M.C.: Maternal and child health nursing, ed. 5, St. Louis, 1983, The C.V. Mosby Co.

Korones, S.B.: High-risk newborn infants: the basis for intensive nursing care, ed, 3, 1981, The C.V. Mosby Co.

Marlow, D.R.: Textbook of pediatric nursing, ed. 5, Philadelphia, 1977, W.B. Saunders Co.

Perez, R.H.: Protocols for perinatal nursing practice, St. Louis, 1981, The C.V. mosby Co.

Pipes, P.L.: Nutrition in infancy and childhood, ed, 2, St. Louis, 1981, The C.V. Mosby Co.

Powell, Ml.: Assessment and management of developmental changes in children, ed. 2, St. Louis, 1981, The C.V. Mosby Co.

Pringle, S.M., and Ramsey, B.: Promoting the health of children: a guide for caretakers and health care professionals, St. Louis, 1982, The C.V. Mosby Co.

Scipien, G.M., et al.: Comprehensive pediatric nursing, ed. 3, New York, 1984, McGraw-Hill Book Co., Inc.

Shirkey, H.C.: Pediatric therapy, ed. 6, St. Louis, 1980, The C.V. Mosby Co.

Spinetta, J.J., et al.: Living with childhood cancer, St. Louis, 1981, The C.V. Mosby Co.

Whaley, L.F., and Wong, D.L.: Essentials of pediatric nursing, St. Louis, 1983, The C.V. Mosby Co.

Whaley, L.F., and Wong, D.L.: Nursing care of infants and children, ed. 2, St. Louis, 1983, The C.V. Mosby Co.

Wong, D.L., and Whaley, L.F.: Clinical handbook of pediatric nursing, St. Louis, 1981, The C.V. Mosby Co.

History and Legal Trends

Creighton, H.: Law every nurse should know, ed. 3, Philadelphia, 1975, W.B. Saunders Co.

George, J.E.: The law and emergency care, St. Louis, 1980, The C.V. Mosby Co.

Gibbon, J.M., and Mathewson, M.L.: Three centuries of Canadian nursing, Toronto, 1947, The Macmillan Co.

Good, S., and Kerr, J.: Contemporary issues in Canadian law for nurses, Toronto, 1973, Holt, Rinehart & Winston.

Hemelt, M.D., and MacKert, M.E.: Dynamics of law in nursing and health care, Reston, Va., 1978, Reston Publishing Co., Inc.

Kelly, L.Y.: Dimensions of professional nursing, ed. 3, New York, 1975, Macmillan Publishing Cp.

Mauksch, I.G., and Miller, M.H.: Implementing change in nursing, St. Louis, 1980, The C.V. Mosby Co.

Muff, J.: Socialization, sexism, and stereotyping: women's issues in nursing, St. Louis, 1982, The C.V. Mosby Co.

Murchison, I., et al.: Legal accountability in the nursing process, ed. 2, St. Louis, 1982, The C.V. Mosby Co.

Murchison, I., and Nichols, T.: Legal foundations of nursing practice, New York, 1970, The Macmillan Co.

Styles, M.M.: On nursing: toward a new endowement, St. Louis, 1982, The C.V. Mosby Co.

Vogt, J.F., et al.: Retaining professional nurses: a planned process, St. Louis, 1983, The C.V. Mosby Co.

Index

Fractures, 236-238
  of hip, 238
  of jaw, 124
  in toddlers, 419-420
Fungi, 24-25

G

Gallbladder, 107
Gametes, formation of, 147
Gas gangrene, 255
Gases
  in circulatory system, 58
  in gastrointestinal system, 112
  in respiratory system, 90-91
Gastric analysis, 121
Gastric gavage, 123
Gastritis, 125-126
Gastrointestinal series, 121
Gastrointestinal system, 105-140
  absorption in, 109
  anatomy and physiology of, 105-111
  chemical principles related to
    active transport, 113
    amino acids, 117
    buffers, 113
    carbohydrates, 113-114
    compounds, 113-117
    diffusion and osmosis, 112
    enzymes, 117
    lipids, 114-115
    nucleoproteins, 116-117
    organic acids, 113
    oxidation and reduction in, 112
    proteins, 115-116
  diagnostic procedures for, 121-124
  digestion in, 108-109
  diseases of
    acute pancreatitis, 128-129
    anorexia nervosa, 139
    appendicitis, 133
    cancer
      of intestines, 136-137
      of mouth, 124-125
      of pancreas, 129-130
    carcinoma
      of liver, 132
      of stomach, 127
    cholecystitis, 127-128
    Crohn's disease, 134
    drugs for, 118-121
    food poisoning, 139-140
    fracture of jaw, 124
    gastritis, 125-126
    hemorrhoids, 137-138
    hepatic cirrhosis, 131-132
    hepatitis, 130-131
    hernias, 138-139
      hiatal, 125
    intestinal obstruction, 135-136
    obesity, 139
    peptic ulcer, 126-127
    peritonitis, 137
    regional enteritis, 133-134
    sprue, 132-133

Gastrointestinal system—cont'd
  diseases of—cont'd
    stomatitis, 124
    ulcerative colitis, 134-135
  functions of, 105
  metabolism in, 109-111
  microorganisms related to, 117-118
  organs in, 106-108
  pharmacology related to disorders of, 118-121
  physical principles related to, 111-112
Gastrointestinal system disorders, pharmacology related to, 118-121
Genes, 148
Genitourinary system, 140-166
  anatomy and physiology of, 140-148
  chemical principles related to, 149
  cleavage in, 147
  and development of individual, 147-148
  diagnostic procedures for, 150
  diseases of
    acute renal failure, 152-154
    adenocarcinoma of kidneys, 155
    bladder trauma, 156-157
    bladder tumors, 156
    chronic renal failure, 154
    cystitis, 151-152
    drugs for, 37-38
    glomerulonephritis, 155-156
    hydronephrosis, 152
    kidney transplantation, 154-155
    renal and ureteral calculi, 152
    urethritis, 157
  and fertilization, 147
  formation of gametes in, 147
  and heredity, 148
  microorganisms related to, 149-150
  nursing procedures for, 150-151
  pharmacology related to disorders of, 37-38
  physical principles related to, 149
  reproductive system; *see* Reproductive system
  urinary system; *see* Urinary system
Glands
  adrenal, 169-170
  hormones of, 167
  location of, 167
  male sex, 144
  mammary, 146
  ovaries, 169
  pancreas, 170-171
  parathyroid, 166
  pineal, 171
  pituitary, 171
  prostate, cancer of, 159
  testes, 169
  thymus, 171
  thyroid, 166
Glaucoma, angle closure, 243
Glomerulonephritis, 155-156
Gonadal function, drugs affecting, 496-497
Gout, 233
Gouty arthritis, 233
Government agencies providing parent-child health services, 499
Graves' disease, 176-177
Gravitation, law of, 56-57, 90

Answer Sheets

Medical-Surgical Nursing

Review Questions 1-160, pp. 260-271

NAME_____ GRADE_____ SEX_____ DATE OF BIRTH_____
       LAST   FIRST   MIDDLE   M OR F   YEAR MONTH DAY

DATE_____ AGE_____ SCHOOL_____ CITY_____
       YEAR MONTH DAY

INSTRUCTOR_____

IDENTIFICATION NUMBER

NAME OF TEST_____

0 ::::: 1 ::::: 2 ::::: 3 ::::: 4 :::::   5 ::::: 6 ::::: 7 ::::: 8 ::::: 9 :::::
0 ::::: 1 ::::: 2 ::::: 3 ::::: 4 :::::   5 ::::: 6 ::::: 7 ::::: 8 ::::: 9 :::::
0 ::::: 1 ::::: 2 ::::: 3 ::::: 4 :::::   5 ::::: 6 ::::: 7 ::::: 8 ::::: 9 :::::
0 ::::: 1 ::::: 2 ::::: 3 ::::: 4 :::::   5 ::::: 6 ::::: 7 ::::: 8 ::::: 9 :::::
BE SURE TO MAKE YOUR MARKS
HEAVY AND BLACK
0 ::::: 1 ::::: 2 ::::: 3 ::::: 4 :::::   5 ::::: 6 ::::: 7 ::::: 8 ::::: 9 :::::
0 ::::: 1 ::::: 2 ::::: 3 ::::: 4 :::::   5 ::::: 6 ::::: 7 ::::: 8 ::::: 9 :::::
ERASE COMPLETELY ANY ANSWERS
YOU WISH TO CHANGE
0 ::::: 1 ::::: 2 ::::: 3 ::::: 4 :::::   5 ::::: 6 ::::: 7 ::::: 8 ::::: 9 :::::
0 ::::: 1 ::::: 2 ::::: 3 ::::: 4 :::::   5 ::::: 6 ::::: 7 ::::: 8 ::::: 9 :::::
0 ::::: 1 ::::: 2 ::::: 3 ::::: 4 :::::   5 ::::: 6 ::::: 7 ::::: 8 ::::: 9 :::::
0 ::::: 1 ::::: 2 ::::: 3 ::::: 4 :::::   5 ::::: 6 ::::: 7 ::::: 8 ::::: 9 :::::

1 1 2 3 4	2 1 2 3 4	3 1 2 3 4	4 1 2 3 4
5 1 2 3 4	6 1 2 3 4	7 1 2 3 4	8 1 2 3 4
9 1 2 3 4	10 1 2 3 4	11 1 2 3 4	12 1 2 3 4
13 1 2 3 4	14 1 2 3 4	15 1 2 3 4	16 1 2 3 4
17 1 2 3 4	18 1 2 3 4	19 1 2 3 4	20 1 2 3 4
21 1 2 3 4	22 1 2 3 4	23 1 2 3 4	24 1 2 3 4
25 1 2 3 4	26 1 2 3 4	27 1 2 3 4	28 1 2 3 4
29 1 2 3 4	30 1 2 3 4	31 1 2 3 4	32 1 2 3 4
33 1 2 3 4	34 1 2 3 4	35 1 2 3 4	36 1 2 3 4
37 1 2 3 4	38 1 2 3 4	39 1 2 3 4	40 1 2 3 4
41 1 2 3 4	42 1 2 3 4	43 1 2 3 4	44 1 2 3 4
45 1 2 3 4	46 1 2 3 4	47 1 2 3 4	48 1 2 3 4
49 1 2 3 4	50 1 2 3 4	51 1 2 3 4	52 1 2 3 4
53 1 2 3 4	54 1 2 3 4	55 1 2 3 4	56 1 2 3 4
57 1 2 3 4	58 1 2 3 4	59 1 2 3 4	60 1 2 3 4
61 1 2 3 4	62 1 2 3 4	63 1 2 3 4	64 1 2 3 4
65 1 2 3 4	66 1 2 3 4	67 1 2 3 4	68 1 2 3 4
69 1 2 3 4	70 1 2 3 4	71 1 2 3 4	72 1 2 3 4
73 1 2 3 4	74 1 2 3 4	75 1 2 3 4	76 1 2 3 4
77 1 2 3 4	78 1 2 3 4	79 1 2 3 4	80 1 2 3 4
81 1 2 3 4	82 1 2 3 4	83 1 2 3 4	84 1 2 3 4
85 1 2 3 4	86 1 2 3 4	87 1 2 3 4	88 1 2 3 4
89 1 2 3 4	90 1 2 3 4	91 1 2 3 4	92 1 2 3 4
93 1 2 3 4	94 1 2 3 4	95 1 2 3 4	96 1 2 3 4
97 1 2 3 4	98 1 2 3 4	99 1 2 3 4	100 1 2 3 4
101 1 2 3 4	102 1 2 3 4	103 1 2 3 4	104 1 2 3 4
105 1 2 3 4	106 1 2 3 4	107 1 2 3 4	108 1 2 3 4
109 1 2 3 4	110 1 2 3 4	111 1 2 3 4	112 1 2 3 4
113 1 2 3 4	114 1 2 3 4	115 1 2 3 4	116 1 2 3 4
117 1 2 3 4	118 1 2 3 4	119 1 2 3 4	120 1 2 3 4
121 1 2 3 4	122 1 2 3 4	123 1 2 3 4	124 1 2 3 4
125 1 2 3 4	126 1 2 3 4	127 1 2 3 4	128 1 2 3 4
129 1 2 3 4	130 1 2 3 4	131 1 2 3 4	132 1 2 3 4
133 1 2 3 4	134 1 2 3 4	135 1 2 3 4	136 1 2 3 4
137 1 2 3 4	138 1 2 3 4	139 1 2 3 4	140 1 2 3 4
141 1 2 3 4	142 1 2 3 4	143 1 2 3 4	144 1 2 3 4
145 1 2 3 4	146 1 2 3 4	147 1 2 3 4	148 1 2 3 4
149 1 2 3 4	150 1 2 3 4	151 1 2 3 4	152 1 2 3 4
153 1 2 3 4	154 1 2 3 4	155 1 2 3 4	156 1 2 3 4
157 1 2 3 4	158 1 2 3 4	159 1 2 3 4	160 1 2 3 4

Continued.

Medical-Surgical Nursing—cont'd

Review Questions 161-320, pp. 271-281

NAME_____ LAST FIRST MIDDLE GRADE_____ SEX___ M OR F DATE OF BIRTH_____ YEAR MONTH DAY

DATE_____ YEAR MONTH DAY AGE___ SCHOOL_____ CITY_____

INSTRUCTOR_____

NAME OF TEST_____

IDENTIFICATION NUMBER

BE SURE TO MAKE YOUR MARKS
HEAVY AND BLACK

ERASE COMPLETELY ANY ANSWERS
YOU WISH TO CHANGE

NAME _____ LAST _____ FIRST _____ MIDDLE _____ GRADE _____ SEX _____ M OR F _____ DATE OF BIRTH _____ YEAR MONTH DAY

DATE _____ YEAR MONTH DAY _____ AGE _____ SCHOOL _____ CITY _____

INSTRUCTOR _____

NAME OF TEST _____

IDENTIFICATION NUMBER

BE SURE TO MAKE YOUR MARKS HEAVY AND BLACK

ERASE COMPLETELY ANY ANSWERS YOU WISH TO CHANGE

| 0 1 2 3 4 5 6 7 8 9 |
| 0 1 2 3 4 5 6 7 8 9 |
| 0 1 2 3 4 5 6 7 8 9 |
| 0 1 2 3 4 5 6 7 8 9 |
| 0 1 2 3 4 5 6 7 8 9 |
| 0 1 2 3 4 5 6 7 8 9 |
| 0 1 2 3 4 5 6 7 8 9 |
| 0 1 2 3 4 5 6 7 8 9 |
| 0 1 2 3 4 5 6 7 8 9 |
| 0 1 2 3 4 5 6 7 8 9 |

321 1 2 3 4	322 1 2 3 4	323 1 2 3 4	324 1 2 3 4
325 1 2 3 4	326 1 2 3 4	327 1 2 3 4	328 1 2 3 4
329 1 2 3 4	330 1 2 3 4	331 1 2 3 4	332 1 2 3 4
333 1 2 3 4	334 1 2 3 4	335 1 2 3 4	336 1 2 3 4
337 1 2 3 4	338 1 2 3 4	339 1 2 3 4	340 1 2 3 4
341 1 2 3 4	342 1 2 3 4	343 1 2 3 4	344 1 2 3 4
345 1 2 3 4	346 1 2 3 4	347 1 2 3 4	348 1 2 3 4
349 1 2 3 4	350 1 2 3 4	351 1 2 3 4	352 1 2 3 4
353 1 2 3 4	354 1 2 3 4	355 1 2 3 4	356 1 2 3 4
357 1 2 3 4	358 1 2 3 4	359 1 2 3 4	360 1 2 3 4
361 1 2 3 4	362 1 2 3 4	363 1 2 3 4	364 1 2 3 4
365 1 2 3 4	366 1 2 3 4	367 1 2 3 4	368 1 2 3 4
369 1 2 3 4	370 1 2 3 4	371 1 2 3 4	372 1 2 3 4
373 1 2 3 4	374 1 2 3 4	375 1 2 3 4	376 1 2 3 4
377 1 2 3 4	378 1 2 3 4	379 1 2 3 4	380 1 2 3 4
381 1 2 3 4	382 1 2 3 4	383 1 2 3 4	384 1 2 3 4
385 1 2 3 4	386 1 2 3 4	387 1 2 3 4	388 1 2 3 4
389 1 2 3 4	390 1 2 3 4	391 1 2 3 4	392 1 2 3 4
393 1 2 3 4	394 1 2 3 4	395 1 2 3 4	396 1 2 3 4
397 1 2 3 4	398 1 2 3 4	399 1 2 3 4	400 1 2 3 4
401 1 2 3 4	402 1 2 3 4	403 1 2 3 4	404 1 2 3 4
405 1 2 3 4	406 1 2 3 4	407 1 2 3 4	408 1 2 3 4
409 1 2 3 4	410 1 2 3 4	411 1 2 3 4	412 1 2 3 4
413 1 2 3 4	414 1 2 3 4	415 1 2 3 4	416 1 2 3 4
417 1 2 3 4	418 1 2 3 4	419 1 2 3 4	420 1 2 3 4
421 1 2 3 4	422 1 2 3 4	423 1 2 3 4	424 1 2 3 4
425 1 2 3 4	426 1 2 3 4	427 1 2 3 4	428 1 2 3 4
429 1 2 3 4	430 1 2 3 4	431 1 2 3 4	432 1 2 3 4
433 1 2 3 4	434 1 2 3 4	435 1 2 3 4	436 1 2 3 4
437 1 2 3 4	438 1 2 3 4	439 1 2 3 4	440 1 2 3 4
441 1 2 3 4	442 1 2 3 4	443 1 2 3 4	444 1 2 3 4
445 1 2 3 4	446 1 2 3 4	447 1 2 3 4	448 1 2 3 4
449 1 2 3 4	450 1 2 3 4	451 1 2 3 4	452 1 2 3 4
453 1 2 3 4	454 1 2 3 4	455 1 2 3 4	456 1 2 3 4
457 1 2 3 4	458 1 2 3 4	459 1 2 3 4	460 1 2 3 4
461 1 2 3 4	462 1 2 3 4	463 1 2 3 4	464 1 2 3 4
465 1 2 3 4	466 1 2 3 4	467 1 2 3 4	468 1 2 3 4
469 1 2 3 4	470 1 2 3 4	471 1 2 3 4	472 1 2 3 4
473 1 2 3 4	474 1 2 3 4	475 1 2 3 4	476 1 2 3 4
477 1 2 3 4	478 1 2 3 4	479 1 2 3 4	480 1 2 3 4

Continued.

Medical-Surgical Nursing—cont'd

Review Questions 481-640, pp. 292-303

NAME_____ LAST FIRST MIDDLE GRADE_____ SEX_____ M OR F DATE OF BIRTH_____ YEAR MONTH DAY

DATE_____ YEAR MONTH DAY AGE_____ SCHOOL_____ CITY_____

INSTRUCTOR_____

IDENTIFICATION NUMBER

NAME OF TEST_____

BE SURE TO MAKE YOUR MARKS HEAVY AND BLACK

ERASE COMPLETELY ANY ANSWERS YOU WISH TO CHANGE

0 1 2 3 4 5 6 7 8 9 (×10 rows)

481 482 483 484
485 486 487 488
489 490 491 492
493 494 495 496
497 498 499 500
501 502 503 504
505 506 507 508
509 510 511 512
513 514 515 516
517 518 519 520
521 522 523 524
525 526 527 528
529 530 531 532
533 534 535 536
537 538 539 540
541 542 543 544
545 546 547 548
549 550 551 552
553 554 555 556
557 558 559 560
561 562 563 564
565 566 567 568
569 570 571 572
573 574 575 576
577 578 579 580
581 582 583 584
585 586 587 588
589 590 591 592
593 594 595 596
597 598 599 600
601 602 603 604
605 606 607 608
609 610 611 612
613 614 615 616
617 618 619 620
621 622 623 624
625 626 627 628
629 630 631 632
633 634 635 636
637 638 639 640

(each question numbered with answer choices 1 2 3 4)

Medical-Surgical Nursing—cont'd

Review Questions 641-800, pp. 304-315

NAME _____ LAST FIRST MIDDLE GRADE_____ SEX _ M OR F DATE OF BIRTH_____ YEAR MONTH DAY

DATE _____ YEAR MONTH DAY AGE_____ SCHOOL_____ CITY_____

INSTRUCTOR_____

NAME OF TEST_____

IDENTIFICATION NUMBER

BE SURE TO MAKE YOUR MARKS HEAVY AND BLACK

ERASE COMPLETELY ANY ANSWERS YOU WISH TO CHANGE

Pediatric Nursing

Review Questions 1-160, pp. 441-452

NAME _____ LAST ___ FIRST ___ MIDDLE ___ GRADE _____ SEX __ M OR F ___ DATE OF BIRTH _____ YEAR MONTH DAY

DATE _____ YEAR MONTH DAY ___ AGE ___ SCHOOL _____ CITY _____

INSTRUCTOR _____

NAME OF TEST _____

BE SURE TO MAKE YOUR MARKS HEAVY AND BLACK

ERASE COMPLETELY ANY ANSWERS YOU WISH TO CHANGE

IDENTIFICATION NUMBER

Continued.

Pediatric Nursing—cont'd

Review Questions 161-200, pp. 453-455

NAME_____ GRADE_____ SEX_____ DATE OF BIRTH_____
LAST   FIRST   MIDDLE   M OR F   YEAR MONTH DAY

DATE_____ AGE_____ SCHOOL_____ CITY_____
YEAR MONTH DAY

INSTRUCTOR_____

NAME OF TEST_____

IDENTIFICATION NUMBER

| 0 | 1 | 2 | 3 | 4 | 5 | 6 | 7 | 8 | 9 |

BE SURE TO MAKE YOUR MARKS HEAVY AND BLACK

ERASE COMPLETELY ANY ANSWERS YOU WISH TO CHANGE

161 1 2 3 4	162 1 2 3 4	163 1 2 3 4	164 1 2 3 4
165 1 2 3 4	166 1 2 3 4	167 1 2 3 4	168 1 2 3 4
169 1 2 3 4	170 1 2 3 4	171 1 2 3 4	172 1 2 3 4
173 1 2 3 4	174 1 2 3 4	175 1 2 3 4	176 1 2 3 4
177 1 2 3 4	178 1 2 3 4	179 1 2 3 4	180 1 2 3 4
181 1 2 3 4	182 1 2 3 4	183 1 2 3 4	184 1 2 3 4
185 1 2 3 4	186 1 2 3 4	187 1 2 3 4	188 1 2 3 4
189 1 2 3 4	190 1 2 3 4	191 1 2 3 4	192 1 2 3 4
193 1 2 3 4	194 1 2 3 4	195 1 2 3 4	196 1 2 3 4
197 1 2 3 4	198 1 2 3 4	199 1 2 3 4	200 1 2 3 4
201 1 2 3 4	202 1 2 3 4	203 1 2 3 4	204 1 2 3 4
205 1 2 3 4	206 1 2 3 4	207 1 2 3 4	208 1 2 3 4
209 1 2 3 4	210 1 2 3 4	211 1 2 3 4	212 1 2 3 4
213 1 2 3 4	214 1 2 3 4	215 1 2 3 4	216 1 2 3 4
217 1 2 3 4	218 1 2 3 4	219 1 2 3 4	220 1 2 3 4
221 1 2 3 4	222 1 2 3 4	223 1 2 3 4	224 1 2 3 4
225 1 2 3 4	226 1 2 3 4	227 1 2 3 4	228 1 2 3 4
229 1 2 3 4	230 1 2 3 4	231 1 2 3 4	232 1 2 3 4
233 1 2 3 4	234 1 2 3 4	235 1 2 3 4	236 1 2 3 4
237 1 2 3 4	238 1 2 3 4	239 1 2 3 4	240 1 2 3 4
241 1 2 3 4	242 1 2 3 4	243 1 2 3 4	244 1 2 3 4
245 1 2 3 4	246 1 2 3 4	247 1 2 3 4	248 1 2 3 4
249 1 2 3 4	250 1 2 3 4	251 1 2 3 4	252 1 2 3 4
253 1 2 3 4	254 1 2 3 4	255 1 2 3 4	256 1 2 3 4
257 1 2 3 4	258 1 2 3 4	259 1 2 3 4	260 1 2 3 4
261 1 2 3 4	262 1 2 3 4	263 1 2 3 4	264 1 2 3 4
265 1 2 3 4	266 1 2 3 4	267 1 2 3 4	268 1 2 3 4
269 1 2 3 4	270 1 2 3 4	271 1 2 3 4	272 1 2 3 4
273 1 2 3 4	274 1 2 3 4	275 1 2 3 4	276 1 2 3 4
277 1 2 3 4	278 1 2 3 4	279 1 2 3 4	280 1 2 3 4
281 1 2 3 4	282 1 2 3 4	283 1 2 3 4	284 1 2 3 4
285 1 2 3 4	286 1 2 3 4	287 1 2 3 4	288 1 2 3 4
289 1 2 3 4	290 1 2 3 4	291 1 2 3 4	292 1 2 3 4
293 1 2 3 4	294 1 2 3 4	295 1 2 3 4	296 1 2 3 4
297 1 2 3 4	298 1 2 3 4	299 1 2 3 4	300 1 2 3 4
301 1 2 3 4	302 1 2 3 4	303 1 2 3 4	304 1 2 3 4
305 1 2 3 4	306 1 2 3 4	307 1 2 3 4	308 1 2 3 4
309 1 2 3 4	310 1 2 3 4	311 1 2 3 4	312 1 2 3 4
313 1 2 3 4	314 1 2 3 4	315 1 2 3 4	316 1 2 3 4
317 1 2 3 4	318 1 2 3 4	319 1 2 3 4	320 1 2 3 4

Maternity Nursing

Review Questions 1-160, pp. 500-512

NAME_____ GRADE_____ SEX_____ DATE OF BIRTH_____
LAST   FIRST   MIDDLE   M OR F   YEAR MONTH DAY

DATE_____ AGE____ SCHOOL_____ CITY_____
YEAR MONTH DAY

INSTRUCTOR_____

NAME OF TEST_____

IDENTIFICATION NUMBER

**BE SURE TO MAKE YOUR MARKS
HEAVY AND BLACK**

**ERASE COMPLETELY ANY ANSWERS
YOU WISH TO CHANGE**

0 1 2 3 4   5 6 7 8 9

Continued.

Maternity Nursing—cont'd

Review Questions 161-200, pp. 512-514

NAME_____ LAST FIRST MIDDLE GRADE_____ SEX _____ M OR F DATE OF BIRTH_____ YEAR MONTH DAY

DATE_____ YEAR MONTH DAY AGE_____ SCHOOL_____ CITY_____

INSTRUCTOR_____

NAME OF TEST_____

IDENTIFICATION NUMBER

0 1 2 3 4 5 6 7 8 9 (repeated rows)

BE SURE TO MAKE YOUR MARKS HEAVY AND BLACK

ERASE COMPLETELY ANY ANSWERS YOU WISH TO CHANGE

161–320 answer grid (choices 1 2 3 4 per question)

Psychiatric Nursing

Review Questions 1-160, pp. 562-574

NAME_____ GRADE_____ SEX_____ DATE OF BIRTH_____
     LAST   FIRST   MIDDLE   M OR F   YEAR MONTH DAY

DATE_____ AGE____ SCHOOL_____ CITY_____
     YEAR MONTH DAY

INSTRUCTOR_____

                 IDENTIFICATION NUMBER

NAME OF TEST_____

**BE SURE TO MAKE YOUR MARKS
HEAVY AND BLACK**

**ERASE COMPLETELY ANY ANSWERS
YOU WISH TO CHANGE**

NAME_____ GRADE_____ SEX _____ DATE OF BIRTH_____
LAST   FIRST   MIDDLE   M OR F   YEAR MONTH DAY

DATE_____ AGE_____ SCHOOL_____ CITY_____
YEAR MONTH DAY

INSTRUCTOR_____

NAME OF TEST_____   IDENTIFICATION NUMBER

**BE SURE TO MAKE YOUR MARKS
HEAVY AND BLACK**

**ERASE COMPLETELY ANY ANSWERS
YOU WISH TO CHANGE**

161	162	163	164
165	166	167	168
169	170	171	172
173	174	175	176
177	178	179	180
181	182	183	184
185	186	187	188
189	190	191	192
193	194	195	196
197	198	199	200
201	202	203	204
205	206	207	208
209	210	211	212
213	214	215	216
217	218	219	220
221	222	223	224
225	226	227	228
229	230	231	232
233	234	235	236
237	238	239	240
241	242	243	244
245	246	247	248
249	250	251	252
253	254	255	256
257	258	259	260
261	262	263	264
265	266	267	268
269	270	271	272
273	274	275	276
277	278	279	280
281	282	283	284
285	286	287	288
289	290	291	292
293	294	295	296
297	298	299	300
301	302	303	304
305	306	307	308
309	310	311	312
313	314	315	316
317	318	319	320

Comprehensive Test 1

Questions 1-120, pp. 625-636

NAME_____ LAST FIRST MIDDLE GRADE_____ SEX_____ M OR F DATE OF BIRTH_____ YEAR MONTH DAY

DATE_____ YEAR MONTH DAY AGE_____ SCHOOL_____ CITY_____

INSTRUCTOR_____

NAME OF TEST_____

BE SURE TO MAKE YOUR MARKS HEAVY AND BLACK

ERASE COMPLETELY ANY ANSWERS YOU WISH TO CHANGE

IDENTIFICATION NUMBER

0 1 2 3 4   5 6 7 8 9
0 1 2 3 4   5 6 7 8 9
0 1 2 3 4   5 6 7 8 9
0 1 2 3 4   5 6 7 8 9
0 1 2 3 4   5 6 7 8 9
0 1 2 3 4   5 6 7 8 9
0 1 2 3 4   5 6 7 8 9
0 1 2 3 4   5 6 7 8 9
0 1 2 3 4   5 6 7 8 9
0 1 2 3 4   5 6 7 8 9

1 1 2 3 4	2 1 2 3 4	3 1 2 3 4	4 1 2 3 4
5 1 2 3 4	6 1 2 3 4	7 1 2 3 4	8 1 2 3 4
9 1 2 3 4	10 1 2 3 4	11 1 2 3 4	12 1 2 3 4
13 1 2 3 4	14 1 2 3 4	15 1 2 3 4	16 1 2 3 4
17 1 2 3 4	18 1 2 3 4	19 1 2 3 4	20 1 2 3 4
21 1 2 3 4	22 1 2 3 4	23 1 2 3 4	24 1 2 3 4
25 1 2 3 4	26 1 2 3 4	27 1 2 3 4	28 1 2 3 4
29 1 2 3 4	30 1 2 3 4	31 1 2 3 4	32 1 2 3 4
33 1 2 3 4	34 1 2 3 4	35 1 2 3 4	36 1 2 3 4
37 1 2 3 4	38 1 2 3 4	39 1 2 3 4	40 1 2 3 4
41 1 2 3 4	42 1 2 3 4	43 1 2 3 4	44 1 2 3 4
45 1 2 3 4	46 1 2 3 4	47 1 2 3 4	48 1 2 3 4
49 1 2 3 4	50 1 2 3 4	51 1 2 3 4	52 1 2 3 4
53 1 2 3 4	54 1 2 3 4	55 1 2 3 4	56 1 2 3 4
57 1 2 3 4	58 1 2 3 4	59 1 2 3 4	60 1 2 3 4
61 1 2 3 4	62 1 2 3 4	63 1 2 3 4	64 1 2 3 4
65 1 2 3 4	66 1 2 3 4	67 1 2 3 4	68 1 2 3 4
69 1 2 3 4	70 1 2 3 4	71 1 2 3 4	72 1 2 3 4
73 1 2 3 4	74 1 2 3 4	75 1 2 3 4	76 1 2 3 4
77 1 2 3 4	78 1 2 3 4	79 1 2 3 4	80 1 2 3 4
81 1 2 3 4	82 1 2 3 4	83 1 2 3 4	84 1 2 3 4
85 1 2 3 4	86 1 2 3 4	87 1 2 3 4	88 1 2 3 4
89 1 2 3 4	90 1 2 3 4	91 1 2 3 4	92 1 2 3 4
93 1 2 3 4	94 1 2 3 4	95 1 2 3 4	96 1 2 3 4
97 1 2 3 4	98 1 2 3 4	99 1 2 3 4	100 1 2 3 4
101 1 2 3 4	102 1 2 3 4	103 1 2 3 4	104 1 2 3 4
105 1 2 3 4	106 1 2 3 4	107 1 2 3 4	108 1 2 3 4
109 1 2 3 4	110 1 2 3 4	111 1 2 3 4	112 1 2 3 4
113 1 2 3 4	114 1 2 3 4	115 1 2 3 4	116 1 2 3 4
117 1 2 3 4	118 1 2 3 4	119 1 2 3 4	120 1 2 3 4
121 1 2 3 4	122 1 2 3 4	123 1 2 3 4	124 1 2 3 4
125 1 2 3 4	126 1 2 3 4	127 1 2 3 4	128 1 2 3 4
129 1 2 3 4	130 1 2 3 4	131 1 2 3 4	132 1 2 3 4
133 1 2 3 4	134 1 2 3 4	135 1 2 3 4	136 1 2 3 4
137 1 2 3 4	138 1 2 3 4	139 1 2 3 4	140 1 2 3 4
141 1 2 3 4	142 1 2 3 4	143 1 2 3 4	144 1 2 3 4
145 1 2 3 4	146 1 2 3 4	147 1 2 3 4	148 1 2 3 4
149 1 2 3 4	150 1 2 3 4	151 1 2 3 4	152 1 2 3 4
153 1 2 3 4	154 1 2 3 4	155 1 2 3 4	156 1 2 3 4
157 1 2 3 4	158 1 2 3 4	159 1 2 3 4	160 1 2 3 4

Comprehensive Test 2

Questions 1-120, pp. 651-662

NAME_____ GRADE_____ SEX_____ DATE OF BIRTH_____
      LAST   FIRST   MIDDLE   M OR F   YEAR MONTH DAY

DATE_____ AGE_____ SCHOOL_____ CITY_____
      YEAR MONTH DAY

INSTRUCTOR_____ IDENTIFICATION NUMBER

NAME OF TEST_____

BE SURE TO MAKE YOUR MARKS
HEAVY AND BLACK

ERASE COMPLETELY ANY ANSWERS
YOU WISH TO CHANGE

(Answer grid: questions 1–160, each with options 1 2 3 4; identification number columns 0–9)

Comprehensive Test 3

Questions 1-120, pp. 676-687

NAME_____ LAST   FIRST   MIDDLE   GRADE_____ SEX_____ M OR F   DATE OF BIRTH_____ YEAR MONTH DAY

DATE_____ YEAR MONTH DAY   AGE_____ SCHOOL_____   CITY_____

INSTRUCTOR_____

NAME OF TEST_____

**BE SURE TO MAKE YOUR MARKS
HEAVY AND BLACK**

**ERASE COMPLETELY ANY ANSWERS
YOU WISH TO CHANGE**

IDENTIFICATION NUMBER

0   1   2   3   4   5   6   7   8   9

(ten rows of identification number bubbles 0–9)

(answer grid, questions 1–160, each with choices 1 2 3 4)

Comprehensive Test 4

Questions 1-120, pp. 702-713

NAME_____ GRADE_____ SEX____ M or F ____ DATE OF BIRTH_____
LAST   FIRST   MIDDLE   YEAR MONTH DAY

DATE_____ AGE_____ SCHOOL_____ CITY_____
YEAR MONTH DAY

INSTRUCTOR_____

NAME OF TEST_____

IDENTIFICATION NUMBER

**BE SURE TO MAKE YOUR MARKS
HEAVY AND BLACK**

**ERASE COMPLETELY ANY ANSWERS
YOU WISH TO CHANGE**

Comprehensive Test 5

Questions 1-120, pp. 728-739

NAME_____ LAST   FIRST   MIDDLE   GRADE_____ SEX___ M OR F   DATE OF BIRTH_____ YEAR MONTH DAY

DATE_____ YEAR MONTH DAY   AGE____ SCHOOL_____   CITY_____

INSTRUCTOR_____

NAME OF TEST_____

**BE SURE TO MAKE YOUR MARKS
HEAVY AND BLACK**

**ERASE COMPLETELY ANY ANSWERS
YOU WISH TO CHANGE**

IDENTIFICATION NUMBER

0	1	2	3	4	5	6	7	8	9

(This is a standardized machine-scored answer sheet. Each numbered item from 1 to 160 has answer bubbles labeled 1, 2, 3, 4 arranged in four columns.)

Comprehensive Test 6

Questions 1-120, pp. 753-765

NAME_____ LAST   FIRST   MIDDLE   GRADE_____ SEX_____ M OR F   DATE OF BIRTH_____ YEAR MONTH DAY

DATE_____ YEAR MONTH DAY   AGE_____ SCHOOL_____   CITY_____

INSTRUCTOR_____

NAME OF TEST_____

IDENTIFICATION NUMBER

BE SURE TO MAKE YOUR MARKS HEAVY AND BLACK

ERASE COMPLETELY ANY ANSWERS YOU WISH TO CHANGE